LARKIN

High-Resolution CT of the Lung

Third Edition

High-Resolution CT of the Lung

Third Edition

W. Richard Webb, M.D.
Professor of Radiology
University of California, San Francisco, School of Medicine
Chief of Thoracic Imaging
University of California, San Francisco, Medical Center
San Francisco, California

Nestor L. Müller, M.D., Ph.D.
Professor and Chairman
Department of Radiology
University of British Columbia
Head, Department of Radiology
Vancouver Hospital and Health Sciences Centre
Vancouver, British Columbia, Canada

David P. Naidich, M.D.
Professor of Radiology
Co-director of Thoracic Imaging
New York University Medical Center/Bellevue Hospital
New York, New York

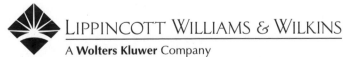
LIPPINCOTT WILLIAMS & WILKINS
A **Wolters Kluwer** Company
Philadelphia · Baltimore · New York · London
Buenos Aires · Hong Kong · Sydney · Tokyo

Acquisitions Editor: Joyce-Rachel John
Developmental Editor: Alexandra T. Anderson
Supervising Editor: Mary Ann McLaughlin
Manufacturing Manager: Colin Warnock
Production Editor: Alyson Langlois, Silverchair Science + Communications
Cover Designer: Christine Jenny
Compositor: Silverchair Science + Communications
Printer: Maple Vail

Library of Congress Cataloging-in-Publication Data

Webb, W. Richard (Wayne Richard), 1945-
   High-resolution CT of the lung / W. Richard Webb, Nestor L. Müller, David P.
Naidich.-- 3rd ed.
      p. ; cm.
   Includes bibliographical references and index.
   ISBN 0-7817-2278-0
      1. Lungs--Tomography. I. Müller, Nestor Luiz, 1948- II. Naidich, David P. III. Title.
   [DNLM: 1. Lung--radiography. 2. Tomography, X-Ray Computed. 3. Lung
Diseases--pathology. WF 600 W368h 2000]
   RC734.T64 W43 2000
   616.2'407572--dc21

                                                                          00-055855

Dedication

To our wives and children:
Teresa, Emma, Clifford, and Andy
Ruth, Alison, and Phillip
Jocelyn and Zachary

Contents

Preface to the First Edition

In his paper "A New Look at Pattern Recognition of Diffuse Pulmonary Disease," Ben Felson (1) reviewed the many problems that are inherent in any attempt to precisely characterize diffuse lung disease on the basis of plain radiographic findings. Although he was a great proponent of pattern recognition and an accomplished master of this technique, he stated in the first sentence of this paper that "the common practice of describing the histologic distribution of pulmonary lesions from their radiographic patterns is often inaccurate." He continued:

> After many years of trying and testing, I have convinced myself that certain patterns of diffuse pulmonary shadows can be distinguished in most patients. Nevertheless I have had considerable difficulty in teaching others how to do it. In fact, a number of respected colleagues who also claim success in pattern recognition often differ with me when viewing the same films. Others even feel that the pattern approach to chest radiography is so unreliable it should be abandoned altogether.
>
> Why the problems?

As indicated by Dr. Felson, and as we review in the introduction to this book, chest radiographs are limited in their ability to characterize lung morphology precisely and to represent the pathological alterations in morphology that occur in the presence of lung disease. High-resolution CT (HRCT), on the other hand, provides the radiologist and clinician with a tool capable of accurately demonstrating gross lung anatomy and accurately characterizing abnormal findings. The correlation between HRCT findings and pathologic findings is excellent and certainly exceeds that possible with plain radiographs. As discussed by Roberta Miller in the Foreword to this book, to the extent that gross pathology can be used to diagnose lung disease, HRCT can as well. In the last five years, HRCT has revolutionized the radiological approach to diagnosing lung disease.

A further advantage of HRCT is that the interpretation of HRCT scans is easier to teach than is the interpretation of chest radiographs. Because of the clarity and precision with which HRCT represents lung anatomy, there is much less individual variation in interpreting HRCT than there is with chest radiographs. It is much easier to recognize HRCT findings as something one has seen before (e.g., a thick-walled bronchus always looks like a thick-walled bronchus), and to understand what they represent. Far fewer HRCT cases must be classified as belonging to the "'I don't know' pattern" (1) than is necessary when interpreting plain films.

In this book, we have limited our discussion of HRCT findings, both normal and abnormal, and the HRCT descriptions of diseases to what is known and described. We have avoided *speculating* as to what the HRCT might look like in patients with one disease or another based on the plain film findings. As indicated above, the notable inaccuracy of plain films would make this a hazardous endeavor.

In answering his own question, "Why the problems?" with plain radiographs, Dr. Felson replied, "I believe inconsistent terminology and certain misconceptions in respect to pathologic alterations are responsible for many of the difficulties" (1). This is a problem we hope to avoid. In this book we will define and name HRCT findings, whenever possible, in relation to specific anatomic structures.

REFERENCE

1. Felson B. A new look at pattern recognition of diffuse pulmonary disease. *AJR* 1979;133:183–189.

Preface

During the past 15 years, high-resolution CT (HRCT) has become an indispensable tool in the evaluation of patients with suspected diffuse pulmonary disease. It is now commonly used in clinical practice to detect and accurately characterize a variety of lung abnormalities. In the 5 years since our Second Edition was published, considerable progress has occurred in the understanding of diffuse lung diseases and their nature, causes, and characteristics. Without doubt, HRCT has played a significant role in this regard.

In this edition, we have incorporated a review of significant recent advances in the reclassification and understanding of lung diseases, including the interstitial pneumonias, and have added discussions of a number of lung diseases not extensively reviewed in the Second Edition, such as lymphoproliferative and eosinophilic lung diseases. Furthermore, chapters on airways diseases and pulmonary vascular diseases supplement those appearing in earlier editions, in recognition of the importance of HRCT in the evaluation of these types of disease. Recent technical advances in obtaining HRCT have also been reviewed, most notably the use of multidetector HRCT.

We have added a number of diagnostic algorithms based on the specific abnormalities observed on HRCT scans. These should prove useful in conceptualizing the most important HRCT findings to look for and the most important decisions to be made in attempting to reach a diagnosis or differential diagnosis.

At the beginning of the book, the Quick Reference guide illustrates the common appearances of the most common diffuse lung diseases. This guide may be of value in the initial differential diagnosis of clinical cases and also is intended to serve as an illustrated index to the detailed descriptions of diseases found elsewhere in the book.

Numerous new illustrations have been provided for the Third Edition, reflecting our increased experience and that of others. In the case of both common and uncommon diseases, we have attempted to illustrate the range of abnormalities that may be encountered in clinical practice. We hope the reader will find these changes helpful.

High-Resolution CT of the Lung

Third Edition

Quick Reference to High-Resolution Computed Tomography Diagnosis of Diffuse Lung Disease

In the following pages, we provide examples of the most common appearances of the most common lung diseases encountered in reading high-resolution computed tomography (HRCT) of the lung. It is our hope that this will serve as a quick reference and an illustrated index to the detailed descriptions of findings found elsewhere in this book, and as a diagnostic aid when a reader is faced with an unfamiliar HRCT appearance.

ACUTE INTERSTITIAL PNEUMONIA (AIP)

(See pages 386–390.)

HRCT Findings

Extensive bilateral ground-glass opacities
Airspace consolidation
Architectural distortion
Consolidation predominantly basilar and dependent

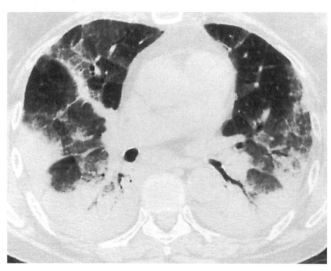 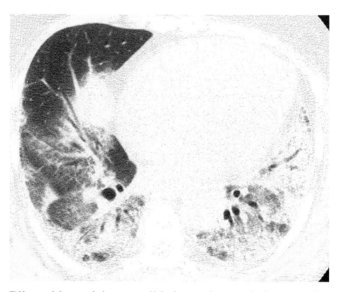

Bilateral consolidation involving posterior lung bases.   Bilateral lower lobe consolidation and ground-glass opacity.

ALLERGIC BRONCHOPULMONARY ASPERGILLOSIS

(See pages 497–513.)

HRCT Findings

Central bronchiectasis
Mucous plugging
High-density mucous plugs
Tree-in-bud
Atelectasis
Mosaic perfusion
Air-trapping on expiration

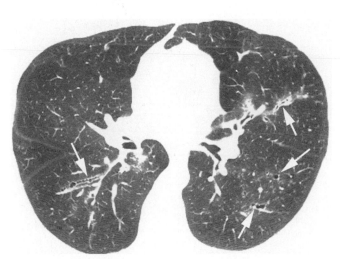

Early disease with mild central bronchiectasis (*arrows*).

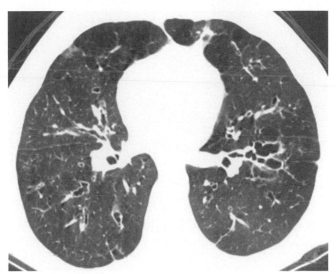

Central bronchiectasis.

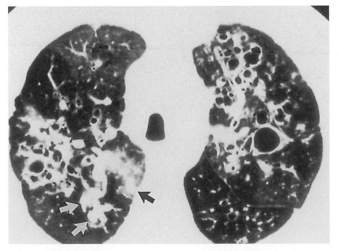

Late disease with bronchiectasis and mucous plugging (*arrows*).

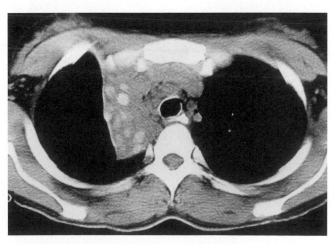

High density mucous plugs with atelectasis.

ALVEOLAR PROTEINOSIS

(See pages 128–144; 390–393.)

HRCT Findings

Patchy ground-glass opacity
Smooth septal thickening in abnormal areas
Crazy-paving
Consolidation
Patchy or geographic distribution

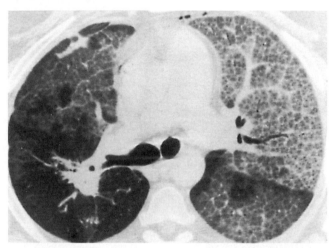

Geographic ground-glass opacity with septal thickening (crazy-paving).

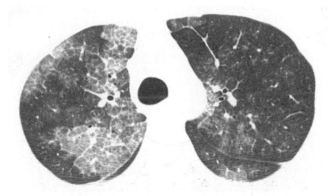

Crazy-paving with a patchy distribution.

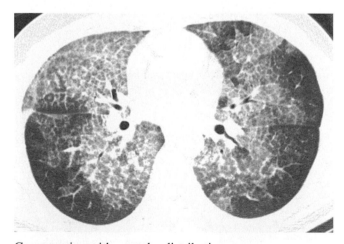

Crazy-paving with a patchy distribution.

ASBESTOSIS AND ASBESTOS-RELATED DISEASE

(See pages 236–251.)

HRCT Findings

Pleural thickening
Subpleural dotlike opacities in early disease
Findings of fibrosis
Honeycombing in advanced disease
Subpleural lines
Parenchymal bands in association with pleural thickening
Earliest abnormalities posterior and basal

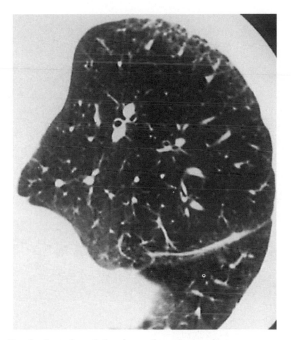

Small subpleural nodules in early asbestosis.

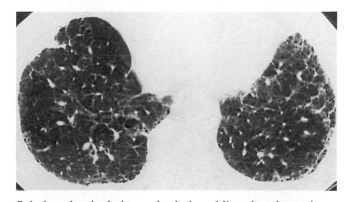

Subpleural reticulation and subpleural lines in asbestosis.

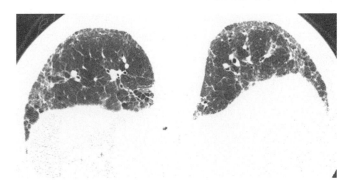

Subpleural intralobular interstitial thickening in asbestosis.

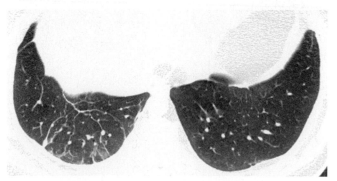

Parenchymal bands associated with pleural disease.

BRONCHIOLITIS OBLITERANS (CONSTRICTIVE BRONCHIOLITIS)

(See pages 529–539.)

HRCT Findings

Bronchiectasis
Mosaic perfusion, usually patchy
Air-trapping on expiration, usually patchy
Air-trapping on expiration with normal inspiratory scans

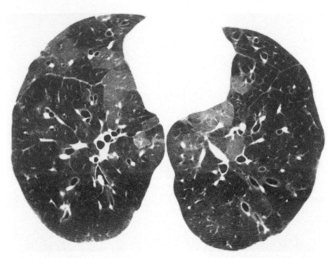

Late disease: extensive bronchiectasis and mosaic perfusion.

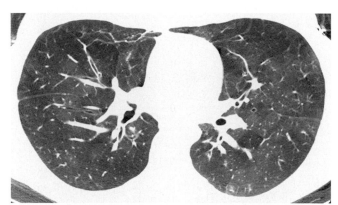

Mild bronchiectasis and mosaic perfusion.

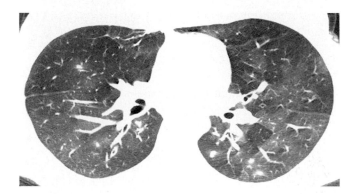

Air-trapping on expiratory scan.

BRONCHIOLITIS OBLITERANS ORGANIZING PNEUMONIA

(See pages 373–378.)

HRCT Findings

Patchy bilateral airspace consolidation
Ground-glass opacity
Subpleural or peribronchovascular distribution, or both
Bronchial wall thickening or dilatation
Centrilobular nodules
Large nodules

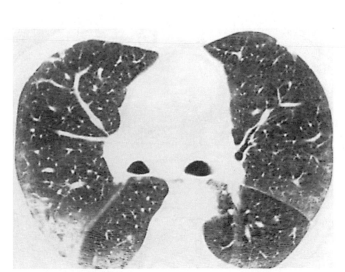

Patchy subpleural ground-glass opacity.

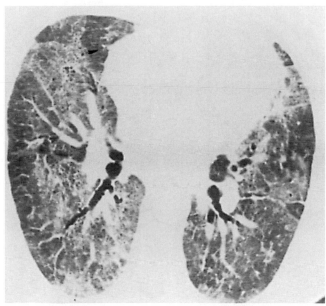

Patchy subpleural consolidation with bronchial dilatation.

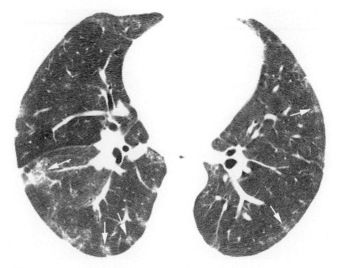

Ill-defined centrilobular nodules (*arrows*).

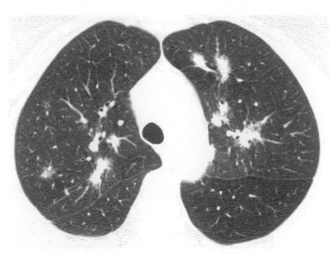

Large irregular nodules.

CHRONIC EOSINOPHILIC PNEUMONIA

(See pages 367–370.)

HRCT Findings

Patchy unilateral or bilateral airspace consolidation
Peripheral, middle and upper-lung predominance
Ground-glass opacity
Subpleural linear opacities

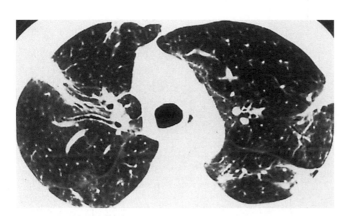

Patchy subpleural consolidation and linear opacities.

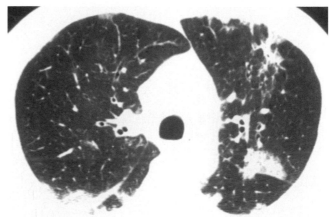

Patchy subpleural consolidation.

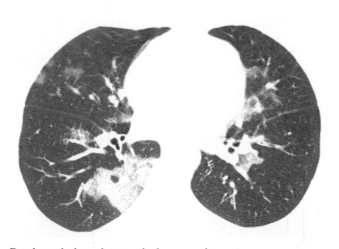

Patchy subpleural ground-glass opacity.

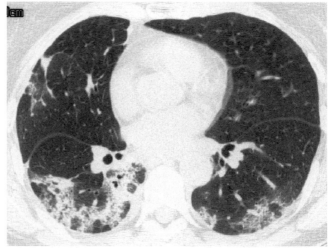

Patchy subpleural ground-glass opacities, consolidation, and linear opacities.

CYSTIC FIBROSIS

(See pages 497–513.)

HRCT Findings

Bronchiectasis, central bronchi and upper lobes involved in all cases
Bronchial wall thickening, right upper lobe first involved
Mucous plugging
Tree-in-bud
Large lung volumes
Areas of atelectasis
Mosaic perfusion
Air-trapping on expiration

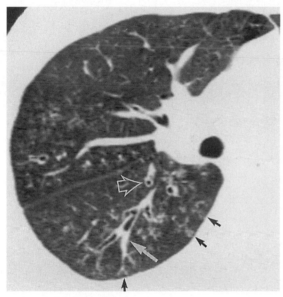

Early disease: bronchial wall thickening (*open arrow*), mucoid impaction (*white arrow*), and tree-in-bud (*small arrows*).

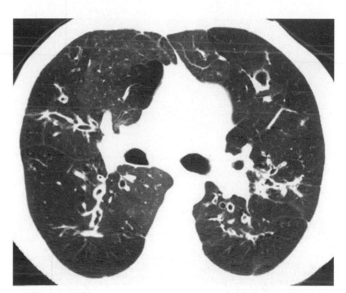

Late disease: central bronchiectasis and mosaic perfusion.

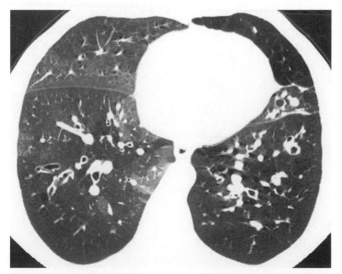

Late disease: bronchiectasis and air trapping on an expiratory scan.

CYTOMEGALOVIRUS PNEUMONIA

(See page 403.)

HRCT Findings

Patchy bilateral ground-glass opacity, consolidation, or both
Reticulation (resolving disease)
Crazy-paving
Centrilobular nodules

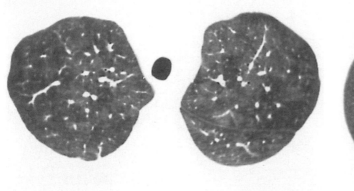

Patchy ground-glass opacity.

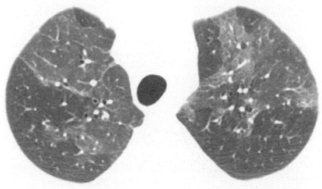

Patchy ground-glass opacity.

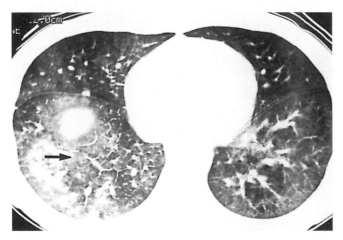

Crazy-paving: patchy ground-glass opacity with septal thickening (*arrow*).

DESQUAMATIVE INTERSTITIAL PNEUMONIA

(See pages 384–385.)

HRCT Findings

Bilateral, patchy ground-glass opacity
Subpleural and basal predominance
Minimal findings of fibrosis (reticulation)

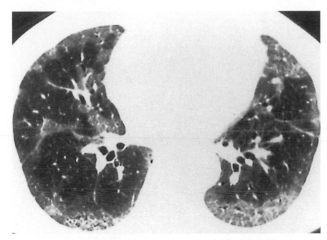 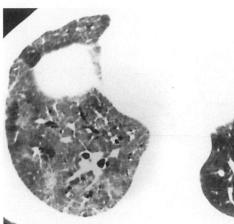 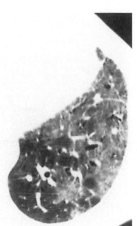

Subpleural ground-glass opacity with mild reticulation.   Subpleural ground-glass opacity.

EMPHYSEMA (CENTRILOBULAR)

(See pages 436–462.)

HRCT Findings

Multiple small, spotty, or centrilobular lucencies
Upper lobe predominance
Lucencies may have thin walls
May be associated with paraseptal emphysema or bullae

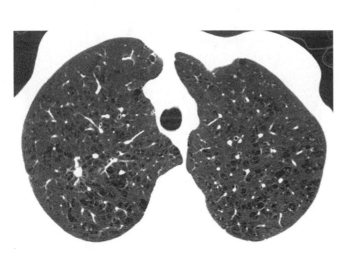

Small lucencies without visible walls.

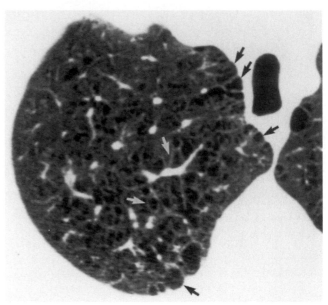

Focal lucencies associated with paraseptal emphysema (*arrows*).

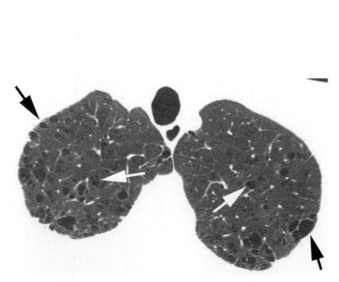

Centrilobular (*white arrows*) and paraseptal emphysema (*black arrows*).

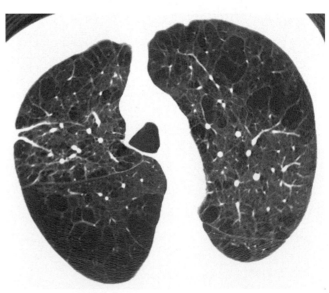

Extensive centrilobular emphysema.

EMPHYSEMA (PANLOBULAR)

(See pages 436–462.)

HRCT Findings

Lucent lung containing small pulmonary vessels
Diffuse or lower lobe predominance
Focal lucencies and bullae less common than with centrilobular emphysema
Bronchiectasis or bronchial wall thickening

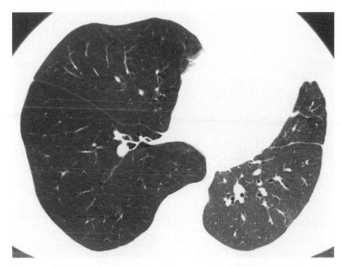

Lucent lung, lower lobe involvement (left lung transplant).

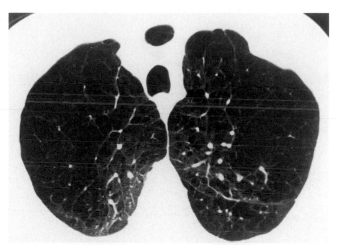

Lucent lung, small pulmonary vessels.

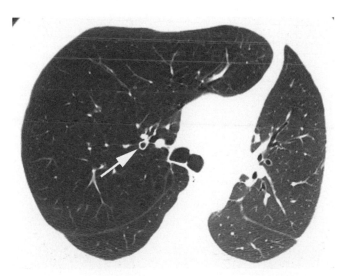

Bronchial wall thickening (*arrow*). Left lung transplant.

EMPHYSEMA (PARASEPTAL)

(See pages 436–462.)

HRCT Findings

Multiple, subpleural lucencies in a single layer, usually smaller than 1 cm
Upper lobe predominance
Thin walls are commonly visible
May be associated with centrilobular emphysema or bullae
Pneumothorax

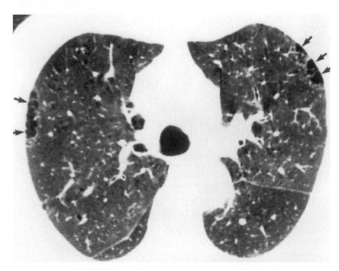

Subpleural lucencies with visible walls (*arrows*).

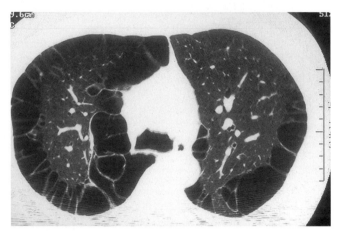

Paraseptal emphysema.

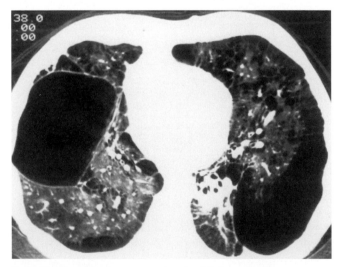

Paraseptal emphysema associated with large bullae.

DIFFUSE PULMONARY HEMORRHAGE

(See pages 408–410.)

HRCT Findings

Ground-glass opacity
Bilateral, patchy, or diffuse
Centrilobular ground-glass opacity
Interlobular septal thickening

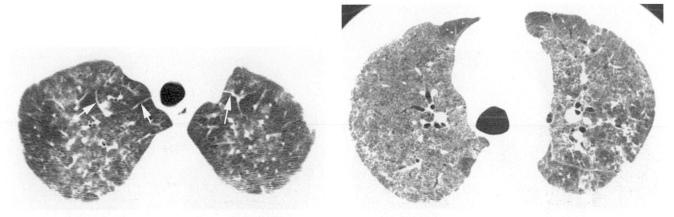

Patchy ground glass opacity with septal thickening (*arrows*). Diffuse ground-glass opacity.

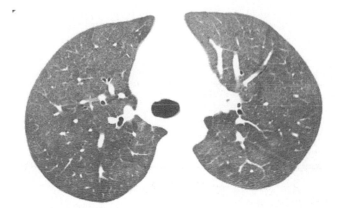

Subtle patchy ground-glass opacity.

HYPERSENSITIVITY PNEUMONITIS (SUBACUTE)

(See pages 356–366.)

HRCT Findings

Patchy or diffuse ground-glass opacity
Small centrilobular nodular opacities
Lobular areas of decreased attenuation (mosaic perfusion)
Combination of ground-glass opacity and patchy air-trapping
Lobular areas of air-trapping on expiratory scans
Findings of fibrosis

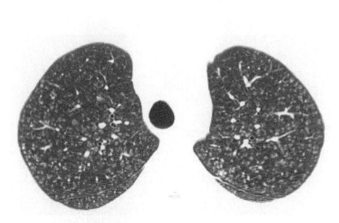

Centrilobular nodules.

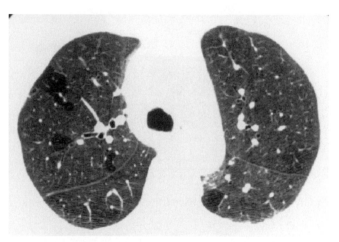

Patchy ground-glass opacity associated with lobular lucencies.

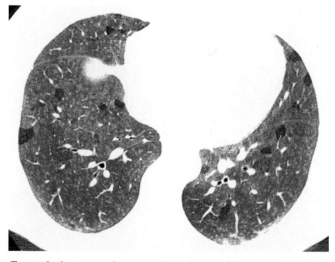

Ground-glass opacity, centrilobular nodules, and lobular lucencies.

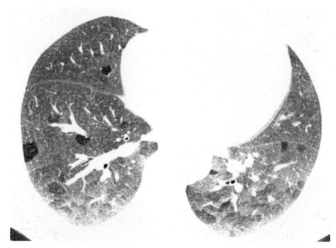

Air-trapping on expiratory scan.

HYPERSENSITIVITY PNEUMONITIS (CHRONIC)

(See pages 356–366.)

HRCT Findings

Findings of fibrosis
Patchy distribution of abnormalities
No zonal predominance of fibrosis

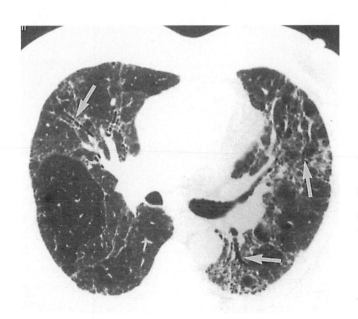

Patchy reticular opacities with traction bronchiectasis (*arrows*).

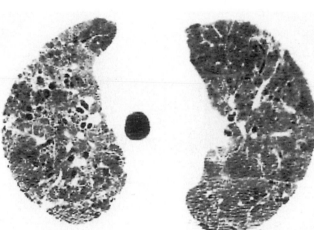

Patchy findings of fibrosis.

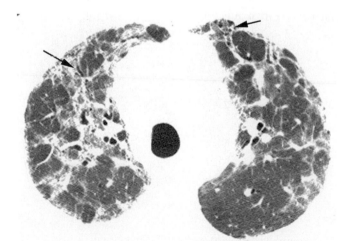

Patchy fibrosis with traction bronchiectasis (*arrows*).

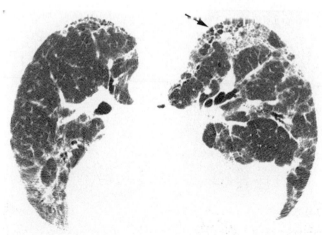

Mild honeycombing (*arrow*).

IDIOPATHIC PULMONARY FIBROSIS (IPF)

(See pages 195–210.)

HRCT Findings

Findings of fibrosis
Honeycombing
Traction bronchiectasis
Ground-glass opacity (unusual except in areas showing fibrosis)
Peripheral, subpleural, lower lung zone, posterior predominance

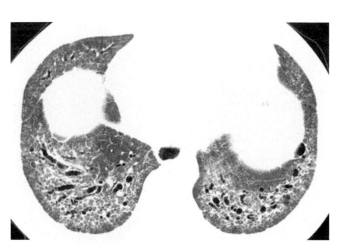

Subpleural intralobular interstitial thickening with traction bronchiectasis.

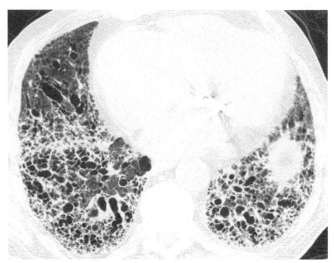

Subpleural, lower lobe honeycombing and traction bronchiectasis.

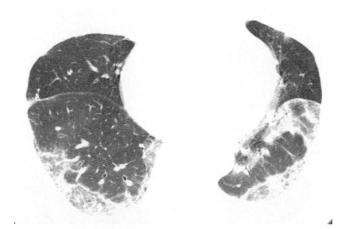

Subpleural ground-glass opacity in active disease.

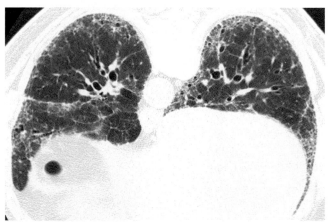

Subpleural intralobular interstitial thickening.

KAPOSI'S SARCOMA (KS)

(See pages 272–274.)

HRCT Findings

Irregular and ill-defined peribronchovascular nodules
Peribronchovascular interstitial thickening
Interlobular septal thickening
Pleural effusions
Lymphadenopathy

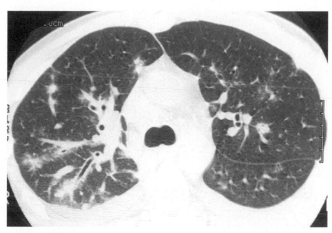

Irregular peribronchovascular infiltration.

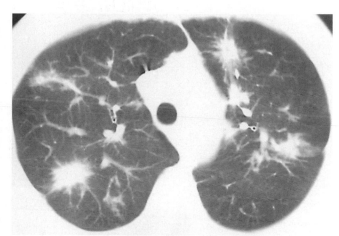

Irregular flame-shaped masses.

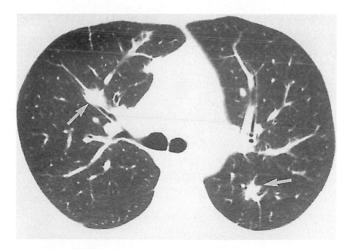

Irregular peribronchovascular nodules (*arrows*).

LANGERHANS CELL HISTIOCYTOSIS

(See pages 145–171; 421–429.)

HRCT Findings

Thick- or thin-walled lung cysts, bizarre shapes
Nodules, usually smaller than 1 to 5 mm, sometimes cavitary
Upper lobe predominance, costophrenic angles spared

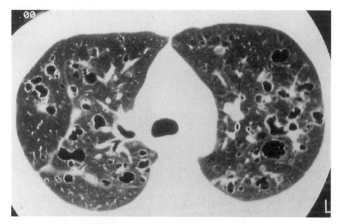

Irregular cysts and nodules.

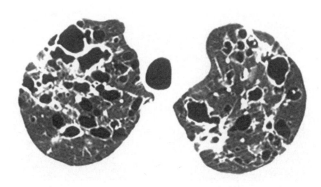

Irregular thick- and thin-walled cysts.

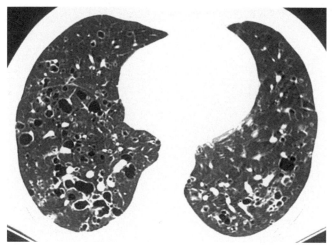

Bases are relatively spared.

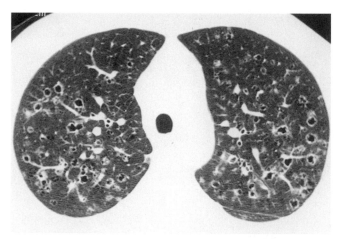

Centrilobular nodules, some cavitary.

LIPOID PNEUMONIA

(See pages 393–396.)

HRCT Findings

Patchy unilateral or bilateral airspace consolidation
Consolidation low in attenuation
Ground-glass opacity
Crazy-paving
Lower lung predominance

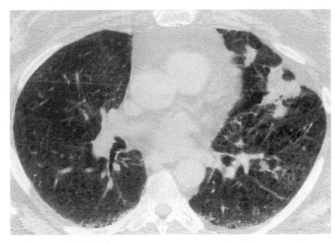

Patchy consolidation.

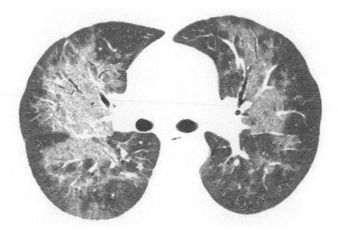

Patchy ground-glass opacity with a crazy-paving appearance.

LYMPHANGIOLEIOMYOMATOSIS

(See pages 145–171; 429–435.)

HRCT Findings

Thin-walled lung cysts
Diffuse distribution
Mild septal thickening or ground-glass opacity
Adenopathy
Small nodules
Pleural effusion

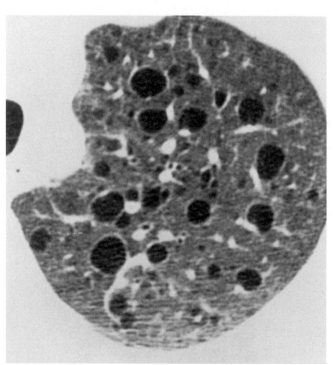

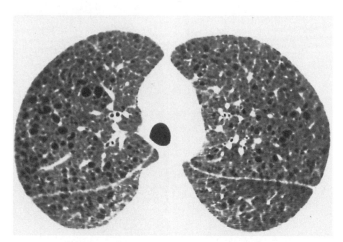

Thin-walled cysts, mild interstitial thickening.

Thin-walled lung cysts, intervening lung normal.

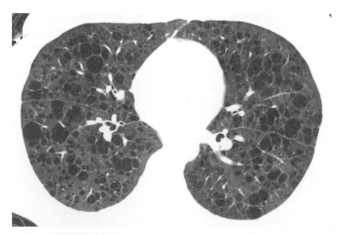

Thin-walled lung cysts.

LYMPHOCYTIC INTERSTITIAL PNEUMONIA (LIP)

(See pages 210–226; 276–277.)

HRCT Findings

Ground-glass opacity
Poorly defined centrilobular nodules
Subpleural nodules
Interlobular septal thickening or nodules
Thickening of peribronchovascular interstitium
Cystic airspaces
Lymph node enlargement

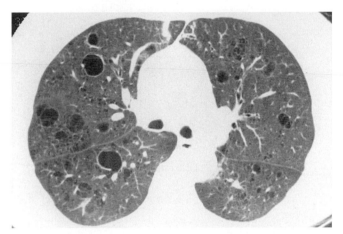

Thin-walled cysts.

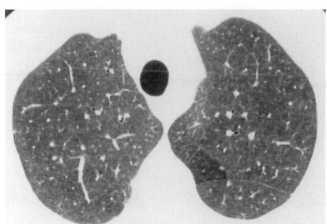

Patchy ground-glass opacity.

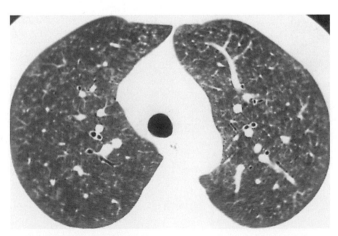

Ill-defined centrilobular nodules.

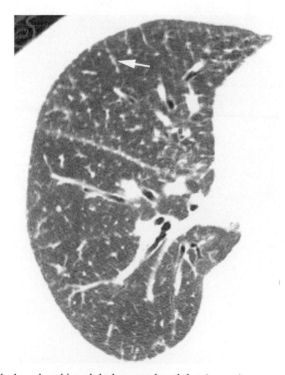

Subpleural and interlobular septal nodules (*arrow*).

LYMPHOMA

(See pages 274–286.)

HRCT Findings

Multiple or solitary nodules
Multiple or localized areas of consolidation
Air bronchograms
Peribronchial distribution
Interstitial infiltration
Pleural effusion

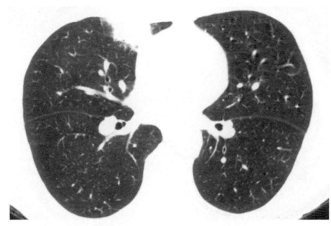

Localized consolidation.

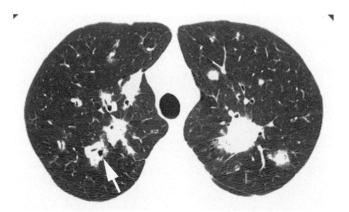

Multiple peribronchial nodules with an air bronchogram (*arrow*).

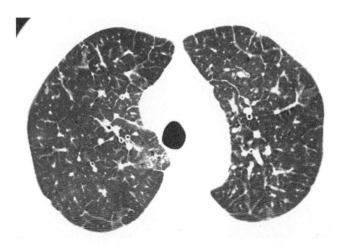

Interlobular septal thickening due to interstitial infiltration.

METASTATIC CARCINOMA (HEMATOGENOUS)

(See pages 267–270.)

HRCT Findings

Well-defined nodules with a uniform distribution
Nodules visible in relation to pleural surfaces
Features of lymphangitic spread of carcinoma may be present

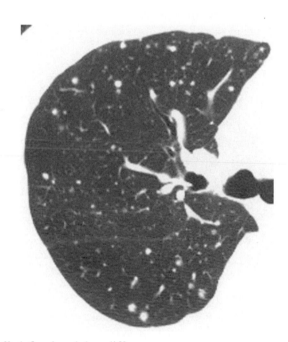

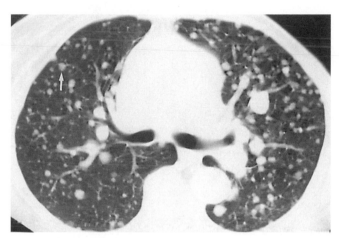

Well-defined nodules, some involving pleural surface (*arrow*).

Well-defined nodules, diffuse.

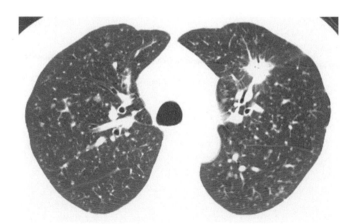

Small, sharply defined, diffuse nodules.

METASTATIC CARCINOMA (LYMPHANGITIC)

(See pages 260–267.)

HRCT Findings

Smooth or nodular peribronchovascular interstitial thickening
Smooth or nodular interlobular septal thickening
Smooth or nodular thickening of fissures
Subpleural nodules
Normal lung architecture; no distortion
Diffuse, patchy, or unilateral distribution
Lymph node enlargement
Pleural effusion

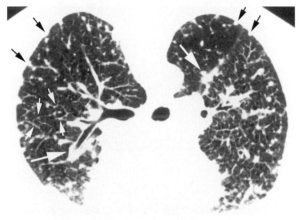

Subpleural nodules (*black arrows*), nodular thickening of septa (*small white arrows*), and peribronchovascular thickening (*large white arrows*).

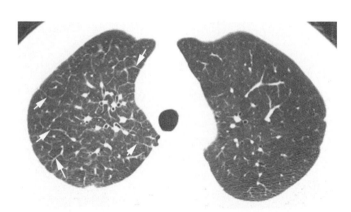

Smooth interlobular septal thickening (*arrows*).

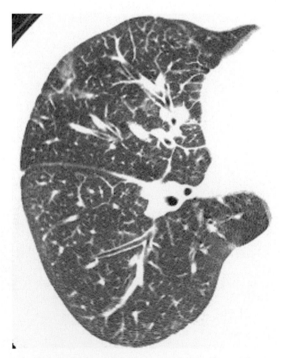

Smooth thickening of septa and peribronchovascular interstitium.

MYCOBACTERIUM AVIUM COMPLEX (MAC) INFECTION

(See pages 325–333.)

HRCT Findings

Bronchiectasis
Small or large nodules
Patchy unilateral or bilateral airspace consolidation
Cavitation, thin- or thick-walled
Tree-in-bud

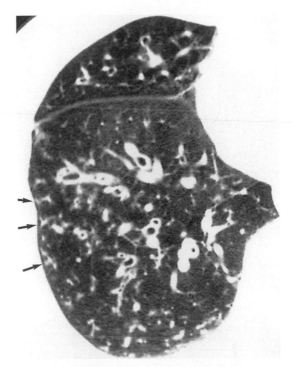

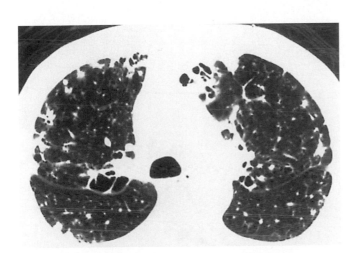

Bronchiectasis and centrilobular nodules.

Bronchiectasis with tree-in-bud (*arrows*).

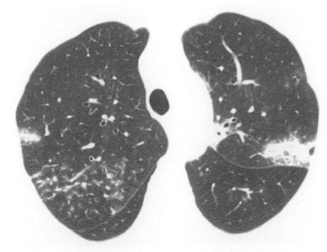

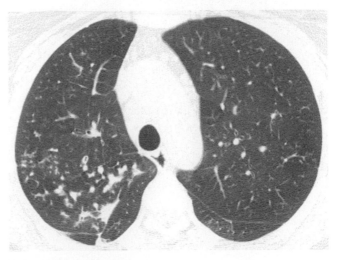

Patchy consolidation with tree-in-bud and nodules.

Large and small nodules.

NONSPECIFIC INTERSTITIAL PNEUMONIA (NSIP)

(See pages 378–381.)

HRCT Findings

Ground-glass opacity
Airspace consolidation
Intralobular linear opacities
Honeycombing (uncommon)
Peripheral and lower lung zone predominance

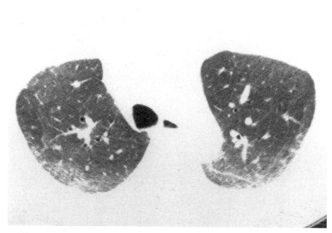

Patchy ground-glass opacities.

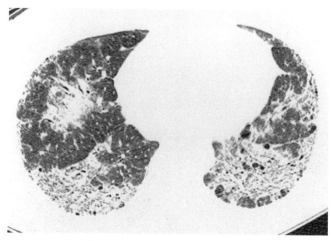

Patchy ground-glass opacity and reticular opacities.

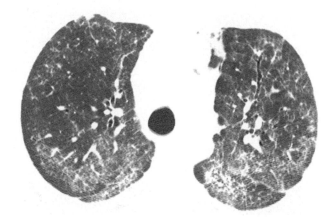

Patchy subpleural ground-glass opacity with reticulation.

PANBRONCHIOLITIS

(See pages 97–128; 529–539.)

HRCT Findings

Tree-in-bud
Bronchiolectasis
Bronchiectasis
Diffuse distribution/basilar predominance
Large lung volumes
Mosaic perfusion
Air-trapping on expiration

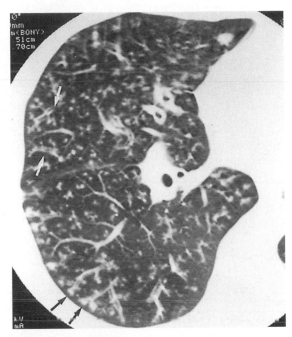

Bronchial wall thickening and tree-in-bud (*arrows*).

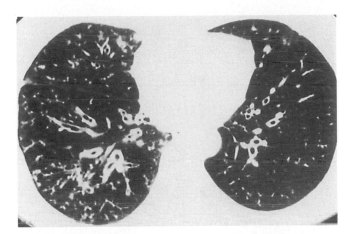

Bronchiectasis, centrilobular nodules, and tree-in-bud.

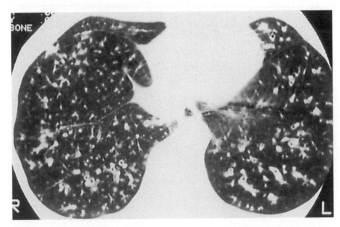

Bronchiolectasis, centrilobular nodules, and tree-in-bud.

PLEXOGENIC ARTERIOPATHY

(See pages 553–562.)

HRCT Findings

Dilatation of main pulmonary artery
Dilatation of central arteries
Variation in size of arteries
Mosaic perfusion (uncommon)

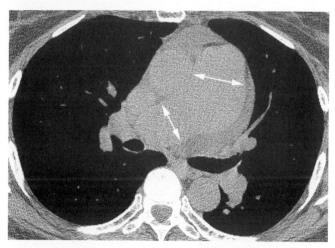

Dilatation of main pulmonary arteries (*arrows*).

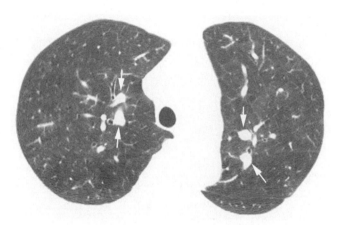

Dilatation of central pulmonary arteries (*arrows*).

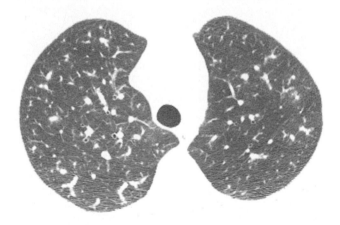

Variation in size of small pulmonary artery branches.

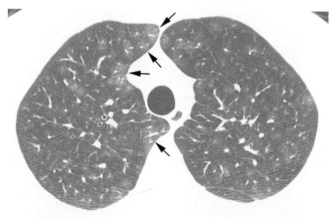

Inhomogeneous lung attenuation due to mosaic perfusion (uncommon).

PNEUMOCYSTIS CARINII PNEUMONIA (PCP)

(See pages 396–403.)

HRCT Findings

Patchy bilateral ground-glass opacity
Central or perihilar distribution in many
Interlobular septal thickening (resolving stage)
Crazy-paving
Thick- or thin-walled, irregular, septated cysts
Pneumothorax
Centrilobular nodules

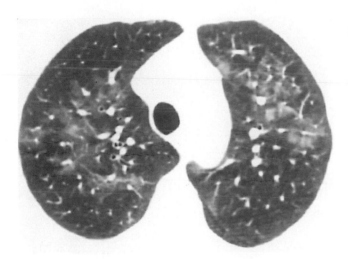

Patchy ground-glass opacity.

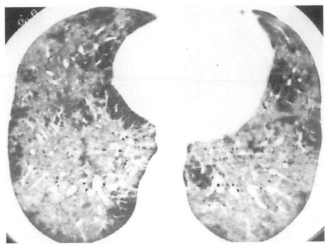

Extensive ground-glass opacity and consolidation.

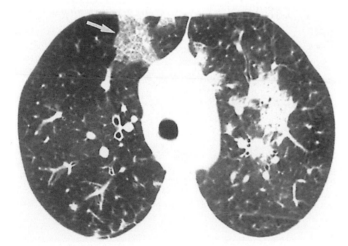

Crazy-paving (*arrow*) and consolidation.

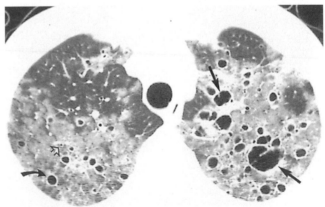

Ground-glass opacity with lung cysts (*arrows*).

PROGRESSIVE SYSTEMIC SCLEROSIS (SCLERODERMA)

(See pages 214–218.)

HRCT Findings

Ground-glass opacity or consolidation
Findings of fibrosis
Peripheral, subpleural, lower lobe, posterior predominance
Pleural thickening or effusion
Small centrilobular nodules (follicular bronchiolitis)
Esophageal dilatation

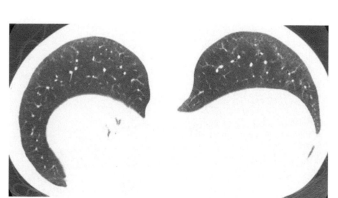

Subpleural ground-glass opacity in active disease.

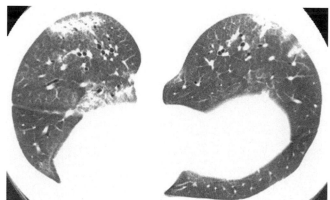

Subpleural consolidation and ground-glass opacity.

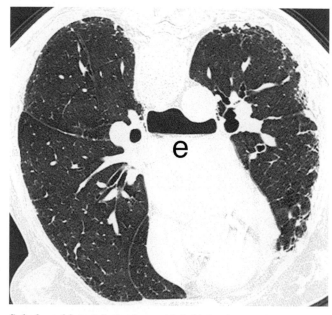

Subpleural intralobular interstitial thickening and esophageal dilatation (e).

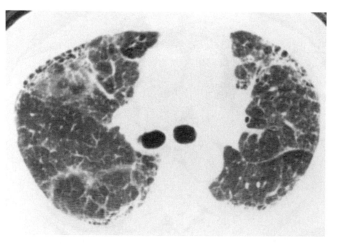

Subpleural honeycombing.

PULMONARY EDEMA

(See pages 72–96; 411–415.)

HRCT Findings

Hydrostatic Edema

Smooth interlobular septal thickening
Patchy ground-glass opacity
Smooth subpleural or fissural thickening
Centrilobular nodules
Dependent, perihilar, or lower lung predominance

Increased Permeability Edema or Acute Respiratory Distress Syndrome

Diffuse or patchy ground-glass opacity or consolidation
Centrilobular opacities
Peripheral distribution

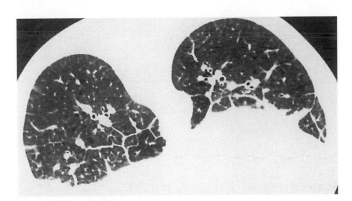

Smooth interlobular septal thickening.

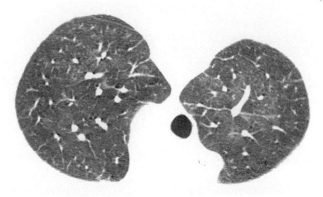

Interlobular septal thickening and ground-glass opacity.

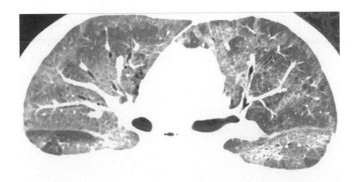

Ground-glass opacity, septal thickening, and pleural effusions.

RESPIRATORY BRONCHIOLITIS-INTERSTITIAL LUNG DISEASE (RB-ILD)

(See pages 382–384.)

HRCT Findings

Centrilobular nodular opacities
Ground-glass opacity
Upper lobe predominance
Findings of fibrosis usually absent

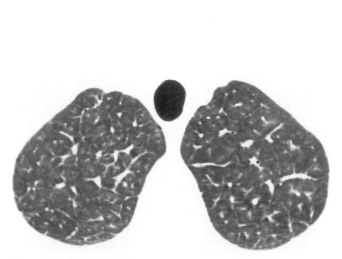

Centrilobular ground-glass opacities.

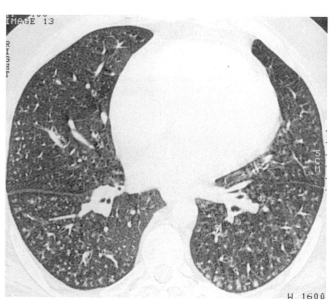

Centrilobular nodular opacities.

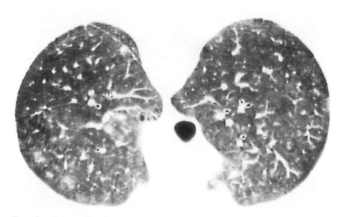

Patchy ground-glass opacity.

RHEUMATOID ARTHRITIS (RA)

(See pages 210–213; 529–539.)

HRCT Findings

Bronchiectasis without fibrosis
Findings of fibrosis
Honeycombing (less common than in IPF)
Ground-glass opacity
Peripheral, subpleural, lower lobe, posterior predominance
Pleural thickening or effusion
Small centrilobular nodules (follicular bronchiolitis)

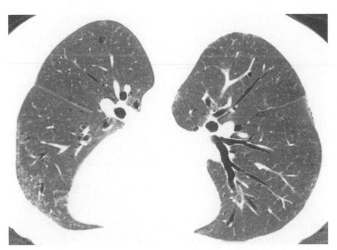

Subpleural nodularity consistent with follicular bronchiolitis.

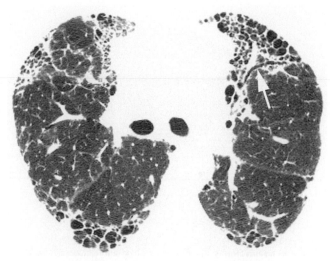

Subpleural honeycombing and traction bronchiectasis (*arrow*).

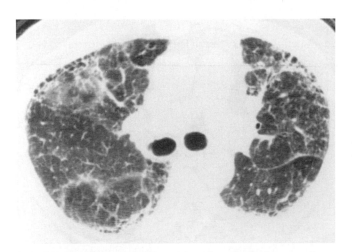

Subpleural reticulation (fibrosis) and ground-glass opacity.

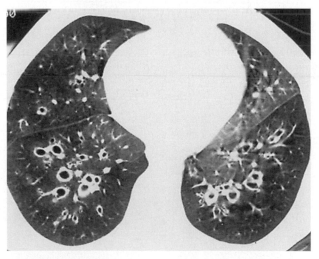

Bronchiectasis and mosaic perfusion.

SARCOIDOSIS

(See pages 286–302.)

HRCT Findings

Smooth or nodular peribronchovascular interstitial thickening
Small, well-defined subpleural nodules (fissures)
Large nodules (larger than 1 cm) or consolidation
Ground-glass opacity
Findings of fibrosis: traction bronchiectasis
Conglomerate masses associated with bronchiectasis
Patchy upper lobe distribution
Lymph node enlargement, usually symmetric

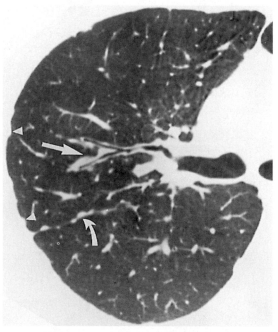

Well-defined nodules adjacent to fissures (*curved arrow*), pleural surface (*arrowheads*), and peribronchovascular interstitium (*large arrow*).

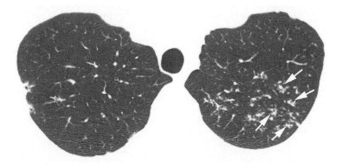

Small nodules in a peribronchovascular location (*arrows*).

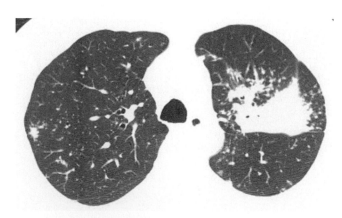

Large confluent mass.

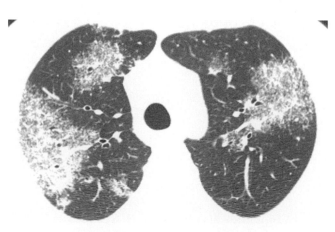

Confluent small nodules with ground-glass opacity.

SARCOIDOSIS: END-STAGE

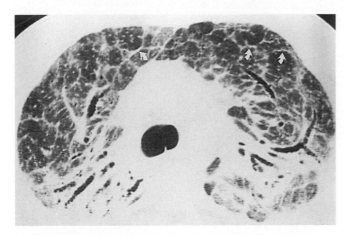

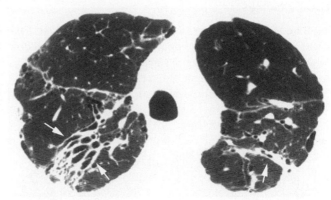

End-stage sarcoidosis with fibrosis, traction bronchiectasis, and irregular septal thickening.

End-stage sarcoidosis with traction bronchiectasis (*arrows*).

SILICOSIS AND COAL WORKER'S PNEUMOCONIOSIS (CWP)

(See pages 303–309.)

HRCT Findings

Small nodules, 2 to 5 mm in diameter, centrilobular and subpleural
Diffuse distribution, with upper lobe and posterior predominance
Conglomerate masses, irregular in shape
Irregular or cicatricial emphysema in silicosis
Lymph node enlargement, calcification

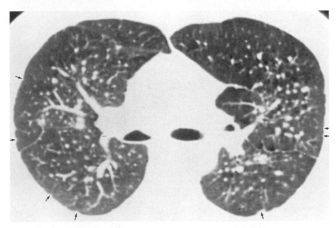

Subpleural (*arrows*) and centrilobular nodules with a posterior upper lobe predominance.

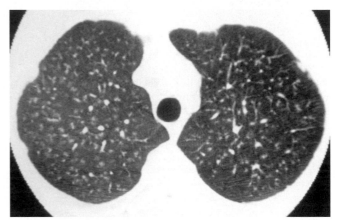

Upper lobe nodules, primarily centrilobular.

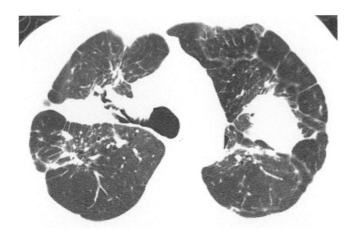

Conglomerate masses of fibrosis and traction bronchiectasis.

SYSTEMIC LUPUS ERYTHEMATOSUS (SLE)

(See pages 218–222.)

HRCT Findings

Findings of fibrosis
Honeycombing (less common than with IPF)
Ground-glass opacity
Peripheral, subpleural, lower lobe, posterior predominance
Bronchiectasis
Pleural thickening or effusion

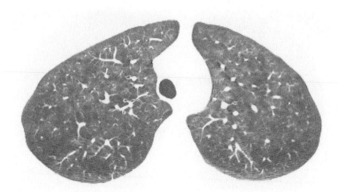

Patchy ground-glass opacity due to lupus pneumonitis.

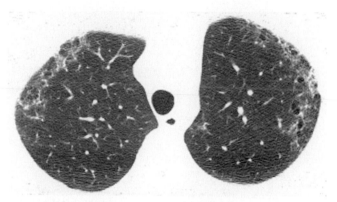

Subpleural reticulation consistent with fibrosis.

TUBERCULOSIS (TB)

(See pages 315–325.)

HRCT Findings

Patchy unilateral or bilateral airspace consolidation
Cavitation, thin- or thick-walled
Scattered centrilobular nodules, tree-in-bud
Small, well-defined nodules, random distribution
Pleural effusion
Low-density hilar/mediastinal lymph nodes

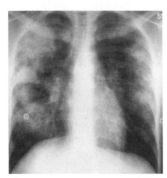
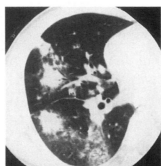

Patchy bilateral consolidation (primary TB).

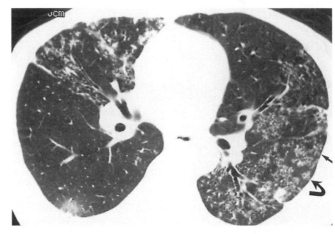

Cavitary lesion with centrilobular nodules and tree-in-bud (*arrows*).

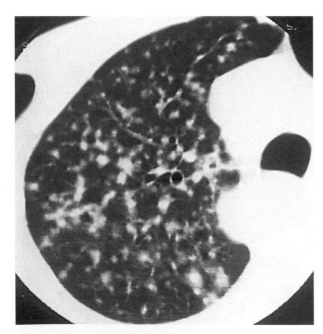

Endobronchial spread of infection with centrilobular nodules.

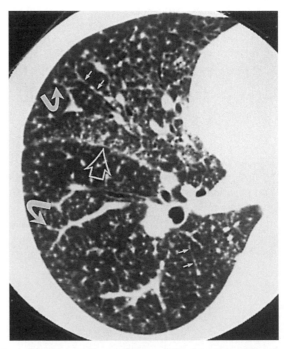

Miliary TB with diffuse small nodules involving the pleural surface (*open arrow*), small vessels (*curved arrows*), and septa (*small arrows*).

CHAPTER 1

Technical Aspects of High-Resolution Computed Tomography

Although the introduction of computed tomography (CT) revolutionized the radiologic diagnosis of chest diseases, the ability of early CT scanners to evaluate pulmonary parenchymal diseases was limited by their resolving power [1]. Specifically, CT obtained with long scan times (18 seconds) and 1-cm collimation provided insufficient anatomic detail to allow a precise evaluation of normal and abnormal pulmonary anatomy, at least to the degree that it would surpass the information available on plain radiographs.

Attempts to improve the resolution of CT for diagnosing lung abnormalities were first described relative to the assessment of focal lung disease and lung nodules. In 1980, Siegelman et al. [2] emphasized the necessity of using 5-mm collimation for the detection of calcification in lung nodules. As thinner collimation became available on commercial scanners, simultaneous with other developments in CT technology, the use of CT for the precise anatomic definition of diffuse lung diseases became possible and was reported by several authors. The first use of the term *high-resolution CT* (HRCT) has been attributed to Todo, Itoh, and others [3],

who described the potential use of this technique for assessing lung disease in 1982. The first reports of HRCT in English date to 1985, including landmark descriptions of HRCT findings by Nakata, Naidich, and Zerhouni [4–6].

HRCT techniques developed since then are capable of imaging the lung with excellent spatial resolution, providing anatomic detail similar to that available from gross pathologic specimens or lung slices [7–10]. HRCT can demonstrate the normal and abnormal lung interstitium and morphologic characteristics of both localized and diffuse parenchymal abnormalities; in this regard, HRCT is clearly superior to plain radiographs and conventional CT. HRCT has become established as an important diagnostic modality and has significantly contributed to our understanding of diffuse lung diseases. In this chapter, we review the CT techniques that are appropriate in obtaining HRCT, spiral HRCT techniques, scan protocols recommended in specific clinical settings, expiratory HRCT, the spatial resolution of HRCT, the radiation dose associated with HRCT, and common HRCT artifacts.

TABLE 1-1. *Summary of HRCT technique*

Recommended
  Collimation: thinnest available collimation (1.0–1.5 mm).
  Reconstruction algorithm: high–spatial frequency or "sharp" algorithm (i.e., GE "bone").
  Scan time: as short as possible (1 sec or less).
  kV(p), 120–140; mA, 240.
  Matrix size: largest available (512 × 512).
  Windows: At least one consistent lung window setting is necessary. Window mean/width values of –600 HU to –700 HU/1,000 HU to 1,500 HU are appropriate. Good combinations are –700/1,000 HU or –600/1,500 HU. Soft-tissue windows of approximately 50/350 HU should also be used for the mediastinum, hila, and pleura.
  Image display: photography of lung windows 12 on 1.
Optional
  kV(p)/mA: Increased kV(p)/mA (i.e., 140/340). Recommended in large patients. Otherwise optional. Reduced mA (low-dose HRCT): 40–80 mA.
  Targeted reconstruction: (15- to 25-cm field of view).
  Windows: Windows may need to be customized; a low-window mean (–800 to –900 HU) is optimal for diagnosing emphysema. For viewing the mediastinum, 50/350 HU is recommended. For viewing pleuro-parenchymal disease, –600/2,000 HU is recommended.
  Image display: Photography of lung windows 6 on 1.

HIGH-RESOLUTION COMPUTED TOMOGRAPHY TECHNIQUE

The HRCT technique attempts to optimize the demonstration of lung anatomy. Although each of the three of us performs HRCT in a slightly different manner, experienced radiologists generally agree as to what technical modifications constitute a "high-resolution" CT study. This section reviews the effect of various technical factors on the appearance of HRCT and summarizes our recommendations for techniques that are either necessary or optional for obtaining an adequate examination.

The most important modifications of CT technique used to increase spatial resolution are the uses of thin collimation and image reconstruction with a high-spatial frequency (sharp) algorithm. Increased kilovolt (peak) [kV(p)] or milliamperes (mA) and targeted image reconstruction may also be used to improve image quality and increase spatial resolution, but these techniques are optional (Table 1-1) [7–13]. The use of appropriate window settings and methods of image display are also necessary to obtain optimal diagnostic images.

Scan Collimation

With thick (7- to 10-mm) collimation, volume averaging within the plane of scan significantly reduces the ability of CT to resolve small structures. Therefore, scanning with the thinnest possible collimation (1- to 1.5-mm) is essential if spatial resolution is to be optimized [4,6,10,11] (Table 1-1). The use of 3- to 5-mm collimation should not be considered for HRCT.

Murata et al. [13] compared the ability of HRCT scans performed with 1.5- and 3-mm collimation to allow the identification of small vessels, bronchi, interlobular septa, and some pathologic findings. With 1.5-mm collimation, greater contrast was evident between vessels and surrounding lung parenchyma, more branches of small vessels were seen, and small bronchi were more often recognizable than with 3-mm collimation [13]. Also, slight increases in lung attenuation (as in early interstitial disease), or decreases in attenuation (as in emphysema) were better resolved with 1.5-mm collimation. On the other hand, the authors concluded that certain pathologic findings, such as thickened interlobular septa, were similarly visible on images with 1.5- and 3-mm collimation [13].

There are several differences in how lung structures are visualized on scans performed with thin collimation compared to more thickly collimated scans. With thin collimation, it is more difficult to follow the courses of vessels and bronchi than it is with 7- to 10-mm collimation. With thick collimation, for example, vessels that lie in the plane of scan look like vessels (i.e., they appear cylindrical or branching) and can be clearly identified as such. With thin collimation, vessels can appear nodular, because only short segments may lie in the plane of scan; this finding may lead to confusion (Fig. 1-1), but with experience, this difficulty is avoided easily.

Also, with thin collimation, the diameter of a vessel that lies in or near the plane of scan can appear larger than it does with 1-cm collimation, because less volume averaging is occurring between the rounded edge of the vessel and the adjacent air-filled lung (Fig. 1-1); thin collimation scans more accurately reflect vessel diameter in this setting, analogous to the better estimation of the diameter of a lung nodule that is possible with thin collimation. Furthermore, with 1-mm collimation, bronchi that are oriented obliquely relative to the scan plane are much better defined than they are with 1-cm collimation, and their wall thicknesses and luminal diameters are more accurately assessed [14]. The diameters of vessels or bronchi that lie perpendicular to the scan plane appear the same with both thin and thick collimation.

Reconstruction Algorithm

The inherent or maximum spatial resolution of a CT scanner is determined by the geometry of the data collecting system and the frequency at which scan data are sampled during the scan sequence [11]. The spatial resolution of the image produced is less than the inherent resolution of the scan system, depending on the reconstruction algorithm that is used, the matrix size, and the field of view (FOV), all of which in turn determine pixel size. In HRCT, these parameters are optimized to increase the spatial resolution of the image.

With conventional body CT, scan data are usually reconstructed with a relatively low–spatial frequency algorithm (e.g., "standard" or "soft-tissue" algorithms), that smoothes the image, reduces visible image noise, and improves the contrast resolution to some degree [12,15]. *Low–spatial frequency* simply means that the frequency of information recorded in the final image is relatively low; it is the same as saying that the algorithm is low-resolution rather than high-resolution.

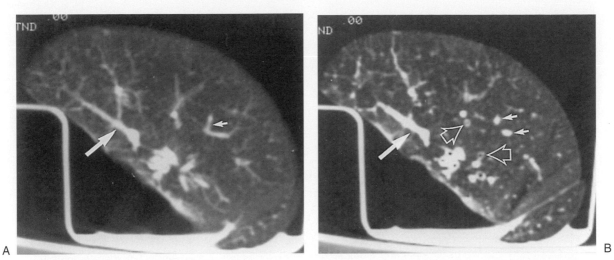

FIG. 1-1. Effects of collimation on resolution. **A:** Conventional CT of a fresh inflated human lung obtained with 1-cm collimation and reconstructed with the standard algorithm. Several cylindrical or branching pulmonary arteries (*small arrow*) are visible. A large pulmonary artery branch (*large arrow*) lies in the plane of scan. **B:** CT at the same level with 1.5-mm collimation; technical parameters and reconstructed algorithm are otherwise identical. Pulmonary arteries seen as branching or cylindrical on the scan obtained using 1-cm collimation appear nodular on the scan with 1.5-mm collimation (*small arrows*). Small bronchi (*open arrows*) are much better seen with thin collimation. Note that the large pulmonary vessel that lies in the plane of scan appears to have a greater diameter with thin collimation (*large arrow*) than it does with 1-cm collimation.

Reconstruction of the image using a high–spatial frequency algorithm—in other words, a high-resolution algorithm (e.g., General Electric "bone" algorithm), reduces image smoothing and increases spatial resolution, making structures appear sharper (Fig. 1-2) [4,11,13]. In one study of HRCT techniques [11], a quantitative improvement in spatial resolution was found when the bone, instead of the standard, algorithm was used to reconstruct scan data (Fig. 1-3); in this study, subjective image quality was also rated more highly with the bone

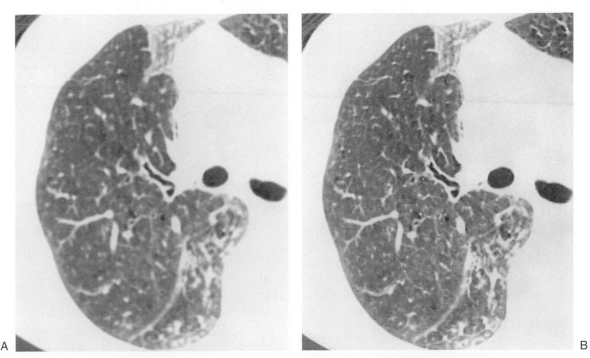

FIG. 1-2. Effect of reconstruction algorithm on resolution. A CT scan obtained with 1.5-mm collimation has been reconstructed using a smoothing (standard) algorithm **(A)** and a sharp (bone) algorithm **(B)**. Lung structures appear much sharper with the bone algorithm.

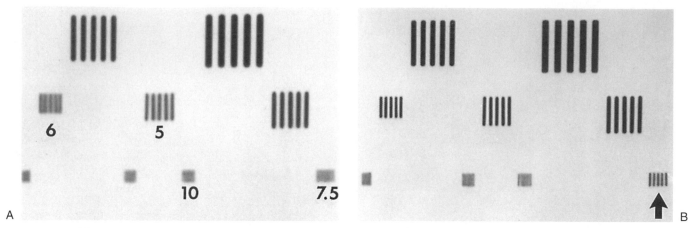

FIG. 1-3. Effect of reconstruction algorithm on spatial resolution. **A:** HRCT of a line-pair phantom obtained with 1.5-mm collimation and reconstructed with the standard algorithm. Numbers indicate the resolution in line pairs per cm. The resolution with this technique is 6-line pairs per cm. **B:** When the same scan is reconstructed using the bone algorithm, spatial resolution improves. Also, in contrast to the scan reconstructed using the standard algorithm, 7.5-line pairs are easily resolved (*arrow*), and edges are considerably sharper. (From Mayo JR, Webb WR, Gould R, et al. High-resolution CT of the lungs: an optimal approach. *Radiology* 1987;163:507, with permission.)

algorithm. In another study of HRCT [13], small vessels and bronchi were better seen when images were reconstructed with the bone algorithm than when the standard algorithm was used. The use of a sharp algorithm has also been recommended for routine chest CT performed using 1-cm collimation, to improve spatial resolution [16].

Using a sharp, or high-resolution, algorithm is a critical element in performing HRCT (Table 1-1) [12,15].

Kilovolt (Peak), Milliamperes, Scan Time, and Low-Dose High-Resolution Computed Tomography

In HRCT, image noise is more apparent than with standard CT. This noise usually appears as a graininess or mottle that can be distracting and may obscure anatomic detail (Fig. 1-4) [11]. High-resolution techniques using a sharp reconstruction algorithm, in addition to increasing image detail, increase the visibility of noise in the CT image [12,15]. Because much of this noise is quantum-related and thus decreases with increased technique (number of photons), increasing the mA or kV(p) used during scanning, or increasing scan time, can reduce noise and improve scan quality (Fig. 1-5) [11]; noise is inversely proportional to the number of photons absorbed (precisely, it is inversely proportional to the square root of the product of the mA and scan time).

Increasing scan time is not generally desirable with lung CT. Because of patient motion, longer scan times can result in an increase in motion-related artifacts. When available, a scan time of 1 second or less is most appropriate for HRCT and is recommended (Table 1-1).

mA and kV(p) can be easily increased when obtaining HRCT, which results in a reduction in visible image noise. In one study [11], a measure of image noise was reduced by approximately 30% when kV(p)/mA were increased from 120/100 to 140/170

(2-second scan time) (Fig. 1-5), and the scans with increased kV(p) and mA settings were rated by observers as being of better quality 80% of the time (Fig. 1-6) [11]. It should also be kept in mind, however, that increasing scan technique also increases the patient's radiation dose [17], although with HRCT, radiation is limited to a few thin scan levels (as discussed below).

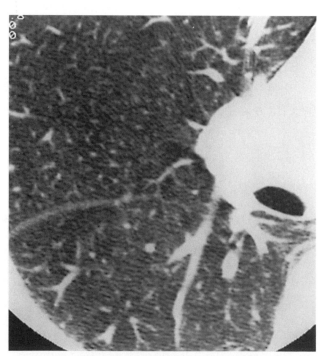

FIG. 1-4. Image noise. Detailed view of an HRCT image of the right lung. The mottled appearance, which is most evident posteriorly, represents image noise. Very thin linear streaks, best seen in the anterior part of the image, represent "aliasing" artifacts.

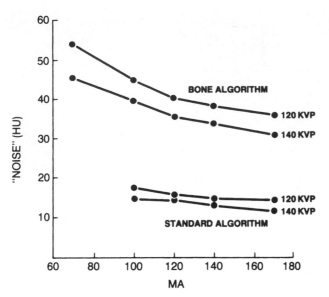

FIG. 1-5. Effect of algorithm, kV(p), and mA on image noise. Graph of HRCT image noise (standard deviation of Hounsfield unit measurements) in an anthropomorphic CT phantom [21] as related to the reconstruction algorithm and scan technique. Noise increases when the bone algorithm is used instead of the standard algorithm. With the bone algorithm, noise decreases approximately 30% with increased kV(p) and mA settings. (From Mayo JR, Webb WR, Gould R, et al. High-resolution CT of the lungs: an optimal approach. *Radiology* 1987;163:507, with permission.)

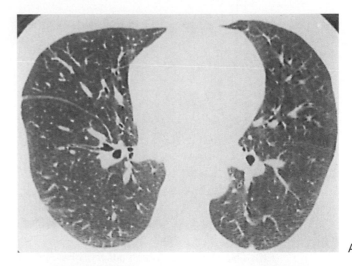

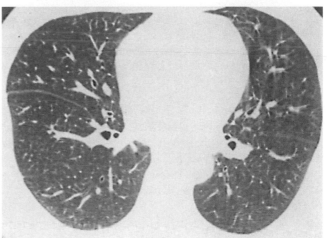

FIG. 1-6. Effect of kV(p) and mA on image noise. HRCT scans obtained with kV(p)/mA settings of 120/100 **(A)** and 140/170 **(B)**. Noise is most evident posteriorly and in the paravertebral regions. Although noise is greater in **A**, the difference is probably not significant clinically. Nonetheless, increasing the kV(p)/mA is optimal. Also note pulsation ("star") artifacts in the left lung on both images and a "double" left major fissure. (From Mayo JR, Webb WR, Gould R, et al. High-resolution CT of the lungs: an optimal approach. *Radiology* 1987;163:507, with permission.)

Although increasing kV(p) and mA reduces image noise, this modification is not generally necessary with current scanners. Adequate diagnostic scans can be obtained in most patients using routine techniques for chest CT [18], although image quality may not be quite as good as when technique is increased. Use of current scanners capable of a 1-second scan time, scan techniques of 120 to 140 kV(p), and mA values of approximately 240 has proven quite satisfactory [19].

Furthermore, the efficacy of low-dose HRCT has been assessed in several studies [20–23]. In a study by Zwirewich et al. [20], scans with 1.5-mm collimation, and 2-second scan time, and at 120 kV(p), were obtained using both 20 mA (low-dose HRCT) and 200 mA (conventional-dose HRCT) at selected levels in the chests of 31 patients. Observers evaluated the visibility of normal structures, various parenchymal abnormalities, and artifacts using both techniques. Low-dose and conventional-dose HRCT were equivalent for the demonstration of vessels, lobular and segmental bronchi, and structures of the secondary pulmonary lobule and in characterizing the extent and distribution of reticular abnormalities, honeycomb cysts, and thickened interlobular septa. However, the low-dose technique failed to demonstrate ground-glass opacity in two of ten cases, and emphysema in one of nine cases, although they were evident but subtle on the usual-dose HRCT. Linear streak artifacts were also more prominent on images acquired with the low-dose technique, but the two techniques were judged equally diagnostic in 97% of cases. The authors concluded that

HRCT images acquired at 20 mA yield anatomic information equivalent to that obtained with 200-mA scans in the majority of patients without significant loss of spatial resolution or image degradation due to streak artifacts.

In a subsequent study [21], the diagnostic accuracies of chest radiographs, low-dose HRCT [80 mA; 120 kV(p), 40 mA, 2 seconds] and conventional-dose HRCT [340 mA; 120 kV(p), 170 mA, 2 seconds] were compared in 50 patients with chronic infiltrative lung disease and ten normal controls. For each HRCT technique, only three images were used, obtained at the levels of the aortic arch, tracheal carina, and 1 cm above the right hemidiaphragm. A correct first-choice diagnosis was made significantly more often with either HRCT technique than with radiography; the cor-

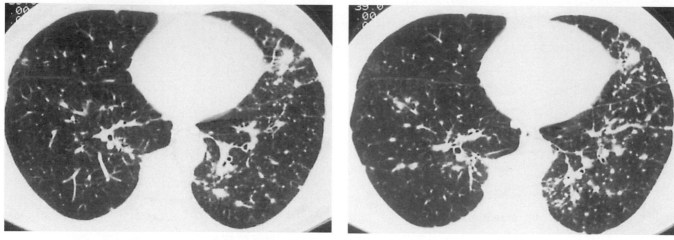

FIG. 1-7. Low-dose **(A)** and conventional-dose **(B)** HRCT in a patient with sarcoidosis. Both techniques demonstrate the presence of small peribronchovascular, septal, and subpleural nodules typical of this disease. Despite the increased noise on the low-dose image, the pattern and extent of abnormalities are equally well seen with both techniques. (From Lee KS, Primack SL, Staples CA, et al. Chronic infiltrative lung disease: comparison of diagnostic accuracies of radiography and low- and conventional-dose thin-section CT. *Radiology* 1994;191:669, with permission.)

rect diagnosis was made in 65% of cases using radiographs, 74% of cases with low-dose HRCT (p <.02), and 80% of conventional HRCT (p <.005). A high confidence level in making a diagnosis was reached in 42% of radiographic examinations, 61% of the low-dose HRCT examinations (p <.01), and 63% of the conventional-dose HRCT examinations (p <.005), and it was correct in 92%, 90%, and 96% of the studies, respectively. Although conventional-dose HRCT was more accurate than low-dose HRCT, this difference was not significant, and both techniques provided quite similar anatomic information (Figs. 1-7 and 1-8) [21].

Majurin et al. [22] compared a variety of low-dose techniques in 45 patients with suspected asbestos-related lung dis-

ease. Of the 37 patients with CT evidence of lung fibrosis, HRCT images obtained with mA as low as 120 (60 mA/2 seconds) clearly showed parenchymal bands, curvilinear opacities, and honeycombing. However, reliable identification of interstitial lines or areas of ground-glass opacity required a minimum technique of 160 mA (80 mA/2 seconds). Furthermore, these authors showed that using the lowest possible dosage (30 mA/2 seconds) HRCT was sufficient only for detecting marked pleural thickening and areas of gross lung fibrosis.

Although optimizing resolution may require the use of increased mA and kV(p), this is optional and uncommonly used with current scanners (Table 1-1). In the majority of patients, diagnostic scans will be obtained without increas-

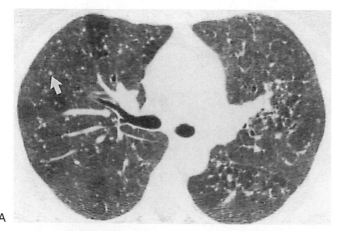
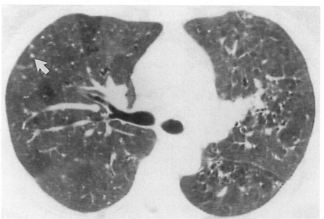

FIG. 1-8. Low-dose **(A)** and conventional-dose **(B)** HRCT in a patient with hypersensitivity pneumonitis. Although noise is much more obvious on the low-dose image, areas of ground-glass opacity and ill-defined nodules (*arrows*) are visible with both techniques. (From Lee KS, Primack SL, Staples CA, et al. Chronic infiltrative lung disease: comparison of diagnostic accuracies of radiography and low- and conventional-dose thin-section CT. *Radiology* 1994;191:669, with permission.)

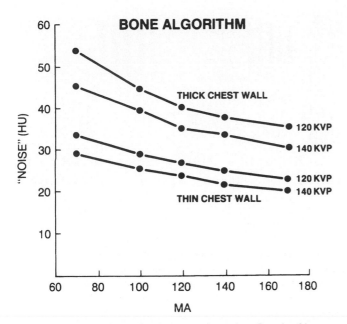

FIG. 1-9. Relationship of noise to patient size. Graph of image noise measured using an anthropomorphic chest phantom [21], with simulated thick and thin chest walls. Noise significantly increases with the thick chest wall. (From Mayo JR, Webb WR, Gould R, et al. High-resolution CT of the lungs: an optimal approach. *Radiology* 1987;163:507, with permission.)

ing scan technique. Because noise is usually a bigger problem in large patients (because more x-ray photons are attenuated by the patient) (Fig. 1-9) and in the posterior part of the scan image (because of photon attenuation by the spine), it would be most important to use increased technical factors when studying large patients or patients with suspected posterior lung disease [11]. Low-dose HRCT should not be routinely used for the initial evaluation of patients with lung disease, although it can be valuable in following patients with a known lung abnormality or in screening large populations at risk for lung disease. Optimal low-dose techniques will likely vary with the clinical setting and indication for the study, and they remain to be established.

Matrix Size, Field of View, and the Use of Targeted Reconstruction

The largest matrix available should be used routinely in image reconstruction, to reduce pixel size [4,11,13]. The largest available matrix is usually 512×512.

Scanning should be performed using an FOV large enough to encompass the patient (e.g., 35 cm). Retrospectively targeting image reconstruction to a single lung instead of the entire thorax, using a smaller FOV, significantly reduces the image pixel size and thus increases spatial reso-

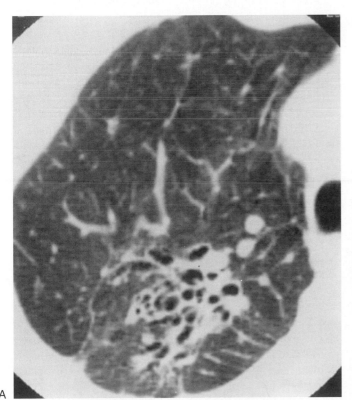

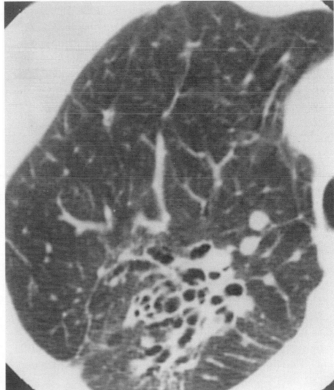

FIG. 1-10. Effect of targeted reconstruction on resolution. **A:** CT image in a patient with end-stage sarcoidosis obtained with a 38-cm field of view (FOV) and 1.5-mm collimation, and reconstructed using the bone algorithm and a 38-cm reconstruction circle. **B:** The same CT scan has been reconstructed using a targeted FOV (15 cm), reducing image-pixel diameter. Image sharpness is improved compared to **A.**

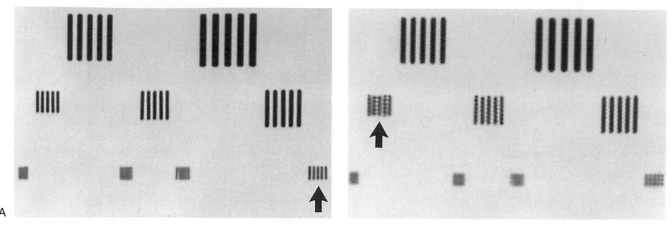

FIG. 1-11. Effect of targeted reconstruction on spatial resolution. **A:** HRCT of a line-pain phantom. The scan was obtained with a 40-cm field of view (FOV), and reconstructed using a targeted FOV of 25 cm. The resolution with this technique is 7.5-line pairs (*arrow*). **B:** The same scan viewed without targeting shows the effects of larger pixel size. Only 6-line pairs can be resolved (*arrow*), and the margins of the lines appear jagged or wavy. (From Mayo JR, Webb WR, Gould R, et al. High-resolution CT of the lungs: an optimal approach. *Radiology* 1987;163:507, with permission.)

lution (Fig. 1-10) [11,18]. For example, with a 40-cm reconstruction circle (FOV) and a 512 × 512 matrix, pixel size measures 0.78 mm. With targeted image reconstruction using a 25-cm FOV, pixel size is reduced to 0.49 mm, and the spatial resolution is correspondingly increased (Fig. 1-11). Using a 15-cm FOV further reduces pixel size to 0.29 mm, but this FOV is usually insufficient to view an entire lung and is not often used clinically. It should be recognized, however, that the improvement in resolution obtainable by targeting is limited by the intrinsic resolution of the detectors. For example, with a General Electric 9800 system, optimal matching of the inherent spatial resolution of the scanner and pixel size occurs at a reconstruction diameter of approximately 13 cm and a pixel size of 0.25 mm [11,12,15]; further reduction in the FOV would be of no benefit in improving spatial resolution.

The use of image targeting, or targeted reconstruction, is often a matter of personal preference. In clinical practice, use of image targeting is uncommon because it requires additional reconstruction time, the raw scan data must be saved until targeting is performed, and additional filming is required to display all the images. Also, with a nontargeted reconstruction, the ability to see both lungs on the same image allows a quick comparison of one lung to the other; this can be quite helpful in diagnosis and is preferred to the marginal increase in resolution achieved with targeting.

Image targeting is considered to be optional (Table 1-1) and is recommended only when optimal resolution is desired.

Window Settings

The window mean and width used for photography have a significant impact on the appearance of the lung parenchyma and the dimensions of visualized structures (Fig. 1-12) [14,24]. If the display technique used is not appropriate, nor-

mal structures can be made to look abnormal, or subtle abnormalities may be overlooked.

The most important window setting to use in photography is the so-called lung window. It should be emphasized that there is no single correct or ideal window setting for the demonstration of lung anatomy on HRCT, and several combinations of window mean and width may be appropriate [25]. Within limits, the precise window width and levels chosen are a matter of personal preference; the values indicated below should serve only as guidelines. However, it is important that a single lung window setting be used consistently in all patients. Unless this is done, it is difficult to compare one case to another, develop an understanding of what appearances are normal and abnormal, and compare sequential examinations in the same patient. Although it is not inappropriate to use some additional window settings in specific cases, depending on what abnormality is being sought, the effects of the variations in window settings on the appearance of the resulting images must be kept in mind.

Level and width settings of approximately –700/1,000 Hounsfield units (HU) are appropriate for a routine lung window (Fig. 1-12). Some authors prefer using a window width of 1,500 HU when viewing the lung, with a window mean of –600 to –700 HU; such settings should also be considered appropriate for routine lung imaging. It should be recognized, however, that an extended window width reduces contrast between lung parenchymal structures, such as vessels, bronchi, and the air-containing alveoli, and may make interstitial structures appear less conspicuous or thinner than they actually are. On the other hand, extended windows may be of some value in detecting abnormalities of overall lung attenuation [26,27] and are also useful in evaluating the relationship of peripheral parenchymal abnormalities to the pleural surfaces. A window width of less than 1,000 HU is not generally appropriate for viewing lung parenchyma, as it unnecessarily increases contrast and may result in an apparent increase in the size of soft-tissue

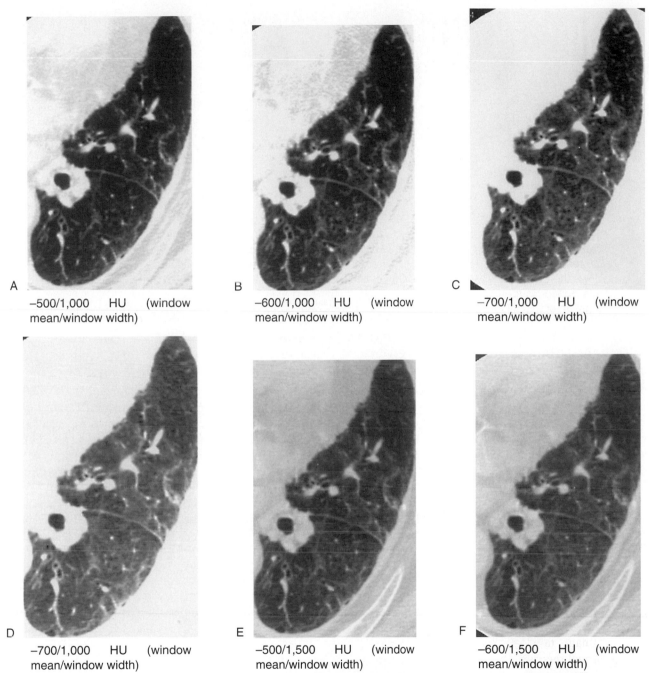

A −500/1,000 HU (window mean/window width)

B −600/1,000 HU (window mean/window width)

C −700/1,000 HU (window mean/window width)

D −700/1,000 HU (window mean/window width)

E −500/1,500 HU (window mean/window width)

F −600/1,500 HU (window mean/window width)

FIG. 1-12. Effects of window mean and width on the appearance of lung and soft tissues in a patient with asbestosis. Window means decrease from left to right. Window widths increase from top to bottom. **A–D:** A window width of 1,000 HU and a window mean of −700 HU **(C)** provides good contrast between soft-tissue structures in the lung (vessels and interstitial abnormalities) and lung parenchyma, allows areas of lung with varying attenuation to be distinguished, and allows air-filled structures (e.g., bronchi, cysts) to be contrasted with lung parenchyma. Abnormal reticular opacities and areas of increased lung and decreased lung attenuation are all visible in **C**. Higher window means **(A)** make lung opacities more difficult to see or make them appear smaller. A lower window mean **(D)** accentuates the visibility of lung opacities and allows air-filled structures to be contrasted with lung parenchyma, but can also make normal lung appear abnormally dense. **E–G:** Wider window settings result in less contrast between soft-tissue lung structures and lung parenchyma. Those images with window levels of −600 and −700 HU **(F,G)** and a width of 1,500 HU provide information comparable to −700/1,000 HU. **H,I:** With a window width of 2,000 HU, much less contrast between normal and abnormal lung regions is visible. However, with this window setting, pleural thickening and calcification are visible. *Continued*

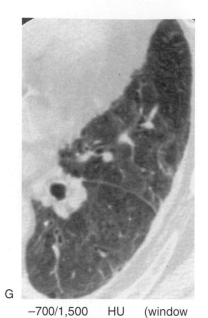

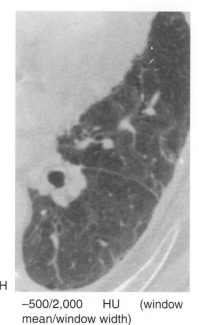

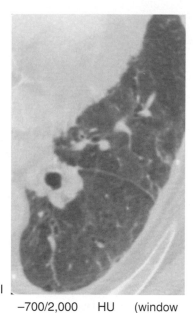

G

−700/1,500 HU (window mean/window width)

H

−500/2,000 HU (window mean/window width)

I

−700/2,000 HU (window mean/window width)

FIG. 1-12. *Continued*

structures. For example, the effect of window mean and level on the HRCT appearance of bronchial walls has been assessed using inflation-fixed lungs [24]. In this study, window widths less than 1,000 HU resulted in a substantial overestimation of bronchial wall thickness, whereas window widths greater than 1,400 HU resulted in an underestimation of bronchial wall thickness (Fig 1-13).

Viewing soft-tissue windows is also important in reading HRCT. Window level/width settings of 50/350 HU or 50/450 HU are best for evaluation of the mediastinum, hila, and

pleura. Mediastinal and pleural abnormalities are sometimes of value in interpreting HRCT of the lung (Table 1-1). For example, the presence of lymph node enlargement, esophageal dilatation, calcification, or pleural thickening may be helpful in making a correct diagnosis of lung disease. When performing an HRCT study, images are routinely displayed using both lung and soft-tissue windows.

As stated, choosing different window levels can be advantageous in individual cases, despite the fact they may not be optimal for all indications (Fig. 1-12). Low-window settings

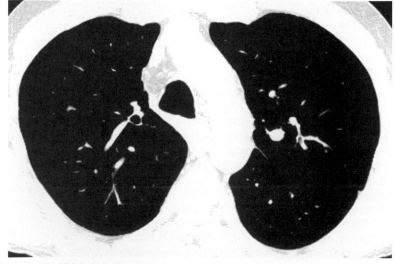

A

−300/500 HU (window mean/window width)

FIG. 1-13. Effects of window mean and width on the visibility of bronchi and vessels in a normal subject. Using a narrow window width (500 HU), a high window mean (e.g., −300 HU) **(A)** makes bronchi and bronchial walls difficult to see, whereas a low window mean (e.g., −900 HU) **(D)** accentuates the apparent thickness of bronchial walls and the diameter of vessels. This effect decreases with increasing window width (i.e., 1,500 HU) **(I–L)**. A window mean of approximately −450 HU and width of 1,000 to 1,400 HU have been shown to be best suited to measuring bronchial wall thickness. *Continued*

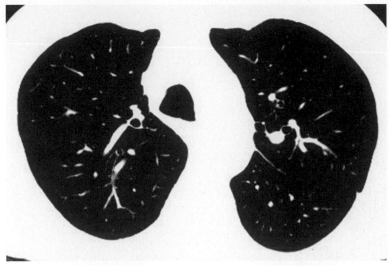

B

−500/500 HU (window mean/window width)

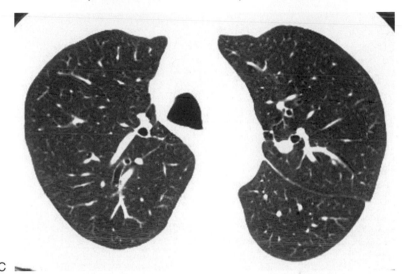

C

−700/500 HU (window mean/window width)

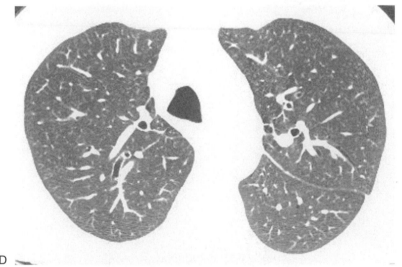

D

−900/500 HU (window mean/window width)

FIG. 1-13. *Continued*

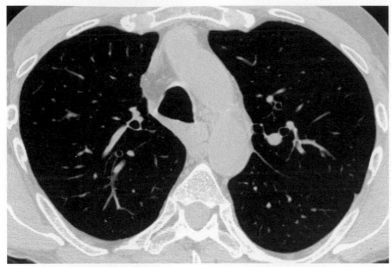

E
−300/1,000 HU (window mean/window width)

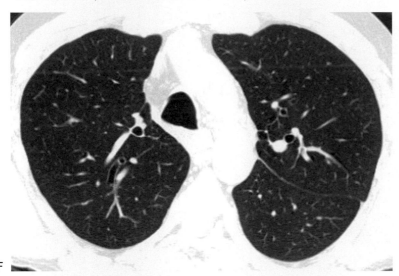

F
−500/1,000 HU (window mean/window width)

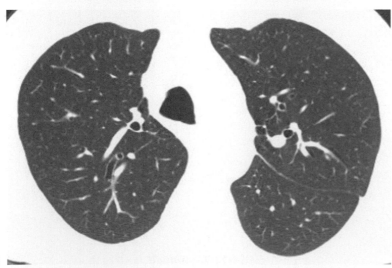

G
−700/1,000 HU (window mean/window width)

FIG. 1-13. *Continued*

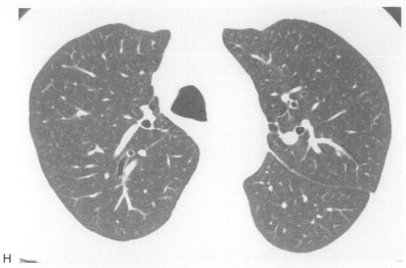

H
−900/1,000 HU (window mean/window width)

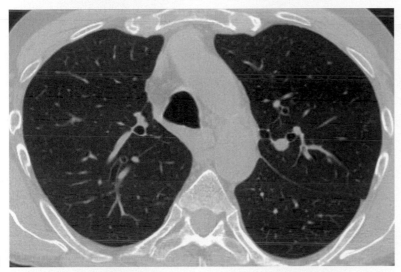

I
−300/1,500 HU (window mean/window width)

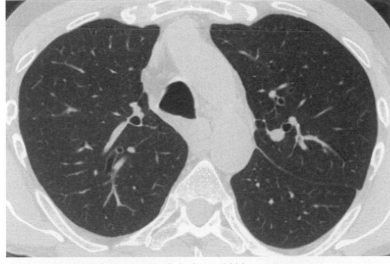

J
−500/1,500 HU (window mean/window width)

FIG. 1-13. *Continued*

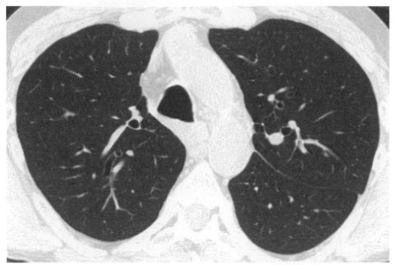

K

−700/1,500 HU (window mean/window width)

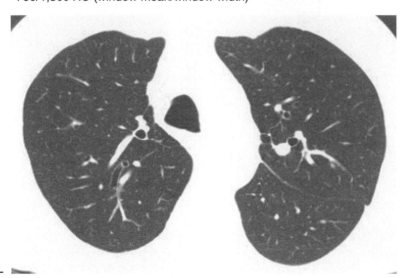

L

−900/1,500 HU (window mean/window width)

FIG. 1-13. *Continued*

(−800 to −900 HU) with narrow-window widths (500 HU) can be valuable in contrasting emphysema or air-filled cystic lesions with normal lung parenchyma. With such a low-window mean, normal lung parenchyma looks gray, whereas areas of emphysema remain black. On the other hand, using this same window to image the lung interstitium would be improper. Such a low-window mean, particularly combined with a narrow-window width, would make the lung interstitium appear much more prominent than it really is and could make a normal case appear abnormal. This window would also result in overestimations of the size of vessels and of bronchial wall thickness.

A window width of 2,000 HU is not generally suitable for viewing lung parenchyma, as contrast is significantly reduced. However, window settings of −500 to −700/2,000 HU may be used and are particularly useful when pleuro-parenchymal abnormalities are being evaluated (Fig. 1-12H and I) [9,18].

Image Photography and Display

Proper photography is important in allowing the images to be interpreted accurately. A 12-on-1 format is acceptable for lung window images. However, large images are much easier to read, and using a 6-on-1 format when photographing lung windows is advantageous, particularly if both lungs are shown on the same slice. A 12-on-1 format is satisfactory for photographing of images reconstructed with a small FOV, and is satisfactory for photographing soft-tissue window images.

Cameras used to photograph CT images for viewing on film are capable of interpolating or smoothing the CT data, producing smaller pixels in the resultant image than are present in the scan itself. A similar process occurs in CT workstations. Although individual CT pixels are clearly visible on close inspection of an unprocessed HRCT image, this is not generally the case when viewing a study on film or on a workstation. In fact, if unprocessed CT images (raw CT pixels) are viewed, the appearance can be disconcerting, and the images may be difficult to read. Cameras are capable of photographing CT scans using a range of settings, from sharp to smooth. If the camera is set on sharp, individual CT pixels will be visible; on a smooth setting, the data are interpolated, and image pixel size is reduced (Fig. 1-14). Although it might seem that a sharp setting would be best for HRCT, this is not the case. Resolution of fine structures is better with a smooth setting, and image interpretation is easier.

The use of an electronic workstation to view HRCT images is helpful and recommended. Scans may be viewed at a larger size than generally possible on film, making small or subtle abnormalities much easier to see. It is also of diagnostic value to toggle rapidly between different preset window settings (e.g., lung window, wide lung window, soft-tissue window) at a given scan level. Having preset windows available is important; in one study assessing the utility of workstation viewing, interpreting HRCT studies with a fixed-window (–500/2,000 HU) setting proved to be more accurate than viewing them with operator-varied window settings [26]. Having preset windows available also markedly reduces the time required to interpret the images.

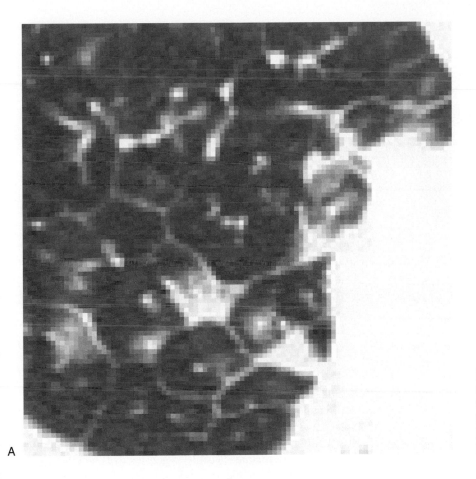

FIG. 1-14. Image interpolation and pixel size. **A:** Actual CT pixels are displayed on this HRCT image in a patient with interlobular septal thickening. The thickening septa have a stair-step appearance, and centrilobular arteries appear square. *Continued*

A

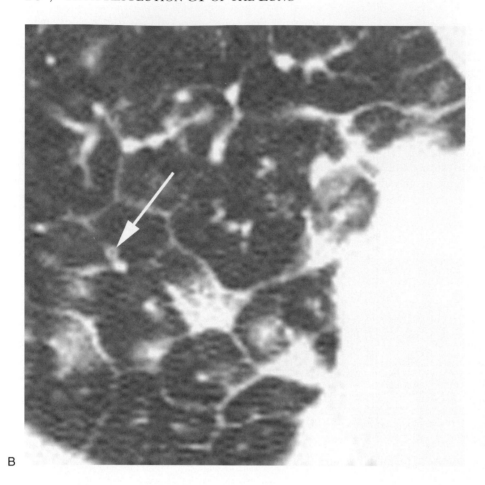

B

FIG. 1-14. *Continued* **B:** With interpolation, the appearance of the image is considerably improved. Note that a small centrilobular bronchiole clearly seen on this image (*arrow*) cannot be recognized on the original image **(A)**.

HIGH-RESOLUTION COMPUTED TOMOGRAPHY EXAMINATION: TECHNICAL MODIFICATIONS

HRCT is usually performed using single slices at spaced intervals. Several technical modifications may be used, depending on the clinical indication for the study. Patient position and scan spacing are most often varied.

Inspiratory Level

Routine HRCT is obtained during suspended full inspiration, which (i) optimizes contrast between normal structures, abnormal soft tissue, and normal aerated lung parenchyma and (ii) reduces transient atelectasis, a finding that may mimic or obscure significant abnormalities. Selected scans obtained during or after forced expiration may also be valuable in diagnosing patients with obstructive lung disease or airway abnormalities. The use of expiratory HRCT is discussed below, and in Chapters 2 and 3.

Patient Position and the Use of Prone Scanning

Scans obtained with the patient supine are adequate in most instances. However, scans obtained with the patient positioned prone are sometimes necessary for diagnosing subtle lung disease. Atelectasis is commonly seen in the dependent lung in both normal and abnormal subjects, resulting in a so-called dependent density or a subpleural line (Fig. 1-15) [28]. These normal findings can closely mimic the appearance of early lung fibrosis, and they can be impossible to distinguish from true pathology on supine scans alone. However, if scans are obtained in both supine and prone positions, dependent density easily can be differentiated from true pathology (Fig. 1-15). Normal dependent density disappears in the prone position (Fig. 1-16); a true abnormality remains visible regardless of whether it is dependent or nondependent (Figs. 1-17 and 1-18).

In a study by Volpe et al. [29], prone scans were considered helpful in 17 of 100 consecutive patients having HRCT. However, it should be pointed out that dependent density results in a diagnostic dilemma only in patients who have normal lungs or subtle lung abnormalities. In patients with obvious abnormalities, such as honeycombing, or who have diffuse lung disease, dependent density is not usually a diagnostic problem. Thus, if the patient being studied has evidence of moderate to severe lung disease on plain radiographs, prone scans are not likely to be needed. On the other hand, if the patient is suspected of having an

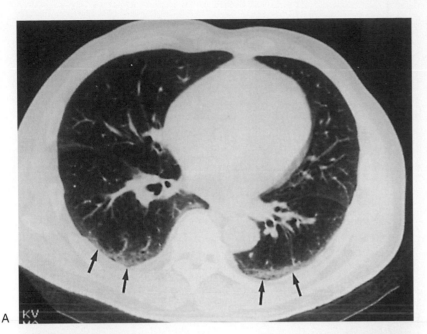

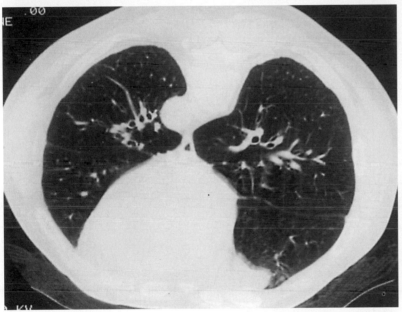

FIG. 1-15. Supine and prone scans with normal "dependent density." **A:** Supine scan in a normal patient shows an ill-defined opacity in the posterior aspect of both lungs (*arrows*). It is impossible to know whether this represents lung disease or is normal atelectasis. **B:** Prone scan done at same level shows no evidence of an abnormality.

interstitial abnormality and the plain radiograph is normal or near normal or the results of chest radiographs are unknown, the supine scan sequence must be closely monitored or prone scans should be obtained. Volpe et al. [29] assessed the usefulness of prone scans in patients who had chest radiographs read as normal, possibly abnormal, or definitely abnormal. Prone HRCT scans were helpful in confirming or ruling out posterior lung abnormalities in 10 of 36 (28%) patients who had normal findings on chest radiographs, five of 18 (28%) patients who had possibly abnormal findings on chest radiographs, and only two of 46 (4%) patients who had definitely abnormal findings on

chest radiographs. The proportion of patients who benefited from prone scans was significantly lower among the patients with abnormal findings on chest radiographs than among the patients with normal ($p = .008$) or possibly abnormal ($p = .02$) findings. The two patients who had abnormal findings on radiographs and in whom CT scans obtained with the patient prone were helpful had minimal radiographic abnormalities.

Some investigators [18,30] obtain HRCT in the prone position only when dependent lung collapse is problematic [31]; however, this approach requires that the scans be closely monitored or that the patient be called back for

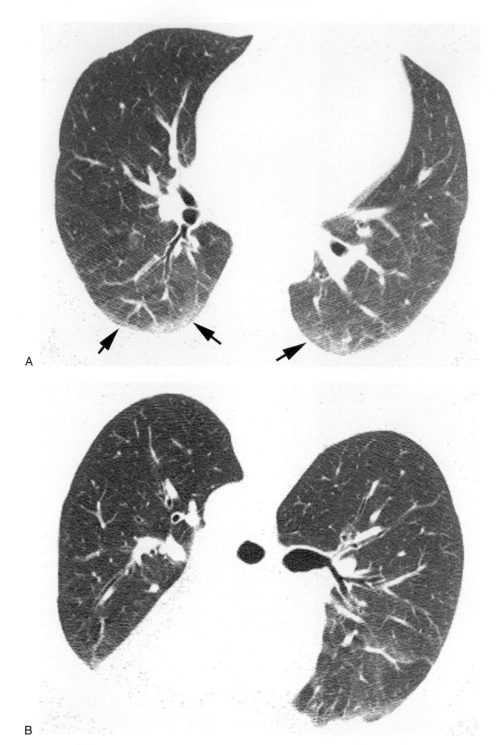

FIG. 1-16. Transient dependent density. **A:** Supine scan shows ill-defined opacity in the posterior lungs (*arrows*). **B:** On a prone image, the posterior lung appears normal. Note some dependent opacity is now visible in the anterior lung.

additional scans. Others use prone scanning routinely; this approach has proved particularly valuable in detecting early lung fibrosis [28,32]. In patients who are suspected of having an airway disease, such as bronchiectasis, or another obstructive lung disease, dependent atelectasis is not usually a diagnostic problem, and prone scans are not usually needed.

Scan Spacing

HRCT is generally performed by obtaining single slices at spaced intervals, from the lung apices to the lung bases during suspended respiration. In this manner, HRCT is intended to "sample" lung anatomy, with the presumptions that a diffuse lung disease will be visible in at least one of the levels sampled

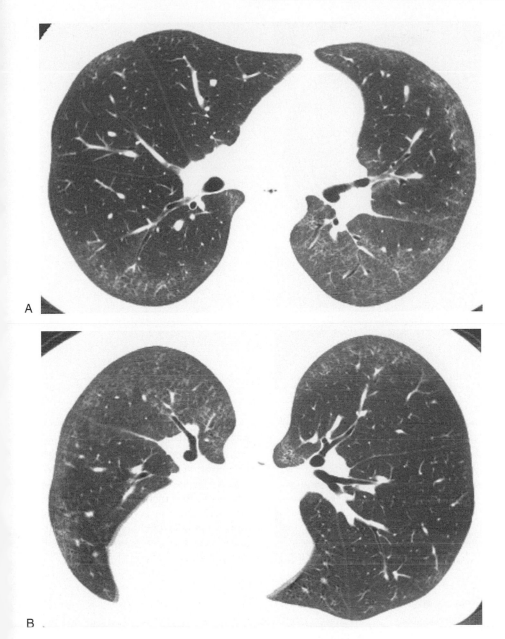

FIG. 1-17. Persistent opacity in the posterior lung in a patient with pulmonary fibrosis. **A:** Supine scan shows ill-defined opacity in the posterior lungs and in a subpleural region anteriorly. **B:** On a prone image, the posterior is unchanged in appearance, indicative of lung disease.

and that the findings seen at the levels scanned will be representative of what is present throughout the lung. These presumptions have proven valid during years of experience with HRCT.

Two fundamentally different approaches to HRCT may be used, at least partially determined by the indications for the examination. The first approach is to obtain HRCT in combination with a conventional CT study, in which the entire thorax is imaged using 7- to 10-mm collimation scans [12,18,30]. This technique is most appropriate when the primary indication for the study is an evaluation of the entire chest, or when the disease being evaluated necessitates comprehensive imaging. For example, even though mediastinal abnormalities are usually visible on HRCT images obtained at spaced intervals, in some patients with both mediastinal and pulmonary abnormalities suspected radiographically, obtaining a conventional

CT study is appropriate. Similarly, in a patient with suspected lymphangitic spread of carcinoma who is having HRCT for diagnosis, obtaining a contrast-enhanced CT would be appropriate to look for or determine the extent of a primary carcinoma. Depending on the indication for the study, either HRCT or conventional CT may be obtained first and monitored to determine the need for additional imaging.

The second approach is to obtain only HRCT images, in lieu of performing a conventional CT examination. Because HRCT is most often obtained to evaluate a patient suspected of having diffuse lung disease [9], and HRCT is optimized for imaging lung parenchyma, obtaining a conventional CT examination is not usually necessary for diagnosis. The great majority of HRCT studies in current clinical practice are obtained in this manner.

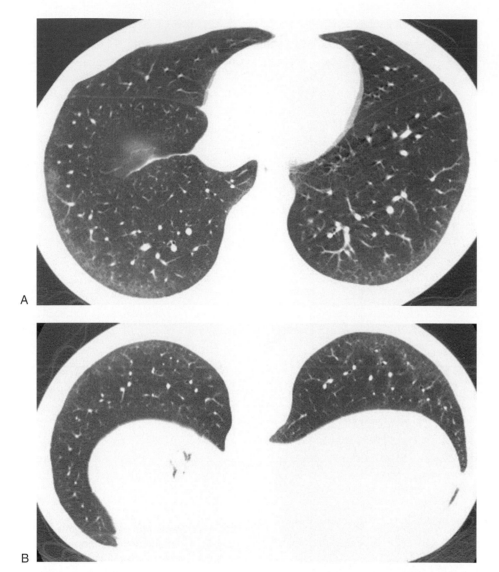

A

B

FIG. 1-18. Persistent posterior lung opacity on prone scans in a patient with scleroderma and interstitial pneumonia. **A:** Supine scan shows ill-defined opacity in the posterior lungs. **B:** On a prone image, the posterior subpleural lung opacity is unchanged in appearance, and the presence of true lung disease can be diagnosed.

We consider scans obtained at 1-cm intervals, from the lung apices to bases, to be the most appropriate routine scanning protocol, allowing a complete sampling of the lung and lung disease regardless of its distribution. Obtaining scans at smaller intervals or obtaining contiguous scans is not usually necessary for diagnosis and would not be desirable because of the increased radiation dose involved. Scanning at 1-cm intervals is currently used by most investigators, although in early reports, HRCT scanning was performed at 2-, 3-, and even 4-cm intervals [9,31]; at three preselected levels [30]; or at one or two levels through the lower lungs [18]. HRCT is performed for a variety of reasons, and to some extent, the number of scans obtained and their levels can vary depending on the clinical indications for the study.

Although obtaining scans at 1-cm intervals is recommended for initial diagnosis, it should be pointed out that in patients with a known disease, a limited number of HRCT images may be sufficient to assess disease extent. In one study [33], the ability of HRCT obtained at three selected levels (*limited HRCT*) to show features of idiopathic pulmonary fibrosis (IPF) was compared to that of HRCT obtained at 10-mm increments (*complete HRCT*). HRCT fibrosis scores strongly correlated with pathology fibrosis scores for the complete ($r = 0.53, p = .0001$) and limited ($r = 0.50, p = .0001$) HRCT examinations. HRCT ground-glass opacity scores correlated with the histologic inflammatory scores on the complete ($r = 0.27, p = .03$) and limited ($r = 0.26, p = .03$) HRCT examinations. As another example, in evaluating patients with asbestos exposure, several investigators have suggested that a limited number of scans should be sufficient for the diagnosis of asbestosis [28,32,34–37]. Obtaining four or five scans near the lung bases has proved to have good sensitivity in patients with suspected asbestosis [38]. Conventional CT combined with a few HRCT images has also been applied to patients with suspected diffuse lung disease and has been shown to be clinically efficacious [30]; HRCT scans obtained at the levels of the aortic arch, carina, and 2 cm above the right hemidiaphragm allow the assessment of the lung regions in which lung biopsies are most frequently performed [12].

In patients who are likely to require prone images, several prone scans can be added to the routine supine sequence obtained with 1-cm scan spacing; a reasonable protocol would

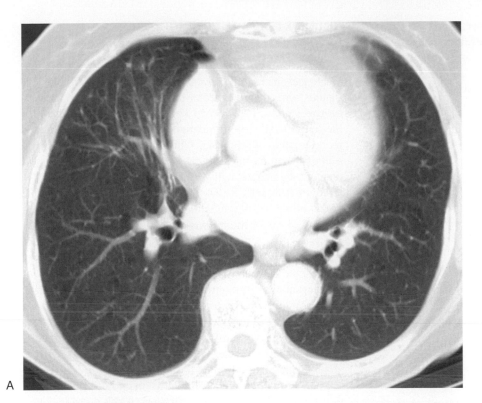

A

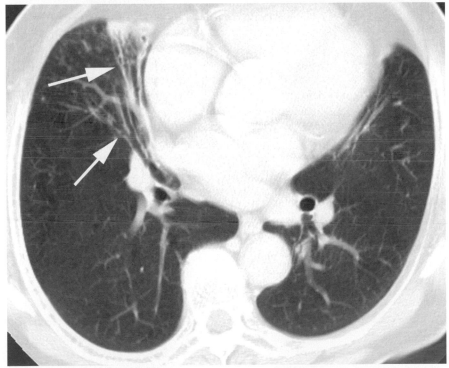

B

FIG. 1-19. Gantry angulation in a patient with right middle lobe bronchiectasis. **A:** HRCT image obtained with the gantry vertical shows bronchial wall thickening in the right middle lobe. **B:** HRCT image obtained with the gantry angulated 20 degrees allows right middle lobe bronchi (*arrows*) to be imaged along their axes.

include additional prone scans at 2- to 4-cm intervals. Alternatively, scans can be obtained at 2-cm intervals from lung apices to bases, in both supine and prone positions. Because the prone and supine images will be slightly different, even if obtained at the same level, the number of images obtained will be equivalent to a supine position scan protocol using 1-cm spacing.

It may be appropriate to customize the number or location of scans, depending on the patient's suspected disease, clinical findings, or the location of plain radiographic abnormalities. For example, if the lung disease being studied predominates in a certain region of lung, as determined by chest radiographs, conventional CT [18], or other imaging studies, it makes sense that more scans should be obtained in the most abnormal area. In patients with suspected asbestosis, it has been recommended that more scans be performed near the diaphragm than in the upper lobes because of the typical basal distribution of this disease, even if the chest radiograph does not suggest an abnormality in this region [28,32].

Some support for this approach has been lent by a paper [39] describing theoretical methods useful in selecting the appropriate number of HRCT images for estimating any quantitative parameter of lung disease; a marked reduction in the number of images necessary for quantification of a desired parameter can be achieved by using a stratified sampling technique based on prior knowledge of the disease distribution.

Gantry Angulation

It has been suggested that, in patients with bronchiectasis, angling the gantry 20 degrees caudally with the patient supine (i.e., the lower gantry is angled toward the feet) improves visibility of the segmental and subsegmental bronchi, particularly in the middle lobe and lingula, by aligning them parallel to the plane of scan (Fig. 1-19) [40]. This technique may be valuable in assessing patients with bronchiectasis [41]. However, in the majority of patients with bronchiectasis, HRCT without gantry angulation is sufficient for diagnosis.

Electrocardiographically Triggered High-Resolution Computed Tomography

HRCT scans obtained in a routine fashion may be degraded by cardiac motion. Several motion-related artifacts may be seen, particularly in the left paracardiac region (see High-Resolution Computed Tomography Artifacts). HRCT scans may be obtained using electrocardiographic (ECG) triggering of scan acquisition in an attempt to reduce these artifacts [42]. In a recent study using a spiral scanner capable of 0.75-second gantry rotation, 500-millisecond HRCT scans, representing a 240-degree rotation of the gantry, were initiated at 50% of the R-R interval. Because of the shorter-than-routine scan time, images were reconstructed using a somewhat smoother algorithm than is usually used for HRCT. In 35 patients, Schoepf et al. [42] found that ECG triggering significantly reduced artifacts caused by cardiac motion, such as distortion of pulmonary vessels, double images, or blurring of the cardiac border, when compared to routine images. Furthermore, in patients with a heart rate of 75 beats per minute or less, ECG triggering significantly improved image quality. It should be noted, however, that this technique was not found to improve diagnostic accuracy.

Use of Contrast Agents

At present, there is no routine indication for the use of contrast agents with HRCT, except when studying a focal lung lesion or solitary nodule [43] or in patients being studied for concomitant vascular disease. Because the lung window settings routinely used for HRCT are intended to accentuate the contrast between air and tissue, vascular opacification is not visible in patients receiving an injection of intravenous contrast. Using a soft-tissue window, opacification of segmental and subsegmental vessels may be seen on HRCT.

VOLUMETRIC HIGH-RESOLUTION COMPUTED TOMOGRAPHY

Volumetric HRCT may be performed using several different techniques, including conventional HRCT with multiple contiguous slices, single detector–row spiral CT, and multidetector-row spiral CT. In each, a volume of lung is examined for the purpose of viewing contiguous slices or the volumetric reconstruction of scan data. With spiral technique, this can be accomplished during a single breath hold, although the volume of lung imaged will vary with the type of scanner.

Volumetric HRCT has several potential advantages. It would allow (i) complete lung imaging, (ii) viewing of contiguous slices for the purpose of better defining lung abnormalities, (iii) a better understanding of the three-dimensional (3D) distribution of abnormalities relative to lung structures, and (iv) the 3D reconstruction of scan data for the purpose of viewing images in nontransaxial planes or obtaining maximum or minimum intensity projections. However, at present, evidence that volumetric imaging improves diagnostic accuracy in patients with diffuse lung disease is limited to several specific situations. Therefore, the use of volumetric HRCT should generally be limited to selected cases.

In an early attempt at volumetric imaging [44], four contiguous HRCT scans were obtained without using spiral technique at each of three locations (the aortic arch, carina, and 2 cm above the right hemidiaphragm) in 50 consecutive patients with interstitial lung disease or bronchiectasis. At each level, the diagnostic information obtainable from the set of four scans was compared to that obtainable from the first scan in the set of four. When the full set of four scans was considered, more findings of disease were identified. The sensitivity of the first scan as compared to the set of four was 84% for the detection of bronchiectasis, 97% for ground-glass opacity, 88% for honeycombing, 88% for septal thickening, and 86% for nodular opacities. However, it is more likely that the improvement in sensitivity found using the set of four scans reflects the number of scans viewed rather than the fact that they were obtained in contiguity.

Other studies have used spiral CT technique with thin collimation and maximum- or minimum-intensity projections (MinIPs) to acquire and display volumetric HRCT data for a slab of lung [45–47]. In this setting, maximum intensity projections (MIPs) have been used primarily for the diagnosis of nodular lung disease. MIP images increase the detection of small lung nodules and can be helpful in demonstrating their anatomic distribution (Fig. 1-20).

Coakley et al. [46] assessed the use of MIP images in the detection of pulmonary nodules by spiral CT. Forty pulmonary nodules of high density were created by placement of 2- and 4-mm beads into the peripheral airways of five dogs. MIP images were generated from overlapped slabs of seven consecutive 3-mm slices, reconstructed at 2-mm intervals and acquired at pitch 2. MIP imaging increased the odds of nodule detection by more than two, when compared to spiral images, and reader confidence for nodule detection was significantly higher with MIP images.

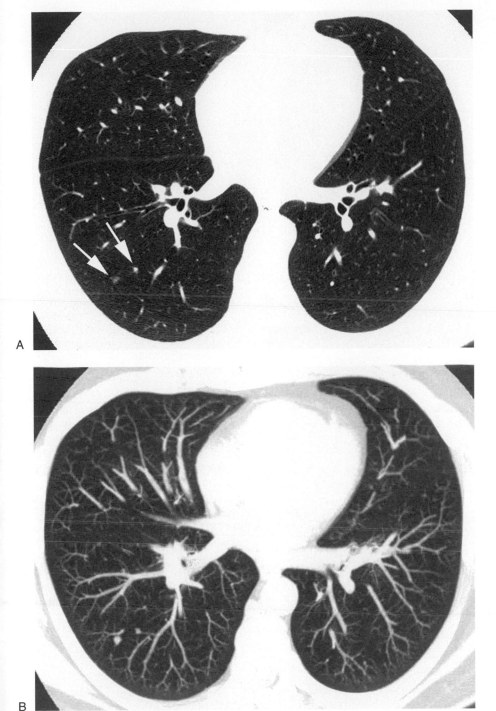

FIG. 1-20. Maximum-intensity projection (MIP) image in a patient with small lung nodules obtained using a multidetector-row spiral CT scanner with 1.25-mm detector width and a pitch of 6. **A:** A single HRCT image shows two small nodules (*arrows*) that are difficult to distinguish from vessels. **B:** An MIP image consisting of eight contiguous HRCT images, including **A**, allows the two small nodules to be easily distinguished from surrounding vessels.

In a study by Bhalla et al. [45], the use of helical HRCT and MIP images was compared in patients with nodular lung disease. Because of the markedly improved visualization of peripheral pulmonary vessels and improved spatial orientation, MIP images were considered superior to helical scans for identifying pulmonary nodules and specifying their location as peribronchovascular or centrilobular, a finding of great value in differential diagnosis.

In another study [47], sliding-thin-slab MIP reconstructions were used in 81 patients with a variety of lung diseases associated with small nodules. In this study, patients were studied using 1- and 8-mm-thick conventional CT and focal spiral CT with generation of 3-, 5- and 8-mm-thick MIP reconstructions. When conventional CT findings were normal, MIPs did not demonstrate additional abnormalities. When conventional CT findings were inconclusive, MIPs enabled detection of micronodules (i.e., nodules 7 mm or less in diameter) involving less than 25% of the lung. When conventional CT scans showed micronodules, MIPs showed the extent and distribution of micronodules and associated

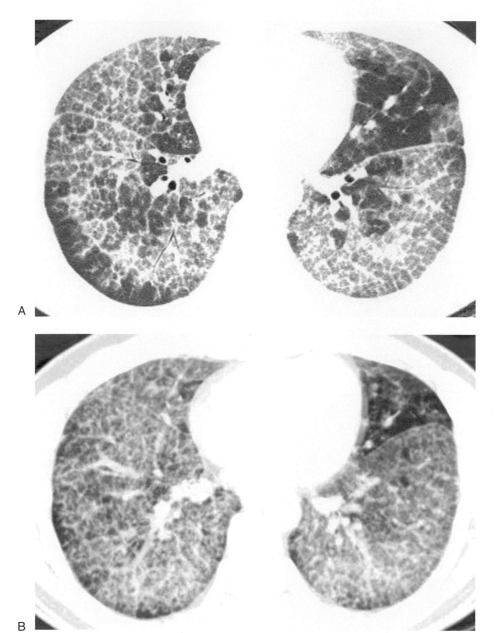

FIG. 1-21. Maximum-intensity projection (MIP) image in a patient with extensive abnormalities due to alveolar proteinosis obtained using a multidetector-row spiral CT scanner with 1.25-mm detector width and a pitch of 6. **A:** A single HRCT image shows a typical patchy distribution of interlobular septal thickening and ground-glass opacity typical of alveolar proteinosis. **B:** An MIP image consisting of five contiguous HRCT images, including **(A)**, results in a confusing superimposition of opacities. Septal thickening is more difficult to diagnose.

bronchiolar abnormalities to better advantage. The sensitivity of MIPs (3-mm-thick MIP, 94%; 5-mm-thick MIP, 100%; 8-mm-thick MIP, 92%) was significantly higher than that of conventional CT (8-mm-thick, 57%; 1-mm-thick, 73%) in the detection of micronodules (p <.001). The authors [47] concluded that sliding-thin-slab MIPs may help to detect micronodular lung disease of limited extent and may be considered a valuable tool in the evaluation of diffuse infiltrative lung disease. On the other hand, in patients with extensive abnormalities, MIPs result in a confusing superimposition of opacities that tends to obscure anatomic detail (Fig. 1-21).

The utility of MinIP images has also been evaluated (Fig. 1-22) [45]. In one study [45], MinIP images were more accurate than routine HRCT scans in identifying (i) the lumina of central airways (Fig. 1-23), (ii) areas of abnormal low attenuation (e.g., emphysema or air-trapping) (Fig. 1-23; see Fig. 7-36), and (iii) ground-glass opacity. In the study by Bhalla et al. [45], when compared to conventional HRCT, volumetric MIP and MinIP images demonstrated additional findings in 13 of 20 (65%) cases. However, although an advantage has been described for volumetric HRCT with MIP or MinIP image reconstruction in demonstrating small nodules of limited extent and subtle areas of increased or decreased lung density, conventional HRCT is advantageous in depicting fine linear structures, such as the walls of dilated small airways and interlobular septa.

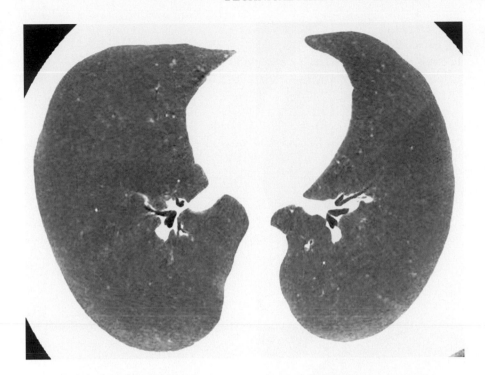

FIG. 1-22. Minimum-intensity projection (MinIP) image in the patient shown in Fig. 1-17A, and at the same anatomic level. Normal lung parenchyma appears relatively homogeneous. Pulmonary vessels disappear on MinIP images.

Single Detector–Row Spiral Computed Tomography

Single detector–row spiral CT scanners have the ability to obtain a volumetric CT data set, with a 1- or 2-cm-thick slab of lung being scanned during a single breath hold, using 1-mm collimation and a pitch of 1. Obtaining scans with a spiral technique results in a small increase in effective slice thickness (compared to scans obtained without table motion), and results in some loss of spatial resolution [48,49], although this effect is minimal with proper technique [50]. Using a pitch of 2 broadens the effective slice thickness by approximately 30% [51,52]. Thus, using 1-mm collimation, effective slice thickness is approximately 1.3 mm. An increase in pitch may also result in some decrease in signal-to-noise ratio, but this is not generally a problem in diagnosis. Although this technique is of potential value in demonstrating the 3D distribution of abnormalities in patients with diffuse lung disease and is an appealing concept, because of the limited volume of lung assessed during a single breath hold, volumetric HRCT using a single detector-row scanner is of considerably more value in assessing patients with focal lung disease or discrete lung nodules [49,53]. The ability to perform this type of thin- or thick-slab volumetric imaging is not a major advantage in assessing most patients with diffuse lung disease; HRCT in patients with suspected diffuse lung disease requires a sampling of lung anatomy in different lung regions, rather than a more detailed volumetric assessment at a few levels.

In general, in patients suspected of having diffuse infiltrative lung disease, HRCT obtained with a single detector–row spiral should be performed without table motion, using thin (1-mm) collimation, scans at spaced intervals, a scan time of 1 second or less, and a high-resolution reconstruction algorithm.

Multidetector-Row Spiral High-Resolution Computed Tomography

Multidetector-row spiral CT scanners make use of multiple adjacent detector rows that acquire scan data simultaneously and may be used independently or in combination to generate images of different thickness. Such scanners typically use high orders of pitch (e.g., 6), and are capable of imaging the entire thorax during a single breath hold with the volumetric reconstruction of thin, high-resolution slices. For example, using one currently available scanner, data may be simultaneously acquired from four 1.25-mm detector rows, with table movement of 7.5 mm per second and a gantry rotation time of 0.8 seconds. Assuming that 25 cm is required for imaging the lungs, volumetric HRCT of the entire lung volume using these parameters would require approximately 27 seconds. Although single detector–row spiral CT does not offer a significant advantage in patients with diffuse lung disease when compared to conventional HRCT performed with individual spaced slices, multidetector-row CT has the potential to fundamentally change the way HRCT is performed, at least in some patients. The volumetric data resulting from this mode of scanning allow near-isotropic imaging and HRCT assessment of lung morphology in a continuous fashion from lung apex to base, the production of MIP and MinIP images at any desired level (Figs. 1-20 through 1-23), and the viewing of the scan volume in non-transaxial planes (Figs. 1-24 through 1-27; see Fig. 7-36).

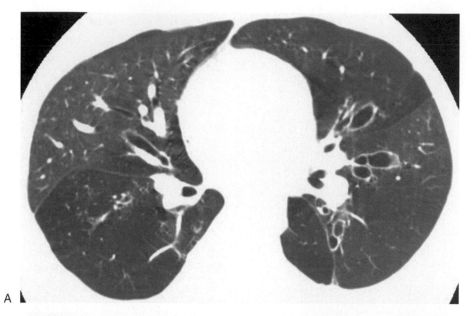

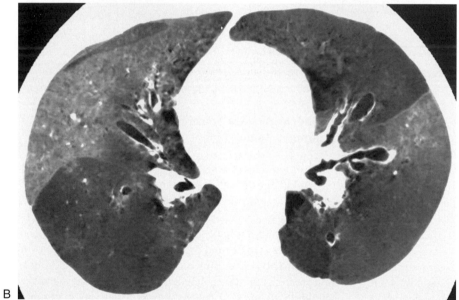

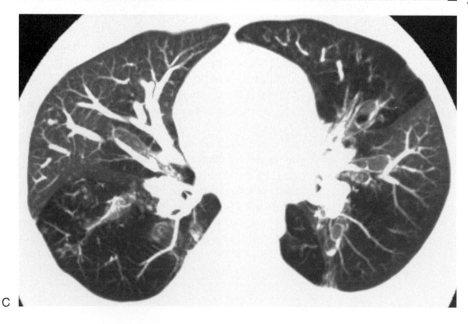

FIG. 1-23. Multidetector-row spiral (HRCT) image with contrast enhancement in a patient with bronchiolitis obliterans and a clinical suspicion of pulmonary embolism. No pulmonary embolism was found. **A:** A single HRCT image obtained with 1.25-mm detector width and a pitch of 6 shows bronchiectasis and patchy lung attenuation with reduced artery size in lucent lung regions due to air-trapping and mosaic perfusion. **B:** A 10-mm-thick minimum-intensity projection image (MinIP) at the same level as **A** accentuates the differences in attenuation between normal lung and lucent lung, but pulmonary arteries cannot be assessed. Bronchiectasis is well seen using MinIP imaging. **C:** A maximum-intensity projection at the same level as **B** shows reduced vessel size in the lucent lung regions. Inhomogeneous lung attenuation is also visible. The bronchiectasis is difficult to see.

The spiral acquisition of HRCT data using this technique results in some broadening of the scan profile, but the effective slice thickness using this technique would still be sufficient for HRCT diagnosis in most cases. With 1.25-mm detector width, effective slice thickness is approximately 1.6 mm when a pitch of 6 (table travel 7.5 mm per gantry rotation) is used. Furthermore, depending on the technique used and how data from the various detector rows are combined, images of different thickness may be produced retrospectively from the same study. Using the protocol described above, in addition to viewing images generated from data acquired by the individual 1.25-mm detectors, data from the detector rows may be combined to produce images representing thicker slices (i.e., 2.5 mm). Thus, this technique enables HRCT and "routine" or thick-section chest imaging to be combined as a single examination, blurring the distinction between these studies.

Combining a volumetric chest CT examination with HRCT by using multidetector-row CT may be of value in patients being studied primarily for diffuse lung disease, for which HRCT would be the examination of choice, and in patients being evaluated for disease usually studied using conventional spiral technique. For example, in patients being evaluated before volume reduction surgery for emphysema or before lung transplantation, volumetric lung imaging might be of value in the diagnosis of associated lung carcinoma, which has an incidence of up to 5% in this patient population, or other significant abnormalities [54]. In patients with hemoptysis, thin and thick image reconstruction may be of value in demonstrating small or large airway disease, respectively. Another advantage of multidetector-row CT would be in patients requiring a "conventional" CT for the diagnosis of thoracic disease, such as evaluation of a lung nodule. In such patients, scan data may be reconstructed with a thickness appropriate for the detection of lung nodules and bronchial abnormalities and for assessment of mediastinal and hilar lymph nodes. At the same time, and without additional scanning, high-resolution images could be reconstructed for the purpose of delineating nodule morphology and attenuation, or for the diagnosis of associated lymphangitic spread.

Similarly, in patients with suspected pulmonary vascular disease, HRCT with contrast enhancement may be obtained using multidetector-row spiral CT, allowing the detailed assessment of both vasculature and pulmonary parenchyma (Figs. 1-23, 1-26, 1-27; see Figs. 9-4, and 9-5). In patients having spiral CT for the diagnosis of acute or chronic pulmonary embolism, scan data can also be reconstructed using thin collimation to look for lung disease that could be associated with similar symptoms (Figs. 1-23 and 1-26).

On the other hand, in patients being assessed using HRCT for known diffuse lung disease, such as IPF, the need for volumetric scanning or thicker slices is less clear, and the additional radiation dose required by volumetric imaging would not seem warranted. Another disadvantage of obtaining vol-

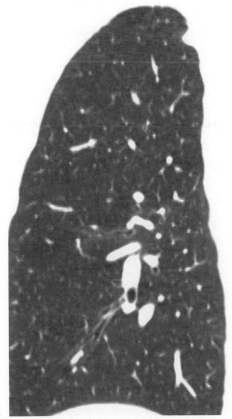
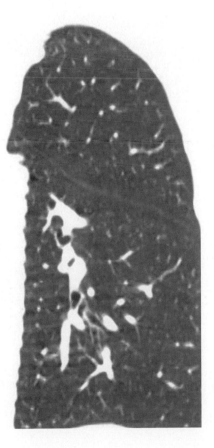

A

FIG. 1-24. Coronal and sagittal image reconstruction from multidetector-row spiral HRCT in a normal subject. **A:** Coronal reconstruction from a multidetector-row spiral CT obtained using 1.25-mm detectors, and a pitch of 6 relative to detector width, during a single breath hold. Small peripheral vessels are visible. The posterior portion of the major fissures are visible as thin stripes of opacity. *Continued*

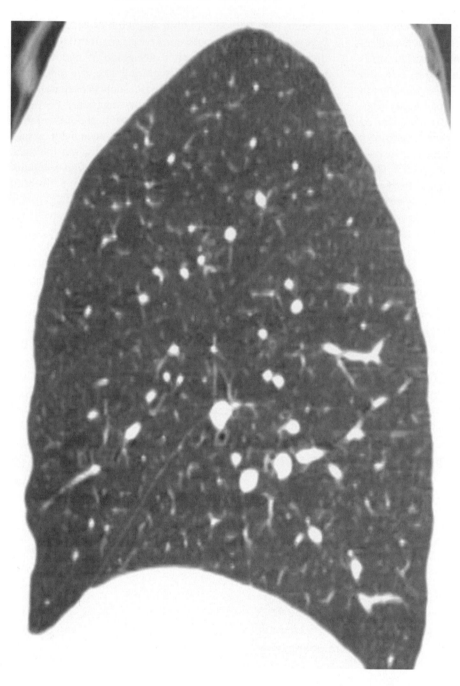

FIG. 1-24. *Continued* B: Parasagittal reconstruction from the same HRCT data set shows the minor and major fissures.

B

umetric HRCT is the large number of images produced. Unless scans are reviewed using a workstation, reading a volumetric study would be cumbersome and would require the use of a large number of films.

Although some patients may be able to hold their breath for a volumetric spiral acquisition using this technique (e.g., 27 seconds), dyspneic patients will not. An advantage of obtaining HRCT with single slices is that a breath hold of 1 second or less is required.

Standardized protocols for performing volumetric multidetector-row HRCT have not been established. However, in patients who may not be able to hold their breath for a complete volumetric study, logic dictates that the scan protocol be modified according to the distribution of the disease suspected. For diseases likely to have a basal predominance, such as IPF, scanning should begin near the diaphragm and proceed in a cephalad direction. In this way, the more important basal lung will be imaged at the beginning of the scan sequence, and if the patient begins to breathe during scanning, only images through the less important upper lobes will be degraded by respiratory motion. For the same reason, in a patient suspected of having a disease with an upper-lobe predominance (e.g., sarcoidosis), it may be appropriate to begin scanning in the lung apices. Because lung movement with respiration is greatest at the lung bases, an alternative approach would be to scan from the bases to apices in all patients. If the patient breathes during the scan, the upper lobes would be less affected. In a dyspneic patient, breaking up the scan sequence into smaller volumes with several breath holds might also be helpful. Experience indicates that using a detector thickness of 1.25 mm and a pitch of 6 (table movement of 7.5 mm per gantry rotation), with reconstruction using a high-resolution algorithm, provides excellent lung detail. Depending on the indication for the study, this may be performed with or without contrast infusion.

With multidetector-row spiral scanners, contiguous HRCT images may also be obtained without table motion, with each detector row acquiring a separate image. Using this technique, clusters of four contiguous scans could be obtained at selected levels (e.g., at 1.5- to 2-cm intervals). The individual scans could be viewed independently, as with conventional HRCT, or could be processed to produce MIP or MinIP images.

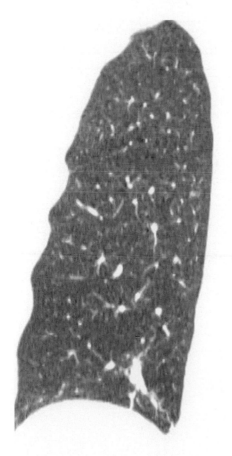
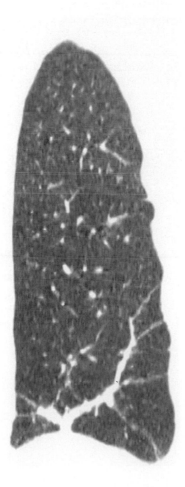

A

FIG. 1-25. Coronal and sagittal image reconstruction from multidetector-row spiral HRCT in a patient with disc atelectasis in the posterior lungs. **A:** Coronal reconstruction from a multidetector-row spiral CT obtained using 1.25-mm detectors, and a pitch of 6 relative to detector width, during a single breath hold. Linear areas of increased attenuation reflect disc atelectasis. **B:** Parasagittal reconstruction shows linear subpleural opacities representing disc atelectasis. *Continued*

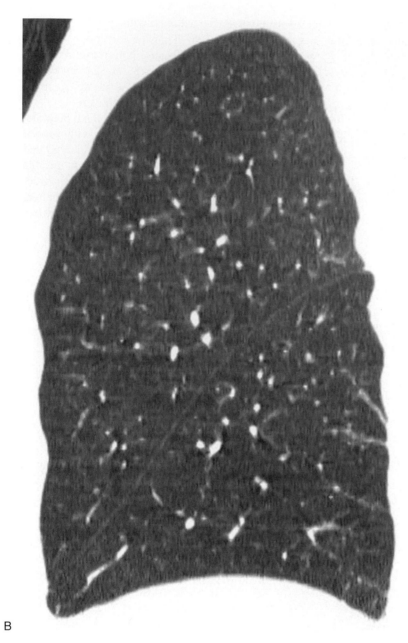

B

FIG. 1-25. *Continued*

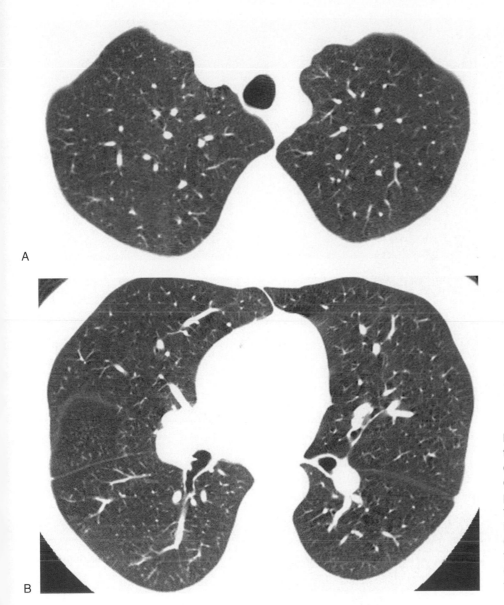

FIG. 1-26. HRCT obtained using multidetector-row HRCT with 1.25-mm detectors and a pitch of 6 relative to detector width, in an AIDS patient with pulmonary hypertension and a differential diagnosis, including chronic pulmonary embolism, vasculitis, and lung disease. Transaxial **(A,B)** and parasagittal reconstructed **(C)** HRCTs obtained during a single breath hold show normal findings. *Continued*

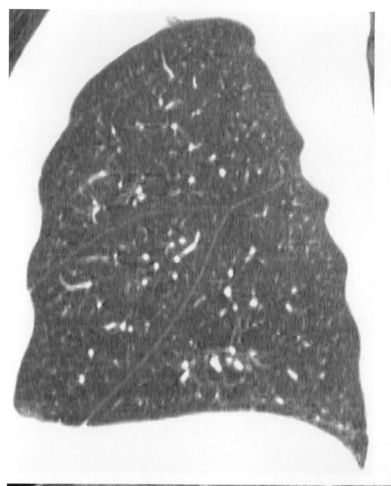

C

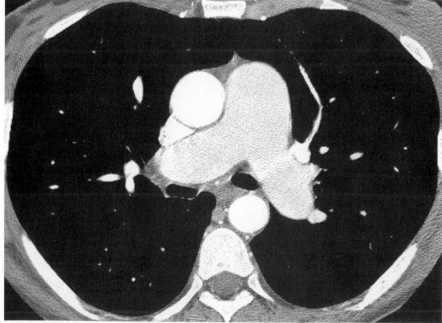

D

FIG. 1-26. *Continued* D: Transaxial image shows enlargement of main pulmonary artery consistent with pulmonary hypertension, but no evidence of pulmonary embolism. The presence of pulmonary hypertension in the absence of pulmonary embolism or lung disease suggests plexogenic arteriopathy.

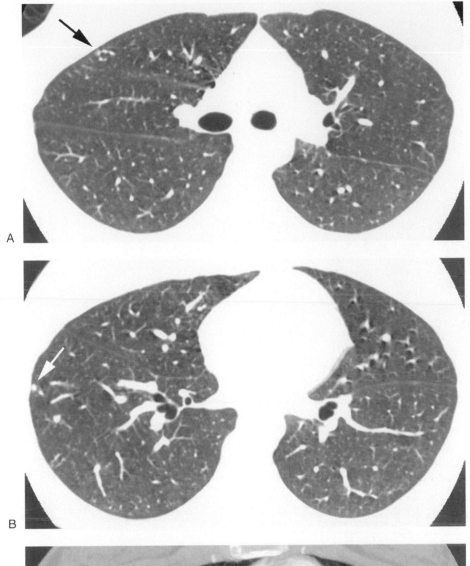

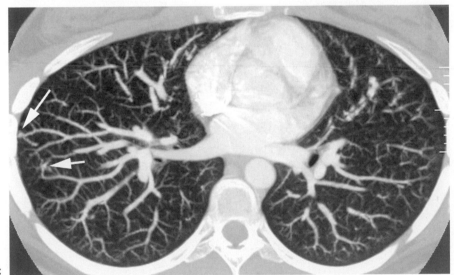

FIG. 1-27. Contrast-enhanced spiral HRCT obtained in a 19-year-old woman with significant hypoxemia. Scans were obtained using multidetector-row HRCT with 1.25-mm detectors and a pitch of 6 relative to detector width. Transaxial **(A,B)** images showed numerous very small subpleural arteriovenous malformations (*arrows*). One-centimeter-thick maximum-intensity projection images in the transaxial **(C,D)** and coronal **(E)** planes show the malformations (*arrows*) and their vascular supply to better advantage. She was subsequently found to have Osler-Weber-Rendu disease. *Continued*

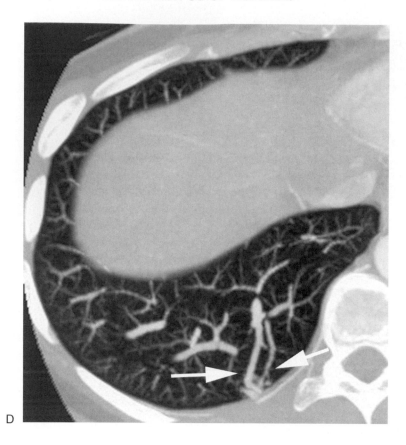

D

FIG. 1-27. *Continued*

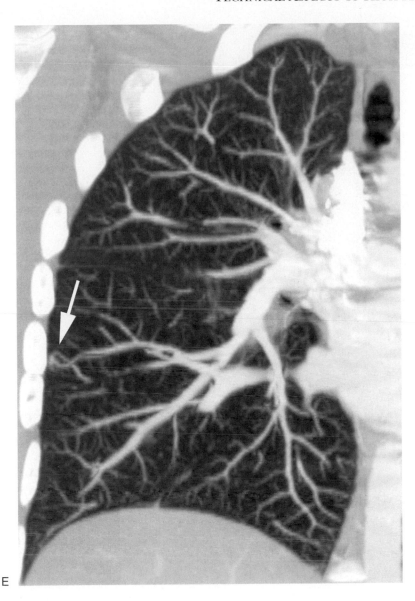

E

FIG. 1-27. *Continued*

EXPIRATORY HIGH-RESOLUTION COMPUTED TOMOGRAPHY

As an adjunct to routine inspiratory images, expiratory HRCT scans have proved useful in the evaluation of patients with a variety of obstructive lung diseases [55,56]. On expiratory scans, focal or diffuse air-trapping may be diagnosed in patients with large or small airway obstruction or emphysema. It has been shown that the presence of air-trapping on expiratory scans (i) correlates to some degree with pulmonary function test abnormalities [57,58], (ii) can confirm the presence of obstructive airway disease in patients with subtle or nonspecific abnormalities visible on inspiratory scans, (iii) allows the diagnosis of significant lung disease in some patients with normal inspiratory scans [59], and (iv) can help distinguish between obstructive disease and infiltrative disease as a cause of inhomogeneous lung opacity seen on inspiratory scans [60].

In most lung regions of normal subjects, lung parenchyma increases uniformly in attenuation during expiration [6,61–65],

but in the presence of air-trapping, lung parenchyma remains lucent on expiration and shows little change in volume. Focal, multifocal, or diffuse air-trapping is visible as areas of abnormally low attenuation on expiratory or postexpiratory CT. On expiratory scans, visible differences in attenuation between normal and obstructed lung regions are visible using standard lung window settings and can be quantitated using regions of interest. Differences in attenuation between normal lung regions and regions that show air-trapping often measure more than 100 HU [66]. Air-trapping visible using expiratory or postexpiratory HRCT has been recognized in patients with various obstructive or airway diseases, such as emphysema [67–69], chronic airways disease [58], asthma [70–72], bronchiolitis obliterans [59,68,73–80], the cystic lung diseases associated with Langerhans histiocytosis and tuberous sclerosis [81], and bronchiectasis [68,82]. It has also proven valuable in demonstrating the presence of bronchiolitis in patients with primarily infiltrative diseases such as hypersensitivity pneumonitis [83,84], sarcoidosis [85,86], and pneumonia.

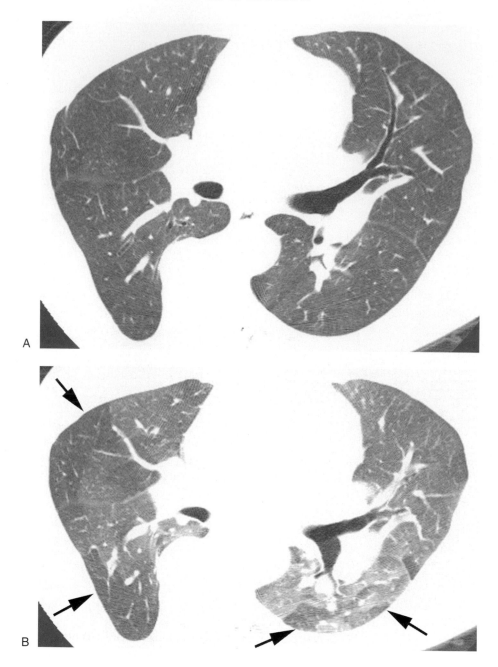

FIG. 1-28. Expiratory air-trapping in a patient with idiopathic scoliosis and normal inspiratory scans. **A:** An inspiratory scan shows homogeneous lung attenuation without evidence of airways disease. **B:** Routine expiratory scan shows patchy air-trapping (*arrows*) indicative of small airways disease.

Some investigators obtain expiratory scans routinely in all patients who have HRCT, whereas others limit their use to patients with inspiratory scan abnormalities or suspected obstructive lung disease [55]. We recommend the routine use of expiratory scans in a patient's initial HRCT evaluation. The functional cause of respiratory disability is not always known before HRCT. Furthermore, even in patients with a known restrictive abnormality on pulmonary function tests, expiratory HRCT may show air-trapping, a finding of potential value in differential diagnosis. Limiting expiratory HRCT to patients with evidence of airway abnormalities on inspiratory scans will result in some missed diagnoses. Expiratory HRCT may show findings of air-trapping in the absence of inspiratory scan abnormalities (Fig. 1-28) [59]. The use of expiratory

scans may be of great value in the follow-up of patients at risk of developing an obstructive abnormality. For example, expiratory scans are valuable in detecting bronchiolitis obliterans in patients being followed for lung transplantation [79,87].

Expiratory HRCT scans may be obtained during suspended respiration after forced exhalation (postexpiratory CT), during forced exhalation (dynamic expiratory CT) [64,68], at a user-selected respiratory level controlled during exhalation with a spirometer (spirometrically triggered expiratory CT), or during other methods [88–93]. Generally, with these techniques, expiratory scans are obtained at selected levels. Three scans, five scans, or scans at 4-cm intervals have been used by different authors. Expiratory imaging may also be performed using spiral technique and 3D volumetric reconstruction

[94,95]. Although not a "high-resolution" technique, this method can be valuable in patients also having HRCT for evaluation of lung disease, particularly emphysema.

Postexpiratory High-Resolution Computed Tomography

Postexpiratory HRCT scans, obtained during suspended respiration after a forced exhalation, are easily performed with any scanner and are most suitable for a routine examination (Fig. 1-28). The primary advantage of this technique is its simplicity. In obtaining expiratory HRCT, the patient is instructed to forcefully exhale and then hold his or her breath for the duration of the single scan. This maneuver is practiced with the patient before the scans are obtained to ensure an adequate level of expiration. Postexpiratory scans can be performed at several predetermined levels (e.g., aortic arch, carina, and lung bases), at 2- to 4-cm intervals, or at levels appearing abnormal on the inspiratory images. Scans at two to five levels have been used by different authors [60,70,71,76,96,97]. Expiratory scans at three selected levels (aortic arch, hila, lower lobes) are generally sufficient for showing significant air-trapping when present, and are used routinely in addition to inspiratory scan series in patients with suspected airways or obstructive lung diseases. Although targeting postexpiratory scans to lung regions that appear abnormal on the inspiratory scans would seem advantageous, using preselected scans allows the same lung regions to be routinely imaged on follow-up examinations and, in some patients, can show air-trapping when inspiratory scans are normal.

Each of the postexpiratory scans is compared to the inspiratory scan that most closely duplicates its level to detect air-trapping. Anatomic landmarks such as pulmonary vessels, bronchi, and fissures are most useful for localizing corresponding levels. Because of diaphragmatic motion occurring with expiration, attempting to localize the same scan levels by using the scout view is difficult and sometimes misleading.

Dynamic Expiratory High-Resolution Computed Tomography

Scans obtained dynamically during forced expiration can be obtained using an electron-beam scanner or a helical scanner. There is some evidence to suggest that a greater increase in lung attenuation occurs with dynamic expiratory imaging than with simple postexpiratory HRCT and that air-trapping consequently is more easily diagnosed.

Dynamic scanning with an electron-beam scanner has been termed *dynamic ultrafast HRCT* [68,81,98,99]. This technique is performed using a scanner capable of obtaining a series of images with a 100-millisecond scan time [500-millisecond interscan delay, 1.5- to 3-mm collimation, 150 kV(p), 650 mA] [68,81,98,100]. In general, when using this technique, a series of ten scans is performed at a single level during a 6-second period, as the patient first inspires and then forcefully exhales. Patients are instructed to breathe in deeply and then breathe out as rapidly as possible (Fig. 1-29).

Images are reconstructed using a high–spatial frequency algorithm. Usually, dynamic CT scan sequences are obtained at several selected levels through the lungs. In papers describing this technique, three levels were used (e.g., at the level of the aortic arch, carina, and lung bases), although the protocol can be varied in individual cases, with imaging limited to a specific region.

During expiration, the diaphragm ascends, and the lungs move cephalad. Lung motion is most significant on scans through the lung bases. Although slightly different regions of the lung are imaged on sequential scans obtained at the same level, the effect of diaphragmatic motion on the assessment of lung attenuation has been regarded as inconsequential [64,68,98]. Little motion-related image degradation is visible on dynamic ultrafast HRCT scans because of the very rapid scan time used [81,100].

Dynamic scans can also be obtained using a spiral or helical CT scanner with a gantry rotation time of 1 second or less. If images are reconstructed using half the scan circle, individual images represent a scan period of one-half second or less. Because of the continuous scanning that is possible with the helical technique, scans can be reconstructed at any point during the scan sequence, thus providing a temporal resolution equivalent or superior to that of dynamic ultrafast HRCT. However, because of the longer time required to obtain each image, some degradation of anatomic detail can be expected on individual images. In performing dynamic expiratory CT, although one or more images obtained during the rapid phases of expiration will show significant motion artifact, images near and at full expiration show little artifact and allow optimal assessment of lung attenuation (Fig. 1-30) [101].

The use of a dynamic spiral technique may be combined with a reduced mA (e.g., 40 mA) so that the sequence of images obtained represents the same radiation dose as that associated with a single expiratory image (see Fig. 2-20). Using such a technique, continuous imaging is performed during 6 seconds, as the patient rapidly exhales. The total radiation dose for the 6-second sequence is equivalent to that of a single scan. Although image quality is reduced using the low-dose technique, images adequate for the diagnosis of air-trapping are obtained. In a group of lung transplant recipients studied using both postexpiratory HRCT and low-dose dynamic expiratory spiral HRCT [101], lung attenuation was noted to increase significantly more with the dynamic technique (204 HU versus 130 HU, $p = .0007$), and in one patient, air-trapping was diagnosed only on the dynamic images.

Using either technique, the dynamic scan sequence is viewed with attention to changes in lung attenuation and regional lung volume during the forced expiration. The images can be evaluated quantitatively or qualitatively, with measurement of lung attenuation during different phases of the respiratory maneuver, calculation of time-attenuation curves, or simple viewing of the serial scans in sequence or in cine mode. Air-trapping is considered to be present when the lung fails to increase normally in attenuation during exhalation [68,81,98]. The image sequence can be analyzed quantitatively as well as

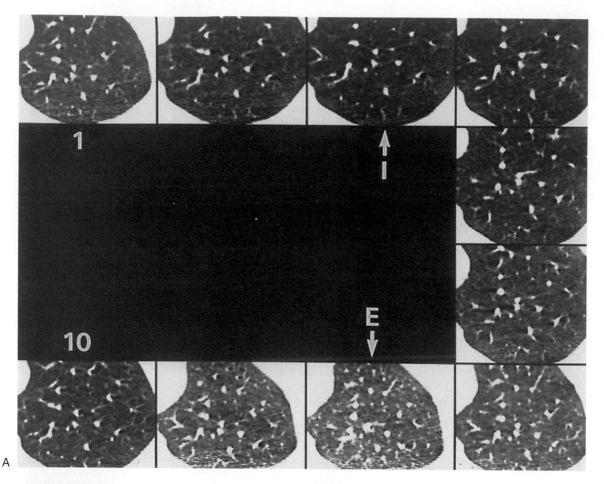

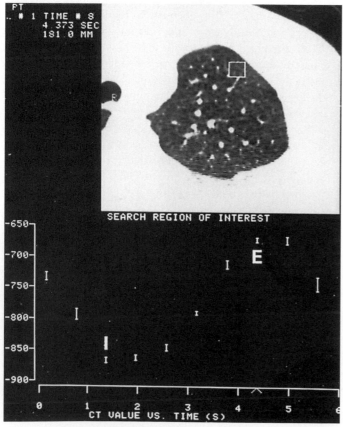

FIG. 1-29. Dynamic expiratory HRCT in a normal subject obtained using an electron-beam scanner. **A:** The ten-image dynamic ultrafast HRCT sequence acquired during a single forced vital capacity maneuver is shown, with the field of view limited to the left upper lobe. These ten 100-millisecond images were obtained at 600-millisecond intervals. They are shown in sequence, in a clockwise fashion, from the left upper corner (1) to the lower left corner (10). Images at full inspiration (I) and full expiration (E) are visible. Note the increase in lung attenuation and decrease in lung volume that occur as the subject exhales. As in most normal subjects, lung attenuation increase on expiration is relatively homogeneous. **B:** A time-attenuation curve is produced by measuring the mean lung attenuation (HU) for a specific region of interest (ROI). In this subject, for an ROI in the anterior lung, attenuation decreases to approximately −870 HU at maximum inspiration (I) and increases in attenuation to −670 HU at maximum expiration (E) for an overall attenuation increase of approximately 200 HU. Each point on the time-attenuation curve represents one image from the dynamic sequence. (From Webb WR, Stern EJ, Kanth N, et al. Dynamic pulmonary CT: findings in normal adult men. *Radiology* 1993;186:117, with permission.)

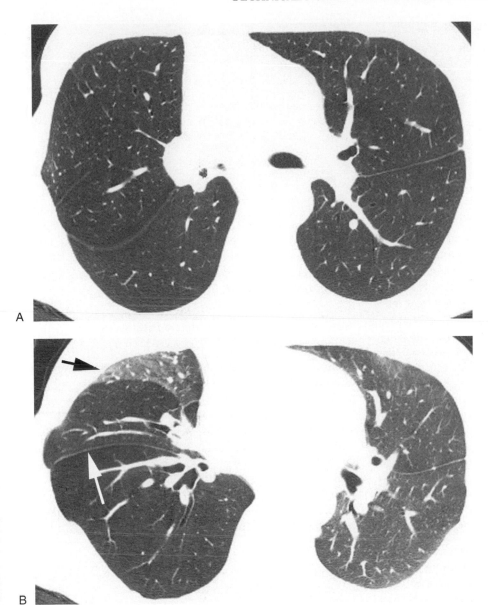

FIG. 1-30. Dynamic expiratory HRCT obtained using a spiral scanner. **A:** In a patient with bilateral lung transplantation, inspiratory HRCT shows stenosis of the bronchus intermedius. The lungs appear normal. **B:** On an image from the expiratory phase, there is marked air-trapping in right middle and lower lobes. Note that the right major fissure (*white arrow*) is bowed forward in comparison to the left major fissure and the inspiratory scan. The right upper lobe (*black arrow*) and left lung increase normally in attenuation.

qualitatively. The mean HU attenuation for a specific region of interest in the lung can be measured and plotted for each scan, producing a time-attenuation curve graphically demonstrating the changes in lung attenuation that have occurred during a single expiration and inspiration (Fig. 1-29B) [81]. This use of dynamic expiratory HRCT is discussed further in Chapters 2 and 3.

Spirometrically Triggered Expiratory High-Resolution Computed Tomography

Spirometrically triggered expiratory HRCT is a technique by which expiratory scanning can be done at specific, reproducible, user-selected lung volumes [88–90,93]. With this technique, the patient breathes through a small hand-held spirometer while positioned on the CT table. Before scanning, a spirometric measurement of the vital capacity is obtained, and trigger level (e.g.,

90% of vital capacity) is chosen. During exhalation, the spirometer and associated microcomputer measure the volume of gas expired and trigger CT after a specific volume is reached. When the trigger signal is generated, air flow is inhibited by closure of a valve attached to the spirometer, and a scanning starts. Two or three different levels in the chest are typically selected and evaluated with respect to lung attenuation at specific lung volumes. Using this method, quantitative assessment of CT images with respect to lung attenuation can be performed with excellent precision [88,89]. This technique may also be used with a spiral scanner or an electron beam scanner [91]. Spirometrically gated or controlled imaging may be particularly valuable in pediatric patients [91]; with inhibition of respiration, respiratory motion artifacts may be avoided. Motion-free inspiratory and expiratory imaging can also be obtained in pediatric patients by using a positive-pressure ventilation device and controlled pauses in spontaneous respiration [92].

Three-Dimensional Expiratory Computed Tomography

The use of helical CT performed with thick collimation (7 to 8 mm) at inspiration and expiration, with 3D reconstruction of the CT data, has also been used to assess lung volume and the extent of emphysema. However, in patients having an HRCT study for diagnosis of a diffuse lung disease, obtaining selected expiratory HRCT scans is generally simpler and preferable to obtaining a spiral CT examination for the diagnosis of air-trapping.

The method of assessing lung attenuation or lung volume using spiral CT has varied with the investigator. Kauczor et al. [94] used helical CT (slice thickness, 8 mm; pitch, 2; increment, 8 mm) with two-dimensional (2D) and 3D postprocessing to assess lung volume at deep inspiration and expiration. 2D and 3D techniques were found to correlate with lung volumes. In another study, 3D volumetric reconstructions of total lung volume at inspiration and at expiration and quantitation of regions of low attenuation (lung attenuation measuring less than −896 HU on inspiratory CT and −790 HU on expiratory CT) were correlated with pulmonary function test results [95]; in this study, an excellent correlation was found between the volume of low-attenuation lung and pulmonary function test findings of obstruction, such as the ratio of forced expiratory volume in 1 sec (FEV_1) to the forced vital capacity.

The use of multidetector-row volumetric HRCT during inspiration and expiration may also be used for the global assessment of lung attenuation, with the advantage that it would also provide anatomic detail.

RECOMMENDED HIGH-RESOLUTION COMPUTED TOMOGRAPHY PROTOCOLS

HRCT may be obtained in a number of different clinical settings, and to some extent the manner in which the examination is obtained is varied according to the diseases suspected. The following protocols are provided as guides, but these may be varied in individual cases.

Suspected Emphysema, Airways, or Obstructive Disease

In patients suspected of having airways or obstructive disease on the basis of clinical, pulmonary function, or plain radiographic findings, HRCT should be obtained at full inspiration, at 1-cm intervals from lung apices to bases, and with the patient supine (Table 1-2); prone scans are not usually needed. This protocol has been recommended specifically for studying patients with suspected bronchiectasis [102]. Scans after expiration obtained at three or more levels are recommended to detect air-trapping. Gantry angulation may be appropriate in selected cases when bronchiectasis is suspected, but it is not recommended as routine [40,41]. Multidetector-row spiral HRCT, using 1- to 1.25-mm detector width would be ideal for assessing this type of abnormality. The assessment of airways disease is discussed in further detail in Chapter 8.

TABLE 1-2. *Scan protocols: suspected emphysema, airways disease, or obstructive lung disease*

Full inspiration
Supine scans with 1-cm spacing from lung apices to bases
Expiratory scans at three or more levels
Options: Gantry angulation for airways disease
      Spiral CT (3-mm collimation; pitch, 1.7–2.0) for airways disease
      Multidetector-row spiral HRCT

In patients with emphysema being evaluated for lung transplantation or volume-reduction surgery, obtaining a routine CT with thick collimation for the detection of lung nodules suspicious for carcinoma is also important. HRCT and volumetric imaging may be combined by using multidetector-row spiral HRCT.

Suspected Fibrotic or Restrictive Disease, or Unknown Lung Disease

In patients suspected of having a fibrotic or restrictive lung disease on the basis of clinical, pulmonary function, or plain radiographic findings, or in patients with an unknown type of respiratory disability, it is also appropriate to obtain HRCT scans at 1-cm intervals with the patient supine. If the chest radiograph appears normal or subtle lung disease is present, or if chest radiographs are unavailable for review, additional prone scans should be obtained, or the scans should be monitored for the presence of problematic dependent opacity (Table 1-3). If the plain radiograph shows a distinct abnormality, prone scans likely will not be needed.

TABLE 1-3. *Scan protocols: suspected restrictive or fibrotic lung disease, or diffuse lung disease of unknown type*

Chest radiograph abnormal
    Full inspiration.
    Supine scans with 1-cm spacing from lung apices to bases.
    Expiratory scans at three or more levels (initial examination only).
Chest radiograph normal or minimally abnormal; chest radiograph unavailable
Option 1
    Full inspiration.
    Scans with 2-cm spacing in both prone and supine positions from lung apices to bases.
    Expiratory scans at three or more levels (initial evaluation only).
Option 2
    Full inspiration.
    Supine scans with 1-cm spacing from lung apices to bases.
    Check scans for "dependent density" and obtain prone scans at appropriate levels if present.
    Expiratory scans at three or more levels (initial evaluation only).

Prone scans at 2-cm intervals, in combination with the supine scans, are recommended when obtaining prone scans routinely; they obviate the need for reviewing plain radiographs or monitoring scans. Scans at 2-cm intervals, in both supine and prone positions, have proven to be a useful protocol for prone and supine imaging and provide the same number of images to review as obtained when scanning a patient with obstructive disease [29] (Table 1-3). In patients having their initial diagnostic evaluation, obtaining expiratory scans at three or more levels is recommended. In a patient with an unknown lung disease, airway obstruction may be the cause of the patient's disability. Furthermore, in a patient with a restrictive or fibrotic disease, the presence of air-trapping visible on expiratory images may be helpful in differential diagnosis [60].

In patients with restrictive disease who are having follow-up HRCT examinations, inspiratory images may be obtained at fewer levels (e.g., at three levels) than are appropriate for the initial examination [33], and expiratory scans are not usually necessary.

Hemoptysis

In patients who present with hemoptysis possibly related to airway abnormalities or an endobronchial lesion, it has been recommended that CT be obtained through the hila using 5-mm collimation with or without spiral technique to allow evaluation of the central bronchi, with HRCT at 1-cm intervals through the remainder of the lung parenchyma to look for bronchiectasis or other airway abnormalities (Table 1-4) [103,104]. Multidetector-row HRCT would also be appropriate in the assessment of patients with hemoptysis, allowing the assessment of both large and small airways disease. Scans may be reconstructed using narrow detector width or by combining detectors to produce thicker scans (see Chapter 8).

Suspected Pulmonary Vascular Disease

Some patients may have symptoms or signs (e.g., hypoxemia, pulmonary hypertension) that may result from lung disease (e.g., emphysema), pulmonary vascular disease (e.g., chronic pulmonary embolism, vasculitis), or a combination of these [105–109]. In such patients, combining HRCT with a contrast-

TABLE 1-5. Scan protocols: suspected pulmonary vascular disease
Full inspiration
HRCT with 1-cm spacing
Expiratory scans at three or more levels (initial evaluation only)
Contrast-enhanced spiral CT
Option: Contrast-enhanced multidetector-row HRCT

enhanced spiral CT may be necessary for diagnosis. The HRCT study is used to detect findings of lung disease or small vessel disease, and the contrast-enhanced spiral CT is used to detect large vessel abnormalities and vascular obstruction.

HRCT obtained at 1-cm intervals in the supine position with expiratory scans would be appropriate (Table 1-5). The spiral CT technique used would depend on the indications. For the diagnosis of chronic pulmonary embolism, although the precise technique varies with the investigator and is beyond the scope of this book, the use of 3-mm collimation and a pitch of 1.7 to 2 during contrast infusion is most appropriate for a single detector–row spiral scanner [110–113]. The use of contrast-enhanced multidetector-row HRCT with 1.25-mm detector width and a pitch of 6 would be ideal for this indication, allowing the detailed assessment of both large and small vessel abnormalities and associated lung disease (Figs. 1-26 and 1-27).

Combined Diagnosis of Diffuse Lung Disease and Focal Abnormalities

Combining conventional CT with HRCT examinations may be of value in patients with a variety of diseases (Table 1-6), but it is particularly important in patients being evaluated before volume-reduction surgery for emphysema or before lung transplantation. In such patients, volumetric lung imaging may be of value in the diagnosis of lung carcinoma, which has an increased incidence in patients with emphysema or lung fibrosis, or other significant focal abnormalities [54]. In patients having single lung transplantation, identification of significant abnormalities localized to one lung may be valuable in allowing the appropriate choice of which lung to remove. Multidetector-row spiral CT would be very useful in this regard.

TABLE 1-4. Scan protocols: hemoptysis
Full inspiration
Supine scans with contiguous 5-mm collimation through the hila
HRCT with 1-cm spacing at other levels
Expiratory scans at three or more levels (initial evaluation only)
Option: Multidetector-row HRCT

TABLE 1-6. Scan protocols: combined diagnosis of diffuse lung disease and focal abnormalities
Full inspiration
HRCT with 1-cm spacing
Prone scans if appropriate
Expiratory scans at three or more levels (initial evaluation only)
Spiral CT with or without contrast infusion
Option: Multidetector-row HRCT

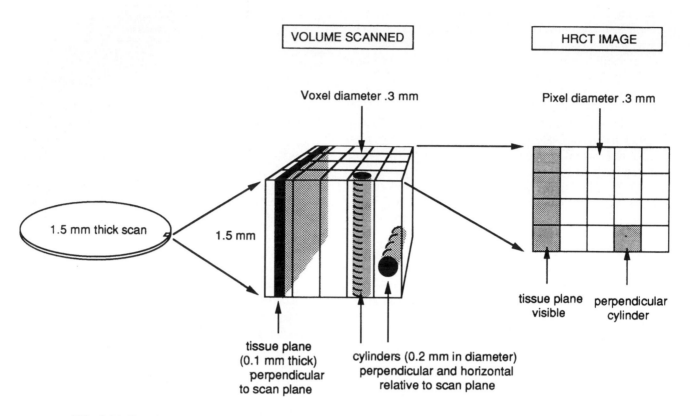

FIG. 1-31. Resolution and size or orientation of structures. The tissue plane, 1 mm thick, and the perpendicular cylinder, 0.2 mm in diameter, are visible on the HRCT scan because they extend through the thickness of the scan volume or voxel. The horizontal cylinder cannot be seen.

SPATIAL RESOLUTION

A fundamental relationship exists between pixel size and the size of structures that can be resolved by CT. For optimal matching of image display to the attainable spatial resolution of the scanner, there should be two pixels for the smallest structure resolved [12]. If a sufficiently small FOV is used with pixel sizes approximating 0.25 mm, current scanners are capable of providing a resolution of 10 to 12 line pairs per cm by using a high-resolution algorithm [11,42].

Structures smaller than the pixel size should be difficult to resolve on HRCT; however, resolution is sometimes possible. Interlobular septa as thin as 0.1 mm and arteries with a diameter of 0.3 mm are sometimes visible on HRCT using a small FOV. The reasons such small structures are visible include the large differences in attenuation between the soft-tissue structures present in the lung and the air-filled alveoli surrounding them, and the use of a high–spatial frequency algorithm for reconstruction, which often results in some edge enhancement.

The ability of HRCT to resolve fine lung structures depends on their orientation relative to the scan plane (Fig. 1-31). Structures measuring 0.1 to 0.2 mm in thickness can be seen if they are largely oriented perpendicular to the scan plane and extend through the thickness of the scan plane or voxel (e.g.,

1.5 mm) [10,11,114,115]. Similarly sized structures (0.1 to 0.2 mm) that are oriented horizontally within the scan plane will not be visible because of volume averaging with the air-filled lung, which occupies most of the thickness of the voxel.

These limitations explain the visibility of various lung structures on HRCT. For example, HRCT allows us to resolve some normal interlobular septa, which represent a plane of tissue approximately 100 to 200 mm or 0.1 to 0.2 mm in thickness, or small vessels that are oriented perpendicular to the scan plane (Fig. 1-31) [10,114,115], whereas vessels or septa lying in the plane of scan are usually visible as discrete structures only if they are larger or thicker than 0.3 to 0.5 mm. Bronchi or bronchioles measuring less than 2 to 3 cm in diameter and having a wall thickness of approximately 0.3 mm are usually invisible in peripheral lung because they have courses that lie roughly in the plane of scan. Bronchi or bronchioles of similar sizes are sometimes visible when oriented perpendicular to the plane of scan.

It should be kept in mind that, although soft-tissue structures can be resolved when they are thinner or smaller than the pixel size, their apparent size in the final HRCT image will be determined, at least partially, by the pixel size and the interpolation algorithm used in the workstation or camera and not by their actual dimensions. This can make the measurement of such small structures on HRCT difficult and prone to inaccuracies.

RADIATION DOSE

HRCT as routinely performed results in a low radiation dose as compared to conventional CT obtained with contiguous 1-cm collimation [116]. Radiation doses at the breast skin surface for patients undergoing conventional chest CT with contiguous 10-mm collimation [140 kV(p), 200 mA] are approximately 20 mGy [117].

Initially, a study of contiguous HRCT scans reported the upper limit of the radiation dose that could be expected using this technique, as measured in the center of a 16-cm plastic phantom [11]. In this study, contiguous HRCT scans resulted in a higher dose than contiguous scans with 10-mm collimation. One-and-one-half–mm scans [120 kV(p), 300 mA] resulted in a dose of 61 mGy, as compared to 55 mGy for contiguous 10-mm collimated scans obtained using the same technique. However, it is important to recognize that the measured radiation dose is affected by scatter and penumbra effects [117]. These effects are greater with contiguous scans than with spaced scans, and it must be kept in mind that HRCT is normally performed using scans spaced at 1- or 2-cm intervals.

In a more recent study [116], the radiation dose to the chest associated with spaced HRCT scans was compared to the radiation dose produced by conventional CT. In this study, using a scan technique of 120 kV(p), 200 mA, and 2 seconds, the mean skin radiation dose was 4.4 mGy for 1.5-mm HRCT scans at 10 mm-intervals, 2.1 mGy for scans at 20-mm intervals, and 36.3 mGy for conventional 10-mm scans at 10-mm intervals. Thus, HRCT scanning at 10- and 20-mm intervals, as done in clinical imaging, results in 12% and 6%, respectively, of the radiation dose associated with conventional CT. It has also been pointed out that obtaining low-dose HRCT (20 mA, 2 seconds) [20] at 20-mm intervals would result in an average skin dose comparable to that administered with chest radiography [116]. This has been confirmed by Lee et al. [21]; the effective radiation dose of low-dose HRCT obtained at three levels with 80 mA is quite similar to that of chest radiographs [118,119].

The use of spiral CT or a multidetector-row spiral CT for volumetric HRCT examination results in a higher radiation dose than conventional HRCT. However, with multidetector-row spiral CT, a volumetric study may be obtained with a radiation dose similar to that of routine chest CT.

HIGH-RESOLUTION COMPUTED TOMOGRAPHY ARTIFACTS

Several confusing artifacts can be seen on HRCT. However, familiarity with their appearances should eliminate potential misdiagnoses [9,11,25,120,121].

Streak Artifacts

Fine streak artifacts that radiate from the edges of sharply marginated, high-contrast structures such as bronchial walls, ribs, or vertebral bodies are common on HRCT. On HRCT,

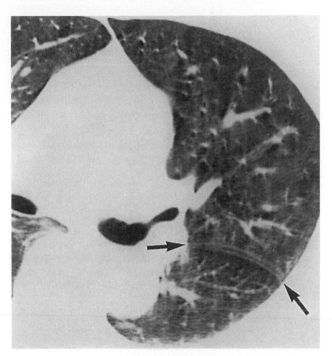

FIG. 1-32. "Double fissure" artifact. The left major fissure (*arrows*) appears to be double. Fine streak artifacts are visible posteriorly. Pulsation artifacts are also visible adjacent to the left heart border.

streak artifacts are often visible as fine, linear, or netlike opacities (Figs. 1-4 and 1-32) that can be seen anywhere but are most commonly found overlying the posterior lung, paralleling the pleural surface and posterior chest wall [11]. Although streak artifacts degrade the image, they do not usually mimic pathology or cause confusion in image interpretation. Streak artifacts are thinner and less dense and have a different appearance than the normal or abnormal interstitium (interlobular septa) visible in this region. Streak artifacts can result from two separate mechanisms—aliasing and correlated noise. Streak artifacts are more evident on scans obtained with low mA [20,25].

Aliasing is a geometric phenomenon that occurs because of undersampling of spatial information and is related to detector spacing and scan collimation [12]. As it is independent of radiation dose, increasing scan technique is of no value in reducing this type of artifact.

Correlated noise has a similar appearance and is most notable in the paravertebral regions, adjacent to the highly attenuating vertebral bodies [12]. This type of artifact is strongly related to radiation dose and can be minimized by increasing kV(p) and mA.

Motion Artifacts

Pulsation or *star artifacts* are commonly visible, particularly at the left lung base, adjacent to the heart (Figs. 1-6, 1-32, and 1-33). With pulsation artifacts, thin streaks radiate from the edges of vessels or other visible structures, which therefore resemble stars, and small areas of apparent lucency may be seen between these streaks. These lucent areas, if not recognized as artifactual, may be mistaken for dilated bronchi [121].

Doubling artifacts. The major fissure, usually on the left (Figs. 1-32 through 1-34), or other parenchymal structures such as vessels and bronchi, may be seen as double because of cardiac pulsation or respiration during the scan [25,120]. This appearance can mimic bronchiectasis (Fig. 1-33). It results when a linear structure, such as the fissure or vessel, is in a slightly different position when scanned by the gantry from opposite directions (180 degrees apart) (Fig. 1-34). As with image noise, these artifacts are much more conspicuous when high-resolution techniques are used, simply because they are more sharply resolved.

Motion-related artifacts can be reduced by ECG gating of scan acquisition [42], by using scanners with very rapid scan times (100 milliseconds) [98], or by spirometrically controlled respiration [91,92].

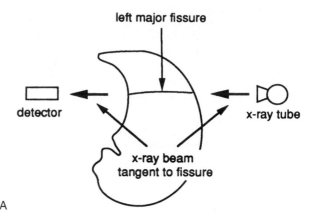

A

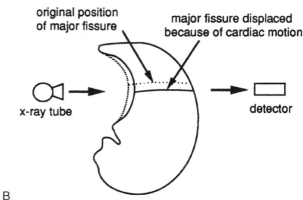

B

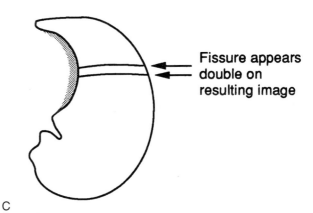

C

FIG. 1-34. Mechanism of "double fissure" artifact. The major fissure is seen by the scanner only when the x-ray beam is tangent to it. If the position of the fissure is slightly altered by cardiac pulsation during the period in which the gantry has rotated 180 degrees **(A,B)**, it appears to be seen in two different locations on the resulting image **(C)**.

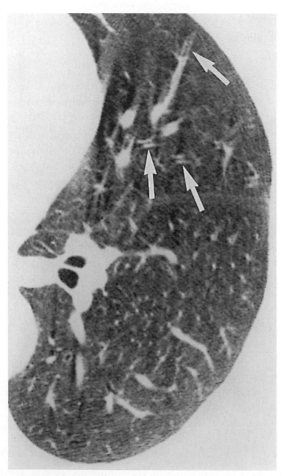

FIG. 1-33. Bronchiectasis artifact ("pseudobronchiectasis"). Several linear structures (*arrows*) appear double, mimicking bronchiectasis.

REFERENCES

1. Naidich DP. Pulmonary parenchymal high-resolution CT: to be or not to be. *Radiology* 1989;171:22–24.
2. Siegelman SS, Zerhouni EA, Leo FP, et al. CT of the solitary pulmonary nodule. *AJR Am J Roentgenol* 1980;135:1–13.
3. Todo G, Itoh H, Nakano Y, et al. [High-resolution CT for the evaluation of pulmonary peripheral disorders]. *Jpn J Clin Radiol* 1982;27:1319–1326.

4. Nakata H, Kimoto T, Nakayama T, et al. Diffuse peripheral lung disease: evaluation by high-resolution computed tomography. *Radiology* 1985;157:181–185.

5. Naidich DP, Zerhouni EA, Hutchins GM, et al. Computed tomography of the pulmonary parenchyma: part 1, distal air-space disease. *J Thorac Imaging* 1985;1:39–53.

6. Zerhouni EA, Naidich DP, Stitik FP, et al. Computed tomography of the pulmonary parenchyma: part 2, interstitial disease. *J Thorac Imaging* 1985;1:54–64.

7. Müller NL, Miller RR. Computed tomography of chronic diffuse infiltrative lung disease: part 1. *Am Rev Respir Dis* 1990;142:1206–1215.

8. Müller NL, Miller RR. Computed tomography of chronic diffuse infiltrative lung disease: part 2. *Am Rev Respir Dis* 1990;142:1440–1448.

9. Webb WR. High-resolution CT of the lung parenchyma. *Radiol Clin North Am* 1989; 27:1085–1097.

10. Zerhouni E. Computed tomography of the pulmonary parenchyma: an overview. *Chest* 1989;95:901–907.

11. Mayo JR, Webb WR, Gould R, et al. High-resolution CT of the lungs: an optimal approach. *Radiology* 1987;163:507–510.

12. Mayo JR. High resolution computed tomography: technical aspects. *Radiol Clin North Am* 1991;29:1043–1049.

13. Murata K, Khan A, Rojas KA, et al. Optimization of computed tomography technique to demonstrate the fine structure of the lung. *Invest Radiol* 1988;23:170–175.

14. Webb WR, Gamsu G, Wall SD, et al. CT of a bronchial phantom: factors affecting appearance and size measurements. *Invest Radiol* 1984;19:394–398.

15. Mayo JR. The high–resolution computed tomography technique. *Semin Roentgenol* 1991;26:104–109.

16. Zwirewich CV, Terriff B, Müller NL. High-spatial-frequency (bone) algorithm improves quality of standard CT of the thorax. *AJR Am J Roentgenol* 1989;153:1169–1173.

17. Naidich DP, Marshall CH, Gribbin C, et al. Low-dose CT of the lungs: preliminary observations. *Radiology* 1990;175:729–731.

18. Murata K, Khan A, Herman PG. Pulmonary parenchymal disease: evaluation with high-resolution CT. *Radiology* 1989;170:629–635.

19. Remy-Jardin M, Giraud F, Remy J, et al. Pulmonary sarcoidosis: role of CT in the evaluation of disease activity and functional impairment and in prognosis assessment. *Radiology* 1994;191:675–680.

20. Zwirewich CV, Mayo JR, Müller NL. Low dose high-resolution CT of lung parenchyma. *Radiology* 1991;180:413–417.

21. Lee KS, Primack SL, Staples CA, et al. Chronic infiltrative lung disease: comparison of diagnostic accuracies of radiography and low- and conventional-dose thin-section CT. *Radiology* 1994;191:669–673.

22. Majurin ML, Varpula M, Kurki T, et al. High-resolution CT of the lung in asbestos-exposed subjects: comparison of low-dose and high-dose HRCT. *Acta Radiol* 1994;35:473–477.

23. Majurin ML, Valavaara R, Varpula M, et al. Low-dose and conventional-dose high resolution CT of pulmonary changes in breast cancer patients treated by tangential field radiotherapy. *Eur J Radiol* 1995;20:114–119.

24. Bankier AA, Fleischmann D, Mallek R, et al. Bronchial wall thickness: appropriate window settings for thin-section CT and radiologic-anatomic correlation. *Radiology* 1996;199:831–836.

25. Primack SL, Remy-Jardin M, Remy J, et al. High-resolution CT of the lung: pitfalls in the diagnosis of infiltrative lung disease. *AJR Am J Roentgenol* 1996;167:413–418.

26. Maguire WM, Herman PG, Khan A, et al. Comparison of fixed and adjustable window width and level settings in the CT evaluation of diffuse lung disease. *J Comput Assist Tomogr* 1993;17:847–852.

27. Remy-Jardin M, Remy J, Giraud F, et al. Computed tomography assessment of ground-glass opacity: semiology and significance. *J Thorac Imaging* 1993;8:249–264.

28. Aberle DR, Gamsu G, Ray CS, et al. Asbestos-related pleural and parenchymal fibrosis: detection with high-resolution CT. *Radiology* 1988;166:729–734.

29. Volpe J, Storto ML, Lee K, et al. High-resolution CT of the lung: determination of the usefulness of CT scans obtained with the patient prone based on plain radiographic findings. *AJR Am J Roentgenol* 1997;169:369–374.

30. Mathieson JR, Mayo JR, Staples CA, et al. Chronic diffuse infiltrative lung disease: comparison of diagnostic accuracy of CT and chest radiography. *Radiology* 1989;171:111–116.

31. Swensen SJ, Aughenbaugh GL, Brown LR. High-resolution computed tomography of the lung. *Mayo Clin Proc* 1989;64:1284–1294.

32. Aberle DR, Gamsu G, Ray CS. High-resolution CT of benign asbestos-related diseases: clinical and radiographic correlation. *AJR Am J Roentgenol* 1988;151:883–891.

33. Kazerooni EA, Martinez FJ, Flint A, et al. Thin-section CT obtained at 10-mm increments versus limited three-level thin-section CT for idiopathic pulmonary fibrosis: correlation with pathologic scoring. *AJR Am J Roentgenol* 1997;169:977–983.

34. Gamsu G, Aberle DR, Lynch D. Computed tomography in the diagnosis of asbestos-related thoracic disease. *J Thorac Imaging* 1989;4:61–67.

35. Friedman AC, Fiel SB, Fisher MS, et al. Asbestos-related pleural disease and asbestosis: a comparison of CT and chest radiography. *AJR Am J Roentgenol* 1988;150:268–275.

36. Friedman AC, Fiel SB, Radecki PD, et al. Computed tomography of benign pleural and pulmonary parenchymal abnormalities related to asbestos exposure. *Semin Ultrasound CT MR* 1990;11:393–408.

37. Staples CA. Computed tomography in the evaluation of benign asbestos-related disorders. *Radiol Clin North Am* 1992;30:1191–1207.

38. Murray K, Gamsu G, Webb WR, et al. High-resolution CT sampling for detection of asbestos-related lung disease. *Acad Radiol* 1995;2:111–115.

39. Henschke CI. Image selection for computed tomography of the chest: a sampling approach. *Invest Radiol* 1992;27:908–911.

40. Remy-Jardin M, Remy J. Comparison of vertical and oblique CT in evaluation of the bronchial tree. *J Comput Assist Tomogr* 1988;12:956–962.

41. Grenier P, Cordeau MP, Beigelman C. High-resolution computed tomography of the airways. *J Thorac Imaging* 1993;8:213–229.

42. Schoepf UJ, Becker CR, Bruening RD, et al. Electrocardiographically gated thin-section CT of the lung. *Radiology* 1999;212:649–654.

43. Swensen SJ, Brown LR, Colby TV, et al. Lung nodule enhancement at CT: prospective findings. *Radiology* 1996;201:447–455.

44. Engeler CE, Tashjian JH, Engeler CM, et al. Volumetric high-resolution CT in the diagnosis of interstitial lung disease and bronchiectasis: diagnostic accuracy and radiation dose. *AJR Am J Roentgenol* 1994;163:31–35.

45. Bhalla M, Naidich DP, McGuinness G, et al. Diffuse lung disease: assessment with helical CT—preliminary observations of the role of maximum and minimum intensity projection images. *Radiology* 1996;200:341–347.

46. Coakley FV, Cohen MD, Johnson MS, et al. Maximum intensity projection images in the detection of simulated pulmonary nodules by spiral CT. *Br J Radiol* 1998;71:135–140.

47. Remy-Jardin M, Remy J, Artaud D, et al. Diffuse infiltrative lung disease: clinical value of sliding-thin-slab maximum intensity projection CT scans in the detection of mild micronodular patterns. *Radiology* 1996;200:333–339.

48. Kalender WA, Seissler W, Klotz E, et al. Spiral volumetric CT with single-breath-hold technique, continuous transport, and continuous scanner rotation. *Radiology* 1990;176:181–183.

49. Vock P, Soucek M. Spiral computed tomography in the assessment of focal and diffuse lung disease. *J Thorac Imaging* 1993;8:283–290.

50. Paranjpe DV, Bergin CJ. Spiral CT of the lungs: optimal technique and resolution compared with conventional CT. *AJR Am J Roentgenol* 1994;162:561–567.

51. Heiken JP, Brink JA, Vannier MW. Spiral (helical) CT. *Radiology* 1993;189:647–656.

52. Polacin A, Kalender WA, Marchal G. Evaluation of section sensitivity profiles and image noise in spiral CT. *Radiology* 1992;185:29–35.

53. Kuriyama K, Tateishi R, Kumatani T, et al. Pleural invasion by peripheral bronchogenic carcinoma: assessment with three-dimensional helical CT. *Radiology* 1994;191:365–369.

54. Kazerooni EA, Chow LC, Whyte RI, et al. Preoperative examination of lung transplant candidates: value of chest CT compared with chest radiography. *AJR Am J Roentgenol* 1995;165:1343–1348.

55. Arakawa H, Webb WR. Expiratory high-resolution CT scan. *Radiol Clin North Am* 1998;36:189–209.

56. Webb WR. Radiology of obstructive pulmonary disease. *AJR Am J Roentgenol* 1997;169:637–647.

57. Chen D, Webb WR, Storto ML, et al. Assessment of air trapping using postexpiratory high-resolution computed tomography. *J Thorac Imaging* 1998;13:135–143.

58. Lucidarme O, Coche E, Cluzel P, et al. Expiratory CT scans for chronic airway disease: correlation with pulmonary function test results. *AJR Am J Roentgenol* 1998;170:301–307.
59. Arakawa H, Webb WR. Air trapping on expiratory high-resolution CT scans in the absence of inspiratory scan abnormalities: correlation with pulmonary function tests and differential diagnosis. *AJR Am J Roentgenol* 1998;170:1349–1353.
60. Arakawa H, Webb WR, McCowin M, et al. Inhomogeneous lung attenuation at thin-section CT: diagnostic value of expiratory scans. *Radiology* 1998;206:89–94.
61. Vock P, Malanowski D, Tschaeppeler H, et al. Computed tomographic lung density in children. *Invest Radiol* 1987;22:627–631.
62. Robinson PJ, Kreel L. Pulmonary tissue attenuation with computed tomography: comparison of inspiration and expiration scans. *J Comput Assist Tomogr* 1979;3:740–748.
63. Millar AB, Denison DM. Vertical gradients of lung density in healthy supine men. *Thorax* 1989;44:485–490.
64. Webb WR, Stern EJ, Kanth N, et al. Dynamic pulmonary CT: findings in normal adult men. *Radiology* 1993;186:117–124.
65. Verschakelen JA, Van Fraeyenhoven L, Laureys G, et al. Differences in CT density between dependent and nondependent portions of the lung: influence of lung volume. *AJR Am J Roentgenol* 1993;161:713–717.
66. Webb WR. High-resolution computed tomography of obstructive lung disease. *Radiol Clin North Am* 1994;32:745–757.
67. Knudson RJ, Standen JR, Kaltenborn WT, et al. Expiratory computed tomography for assessment of suspected pulmonary emphysema. *Chest* 1991;99:1357–1366.
68. Stern EJ, Webb WR, Gamsu G. Dynamic quantitative computed tomography: a predictor of pulmonary function in obstructive lung diseases. *Invest Radiol* 1994;29:564–569.
69. Kitahara Y, Takamoto M, Maruyama M, et al. Differential diagnosis of pulmonary emphysema using the CT index: LL%. *Nippon Kyobu Shikkan Gakkai Zasshi* 1989;27:689–695.
70. Newman KB, Lynch DA, Newman LS, et al. Quantitative computed tomography detects air trapping due to asthma. *Chest* 1994;106:105–109.
71. Park CS, Müller NL, Worthy SA, et al. Airway obstruction in asthmatic and healthy individuals: inspiratory and expiratory thin-section CT findings. *Radiology* 1997;203:361–367.
72. Lynch DA. Imaging of asthma and allergic bronchopulmonary mycosis. *Radiol Clin North Am* 1998;36:129–142.
73. Garg K, Lynch DA, Newell JD, et al. Proliferative and constrictive bronchiolitis: classification and radiologic features. *AJR Am J Roentgenol* 1994;162:803–808.
74. Padley SPG, Adler BD, Hansell DM, et al. Bronchiolitis obliterans: high-resolution CT findings and correlation with pulmonary function tests. *Clin Radiol* 1993;47:236–240.
75. Moore ADA, Godwin JD, Dietrich PA, et al. Swyer-James syndrome: CT findings in eight patients. *AJR Am J Roentgenol* 1992;158:1211–1215.
76. Marti-Bonmati L, Ruiz PF, Catala F, et al. CT findings in Swyer-James syndrome. *Radiology* 1989;172:477–480.
77. Sweatman MC, Millar AB, Strickland B, et al. Computed tomography in adult obliterative bronchiolitis. *Clin Radiol* 1990;41:116–119.
78. Aquino SL, Webb WR, Golden J. Bronchiolitis obliterans associated with rheumatoid arthritis: findings on HRCT and dynamic expiratory CT. *J Comput Assist Tomogr* 1994;18:555–558.
79. Leung AN, Fisher K, Valentine V, et al. Bronchiolitis obliterans after lung transplantation: detection using expiratory HRCT. *Chest* 1998;113:365–370.
80. Yang CF, Wu MT, Chiang AA, et al. Correlation of high-resolution CT and pulmonary function in bronchiolitis obliterans: a study based on 24 patients associated with consumption of *sauropus androgynus*. *AJR Am J Roentgenol* 1997;168:1045–1050.
81. Stern EJ, Webb WR, Golden JA, et al. Cystic lung disease associated with eosinophilic granuloma and tuberous sclerosis: air trapping at dynamic ultrafast high-resolution CT. *Radiology* 1992;182:325–329.
82. Hansell DM, Wells AU, Rubens MB, et al. Bronchiectasis: functional significance of areas of decreased attenuation at expiratory CT. *Radiology* 1994;193:369–374.
83. Hansell DM, Wells AU, Padley SP, et al. Hypersensitivity pneumonitis: correlation of individual CT patterns with functional abnormalities. *Radiology* 1996;199:123–128.
84. Small JH, Flower CD, Traill ZC, et al. Air-trapping in extrinsic allergic alveolitis on computed tomography. *Clin Radiol* 1996;51:684–688.
85. Hansell DM, Milne DG, Wilsher ML, et al. Pulmonary sarcoidosis: morphologic associations of airflow obstruction at thin-section CT. *Radiology* 1998;209:697–704.
86. Gleeson FV, Traill ZC, Hansell DM. Evidence of expiratory CT scans of small-airway obstruction in sarcoidosis. *AJR Am J Roentgenol* 1996;166:1052–1054.
87. Worthy SA, Park CS, Kim JS, et al. Bronchiolitis obliterans after lung transplantation: high resolution CT findings in 15 patients. *AJR Am J Roentgenol* 1997;169:673–677.
88. Kalender WA, Rienmuller R, Seissler W, et al. Measurement of pulmonary parenchymal attenuation: use of spirometric gating with quantitative CT. *Radiology* 1990;175:265–268.
89. Kalender WA, Fichte H, Bautz W, et al. Semiautomatic evaluation procedures for quantitative CT of the lung. *J Comput Assist Tomogr* 1991;15:248–255.
90. Lamers RJ, Thelissen GR, Kessels AG, et al. Chronic obstructive pulmonary diseases. evaluation with spirometrically controlled CT lung densitometry. *Radiology* 1994;193:109–113.
91. Robinson TE, Leung AN, Moss RB, et al. Standardized high-resolution CT of the lung using a spirometer-triggered electron beam CT scanner. *AJR Am J Roentgenol* 1999;172:1636–1638.
92. Long FR, Castile RG, Brody AS, et al. Lungs in infants and young children: improved thin-section CT with a noninvasive controlled-ventilation technique—initial experience. *Radiology* 1999;212:588–593.
93. Beinert T, Behr J, Mehnert F, et al. Spirometrically controlled quantitative CT for assessing diffuse parenchymal lung disease. *J Comput Assist Tomogr* 1995;19:924–931.
94. Kauczor HU, Heussel CP, Fischer B, et al. Assessment of lung volumes using helical CT at inspiration and expiration: comparison with pulmonary function tests. *AJR Am J Roentgenol* 1998;171:1091–1095.
95. Mergo PJ, Williams WF, Gonzalez-Rothi R, et al. Three-dimensional volumetric assessment of abnormally low attenuation of the lung from routine helical CT: inspiratory and expiratory quantification. *AJR Am J Roentgenol* 1998;170:1355–1360.
96. Lee ES, Gotway MB, Reddy GP, et al. Expiratory high-resolution CT: accuracy for the diagnosis of early bronchiolitis obliterans following lung transplantation. *Radiology* (in press).
97. Lee KW, Chung SY, Yang I, et al. Correlation of aging and smoking with air trapping at thin-section CT of the lung in asymptomatic subjects. *Radiology* 2000;214:831–836.
98. Stern EJ, Webb WR. Dynamic imaging of lung morphology with ultrafast high-resolution computed tomography. *J Thorac Imaging* 1993;8:273–282.
99. Stern EJ, Webb WR, Warnock ML, et al. Bronchopulmonary sequestration: dynamic, ultrafast, high-resolution CT evidence of air trapping. *AJR Am J Roentgenol* 1991;157:947–949.
100. Lynch DA, Brasch RC, Hardy KA, et al. Pediatric pulmonary disease: assessment with high-resolution ultrafast CT. *Radiology* 1990;176:243–248.
101. Gotway MB, Lee ES, Reddy GP, et al. Low-dose, dynamic expiratory high-resolution CT using a spiral scanner. *J Thorac Imaging* (in press).
102. Grenier P, Maurice F, Musset D, et al. Bronchiectasis: assessment by thin-section CT. *Radiology* 1986;161:95–99.
103. Naidich DP, Funt S, Ettenger NA, et al. Hemoptysis: CT-bronchoscopic correlations in 58 cases. *Radiology* 1990;177:357–362.
104. Set PAK, Flower CDR, Smith IE, et al. Hemoptysis: comparative study of the role of CT and fiberoptic bronchoscopy. *Radiology* 1993;189:677–680.
105. Bergin CJ, Rios G, King MA, et al. Accuracy of high-resolution CT in identifying chronic pulmonary thromboembolic disease. *AJR Am J Roentgenol* 1996;166:1371–1377.
106. King MA, Ysrael M, Bergin CJ. Chronic thromboembolic pulmonary hypertension: CT findings. *AJR Am J Roentgenol* 1998;170:955–960.
107. Lee KN, Lee HJ, Shin WW, et al. Hypoxemia and liver cirrhosis (hepatopulmonary syndrome) in eight patients: comparison of the central and peripheral pulmonary vasculature. *Radiology* 1999;211:549–553.
108. Sherrick AD, Swensen SJ, Hartman TE. Mosaic pattern of lung attenuation on CT scans: frequency among patients with pulmonary artery hypertension of different causes. *AJR Am J Roentgenol* 1997;169:79–82.

109. Connolly B, Manson D, Eberhard A, et al. CT appearance of pulmonary vasculitis in children. *AJR Am J Roentgenol* 1996; 167:901–904.
110. Drucker EA, Rivitz SM, Shepard JA, et al. Acute pulmonary embolism: assessment of helical CT for diagnosis. *Radiology* 1998;209:235–241.
111. Mayo JR, Remy-Jardin M, Müller NL, et al. Pulmonary embolism: prospective comparison of spiral CT with ventilation-perfusion scintigraphy. *Radiology* 1997;205:447–452.
112. Remy-Jardin M, Remy J, Artaud D, et al. Spiral CT of pulmonary embolism: technical considerations and interpretive pitfalls. *J Thorac Imaging* 1997;12:103–117.
113. Rubin GD, Goodman LR, Lipchik RJ, et al. Helical CT for the detection of acute pulmonary embolism: experts debate. *J Thorac Imaging* 1997;12:81–102.
114. Webb WR, Stein MG, Finkbeiner WE, et al. Normal and diseased isolated lungs: high-resolution CT. *Radiology* 1988;166:81–87.
115. Murata K, Itoh H, Todo G, et al. Centrilobular lesions of the lung: demonstration by high-resolution CT and pathologic correlation. *Radiology* 1986;161:641–645.
116. Mayo JR, Jackson SA, Müller NL. High-resolution CT of the chest: radiation dose. *AJR Am J Roentgenol* 1993;160:479–481.
117. Evans SH, Davis R, Cooke J, et al. A comparison of radiation doses to the breast in computed tomographic chest examinations for two scanning protocols. *Clin Radiol* 1989;40:45–46.
118. Reuter FG, Conway BJ, McCrohan ML, et al. Average radiation exposure values for three diagnostic radiographic examinations. *Radiology* 1990;177:341–345.
119. Müller NL. Clinical value of high-resolution CT in chronic diffuse lung disease. *AJR Am J Roentgenol* 1991;157:1163–1170.
120. Mayo JR, Müller NL, Henkelman RM. The double-fissure sign: a motion artifact on thin-section CT scans. *Radiology* 1987;165:580–581.
121. Tarver RD, Conces DJ, Godwin JD. Motion artifacts on CT simulate bronchiectasis. *AJR Am J Roentgenol* 1988;151:1117–1119.

CHAPTER 2

Normal Lung Anatomy

The accurate interpretation of high-resolution computed tomography (HRCT) images requires a detailed understanding of normal lung anatomy and of the pathologic alterations in normal lung anatomy occurring in the presence of disease [1–4]. In this chapter, only those aspects of lung anatomy that are important in using and interpreting HRCT are reviewed.

LUNG INTERSTITIUM

The lung is supported by a network of connective tissue fibers called the lung *interstitium*. Although the lung interstitium is not generally visible on HRCT in normal patients, interstitial thickening is often recognizable. For the purpose of interpretation of HRCT and identification of abnormal findings, the interstitium can be thought of as having several components (Fig. 2-1) [5].

The peribronchovascular interstitium is a system of fibers that invests bronchi and pulmonary arteries (Fig. 2-1). In the perihilar regions, the peribronchovascular interstitium forms a strong connective tissue sheath that surrounds large bronchi and arteries [6]. The more peripheral continuum of this interstitial fiber system, which is associated with small centrilobular bronchioles and arteries, may be termed the centrilobular interstitium (Fig. 2-1). Taken together, the peribronchovascular interstitium and centrilobular interstitium correspond to the "axial fiber system" described by Weibel, which extends peripherally from the pulmonary hila to the level of the alveolar ducts and sacs [5].

The subpleural interstitium is located beneath the visceral pleura; it envelops the lung in a fibrous sac from which connective tissue septa penetrate into the lung parenchyma (Fig. 2-1). These septa include the interlobular septa, which are described in detail below. The subpleural interstitium and interlobular septa are parts of the "peripheral fiber system" described by Weibel [5].

The intralobular interstitium is a network of thin fibers that forms a fine connective tissue mesh in the walls of alveoli and thus bridges the gap between the centrilobular interstitium in the center of lobules and the interlobular septa and subpleural interstitium in the lobular periphery (Fig. 2-1). Together, the intralobular interstitium, peribronchovascular interstitium, centrilobular interstitium, subpleural interstitium, and interlobular septa form a continuous fiber skeleton for the lung (Fig. 2-1). The intralobular interstitium corresponds to the "septal fibers" described by Weibel [5].

LARGE BRONCHI AND ARTERIES

Within the lung parenchyma, the bronchi and pulmonary artery branches are closely associated and branch in parallel. As indicated in the previous section, they are encased by the peribronchovascular interstitium, which extends from the pulmonary hila into the peripheral lung. Because some lung diseases produce thickening of the peribronchovascular interstitium in the central or perihilar lung, in relation to large bronchi and pulmonary vessels it is important to be aware of the normal HRCT appearances of the perihilar bronchi and pulmonary vessels.

When imaged at an angle to their longitudinal axis, central pulmonary arteries normally appear as rounded or elliptic opacities on HRCT, accompanied by uniformly thin-walled bronchi of similar shape (Fig. 2-2). When imaged along their axis, bronchi and vessels should appear roughly cylindrical or show slight tapering as they branch, depending on the length of the segment that is visible; tapering of a vessel or bronchus is most easily seen when a long segment is visible.

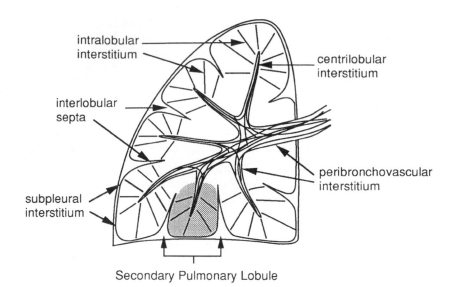

intralobular interstitium

centrilobular interstitium

interlobular septa

peribronchovascular interstitium

subpleural interstitium

Secondary Pulmonary Lobule

FIG. 2-1. Components of the lung interstitium. Taken together, the peribronchovascular interstitium and centrilobular interstitium correspond to the "axial fiber system" described by Weibel [5]. The subpleural interstitium and interlobular septa correspond to Weibel's "peripheral fiber system." The intralobular interstitium is roughly equivalent to the "septal fibers" described by Weibel.

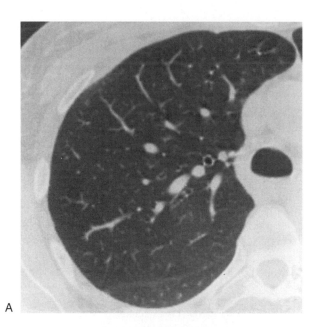

A

FIG. 2-2. Normal appearances of large bronchi and arteries photographed with window settings of –600/2,000 HU **(A)** and –700/1,000 HU **(B)**. The diameters of vessels and their neighboring bronchi are approximately equal. The outer walls of bronchi and pulmonary vessels are smooth and sharply defined. Bronchi are usually invisible within the peripheral 2 cm of lung, despite the fact that vessels are well seen in this region.

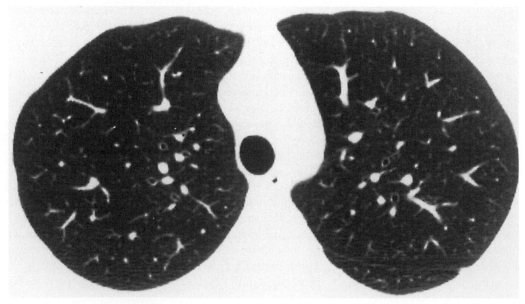

B

TABLE 2-1. *Relation of airway diameter to wall thickness*

Airway	Diameter (mm)	Wall thickness (mm)
Lobular and segmental bronchi	5–8	1.5
Subsegmental bronchi/ bronchiole	1.5–3.0	0.2–0.3
Lobular bronchiole	1	0.15
Terminal bronchiole	0.7	0.1
Acinar bronchiole	0.5	0.05

Modified from Weibel ER. High resolution computed tomography of the pulmonary parenchyma: anatomical background. Presented at: Fleischner Society Symposium on Chest Disease; 1990; Scottsdale, AZ.

The diameter of an artery and its neighboring bronchus should be approximately equal, although vessels may appear slightly larger than their accompanying bronchi, particularly in dependent lung regions. Although the presence of bronchi larger than their adjacent arteries is often assumed to indicate bronchial dilatation, or bronchiectasis, bronchi may appear larger than adjacent arteries in a significant number of nor-mal subjects. In an HRCT study of normal subjects, Lynch et al. [7] compared the internal diameters of lobular, segmental, subsegmental, and smaller bronchi to those of adjacent artery branches. Nineteen percent of bronchi had an internal bronchial diameter longer than the artery diameter, and 59% of normal subjects showed at least one such bronchus. Furthermore, a bronchus may appear larger than the adjacent artery branches if the scan traverses an undivided bronchus near its branch point, and its accompanying artery has already branched. In this situation, two artery branches may be seen to lie adjacent to the "dilated" bronchus.

The outer walls of visible pulmonary artery branches form a smooth and sharply defined interface with the surrounding lung, whether they are seen in cross section or along their length. The walls of large bronchi, outlined by lung on one side and air in the bronchial lumen on the other, should appear smooth and of uniform thickness. Thickening of the peribronchial and perivascular interstitiums can result in irregularity of the interface between arteries and bronchi and the adjacent lung [4,6,8].

Assessment of bronchial wall thickness on HRCT is quite subjective and is dependent on the window settings used [7]. Also, because the apparent thickness of the bronchial wall represents not only the wall itself, but the surrounding peribronchovascular interstitium as well, peribronchovascular interstitial thickening can result in apparent bronchial wall thickening (so-called peribronchial cuffing) on HRCT.

The wall thickness of conducting bronchi and bronchioles is approximately proportional to their diameter, at least for bronchi distal to the segmental level. In general, the thickness of the wall of a bronchus or bronchiole less than 5 mm in diameter should measure from one-sixth to one-tenth of its diameter (Table 2-1) [9]; however, precise measurement of the wall thickness of small bronchi or bronchioles is difficult, as wall thickness approximates pixel size.

Because bronchi taper and become thinner-walled as they branch, they become more difficult to see as they become more peripheral. Bronchi less than 2 mm in diameter are not normally visible on HRCT, and bronchioles within 2 cm of the pleural surface tend to be inconspicuous (Figs. 2-2 and 2-3) [10,11]. It is rare for normal bronchioles to be visible within 1 cm of the pleural surface [12,13].

SECONDARY PULMONARY LOBULE

The secondary pulmonary lobule as defined by Miller refers to the smallest unit of lung structure marginated by connective tissue septa [9,14]. Secondary lobules are easily visible on the surface of the lung because of these septa (Fig. 2-4) [9,15]. The terms secondary pulmonary lobule, secondary lobule, and pulmonary lobule are often used interchangeably, and are used as synonyms in this book. The term primary pulmonary lobule has also been used by Miller to describe a much smaller lung unit associated with a single alveolar duct [16,17], but this designation is not in common use.

Secondary pulmonary lobules are irregularly polyhedral in shape and somewhat variable in size, measuring approxi-

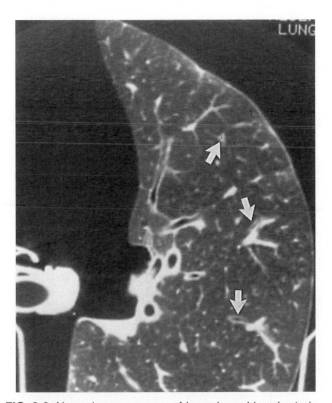

FIG. 2-3. Normal appearances of large bronchi and arteries. In an isolated lung, the smallest bronchi visible (*arrows*) measures 2 to 3 mm in diameter. Bronchi and bronchioles are not visible within the peripheral 1 cm of lung, although the artery branches that accompany these bronchi are sharply seen. (Note: The "isolated" lungs illustrated in this volume are fresh lungs obtained at autopsy and scanned while inflated with air at a pressure of approximately 30 cm of water [10].)

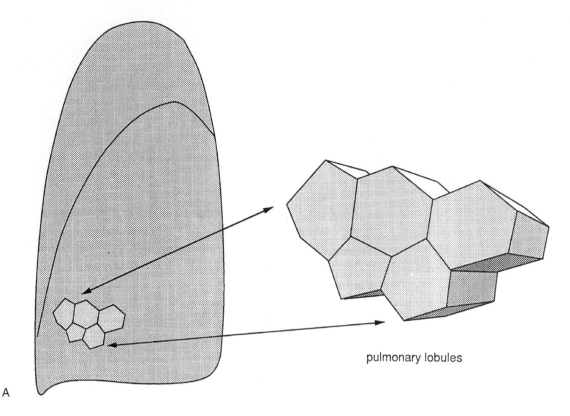

A

pulmonary lobules

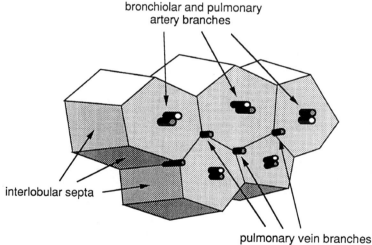

bronchiolar and pulmonary
artery branches

interlobular septa

pulmonary vein branches

B

FIG. 2-4. Pulmonary lobular anatomy. **A:** Pulmonary lobules that are irregularly polyhedral or conical in shape are often visible on the surface of the lung, as shown in this diagram of five lobules visible on the posterior surface of the left lung. **B:** Lobules are supplied by small bronchiolar and pulmonary artery branches, which are central in location, and are variably marginated by connective tissue interlobular septa that contain pulmonary vein and lymphatic branches.

mately 1 to 2.5 cm in diameter in most locations (Fig. 2-5) [5,9,15,18,19]. In one study, the average diameter of pulmonary lobules measured in several adults ranged from 11 to 17 mm [19]. Each secondary lobule is supplied by a small bronchiole and pulmonary artery, and is variably marginated, in different lung regions, by connective tissue interlobular septa containing pulmonary vein and lymphatic branches [16].

Secondary pulmonary lobules are made up of a limited number of pulmonary acini, usually a dozen or fewer, although the reported number varies considerably in different studies (Fig. 2-5A) [20,21]; in a study by Nishimura and Itoh [22], the number of acini counted in lobules of varying sizes ranged from three to 24. A pulmonary acinus is defined as the portion of the lung parenchyma distal to a terminal bronchiole and supplied by a first-order respiratory bronchiole or bronchioles [23]. Because respiratory bronchioles are the largest airways that have alveoli in their walls, an acinus is the largest lung unit in which all airways participate in gas exchange. Acini are usually described as ranging from 6 to 10 mm in diameter [19,24].

As indicated at the beginning of this section, Miller has defined the secondary lobule as the smallest lung unit marginated by connective tissue septa. Reid has suggested an alternate definition of the secondary pulmonary lobule, based on the branching pattern of peripheral bronchioles, rather than the presence and location of connective tissue septa (Fig. 2-6) [16,21,23]. On bronchograms, small bronchioles can be seen to arise at intervals of 5 to 10 mm from larger airways

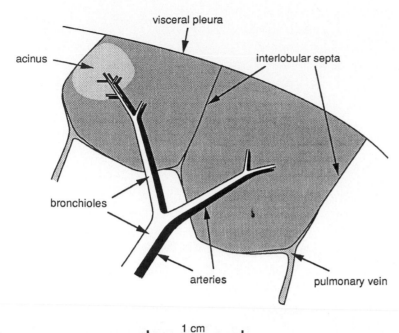

A

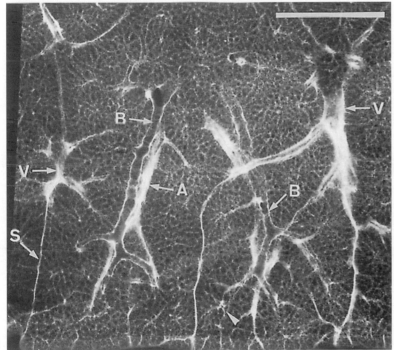

B

FIG. 2-5. A: Anatomy of the secondary pulmonary lobule, as defined by Miller. Two adjacent lobules are shown in this diagram. **B:** Radiographic anatomy of the secondary pulmonary lobule. Radiograph of a 1-mm lung slice taken from the lower lobe. Two well-defined secondary pulmonary lobules are visible. Lobules are marginated by thin interlobular septa (S) containing pulmonary vein (V) branches. Bronchioles (B) and pulmonary arteries (A) are centrilobular. Bar = 1 cm. (Reprinted from Itoh H, Murata K, et al. Diffuse lung disease: pathologic basis for the high-resolution computed tomography findings. *J Thorac Imaging* 1993;8:176, with permission.)

(the so-called centimeter pattern of branching); these small bronchioles then show branching at approximately 2-mm intervals (the "millimeter pattern") [23]. Airways showing the millimeter pattern of branching are considered by Reid to be intralobular, with each branch corresponding to a terminal bronchiole [21]. Lobules are considered to be the lung units supplied by 3 to 5 "millimeter pattern" bronchioles. Although Reid's criteria delineate lung units of approximately equal size, about 1 cm in diameter and containing 3 to 5 acini, it should be noted that this definition does not necessarily describe lung units equivalent to secondary lobules as defined by Miller and marginated by interlobular septa (Fig. 2-6) [21,22], although a small Miller's lobule can be the same as a Reid's lobule. Miller's definition is most applicable to the interpretation of HRCT and is widely accepted by pathologists, because interlobular septa are visible on histologic sections [22]. In this book, we use the term secondary pulmonary lobule to refer to a lobule as defined by Miller.

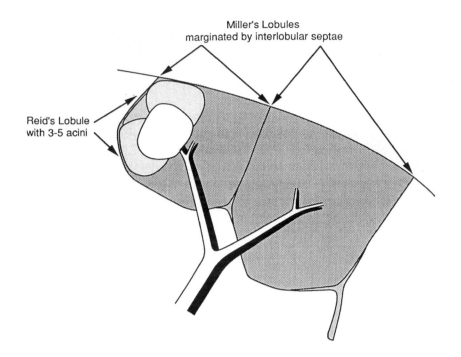

Miller's Lobules
marginated by interlobular septae

Reid's Lobule
with 3-5 acini

FIG. 2-6. Relative size and relationships of "Miller's lobule" and "Reid's lobule."

Anatomy of the Secondary Lobule and Its Components

An understanding of secondary lobular anatomy and the appearances of lobular structures is key to the interpretation of HRCT. HRCT can show many features of the secondary pulmonary lobule in normal and abnormal lungs, and many lung diseases, particularly interstitial diseases, produce characteristic changes in lobular structures [3,4,8,10,11,25,26]. Heitzman has been instrumental in emphasizing the importance of the secondary pulmonary lobule in the radiologic diagnosis of lung disease [15,16,27].

As discussed in Chapter 1, the visibility of normal lobular structures on HRCT is related to their size and orientation relative to the plane of scan, although size is most important (Fig. 2-7). Generally, the smallest structures visible on HRCT range from 0.3 to 0.5 mm in thickness; thinner structures, measuring 0.1 to 0.2 mm, are occasionally seen.

For the purposes of the interpretation of HRCT, the secondary lobule is most appropriately conceptualized as having three principal parts or components:

1. Interlobular septa and contiguous subpleural interstitium
2. Centrilobular structures
3. Lobular parenchyma and acini

Interlobular Septa

Anatomically, secondary lobules are marginated by connective tissue interlobular septa, which extend inward from the pleural surface (Figs. 2-4 and 2-5). These septa are part of the peripheral interstitial fiber system described by Weibel (Fig. 2-1) [5], which extends over the surface of the lung beneath the vis-

ceral pleura. Pulmonary veins and lymphatics lie within the connective tissue interlobular septa that marginate the lobule.

It should be emphasized that not all interlobular septa are equally well defined. The interlobular septa are thickest and most numerous in the apical, anterior, and lateral aspects of the upper lobes, the anterior and lateral aspects of the middle lobe and lingula, the anterior and diaphragmatic surfaces of the lower lobes, and along the mediastinal pleural surfaces [28]; thus, secondary lobules are best defined in these regions. Septa measure approximately 100 μm (0.1 mm) in thickness in a subpleural location [3,5,10,11]. Within the central lung, interlobular septa are thinner and less well defined than peripherally, and lobules are more difficult to identify in this location.

Peripherally, interlobular septa measuring 100 μm or 0.1 mm in thickness are at the lower limit of HRCT resolution [11], but nonetheless they are often visible on HRCT scans performed in vitro [10]. On in vitro HRCT, interlobular septa are often visible as very thin, straight lines of uniform thickness that are usually 1 to 2.5 cm in length and perpendicular to the pleural surface (Figs. 2-7 and 2-8). Several septa in continuity can be seen as a linear opacity measuring up to 4 cm in length (Fig. 2-9) [10].

On clinical scans in normal patients, interlobular septa are less commonly seen and are seen less well than they are in studies of isolated lungs. A few septa are often visible in the lung periphery in normal subjects, but they tend to be inconspicuous (Fig. 2-10); normal septa are most often seen anteriorly and along the mediastinal pleural surfaces [4,29]. When visible, they are usually seen extending to the pleural surface. In the central lung, septa are thinner than they are peripherally and are infrequently seen in normal subjects (Fig. 2-9); often, interlobular septa that are clearly defined in this region are abnormally thickened. Occasionally, when interlobular septa are not clearly

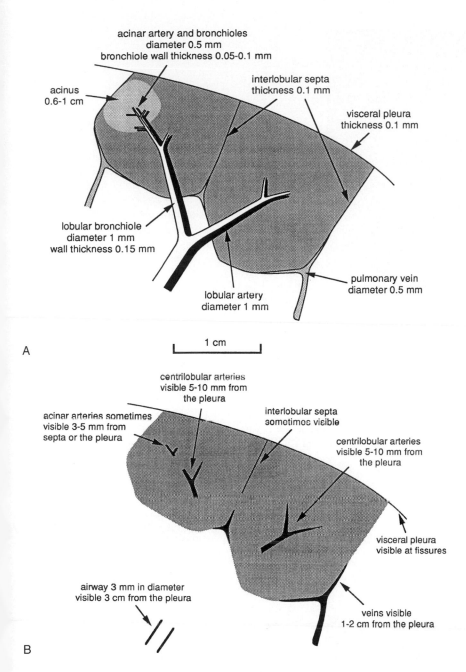

acinar artery and bronchioles
diameter 0.5 mm
bronchiole wall thickness 0.05-0.1 mm

interlobular septa
thickness 0.1 mm

acinus
0.6-1 cm

visceral pleura
thickness 0.1 mm

lobular bronchiole
diameter 1 mm
wall thickness 0.15 mm

pulmonary vein
diameter 0.5 mm

lobular artery
diameter 1 mm

1 cm

A

centrilobular arteries
visible 5-10 mm from
the pleura

acinar arteries sometimes
visible 3-5 mm from
septa or the pleura

interlobular septa
sometimes visible

centrilobular arteries
visible 5-10 mm from
the pleura

visceral pleura
visible at fissures

airway 3 mm in diameter
visible 3 cm from the pleura

veins visible
1-2 cm from the pleura

B

FIG. 2-7. Dimensions of secondary lobular structures **(A)** and their visibility on HRCT **(B)**.

visible, their locations can be inferred by locating septal pulmonary vein branches, approximately 0.5 mm in diameter. Veins can sometimes be seen as linear (Fig. 2-10B), arcuate, or branching structures (Fig. 2-10C–E), or as a row or chain of dots surrounding centrilobular arteries and approximately 5 to 10 mm from them. Pulmonary veins may also be identified by their pattern of branching; it is common for small veins to arise at nearly right angles to a much larger main branch.

Centrilobular Region and Centrilobular Structures

The central portion of the lobule, referred to as the centrilobular region or lobular core [16], contains the pulmonary artery and bronchiolar branches that supply the lobule, as well as some supporting connective tissue (the centrilobular

interstitium described previously) [3,5,9–11]. It is difficult to precisely define lobules in relation to the bronchial or arterial trees; lobules do not arise at a specific branching generation or from a specific type of bronchiole or artery [9].

Branching of the lobular bronchiole and artery is irregularly dichotomous [22]. When they divide, they generally divide into two branches. Most often, they divide into two branches of different sizes, (one branch being nearly the same size as the one it arose from, and the other being smaller) (Fig. 2-5B). Thus, on bronchograms, arteriograms, or HRCT, there often appears to be a single dominant bronchiole or artery in the center of the lobule, which gives off smaller branches at intervals along its length.

The HRCT appearances and visibility of centrilobular structures are determined primarily by their size (Fig. 2-7). Second-

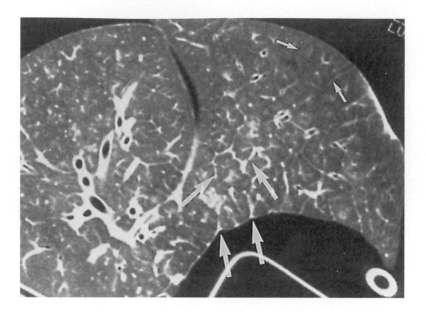

FIG. 2-8. Interlobular septa in an isolated lung. Some thin, normal interlobular septa (*small arrows*) are faintly visible in the peripheral lung. Interlobular septa along the mediastinal pleural surface (*large arrows*) are slightly thickened by edema fluid and are more easily seen. Note that a very thin line is visible at the pleural surfaces and in the lung fissure, similar in appearance and thickness to the normal interlobular septa. This line represents the subpleural interstitial compartment and visceral pleura. (From Webb WR, Stein MG, et al. Normal and diseased isolated lungs: high-resolution CT. *Radiology* 1988;166:81, with permission.)

ary lobules are supplied by arteries and bronchioles measuring approximately 1 mm in diameter, whereas intralobular terminal bronchioles and arteries measure approximately 0.7 mm in diameter, and acinar bronchioles and arteries range from 0.3 to 0.5 mm in diameter. Arteries of this size can be easily resolved using the HRCT technique [10,11].

On clinical scans, a linear, branching, or dotlike opacity frequently seen within the center of a lobule, or within a centimeter of the pleural surface, represents the intralobular artery branch or its divisions (Figs. 2-10C–E, 2-11, and 2-12) [3,10,11]. The smallest arteries resolved extend to within 3 to 5 mm of the pleural surface or lobular margin and are as small as 0.2 mm in diameter [3,10,11]. The visible centrilob-

ular arteries are not seen to extend to the pleural surface in the absence of atelectasis (Fig. 2-13).

Regarding the visibility of bronchioles in the lungs of normal patients, it is necessary to consider bronchiolar wall thickness rather than bronchiolar diameter. For a 1-mm bronchiole supplying a secondary lobule, the thickness of its wall measures approximately 0.15 mm; this is at the lower limit of HRCT resolution. The wall of a terminal bronchiole measures only 0.1 mm in thickness, and that of an acinar bronchiole only 0.05 mm, both of which are below the resolution of HRCT technique for a tubular structure (Fig. 2-7). In one in vitro study, only bronchioles having a diameter of 2 mm or more or having a wall thickness of more than 100

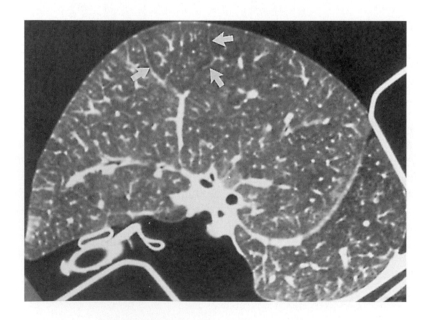

FIG. 2-9. Interlobular septa in continuity in an isolated lung. On HRCT, long interlobular septa (*arrows*) can be seen marginating several secondary lobules. The septa in this lung are slightly thickened by fluid. Septa are well seen peripherally, but note that the septa and, therefore, secondary lobules are less well defined in the central lung. (From Webb WR, Stein MG, et al. Normal and diseased isolated lungs: high-resolution CT. *Radiology* 1988;166:81, with permission.)

μm (0.1 mm) were visible using HRCT [11]; and resolution is certainly less than this on clinical scans. It is important to remember that on clinical HRCT, intralobular bronchioles are not normally visible, and bronchi or bronchioles are rarely seen within 1 cm of the pleural surface (Figs. 2-11 and 2-12) [12,13].

Lobular (Lung) Parenchyma

The substance of the secondary lobule, surrounding the lobular core and contained within the interlobular septa, consists of functioning lung parenchyma—namely, alveoli and the associated pulmonary capillary bed—supplied by small airways and branches of the pulmonary arteries and veins. This parenchyma is supported by a connective tissue stroma, a fine network of very thin fibers within the alveolar septa called the intralobular interstitium (Fig. 2-1) [5,9], which is normally invisible. On HRCT, the lobular parenchyma should be of greater opacity than air (Fig. 2-14), but this difference may vary with window settings (see Chapter 1). Some small intralobular vascular branches are often visible.

It should be emphasized that all three interstitial fiber systems described by Weibel (axial, peripheral, and septal) are represented at the level of the pulmonary lobule (Fig. 2-1), and abnormalities in any can produce recognizable lobular abnormalities on HRCT [10]. Axial (centrilobular) fibers surround the artery and bronchiole in the lobular core, peripheral fibers making up the interlobular septa marginate the lobule, and septal fibers (the intralobular interstitium) extend throughout the substance of the lobule in relation to the alveolar walls.

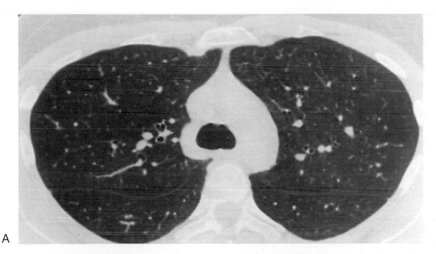

A

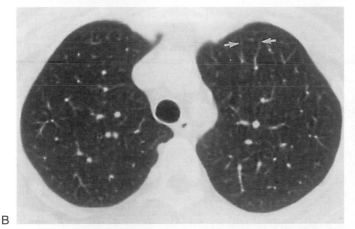

B

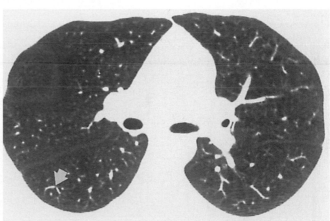

C

FIG. 2-10. Normal HRCT in different subjects. **A:** HRCT in a normal subject; window mean/width:-600/ 2,000 HU. Interlobular septa are inconspicuous, and those few that are visible are very thin. The major fissures appear as thin, sharply defined lines. **B:** Two pulmonary vein branches (*arrows*) marginate a pulmonary lobule in the anterior lung, but the interlobular septa surrounding this lobule are very thin and difficult to see. The centrilobular artery lies equidistant between the veins. **C:** HRCT in a normal subject (–700/1,000 HU) shows few interlobular septa. A venous arcade (*arrow*) is visible in the lower lobe, with the centrilobular artery visible as a dot centered in the arcade. *Continued*

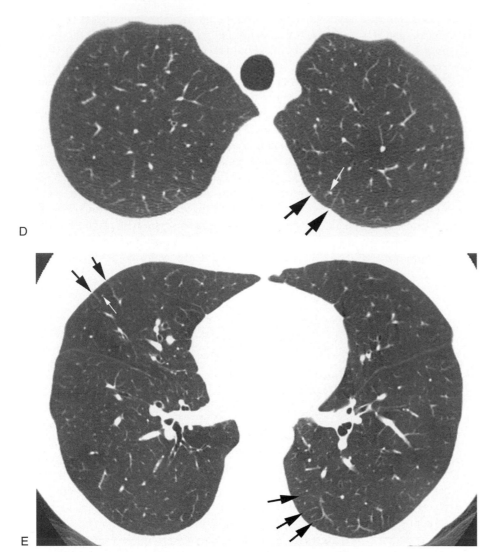

D

E

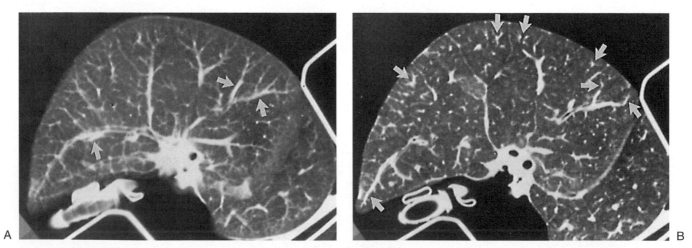

A

B

FIG. 2-10. *Continued* D: HRCT through the upper lobes in a normal subject (−700/1,000 HU). Normal interlobular septa (*black arrows*) are visible. The centrilobular artery (*white arrow*) is centered between them. E: In the same patient as D, a scan through the lower lobes shows normal pulmonary vein branches (*black arrows*) marginating pulmonary lobules. The centrilobular artery branches (*white arrow*) are visible as a rounded dot between the veins.

FIG. 2-11. Centrilobular anatomy in an isolated lung. A: On a CT scan obtained with 1-cm collimation, pulmonary artery branches (*arrows*) with their accompanying bronchi can be identified. B: On an HRCT scan at the same level, interlobular septa can be seen marginating one or more lobules (Fig. 2-9). Pulmonary artery branches (*arrows*) can be seen extending into the centers of pulmonary lobules, but intralobular bronchioles are not visible. The last visible branching point of pulmonary arteries is approximately 1 cm from the pleural surface. Bronchi are invisible within 2 or 3 cm of the pleural surface. (From Webb WR, Stein MG, et al. Normal and diseased isolated lungs: high-resolution CT. *Radiology* 1988;166:81, with permission.)

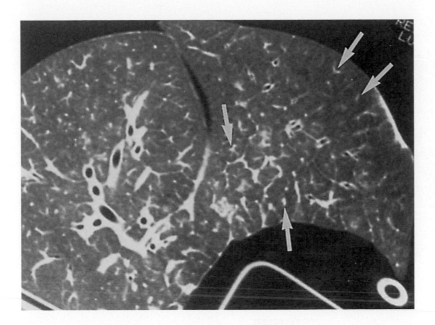

FIG. 2-12. Centrilobular anatomy in an isolated lung. Lobular core anatomy in an isolated lung. Branching pulmonary arteries (*arrows*) are visible within 1 cm of the pleural surface, but intralobular bronchioles are invisible. In the central lung, centrilobular arteries appear dotlike or as a branching structure. (From Webb WR, Stein MG, et al. Normal and diseased isolated lungs: high-resolution CT. *Radiology* 1988;166:81, with permission.)

Pulmonary Acinus

Pulmonary acini are not normally visible on HRCT [22]. As with lobules, acini vary in size. They are usually described as ranging from 6 to 10 mm in diameter and have been measured as averaging 7 to 8 mm in diameter in adults [19,24]. As indicated above, secondary pulmonary lobules defined by the presence of connective tissue interlobular septa usually consist of a dozen or fewer pulmonary acini (Fig. 2-5A) [9,19,20,24].

First-order respiratory bronchioles and the acinar artery branch measure approximately 0.5 mm in diameter (Fig. 2-7A); thus, intralobular acinar arteries are large enough to be seen on HRCT in some normal subjects [5,9,19,24]. Murata [11] has shown that pulmonary artery branches as small as 0.2 mm, associated with a respiratory bronchiole and thus acinar in nature, are visible on HRCT and extend to within 3 to 5 mm of the lobular margins or pleural surface (Fig. 2-7).

Lobular Anatomy and the Concept of Cortical and Medullary Lung

At least partially based on differences in lobular anatomy, it has been suggested that the lung can be divided into a peripheral cortex and a central medulla [16,30]. Although these terms are not in general use, the concept of cortical and medullary lung regions is useful in highlighting differences in lung anatomy and the varying appearances of secondary pulmonary lobules in the peripheral and central lung regions [31]. It also serves to emphasize some anatomic (and perhaps physiologic) differences between the peripheral and central lung that are useful in predicting the HRCT distribution of some lung diseases [32].

Peripheral or Cortical Lung

Cortical lung can be conceived of as consisting of two or three rows or tiers of well-organized and well-defined secondary pulmonary lobules, which together form a layer 3 to 4 cm in thickness at the lung periphery and along the lung surfaces adjacent to fissures (Fig. 2-15) [16,30]. The pulmonary lobules in the lung cortex are relatively large in size and are marginated by interlobular septa that are thicker and better defined than in other parts of the lung; thus, cortical lobules tend to be better defined than those in the central or medullary lung. Bronchi and pulmonary vessels in the lung cortex are relatively small; although cortical arteries and veins are visible on HRCT, bronchi and bronchioles are uncommonly visible. This contrasts with the anatomy of medullary lung, in which large vessels and bronchi are visible.

Lobules in the lung cortex tend to be relatively uniform in appearance and can be conceived of as being similar to the stones in a Roman arch: all of similar size and shape (Fig. 2-15) [30]. They can appear cuboid or be shaped like a truncated cone or pyramid [16]. However, it should be remembered that the size, shape, and appearance of pulmonary lobules as seen on HRCT are significantly affected by the orientation of the scan plane relative to the central and longitudinal axes of the lobules. A single scan typically traverses different parts of adjacent lobules (Figs. 2-8 and 2-9), resulting in widely varying appearances of the lobules, despite the fact that they are all of similar size and shape.

Central or Medullary Lung

Pulmonary lobules in the central or medullary lung are smaller and more irregular in shape than in the cortical lung and are marginated by interlobular septa that are thinner and less well defined. When visible, medullary lobules may appear hexagonal or polygonal in shape, but well-defined lobules are uncommonly seen in normals. In contrast with the peripheral lung, perihilar vessels and bronchi in the lung medulla are large and easily seen on HRCT.

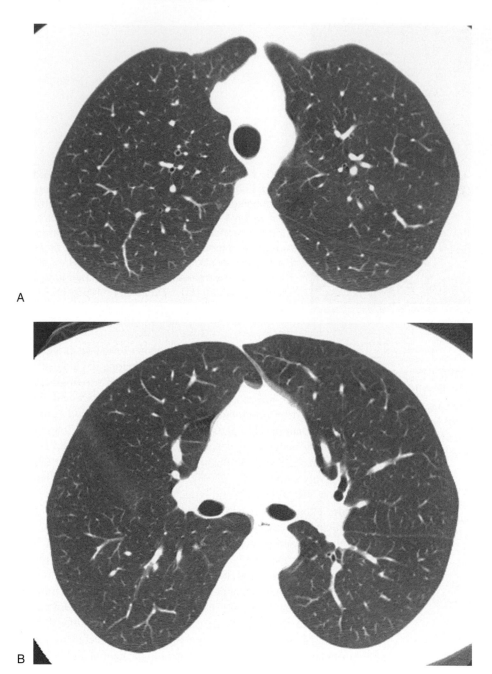

FIG. 2-13. Normal lobular anatomy. HRCT (−700/1,000 HU) at two levels **(A, B)** in a normal subject shows artery branches extending to within 1 cm of the pleural surface. The arteries do not reach the pleura.

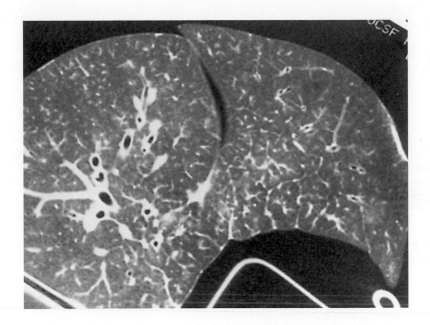

FIG. 2-14. Normal appearance of the lobular parenchyma. The lung parenchyma should appear to be homogeneously denser than air in the bronchi or, as in this isolated lung, denser than room air surrounding the specimen. The relative opacities of lung and air depend on the window settings.

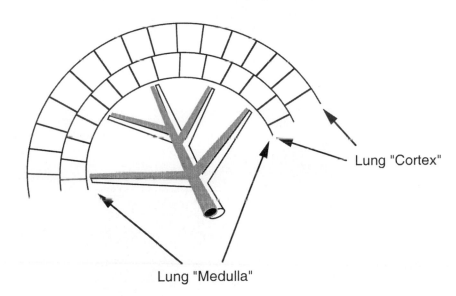

Lung "Cortex"

Lung "Medulla"

FIG. 2-15. Corticomedullary differentiation in the lung. The lung cortex is composed of one or two rows or tiers of well-organized and well-defined secondary pulmonary lobules 3 to 4 cm in thickness. The pulmonary lobules in the lung cortex tend to be well defined and relatively large, and can be conceived of as being similar to the stones in a Roman arch: all of similar size and shape. The cortical airways and vessels are small, usually less than 2 to 3 mm in diameter.

SUBPLEURAL INTERSTITIUM AND PLEURAL SURFACES

Diffuse infiltrative lung diseases involving the subpleural interstitium or pleura can result in abnormalities visible at the pleural surfaces.

Subpleural Interstitium and Visceral Pleura

The visceral pleura consists of a single layer of flattened mesothelial cells that is subtended by layers of fibroelastic connective tissue; it measures 0.1 to 0.2 mm in thickness [33,34]. The connective tissue component of the visceral pleura is generally referred to on HRCT as the subpleural interstitium, and is part of the "peripheral" interstitial fiber network described by Weibel (Fig. 2-1) [5]. The subpleural interstitium contains small vessels, which are involved in the formation of pleural fluid, and lymphatic branches. Interstitial lung diseases that affect the interlobular septa or result in lung fibrosis often result in abnormalities of the subpleural interstitium.

Abnormalities of the subpleural interstitium can be recognized over the costal surfaces of the lung, but are more easily seen in relation to the major fissures, at which two layers of the visceral pleura and subpleural interstitium come in contact. In contrast to conventional CT, in which the obliquely oriented major fissures are usually seen as broad bands of increased or decreased opacity, these fissures are consistently visualized on HRCT as continuous, smooth, and very thin linear opacities. Normal fissures are

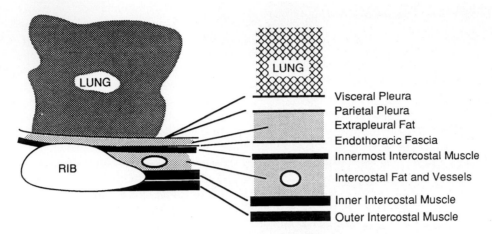

Visceral Pleura
Parietal Pleura
Extrapleural Fat
Endothoracic Fascia
Innermost Intercostal Muscle

Intercostal Fat and Vessels

Inner Intercostal Muscle
Outer Intercostal Muscle

FIG. 2-16. Anatomy of the pleural surfaces and chest wall.

less than 1 mm thick, smooth in contour, uniform in thickness, and sharply defined (Figs. 2-2A, 2-10A, and 2-13). The visceral pleura and subpleural interstitium along the costal surfaces of lung are not visible on HRCT in normal subjects.

Parietal Pleura

The parietal pleura, as with the visceral pleura, consists of a mesothelial cell membrane in association with a thin layer of connective tissue. The parietal pleura is somewhat thinner than the visceral pleura, measuring approximately 0.1 mm [33,34]. External to the parietal pleura is a thin layer of loose areolar connective tissue or extrapleural fat, which separates the pleura from the fibroelastic endothoracic fascia and lines the thoracic cavity (Fig. 2-16); the endothoracic fascia is approximately 0.25 mm thick [34,35]. External to the endothoracic fascia are the innermost intercostal muscles and ribs. The innermost intercostal muscles pass between adjacent ribs but do not extend into the paravertebral regions.

As stated in Chapter 1, window level/width settings of 50/350 Hounsfield units (HU) are best for evaluating the parietal pleura and adjacent chest wall. Images at a level of –600 HU with an extended window width of 2,000 HU are also useful in evaluating the relationship of peripheral parenchymal abnormalities to the pleural surfaces [3,36].

On HRCT in normal patients, the innermost intercostal muscles are often visible as 1- to 2-mm-thick stripes (the intercostal stripes) of soft-tissue opacity at the lung–chest wall interface, passing between adjacent rib segments in the anterolateral, lateral, and posterolateral thorax (Fig. 2-17). The parietal pleura is too thin to see on HRCT along the costal pleural surfaces, even in combination with the visceral pleura and endothoracic fascia [37]. However, in the paravertebral regions, the innermost intercostal muscle is anatomically absent, and a very thin line (the

paravertebral line) is sometimes visible at the interface between lung and paravertebral fat or rib (Fig. 2-18) [37]. This line probably represents the combined thickness (0.2 to 0.4 mm) of the normal pleural layers and endothoracic fascia.

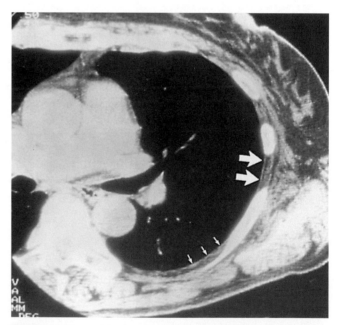

FIG. 2-17. Normal intercostal stripe. On high-resolution CT in a normal subject, the intercostal stripe is visible as a thin white line (*large arrows*). Although it represents the combined thickness of visceral and parietal pleurae, the fluid-filled pleural space, endothoracic fascia, and innermost intercostal muscle, it primarily represents the innermost intercostal muscle. The intercostal stripe is seen as separate from the more external layers of the intercostal muscles because of a layer of intercostal fat. Posteriorly, the intercostal stripe (*small arrows*) is visible anterior to the lower edge of a rib.

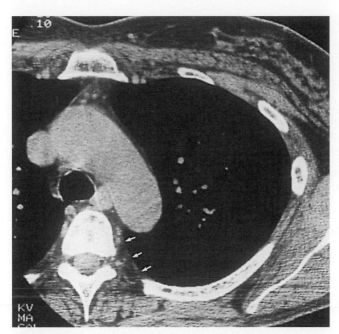

FIG. 2-18. The paravertebral line. In the paravertebral regions (*arrows*), the innermost intercostal muscle is absent, and, at most, a very thin line (the paravertebral line) is present at the lung–chest wall interface. As in this case, a distinct line may not be seen.

HIGH-RESOLUTION COMPUTED TOMOGRAPHY MEASUREMENT OF LUNG ATTENUATION

Generally speaking, lung attenuation appears relatively homogeneous on HRCT scans obtained at full inspiration. Measurements of lung attenuation in normal subjects usually range from –700 to –900 HU, corresponding to lung densities of approximately 0.300 to 0.100 g per mL, respectively [38,39]. In a study by Lamers et al. [40], with HRCT obtained using spirometric control of lung volume, the mean lung attenuation measured in 20 healthy subjects at 90% of vital capacity was –859 HU [standard deviation (SD), 39] in the upper lung zones and –847 (SD, 34) in the lower lung zones. A mean lung density of –866 ± 16 HU (range –983 to –824 HU) was found by Gevenois et al. [41] in a study of 42 healthy subjects (21 men, 21 women) from 23 to 71 years of age. In this study, no significant correlation between mean lung density and age was found, but a significant correlation between the total lung capacity, expressed as absolute values and mean lung density was found. A study by Chen et al. [42] of 13 patients with normal pulmonary function tests showed an average lung attenuation of –814 ± 24 HU on HRCT when the entire cross section of lung was used for measurement and an attenuation of –829 ± 21 HU (range, –858 to –770 HU) using three small regions of interest placed in anterior, middle, and posterior lung regions.

An attenuation gradient is normally present, with the most dependent lung regions being the densest, and the least dependent lung regions being the least dense. This gradient is largely caused by regional differences in blood and gas volume that, in turn, are determined by gravity, mechanical stresses on the lung, and intrapleural pressures [36,38]. Differences in attenuation between anterior and posterior lung have been measured in supine patients, and values generally range from 50 to 100 HU [38,43,44], although gradients of more than 200 HU have been reported [43]. The anteroposterior attenuation gradient was found to be nearly linear and was present regardless of whether the subject was supine or prone [43].

Genereux measured anteroposterior attenuation gradients at three levels (aortic arch, carina, and above the right hemidiaphragm) in normal subjects [44]. An anteroposterior attenuation gradient was found at all levels, although the gradient was larger at the lung bases than in the upper lung; the anteroposterior gradient averaged 36 HU at the aortic arch, 65 HU at the carina, and 88 HU at the lung bases. The attenuation gradient was even larger if only cortical lung was considered. Within cortical lung, the attenuation differences at the three levels studied were 45, 81, and 113 HU, respectively.

Vock et al. [38] analyzed CT-measured pulmonary attenuation in children. In general, lung attenuation in children is greater than in adults [38,43], but anteroposterior attenuation gradients were similar to those found in adults, averaging 56 HU at the subcarinal level.

Although most authors have reported that normal anteroposterior lung attenuation gradients are linear, with attenuation increasing gradually from anterior to posterior lung, the lingula and superior segments of the lower lobes can appear relatively lucent in many normal subjects [45]; focal lucency in these segments should be considered a normal finding. Although the reason is unclear, these slender segments may be less well ventilated than adjacent lung and therefore less well perfused, or some air-trapping may be present.

NORMAL EXPIRATORY HIGH-RESOLUTION COMPUTED TOMOGRAPHY

Expiratory HRCT is generally performed to detect air-trapping in patients with a small airway obstruction or emphysema. On expiratory HRCT, changes in the lung attenuation, cross-sectional area [46], and appearance of airways are typical [47]. Air-trapping of limited extent may also be seen in normals.

Lung Attenuation Changes

Lung parenchyma normally increases in CT attenuation as lung volume is reduced during expiration. This change can generally be recognized on HRCT as an increase in lung opacity (Figs. 2-19 through 2-21; see Figs. 1-28 through 1-30) [8,38,43,48–50]. Robinson and Kreel [49] found significant inverse correlations between lung volumes determined spirometrically and CT-measured lung attenuation, for the whole

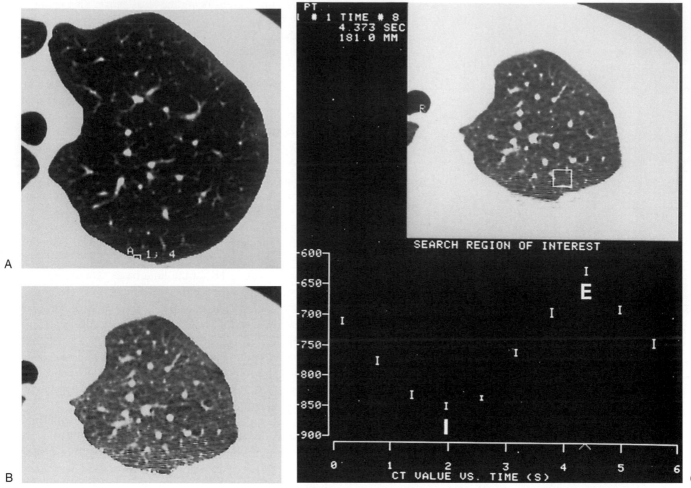

FIG. 2-19. Normal dynamic expiratory HRCT. Inspiratory **(A)** and expiratory **(B)** images from a sequence of ten scans obtained during forced expiration in a normal subject. Lung attenuation increases and cross-sectional lung area decreases on the expiratory scan. **C:** A region of interest has been positioned in the posterior lung, and a time-attenuation curve calculated for this region of interest shows an increase in attenuation from −850 HU to −625 HU from maximal inspiration (I) to maximal expiration (E). Each point on the time density curve represents one image from the dynamic sequence.

lung ($r = -0.680$, $p > .0005$) and for anterior, middle, and posterior lung zones considered individually.

The mean attenuation change between full inspiration and expiration ranges from 80 to 300 HU regardless of the expiratory technique used [8,38,40,45,50]. In a study of young, normal volunteers, an increase in lung attenuation averaging 200 HU was consistently seen during forced expiration, but the increase was variable and ranged from 84 to 372 HU [45]. In a study by Chen et al. [42] of patients with normal pulmonary function tests, the average lung attenuation increase on postexpiratory HRCT was 144 ± 47 HU (range, 85 to 235 HU) when three small regions of interest placed in different lung regions were used for measurement and 149 ± 54 HU when the entire cross section of lung was used for measurement. Average lung attenuation on postexpiratory HRCT was −685 HU ± 51 (range, −763 to −580 HU) using three regions of interest and −665 ± 80 HU for the entire cross section of

lung [42]. According to Kalender et al., using spirometrically triggered CT [51], a 10% change in vital capacity resulted, on average, in a change of approximately 16 HU, and estimates of lung attenuation at 0% and 100% of vital capacity were −730 HU and −895 HU, respectively. In a study by Lamers et al. [40], with HRCT obtained using spirometric control of lung volume, the mean lung attenuation in 20 healthy subjects measured in the upper lung zones at 90% of vital capacity was −859 HU (SD, 39), whereas at 10% of vital capacity, it was −786 HU (SD, 39). In the lower lung zones, lung attenuation increased from -847 HU (SD, 34) at 90% of vital capacity to −767 HU (SD, 56) at 10% of vital capacity. In a study of spirometrically gated HRCT [52] at 20%, 50%, and 80% of vital capacity, mean lung attenuation measured −747, −816, and −855 HU, respectively. Millar et al. [48] calculated the physical density of lung at full inspiration and expiration, based on the assumption that physical density had

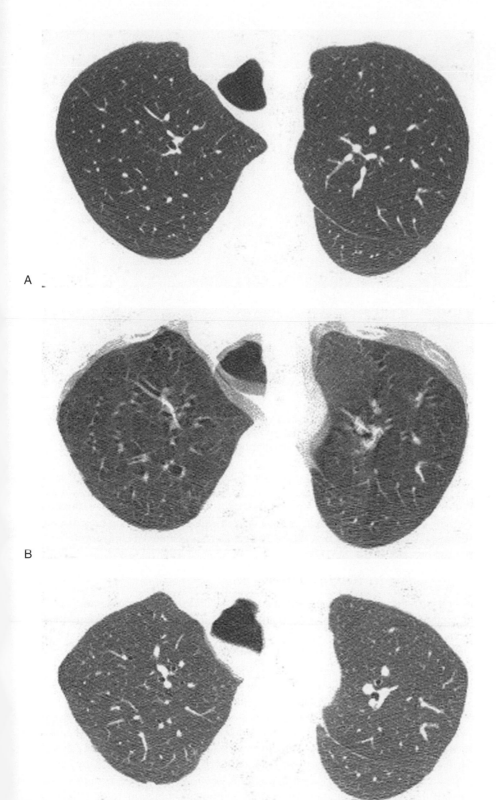

A

B

C

FIG. 2-20. Dynamic inspiratory **(A)** and expiratory **(B–C)** HRCT in a normal subject, obtained with low (40) mA. On the inspiratory scan **(A)**, lungs appear homogeneous in attenuation. Lung attenuation measured −875 HU in the posterior right lung. During rapid expiration **(B)**, image quality is degraded by respiratory motion. On a scan at maximum expiration **(C)**, lung decreases in volume and increases in attenuation. Posterior dependent lung increases in attenuation to a greater degree than anterior nondependent lung, now measuring −750 HU. Note some anterior bowing of the posterior tracheal membrane, typical of expiratory images.

linear relation to radiographic density (physical density = 1 − CT attenuation in HU/1,000) [53]. Using this method, peripheral lung tissue density was measured as 0.0715 g per cm³ (SD, 0.017) at full inspiration and 0.272 g per cm³ (SD, 0.067) at end expiration. Using dynamic expiratory HRCT, a greater increase in lung attenuation may be seen than with static imaging.

In children, the CT attenuation of lung parenchyma is higher than in adults and decreases with age [38,43]. Attenuation increases seen with expiration are similar to those found

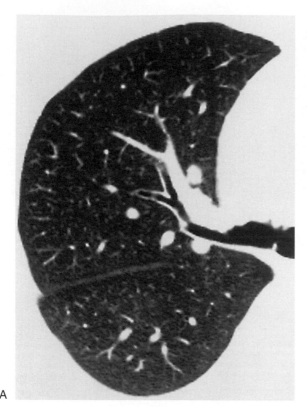
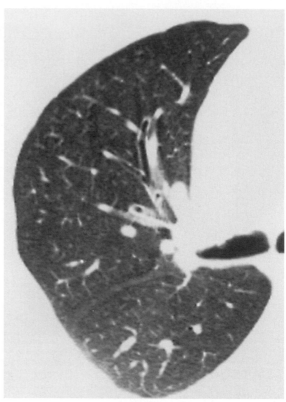

A

B

FIG. 2-21. Inspiratory **(A)** and postexpiratory **(B)** HRCT in a normal subject. On the expiratory scan, lung increases in attenuation. Posterior dependent lung increases in attenuation to a greater degree than anterior nondependent lung.

in adults. Ringertz et al. [54], using ultrafast CT, measured the CT attenuation of children younger than 2.5 years during quiet respiration; the average CT lung attenuation was –551 (SD, 106) on inspiration and –435 HU (SD, 103) on expiration. Vock et al. [38] measured the lung attenuation changes in children ranging in age from 9 to 18 years. Mean lung attenuation at full inspiration and full expiration measured –804 HU and –646 HU, respectively. The anteroposterior attenuation differences were similar to those seen in adults, averaging 56 HU at the subcarinal level, and increased with maximal expiration and increased during expiration [38].

Usually, dependent lung regions show a greater increase in lung attenuation during expiration than do nondependent lung regions irrespective of the patient's position [8,43,45,49,50,55]. As a result, the anteroposterior attenuation gradients normally seen on inspiration are significantly greater on expiratory scans (Fig. 2-21) [38,49,50]; the increase in the anterior-to-posterior attenuation gradient after expiration has been reported to range from 47 to 130 HU in different studies [8,38,45,50]. Furthermore, the expiratory lung attenuation increase in dependent lung regions is greater in the lower lung zones than in the middle and upper zones, probably due to greater diaphragmatic movement or greater basal blood volume [45]. The sum of these changes may be recognizable as increased attenuation or dependent density on supine scans at low lung volume. Although using measure-

ments of attenuation gradients on inspiration and expiration has been investigated as a method of diagnosing lung disease [8,48,56], this technique has not assumed a clinical role.

Normal Air-Trapping

In many normal subjects, areas of air-trapping are visible on expiratory scans (Figs. 2-22 and 2-23); in these regions, lung does not increase normally in attenuation and appears relatively lucent. This appearance is most typically seen in the superior segments of the lower lobes or in the anterior middle lobe or lingula, or it involves individual pulmonary lobules, particularly in the lower lobes [45,57]; it is limited to a small proportion of lung volume. In a study by Chen et al. [42], focal areas of air-trapping, including the superior segments of the lower lobes, were visible in 61% of patients having normal pulmonary function tests. In a study by Lee et al. [57], air-trapping was seen in 52% of 82 asymptomatic subjects with normal pulmonary function tests. The frequency of air-trapping increased with age ($p < .05$), being seen in 23% of patients aged 21 to 30 years, 41% of those aged 31 to 40 years, 50% aged 41 to 50 years, 65% aged 51 to 60 years, and 76% of those older than 61 years. In another study, discounting the superior segments and air-trapping involving less than two contiguous or five noncontiguous pulmonary lobules, air-trapping was not seen on expiratory

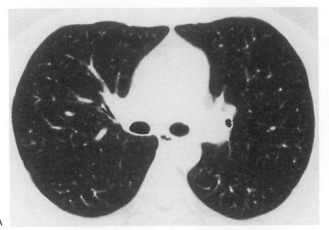
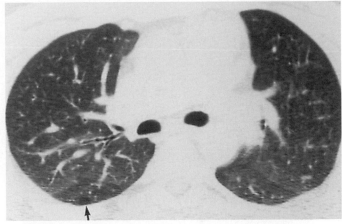

A   B

FIG. 2-22. Inspiratory **(A)** and postexpiratory **(B)** HRCT in a normal subject. On the expiratory scan, there is relative lucency in the superior segments of the lower lobes, posterior to the major fissures. This appearance is normal. Also, focal air-trapping is present in a single lobule (*arrow*) in the posterior right lung. Note slight anterior bowing of the posterior right bronchus intermedius. This may be seen in some patients on expiration.

scans in ten healthy nonsmokers, although it was visible in 40% of patients with suspected chronic airways disease who had normal pulmonary function tests [58]. Normal air-trapping is discussed in greater detail in Chapter 3.

Changes in Cross-Sectional Lung Area

The reduction in cross-sectional lung area occurring with expiration has been assessed in several studies and usually ranges from 40% to 50%. In a study of dynamic expiratory HRCT, Webb et al. [45] determined the percent decrease in lung cross-sectional area from full inspiration to full expiration in ten normal volunteers. The area change ranged from 14.8% to 61.3% for all subjects, subject positions, and lung regions. The greatest percentage decrease in cross-sectional area during exhalation occurred in the upper lung zones. This value averaged 51.3% (SD, 6.7) in the supine position and 43.1% (SD, 10.2) in the prone position. The percentage decrease in lung cross-sectional area was least at the lung bases, averaging 30.9% (SD, 7.5) in the supine position and 25.2% (SD, 5) in the prone position. The average area changes for the midlung regions were intermediate between those of upper and lower lung zones, measuring 38.9% (SD, 7.4) in the supine position and 36.7% (SD, 5.3) in the prone position. Similarly, in a study by Lucidarme et al. [58], cross-sectional lung area decreased by an average of 43% (range, 34% to 57%) in a group of ten normal volunteers. Mitchell et al. [46] measured lung area on inspiratory and end expiratory scans at the level of the carina in 78 normal subjects. The percentage change in area from inspiration to expiration averaged 55% (SD, 8.7%).

Changes in cross-sectional lung area during expiration can be related to changes in lung attenuation as shown on HRCT. Simply stated, attenuation increases at the same time that cross-sectional lung area decreases during expiration (Fig.

2-19). For example, Robinson and Kreel [49] found a significant inverse correlation between the expiratory change in cross-sectional lung area measured on CT and changes in CT-measured lung attenuation ($r = -0.793$, $p > .0005$). In a study using dynamic expiratory HRCT [45], a correlation between cross-sectional lung area and lung attenuation was found for each of three lung regions evaluated (upper lung, $r = 0.51$, $p = .03$; midlung, $r = 0.58$, $p = .01$; lower lung, $r = 0.51$, $p = .05$). The lower lung zone showed a greater attenuation increase for a given area change; this phenomenon likely reflects the much-greater effect of diaphragmatic elevation on basal lung attenuation than occurs in the upper lungs.

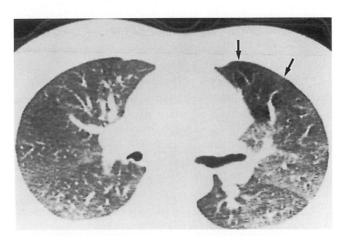

FIG. 2-23. Dynamic expiratory HRCT in a normal subject showing air-trapping in the anterior lingula (*arrows*) and relative lucency posterior to the left major fissure. Pulmonary lobules in the lung medulla are smaller and less well defined than in the periphery. However, vessels and bronchi in the lung medulla are large and easily seen on HRCT. Note anterior bowing of the posterior wall of the right bronchus.

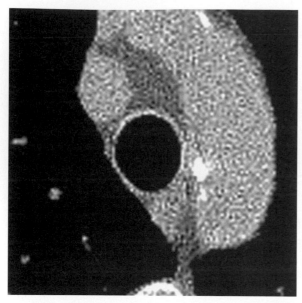
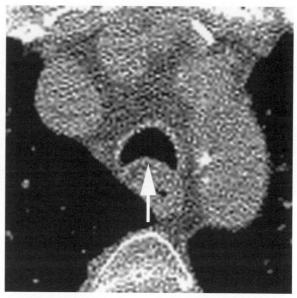

A   B

FIG. 2-24. Normal HRCT appearances of the trachea on inspiratory **(A)** and expiratory **(B)** scans. **A:** On an inspiratory scan shown at a tissue window setting, the trachea appears elliptic. **B:** After forced expiration, there is marked anterior bowing of the posterior tracheal membrane (*arrow*) resulting in a decreased anteroposterior diameter. There is little side-to-side narrowing of the tracheal lumen.

Changes in Airway Morphology

The intrathoracic trachea shows significant changes in cross-sectional area, anteroposterior diameter, and transverse diameter from full inspiration to full expiration (Figs. 2-20 and 2-24). In a study using ultrafast dynamic CT in ten healthy men [56], the mean cross-sectional area of the trachea decreased 35% during forced vital capacity maneuver (range, 11% to 61%; SD, 18). The anteroposterior diameter decreased from a mean of 19.6 mm (range, 16.1 to 23.2 mm; SD, 2.3) to 13.3 mm (range, 8.3 to 18.0 mm; SD, 3.5), for a mean decrease of 32%. This change is largely due to an invagination of the posterior tracheal membrane, a finding that is useful in confirming that an adequate expiration has occurred on expiratory CT (Fig. 2-24). The transverse diameter shows less change with expiration; in this study, it decreased from a mean of 19.4 mm (range, 15.2 to 25.3 mm; SD, 2.7) to a mean of 16.9 mm (range, 12.3 to 20.5 mm; SD, 2.6), for a mean decrease of 13%. The change of cross-sectional area correlated strongly with the changes in the anteroposterior and transverse diameters of the trachea ($r = 0.88, 0.92; p = .0018, .0002$, respectively). The shape of the normal trachea is round or elliptic on inspiration and horseshoe-shaped during and at the end of a full expiration, as the posterior tracheal membrane bows anteriorly.

Morphologic changes in the appearances of bronchi during respiration have not been studied systematically. In our experience, the cross-sectional area of main and lobular bronchi appears slightly reduced on full expiration; some invagination of the posterior wall of the right main bronchus or bronchus intermedius sometimes occurs during forced expiration (Figs. 2-22 and 2-23). Because slightly different levels are usually imaged on the inspiratory and expiratory scans, comparing individual bronchi or specific bronchial levels is often difficult.

REFERENCES

1. Müller NL, Miller RR. Computed tomography of chronic diffuse infiltrative lung disease: part 1. *Am Rev Respir Dis* 1990;142:1206–1215.
2. Müller NL, Miller RR. Computed tomography of chronic diffuse infiltrative lung disease: part 2. *Am Rev Respir Dis* 1990;142:1440–1448.
3. Webb WR. High-resolution CT of the lung parenchyma. *Radiol Clin North Am* 1989;27:1085–1097.
4. Zerhouni E. Computed tomography of the pulmonary parenchyma: an overview. *Chest* 1989;95:901–907.
5. Weibel ER. Looking into the lung: What can it tell us? *AJR Am J Roentgenol* 1979;133:1021–1031.
6. Murata K, Takahashi M, Mori M, et al. Peribronchovascular interstitium of the pulmonary hilum: normal and abnormal findings on thin-section electron-beam CT. *AJR Am J Roentgenol* 1996;166:309–312.
7. Lynch DA, Newell JD, Tschomper BA, et al. Uncomplicated asthma in adults: comparison of CT appearance of the lungs in asthmatic and healthy subjects. *Radiology* 1993;188:829–833.
8. Zerhouni EA, Naidich DP, Stitik FP, et al. Computed tomography of the pulmonary parenchyma: part 2. Interstitial disease. *J Thorac Imaging* 1985;1:54–64.
9. Weibel ER, Taylor CR. Design and structure of the human lung. In: Fishman AP, ed. *Pulmonary diseases and disorders*. New York: McGraw-Hill, 1988:11–60.
10. Webb WR, Stein MG, Finkbeiner WE, et al. Normal and diseased isolated lungs: high-resolution CT. *Radiology* 1988;166:81–87.
11. Murata K, Itoh H, Todo G, et al. Centrilobular lesions of the lung: demonstration by high-resolution CT and pathologic correlation. *Radiology* 1986;161:641–645.
12. Kim JS, Müller NL, Park CS, et al. Cylindrical bronchiectasis: diagnostic findings on thin-section CT. *AJR Am J Roentgenol* 1997;168:751–754.

13. Kang EY, Miller RR, Müller NL. Bronchiectasis: comparison of pre-operative thin-section CT and pathologic findings in resected specimens. *Radiology* 1995;195:649–654.

14. Miller WS. *The lung.* Springfield, IL: Charles C Thomas Publisher, 1947:39–42.

15. Heitzman ER, Markarian B, Berger I, et al. The secondary pulmonary lobule: a practical concept for interpretation of radiographs: II. Application of the anatomic concept to an understanding of roentgen pattern of in disease states. *Radiology* 1969;93:514–520.

16. Heitzman ER, Markarian B, Berger I, et al. The secondary pulmonary lobule: a practical concept for interpretation of radiographs: I. Roentgen anatomy of the normal secondary pulmonary lobule. *Radiology* 1969;93:508–513.

17. Miller WS. *The lung.* Springfield, IL: Charles C Thomas Publisher, 1947:203.

18. Raskin SP. The pulmonary acinus: historical notes. *Radiology* 1982;144:31–34.

19. Osborne DR, Effmann EL, Hedlund LW. Postnatal growth and size of the pulmonary acinus and secondary lobule in man. *AJR Am J Roentgenol* 1983;140:449–454.

20. Weibel ER. High resolution computed tomography of the pulmonary parenchyma: anatomical background. Presented at: Fleischner Society Symposium on Chest Disease; 1990. Scottsdale, AZ.

21. Reid L. The secondary pulmonary lobule in the adult human lung, with special reference to its appearance in bronchograms. *Thorax* 1958;13:110–115.

22. Itoh H, Murata K, Konishi J, et al. Diffuse lung disease: pathologic basis for the high-resolution computed tomography findings. *J Thorac Imaging* 1993;8:176–188.

23. Reid L, Simon G. The peripheral pattern in the normal bronchogram and its relation to peripheral pulmonary anatomy. *Thorax* 1958;13:103–109.

24. Gamsu G, Thurlbeck WM, Fraser RG, et al. Peripheral bronchographic morphology in the normal human lung. *Invest Radiol* 1971;6:161–170.

25. Bergin C, Roggli V, Coblentz C, et al. The secondary pulmonary lobule: normal and abnormal CT appearances. *AJR Am J Roentgenol* 1988;151:21–25.

26. Hruban RH, Meziane MA, Zerhouni EA, et al. High resolution computed tomography of inflation fixed lungs: pathologic-radiologic correlation of centrilobular emphysema. *Am Rev Respir Dis* 1987;136:935–940.

27. Heitzman ER. Subsegmental anatomy of the lung. In: *The lung: radiologic-pathologic correlations,* 2nd ed. St. Louis: Mosby, 1984:42–49.

28. Reid L, Rubino M. The connective tissue septa in the foetal human lung. *Thorax* 1959;14:3–13.

29. Aberle DR, Gamsu G, Ray CS, et al. Asbestos-related pleural and parenchymal fibrosis: detection with high-resolution CT. *Radiology* 1988;166:729–734.

30. Fleischner FG. The butterfly pattern of pulmonary edema. In: *Frontiers of pulmonary radiology.* New York: Grune & Stratton, 1969:360–379.

31. Genereux GP. The Fleischner lecture: computed tomography of diffuse pulmonary disease. *J Thorac Imaging* 1989;4:50–87.

32. Gurney JW. Cross-sectional physiology of the lung. *Radiology* 1991;178:1–10.

33. Agostoni E, Miserocchi G, Bonanni MV. Thickness and pressure of the pleural liquid in some mammals. *Respir Phys* 1969;6:245–256.

34. Bernaudin J-F, Fleury J. Anatomy of the blood and lymphatic circulation of the pleural serosa. In: *The pleura in health and disease.* New York: Marcel Dekker, 1985:101–124.

35. Policard A, Galy P. *La Plevre.* Paris: Masson, 1942:23–33.

36. Murata K, Khan A, Herman PG. Pulmonary parenchymal disease: evaluation with high-resolution CT. *Radiology* 1989;170:629–635.

37. Im JG, Webb WR, Rosen A. Costal pleura: appearances at high-resolution CT. *Radiology* 1989;171:125–131.

38. Vock P, Malanowski D, Tschaeppeler H, et al. Computed tomographic lung density in children. *Invest Radiol* 1987;22:627–631.

39. Millar AB, Denison DM. Vertical gradients of lung density in supine subjects with fibrosing alveolitis or pulmonary emphysema. *Thorax* 1990;45:602–605.

40. Lamers RJ, Thelissen GR, Kessels AG, et al. Chronic obstructive pulmonary diseases. evaluation with spirometrically controlled CT lung densitometry. *Radiology* 1994;193:109–113.

41. Gevenois PA, Scillia P, de Maertelaer V, et al. The effects of age, sex, lung size, and hyperinflation on CT lung densitometry. *AJR Am J Roentgenol* 1996;167:1169–1173.

42. Chen D, Webb WR, Storto ML, et al. Assessment of air trapping using postexpiratory high-resolution computed tomography. *J Thorac Imaging* 1998;13:135–143.

43. Rosenblum LJ, Mauceri RA, Wellenstein DE, et al. Density patterns in the normal lung as determined by computed tomography. *Radiology* 1980;137:409–416.

44. Genereux GP. Computed tomography and the lung: review of anatomic and densitometric features with their clinical application. *J Can Assoc Radiol* 1985;36:88–102.

45. Webb WR, Stern EJ, Kanth N, et al. Dynamic pulmonary CT: findings in normal adult men. *Radiology* 1993;186:117–124.

46. Mitchell AW, Wells AU, Hansell DM. Changes in cross-sectional area of the lungs on end expiratory computed tomography in normal individuals. *Clin Radiol* 1996;51:804–806.

47. Arakawa H, Webb WR. Expiratory high-resolution CT scan. *Radiol Clin North Am* 1998;36:189–209.

48. Millar AB, Denison DM. Vertical gradients of lung density in healthy supine men. *Thorax* 1989;44:485–490.

49. Robinson PJ, Kreel L. Pulmonary tissue attenuation with computed tomography: comparison of inspiration and expiration scans. *J Comput Assist Tomogr* 1979;3:740–748.

50. Verschakelen JA, Van Fraeyenhoven L, Laureys G, et al. Differences in CT density between dependent and nondependent portions of the lung: influence of lung volume. *AJR Am J Roentgenol* 1993;161:713–717.

51. Kalender WA, Rienmuller R, Seissler W, et al. Measurement of pulmonary parenchymal attenuation: use of spirometric gating with quantitative CT. *Radiology* 1990;175:265–268.

52. Beinert T, Behr J, Mehnert F, et al. Spirometrically controlled quantitative CT for assessing diffuse parenchymal lung disease. *J Comput Assist Tomogr* 1995;19:924–931.

53. Denison DM, Morgan MDL, Millar AB. Estimation of regional gas and tissue volumes of the lung in supine man using computed tomography. *Thorax* 1986;41:620–628.

54. Ringertz HG, Brasch RC, Gooding CA, et al. Quantitative density-time measurements in the lungs of children with suspected airway obstruction using ultrafast CT. *Pediatr Radiol* 1989;19:366–370.

55. Stern EJ, Webb WR. Dynamic imaging of lung morphology with ultrafast high-resolution computed tomography. *J Thorac Imaging* 1993;8:273–282.

56. Stern EJ, Graham CM, Webb WR, et al. Normal trachea during forced expiration: dynamic CT measurements. *Radiology* 1993;187:27–31.

57. Lee KW, Chung SY, Yang I, et al. Correlation of aging and smoking with air trapping at thin-section CT of the lung in asymptomatic subjects. *Radiology* 2000;214:831–836.

58. Lucidarme O, Coche E, Cluzel P, et al. Expiratory CT scans for chronic airway disease: correlation with pulmonary function test results. *AJR Am J Roentgenol* 1998;170:301–307.

High-Resolution Computed Tomography Findings of Lung Disease

The detection and diagnosis of diffuse lung disease using high-resolution computed tomography (HRCT) are based on the recognition of specific abnormal findings [1–4]. In this chapter, we review a number of HRCT findings of value in the differential diagnosis of diffuse lung disease.

First, a word about terminology. In the past, different terms have been used by authors to describe similar or iden-

tical HRCT abnormalities, which has led to confusion and difficulty in comparing one study to another [5]. In this book, whenever possible, we name and define HRCT findings on the basis of their specific corresponding anatomic abnormalities, as there is a close correlation in many instances between these findings and pathologic or histologic lung abnormalities. Furthermore, the terms used comply with those recommended by the Nomenclature Committee of the Fleischner Society [6]. Nonspecific, descriptive, or nonanatomic terms have been avoided, unless the HRCT findings themselves are nonspecific and cannot be related to particular anatomic abnormalities, or unless a descriptive term is particularly helpful in understanding and recognizing the specific abnormal finding. Several of these colorful terms have become indispensable parts of the HRCT lexicon. For easy reference, an illustrated glossary of many of these terms is provided at the end of this book.

Generally, HRCT findings of lung disease can be classified into four large categories based on their appearances. These are (i) linear and reticular opacities, (ii) nodules and nodular opacities, (iii) increased lung opacity, and (iv) abnormalities associated with decreased lung opacity, including cystic lesions, emphysema, and airway abnormalities.

LINEAR AND RETICULAR OPACITIES

Thickening of the interstitial fiber network of the lung by fluid or fibrous tissue, or because of interstitial infiltration by cells or other material, primarily results in an increase in linear or reticular lung opacities as seen on HRCT. Linear or reticular opacities may be manifested by the interface sign, peribronchovascular interstitial thickening, interlobular septal thickening, parenchymal bands, subpleural interstitial thickening, intralobular interstitial thickening, honeycombing, irregular linear opacities, and subpleural lines (Fig. 3-1).

Interface Sign

The presence of irregular interfaces between the aerated lung parenchyma and bronchi, vessels, or visceral pleural surfaces has been termed the *interface sign* by Zerhouni et al. [4,7] (Fig. 3-2). The interface sign is nonspecific, and is commonly seen in patients with an interstitial abnormality, regardless of its cause. In the original description of the interface sign, this finding was visible in 89% of patients with interstitial lung disease [7].

The interface sign is generally associated with an increase in lung reticulation; the presence of thin linear opacities contacting the bronchi, vessels, or pleural surfaces is responsible for their having an irregular or spiculated appearance on HRCT. These linear opacities represent thickened interlobular septa, thickened intralobular interstitial fibers, or irregular scars (Fig. 3-1). The interface sign is most frequently visible in patients with fibrotic lung disease, and Nishimura et al. [8] reported the presence of irregular pleural surfaces and irregular vessel margins in 94% and 98%, respectively, of patients with idiopathic pulmonary fibrosis. In virtually all cases showing the interface sign, other, more specific, abnormal findings will also be visible on HRCT.

Peribronchovascular Interstitial Thickening

Central bronchi and pulmonary arteries are surrounded and enveloped by a strong connective tissue sheath, termed the *peribronchovascular interstitium,* extending from the level of the pulmonary hila into the peripheral lung. In the lung periph-

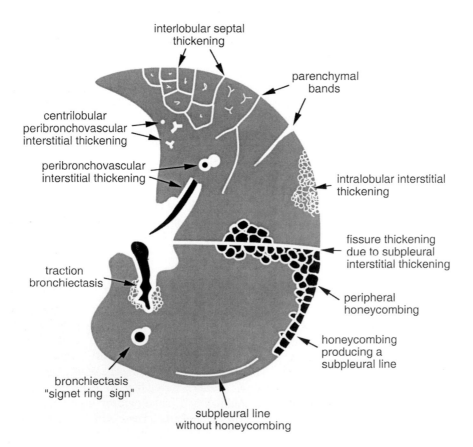

FIG. 3-1. Linear and reticular opacities visible on HRCT.

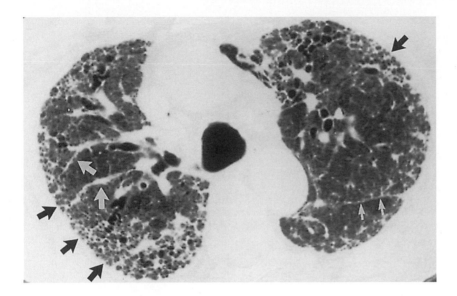

FIG. 3-2. The interface sign. In this patient with idiopathic pulmonary fibrosis and honeycombing, irregular interfaces are visible between the aerated lung parenchyma and structures such as vessels (*large white arrows*), fissures (*small white arrows*), and the visceral pleural surfaces (*black arrows*). This finding is commonly seen in patients with an interstitial abnormality, regardless of its cause, but is most frequent in patients with abnormal reticular opacities and fibrosis.

ery, the peribronchovascular interstitium surrounds centrilobular arteries and bronchioles, and, more distally, supports the alveolar ducts and alveoli (see Fig. 2-1) [9]. The peribronchovascular interstitium is also termed the *axial interstitium* by Weibel [10]. Thickening of the perihilar peribronchovascular interstitium occurs in many diseases that cause a generalized interstitial abnormality [3,11–13]. Peribronchovascular interstitial thickening is common in patients with lymphangitic spread of carcinoma [11,12,14]; lymphoma [15]; leukemia [16]; lymphoproliferative disease such as lymphocytic interstitial pneumonia (LIP) [17–19]; interstitial pulmonary edema; diseases that result in a perilymphatic distribution of nodules (e.g., sarcoidosis) [20]; and in many diseases that result in pulmonary fibrosis, particularly sarcoidosis, which has a propensity to involve the peribronchovascular interstitium (Table 3-1) [21]. Peribronchovascular interstitial thickening has also been reported in as many as 65% of patients with nonspecific interstitial pneumonia (NSIP) [22] and 19% of patients with chronic hypersensitivity pneumonitis [23].

Because the thickened peribronchovascular interstitium cannot be distinguished from the underlying opacity of the bronchial wall or pulmonary artery, this abnormality is usually perceived on HRCT as an increase in bronchial wall thickness or an increase in diameter of pulmonary artery branches (Fig. 3-3) [11]. Apparent bronchial wall thickening is the easier of these two findings to recognize. This finding is exactly equivalent to "peribronchial cuffing" seen on plain chest radiographs in patients with an interstitial abnormality. In patients with pulmonary interstitial emphysema, air is commonly seen within the peribronchovascular interstitium, outlining vessels and bronchi (Fig. 3-3D) [24–26].

Thickening of the peribronchovascular interstitium can appear smooth, nodular, or irregular in different diseases (Fig. 3-3) (Table 3-1) [9]. Smooth peribronchovascular interstitial thickening is most typical of patients with lymphangitic spread of carcinoma or lymphoma (Fig. 3-4) and interstitial pulmonary edema [27,28] but can be seen in patients with fibrotic lung disease as well. Nodular thickening of the peribronchovascular

TABLE 3-1. *Differential diagnosis of peribronchovascular interstitial thickening*	
Diagnosis	Comments
Lymphangitic carcinomatosis, lymphoma, leukemia	Common; smooth or nodular; may be the only abnormality
Lymphoproliferative disease (e.g., lymphocytic interstitial pneumonia)	Smooth or nodular; other abnormalities typically present
Pulmonary edema	Common; smooth
Sarcoidosis	Common; usually nodular or irregular; conglomerate masses of fibrous tissue with bronchiectasis typical in end stage
Idiopathic pulmonary fibrosis or other cause of usual interstitial pneumonia	Common; often irregular; associated with traction bronchiectasis; other findings of fibrosis predominate
Nonspecific interstitial pneumonia	With findings of ground-glass opacity and reticulation
Silicosis/coal worker's pneumoconiosis, talcosis	Conglomerate masses
Hypersensitivity pneumonitis (chronic)	Sometimes visible; often irregular; associated with traction bronchiectasis

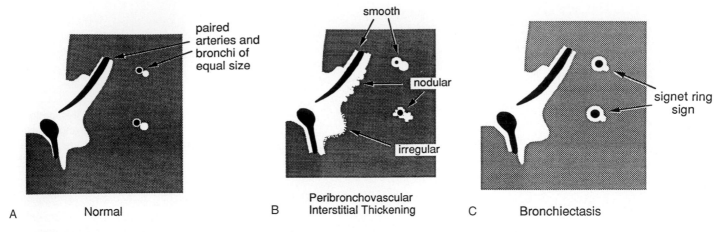

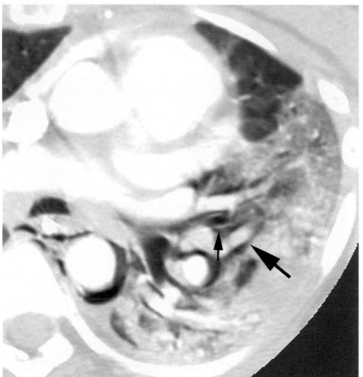

FIG. 3-3. Differentiation of peribronchovascular interstitial thickening and bronchiectasis. **A:** In a normal subject, bronchi are uniformly thin-walled and appear approximately equal in diameter to adjacent pulmonary arteries. **B:** In the presence of peribronchovascular interstitial thickening, there appears to be an increase in bronchial wall thickness and a corresponding increase in diameter of pulmonary artery branches. The contours of the bronchi and vessels can appear smooth, nodular, or irregular in different diseases. **C:** In bronchiectasis, bronchi are usually thick-walled and appear larger than adjacent pulmonary arteries. This can result in the so-called signet ring sign. **D:** CT with 3-mm collimation in a patient with pulmonary interstitial emphysema. Air is visible within the peribronchovascular interstitial sheath, outlining pulmonary arteries (*large black arrow*) and bronchi (*small black arrow*). Air also surrounds pulmonary veins.

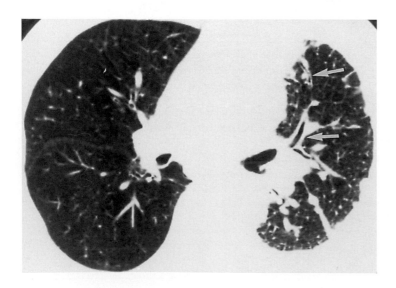

FIG. 3-4. Peribronchovascular interstitial thickening. In a patient with unilateral lymphangitic spread of carcinoma involving the left lung, there is smooth thickening of the peribronchovascular interstitium manifested by peribronchial cuffing (*arrows*); this appearance is easily contrasted with that of normal bronchi in the right lung. Note that the left-sided pulmonary artery branches appear similar in diameter to the cuffed bronchi because the thickened interstitium surrounds them as well. Small intrapulmonary vessels on the left also appear more prominent than those on the normal side because of perivascular interstitial thickening. Interlobular septal thickening and subpleural nodules are also visible on the left. Subpleural interstitial thickening results in nodular thickening of the left major fissure.

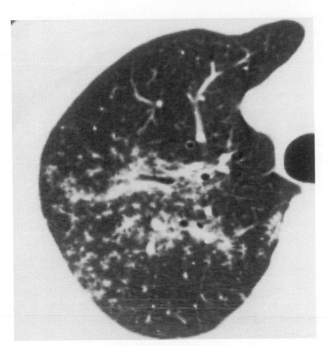

FIG. 3-5. Nodular peribronchovascular interstitial thickening in a patient with sarcoidosis. Numerous small nodules surround central bronchi and vessels.

interstitium is particularly common in sarcoidosis (Fig. 3-5) and lymphangitic spread of carcinoma. The presence of irregular peribronchovascular interstitial thickening, as an example of the interface sign, is most frequently seen in patients with peribronchovascular and adjacent lung fibrosis. Extensive peribronchovascular fibrosis can also result in the presence of large conglomerate masses of fibrous tissue (Fig. 3-6). This can occur in patients with sarcoidosis [20], silicosis, tuberculosis, and talcosis and is discussed in greater detail in the section Conglomerate Nodules or Masses in Diffuse Lung Disease.

Peribronchovascular interstitial thickening is easy to diagnose if it is of a marked degree, in which bronchial walls appear several millimeters thick or bronchovascular structures show evidence of the interface sign or nodules. However, the diagnosis of minimal peribronchovascular thickening can be difficult and quite subjective, particularly if the abnormality is diffuse and symmetric. Although the thickness of the wall of a normal bronchus should measure from one-sixth to one-tenth of its diameter [29], there are no reliable criteria as to what represents the upper limit of normal for the combined thickness of bronchial wall and the surrounding interstitium [30]. Furthermore, these measurements vary depending on the lung window chosen, and too low a window mean can make normal bronchi or vessels appear abnormal (see Fig. 1-13) However, in many patients with peribronchovascular interstitial thickening, and particularly in patients with lymphangitic spread of carcinoma and sarcoidosis, this abnormality is unilateral or patchy, sparing some areas of lung. In such patients, normal and abnormal lung regions easily can be contrasted (Fig. 3-4). As a rule, bronchial walls in corresponding regions of one or both lungs should be similar in thickness.

In patients with lung fibrosis and peribronchovascular interstitial thickening, bronchial dilatation is commonly present and results from traction by fibrous tissue on the bronchi walls. This is termed *traction bronchiectasis* (Figs. 3-1 and 3-6); it typically results in irregular bronchial dilatation that appears varicose or corkscrewed [31,32]. Traction bronchiectasis usually involves the segmental and subsegmental bronchi and is most commonly visible in the perihilar regions in patients with significant lung fibrosis [20,33]. It can also affect small peripheral bronchi or bronchioles, an occurrence termed *traction bronchiolectasis*.

Bronchial wall thickening occurring in patients with true bronchiectasis produces an abnormality that closely mimics the HRCT appearance of peribronchovascular interstitial thickening. However, airway diseases and interstitial diseases can usually be distinguished on the basis of symptoms or pulmonary function abnormalities, and confusion between these two is not often a problem in clinical diagnosis. In addition, several HRCT findings allow these two entities to be differentiated (Fig. 3-3). First, peribronchovascular interstitial thickening is often associated with other findings of interstitial disease, such as septal thickening, honeycomb-

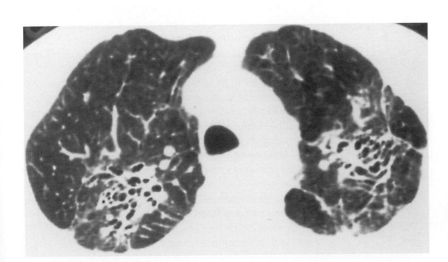

FIG. 3-6. Peribronchovascular interstitial thickening in end-stage sarcoidosis, with conglomerate masses of fibrous tissue surrounding central vessels and bronchi. Bronchi appear dilated and thick walled because of surrounding fibrosis and traction bronchiectasis. Note that vessels and bronchi appear to be of similar diameter.

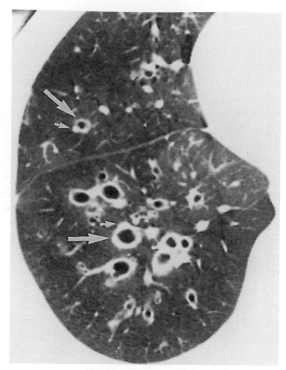

FIG. 3-7. Bronchiectasis with the signet ring sign. Thick-walled and dilated bronchi (*large arrows*) appear larger than the adjacent pulmonary artery branches (*small arrows*). This appearance is termed the *signet ring sign* and is typical of bronchiectasis.

ing, or the interface sign, whereas bronchiectasis usually is not. Second, in patients with bronchiectasis, the abnormal thick-walled and dilated bronchi often appear much larger than the adjacent pulmonary artery branches (Fig. 3-7). This results in the appearance of large ring shadows, each associated with a small, rounded opacity, a finding that has been termed the *signet ring sign*, and is considered to be diagnostic of bronchiectasis [34–38]. In patients with peribronchovascular interstitial thickening, on the other hand, the size

relationship between the bronchus and artery is maintained, and they appear to be of approximately equal size. The diagnosis and appearances of bronchiectasis is discussed in greater detail in the section Bronchiectasis and in Chapter 8.

Diseases that cause peribronchovascular interstitial thickening often result in prominence of the centrilobular artery, which normally appears as a dot, Y-shaped, or X-shaped branching opacity. This finding reflects thickening of the intralobular component of the peribronchovascular interstitium, also termed the *centrilobular interstitium* (see Fig. 2-1) [3,7,12,39]. On HRCT, a linear, branching, or dotlike centrilobular opacity may be seen (Fig. 3-1).

Thickening of the centrilobular interstitium is usually associated with interlobular septal thickening or intralobular interstitial thickening (Fig. 3-1) but sometimes occurs as an isolated abnormality. Centrilobular interstitial thickening is common in patients with lymphangitic spread of carcinoma or lymphoma [11,12] and interstitial pulmonary edema [28,40]. In patients with lung fibrosis, centrilobular interstitial thickening is common but almost always associated with honeycombing or intralobular lines.

Interlobular Septal Thickening

On HRCT, numerous clearly visible interlobular septa almost always indicate the presence of an interstitial abnormality; only a few septa should be visible in normal patients. Septal thickening can be seen in the presence of interstitial fluid, cellular infiltration, or fibrosis.

Within the peripheral lung, thickened septa 1 to 2 cm in length may outline part of or an entire lobule and are usually seen extending to the pleural surface, being roughly perpendicular to the pleura (Figs. 3-1, 3-8, and 3-9) [3,4,11,12, 39,41–43]. Lobules at the pleural surface may have a variety of appearances, but they are often longer than they are wide, resembling a cone or truncated cone. Within the central lung, thickened septa outline lobules that are 1 to 2.5 cm in diameter and appear polygonal, or sometimes hexagonal, in shape

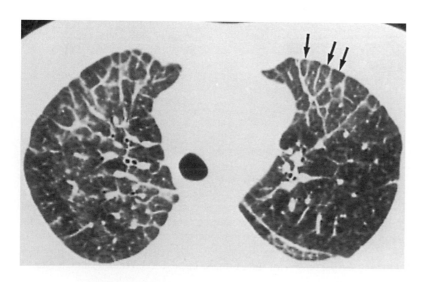

FIG. 3-8. Interlobular septal thickening in a patient with lymphangitic spread of carcinoma. Diffuse interlobular septal thickening outlines numerous pulmonary lobules. Those visible in the peripheral lung may appear to be of various sizes and shapes, depending at least partially on the relationship of the lobule to the plane of scan. However, many lobules are conical in shape (*arrows*). In the more central lung, lobules appear more hexagonal or polygonal. The branching or dotlike intralobular vessel is often visible. The septal thickening in this case is primarily smooth in contour, although nodularity is seen in several regions, particularly adjacent to the left major fissure. Long septa that marginate several lobules have been termed *parenchymal bands*. The presence of multiple thickened septa form "peripheral" or "polygonal arcades."

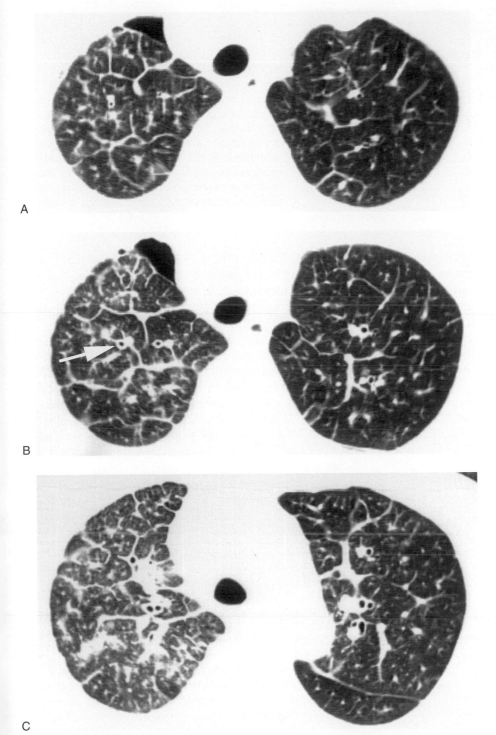

A

B

C

FIG. 3-9. A–C: Interlobular septal thickening in a patient with lymphangitic spread of breast carcinoma. Diffuse, smooth interlobular septal thickening outlines numerous pulmonary lobules, primarily in the right lung. In addition to septal thickening, there is increased prominence of the peribronchovascular interstitium most easily recognized as bronchial wall thickening (*arrow*, **B**). A small pneumothorax is visible on the right because of a recent thoracentesis.

(Figs. 3-8 and 3-9). Lobules delineated by thickened septa commonly contain a visible dotlike or branching centrilobular pulmonary artery. The characteristic relationship of the interlobular septa and centrilobular artery is often of value in identifying each of these structures.

Thickened interlobular septa also may be described using the terms *septal lines* or *septal thickening* (Figs. 3-8 through 3-10) [6], and are preferred to terms such as *peripheral lines*, *short lines*, and *interlobular lines* [12,39,44]. Similarly, although

thickened septa outlining one or more pulmonary lobules have been described as producing a "large reticular pattern" [4,7] or "polygons" [45], and, if they can be seen contacting the pleural surface, as "peripheral arcades" or "polygonal arcades" [12], the terms *interlobular septal thickening, septal thickening*, and *septal lines* are considered more appropriate in describing these appearances [5,6].

Thickening of the interlobular septa is commonly seen in patients with interstitial lung disease. When visible as a pre-

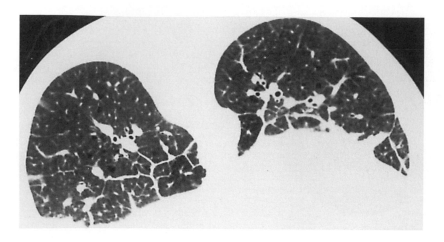

FIG. 3-10. Interlobular septal thickening resulting from pulmonary edema. Prone HRCT shows thickening of numerous interlobular septa in the dependent lung and over the pleural surfaces. Septa within the dependent lung are thickest. Centrilobular arteries appear prominent within most of the lobules surrounded by thickened septa, a finding that reflects thickening of the centrilobular interstitium. Peribronchovascular interstitial thickening is also present.

dominant feature, however, it has a limited differential diagnosis (Table 3-2). Septal thickening can be smooth, nodular, or irregular in contour in different pathologic processes [46]. Smooth septal thickening is seen in patients with pulmonary edema or hemorrhage (Fig. 3-10) [28,47,48], lymphangitic spread of carcinoma (Figs. 3-8 and 3-9) [11,12,49], lymphoma, leukemia, interstitial infiltration associated with amyloidosis [50], and some pneumonias, and in a small percentage of patients with pulmonary fibrosis. Smooth septal thickening may also be seen in association with ground-glass opacity, a pattern termed *crazy-paving*; this pattern is typical of alveolar proteinosis (Fig. 3-11) but has a long differential diagnosis which is reviewed elsewhere [51–55]. Nodular or "beaded" septal thickening occurs in lymphangitic spread of carcinoma or lymphoma (Figs. 3-12 and 3-13) [11,12,49], sarcoidosis, silicosis or coal worker's pneumoconiosis (CWP)

[20,21,56–58], LIP [17–19], and amyloidosis [50,59]. In patients who have interstitial fibrosis, septal thickening visible on HRCT is often irregular in appearance (Figs. 3-14 through 3-16) [32]. A simple algorithm (Algorithm 1) based on the recognition of these findings may be used for diagnosis.

Pulmonary disease occurring predominantly in relation to interlobular septa and the periphery of lobules has been termed *perilobular* [60,61]. Johkoh et al. [55,61] have emphasized that a perilobular distribution of disease may reflect abnormalities of the peripheral alveoli and subpleural interstitium in addition to thickening of interlobular septa.

Although interlobular septal thickening can be seen on HRCT in association with fibrosis and honeycombing [44], it is not usually a predominant feature [8,42,62]. Generally speaking, in the presence of significant fibrosis and honeycombing, distortion of lung architecture makes the recognition

TABLE 3-2. *Differential diagnosis of interlobular septal thickening*

Diagnosis	Comments
Lymphangitic carcinomatosis, lymphoma, leukemia	Common; predominant finding in most; usually smooth; sometimes nodular
Lymphoproliferative disease (e.g., lymphocytic interstitial pneumonia)	Smooth or nodular; other abnormalities (i.e., nodules) typically present
Pulmonary edema	Common; predominant finding in most; smooth; ground-glass opacity can be present
Pulmonary hemorrhage	Smooth; associated with ground-glass opacity
Pneumonia (e.g., viral, *Pneumocystis carinii*)	Smooth; associated with ground-glass opacity
Sarcoidosis	Common; usually nodular or irregular; conglomerate masses of fibrous tissue with bronchiectasis typical in end stage
Idiopathic pulmonary fibrosis or other cause of usual interstitial pneumonia	Sometimes visible but not common; appears irregular; intralobular thickening and honeycombing usually predominate
Nonspecific interstitial pneumonia	With findings of ground-glass opacity and reticulation
Silicosis/coal worker's pneumoconiosis; talcosis	Occasionally visible; nodular when active; irregular in end-stage disease
Asbestosis	Sometimes visible; irregular
Hypersensitivity pneumonitis (chronic)	Uncommon; irregular reticular opacities and honeycombing usually predominate
Amyloidosis	Smooth or nodular

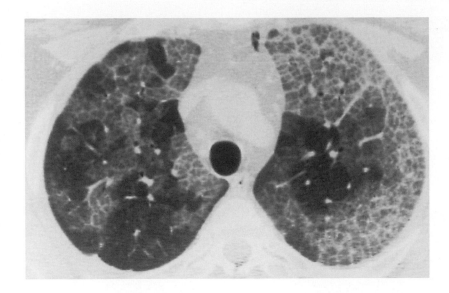

FIG. 3-11. Interlobular septal thickening in alveolar proteinosis. Thickened septa are associated with ground-glass opacity. This appearance is typical of alveolar proteinosis.

of thickened septa difficult (Fig. 3-15). Among patients with pulmonary fibrosis and "end-stage" lung disease, the presence of interlobular septal thickening on HRCT is most frequent in patients with sarcoidosis (Fig. 3-16) (56% of patients) and is less common in those with usual interstitial pneumonia (UIP) of various causes (Fig. 3-17), asbestosis, and hypersensitivity pneumonitis [62]. The frequency of septal thickening and fibrosis in patients with sarcoidosis reflects the tendency of active sarcoid granulomas to involve the interlobular septa. In patients with idiopathic pulmonary fibrosis (IPF) or UIP of another cause, the appearance of irregular septal thickening correlates with the presence of fibrosis predominantly affecting the periphery of the secondary lobule [8].

Parenchymal Bands

The term *parenchymal band* has been used to describe a nontapering, reticular opacity, usually several millimeters in thickness and from 2 to 5 cm in length, seen in patients with atelectasis, pulmonary fibrosis, or other causes of interstitial thickening (Figs. 3-1, 3-16, and 3-18) [6,39,63]. A parenchymal band is often peripheral and generally contacts the pleural surface, which may be thickened and retracted inward.

In some patients, these bands represent contiguous thickened interlobular septa and have the same significance and differential diagnosis as septal thickening [44]. When parenchymal bands can be identified as thickened septa (Figs. 3-16 and 3-18), the use of a separate term to describe this finding is unjustified; the term *septal thickening* should suffice.

However, parenchymal bands visible on HRCT can also represent areas of peribronchovascular fibrosis, coarse scars, or atelectasis associated with lung infiltration or pleural fibrosis (Figs. 3-19 through 3-21) [44,64]. These nonseptal bands are often several millimeters thick and irregular in contour and are associated with significant distortion of adjacent lung parenchyma and bronchovascular structures [65].

Parenchymal bands have been reported as most common in patients with asbestos-related lung and pleural disease (Fig. 3-21), sarcoidosis with interstitial fibrosis (Figs. 3-16 and 3-18) [20], silicosis associated with progressive massive

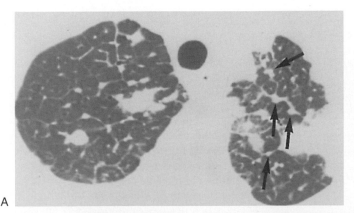
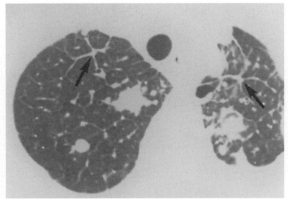

A   B

FIG. 3-12. "Beaded" or nodular septal thickening with lymphangitic spread of carcinoma. **A,B:** Generalized septal thickening is associated with some nodularity (*arrows*); this has been termed the *beaded septum sign*. Septa are well defined. Several large nodules are also visible in the lung. This is a common appearance in patients with lymphangitic spread of carcinoma.

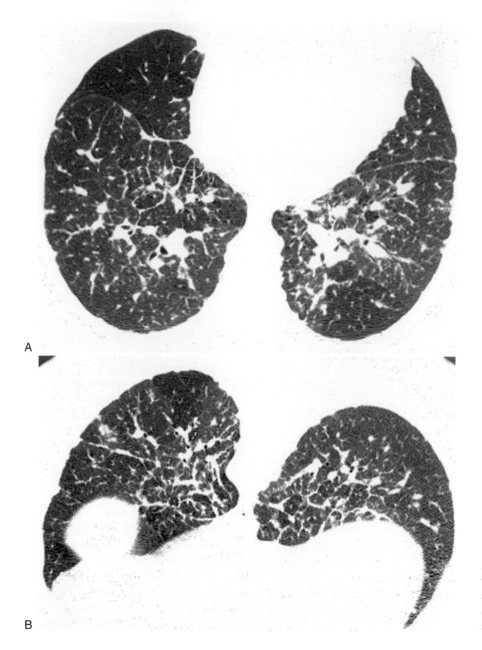

A

B

FIG. 3-13. Nodular septal thickening in a patient with sarcoidosis. Septal thickening at the lung bases is associated with a distinct nodularity on supine (A) and prone (B) scans. In patients with sarcoidosis, this appearance correlates with the presence of septal granulomas.

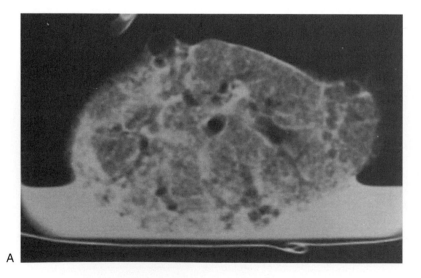

A

FIG. 3-14. Pulmonary fibrosis in an isolated inflated lung specimen. Scans performed with 1-cm collimation and conventional technique (A) and with HRCT technique (B). On the HRCT scan, a lobule at the lung surface is well shown. It is marginated with irregularly thickened interlobular septa (*small arrows*). Intralobular interstitial thickening is visible as a fine network of lines. The intralobular bronchiole is also visible (*white arrow*). The subpleural interstitium is thickened. These findings are not clearly shown with conventional technique. (B from Webb WR. HRCT of the lung parenchyma. *Radiol Clin North Am* 1989;27:1085, with permission.) *Continued*

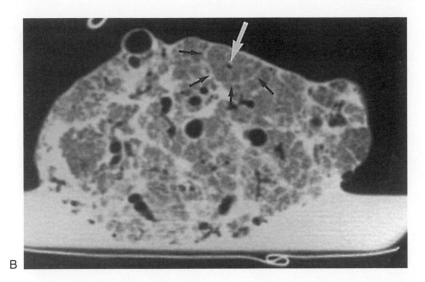

FIG. 3-14. *Continued*

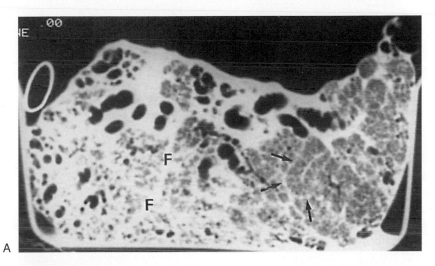

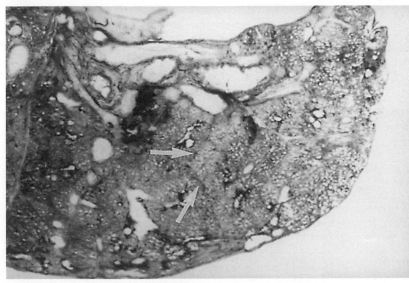

FIG. 3-15. HRCT of pulmonary fibrosis in an isolated inflated lung. The HRCT **(A)** and the corresponding lung section **(B)** are shown for comparison. Typical HRCT findings of fibrosis include interlobular septal thickening that is irregular in contour (*arrows*) and subpleural interstitial thickening shown at the lung surfaces and adjacent to the major fissure (F). (From Webb WR, Stein MG, et al. Normal and diseased isolated lungs: HRCT. *Radiology* 1988;166:81, with permission.)

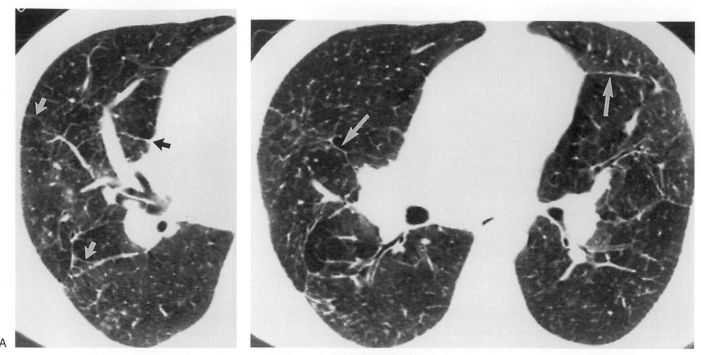

FIG. 3-16. Interlobular septal thickening and parenchymal bands in a patient with end-stage sarcoidosis. **A:** Septa (*arrows*) appear irregular in contour, a finding usually associated with fibrosis. **B:** Longer lines (*arrows*) are parenchymal bands. As in this patient, these often represent several contiguous thickened septa. Lung distortion is also present, indicative of fibrosis.

fibrosis and conglomerate masses, and tuberculosis (Table 3-3). In patients with asbestos exposure, multiple parenchymal bands are common; in one study [39], multiple parenchymal bands were seen in 66% of asbestos-exposed patients. In patients with asbestos-related disease, parenchymal bands can reflect thickened interlobular septa, indicating pulmonary fibrosis, or, more often, areas of atelectasis and focal scarring occurring in association with pleural plaques. In asbestos-exposed patients, parenchymal bands are frequently associated with areas of thickened pleura and have a basal predominance [39,64].

Subpleural Interstitial Thickening

Usually, thickening of the interlobular septa within the peripheral lung is associated with thickening of the subpleural interstitium [3,4]; both the septa and the subpleural interstitium are part of the peripheral interstitial fiber system described by Weibel (see Fig. 2-1) [10]. Subpleural interstitial thickening can be difficult to recognize in locations where the lung contacts the chest wall or mediastinum but is easy to see adjacent to the major fissures (Figs. 3-1, 3-4, 3-8, and 3-22). Because two layers of the subpleural interstitium are seen adjacent to

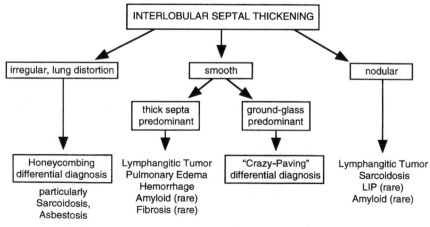

ALGORITHM 1

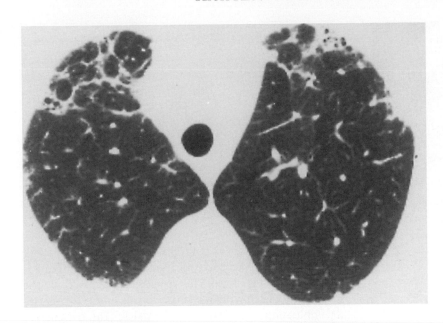

FIG. 3-17. Interlobular septal thickening in a patient with rheumatoid lung disease. Numerous irregularly thickened septa are visible in the anterior right lung.

each other in this location, any subpleural abnormality appears twice as abnormal as it does elsewhere. Thus, thickening of the fissure visible on HRCT often represents subpleural interstitial thickening. If the thickening is smooth, it may be difficult to distinguish from fissural fluid. If the interface sign is present and the thickening is irregular in appearance (Fig. 3-22) [4,7], or if the thickening is nodular (Figs. 3-4 and 3-8), an interstitial abnormality is more easily diagnosed.

In general, the differential diagnosis of subpleural interstitial thickening is the same as that of interlobular septal thickening, although subpleural interstitial thickening is more common than septal thickening in patients with IPF or UIP

of any cause (Table 3-2). The presence of subpleural interstitial fibrosis with irregular or "rugged" pleural surfaces has been reported by Nishimura et al. [8] as a common finding in IPF, correlating with the presence of fibrosis predominantly affecting the lobular periphery; this finding was present in 94% of the cases of IPF that he studied. A subpleural predominance of fibrosis can also be seen in patients with collagen-vascular diseases and drug-related fibrosis [66].

Nodular thickening of the subpleural interstitium can also be seen (Fig. 3-4), and it has the same differential diagnosis as nodular septal thickening [57]. Remy-Jardin et al. [57] have reported the appearance of *subpleural micronodules*, defined

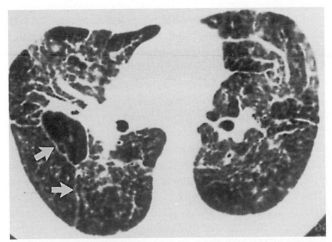

FIG. 3-18. Pulmonary fibrosis and parenchymal bands in a patient with sarcoidosis. Irregular septal thickening is present with distortion of lung architecture. Long confluent septa or parenchymal bands (*arrows*) are present bilaterally. Peribronchovascular interstitial thickening also results in prominence of the bronchi and pulmonary vessels. The pleural surfaces and the walls of vessels and bronchi appear irregular.

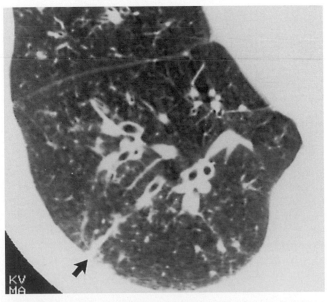

FIG. 3-19. Thick parenchymal band (*arrow*) represents a coarse scar in the peripheral lung. Also note thickening of the bronchial walls because of peribronchovascular fibrosis.

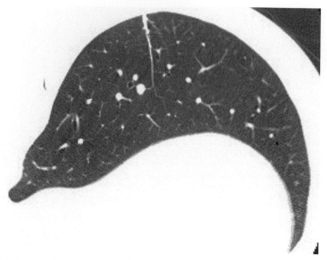

FIG. 3-20. Parenchymal band in a patient with otherwise normal lungs. This likely represents an isolated scar.

as 7 mm or less in diameter, on HRCT in patients with sarcoidosis, CWP, lymphangitic spread of carcinoma, and LIP, and in a small percentage of normal subjects. Subpleural nodules are described further in the section Perilymphatic Distribution.

Intralobular Interstitial Thickening

Thickening of the intralobular interstitium (see Fig. 2-1) results in a fine reticular pattern as seen on HRCT, with the lines of opacity separated by a few millimeters [32]. Lung

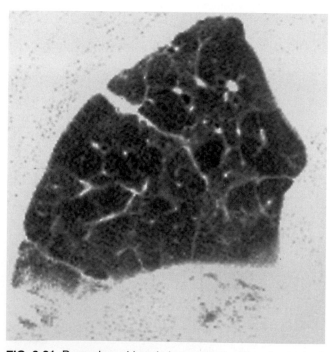

FIG. 3-21. Parenchymal bands in a patient with asbestosis. A prone scan shows both thick and thin bands. Most correspond to thickened septa.

TABLE 3-3. *Differential diagnosis of parenchymal bands*

Diagnosis	Comments
Asbestosis	Multiple parenchymal bands common; smooth; associated with thickened pleura
Sarcoidosis	Common; associated with septal thickening
Silicosis/coal worker's pneumoconiosis	In association with progressive massive fibrosis and emphysema
Tuberculosis	Associated with scarring

regions showing this finding characteristically have a fine lace- or netlike appearance that is easy to recognize (Figs. 3-1 and 3-23 through 3-26). This appearance is nonspecific and may be associated with interstitial fibrosis or diffuse interstitial infiltration in the absence of fibrosis. The presence of intralobular interstitial thickening can also be described using the term *intralobular lines* [6]. This finding is responsible for the "small reticular pattern" described by Zerhouni [7].

In patients with intralobular interstitial thickening resulting from fibrosis, intralobular bronchioles may be visible in the peripheral lung. This results from a combination of their dilatation (i.e., traction bronchiolectasis) and thickening of the peribronchiolar interstitium that surrounds them (Figs. 3-1, 3-23, and 3-24) [8,32]. Traction bronchiectasis, dilatation of large bronchi occurring because of fibrosis, may also be seen (Figs. 3-27 and 3-28). Interlobular septal thickening may or may not be present in patients who have intralobular interstitial thickening; when thickened septa are visible, they usually appear irregular. The pleural surfaces also appear irregular in the presence of intralobular interstitial thickening.

Intralobular interstitial thickening as perceived on HRCT reflects thickening of the distal peribronchovascular interstitial tissues and the intralobular interstitium. As an isolated finding, it is most commonly seen in patients with pulmonary fibrosis (Figs. 3-23 through 3-28) (Table 3-4). In patients who have IPF or other causes of UIP, such as rheumatoid arthritis, scleroderma, or other collagen-vascular diseases, fibrosis tends to predominantly involve alveoli in the periphery of acini, resulting in a "peripheral acinar distribution" of interstitial fibrosis [8,66]; this histologic finding correlates with the presence of intralobular lines on HRCT. In addition, the HRCT pattern of intralobular interstitial thickening can reflect the presence of very small honeycomb cysts or dilated bronchioles associated with surrounding lung fibrosis. Nishimura et al. [8] reviewed 46 cases of IPF with UIP, correlating findings on CT with appearances of lung histology from open biopsy specimens or autopsy. Visibility of centrilobular bronchioles in association with a fine reticulation or increased lung attenuation was found in 96% of cases, indicating the presence of bronchiolar dilatation, fibrosis, and "microscopic" honeycombing, with dilated bronchioles or small cysts measuring approximately 1 mm in diameter [8]. Intral-

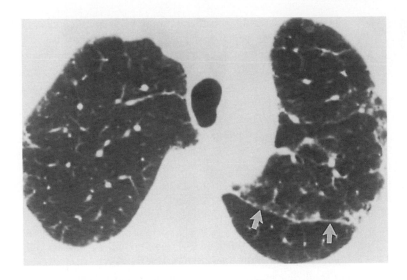

FIG. 3-22. Subpleural interstitial thickening in a patient with pulmonary fibrosis. Apparent thickening of the left major fissure (*arrows*) reflects irregular thickening of the subpleural interstitium. This finding is easiest to recognize adjacent to the fissures.

obular lines, resulting in a fine reticular pattern, can also be seen in patients with NSIP [22,67–69]. In this entity, the appearance of intralobular lines or irregular linear opacities correlated with the presence of interstitial fibrosis and was often associated with bronchial or bronchiolar dilatation

(traction bronchiectasis or bronchiolectasis) [22]. In a study of HRCT appearances of various idiopathic interstitial pneumonias, intralobular lines were visible in 97% of patients with UIP, 93% of patients with NSIP, 78% of patients with desquamative interstitial pneumonia (DIP), 71% of patients with

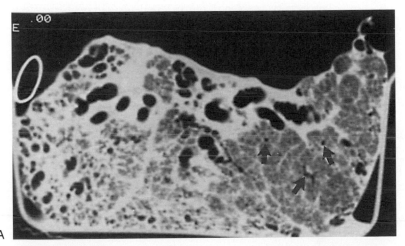

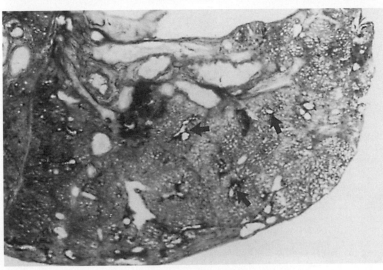

FIG. 3-23. Intralobular interstitial thickening in an isolated lung with pulmonary fibrosis. This is the same specimen as shown in Figure 3-15. A fine network of lines within visible lobules produces a "spider-web" or "netlike" appearance **(A)**. This abnormality contributes to the appearance of irregular interfaces (the "interface sign") at the edges of various structures such as arteries and bronchi. Intralobular bronchioles (*arrows*, **A** and **B**) are visible because of a combination of increased attenuation of surrounding lung, thickening of the peribronchiolar interstitium, and dilatation of the bronchiole that occur as a result of fibrosis. (From Webb WR, Stein MG, et al. Normal and diseased isolated lungs: HRCT. *Radiology* 1988;166:81, with permission.)

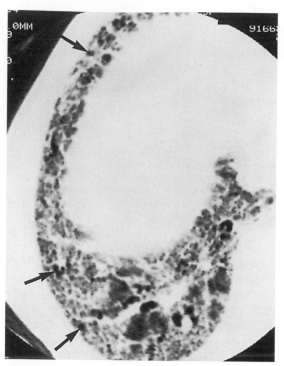

FIG. 3-24. Intralobular interstitial thickening in a patient with idiopathic pulmonary fibrosis. A fine network of lines is visible. Intralobular bronchioles (*arrows*) are visible throughout the peripheral lung as a result of fibrosis and traction bronchiolectasis.

bronchiolitis obliterans organizing pneumonia (BOOP), and 70% of patients with acute interstitial pneumonia (AIP) [67].

Intralobular interstitial thickening can also be seen in the absence of significant fibrosis in patients with a variety of infiltrative lung diseases. When this is the case, traction bronchiectasis or other manifestations of fibrosis are absent.

Intralobular interstitial thickening may be seen in association with interlobular septal thickening in patients with diseases such as lymphangitic spread of carcinoma [11] and pulmonary edema (Algorithm 2). The differential diagnosis of this is identical to that of interlobular septal thickening. Intralobular lines may also be seen in patients with ground-glass opacity or the pattern of crazy-paving, in association with diseases such as pulmonary hemorrhage, some pneumonias (e.g., *Pneumocystis carinii*, cytomegalovirus), and alveolar proteinosis (Fig. 3-11).

Honeycombing

Extensive interstitial and alveolar fibrosis that results in alveolar disruption and bronchiolectasis produces the classic and characteristic appearance of *honeycombing* or *honeycomb lung*. Pathologically, honeycombing is defined by the presence of small air-containing cystic spaces, generally lined by bronchiolar epithelium and having thickened walls composed of dense fibrous tissue. Honeycombing indicates the presence of end-stage lung and can be seen in many diseases leading to end-stage pulmonary fibrosis (Table 3-5) [62,70].

Honeycombing produces a characteristic cystic appearance on HRCT that allows a confident diagnosis of lung fibrosis [32,42]. On HRCT, the cystic spaces of honeycombing usually average 1 cm in diameter, although they can range from several millimeters to several centimeters in size; they are characterized by clearly definable walls 1 to 3 mm in thickness [32,42] (Figs. 3-1, 3-2, 3-29, and 3-30). The cysts are air-filled and appear lucent in comparison to normal lung parenchyma. Adjacent honeycomb cysts typically share walls. Although there is some overlap between the appearances of fine honeycombing and intralobular interstitial thickening, if the spaces between the lines (i.e., the cysts) appear to be air-filled (i.e., black), rather than having the density of lung parenchyma, honeycombing is present.

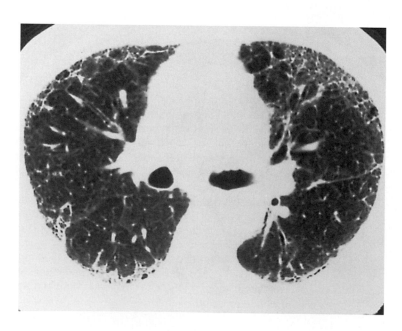

FIG. 3-25. Intralobular interstitial thickening in a patient with idiopathic pulmonary fibrosis. A fine network of lines in the anterior left lung reflects intralobular interstitial thickening.

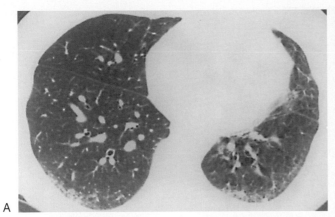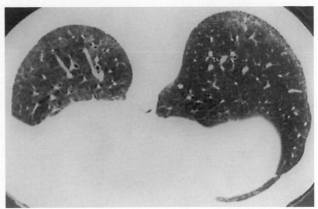

A   B

FIG. 3-26. Intralobular interstitial thickening in a patient with idiopathic pulmonary fibrosis. **A:** On a supine scan, an ill-defined increase in opacity is visible posteriorly. This would be difficult to diagnose as abnormal with certainty on this scan alone. **B:** In the prone position, a very fine reticular or weblike pattern is visible posteriorly in the peripheral lung, along with a few thickened septa. This appearance is typical of intralobular interstitial thickening. The peripheral distribution is characteristic of idiopathic pulmonary fibrosis.

Honeycombing has been described by Zerhouni and associates as producing an "intermediate reticular pattern" to distinguish it from the larger pattern seen with interlobular septal thickening and the smaller pattern visible with intralobular interstitial thickening [7].

Honeycomb cysts often predominate in the peripheral and subpleural lung regions regardless of their cause, and perihilar lung can appear normal despite the presence of extensive peripheral abnormalities (Figs. 3-30 through 3-33). Subpleural honeycomb cysts typically occur in several contiguous layers

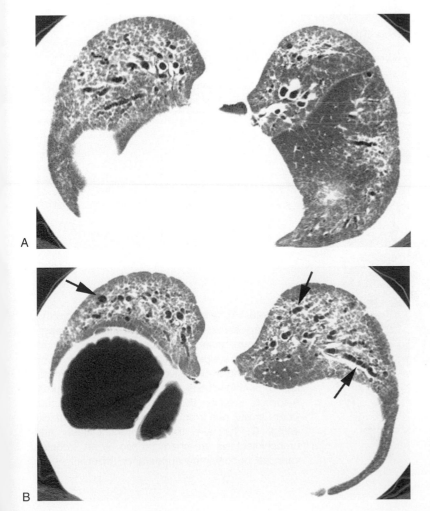

A

B

FIG. 3-27. Prone scans in a patient with idiopathic pulmonary fibrosis. **A:** Abnormal reticulation represents intralobular interstitial thickening. **B:** At a lower level, traction bronchiectasis and bronchiolectasis (*arrows*) are easily seen.

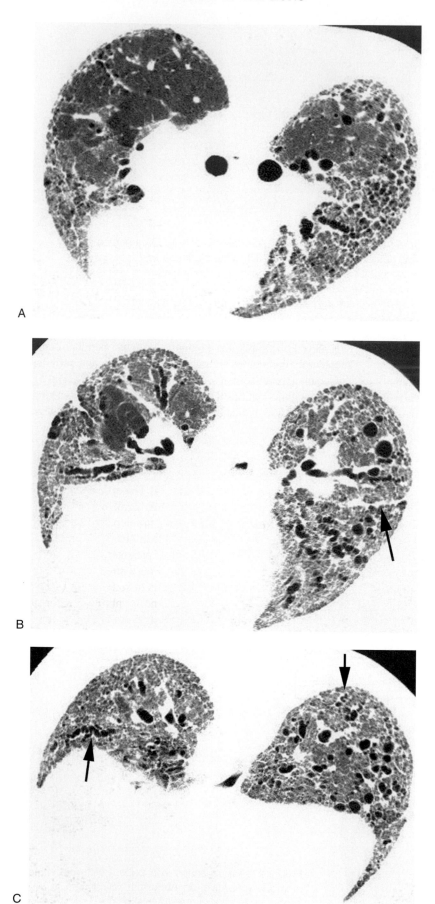

FIG. 3-28. Prone scans in a patient with idiopathic pulmonary fibrosis. **A:** Abnormal reticulation representing intralobular interstitial thickening predominates in the subpleural lung. **B:** At a lower level, fibrosis is more extensive. Traction bronchiectasis and bronchiolectasis are predominant features. Also note irregular thickening of the major fissure (*large arrow*) and irregular interlobular septal thickening. **C:** Typically, traction bronchiectasis and bronchiolectasis are characterized by an irregular, varicose, or corkscrew appearance (*arrows*).

TABLE 3-4. *Differential diagnosis of intralobular interstitial thickening*

Diagnosis	Comments
Idiopathic pulmonary fibrosis or other cause of usual interstitial pneumonia	Common (97%); often associated with honeycombing
Hypersensitivity pneumonitis (chronic)	Common; associated with other findings of fibrosis
Asbestosis	Common; associated with other findings of fibrosis
Nonspecific interstitial pneumonia	Common (93%); ground-glass opacity commonly visible
Other idiopathic interstitial pneumonia (i.e., desquamative interstitial pneumonia, bronchiolitis obliterans organizing pneumonia, acute interstitial pneumonia)	Common (70%); other findings (i.e., ground-glass opacity, consolidation also present)
Lymphangitic carcinomatosis; lymphoma; leukemia	Smooth or nodular; associated with septal thickening
Pulmonary edema	Smooth; associated with septal thickening and ground-glass opacity
Pulmonary hemorrhage	Smooth; associated with septal thickening and ground-glass opacity
Pneumonia (e.g., viral, *Pneumocystis carinii*)	Smooth; associated with septal thickening and ground-glass opacity
Alveolar proteinosis	Smooth; associated with septal thickening and ground-glass opacity

(Figs. 3-31 through 3-33). This finding can allow honeycombing to be distinguished from subpleural emphysema (paraseptal emphysema); in paraseptal emphysema, subpleural cysts usually occur in a single layer. Lung consolidation in a patient with emphysema can mimic the appearance of honeycombing.

Honeycombing is often associated with other findings of lung fibrosis, such as architectural distortion, intralobular interstitial thickening, traction bronchiectasis, traction bronchiolectasis, irregular subpleural interstitial thickening, and irregular linear opacities (Fig. 3-29). On the other hand, significant interlobular septal thickening is not commonly visible in association with honeycombing, except in patients with sarcoidosis [62]. In patients with HRCT findings of septal thickening, the presence of honeycombing distinguishes fibrosis from other causes of reticulation, such as pulmonary edema or lymphangitic spread of carcinoma.

The visible presence of honeycombing on HRCT is indicative of significant lung fibrosis and in most cases should lead to a diagnosis of UIP and a consideration of its most common causes, including IPF (Fig. 3-32); collagen-vascular diseases, most notably rheumatoid arthritis (Fig. 3-33) and scleroderma; asbestosis; and drug-related fibrosis. However, other diseases may also result in honeycombing that is visible on HRCT. In a survey of patients with end-stage lung [62], subpleural honeycombing was present in 96% of patients with UIP associated with IPF or rheumatoid arthritis, in 100% of asbestosis patients, in 44% of those with sarcoidosis, and in 75% of those with hypersensitivity pneumonitis (Table 3-5). Honeycombing is relatively uncommon in patients with NSIP [22,68,69]. In a study of HRCT appearances of proven cases of idiopathic interstitial pneumonias, honeycombing was visible in 71% of patients with UIP, 39% of patients with DIP, 30% of patients with AIP, 26% of patients with NSIP, and 13% of patients with BOOP [67].

The distribution of honeycombing is of some value in differential diagnosis (Algorithm 3). Honeycombing in patients with IPF and asbestosis is usually most severe in the subpleu-

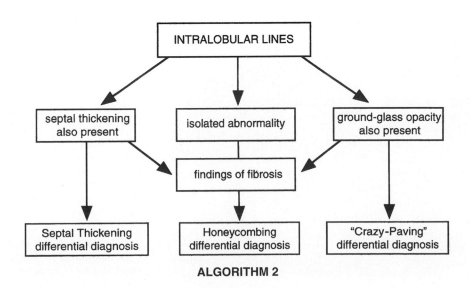

ALGORITHM 2

TABLE 3-5. *Differential diagnosis of honeycombing*

Diagnosis	Comments
Idiopathic pulmonary fibrosis or other cause of usual interstitial pneumonia such as collagen-vascular disease	Common (70%); peripheral, basal, and subpleural predominance
Asbestosis	Common in advanced disease; peripheral, basal, and subpleural predominance
Hypersensitivity pneumonitis (chronic)	Common in advanced disease; may be peripheral, patchy, or diffuse; midlung predominance common
Sarcoidosis	A few percent of cases; may be peripheral or patchy; upper lung predominance common
Nonspecific interstitial pneumonia	Uncommon (10–20%); other findings usually predominate
Other idiopathic interstitial pneumonia (i.e., desquamative interstitial pneumonia, bronchiolitis obliterans organizing pneumonia, acute interstitial pneumonia)	Uncommon (10–20%); other findings usually predominate
Silicosis/coal worker's pneumoconiosis	Uncommon

ral lung regions and at the lung bases. The honeycombing in chronic hypersensitivity pneumonitis may be most marked in the subpleural lung regions, but is more often patchy in distribution, and tends to be most severe in the midlung zones with relative sparing of the lung bases [23,62]. Honeycomb-

ing in sarcoidosis may have an upper lobe predominance. In patients who have pulmonary fibrosis resulting from adult respiratory distress syndrome (ARDS) [71], findings of fibrosis on follow-up HRCT had a striking anterior distribution (see Fig. 6-76) . This distribution of reticular opacities and

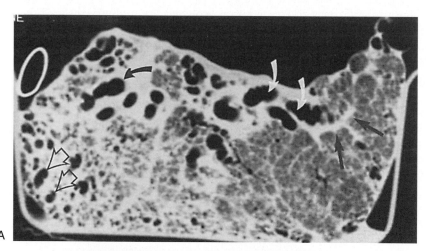

A

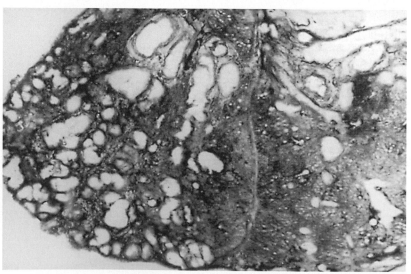

B

FIG. 3-29. Honeycombing and traction bronchiectasis in the patient with pulmonary fibrosis shown in Figs. 3-15 and 3-23. Large honeycomb cysts present in the posterior lung result in cystic spaces ranging up to several centimeters in diameter (*open arrows*, **A**). They are characterized by thick, clearly definable, fibrous walls, and are easily identified in the corresponding lung section **(B)**. Traction bronchiectasis (*curved arrows*, **A**) also reflects extensive fibrosis, and is often seen in patients with honeycombing. The edges of pulmonary vessels (*solid arrows*, **A**) appear irregular because of surrounding fibrosis. (From Webb WR, Stein MG, et al. Normal and diseased isolated lungs: HRCT. *Radiology* 1988;166:81, with permission.)

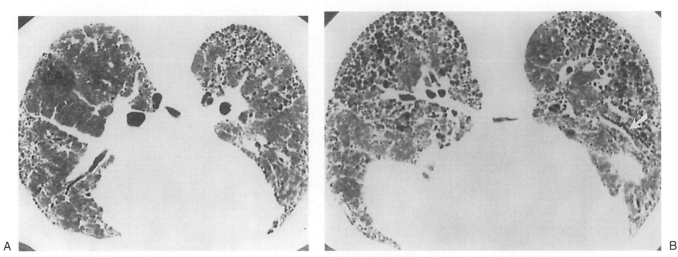

FIG. 3-30. Honeycombing in a patient with idiopathic pulmonary fibrosis (**A,B**; prone HRCT). Honeycombing results in cysts of varying sizes, which have a peripheral predominance. The cysts have thick and clearly definable walls. In areas of honeycombing, lobular anatomy cannot be resolved because of architectural distortion. In less abnormal areas, some septal thickening can be seen. Vessels and bronchi have irregular interfaces, and bronchial irregularity (*arrow*) indicates traction bronchiectasis (**B**). Findings of honeycombing are more severe at the lung bases (**B**).

lung fibrosis is unusual in other diseases. Lung fibrosis limited to anterior lung regions probably reflects the fact that patients with ARDS typically develop posterior lung atelectasis and consolidation during the acute phase of their disease; it is thought that consolidation protects the posterior lung regions from the effects of mechanical ventilation, including high ventilatory pressures and high oxygen tension [71].

In the majority of patients who present with clinical features of UIP, the presence of a predominantly subpleural and basal distribution of fibrosis on HRCT can be sufficiently characteristic to obviate biopsy, especially in patients in whom HRCT shows no evidence suggesting disease activity [72,73]. HRCT findings, including the presence of honeycombing with a subpleural and basal

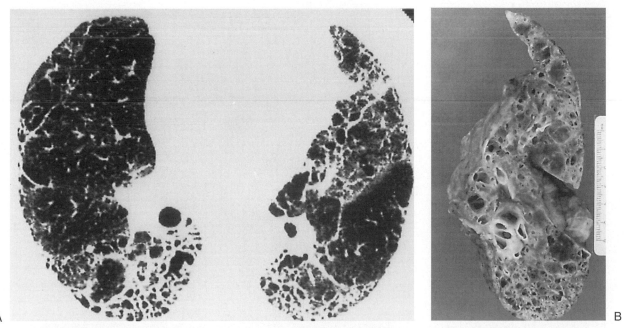

FIG. 3-31. Honeycombing in idiopathic pulmonary fibrosis. **A:** HRCT shows honeycomb cysts to predominate in the peripheral and subpleural regions. Note that the cysts occur in several layers. **B:** The resected left lung in this patient sectioned at the level of the HRCT shown in **A**, shows the honeycomb cysts, which are most extensive in the posterior and peripheral lung.

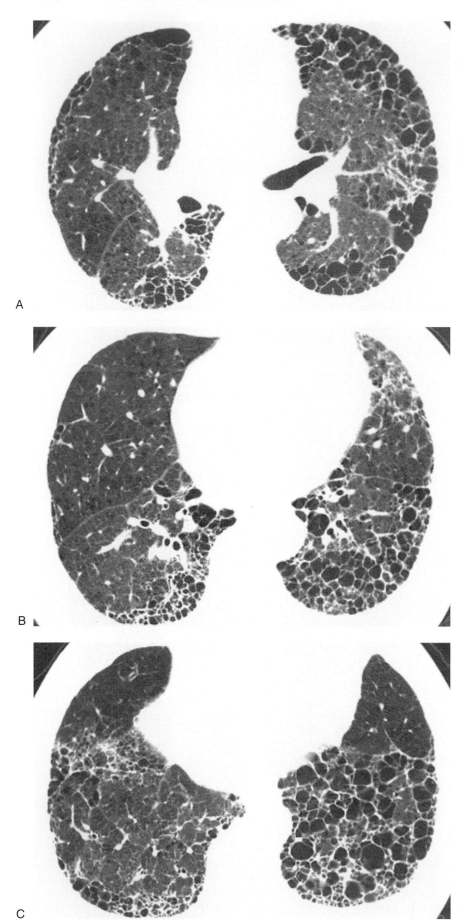

FIG. 3-32. A–C: Honeycombing in idiopathic pulmonary fibrosis. HRCT shows honeycomb cysts with a distinct predominance in the peripheral and subpleural regions. The cysts occur in several layers at the pleural surface, and the largest cysts are slightly larger than 1 cm in diameter. A basal predominance is also noted, and this is typical of idiopathic pulmonary fibrosis and most other causes of honeycombing. As in this case, some asymmetry is not uncommon.

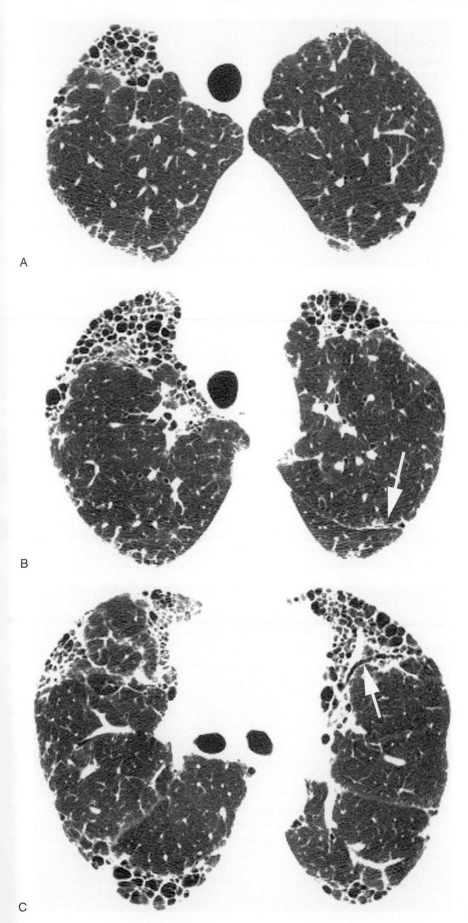

FIG. 3-33. A–C: Honeycombing in rheumatoid lung disease. HRCT shows honeycomb cysts with a distinct subpleural predominance. The cysts are generally smaller than 1 cm in diameter and share walls. Other findings of fibrosis include irregular thickening of the left major fissure (*arrow*, **B**), and traction bronchiectasis (*arrow*, **C**).

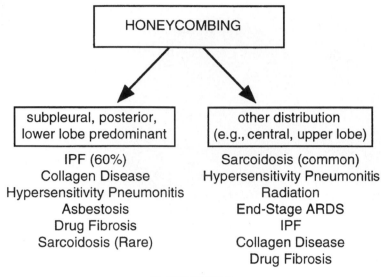

ALGORITHM 3

predominance, have been shown to be highly accurate in making this diagnosis [62,74–80]; a confident first-choice diagnosis of UIP was made in 77% to 89% of cases in these studies. However, a definite diagnosis of UIP cannot be made using HRCT. In a study by Johkoh et al. [67] of 129 patients with idiopathic interstitial pneumonia, admittedly including atypical cases requiring biopsy for diagnosis, a combination of honeycombing with a basal predominance was found in 59% of patients with UIP, 26% of patients with DIP, 22% of patients with NSIP, and 4% of patients with BOOP.

Irregular Linear Opacities

Irregular linear opacities 1- to 3-mm thick that cannot be characterized as representing parenchymal bands, peribronchovascular interstitial thickening, interlobular septal thickening, intralobular lines, or honeycombing are often visible in patients with interstitial disease, usually representing irregular areas of fibrosis (Fig. 3-34) [6]. These are nonspecific and may be seen in a variety of diseases, including UIP and NSIP [22,67–69]. In patients who have UIP and its various causes, irregular linear opacities may be seen instead of honeycombing; in patients with NSIP, they are more common than honeycombing.

Subpleural Lines

A curvilinear opacity a few millimeters or less in thickness, less than 1 cm from the pleural surface and paralleling the pleura, is termed a *subpleural line* [6]. It is a nonspecific indicator of atelectasis, fibrosis, or inflammation. It was first described in patients with asbestosis [81],

and was termed a *subpleural curvilinear shadow.* It was originally suggested that a subpleural line reflects the presence of fibrosis associated with honeycombing [81], and in some patients, a confluence of honeycomb cysts can result in a somewhat irregular subpleural line (Figs. 3-35 through 3-37).

A subpleural line is much more common in patients who have asbestosis than in those who have IPF or other causes of UIP [75]. Indeed, the presence of a subpleural line in nondependent lung has been reported in as many as 41% of patients with clinical findings of asbestosis [39]. However, the presence of this finding is nonspecific and can be seen in a variety of lung diseases (Fig. 3-1). The presence of a subpleural line has also been reported as common in patients with scleroderma who have interstitial disease [82,83].

A subpleural line also has been reported to occur as a result of the confluence of peribronchiolar interstitial abnormalities in patients with asbestosis, representing early fibrosis with associated alveolar flattening and collapse [44]. In these patients, honeycombing was not present. Also, in patients with asbestos exposure, a subpleural line may be seen adjacent to focal pleural thickening or plaques. These most likely represent focal atelectasis.

A subpleural line can also be seen in normal patients as a result of atelectasis within the dependent lung (e.g., the posterior lung when the patient is positioned supine) (Fig. 3-38); the presence of dependent atelectasis has been confirmed experimentally [84]. Also, a thicker, less-well-defined subpleural opacity, a so-called dependent density [39], can also be seen in normal subjects as a result of volume loss. Such normal posterior lines or opacities are transient and disap-

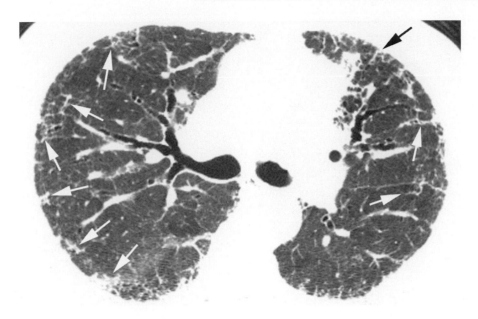

FIG. 3-34. Irregular linear opacities (*arrows*) in a patient with pulmonary fibrosis related to treatment with methotrexate. Irregular lines may be seen in various diseases resulting in fibrosis. These are nonspecific, but in a subpleural location as in this patient are suggestive of usual interstitial pneumonia or nonspecific interstitial pneumonia.

pear in the prone position. In a study by Aberle and associates [39] of patients with asbestos exposure, neither transient subpleural lines nor transient dependent densities correlated with the clinical suspicion of pulmonary fibrosis.

In patients with early interstitial lung disease, there may be a greater tendency for atelectasis to develop in the peripheral lung, resulting in the appearance of a subpleural line. As such, the presence of this abnormality could reflect an increased closing volume (i.e., an increased tendency for the lung to collapse) that is known to occur as a result of early interstitial lung disease. In the presence of appropriate treatment, such a finding might disappear (Fig. 3-39). The association of platelike atelectasis at the junction of "cortical" and "medullary" lung regions, air-trapping in the lung peripheral to the atelectasis, and decreased compliance of lung because of interstitial infiltration was first reported by Kubota et al. [85]. In addition, in some patients with asbestos exposure, a subpleural line may be seen adjacent to pleural plaques, representing focal atelectasis.

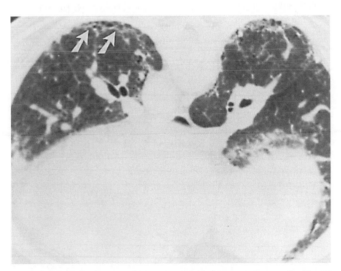

FIG. 3-35. Subpleural line in a patient with asbestosis. An ill-defined subpleural line (*arrows*) on a prone scan reflects subpleural fibrosis and honeycombing. Other findings of pulmonary fibrosis are also present.

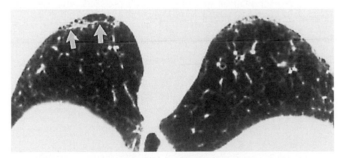

FIG. 3-36. Subpleural line (*arrows*) in a patient with rheumatoid lung disease and fibrosis, shown on a prone scan. Small honeycomb cysts are associated.

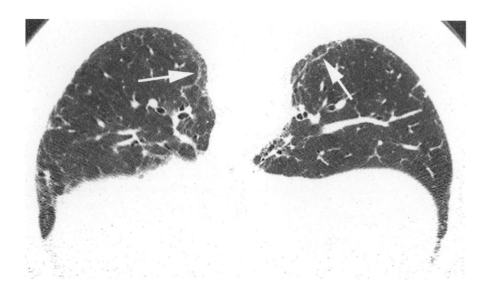

FIG. 3-37. Bilateral subpleural lines (*arrows*) in a patient with early idiopathic pulmonary fibrosis.

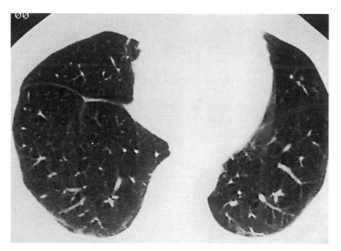

FIG. 3-38. Dependent atelectasis resulting in a posterior subpleural line. An ill-defined subpleural line is present posteriorly. No other findings of fibrosis are present, and this line disappeared in the prone position.

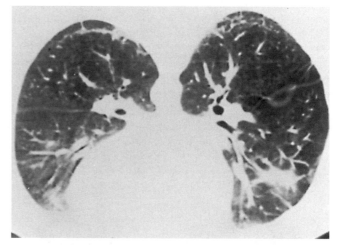

FIG. 3-39. Subpleural line that resolved after treatment in a patient with idiopathic pulmonary fibrosis. In the prone position, bilateral nontransient subpleural lines appear to represent fibrosis. Several small lucencies peripheral to them appear to represent areas of lung destruction or honeycombing. However, all of these findings cleared after treatment with steroids. This appearance may reflect atelectasis and air-trapping within the peripheral lung, occurring as a result of an increased closing volume (i.e., an increased tendency for lung collapse).

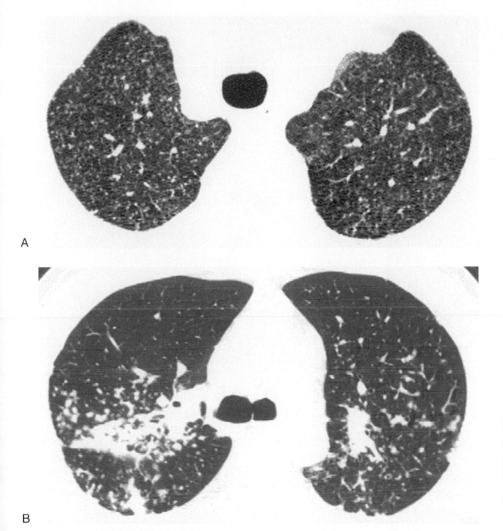

A

B

FIG. 3-40. Interstitial nodules. **A:** Very small nodules are easily visible in a patient with miliary tuberculosis. **B:** In a patient with sarcoidosis, nodules a few millimeters in diameter are sharply marginated and of soft-tissue attenuation. In regions of confluence, the nodules obscure vessels.

NODULES AND NODULAR OPACITIES

The term *nodule* is defined as a rounded opacity, at least moderately well-defined, and no more than 3 cm in diameter [6]. An approach to the HRCT assessment and differential diagnosis of multiple nodular opacities is based on a consideration of their size (small or large), appearance (well-defined or ill-defined), attenuation (soft-tissue or ground-glass opacity), and distribution.

Small Nodules

In this book, the term *small nodule* is used to define a rounded opacity smaller than 1 cm in diameter, whereas *large nodule* is used to refer to nodules 1 cm or larger in diameter. Some authors have used *micronodule* to describe nodules that are either smaller than 3 mm [77] or smaller than 7 mm in diameter [57,86]. The Nomenclature Committee of the Fleischner Society [6] recommends that "micronodule" be used to refer to nodules no larger than 7 mm in diameter. It is not clear that a distinction between a small nodule and a micronodule is of value in differential diagnosis [77].

Differences in the appearances of nodules that are predominantly interstitial or predominantly airspace in origin have been emphasized by several authors. Nodules considered to be interstitial are usually well-defined despite their small size (Fig. 3-40). Nodules as small as 1 to 2 mm in diameter can be detected on HRCT in patients with interstitial diseases such as miliary tuberculosis (Fig. 3-40A) [43,87–89], sarcoidosis (Fig. 3-40B) [13,21,56,60,90,91], Langerhans histiocytosis [92,93], silicosis and CWP [57,58,76,94,95], and metastatic tumor [4,49,96]. Interstitial nodules usually appear to be of soft-tissue attenuation and obscure the edges of vessels or other structures that they touch (Fig. 3-40B) [97–101].

Airspace nodules, on the other hand, are more likely to be ill-defined [3,43,102–104]; they can be of homogeneous soft-tissue attenuation (Figs. 3-41 and 3-42) or hazy and less dense than adjacent vessels (so-called ground-glass opacity) (Fig. 3-43). A cluster or rosette of small nodules can also be seen in patients who have airspace disease [102]. Airspace nodules have also been termed *acinar nodules* because they approximate the size of acini, but these nodules are not acinar histologically and instead tend to be centrilobular and peribronchiolar [103]; *ill-defined nodule* or *airspace nodule* is a preferable term.

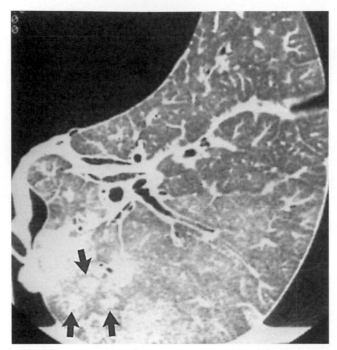

FIG. 3-41. Airspace nodules in an isolated lung. In this patient, centrilobular nodules (*arrows*) representing airspace pulmonary edema are visible in the posterior lung. These are larger and less well defined than interstitial nodules. (From Webb WR. HRCT of the lung parenchyma. *Radiol Clin North Am* 1989;27:1085, with permission.)

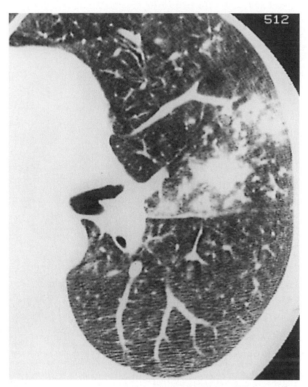

FIG. 3-42. Airspace nodules in a patient with a lobular pneumonia. The nodules are of soft-tissue opacity and obscure vessels. They are centrilobular in location and spare the subpleural lung peripherally and adjacent to the fissures. The small lucency seen within several of the nodules may reflect the centrilobular bronchiole. (From Webb WR. HRCT of the lung parenchyma. *Radiol Clin North Am* 1989;27:1085, with permission.)

Despite these differences in appearance, a distinction between interstitial and airspace nodules on the basis of HRCT findings can be quite difficult, and, in fact, is somewhat arbitrary, because many nodular diseases affect both the interstitial and alveolar compartments histologically.

The distribution or location of small nodules is generally of more value in differential diagnosis than their appearance, although both are usually taken into account (Table 3-6). In different conditions, small nodules can appear perilymphatic in distribution, randomly distributed, or predominantly centrilobular. Although there may be some overlap between these appearances, in most cases, a predominant distribution of nodules is evident on HRCT [105,106].

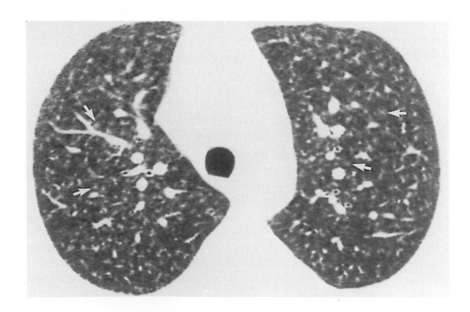

FIG. 3-43. Airspace nodules in bronchiolitis obliterans organizing pneumonia. Small, ill-defined ground-glass opacity nodules (*arrows*) are visible diffusely. Some can be seen to be centrilobular.

TABLE 3-6. *Differential diagnosis and characteristics of small nodules*

Disease	Distribution	Size (mm)	Appearance	Comments
Sarcoidosis	PL, occ R	≥1	W/ID, ST ± CALC	Subpleural, peribronchovascular; often patchy and asymmetric
Silicosis	PL, CL	≥1	WD, ST ± CALC	CL, subpleural, symmetric; posterior upper lobe predominance
Lymphangitic carcinoma	PL	≥1	WD, ST	Septal, peribronchovascular; may be patchy or unilateral
Amyloidosis	PL	≥1	WD, ST ± CALC	Predominantly septal, subpleural
Lymphocytic interstitial pneumonia	PL, CL	1–5	W/ID, ST, or GGO	May mimic lymphangitic spread when PL or hypersensitivity when CL; cysts may also be present
Miliary infection	R	1–5	WD, ST	Diffuse and uniform involvement
Hematogenous metastases	R	≥1	WD, ST	May overlap with appearance of lymphangitic spread
Endobronchial spread of infection (e.g., tuberculosis)	CL	≥3	W/ID, ST	Tree-in-bud common; patchy or diffuse; may be confluent
Viral pneumonia (e.g., cytomegalovirus)	CL	≥3	ID, GGO	Nodules of similar size surrounding small vessels
Airway disease (e.g., cystic fibrosis)	CL	≥3	W/ID, ST	Tree-in-bud common; patchy; bronchiectasis common
Panbronchiolitis	CL	≥3	W/ID, ST	Tree-in-bud common; bronchiectasis common
Allergic bronchopulmonary aspergillosis	CL	≥3	W/ID, ST	Tree-in-bud common; bronchiectasis common
Hypersensitivity pneumonitis	CL	>3	ID, GGO	Nodules of similar size surrounding small vessels
Langerhans histiocytosis	CL, occ R	≥3	WD, ST	Cysts may also be present
Bronchiolitis obliterans organizing pneumonia	CL	≥3	W/ID, ST, or GGO	Patchy or diffuse; peripheral predominance; consolidation
Bronchiolitis obliterans	CL	≥3	ID, GGO	Nodules uncommon; tree-in-bud rare
Respiratory bronchiolitis	CL	≥3	ID, GGO	Patchy GGO also common
Asbestosis	CL	2–3	W/ID, ST, or GGO	Early finding; basal, subpleural predominance; also reticular opacities
Follicular bronchiolitis	CL	≥1	WD, ST	Manifestation of collagen diseases, acquired immunodeficiency syndrome; branching appearance common
Endobronchial spread of tumor	CL	≥3	WD, ST	Patchy or diffuse; consolidation may be present; tree-in-bud rare
Edema, hemorrhage	CL	≥3	ID, GGO	± Septal thickening
Vasculitis	CL	≥3	ID, GGO	Talcosis; collagen disease
Metastatic calcification	CL	≥3	ID, GGO, or CALC	± Visible CALC on tissue window scans; upper lobe predominance

CALC, calcification; CL, centrilobular; GGO, ground-glass opacity; ID, ill defined; occ, occasionally; PL, perilymphatic; R, random; ST, soft-tissue attenuation; WD, well defined; W/ID, well or ill defined.

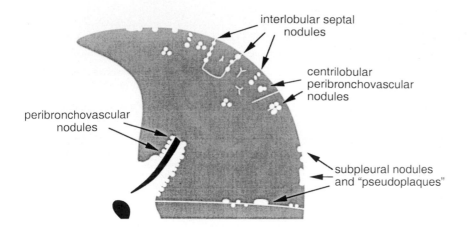

FIG. 3-44. Appearance of small nodules with a perilymphatic distribution. Nodules predominate in relation to the perihilar peribronchovascular interstitium, centrilobular interstitium, interlobular septa, and subpleural regions. Conglomerate subpleural nodules can form pseudoplaques.

Perilymphatic Distribution

Several diseases are characteristically associated with nodules occurring predominantly in relation to pulmonary lymphatics. These diseases have been termed *lymphatic* or *perilymphatic* [57,66] (Table 3-6). In patients with a perilymphatic distribution, both histologically and on HRCT, nodules predominate in relation to (i) the perihilar peribronchovascular interstitium, (ii) the interlobular septa, (iii) the subpleural regions, and (iv) the centrilobular interstitium. This pattern is most typical in patients with sarcoidosis, silicosis and CWP, and lymphangitic spread of carcinoma (Fig. 3-44) [20].

Subpleural nodules are usually seen in patients with a perilymphatic distribution of nodules. These are most easily recognized in relation to the fissures, where they can be easily distinguished from pulmonary vessels (Figs. 3-45 through 3-47). Subpleural nodules have been reported in approximately 80% of patients with silicosis or CWP, and at least 50% of patients with sarcoidosis, and are also common with lymphangitic spread of carcinoma [57]. Confluent subpleural nodules can result in the appearance of *pseudoplaques*: linear areas of subpleural opacity several millimeters in thickness that mimic the appearance of asbestos-related parietal pleural plaques (Figs. 3-44, 3-46, and 3-47). The presence of pseudoplaques in these diseases correlates significantly with the profusion of subpleural nodules [57].

Although sarcoidosis, silicosis and CWP, and lymphangitic spread of carcinoma all have a perilymphatic distribution of nodules, these diseases usually show different patterns of involvement of the perilymphatic interstitium. HRCT findings allow their differentiation in most cases.

Sarcoidosis

In nearly all patients with sarcoidosis, HRCT shows nodules ranging in size from several millimeters to 1 cm or more in diameter [20,21,56]. The nodules often appear sharply defined despite their small size, but they can be ill-defined (Figs. 3-40B and 3-45 through 3-48). Nodules are most frequently seen in relationship to the perihilar peribronchovascular intersti-

tium (Fig. 3-5), the subpleural interstitium, and small vessels; histologically small clusters of granulomas are visible in these locations (Figs. 3-45 through 3-47) [21,56,97]. A preponderance of nodules in relation to the major fissures and central bronchi and vessels is very typical of sarcoidosis. Nodules recognizable as centrilobular or septal in location are less frequently seen on HRCT (Figs. 3-13 and 3-45) [107], but they also correlate with typical histologic abnormalities. Large nodules measuring from 1 to 4 cm in diameter are seen in 15% to 25% of patients (Figs. 3-47 and 3-48) [21,98,99] and represent masses of granulomatous lesions, each granuloma being less than 0.4 millimeters in diameter [97]. These large nodules tend to have irregular margins (Fig. 3-48). Nodules can cavitate, but this is uncommon; Grenier et al. [77] reported this finding in only 3% of cases. Occasionally, nodules visible on HRCT represent nodular areas of fibrosis rather than active granulomas [56]. An upper-lobe predominance of nodules is common in sarcoidosis [57]. The lung is characteristically involved in a patchy fashion, with groups of granulomas occurring in some regions of lung, whereas other regions appear normal (Fig. 3-47). Asymmetry is very common.

Silicosis

Silicosis and CWP are associated with the presence of small, well-defined nodules, usually measuring from 2 to 5 mm in diameter, which predominantly appear centrilobular and subpleural in location on HRCT (Fig. 3-49) [57,58,94,95,100]. These correlate with areas of fibrosis surrounding centrilobular respiratory bronchioles and involving the subpleural interstitium caused by the accumulation of particulate material in these regions [57,95]. Parenchymal nodules are visible in 80% of patients with CWP, whereas subpleural nodules are seen in 87% [57,58]. Nodules occurring in relation to the peribronchovascular interstitium and thickened interlobular septa are less frequent and less conspicuous than in patients with sarcoidosis or lymphangitic spread of tumor. Also, nodules appear more evenly distributed than in patients with sarcoidosis; they are present diffusely, bilaterally, and symmetrically, but in patients with mild silico-

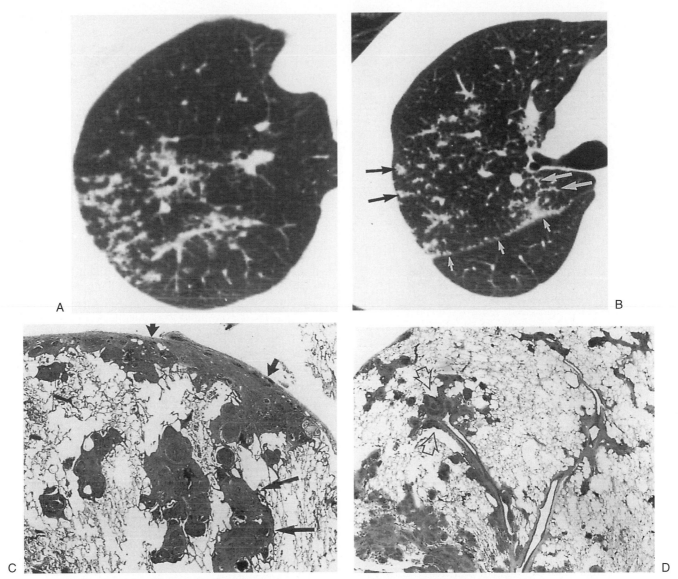

FIG. 3-45. Sarcoidosis showing a perilymphatic distribution on HRCT and open lung biopsy. **A:** HRCT through the upper lobe shows small nodules in relation to the peribronchovascular regions and small vessels. Vessels and bronchi show a nodular appearance. **B:** At a lower level, small nodules are seen in the subpleural regions along the fissure (*small white arrows*), in the centrilobular regions (*black arrows*), and interlobular septa (*long white arrows*). **C,D:** Open lung biopsy shows that the small nodules correspond to groups of granulomas that are subpleural (**C**, *short arrows*), septal (**C**, *long arrows*), and centrilobular and peribronchiolar (**D**, *open arrows*).

sis or CWP are usually visible only in the upper lobes. A posterior predominance of nodules is often present [58,94]. In patients who have silicosis, the nodules can calcify.

Lymphangitic Spread of Tumor

In patients with lymphangitic spread of tumor, when nodules are visible, they are most often visible within the thickened peribronchovascular interstitium and interlobular septa (Figs. 3-12 and 3-50 through 3-52) [7,11,12,14,49,76]. Peribronchovascular and subpleural nodules are typically not as profuse as in patients with sarcoidosis. Septal thickening results in the appearance of a "beaded" septum (Figs. 3-12 and 3-50 through 3-52) [13,49,101]. In an HRCT study of postmortem lung specimens [49], 19 of 22 cases with interstitial pulmonary metastases showed the appearance of "beaded" or nodular septal thickening on HRCT. The beaded septa corresponded directly to the presence of tumor growing in pulmonary capillaries, lymphatics, and septal interstitium. In this study [49], beaded septa were not noted in any of the specimens of patients with pulmonary edema, fibrosis, or in normal lungs. In patients with lymphangitic carcinomatosis, the abnormalities may be unilateral, patchy, bilateral, or symmetric.

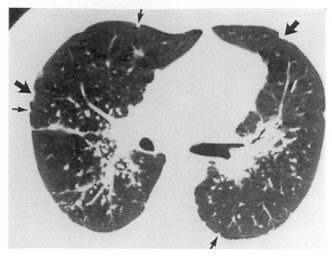

FIG. 3-46. Sarcoidosis with a perilymphatic distribution of nodules. Numerous small nodules are seen in relation to the perihilar, bronchovascular interstitium. Bronchial walls appear irregularly thickened. Subpleural nodules (*small arrows*) are also seen bordering the costal pleural surfaces and right major fissure. This appearance is virtually diagnostic of sarcoidosis. Clusters of subpleural granulomas (*large arrows*) have been termed *pseudoplaques*.

A perilymphatic distribution of nodules also may be seen in other diseases, but these are uncommon. In patients with *diffuse amyloidosis*, interstitial thickening with nodularity visible in relation to vessels, bronchi, interlobular septa, and the subpleural interstitium has been reported (Fig. 3-53; see Fig. 5-59) [50,106]. In smokers, a few small subpleural and centrilobular nodules can be seen, probably related to the presence of fibrosis and accumulated particulate material in the peribronchial regions and at the bases of interlobular septa, and related to pathways of lymphatic drainage [108,109]. LIP, occurring primarily in patients with dysproteinemia; autoimmune disease, particularly Sjögren's syndrome; multicentric Castleman's disease; and in patients with acquired immunodeficiency syndrome (AIDS), can result in the presence of lymphocytic and plasma cell infiltrates in relation to the peribronchovascular interstitium and interlobular septa, and in the subpleural and centrilobular regions [110–113]. On HRCT, LIP may result in a variety of appearances [17,19, 114], but in some patients, it closely mimics the appearance of lymphangitic spread of carcinoma, with subpleural, peribronchovascular, and septal nodules (Fig. 3-54).

Random Distribution

Small nodules that appear randomly distributed in relation to structures of the secondary lobule and lung are often seen in patients with miliary tuberculosis (Fig. 3-55) [88,89], miliary fungal infections, and hematogenous metastases [66] (Table 3-6). As with a perilymphatic distribution, the nodules can be seen in relation to the pleural surfaces, small vessels, and interlobular septa but do not appear to have a consistent or predominant relationship to any of these. On HRCT, a uniform distribution of nodules throughout the lung, without respect for anatomic structures, is most typical. Lung involvement tends to be bilateral and symmetric; a patchy distribution of nodules, as is often seen in patients with a perilymphatic pattern, is atypical.

In miliary tuberculosis (Fig. 3-55) or fungal infections (Fig. 3-56), the nodules tend to be well-defined and up to several millimeters in diameter [89]. Hematogenous metastases also tend to be well-defined (Fig. 3-57) [115]. As with miliary tuberculosis, the nodules can be seen in relation to small vessels in some locations, a fact that likely reflects their mode of dissemination. Although random in distribution, they have a recognized tendency to predominate in the lung periphery and at the lung bases [115]. An appearance of small well-defined and ill-defined random nodules has also been reported with varicella-zoster pneumonia [116].

In a study correlating HRCT and pathologic findings in patients with metastatic tumor [115], nodules less than 3 mm in diameter had no consistent relationship to lobular structures. Eleven percent of nodules were seen in relation to the centrilobular pulmonary arteries, 21% were related to interlobular septa, and 68% were located in-between. On examination of specimen radiographs and pathology, a similar distribution was noted. Nodules resulting from hematogenous metastasis are characteristically well-defined. Some overlap between a random pattern and a perilymphatic pattern may be seen in patients with metastatic tumor.

When numerous, nodules in patients with sarcoidosis (Fig. 3-58), Langerhans histiocytosis (Fig. 3-59), or silicosis may appear to be randomly and diffusely distributed [66] and may be difficult to distinguish from the nodules of miliary infection or metastases.

Centrilobular Distribution

Nodules limited to the centrilobular regions can also be seen (Fig. 3-60). Centrilobular nodules can reflect the presence of either interstitial or airspace abnormalities, and the histologic correlations reported to occur in association with centrilobular nodules vary with the disease entity [107]. Centrilobular nodules may be dense and of homogeneous opacity, or of ground-glass opacity (Figs. 3-61 and 3-62), and may range from a few millimeters to a centimeter in size. Either a single centrilobular nodule or a centrilobular rosette of nodules may be visible [43,102,103]. Although they are often ill-defined, this is not always the case. Because of the similar size of secondary lobules, centrilobular nodules often appear to be evenly spaced. They may appear patchy or diffuse in different diseases. The finding of "tree-in-bud," representing impaction of centrilobular bronchioles by fluid, mucus, or pus and often appearing as a branching opacity in the peripheral lung (Fig. 3-63), may be present in patients with a centrilobular distribution of nodules. Tree-in-bud almost always indicates the presence of bronchiolar infection. The appearance and significance of tree-in-bud are discussed in detail later.

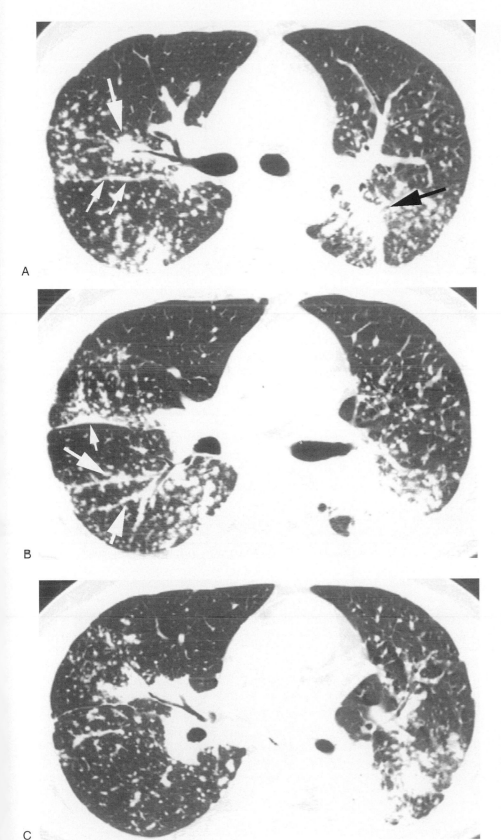

FIG. 3-47. A–C: HRCT at three levels in a patient with sarcoidosis and a typical perilymphatic distribution of nodules. Numerous nodules are predominant in relation to the major fissure (*small arrows*) and perihilar bronchovascular interstitium (*large arrows*). Subpleural nodules and pseudoplaques are also seen bordering the costal pleural surfaces. Confluence of granulomas in the left lower lobe (**B** and **C**) results in consolidation or large masses. As in this patient, lung involvement in patients with sarcoidosis is often patchy, with some areas appearing relatively normal.

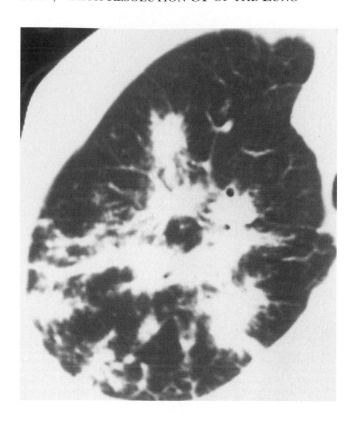

FIG. 3-48. Large peribronchovascular nodules in a patient with sarcoidosis, representing clusters of granulomas. These have irregular margins. Small nodules are also visible.

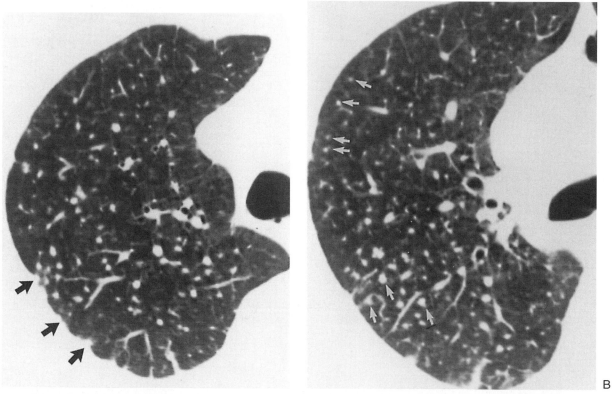

A

B

FIG. 3-49. A,B: Perilymphatic nodules in a patient with silicosis. Nodules predominate in the subpleural (**A**, *black arrows*) and centrilobular (**B**, *white arrows*) regions. In patients with silicosis, peribronchovascular nodules are less frequent than in sarcoidosis, and the nodules appear more evenly distributed. The nodules often predominate posteriorly and in the upper lobes in patients with this disease. (Courtesy of Raymond Glyn Thomas, M.D., The Rand Mutual Hospital, Johannesburg, South Africa.)

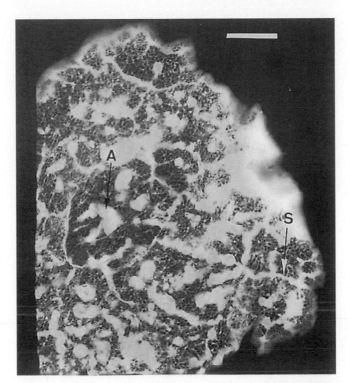

FIG. 3-50. Radiograph of a 1-mm–thick lung slice in a patient with lymphangitic spread of tumor. Note the nodular thickening of interlobular septa (S), and the centrilobular interstitium surrounding arteries (A). Bar = 1 cm. (Courtesy of Harumi Itoh, M.D., Chest Disease Research Institute, Kyoto University, Kyoto, Japan.)

Centrilobular nodules are usually separated from the pleural surfaces, fissures, and interlobular septa by a distance of several millimeters. In the lung periphery, the nodules are usually centered 5 to 10 mm from the pleural surface, a fact that reflects their centrilobular origin (Figs. 3-61 and 3-62). They are not usually seen occurring in relation to interlobular septa or the pleural surfaces, as do random or perilymphatic nodules, and the subpleural lung is typically spared. This difference can be particularly valuable in distinguishing diffuse centrilobular nodules from diffuse random nodules. Although centrilobular nodules, when large, may touch the pleural surface, they do not appear to arise at the pleural surface.

The term *centrilobular nodule* is best thought of as indicating that the nodule is related to *centrilobular structures*, such as small vessels, even if they cannot be precisely localized to the lobular core (Figs. 3-41 through 3-43, 3-61, and 3-62). Indeed, in some cases, centrilobular nodules can be correctly identified by noting their association with small pulmonary artery branches. It is typical for centrilobular nodules to appear perivascular on HRCT, surrounding or obscuring the smallest visible pulmonary arteries (Fig. 3-62). In occasional cases, the air-filled centrilobular bronchiole can be recognized as a rounded lucency within a centrilobular nodule (Figs. 3-42, 3-64, and 3-65).

As indicated above, centrilobular nodules can be seen in patients having a perilymphatic distribution of disease. Pulmonary lymphatics are located in the peribronchovascular interstitial compartment in the centrilobular region. However, in patients with a perilymphatic distribution, nodules will also be seen in other locations (i.e., subpleural regions or interlobular septa). Sarcoid granulomas are typically distributed along lymphatics in the peribronchovascular interstitial space both in the perihilar regions and lobular core (Fig. 3-45) [56,57,60]. In some cases, centrilobular clusters of granulomas are a predominant feature of the disease, but nodules involving the subpleural regions are also present in most cases. Small centrilobular nodules are also characteristic of both silicosis and CWP [58,95]. In patients with silicosis, early lesions are centrilobular and peribronchiolar; the

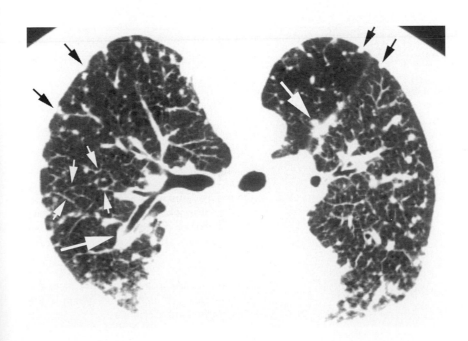

FIG. 3-51. Lymphangitic spread of carcinoma. A prone HRCT shows peribronchovascular nodules (*large white arrows*) giving a nodular appearance to pulmonary artery branches, nodular interlobular septal thickening (*small white arrows*), and subpleural nodules (*black arrows*).

nodules are a few millimeters in diameter and consist of layers of lamellated connective tissue. Subpleural nodules are also typically present (Fig. 3-49). The characteristic lesion of CWP is the so-called coal macule, which consists of a focal accumulation of coal dust surrounded by a small amount of fibrous tissue, occurring in a centrilobular, peribronchiolar location. In patients with lymphangitic spread of carcinoma, although interlobular septal thickening is usually a predominant feature of the disease, centrilobular peribronchovascular interstitial thickening or nodules are commonly seen (Fig. 3-50) [107]. Other findings include thickening of the peribronchovascular interstitium in the perihilar lung.

LIP or follicular bronchiolitis in AIDS patients can result in the presence of ill-defined centrilobular opacities. LIP is associated with a lymphocytic and plasma cell infiltrate in relation to lymphatics; it may predominate in the centrilobular regions or mimic the appearance of lymphangitic spread of carcinoma.

Nodules limited to centrilobular regions (i.e., a centrilobular distribution) can be seen in patients with a variety of diseases that primarily affect centrilobular bronchioles or arteries and result in inflammation, infiltration, or fibrosis of the surrounding interstitium and alveoli (Table 3-6) [66,107]. The differential diagnosis of this appearance is long. Diseases

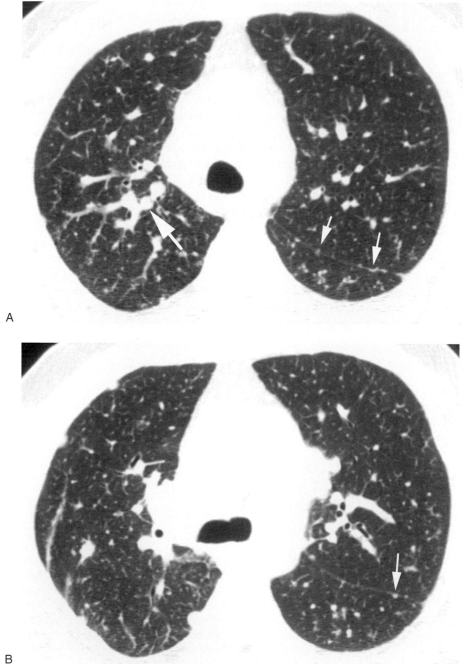

A

B

FIG. 3-52. Lymphangitic spread of thyroid carcinoma. HRCT at three levels **(A–C)** shows subpleural nodules along the fissures (*small arrows*) and peribronchovascular nodules (*large arrow*) resulting in a nodular appearance of pulmonary artery branches. Interlobular septal thickening is inconspicuous in this patient. Subpleural nodules are easy to see in the periphery. Note the presence of right hilar lymph node enlargement. *Continued*

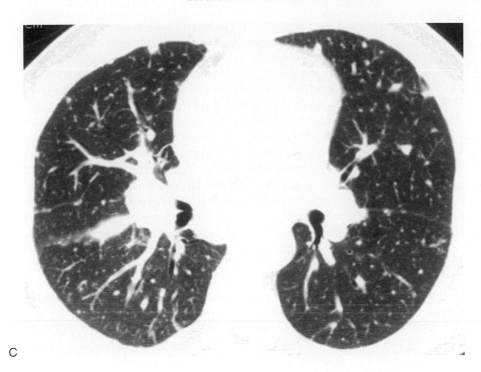

C
FIG. 3-52. *Continued*

resulting in this appearance may be classified as bronchiolar and peribronchiolar or vascular and perivascular.

Bronchiolar and Peribronchiolar Diseases

Bronchiolar diseases secondarily involving the peribronchiolar interstitium or alveoli, or both, are the most frequent causes of centrilobular opacities seen on HRCT. Their histologic correlates and HRCT appearances vary with the nature of the disease. The differential diagnosis of airway diseases associated with centrilobular abnormalities includes the following entities:

Endobronchial Spread of Tuberculosis, Nontuberculous Mycobacteria, and Other Granulomatous Infections. Bronchogenic dissemination of infection can occur in patients with active tuberculosis and nontuberculous mycobacterial disease (Figs. 3-66 through 3-69) [43,60,65,103,117,118]. Nodules, or clusters of nodules, that reflect peribronchiolar consolidation or granuloma formation are common, visible on HRCT in as many as 97% of patients with active tuberculosis, and are also common in patients with nontuberculous mycobacterial infection [118,119]. Bronchioles filled with infected material can also result in the appearance of a tree-in-bud (Fig. 3-66) [65]. Fungal infections may result

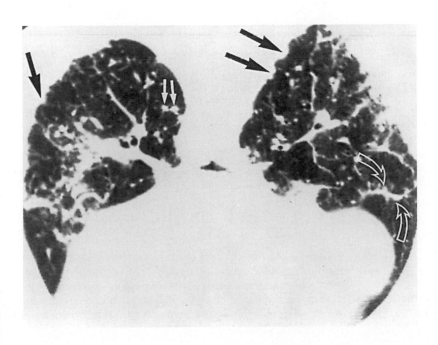

FIG. 3-53. Amyloidosis with perilymphatic nodules. Small subpleural nodules (*large arrows*) and interlobular septal nodules (*small arrows*) were found on biopsy to represent small nodular deposits of amyloid. Nodules are also seen along the right major fissure (*open arrows*).

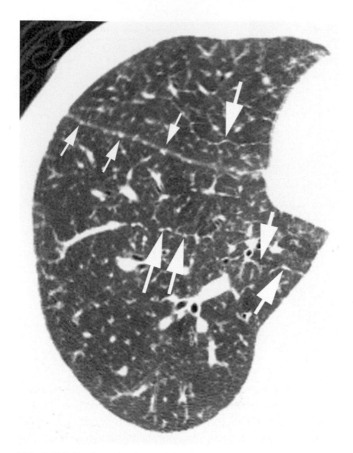

FIG. 3-54. Perilymphatic nodules in an acquired immunodeficiency syndrome patient with lymphocytic interstitial pneumonia. Small subpleural nodules (*small arrows*) are visible along the major fissure. Nodules within interlobular septa (*large arrows*) are also visible.

in similar findings [120]. Specifically, *Aspergillus bronchiolitis* and bronchopneumonia (airway invasive aspergillosis) are characterized by patchy consolidation, centrilobular nodules, and the finding of a tree-in-bud (see Figs. 5-88 and 5-89) [121,122].

Bronchopneumonia. Bronchopneumonia resulting from various organisms, most commonly bacteria, is associated with the presence of bronchial and peribronchiolar inflammatory exudates, which also involve surrounding alveoli. HRCT findings are quite similar to those of endobronchial spread of tuberculosis (Figs. 3-42, 3-64, 3-65, 3-70, and 3-71) [3,60,102]. Viral infections and *P. carinii* pneumonia can also result in the appearance of centrilobular nodules (see Fig. 6-52).

Infectious Bronchiolitis. Infectious bronchiolitis is seen most often in children, and presents with fever, dyspnea, and wheezing. It is often due to respiratory syncytial virus, although other viruses and bacteria, particularly mycoplasma, may be involved. Centrilobular nodules or tree-in-bud may be visible [123].

Cystic Fibrosis. In patients with cystic fibrosis, thick-walled, mucus- or pus-filled bronchioles are seen as rounded or branching centrilobular opacities (i.e., tree-in-bud), usually in association with central bronchiectasis (Figs. 3-63 and 3-72) [60,124,125]. The centrilobular bronchiolar abnormalities can be an early finding and can be patchy in distribution.

Bronchiectasis. Findings similar to those of cystic fibrosis can be seen in patients with chronic bronchiectasis of any cause, including congenital immunodeficiency states, ciliary dysmotility syndrome, and the syndrome of yellow nails and lymphedema (Figs. 3-73 and 3-74).

Panbronchiolitis. In patients with Asian panbronchiolitis, aggregates of histiocytes, lymphocytes, and plasma cells infiltrate the walls of respiratory bronchioles and extend into the peribronchiolar tissues. HRCT can show (i) prominent branching centrilobular opacities representing dilated bronchioles with inflammatory bronchiolar wall thickening and abundant intraluminal secretions, (ii) bronchiolar dilatation that tends to occur late in the disease process [126–128] and is typically proximal to the nodular peribronchiolar opacities, and (iii) centrilobular nodules that reflect bronchiolar and peribronchiolar inflammation and fibrosis (Fig. 3-75) [127].

Asthma and Allergic Bronchopulmonary Aspergillosis. Patients with asthma and allergic bronchopulmonary aspergillosis may develop mucoid impaction of centrilobular bronchioles visible as centrilobular opacities. These are more common in patients with allergic bronchopulmonary aspergillosis (93%) than in those who have asthma (28%) [129].

Hypersensitivity Pneumonitis. An immunologic response to a variety of inhaled allergens in sensitized persons, subacute hypersensitivity pneumonitis (extrinsic allergic alveolitis) is characterized by a peribronchiolar and perivascular lymphocytic and plasma cell infiltrate with formation of poorly defined granulomas [130]. There may be associated plugs of granulation tissue within bronchiolar lumens (bronchiolitis obliterans). Centrilobular nodules of ground-glass opacity seen on HRCT are typical (Figs. 3-61 and 3-62), reflecting the histologic abnormality [130–133].

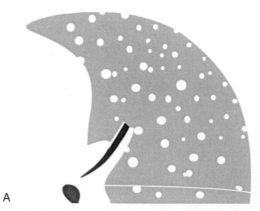

FIG. 3-55. A: Appearance of small nodules with a random distribution. Although some nodules can be seen in relation to interlobular septa, vessels, or the pleural surfaces, nodules do not appear to have a consistent or predominant relationship to any of these structures. A uniform distribution is most typical. *Continued.*

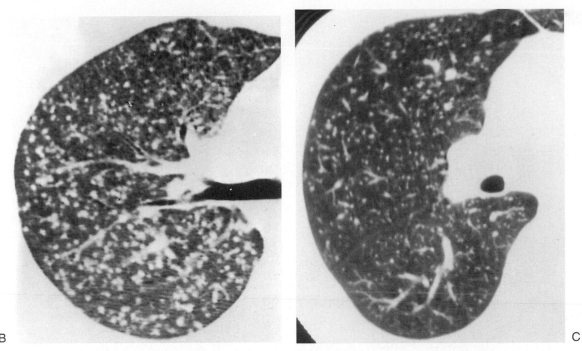

B

C

FIG. 3-55. *Continued* B: Miliary tuberculosis with small nodules. Nodules a few millimeters in diameter have a random distribution and appear widely and evenly distributed throughout the lung. Some nodules can be seen in relation to small vessels, the pleural surfaces, and the interlobar fissure, but the nodules do not predominate in relation to these structures. (From Im JG, Itoh H, et al. Pulmonary tuberculosis: CT findings—early active disease and sequential change with antituberculous therapy. *Radiology* 1993;186:653, with permission.) **C:** In another patient with miliary tuberculosis, the nodules are smaller than those shown in **B**. The nodules are widely dispersed. (Courtesy of Shin-Ho Kook, M.D., Koryo General Hospital, Seoul, South Korea.)

Langerhans Histiocytosis. Initially, granulomas form in the peribronchiolar tissues and adjacent alveolar interstitium. Mononuclear Langerhans cells are present in the early stages of the disease; later, the cellular response diminishes and fibrosis dominates. Centrilobular nodules on HRCT reflect the peribronchiolar abnormality (Fig. 3-59) [93]. Later in the course of the disease, cavitation of nodules, cyst formation, and centrilobular bronchiolectasis can be seen.

Bronchiolitis Obliterans Organizing Pneumonia. BOOP, also known as *cryptogenic organizing pneumonia* (COP) or simply *organizing pneumonia*, is characterized by the presence of inflammatory cells lining the walls of the terminal and respiratory bronchioles with plugs of granulation tissue within airway lumen and organizing pneumonia. Because the organizing pneumonia is distributed in the peribronchiolar airspaces, centrilobular opacities can be present in patients

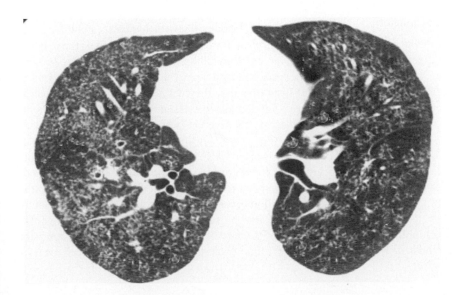

FIG. 3-56. Miliary coccidioidomycosis with numerous very small nodules that have a random distribution.

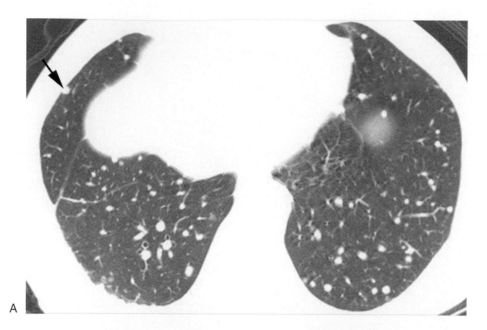

A

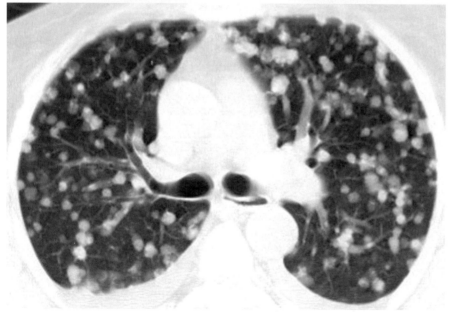

B

FIG. 3-57. Hematogenous metastases from a rectal carcinoma. **A:** HRCT obtained in a patient with an abnormal chest radiograph and no known tumor. Multiple small, well-defined nodules are visible, with involvement of the peripheral pleural surfaces (*arrow*). The overall pattern of distribution is random. **B:** Spiral CT obtained 6 months later following diagnosis of the patient's tumor shows progression of the metastases. A random distribution, with diffuse and uniform lung involvement is well demonstrated.

with BOOP (Figs. 3-76 and 3-77). Frank consolidation or larger areas of ground-glass opacity, however, are more common [134,135]. Tree-in-bud may occasionally be seen [123].

Bronchiolitis Obliterans. Bronchiolitis obliterans, also known as *constrictive bronchiolitis*, is characterized primarily by concentric bronchiolar and peribronchiolar fibrosis and luminal narrowing or obliteration. In an acute phase, ill-defined centrilobular nodules may sometimes be seen, reflecting peribronchiolar inflammation [107,136,137]. In the later obliterative stage, centrilobular opacities occasionally may be seen, but they are not a common feature of this disease [60]. Airway obstruction with air-trapping is much more frequent.

Respiratory Bronchiolitis. Respiratory bronchiolitis is thought to represent a nonspecific reaction to inhaled irri-

tants, usually in association with cigarette smoking; it is almost always seen in smokers. Inflammation of the respiratory bronchioles, with filling of the bronchioles by brown-pigmented macrophages, plasma cells, and lymphocytes is present histologically. In symptomatic patients, macrophages and inflammatory cells extend into the peribronchiolar airspaces and alveolar walls. When associated with symptoms, the term *respiratory bronchiolitis-interstitial lung disease* is used. HRCT findings in symptomatic patients include multifocal ground-glass opacities with a centrilobular distribution that reflects the peribronchiolar nature of this disease (see Figs. 6-34 and 6-35) [109,138–140]. Patchy opacities can also be seen. Distinct centrilobular opacities may be seen in patients who use inhalational drugs—for example, so-called crack lung.

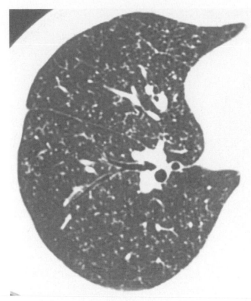

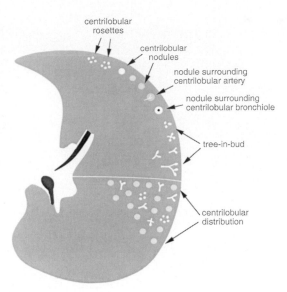

FIG. 3-58. Diffuse sarcoidosis with a random distribution of nodules. Very small nodules are seen in relation to the major fissure, but the overall distribution is diffuse and uniform. Findings typical of sarcoidosis, such as a patchy distribution or a predominance of nodules in relation to peribronchovascular regions, are not seen. (Courtesy of Luigia Storto, Chieti, Italy.)

Cigarette Smoking. A few small subpleural and centrilobular nodules can be seen in subjects who smoke or have a history of smoking. Ill-defined centrilobular nodules have been reported in as many as 12% to 27% of smokers studied using HRCT, reflecting the presence of bronchiolectasis and peribronchiolar fibrosis [108,109], although in our experience, this is not a common finding.

Aspiration. Aspiration of a variety of materials, including gastric contents, water, or blood, associated with a variable

FIG. 3-60. HRCT appearances of centrilobular nodules. Centrilobular nodules are usually separated from the interlobular septa and pleural surfaces by a distance of several millimeters; in the lung periphery, the nodules are usually centered 5 to 10 mm from the pleural surface. Also, centrilobular nodules may be associated with small pulmonary artery branches. Because of the similar size of secondary lobules, centrilobular nodules often appear to be evenly spaced. Although they are often ill defined, this is not always the case. Either a single centrilobular nodule or a centrilobular rosette of nodules may be seen. In occasional cases, the air-filled centrilobular bronchiole can be recognized as a rounded lucency within a centrilobular nodule. Tree-in-bud may be seen in patients with a centrilobular distribution, representing impaction of centrilobular bronchioles.

inflammatory response may result in ill-defined centrilobular opacities [136,137].

Asbestosis. In patients with early asbestosis, the histologic abnormality is nearly identical to that seen in patients

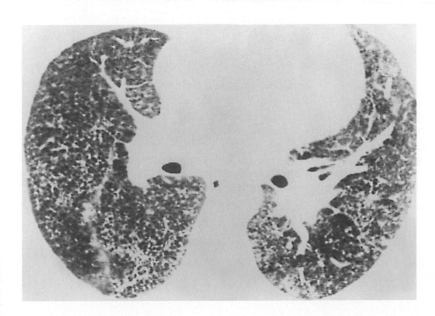

FIG. 3-59. Langerhans histiocytosis with small nodules. Small nodules, best seen in the paravertebral regions, are numerous and have a random distribution.

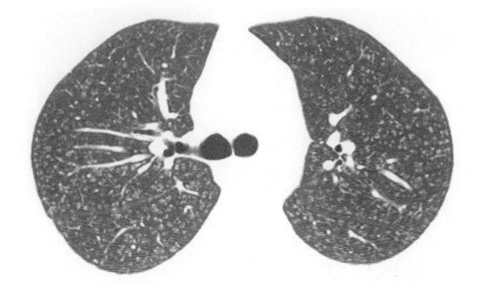

FIG. 3-61. Ill-defined centrilobular nodules and rosettes in a patient with hypersensitivity pneumonitis. The nodules are separated from the pleural surfaces and fissures by a distance of several millimeters. As is typical, the nodules often appear to be evenly spaced and, in this case, are diffusely distributed. This is a common appearance in hypersensitivity pneumonitis.

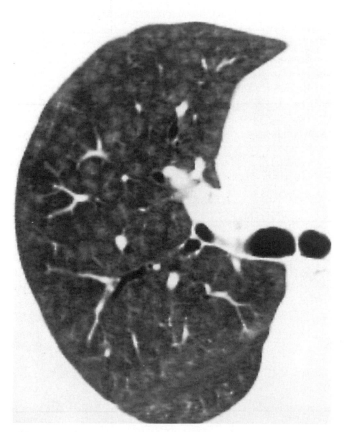

FIG. 3-62. Centrilobular nodules of ground-glass opacity in a patient with hypersensitivity pneumonitis. The ill-defined opacities are visible in relation to small vascular branches throughout the lung. The most peripheral nodules are centered 5 to 10 mm from the pleural surface. The subpleural lung region appears spared.

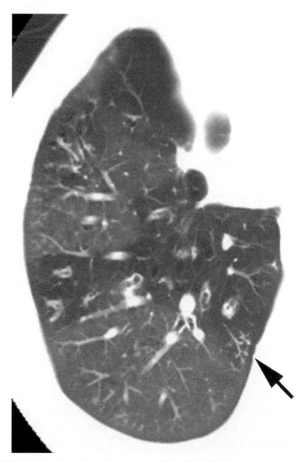

FIG. 3-63. Centrilobular tree-in-bud (*arrow*) in a patient with cystic fibrosis and chronic airway infection. Also note bronchial wall thickening and inhomogeneous lung attenuation due to airways obstruction and air-trapping with mosaic perfusion.

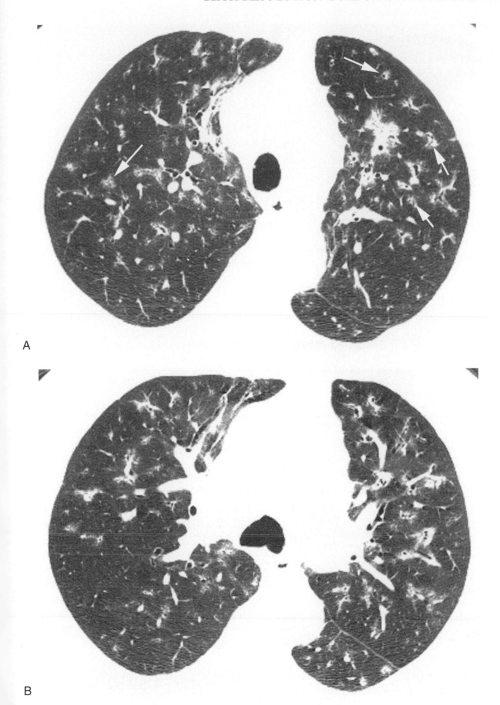

A

B

FIG. 3-64. A,B: Ill-defined centrilobular nodules in a patient with chronic airways disease and bronchopneumonia. A number of the ill-defined nodules surround an air-filled bronchus or bronchiole (*arrows*).

with respiratory bronchiolitis, but asbestos fibers can be identified in the peribronchiolar tissues. Fiber deposition in the respiratory bronchioles results in a peribronchiolar cellular response and fibrosis that eventually extends to involve the contiguous airspaces and alveolar interstitium. Ill-defined centrilobular opacities have been reported on HRCT in as many as half of patients with early asbestosis (see Figs. 4-46 and 4-47) [141]. Nodules predominate posteriorly and at the lung bases, probably due to the gravitational effects of fiber deposition [44,141]. Other inhaled inorganic materials can result in similar histologic and imaging abnormalities.

Follicular Bronchiolitis. This entity, defined as lymphoid hyperplasia of bronchus-associated lymphoid tissue, is characterized by hyperplastic lymphoid follicles along the walls of centrilobular bronchioles. It may be seen in patients with collagen-vascular diseases, particularly rheumatoid arthritis or AIDS, and is related histologically to LIP. Small, well-defined centrilobular nodules, often smaller than 3 mm in diameter, are invariably seen, and large airway abnormalities and peribronchial nodules may also be present (see Figs. 4-21 and 5-14) [120,142–144].

Endobronchial Spread of Neoplasm. Centrilobular nodules can be seen in bronchioloalveolar carcinoma (see Fig. 5-

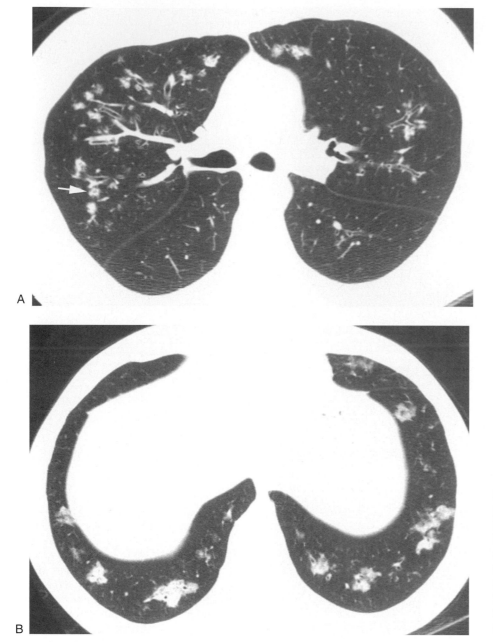

A

B

FIG. 3-65. Centrilobular nodules in a patient with bronchopneumonia. **A:** Scattered ill-defined nodules represent peribronchiolar consolidation and may contain a visible bronchiole (*arrow*). **B:** At the lung bases, consolidated lobules surround air-filled bronchioles in several locations. Bronchopneumonia is also termed *lobular pneumonia* because of this appearance.

11) or tracheobronchial papillomatosis (Fig. 3-78) when endobronchial spread of tumor occurs [145,146]. These can be well-defined or ill-defined. Large airway papillomas or cystic lesions may also be visible in patients with tracheobronchial papillomatosis.

Vascular and Perivascular Diseases

Vascular pathology, either localized to the walls of arteries or to perivascular tissues, can cause centrilobular abnormality. Because airways are not involved, bronchiolectasis and tree-in-bud are absent, although if the cellular response extends into the peribronchiolovascular interstitium, apparent bronchiolar wall thickening may result.

Pulmonary Edema. Mild cases of edema may show hazy, ill-defined centrilobular opacities (see Figs. 6-71 and 6-72) [28,40,103]. Increased prominence of the centrilobular artery resulting from perivascular interstitial thickening is also commonly visible (Figs. 3-10 and 3-41). Septal thickening is variably associated, but in some patients, centrilobular opacities predominate. Pleural effusion may also be present.

Vasculitis. Processes resulting in a vascular and perivascular inflammatory response, including vasculitis and reaction to injected substances, such as talc [95,107,147], can result in ill-defined centrilobular opacities on HRCT. Connolly et al. [148] reported hazy or fluffy centrilobular, perivascular opacities in eight children with vasculitis,

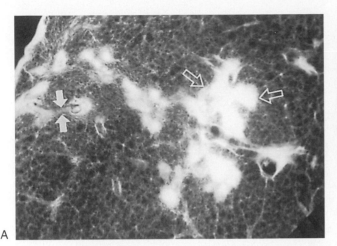
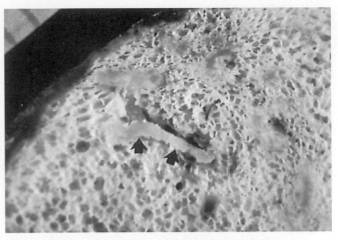

A

B

FIG. 3-66. Centrilobular nodules and tree-in-bud in a patient with tuberculosis. **A:** Radiograph of a resected lung in a patient with endobronchial spread of tuberculosis, shows a branching centrilobular opacity (*solid arrows*), and rosettes of small nodular opacities producing a tree-in-bud appearance (*open arrows*). **B:** On pathologic examination, the branching centrilobular opacity represents caseous material filling bronchioles and alveolar ducts (*arrows*). (From Im JG, Itoh H, et al. Pulmonary tuberculosis: CT findings—early active disease and sequential change with antituberculous therapy. *Radiology* 1993;186:653, with permission.)

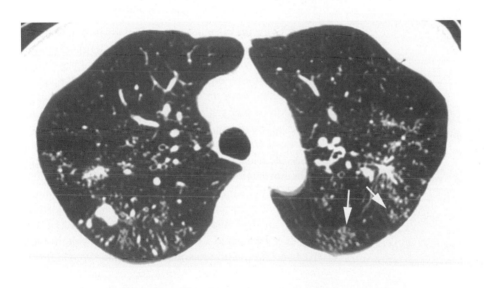

FIG. 3-67. Centrilobular nodules and rosettes in a patient with endobronchial spread of tuberculosis. Multiple small nodules occurring in clusters (*arrows*) are common in patients with this disease. The nodules, being centrilobular, spare the pleural surfaces.

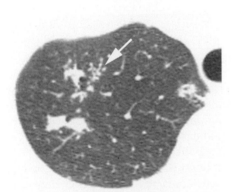
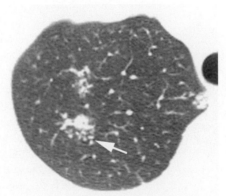
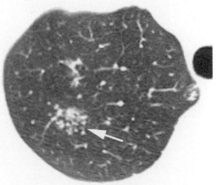

A–C

FIG. 3-68. A–C: Centrilobular rosettes and tree-in-bud in a patient with endobronchial spread of tuberculosis. Multiple small nodules occurring in clusters and the appearance of tree-in-bud (*arrows*) are seen in association with several larger nodules in the right lung apex. The appearance of tree-in-bud almost always indicates infection. *Mycobacterium tuberculosis* was found in this patient's sputum.

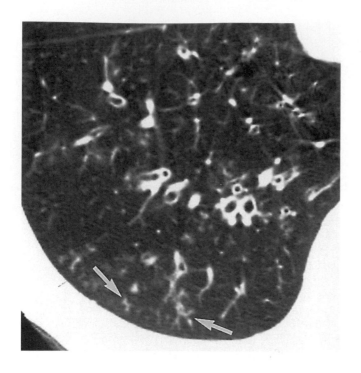

FIG. 3-69. Nontuberculous mycobacterial infection with endobronchial spread. Coned view of the right lower lobe in a patient with chronic obstructive lung disease and *Mycobacterium avium-intracellulare* complex infection on sputum cultures. Central bronchi are dilated and thick walled; centrilobular bronchioles are also dilated, and have a tree-in-bud appearance (*arrows*). (From Gruden JF, Webb WR, et al. Centrilobular opacities in the lung on HRCT: diagnostic considerations and pathologic correlation. *AJR Am J Roentgenol* 1994;162:569, with permission.)

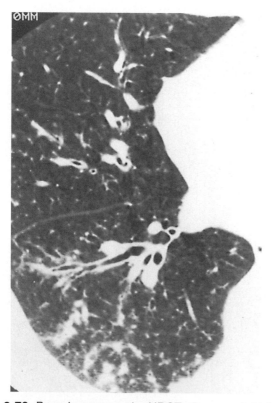

FIG. 3-70. Bronchopneumonia. HRCT shows a right lower lobe bronchopneumonia with ill-defined centrilobular nodules and bronchiolar dilatation. Lower lobe bronchi also appear thick walled.

including five with Wegener's granulomatosis, one with systemic lupus erythematosus, one with scleroderma-polymyositis overlap syndrome, and one with Churg-Strauss syndrome. In these eight children, centrilobular opacities were associated with the onset of active disease or with an exacerbation of preexisting disease. In four of five patients, this abnormality disappeared on treatment.

Pulmonary Hemorrhage. Ill-defined centrilobular nodules may occasionally be seen in patients with acute pulmonary hemorrhage [149]. In children with idiopathic pulmonary hemorrhage, also known as *idiopathic pulmonary hemosiderosis*, recurrent episodes of pulmonary hemorrhage may result in ill-defined centrilobular nodules [121]. This finding may be related to deposition of hemosiderin-laden macrophages in relation to small vessels and bronchioles.

Metastatic Calcification. Metastatic calcification is described in detail in the section Metastatic Calcification. Calcium deposits typically involve the interstitium and alveolar septa in a centrilobular perivascular distribution. Ill-defined nodules of ground-glass opacity or obvious calcifications may be seen. These may be lobular or centrilobular (Fig. 3-106) [150,151].

Pulmonary Hypertension. Cholesterol granulomas may be seen in a centrilobular location in patients with pulmonary hypertension. In one study, histopathologic evidence of cholesterol granulomas was found in five (25%) of 20 patients with severe pulmonary hypertension [152]. In three of these five patients, the granulomas manifested on HRCT as small centrilobular nodules. These may also occur in patients with endogenous lipoid pneumonia and alveolar proteinosis. In patients with pulmonary hypertension and capillary hemangiomatosis, ill-defined centrilobular nodules may also be seen (see Fig. 9-9) [153].

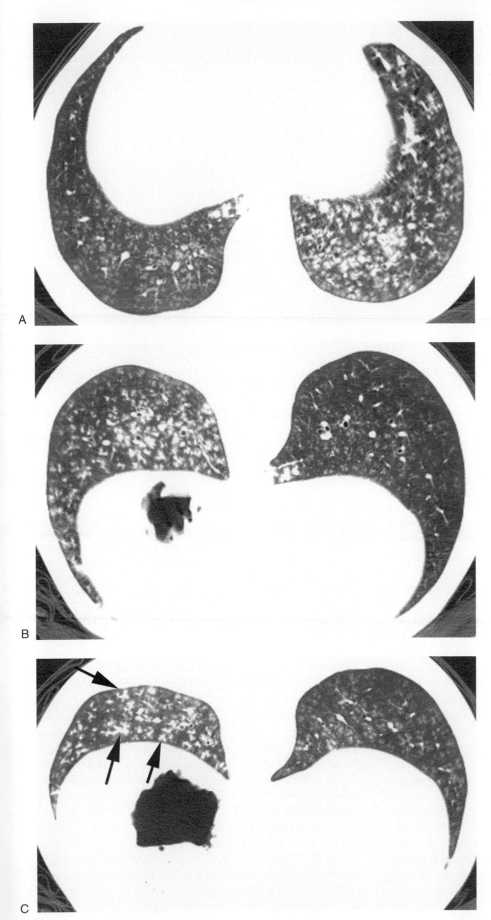

FIG. 3-71. Supine **(A)** and prone **(B and C)** HRCT in a patient with bronchopneumonia due to *Haemophilus influenzae*. Ill-defined centrilobular nodules are visible bilaterally, with a predominance on the left. An appearance of tree-in-bud is visible in many locations (*arrows*, **C**).

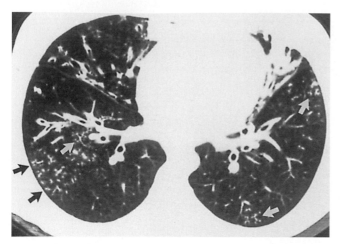

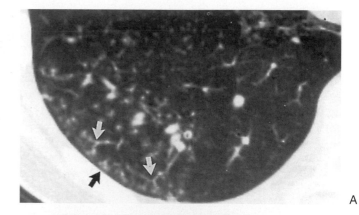

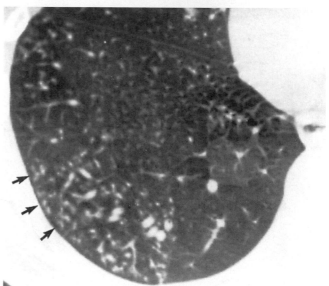

FIG. 3-72. Centrilobular bronchiolar abnormality with tree-in-bud in a patient with cystic fibrosis. Fluid, mucus, or pus-filled centrilobular bronchioles result in a tree-in-bud appearance in several lung regions (*arrows*). These are associated with findings of bronchiectasis.

FIG. 3-73. A,B: Centrilobular bronchiolar abnormality and tree-in-bud in a patient with yellow nails and lymphedema syndrome and chronic bronchial sepsis. A tree-in-bud appearance and small well-defined centrilobular nodules (*arrows*) are visible in the posterior right lower lobe. These reflect the presence of pus-filled centrilobular bronchioles. This appearance is easily contrasted with the appearance of normal lung more medially.

Centrilobular Distribution with Tree-in-Bud

A centrilobular distribution of nodular opacities may be associated with an important finding, termed *tree-in-bud*, which is of great value in differential diagnosis (Table 3-6) [65,107,136,137,154]. The finding of tree-in-bud reflects the presence of dilated centrilobular bronchioles, their lumina impacted with mucus, fluid, or pus, and often associated with peribronchiolar inflammation. Because of the branching pattern of the dilated bronchiole and the presence of ill-defined nodules of peribronchiolar inflammation, its appearance has been likened to a budding or fruiting tree [65,126], or the children's toy jacks [154] (Figs. 3-60, 3-63, 3-66, 3-68, 3-69, 3-71 through 3-75, 3-79, and 3-80). The term *budding tree* has also been used to describe the appearance of small airway filling on bronchography [155].

On HRCT, the finding of tree-in-bud is usually easy to recognize, but several different appearances may be seen alone or in combination. In the lung periphery, tree-in-bud may be associated with a typical branching appearance, with the most peripheral branches or nodular opacities being several millimeters from the pleural surface. Tree-in-bud may also appear as a centrilobular cluster of nodules, depending on the relationship of the bronchiole to the plane of scan. If the centrilobular bronchiole is sectioned across its axis, as is typical in the costophrenic angles, the impacted bronchiole may appear to be a single, well-defined, centrilobular nodule a few millimeters in diameter.

Abnormal bronchioles producing a tree-in-bud pattern can usually be distinguished from normal centrilobular vessels by their more irregular appearance, a lack of tapering, and a knobby or bulbous appearance at the tips of small branches (Figs. 3-79 and 3-80). Normal centrilobular arteries are considerably thinner than the branching bronchioles seen in patients with this finding, and are much less conspicuous.

Furthermore, because tree-in-bud is often patchy in distribution, it is easy to contrast its appearance with that of adjacent normal lung regions.

Tree-in-bud is not usually the only abnormal finding visible on HRCT. Bronchiolar dilatation and wall thickening can sometimes be seen in association with tree-in-bud if the dilated bronchioles are air-filled; normal bronchioles should not be visible in the peripheral 1 cm of lung. Tree-in-bud may also be associated with ill-defined centrilobular nodules representing areas of inflammation (Fig. 3-71). Large airway abnormalities with wall thickening or bronchiectasis are also often present (Fig. 3-72) [107]. For example, in a study by Aquino et al. [137], 26 (96%) of 27 patients showing tree-in-bud on HRCT also showed bronchiectasis or bronchial wall thickening.

The finding of tree-in-bud is indicative of small airways disease. Furthermore, a tree-in-bud appearance is associated

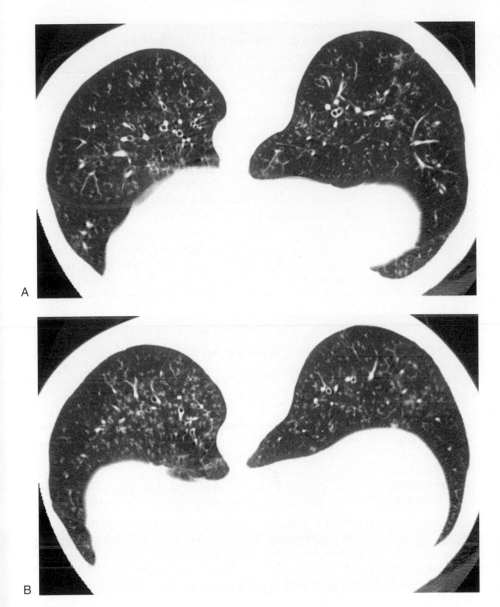

FIG. 3-74. A,B: Prone scans in a patient with chronic bronchiectasis and small airway infection. Small centrilobular nodules, rosettes, and tree-in-bud are visible throughout the lower lobes.

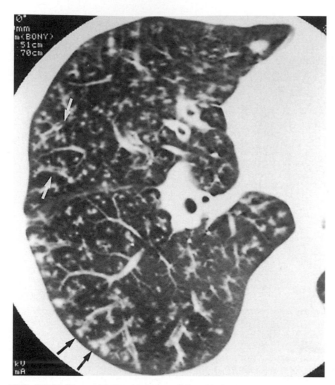

FIG. 3-75. Bronchiolar abnormalities in Asian panbronchiolitis. Dilated and thick-walled bronchioles (*white arrows*) are seen in association with a tree-in-bud appearance (*black arrows*) and multiple centrilobular nodules. These findings correlate pathologically with the presence of dilated bronchioles, inflammatory bronchiolar wall thickening, abundant intraluminal secretions, and peribronchiolar inflammation. (Courtesy of Harumi Itoh, M.D., Chest Disease Research Institute, Kyoto University, Kyoto, Japan.)

with airway infection in the large majority of cases, although it may also be seen in patients with mucoid impaction of centrilobular bronchioles in absence of infection and in some patients with bronchiolar wall infiltration [142]. In a study by Aquino et al. [137], 25% of patients with bronchiectasis and 18% of patients with infectious bronchitis showed tree-in-bud, but this finding was not visible in patients with other diseases involving the airways, such as emphysema, respiratory bronchiolitis, bronchiolitis obliterans, BOOP, or hypersensitivity pneumonitis. Similarly, in patients with active tuberculosis, a tree-in-bud appearance was visible in 72% of patients in one study [65], correlating with the presence of solid caseous material within terminal and respiratory bronchioles (Fig. 3-66). In patients with Asian panbronchiolitis, prominent, branching centrilobular opacities represent dilated bronchioles with inflammatory bronchiolar wall thickening and abundant intraluminal secretions (Fig. 3-75) [126,127].

Thus, in patients with a centrilobular distribution of nodules, if tree-in-bud can be recognized, the differential diagnosis is limited. Among the larger group of diseases causing centrilobular nodules listed in the previous paragraph, tree-in-bud may be seen in patients with endobronchial spread of

tuberculosis [65] or nontuberculous mycobacteria [107], bronchopneumonia, infectious bronchiolitis [123], cystic fibrosis [124], bronchiectasis of any cause [107,136,137], and Asian panbronchiolitis [126,127]. It may also be seen in airway diseases that result in the accumulation of mucus within small bronchi, such as asthma or allergic bronchopulmonary aspergillosis [136], but this finding is less frequent. It is rarely seen in patients with constrictive bronchiolitis, presumably related to impaction of bronchioles [136]. An appearance resembling tree-in-bud has been reported in patients with follicular bronchiolitis, an entity in which hyperplasia of lymphoid follicles occurs in relation to centrilobular airways; it is seen in association with collagen-vascular disease or AIDS [142]. Bronchioloalveolar carcinoma may occasionally show tree-in-bud, although nodules are more typical [146]. In some patients with sarcoidosis, nodules occurring in relation to centrilobular arteries may mimic the appearance of tree-in-bud, although other typical features of sarcoidosis are usually present [107,136].

Algorithmic Approach to Nodule Localization and Diagnosis

A simple algorithm may be used to help localize small nodules as perilymphatic, random, or centrilobular and classify them for the purposes of differential diagnosis (Algorithm 4) [156]. Distinguishing these three distributions is most easily accomplished by looking first for pleural nodules and nodules arising in relation to the fissures.

If subpleural nodules are absent, the pattern is centrilobular. Keep in mind that large centrilobular nodules may touch the pleura but do not appear to arise from it; nodules a few millimeters in diameter that touch the pleura are not centrilobular. If a centrilobular distribution is present, the finding of tree-in-bud should be sought. The differential diagnosis of centrilobular nodules unassociated with tree-in-bud is long and includes airway abnormalities and vascular abnormalities. If tree-in-bud is present, then nearly all cases will represent airway disease, which is infectious in nature.

If numerous subpleural or fissural nodules are present, then the pattern is either perilymphatic or random. These two patterns are distinguished by looking at the distribution of other nodules. If they are patchy in distribution, and particularly if a distinct predominance is noted relative to the peribronchovascular interstitium, interlobular septa, or subpleural regions, then the nodules are perilymphatic. If the nodules are distributed in a diffuse and uniform manner, the pattern is random.

The presence of a few subpleural nodules is nonspecific and may be seen regardless of the pattern. A few subpleural nodules that look different than the other visible nodules (i.e., smaller, denser, or better defined) are likely unrelated to the patient's disease and should be ignored, whereas subpleural nodules that appear similar to other visible nodules are of potential significance in differential diagnosis. If a few subpleural nodules are visible, a determination of the

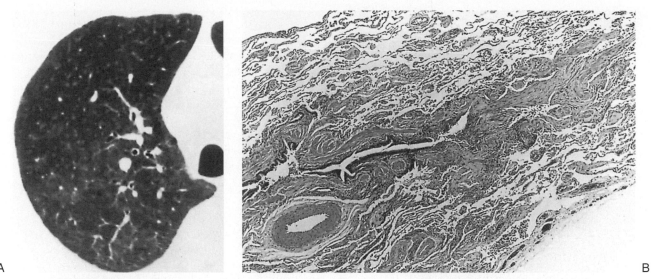

FIG. 3-76. Bronchiolitis obliterans organizing pneumonia (BOOP) with ill-defined centrilobular nodules. **A:** Multifocal areas of ill-defined opacity are present in the right upper lobe. Note that small pulmonary artery branches are partially obscured by the centrilobular opacities. **B:** Open lung biopsy showed features of BOOP. Bronchioles are compressed and occluded by granulation tissue; organizing pneumonia and loose connective tissue are also present, surrounding the bronchioles. (From Gruden JF, Webb WR, et al. Centrilobular opacities in the lung on HRCT: diagnostic considerations and pathologic correlation. *AJR Am J Roentgenol* 1994;162:569, with permission.)

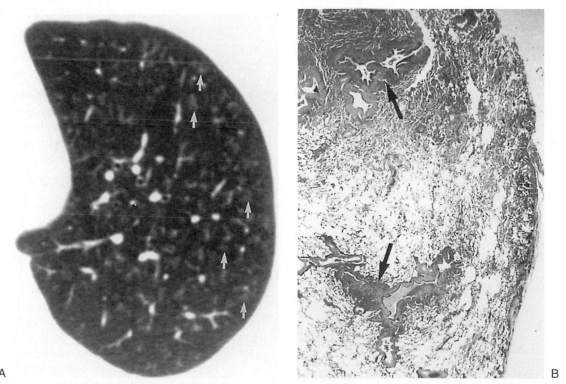

FIG. 3-77. Bronchiolitis obliterans organizing pneumonia with centrilobular opacities. **A:** Ill-defined nodular opacities (*arrows*) are scattered throughout the left upper lobe in this patient who had received an allogenic bone marrow transplant several years previously. Their centrilobular location can be inferred in that they surround small artery branches. **B:** Open lung biopsy shows bronchioles (*arrows*) partially occluded by plugs of granulation tissue. Inflammation surrounding the bronchioles probably accounts for the opacities seen on HRCT. (From Gruden JF, Webb WR, et al. Centrilobular opacities in the lung on HRCT: diagnostic considerations and pathologic correlation. *AJR Am J Roentgenol* 1994;162:569, with permission.)

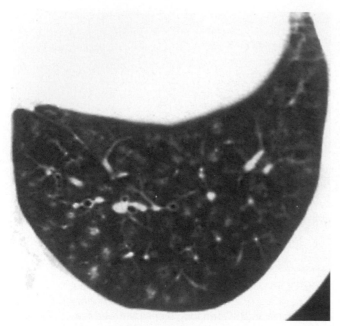

FIG. 3-78. Endobronchial spread of tracheobronchial papillomatosis. Multiple small, ill-defined, centrilobular nodules are present in the posterior left lower lobe. Many appear to be approximately 1 cm from the pleural surface or are related to small vessels.

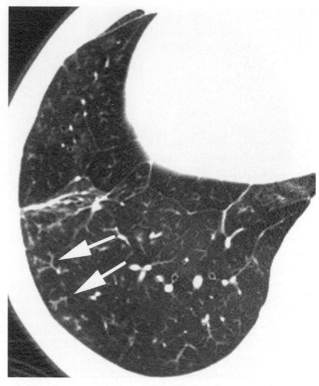

FIG. 3-79. Tree-in-bud in a patient with airway infection. Branching, impacted, pus-filled bronchioles (*arrows*) are visible in the peripheral lung. A parenchymal band seen more anteriorly represents focal atelectasis.

distribution and differential diagnosis should generally be based on other findings, such as tree-in-bud (i.e., centrilobular airways disease), patchy distribution (i.e., perilymphatic or centrilobular disease), predominant involvement of the peribronchovascular interstitium or interlobular septa (i.e., perilymphatic), or nodules of ground-glass opacity (centrilobular).

Accuracy of High-Resolution Computed Tomography in Nodule Localization

HRCT is accurate in localizing nodules according to their anatomic distribution, thus limiting the differential diagnosis. In a study by Gruden et al. [105], the interobserver vari-

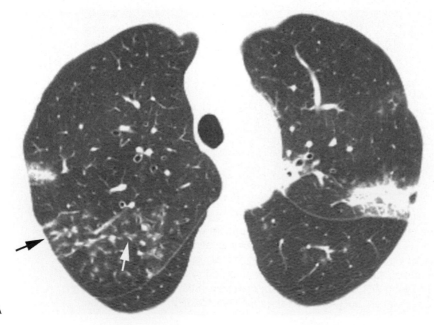

FIG. 3-80. Tree-in-bud in a patient with *Mycobacterium avium* complex infection. **A:** In addition to patchy consolidation, branching centrilobular structures (*arrows*) in the right lung are typical of tree-in-bud, and strongly suggest the presence of infection. Tree-in-bud can be distinguished from normal branching arteries because of their more irregular appearance, lack of tapering, and a knobby or bulbous appearance. *Continued*

A

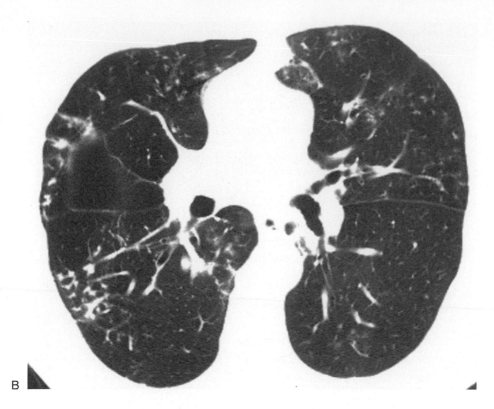

FIG. 3-80. *Continued* **B:** At a lower level, centrilobular nodules and tree-in-bud are visible in several locations.

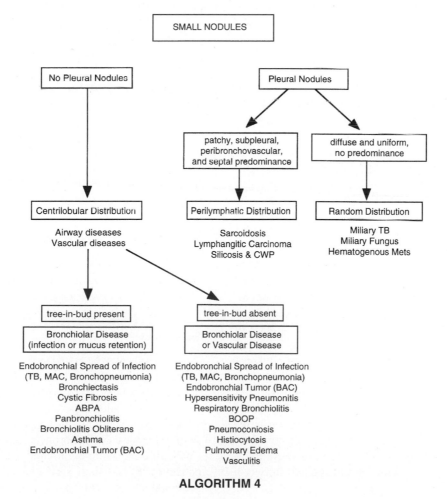

ALGORITHM 4

TABLE 3-7. *Differential diagnosis of large nodules and masses*

Diagnosis	Comments
Sarcoidosis	Common; upper lobe and peribronchovascular predominance; confluent masses of granulomas (active disease) or fibrous tissue (end-stage disease)
Silicosis/coal worker's pneumoconiosis	Common in advanced disease; upper lobe; associated with surrounding emphysema
Talcosis	Conglomerate masses of fibrous tissue; upper lobe and perihilar predominance; high-attenuation common
Langerhans histiocytosis	Large nodules in 20%
Metastatic carcinoma	Peripheral and basal predominance common
Diffuse bronchioloalveolar carcinoma	Large nodules in 30%; ill defined; basal predominance
Lymphoma	Commonly contain air bronchograms
Lymphoproliferative disease	Large nodules common; air bronchograms; often peribronchovascular or subpleural
Bronchiolitis obliterans organizing pneumonia	Uncommon
Wegener's granulomatosis	Common manifestation; cavitation common
Churg-Strauss syndrome	Cavitation may be present
Amyloidosis	Smooth or lobulated; cavitation in 20%
Infection	Fungal infection in immunosuppressed patient
Rounded atelectasis	Associated with asbestos pleural disease

ability and accuracy of the algorithm described (i.e., Algorithm 4) was assessed; four experienced chest radiologists independently evaluated HRCT images in 58 patients with nodular lung disease [105]. Nodules were classified as perilymphatic, random, centrilobular, or associated with tree-in-bud and small airways disease. The observers were correct in 218 (94%) of 232 localizations in the 58 cases. Three of four observers agreed in 56 (97%) of 58 cases, and all four observers agreed in 79% (46 of 58) of the cases. The most noteworthy source of error and of disagreement between observers was the confusion of perilymphatic and small airways disease–associated nodules in a small number of cases.

In another study [106], HRCT findings were compared to those from pathologic examination in 40 consecutive patients with diffuse micronodular lung disease. HRCT scans were analyzed with particular attention to the location of nodules (i.e., centrilobular, perilymphatic, and random) and their zonal distribution. HRCT scans showed centrilobular nodules in patients with diffuse panbronchiolitis (n = 4), infectious bronchiolitis (n = 4), hypersensitivity pneumonitis (n = 3), endobronchial spread of tuberculosis (n = 3), pneumoconiosis (n = 1), primary lymphoma of the lung (n = 1), and foreign body–induced necrotizing vasculitis (n = 1). They demonstrated perilymphatic nodules in patients with pneumoconiosis (n = 5), sarcoidosis (n = 2), and amyloidosis (n = 2). HRCT demonstrated micronodules of random distribution in the patients with miliary tuberculosis (n = 9) and pulmonary metastasis (n = 5). An upper- and middle-zonal predominance was seen in patients with sarcoidosis and in two of six patients with pneumoconiosis.

Large Nodules and Masses

The term *large nodule* is used in this book to refer to rounded opacities that are 1 cm or more in diameter. The term *mass* is generally used to describe nodular lesions larger than 3 cm in diameter [6,157]. Nodules approximating 1 cm may be seen in many small nodular lung diseases and are nonspecific. Furthermore, in patients with small nodular diseases, larger nodules or masses may sometimes be seen, representing conglomerate masses; these are common in sarcoidosis, silicosis, and talcosis (Table 3-7). Some diffuse lung diseases result in large nodules as a primary manifestation of the disease (Table 3-7).

Conglomerate Nodules or Masses in Diffuse Lung Disease

In patients who have diseases characterized by small nodules, conglomeration or confluence of nodules can result in large nodular or masslike opacities [90].

Sarcoidosis

Sarcoidosis may be associated with the presence of confluent nodules larger than 1 cm in diameter in half of all sarcoidosis patients [77]. In our experience, these predominate in the upper lobes and the peribronchovascular regions (Figs. 3-48 and 3-81). These nodules or masses are often irregular in shape, surround central bronchi and vessels, and can show small, discrete nodules at their periphery (Fig. 3-81). In patients with end-stage sarcoidosis, it is not uncommon to see conglomerate masses in the upper lobes associated with

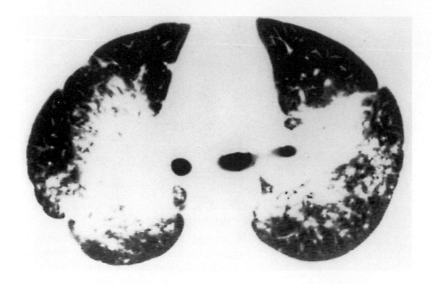

FIG. 3-81. Conglomerate masses of nodules in a patient with sarcoidosis. These masses, which surround central bronchi and vessels, show small discrete nodules at their margins.

central crowding of vessels and bronchi as a result of peribronchovascular fibrosis (Figs. 3-6 and 3-82). Traction bronchiectasis is often visible within the masses of fibrous tissue, and posterior displacement of upper lobe bronchi is commonly present. Adjacent areas of emphysema or bullae are visible in some cases. Similar upper lobe masses associated with bronchiectasis have been reported in patients with tuberculosis and are most frequent after treatment [65].

Silicosis

Patients who have silicosis and coal workers who have complicated pneumoconiosis or progressive massive fibrosis also show conglomerate masses in the upper lobes, but these are typically of homogeneous opacity and tend to be unassociated with visible traction bronchiectasis, as seen in sarcoidosis (Fig. 3-83) [58,94]. Also, areas of emphysema peripheral to the conglomerate masses are

common. This finding is present in as many as 48% of patients with CWP [58].

Talcosis

An appearance of progressive massive fibrosis very similar to that occurring in patients with silicosis or sarcoidosis can be seen in intravenous drug users who develop talcosis from injection of talc-containing substances [147]. The fibrotic masses can show high attenuation at soft-tissue windows, indicating the presence of talc (see Fig. 5-58). A perihilar and upper lobe predominance has been reported.

Langerhans Histiocytosis

Large nodules have been seen in as many as 24% of patients with Langerhans histiocytosis, although masses are not generally seen in this disease [77].

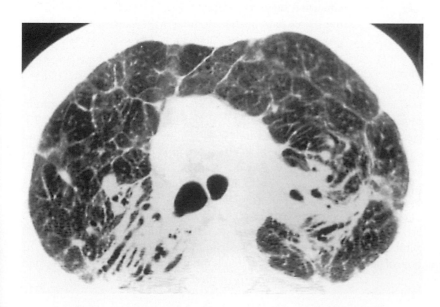

FIG. 3-82. Sarcoidosis with peribronchovascular fibrosis associated with traction bronchiectasis. Volume loss, interlobular septal thickening, and parenchymal bands are also evident.

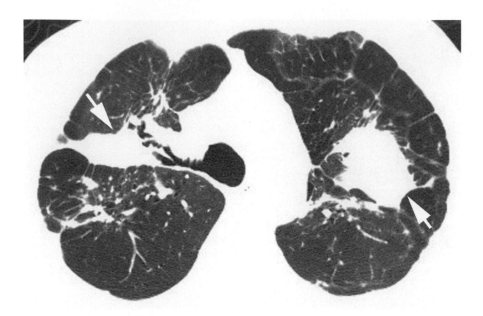

FIG. 3-83. Conglomerate masses of fibrosis in silicosis. Central areas of peribronchovascular fibrosis (*arrows*) are associated with small nodules, typical of silicosis, and distortion of lung architecture.

Large Nodules in Diffuse Infiltrative Lung Diseases

Several subacute or chronic infiltrative lung diseases may be characterized by large nodules as the primary manifestation of disease.

Metastatic Carcinoma

Metastatic carcinoma commonly results in large nodules or masses [146,158,159]. They may be well-defined or ill-defined, and they typically have a peripheral and basal predominance. Large nodules or masses may sometimes be seen in patients with neoplasms being assessed using HRCT, but spiral CT is more appropriate if large nodules are visible on chest radiographs. Primary lung cancer presenting as a large solitary nodule or mass may sometimes be associated with other findings evaluated using HRCT, such as lymphangitic spread of carcinoma.

Diffuse Bronchioloalveolar Carcinoma

Diffuse bronchioloalveolar carcinoma shows a pattern of multiple nodules, up to 3 cm in size, in approximately 30% of cases [146]. Half of the cases have a peripheral or lower lobe predominance. Nodules are most often ill-defined or associated with a halo sign. Cavitation of nodules is sometimes present.

Lymphoma

Lymphoma involving the lung most commonly results in airspace consolidation (66% of cases) and large nodules (41% of cases) [114], often ill-defined and sometimes containing air bronchograms [160]. In most instances, spiral CT, rather than HRCT, is most appropriate in evaluation of a patient with lymphoma [15,161].

Lymphoproliferative Disorders

Lymphoproliferative disorders, often associated with the Epstein-Barr virus, may range from benign lymphoid hyperplasia to high-grade lymphoma and occur in immunosuppressed patients (e.g., those with AIDS, congenital immune deficiency, or receiving immunosuppressive therapy). The most common CT manifestation consists of multiple nodules, 2 to 4 cm in diameter, frequently in a predominantly peribronchovascular or subpleural distribution [162]. In a review of 246 patients who had lung transplantation [163], nine patients (4%) were diagnosed with posttransplantation lymphoproliferative disorders. The most common abnormality visible on CT was the presence of multiple, well-defined pulmonary nodules ranging up to 3 cm in diameter. These nodules, when multiple, had basilar and peripheral predominance. Other abnormal features included hilar or mediastinal adenopathy. Three patients had nodules with a surrounding area of ground-glass opacity ("halo sign").

Bronchiolitis Obliterans Organizing Pneumonia

Multiple large nodules or masses are an uncommon manifestation of BOOP, but may be seen (see Fig. 6-30) [164]. Akira et al. [164] reviewed the HRCT scans and clinical records of 59 consecutive patients with histologically proven BOOP; 12 patients had multiple large nodules or masses. Of 60 lesions found in the 12 patients, 53 (88%) had an irregular margin, 27 (45%) had an air bronchogram, 23 (38%) had a pleural tail, and 21 (35%) had a spiculated margin. Ancillary findings included focal thickening of the interlobular septa in five (42%) of the 12 patients, pleural thickening in four (33%) patients, and parenchymal bands in three (25%) patients.

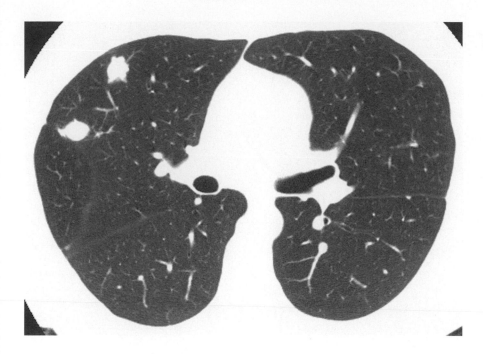

FIG. 3-84. Large lung nodules in Wegener's granulomatosis. These are nonspecific in appearance.

Wegener's Granulomatosis

Wegener's granulomatosis is typically manifested by multiple nodules that are usually limited in number, range in size from a few millimeters to 10 cm in diameter, have no zonal predominance, and have a random distribution (Fig. 3-84) [165–167]. Masses may also appear peribronchial or peribronchovascular in distribution [168]. In a study of ten patients [167], CT scans revealed multiple pulmonary nodules in seven patients and a single nodule in one. The nodules ranged in diameter from 2 mm to 7 cm, and most had irregular margins. Ill-defined centrilobular nodules, likely reflecting the presence of vasculitis, have also been reported [148]. Cavitation of nodules is common, being present in all nodules larger than 2 cm in one study [167]; the cavity walls are often thick and irregular or shaggy, although thin-walled cavities may also be seen. Consolidation may also be associated, usually related to pulmonary hemorrhage.

Churg-Strauss Syndrome

Churg-Strauss syndrome is most often characterized by parenchymal opacification (consolidation or ground-glass attenuation), but pulmonary nodules may be present with or without cavitation [169].

Amyloidosis

Large pulmonary nodules are common in patients with localized amyloidosis [170], ranging in size from 8 mm to 3 cm [59]. Nodules may be solitary (60% of cases) or multiple, with a smooth or lobular contour, and are often subpleural or peripheral. Calcification may occur (20% of cases) [59].

Infections

Infections, particularly in immunosuppressed patients and usually representing a fungus, may be manifested by multiple large nodules or masses. Nodules are often ill-defined and may be associated with cavitation, air bronchograms, or a surrounding halo of ground-glass opacity (i.e., the "halo sign"). In a study of immunosuppressed patients with fever, large nodules shown on CT predicted the presence of a fungal infection [171]. Invasive aspergillosis is most common in neutropenic patients, typically showing scattered nodules that are often associated with vessels, the halo sign, and cavitation during later stages of the infection [172]. Although the halo sign can be associated with a variety of infectious processes, including tuberculosis [173], candidiasis, *Legionella pneumonia*, cytomegalovirus, or herpes simplex [174] in a neutropenic patient, it should suggest invasive aspergillosis [175].

Rounded Atelectasis

Rounded atelectasis represents a focal, collapsed, and often folded region of lung [64,176–178]. It almost always occurs in association with ipsilateral pleural disease and typically contacts the pleural surface. Rounded atelectasis occurs most commonly in the paravertebral regions of the posterior lung and may be bilateral. Bending or bowing of adjacent bronchi and arteries toward the area of atelectasis because of volume loss or folding of lung is characteristic. This appearance has been likened to a comet tail. Air bronchograms within the mass can sometimes be seen. In the presence of pleural disease and these typical findings, the diagnosis can usually be suggested. Focal fibrotic masses, usually irregular in shape, have been described as occurring

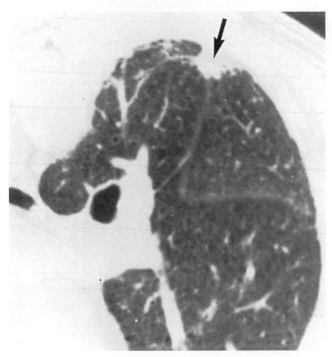

FIG. 3-85. Peripheral fibrotic mass in a patient with pulmonary fibrosis. The focal fibrotic mass (*arrow*) is irregular in shape and associated with other findings of fibrosis.

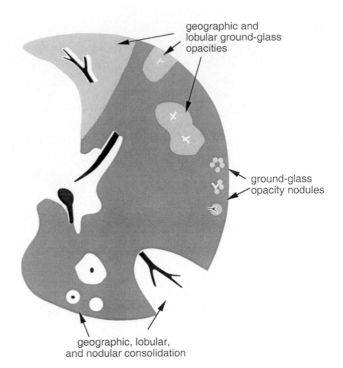

FIG. 3-86. HRCT appearances of increased lung opacity. Ground-glass opacity does not result in obscuration of underlying vessels, whereas consolidation does. Both can be associated with air bronchograms and can be nodular, lobular, or patchy and geographic.

in the peripheral lung in relation to pleural abnormalities in patients with asbestos exposure [64]. These represent focal areas of scarring or rounded atelectasis (Fig. 3-85).

INCREASED LUNG OPACITY

Increased lung opacity, or parenchymal opacification, is a common finding on HRCT in patients with chronic lung disease. Increased lung opacity is generally described as being ground-glass opacity or consolidation [5,6,157] (Fig. 3-86). Lung calcification may also result in increased attenuation.

Ground-Glass Opacity

Ground-glass opacity, or *ground-glass attenuation*, is a nonspecific term referring to the presence on HRCT of a hazy increase in lung opacity that is not associated with obscuration of underlying vessels (Figs. 3-86 and 3-87); if vessels are obscured, the term *consolidation* is generally used [5,6,157]. This finding can reflect the presence of a number of diseases and can be seen in patients with minimal airspace disease (Fig. 3-88), interstitial thickening (Fig. 3-89), or both [3,73,135,179–183].

Ground-glass opacity results from the volume averaging of morphologic abnormalities too small to be clearly resolved by HRCT [73,181–183]. It can reflect the presence of minimal thickening of the "septal" or alveolar interstitium, thickening of alveolar walls, or the presence of cells or fluid partially filling the alveolar spaces. Ground-glass opac-

ity has been seen in patients with histologic findings of mild or early interstitial inflammation or infiltration [72,135]. Also, when a small amount of fluid is present within the alveoli, as can occur in the early stages of an airspace filling disease, the fluid tends to layer against the alveolar walls and is indistinguishable on HRCT from alveolar wall thickening [102]. In a study comparing the results of lung biopsy with HRCT in 22 patients who showed ground-glass opacity, 14%

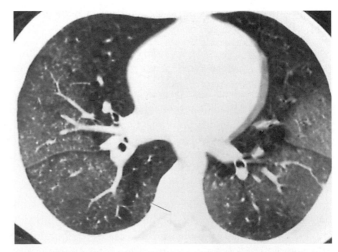

FIG. 3-87. Ground-glass opacity in a 16-year-old boy with Goodpasture's syndrome and pulmonary hemorrhage.

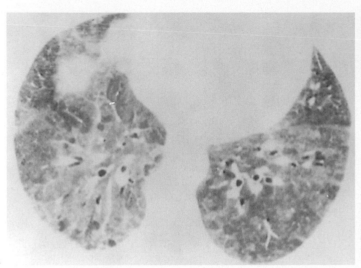
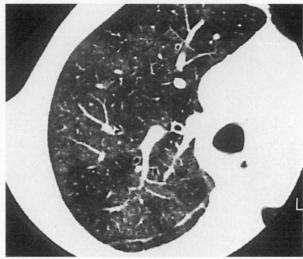

A

B

FIG. 3-88. *Pneumocystis carinii* pneumonia with ground-glass opacity. **A:** In one patient, ground-glass opacity is extensive but patchy in distribution. **B:** In another patient, who had a normal chest radiograph, minimal patchy ground-glass opacity is visible.

had diseases primarily affecting airspaces, 32% had a mixed interstitial and airspace abnormality, and 54% had a primarily interstitial abnormality [135]. The term *ground-glass opacity* may also be used to refer to increased lung density resulting from increased capillary blood volume, although this is better termed *mosaic perfusion* if the etiology of the lung attenuation abnormality is known [6]. The appearance of mosaic perfusion is described below.

Ground-glass opacity is difficult to recognize if it is of minimal severity and diffuse in distribution, involving all of the lung to an equal degree. However, this abnormality is almost always patchy in distribution, affecting some lung regions whereas others appear to be spared; this "geographic" appearance of the lung parenchyma makes it easier to detect and diagnose with confidence (Figs. 3-89 through 3-91). In some patients, entire lobules may appear abnormally dense, whereas adjacent lobules appear normal. In others, the abnormal ground-glass opacities are centrilobular and peribronchiolar in location (Fig. 3-62), resulting in the appearance of ill-defined centrilobular nodules [3,43,102,104,130,184]. Ground-glass opacity can involve individual segments and lobes, can involve nonsegmental regions of lung (Fig. 3-92), or may be diffuse (Fig. 3-93). The presence of air-filled bronchi that appear "too black" within an area of lung can also be a clue as to the presence of ground-glass opacity (Figs. 3-92 and 3-93A); this dark bronchus appearance is essentially that of an air bronchogram.

Significance and Differential Diagnosis of Ground-Glass Opacity

Ground-glass opacity is a highly significant finding, as it often indicates the presence of an ongoing, active, and potentially treatable process. In patients with acute symptoms, the association of ground-glass opacity with active disease is very high. For example, in patients with AIDS and acute respiratory distress, ground-glass opacity visible on HRCT accurately predicts the presence of *P. carinii* pneumonia [156].

In patients who have subacute or chronic symptoms, ground-glass opacity also indicates the likelihood of active disease, although in this setting fibrosis may also result in this finding. Of the 22 patients with ground-glass opacity studied by Leung et al. [135], 18 (82%) were considered to have active or potentially reversible disease on lung biopsy. In a similar study by Remy-Jardin et al. [72], HRCT findings were correlated with histology at 37 biopsy sites in 26 patients. In 24 (65%) of the 37 biopsies, they found that ground-glass opacity corresponded to the presence of inflammation that exceeded or was equal to fibrosis in degree. In eight biopsies (22%), inflammation was present but fibrosis predominated, whereas in the remaining five (13%), fibrosis was the sole histologic finding. Because of its association with active lung disease, the presence of ground-glass opacity often leads to further diagnostic evaluation, including lung biopsy, depending on the clinical status of the patient. Also, when a lung biopsy is performed, areas of ground-glass opacity can be targeted by the surgeon or bronchoscopist. Because such areas are most likely to be active, they are most likely to yield diagnostic material.

Because ground-glass opacity can reflect the presence of either fibrosis or inflammation, one should be careful to diagnose an active process only when ground-glass opacity is unassociated with HRCT findings of fibrosis or is the predominant finding (Figs. 3-90 through 3-94). If ground-glass opacity is seen only in lung regions that also show significant HRCT findings of fibrosis, such as traction bron-

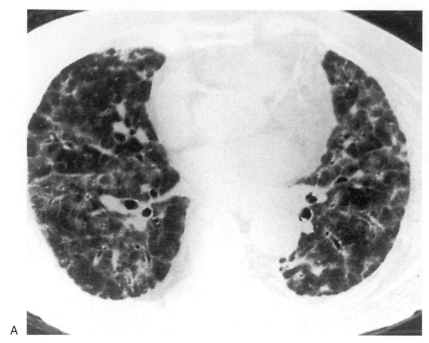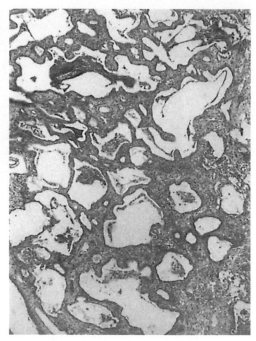

A   B

FIG. 3-89. Ground-glass opacity associated with interstitial fibrosis. **A:** HRCT shows patchy areas of ground-glass opacity. **B:** Biopsy specimen shows the abnormality to consist of alveolar wall thickening and fibrosis, with little airspace abnormality. (From Leung AN, Miller RR, et al. Parenchymal opacification in chronic infiltrative lung diseases: CT-pathologic correlation. *Radiology* 1993;188:209, with permission.)

chiectasis or honeycombing, it is most likely that fibrosis will be the predominant histologic abnormality (Figs. 3-89 and 3-95). For example, in a study by Remy-Jardin et al. [72], patients showing traction bronchiectasis or bronchiolectasis on HRCT in regions of ground-glass opacity all had fibrosis on lung biopsy. On the other hand, in patients without traction bronchiectasis in areas of ground-glass opacity, 92% were found to have active inflammatory disease on lung biopsy.

A large number of diseases can be associated with ground-glass opacity on HRCT. In many, this reflects the presence of similar histologic reactions in the early or active stages of disease, with inflammatory exudates involving the alveolar septa and alveolar spaces, although this pattern can be the result of a variety of pathologic processes.

When considering the differential diagnosis of ground-glass opacity, it is important to know whether the patient's symptoms are acute, subacute, or chronic (Table 3-8). Among those causes of ground-glass opacity typically having an acute presentation are AIP (see Figs. 6-40 through 6-43) [185] or other causes of diffuse alveolar damage (Fig. 3-92), or the adult respiratory distress syndrome (ARDS); pulmonary edema of various causes (see Figs. 6-73 and 6-74) [27,28]; pulmonary hemorrhage (Fig. 3-87) [149]; pneumonias of all types, but particularly *P. carinii* pneumonia (Figs. 3-88 and 3-93) [27,156,186–188] (Fig. 3-58), viral pneumonias (e.g., cytomegalovirus) (see Fig.

6-62) [189], and mycoplasma pneumonia (see Fig. 6-65) [190]; acute eosinophilic pneumonia [191]; and early radiation pneumonitis [33,184,192].

The most common causes of ground-glass opacity in patients having subacute or chronic symptoms (Table 3-8) include interstitial pneumonias such as NSIP or UIP (Fig.

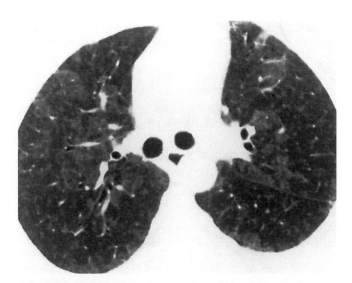

FIG. 3-90. Patchy areas of subtle ground-glass opacity in a patient with hypersensitivity pneumonitis.

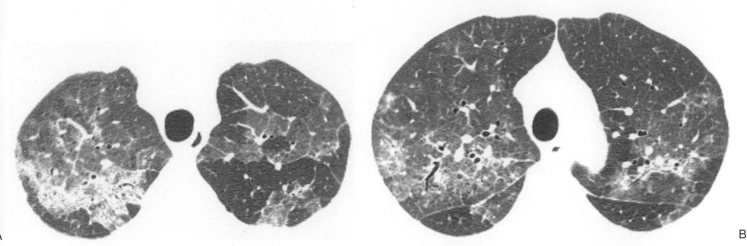

FIG. 3-91. A,B: Patchy ground-glass opacity associated with hypersensitivity pneumonitis. Abnormalities had an upper lobe predominance.

3-94), either idiopathic or associated with specific diseases, such as scleroderma or other collagen-vascular diseases [22,69,72,135,143]; DIP [193]; respiratory bronchiolitis interstitial lung disease (RB-ILD) (see Figs. 6-34 and 6-35) [109,138,139]; hypersensitivity pneumonitis (Figs. 3-90 and 3-91) [72,130–132]; BOOP (Fig. 3-100) [72,135]; chronic eosinophilic pneumonia [55]; Churg-Strauss syndrome [169]; lipoid pneumonia [194]; bronchioloalveolar carcinoma [195]; sarcoidosis (see Figs. 5-40 and 5-41) [56,72,90,135,196]; and alveolar proteinosis (Figs. 3-11 and 3-96) [51–53,197].

In patients with ground-glass opacity, the nature of the histologic abnormalities associated with this finding varies according to the typical histologic features of the disease; no specific histology is associated with this finding (Table 3-9) [97,109,130,135,198,199]. In patients with UIP due to IPF,

NSIP, scleroderma, or other collagen-vascular diseases, a number of studies have correlated the presence of ground-glass opacity on HRCT with biopsy results, response to treatment, and patient survival [8,73,143,179,182,183,193,200–202]. In histologic studies of patients with interstitial pneumonia, ground-glass opacity has been shown to be associated with the presence of alveolar wall or intraalveolar inflammation in most. For example, in a study of scleroderma patients by Wells et al. [182], increased opacity on HRCT correlated with predominant inflammation on biopsy in four of seven cases, whereas reticulation on HRCT indicated fibrosis in 12 of 13 [182]. In another study, of 14 patients with IPF and ground-glass opacity on HRCT, 12 had inflammation on biopsy [135]. In patients with UIP, ground-glass opacity is associated with alveolar septal inflammation, varying numbers of intraalveolar histiocytes, and varying degrees of fibro-

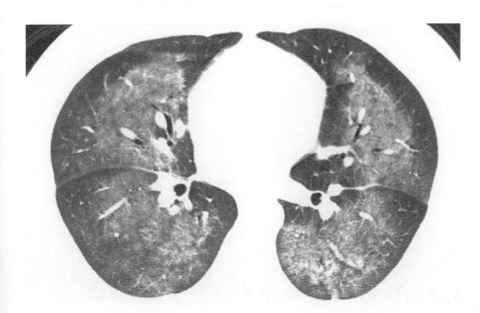

FIG. 3-92. Extensive perihilar ground-glass opacity associated with acute lung injury and diffuse alveolar damage related to smoking cocaine. This abnormality was transient and cleared within 2 weeks.

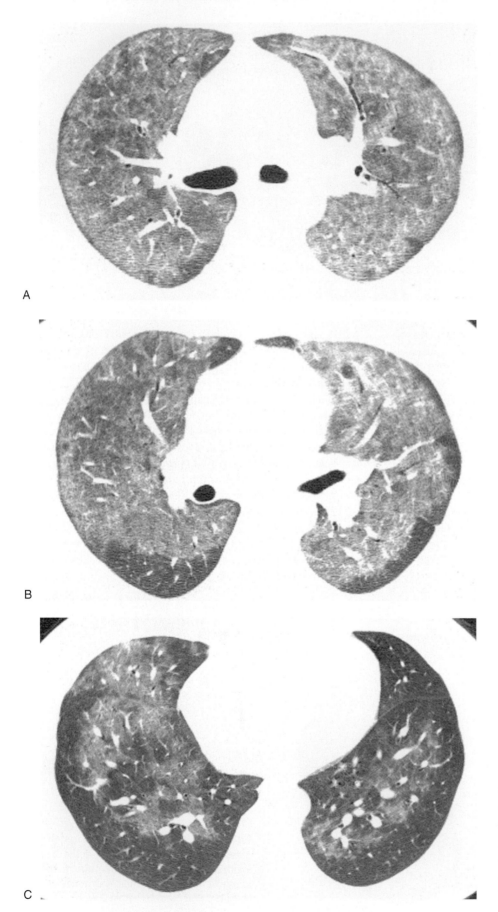

A

B

C

FIG. 3-93. A–C: HRCT at three levels in a patient with *Pneumocystis carinii* pneumonia associated with acquired immunodeficiency syndrome. Diffuse ground-glass opacity predominates in the upper lobes and perihilar regions **(A)**. In the lower lobes **(C)**, ground-glass opacity is more patchy in distribution.

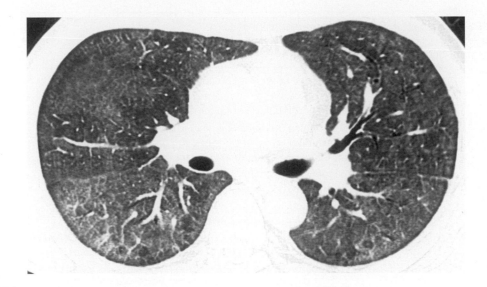

FIG. 3-94. Patchy ground-glass opacity in a patient with nonspecific interstitial pneumonia. A posterior and subpleural predominance is present. Findings of fibrosis, such as traction bronchiectasis, are absent.

sis; ground-glass opacity in patients with DIP largely reflects the presence of macrophages within alveoli [8,135,182,193].

Crazy-Paving Pattern

In some patients with ground-glass opacity visible on HRCT, superimposition of a reticular pattern results in an appearance termed *crazy-paving* [51]. This pattern was first recognized in patients with pulmonary alveolar proteinosis (PAP) (Figs. 3-11 and 3-96) [51] and is quite typical of PAP, but may also be seen in patients with a variety of other diseases [54,55]. In patients with crazy-paving, ground-glass opacity may reflect the presence of airspace or interstitial abnormalities; the reticular opacities may represent interlobular septal thickening, thickening of the intralobular interstitium, irregular areas of fibrosis, or a preponderance of an airspace-filling process at the periphery of lobules or acini [55].

The differential diagnosis of crazy-paving includes diseases considered to be primarily airspace or interstitial and mixed (Table 3-10) [54,55]. These include PAP (Fig. 3-96) [51,53]; pulmonary edema [28]; pulmonary hemorrhage (Fig. 3-97) [149]; ARDS [54]; AIP; diffuse alveolar damage; pneumonias due to *P. carinii* (Fig. 3-98), virus (e.g., cytomegalovirus) (Fig. 3-99), mycoplasma, bacteria, and tuberculosis; BOOP (Fig. 3-100); chronic eosinophilic pneumonia; acute eosinophilic pneumonia [191]; Churg-Strauss syndrome [169], radiation pneumonitis [33], or drug-related pneumonitis; bronchioloalveolar carcinoma (Fig. 3-101) [195]; and lipoid pneumonia [194]. Clearly, the differential diagnosis of a crazy-paving pattern must be based on a consideration of clinical as well as HRCT findings, and knowledge of whether symptoms are acute or chronic (Table 3-10).

In the study by Johkoh et al. [55] of 46 patients showing the crazy-paving pattern on HRCT, the most common causes included ARDS (n = 8), bacterial pneumonia (n = 7),

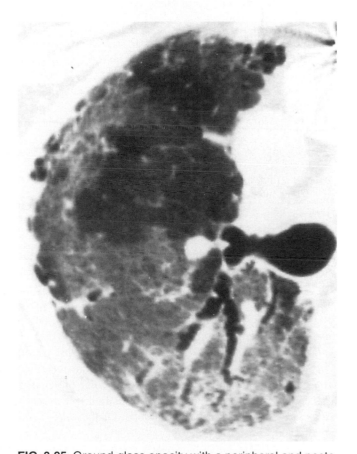

FIG. 3-95. Ground-glass opacity with a peripheral and posterior predominance in a patient with idiopathic pulmonary fibrosis. In addition to the increased lung opacity, there is evidence of increased reticulation, traction bronchiectasis, and some subpleural honeycombing. These findings indicate the presence of fibrosis. End-stage fibrosis was found on biopsy, without evidence of active disease.

TABLE 3-8. *Differential diagnosis of ground-glass opacity*

Diagnosis	Course	Comments
Acute interstitial pneumonia; adult respiratory distress syndrome	Acute	Always present; consolidation common; patchy or diffuse
Pulmonary edema	Acute	Diffuse or centrilobular; septal thickening sometimes present
Pulmonary hemorrhage	Acute	Patchy or diffuse; septal thickening sometimes present
Pneumonia (e.g., *Pneumocystis carinii*, viral, *Mycoplasma* pneumonias)	Acute	Common; diffuse or patchy; centrilobular nodules; consolidation or septal thickening may also be present
Acute eosinophilic pneumonia	Acute	Diffuse; respiratory failure common
Radiation pneumonitis	Acute	Extent usually corresponds to radiation ports
Nonspecific interstitial pneumonia	Subacute, chronic	Common; patchy; subpleural; reticular opacities often associated; multiple causes including collagen diseases
Usual interstitial pneumonia and idiopathic pulmonary fibrosis	Subacute, chronic	Common in association with findings of fibrosis; uncommon as an isolated finding; subpleural and basal predominance
Desquamative interstitial pneumonia	Subacute, chronic	Always present; diffuse or patchy; findings of fibrosis less common than in usual interstitial pneumonia
Respiratory bronchiolitis interstitial lung disease	Subacute, chronic	Always present; patchy and localized; may be centrilobular; fibrosis uncommon
Hypersensitivity pneumonitis	Subacute, chronic	Very common; patchy or nodular; can be centrilobular; consolidation and air-trapping may also be present
Bronchiolitis obliterans organizing pneumonia	Subacute, chronic	Common; consolidation may also be present; often predominant in peripheral regions; can be nodular
Chronic eosinophilic pneumonia	Subacute, chronic	Consolidation more common; patchy or nodular; peripheral predominance
Churg-Strauss syndrome	Subacute, chronic	Consolidation also present; nodular
Bronchioloalveolar carcinoma (diffuse)	Subacute, chronic	Diffuse, patchy, or centrilobular; consolidation common
Lipoid pneumonia	Subacute, chronic	Patchy or lobular; low-attenuation consolidation may be present
Sarcoidosis	Subacute, chronic	Uncommon manifestation due to confluence of very small granulomas
Alveolar proteinosis	Subacute, chronic	Very common; patchy or diffuse; septal thickening common; fibrosis rare

AIP (n = 5), and, despite its rarity, alveolar proteinosis (n = 5). Of these common causes of crazy-paving, it is worth noting that only PAP presents with subacute or chronic symptoms, and ARDS, bacterial pneumonia, and AIP are not commonly studied using HRCT in clinical practice. Also, the highest prevalences of crazy-paving in this study were seen in PAP (100%), diffuse alveolar damage (67%), AIP (31%), and ARDS (21%) [55].

In a prospective study of patients showing this pattern [54], a variety of causes of crazy-paving were identified. These included *P. carinii* pneumonia, alveolar proteinosis, UIP, pulmonary hemorrhage, acute radiation pneumonitis, ARDS, and drug-induced pneumonitis. Of these, *P. carinii* pneumonia was most common.

Algorithmic Approach to the Diagnosis of Ground-Glass Opacity

If ground-glass opacity is associated with significant reticulation, the reticular pattern should be identified (Algorithm 5). If honeycombing or traction bronchiectasis is present in areas of increased attenuation, fibrosis is very likely present, and the differential diagnosis is that of honeycombing. If the reticular pattern is that of interlobular septal thickening, crazy-paving is present (Table 3-10). If the only reticular pattern present is that of intralobular interstitial thickening, fibrosis is likely present if opacities are peripheral and subpleural (i.e., as in IPF), but the pattern is nonspecific. Ground-glass opacity unassociated with reticulation, as with crazy-paving, likely represents active disease. In this situation, a specific diagnosis is difficult to make, but the differential diagnosis is based, at least to some extent, on the distribution of abnormalities, and, as indicated above, the presence of acute, subacute, or chronic symptoms. Ground-glass opacity with a patchy or peripheral distribution is most likely due to active interstitial pneumonia (NSIP, UIP, and DIP), eosinophilic pneumonia, hypersensitivity pneumonitis, BOOP, alveolar proteinosis, sarcoidosis, pulmonary edema, or hemorrhage. The differential diagnosis of a centrilobular nodular distribution of ground-glass opacity includes hypersensitivity pneumoni-

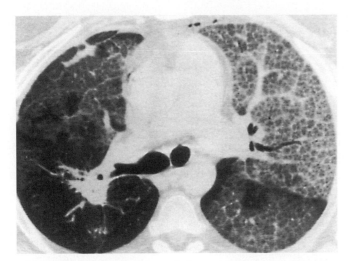

FIG. 3-96. Geographic ground-glass opacities in association with interlobular septal thickening, characteristic of alveolar proteinosis. This pattern, characterized by the association of ground-glass opacity and interlobular septal thickening or reticulation, is termed *crazy-paving.*

tis, BOOP, LIP, cytomegalovirus and *P. carinii* pneumonia, and vasculitis. Diffuse and extensive ground-glass opacity may be seen with hypersensitivity pneumonitis, *P. carinii* pneumonia, cytomegalovirus pneumonia, pulmonary edema, pulmonary hemorrhage, ARDS, and AIP.

Pitfalls in the Diagnosis of Ground-Glass Opacity

There are several potential pitfalls in the recognition and diagnosis of ground-glass opacity. First, it is important to keep in mind that because ground-glass opacity reflects the volume averaging of subtle morphologic abnormalities, the thicker the collimation used for scanning, the more likely volume averaging will occur, regardless of the nature of the anatomic abnormality present. Thus, ground-glass opacity should be diagnosed only on scans obtained with thin collimation.

The diagnosis of ground-glass opacity is largely subjective and based on a qualitative assessment of lung attenuation [181]. The use of lung attenuation measurements to determine the presence of increased lung density in patients with ground-glass opacity is difficult because of the variations in attenuation measurements that are known to be associated with gravitational density gradients in the lung, the level of inspiration, and fluctuations that occur as a result of patient size, position, chest wall thickness, and kilovolt peak [kV(p)]. Using consistent window settings for the interpretation of HRCT is very important. Using too low a window mean in conjunction with a relatively narrow window width can give the appearance of a diffuse ground-glass abnormality [181]. In addition, using a wider window width than one is accustomed to without changing window mean can give the impression of increased lung attenuation. In assessing the attenuation of lung parenchyma, it is often helpful to compare its appearance to that of air in the trachea or bronchi; if tracheal air appears gray instead of black, then increased attenuation or "grayness" of the lung parenchyma may not be significant.

Also, as previously indicated, increased lung opacity is commonly seen in the dependent lung on HRCT largely as a result of volume loss in the dependent lung parenchyma; this is so-called dependent density [39]. This can result in a stripe of ground-glass opacity several centimeters thick in the posterior lung of supine patients; prone scans allow this transient finding to be distinguished from a true abnormality. Similarly, on expiration, because of a reduction of the amount of air within alveoli, lung regions increase in attenuation and can mimic the appearance of ground-glass opacity resulting from lung disease.

TABLE 3-9. *Histologic abnormalities associated with ground-glass opacity* [22,97,109,130,135,138,198,199]

Diagnosis	Histologic findings
Usual interstitial pneumonia	Alveolar septal inflammation; intraalveolar cellular infiltrate; fibrosis
Nonspecific interstitial pneumonia	Alveolar septal inflammation; intraalveolar cellular infiltrate; fibrosis
Desquamative interstitial pneumonia	Alveolar macrophages; interstitial inflammatory infiltrate; mild fibrosis
Respiratory bronchiolitis	Pigment-containing alveolar macrophages
Acute interstitial pneumonia	Interstitial inflammatory exudate; edema; diffuse alveolar damage with hyaline membranes
Hypersensitivity pneumonitis	Alveolitis; interstitial infiltrates; poorly defined granulomas; cellular bronchiolitis
Bronchiolitis obliterans organizing pneumonia	Alveolar septal inflammation; alveolar cellular desquamation
Eosinophilic pneumonia	Eosinophilic interstitial infiltrate; alveolar eosinophils and histiocytes
Pneumocystis carinii pneumonia	Alveolar inflammatory exudate; alveolar septal thickening
Sarcoidosis	Largely due to numerous small granulomas; alveolitis less important
Alveolar proteinosis	Intraalveolar lipoproteinaceous material

TABLE 3-10. *Differential diagnosis of crazy-paving*

Diagnosis	Course	Comments
Acute interstitial pneumonia; adult respiratory distress syndrome	Acute	Consolidation common; patchy or diffuse
Pulmonary edema	Acute	Common
Pulmonary hemorrhage	Acute	Patchy or diffuse
Pneumonia (e.g., *Pneumocystis carinii*, viral, *Mycoplasma*, bacterial pneumonias)	Acute	Common; diffuse or patchy; centrilobular nodules; consolidation
Acute eosinophilic pneumonia	Acute	Rare
Radiation pneumonitis	Acute	Extent usually corresponds to radiation ports
Alveolar proteinosis	Subacute, chronic	Always present; patchy or diffuse; geographic
Nonspecific interstitial pneumonia	Subacute, chronic	Patchy; subpleural
Usual interstitial pneumonia and idiopathic pulmonary fibrosis	Subacute, chronic	Uncommon cause; subpleural
Hypersensitivity pneumonitis	Subacute, chronic	Very common; patchy or nodular; can be centrilobular; consolidation and air-trapping may also be present
Bronchiolitis obliterans organizing pneumonia	Subacute, chronic	Common; consolidation may also be present; often predominant in peripheral regions; can be nodular
Chronic eosinophilic pneumonia	Subacute, chronic	Consolidation more common; patchy; peripheral predominance
Churg-Strauss syndrome	Subacute, chronic	Consolidation also present; nodular
Lipoid pneumonia	Subacute, chronic	Patchy or lobular; low-attenuation consolidation may be present
Bronchioloalveolar carcinoma (diffuse)	Subacute, chronic	Diffuse, patchy, or centrilobular; consolidation nodules common

Furthermore, in patients who have emphysema or other causes of lung hyperlucency, such as airways obstruction and air-trapping, normal lung regions can appear relatively dense, thus mimicking the appearance of ground-glass opacity. This pitfall can usually be avoided if consistent window settings are used for interpretation of scans, and the interpreter is accustomed to the appearances of normal lung, lung of increased attenuation, and lung of decreased attenuation. Also, dark bronchi or air bronchograms will not be seen within the relatively dense, normal lung regions, as they are in patients with true ground-glass opacity. The use of expiratory HRCT can also be of value in distinguishing the presence of heterogeneous lung attenuation resulting from emphysema or air-trapping from that representing ground-glass opacity. This is described further in the section Inhomogeneous Lung Opacity.

Consolidation

Increased lung attenuation with obscuration of underlying pulmonary vessels is referred to as *consolidation* (Figs. 3-86 and 3-102 through 3-104) [5,157]; air bronchograms may be present. HRCT has little to add to the diagnosis of patients with clear-cut evidence of consolidation visible on chest radiographs. However, HRCT can allow the detection of consolidation before it becomes diagnosable radiographically. Some evidence of consolidation can be seen in patients with a variety of diffuse lung diseases.

By definition, diseases that produce consolidation are characterized by a replacement of alveolar air by fluid, cells, tissue, or some other substance [102,157,197]. Most are associated with airspace filling, but diseases that produce an extensive, confluent interstitial abnormality, such as UIP or sarcoidosis, can also result in this finding [20,135]. Airspace nodules or focal areas of ground-glass opacity are often seen in association with areas of frank consolidation. Patients who show consolidation in association with another pattern, such as small nodules, should be diagnosed using the other pattern. In such patients, consolidation probably represents confluent disease.

Areas of consolidation are common in patients with diffuse lung disease regardless of the diagnosis and generally may be discounted. The differential diagnosis of consolidation overlaps that listed for ground-glass opacity (Table 3-8), and, in fact, many of the diseases listed in Table 3-8 can show a mixture of both findings. Consolidation representing the predominant abnormality has a limited differential diagnosis (Table 3-11). The differential diagnosis of consolidation includes pneumonia of different causes including *P. carinii* pneumonia [102,187], BOOP (Fig. 3-102) [134,203], eosinophilic pneumonia (Figs. 3-103 and 3-104) [204], hypersensitivity pneumonitis [132], radiation pneumonitis [33,184, 192,205,206], bronchioloalveolar carcinoma and lymphoma [102,135,146], UIP [135,179], alveolar proteinosis [52], AIP [185], sarcoidosis [98], drug reactions [207], pulmonary edema, and ARDS [102].

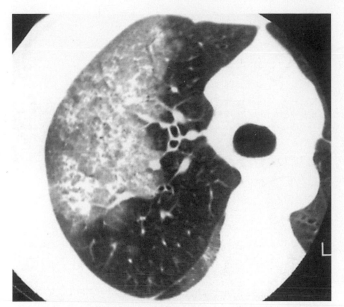

FIG. 3-97. Ground-glass opacity in a patient with pulmonary hemorrhage. Vessels are visible within the area of opacity, as are areas of reticulation. The reticular opacities appear to represent thickening of the intralobular interstitium.

Lung diseases causing consolidation can have widely differing appearances and distributions depending on the nature of the pathologic process responsible (Algorithm 6). Lobular consolidation is often due to infection, although consolidation due to bronchioloalveolar carcinoma and alveolar proteinosis can also have a lobular predominance. Diffuse consolidation is most typical of pneumonia, bronchioloalveolar carcinoma, ARDS, AIP, pulmonary edema, and pulmonary hemorrhage. A subpleural distribution is most suggestive of eosinophilic pneumonia and BOOP but may also be seen with UIP and NSIP. Chronic lung diseases that result in consolidation often involve the lung in a patchy fashion. Patchy consolidation can show a nonanatomic and nonsegmental distribution, but can also be panlobular (Fig. 3-65B) or can appear nodular and centrilobular on HRCT [3,60,65,102]. Eosinophilic pneumonia, BOOP, bronchioloalveolar carcinoma, and bronchopneumonia may show this appearance. A *panlobular distribution*— that is, uniform involvement of secondary pulmonary lobules by the pathologic process [60]—is typical of diseases producing airspace consolidation, such as bronchopneumonia or lobular pneumonia (Fig. 3-65) [65], but it can be seen in a variety of diffuse interstitial diseases characterized by ground-glass opacity and is nonspecific.

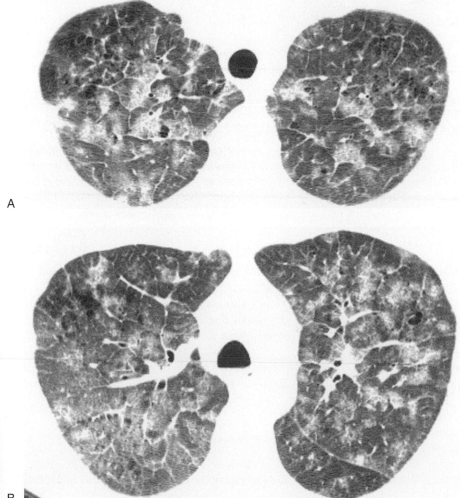

FIG. 3-98. A,B: *Pneumocystis carinii* pneumonia in an immunosuppressed patient with leukemia. Patchy areas of ground-glass opacity are associated with distinct interlobular septal thickening.

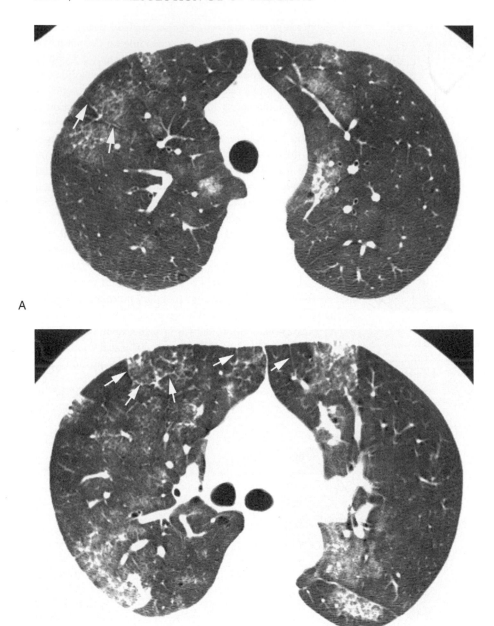

A

B

FIG. 3-99. A,B: Pneumonia due to respiratory syncytial virus. HRCT at two levels shows patchy ground-glass opacity associated with some interlobular septal thickening (*arrows*).

Lung Calcification and Lung Attenuation Greater than Soft Tissue

Multifocal lung calcification, often associated with lung nodules, has been reported in association with infectious granulomatous diseases such as tuberculosis [65], sarcoidosis (Fig. 3-105) [57], silicosis [57,58], amyloidosis [50], and fat embolism associated with ARDS [208]. Diffuse and dense lung calcification can be seen in the presence of metastatic calcification, disseminated pulmonary ossification, or alveolar microlithiasis. Increased attenuation can be seen in patients with talcosis [147] associated with fibrotic masses, although this may represent the injected material rather than calcification. Diffuse, increased lung attenuation in the absence of calcification can be seen as a result of amiodarone lung toxicity.

Disseminated pulmonary ossification is a rare condition in which very small deposits of mature bone form within the lung parenchyma [209]. It can be associated with chronic heart disease, such as mitral stenosis, or chronic interstitial fibrosis, such as IPF or asbestosis, or be related to drugs. Such calcification is usually invisible on chest radiographs and on HRCT.

Metastatic Calcification

Deposition of calcium within the lung parenchyma (metastatic calcification) can occur due to hypercalcemia in patients

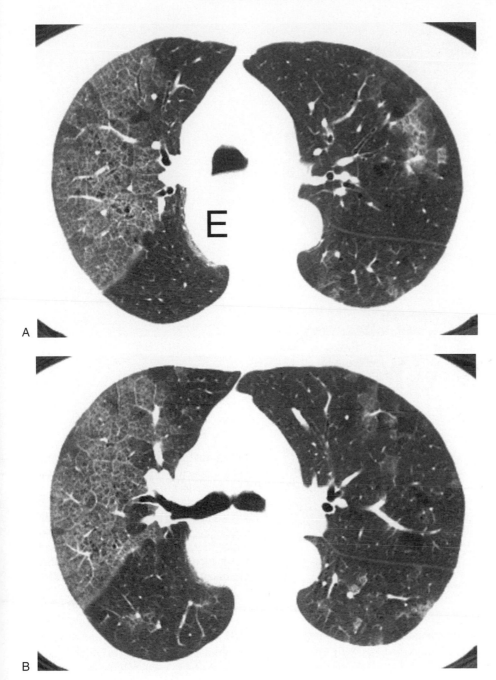

FIG. 3-100. A,B: Patchy areas of ground-glass opacity and interlobular septal thickening (crazy-paving) in a patient with bronchiolitis obliterans organizing pneumonia associated with aspiration. Note the presence of a dilated fluid-filled esophagus (E).

with abnormal calcium and phosphate metabolism and is most common in patients with chronic renal failure and secondary hyperparathyroidism (Fig. 3-106) [150,151,210]. Metastatic calcification is typically interstitial, involving the alveolar septa, bronchioles, and arteries, and can be associated with secondary lung fibrosis. Plain radiographs are relatively insensitive in detecting this calcification, whereas HRCT can show calcification in the absence of radiographic findings. Calcifications can be focal, centrilobular, or diffuse (Fig. 3-106). Ground-glass opacities with a centrilobular distribution have been reported in association with metastatic calcification [150].

Hartman et al. [151] reviewed the chest radiographs and CT and HRCT scans of seven patients with hypercalcemia

and biopsy-proven metastatic calcification. In five patients, the radiographic findings were nonspecific, consisting of poorly defined nodular opacities and patchy areas of parenchymal consolidation, whereas in two patients calcified nodules were visible. CT and HRCT findings consisted of numerous fluffy and poorly defined nodules measuring 3 to 10 mm in diameter. The nodules primarily involved the upper lobes in three patients, were diffuse in three, and were predominant in the lower lung zones in one. Areas of ground-glass opacity were present in three of the seven patients, and patchy areas of consolidation were present in two. Calcification of some or all of the nodules was seen on CT in four of the seven patients.

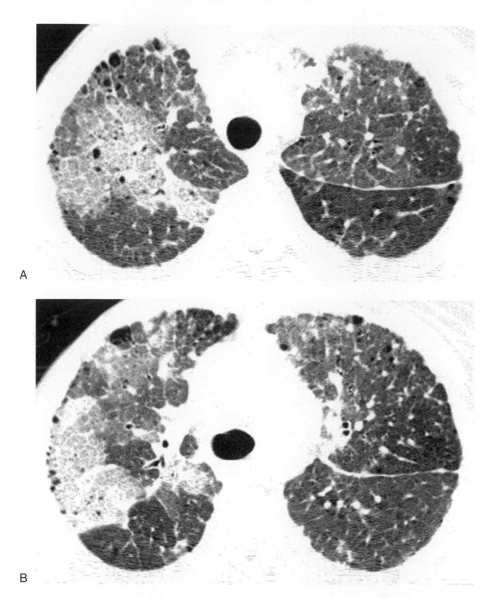

A

B

FIG. 3-101. A,B: Patchy areas of ground-glass opacity and interlobular septal thickening in a patient with diffuse bronchioloalveolar carcinoma. Nodules within the left lung and nodular thickening of the subpleural interstitium adjacent to the left major fissure also reflect tumor spread. Focal lucencies within the upper lobes are caused by underlying emphysema.

Six of the seven patients also had evidence of calcification in the vessels of the chest wall, and one had calcification of the left atrial wall.

Alveolar Microlithiasis

The HRCT appearances of several patients with pulmonary alveolar microlithiasis have been reported, corresponding closely to pathologic findings in this disease [211–213]. Alveolar microlithiasis is characterized by widespread intraalveolar calcifications, representing so-called microliths or calcospheres. HRCT shows a posterior and lower lobe predominance of the calcifications, with a high concentration in the subpleural parenchyma and in association with bronchi and vessels (Fig. 3-107). A perilobular and centrilobular distribution of the calcifications may be seen, or calcifications may be associated with interlobular septa. Intraparenchymal cysts or paraseptal emphy-

sema may be associated [211,212]. In children or patients with early disease, ground-glass opacity or reticulation may be the predominant finding, with calcification being inconspicuous [213].

Amiodarone Pulmonary Toxicity

Amiodarone is a triiodinated drug used to treat refractory tachyarrhythmias. It accumulates in lung, largely within macrophages and type-2 pneumocytes, where it forms lamellar inclusion bodies and has a very long half-life. In some patients, accumulation of the drug results in pulmonary toxicity with interstitial pneumonia and fibrosis, although the mechanisms of disease are unclear. CT in patients with amiodarone can show high-attenuation areas of consolidation or high-attenuation nodules or masses, sometimes in association with an abnormal reticulation or ground-glass opacity (Fig. 3-108) [207,214]. High-attenuation consolidation or masses

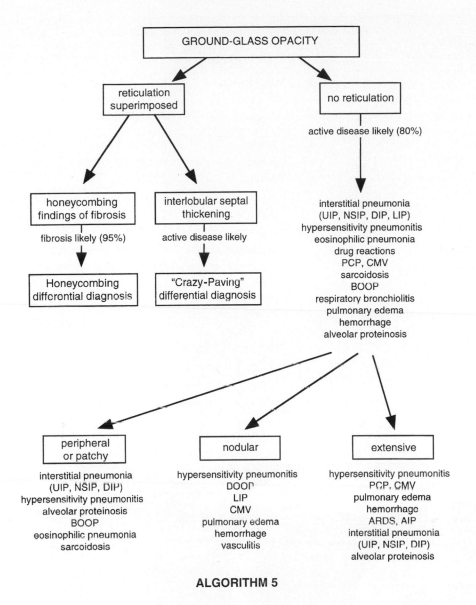

ALGORITHM 5

were seen in 8 of 11 patients in one series [214], correlating with the presence of numerous foamy macrophages in the interstitium and alveolar spaces. Unconsolidated lung parenchyma does not appear abnormally dense. Because the drug also accumulates in the liver and spleen, these also appear abnormally dense on scans obtained through the lung bases.

Heavy Metal Pneumoconiosis

Inhalation of radiodense material, such as iron oxide, tin, and barium, may result in dense pulmonary lesions. The HRCT appearance of dense lung lesions secondary to inhaled iron oxide has been reported in welders [215].

TABLE 3-11. *Differential diagnosis of consolidation*

Diagnosis	Course	Comments
Pneumonia (e.g., bacterial, *Pneumocystis carinii*, viral, *Mycoplasma* pneumonias)	Acute	Patchy, nodular, lobular, or diffuse depending on the organism
Acute interstitial pneumonia; acute respiratory distress syndrome	Acute	Patchy or diffuse
Pulmonary edema	Acute	Diffuse
Pulmonary hemorrhage	Acute	Patchy or diffuse
Acute eosinophilic pneumonia	Acute	Diffuse
Radiation pneumonitis	Acute	Extent usually corresponds to radiation ports
Bronchiolitis obliterans organizing pneumonia	Subacute, chronic	Common; peripheral; can be masslike
Chronic eosinophilic pneumonia	Subacute, chronic	Patchy or nodular; peripheral
Churg-Strauss syndrome	Subacute, chronic	Consolidation also present; nodular
Bronchioloalveolar carcinoma (diffuse)	Subacute, chronic	Diffuse, patchy, or nodular
Lymphoma	Subacute, chronic	Diffuse, patchy, or nodular
Nonspecific interstitial pneumonia	Subacute, chronic	Patchy; subpleural
Usual interstitial pneumonia and idiopathic pulmonary fibrosis	Subacute, chronic	Subpleural and basal predominance
Hypersensitivity pneumonitis	Subacute, chronic	Patchy; ground-glass opacity more common
Lipoid pneumonia	Subacute, chronic	Patchy or lobular; low-attenuation consolidation
Sarcoidosis	Subacute, chronic	Confluence of very small granulomas
Alveolar proteinosis	Subacute, chronic	Ground-glass opacity more common

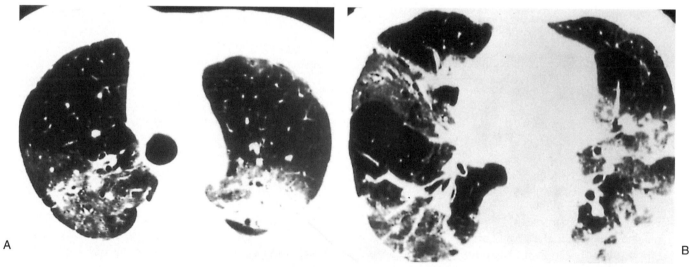

A

B

FIG. 3-102. A,B: Bronchiolitis obliterans organizing pneumonia with patchy areas of consolidation and ground-glass opacity. A peripheral distribution is typical.

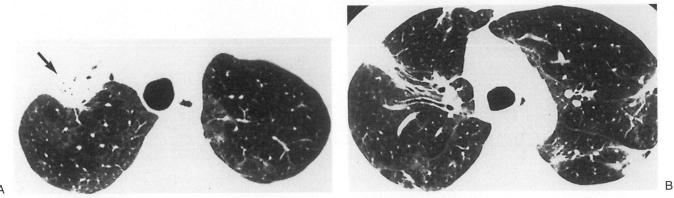

FIG. 3-103. Eosinophilic pneumonia with focal areas of consolidation and ground-glass opacity. As in patients with bronchiolitis obliterans organizing pneumonia, a peripheral distribution is typical. Note the presence of air bronchograms and obscuration of vessels in the apical opacity (*arrow*).

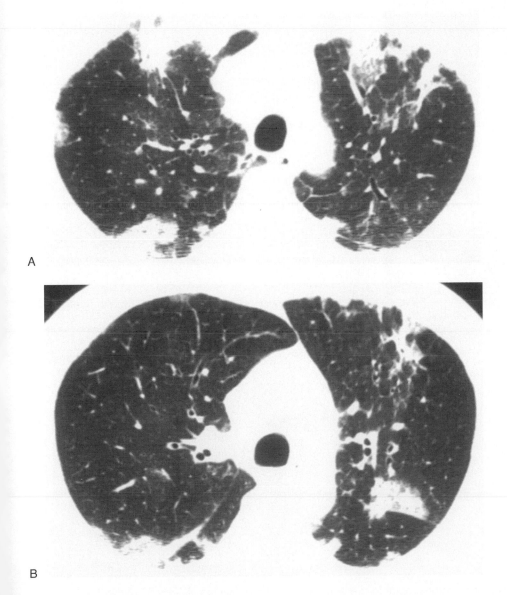

FIG. 3-104. A,B: Eosinophilic pneumonia with focal areas of consolidation having a peripheral and subpleural distribution.

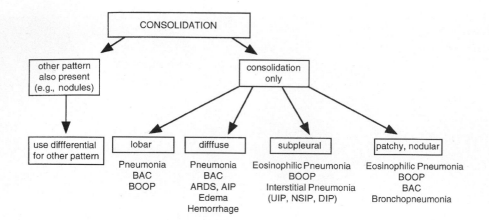

ALGORITHM 6

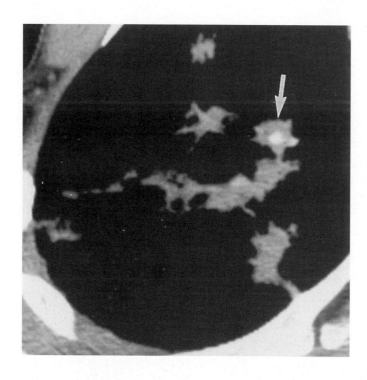

FIG. 3-105. Calcification (*arrow*) within nodular lung disease in a patient with sarcoidosis.

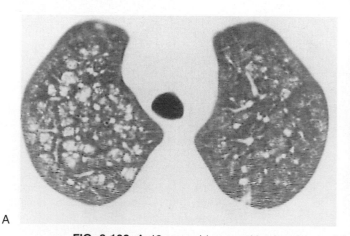

A

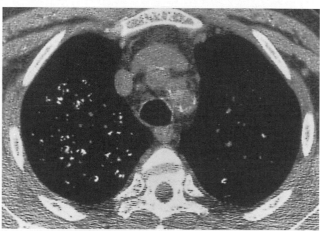

B

FIG. 3-106. A 42-year-old man with chronic renal failure and metastatic calcification. **A:** HRCT shows nodular areas of opacity that appear centrilobular, as well as some ground-glass opacities. **B:** Soft-tissue window scan shows multiple areas of calcification within these opacities.

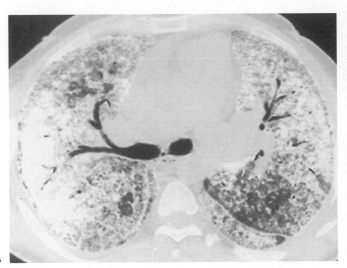
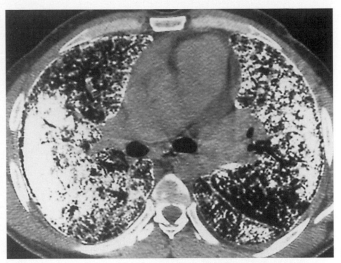

FIG. 3-107. HRCT in a patient with alveolar microlithiasis, with lung **(A)** and soft-tissue **(B)** windows. Calcifications that are very small and diffuse show a subpleural predominance. (Courtesy of Joseph Cherian, M.D., Al-Sabah Hospital, Kuwait.)

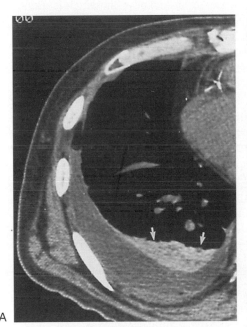
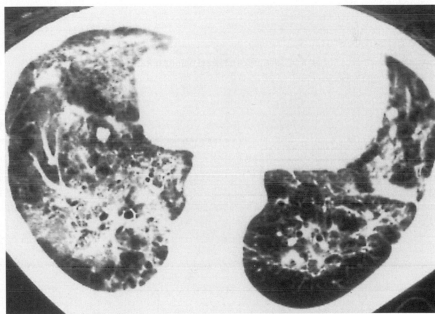

FIG. 3-108. HRCT in pulmonary amiodarone toxicity. **A:** On an unenhanced HRCT, a focal area of dense lung consolidation is present in the posterior lung. A pleural effusion is also visible, due to cardiac decompensation. **B:** In another patient with amiodarone toxicity, a lung window scan shows areas of ground-glass opacity, consolidation, nodular opacities, and abnormal reticulation. The high attenuation cannot be appreciated with this window setting.

DECREASED LUNG OPACITY, CYSTS, AND AIRWAY ABNORMALITIES

A variety of abnormalities result in decreased lung attenuation or air-filled cystic lesions on HRCT. These include honeycombing, lung cysts, emphysema, bullae, pneumatoceles, cavitary nodules, bronchiectasis, mosaic perfusion, and air-trapping due to airways disease (Fig. 3-109). In most cases, these can be readily distinguished on the basis of HRCT findings [216].

Honeycombing

In patients with interstitial fibrosis, alveolar disruption, dilatation of alveolar ducts, and bronchiolar dilatation result in the formation of honeycomb cysts [8,217]. These cysts

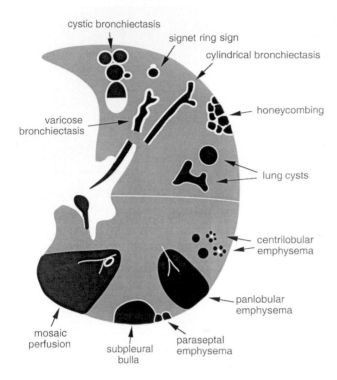

FIG. 3-109. HRCT appearances of decreased lung opacity, cystic abnormalities, emphysema, bronchiectasis, and mosaic perfusion.

have fibrous walls and are lined by bronchiolar epithelium. On HRCT, honeycombing is characterized by the presence of air-filled, cystic spaces, several millimeters to several centimeters in diameter, which often predominate in a peripheral and subpleural location, occur in several layers, and are char-

acterized by clearly definable walls 1- to 3-mm in thickness [32,42] (Figs. 3-29, 3-31, 3-32, and 3-110 through 3-112). In contradistinction to the lung cysts seen in patients with lymphangiomyomatosis (LAM), Langerhans histiocytosis and LIP, and the lucencies seen in patients with centrilobular emphysema, honeycomb cysts tend to share walls. The presence of honeycombing on HRCT indicates the presence of severe fibrosis.

Large cystic spaces, several centimeters in diameter, can be associated with honeycombing, mimicking the appearance of bullae (Figs. 3-111 and 3-112). These large cysts tend to predominate in the upper lobes, but they may be seen at the lung bases as well. They often have a subpleural predominance. These large honeycomb cysts decrease in size on expiratory scans [218,219].

Lung Cysts

On HRCT, the term *lung cyst* is used to refer to a well-defined, rounded, and circumscribed lesion, with a wall that may be uniform or varied in thickness but which is usually thin (less than 3 mm thick) [216]. It usually contains air but may also contain liquid, semisolid, or solid material [6,216]. Lung cysts are also defined as having a wall composed of one of a variety of cellular elements, usually fibrous or epithelial in nature [157]. For example, in patients with end-stage pulmonary fibrosis, honeycomb cysts are lined by bronchiolar epithelium; on the other hand, in patients with LAM, the cysts are lined by abnormal spindle cells resembling smooth muscle. This term is not usually used to describe airspaces in patients with emphysema. The term *cystic airspace* may be used to describe a peripheral air-containing lesion surrounded by a wall of variable thickness, that may be thin, as in LAM or thick as in honeycombing [6].

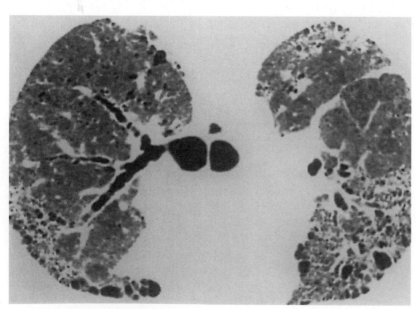

A

FIG. 3-110. Honeycombing in a patient with idiopathic pulmonary fibrosis. **A,B:** On HRCT, honeycombing cysts have clearly definable walls a few millimeters in thickness. In areas of honeycombing, lobular anatomy cannot be resolved because of architectural distortion. Bronchial irregularity and traction bronchiectasis (*arrows,* **B**) are often present in patients with severe fibrosis and may be difficult to distinguish from honeycombing. *Continued*

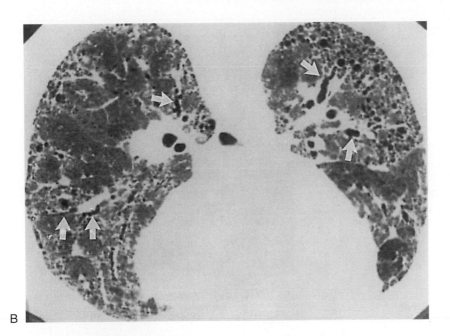

B

FIG. 3-110. *Continued*

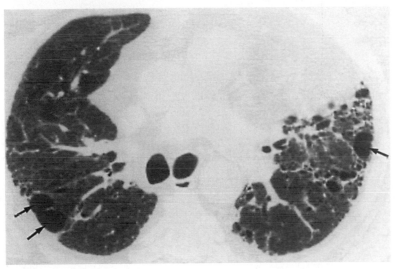

FIG. 3-111. Honeycombing with large lung cysts. In a patient with idiopathic pulmonary fibrosis, peripheral honeycombing, traction bronchiectasis, and several large lung cysts (*arrows*) are visible.

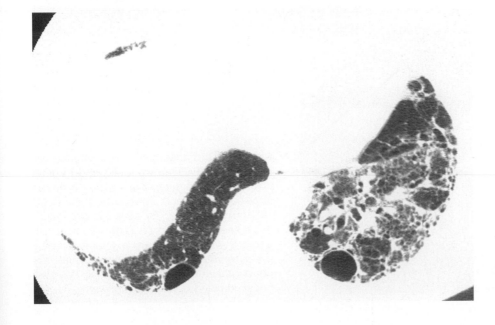

FIG. 3-112. Idiopathic pulmonary fibrosis with asymmetric honeycombing and large lung cysts. Peripheral honeycombing and irregular reticular opacities are associated with large lung cysts. These are predominantly subpleural in location.

TABLE 3-12. *Differential diagnosis of cystic lung disease*

Diagnosis	Comments
Lymphangiomyomatosis (LAM)	Cysts usually round and relatively uniform in size and shape; diffuse lung involvement; almost exclusively in women
Langerhans histiocytosis	Cysts have unusual shapes; larger and more numerous in lung apices; costophrenic angles usually spared; small nodules may be present
Lymphocytic interstitial pneumonitis	Less numerous than in LAM or histiocytosis; nodules may be associated
Bullae	Subpleural distribution in most cases; single layer at the pleural surface; centrilobular emphysema may be present
Pneumatoceles	Scattered; patchy distribution; limited in number; findings of pneumonia
Honeycombing	Subpleural predominance; multiple layers at the pleural surface; cysts share walls; findings of fibrosis
Cystic bronchiectasis	Clustered or perihilar distribution; air-fluid levels may be present

LAM, Langerhans histiocytosis, and LIP often produce multiple lung cysts, whose appearance on HRCT is usually quite distinct from that of honeycombing (Table 3-12) [17,18,92, 93,220–225]. The cysts have a thin but easily discernible wall in most instances, ranging up to a few millimeters in thickness (Figs. 3-113 through 3-118). Associated findings of fibrosis are usually absent or much less conspicuous than they are in patients with honeycombing and end-stage lung disease. In LAM, Langerhans histiocytosis, and LIP, the cysts are usually interspersed within areas of normal-appearing lung.

In patients with Langerhans histiocytosis, the cysts can have bizarre shapes because of the fusion of several cysts, or perhaps because they represent ectatic and thick-walled bronchi (Figs. 3-113 through 3-115). Although confluent cysts can also be seen with LAM, they are less common; in patients with LAM, cysts generally appear rounder and more uniform in size than those seen with histiocytosis (Figs. 3-116 through 3-118). Multiple thin-walled lung cysts are also seen in patients with LIP (see Figs. 5-19 and 5-61)

[17,18,225]. In one study of 22 patients with LIP, cystic airspaces were seen in 15; other findings included small subpleural nodules, centrilobular nodules, interlobular septal thickening, and ground-glass attenuation [17].

As described above, the term *lung cyst* refers to a specific type of cystic space within the lung parenchyma. If possible, lung cysts should be distinguished from other air-containing spaces, such as emphysematous bullae, blebs, and pneumatoceles, which are described in the paragraphs that follow.

Emphysema

Emphysema is defined as a permanent, abnormal enlargement of airspaces distal to the terminal bronchiole and accompanied by the destruction of the walls of the involved airspaces [216]. Emphysema can be accurately diagnosed using HRCT [32,43,96,226–228] and results in focal areas of very low attenuation that can be easily con-

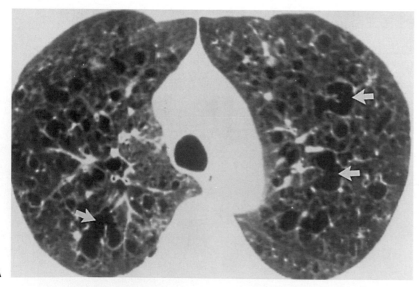

FIG. 3-113. Langerhans histiocytosis with lung cysts. HRCT at two levels show numerous thin-walled lung cysts. The cysts are larger and most numerous in the upper lobes **(A)** than in the lower **(B)**, as is characteristic of this disease. Some cysts (*arrows*) are confluent, branching, or irregular in shape. Note that the intervening lung appears normal. The peripheral predominance commonly seen with honeycombing is absent. *Continued*

A

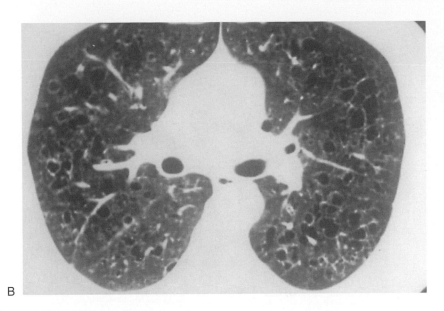

B

FIG. 3-113. *Continued*

trasted with surrounding higher-attenuation normal lung parenchyma if sufficiently low-window means [−600 to −800 Hounsfield units (HU)] are used (Figs. 3-119 through 3-123 and 3-125 through 3-129). Although some types of emphysema can have walls visible on HRCT, these are usually inconspicuous.

In many patients, it is possible to classify the type of emphysema on the basis of its HRCT appearance [32,43]. *Centrilobular* (*proximal* or *centriacinar*) *emphysema* is characterized on HRCT by the presence of multiple small lucencies that predominate in the upper lobes and, in some subjects or regions, may appear centrilobular (Figs. 3-109 and 3-119 through 3-123). Even if the centrilobular location of these lucencies is not visible, a spotty distribution is typical of centrilobular emphysema (Figs. 3-121 through 3-123). In most cases, the areas of low attenuation seen on HRCT in patients with centrilobular emphysema lack a visible wall, although very thin walls are occasionally visible and are related to areas of fibrosis (Fig. 3-122). In severe cases, the areas of centrilobular emphysema may become confluent.

Panlobular (*panacinar*) *emphysema* typically results in an overall decrease in lung attenuation and a reduction in size of pulmonary vessels, without the focal areas of lucency typically seen in patients with centrilobular emphysema (Fig. 3-124). Areas of panlobular emphysema typically lack visible walls. This form of emphysema has been aptly described as a diffuse simplification of lung architecture. Severe or confluent centrilobular emphysema can mimic this appearance (Figs. 3-125 and 3-126).

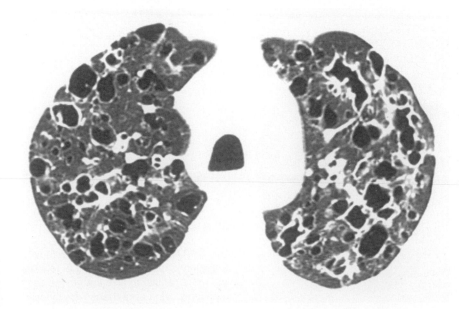

FIG. 3-114. HRCT in a man with Langerhans histiocytosis. The cysts vary in size, and many are irregular in shape. These findings are typical of this disease. (Courtesy of Marcia McCowin, San Francisco, CA.)

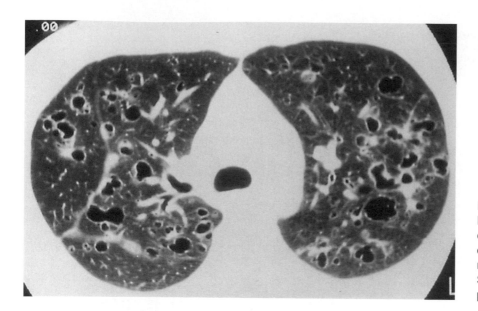

FIG. 3-115. HRCT in a patient with cystic lung disease typical of Langerhans histiocytosis. Multiple lung cysts, many bifurcating or complex, are interspersed within normal-appearing lung. (Courtesy of Shin-Ho Kook, M.D., Koryo General Hospital, Seoul, Korea.)

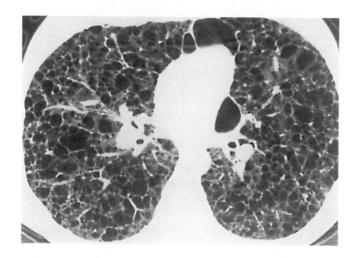

FIG. 3-116. HRCT in a patient with tuberous sclerosis and lymphangiomyomatosis. Cystic airspaces have clearly defined walls measuring up to 2 mm in thickness.

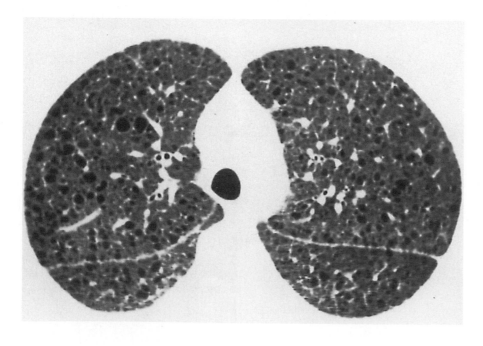

FIG. 3-117. HRCT in a woman with lymphangiomyomatosis. Cysts are rounder and more regular in size than those seen in patients with Langerhans histiocytosis.

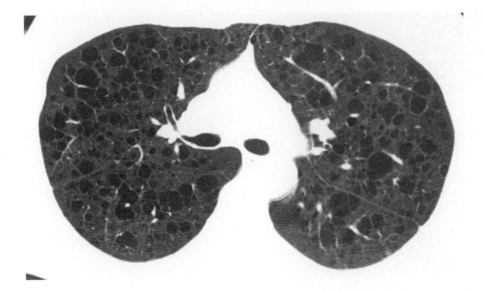

FIG. 3-118. HRCT in a young woman with lymphangiomyomatosis associated with tuberous sclerosis. Cysts are round and very thin walled. Intervening lung parenchyma appears normal.

Paraseptal (distal acinar) emphysema results in the presence of subpleural lucencies, which often share very thin walls that are visible on HRCT; paraseptal emphysema can be seen as an isolated abnormality but is often associated with centrilobular emphysema (Figs. 3-127 through 3-129).

Irregular airspace enlargement, previously known as *irregular* or *cicatricial emphysema*, can be seen in association with fibrosis, as in patients with silicosis and progressive massive fibrosis or sarcoidosis (see Fig. 5-47) [95,229].

Bullous emphysema does not represent a specific histologic entity but represents emphysema characterized primarily by large bullae (Fig. 3-129) [230]. It is often associated with centrilobular and paraseptal emphysema. These types of emphysema and their HRCT appearances are further described in Chapter 7.

Paraseptal Emphysema versus Honeycombing

The appearance of paraseptal emphysema may mimic that of honeycombing in some cases, although a careful consideration of anatomic findings usually allows them to be distinguished. In patients with paraseptal emphysema, areas of lung destruction are typically marginated by thin linear opacities extending to the pleural surface. These linear opacities often correspond to interlobular septa, sometimes thickened by minimal fibrosis (Figs. 3-109 and 3-127 through 3-129). Areas of paraseptal emphysema usually occur in a single layer at the pleural surface, predominate in the upper lobes, and may be associated with other findings of emphysema such as large subpleural bullae, but are typically unassociated with significant fibrosis. Honeycomb cysts are usually

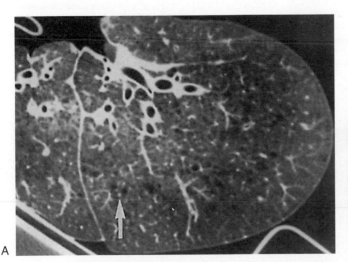

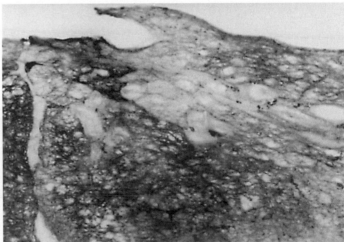

A   B

FIG. 3-119. Isolated inflated lung from a patient with centrilobular emphysema. **A:** Small lucencies without identifiable walls are present. Some lucencies are seen to cluster around a centrilobular artery (*arrow*). This appearance is typical of centrilobular emphysema. **B:** On the corresponding lung section, the small centrilobular foci of destruction are clearly seen. (From Webb WR, Stein MG, et al. Normal and diseased isolated lungs: HRCT. *Radiology* 1988;166:81, with permission.)

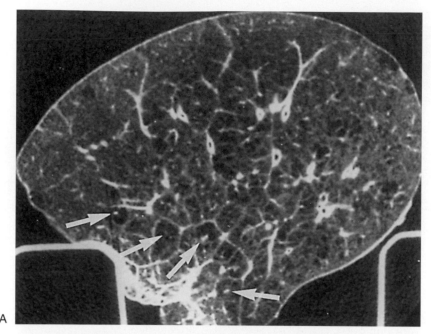

A

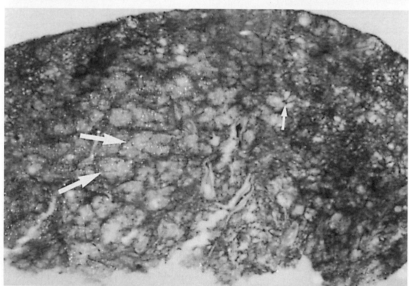

B

FIG. 3-120. Centrilobular emphysema in an isolated lung. **A:** More severe, but patchy, emphysema is visible on the HRCT. The areas of destruction cluster about the centrilobular arteries (*arrows*). (From Webb WR, Stein MG, et al. Normal and diseased isolated lungs: HRCT. *Radiology* 1988;166:81, with permission.) **B:** On the pathologic specimen, some lobules (*large arrows*) show extensive destruction. In some, the centrilobular artery remains visible (*small arrow*) within the area of emphysema.

smaller, occur in several layers in the subpleural lung, tend to predominate at the lung bases, and are associated with disruption of lobular architecture and other findings of fibrosis, such as traction bronchiectasis. In occasional patients, emphysema and honeycombing coexist. In such cases, emphysema usually predominates in the upper lobes and central or subpleural lung, whereas honeycombing predominates at the bases and in the subpleural lung regions (Fig. 3-130). The HRCT appearance, however, may be confusing.

Centrilobular Emphysema versus Lung Cysts

In many patients with centrilobular emphysema, the focal areas of lucency that characterize this condition lack visible walls; lung cysts, on the other hand, have walls recognizable on HRCT. However, in some patients with centrilobular emphysema, areas of lung destruction show very thin walls on HRCT, mimicking the appearance of lung cysts. These walls likely reflect the presence of minimal lung fibrosis or compressed adjacent lung parenchyma and are usually less well-defined than those seen in patients with cystic lung disease. Also, lung cysts often appear larger than areas of centrilobular emphysema, which usually range from several millimeters to 1 cm. In patients with centrilobular emphysema, lucencies can often be seen involving only one part of an otherwise normal-appearing secondary lobule (Fig. 3-109); this appearance is diagnostic.

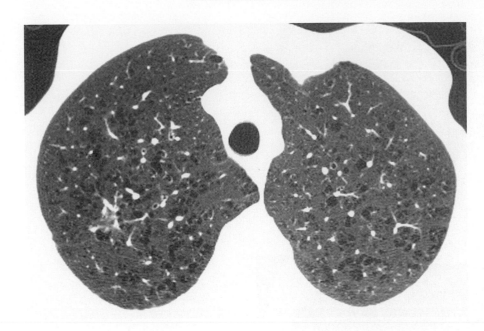

FIG. 3-121. Centrilobular emphysema on HRCT. Spotty areas of lucency predominate in the upper lobes. This appearance is typical and diagnostic. The small areas of emphysema lack visible walls.

Bullae and Blebs

Emphysematous bullae are well seen using HRCT. A *bulla* has been defined as a sharply demarcated area of emphysema measuring 1 cm or more in diameter and possessing a thin epithelialized wall that is usually no thicker than 1 mm (Figs. 3-128 and 3-129) [6,157]. Although it is not always possible to distinguish a bulla from a lung cyst, bullae are uncommon as isolated findings, except in the lung apices, and are usually associated with evidence of extensive centrilobular or paraseptal emphysema. Subpleural bullae are often associated with areas of paraseptal emphysema. When emphysema is associated with predominant bullae, it may be termed *bullous emphysema* [230].

On HRCT, bullae show a distinct wall that usually appears approximately 1-mm thick. Bullae can range up to 20 cm in diameter but are usually between 2 and 8 cm in diameter. Bullae can be seen in a subpleural location or within the lung parenchyma, but subpleural bullae appear more frequently. In patients with bullous emphysema, bullae are often asymmetric, with one lung being involved to a greater degree [230].

The term *bleb* is used pathologically to refer to a gas-containing space within the visceral pleura [157]. Radiographically, this term is sometimes used to describe a focal thin-walled lucency contiguous with the pleura, usually at the lung apex. However, the distinction between bleb and bulla is of little practical significance and is seldom justified. The term *bulla* is preferred [157].

Pneumatocele

Pneumatocele is defined as a thin-walled, gas-filled space within the lung, usually occurring in association with acute pneumonia and almost invariably transient [157]. Pneumato-cele has an appearance similar to lung cyst or bulla on HRCT and cannot be distinguished on the basis of HRCT findings. The association of such an abnormality with acute pneumonia, particularly resulting from *P. carinii* or *Staphylococcus*, would suggest the presence of a pneumatocele, but a spectrum of cystic abnormalities can be seen in such patients (Figs. 3-131 and 3-132) [231–233]. The association of lung cysts or bullae with *P. carinii* pneumonia is discussed in Chapter 6.

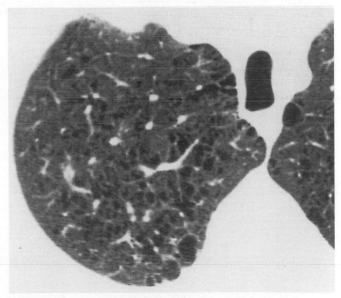

FIG. 3-122. Centrilobular emphysema on HRCT. Spotty areas of lucency predominate in the upper lobes. This appearance is typical and diagnostic. Some of the areas of emphysema have very thin walls, likely reflecting the presence of associated fibrosis.

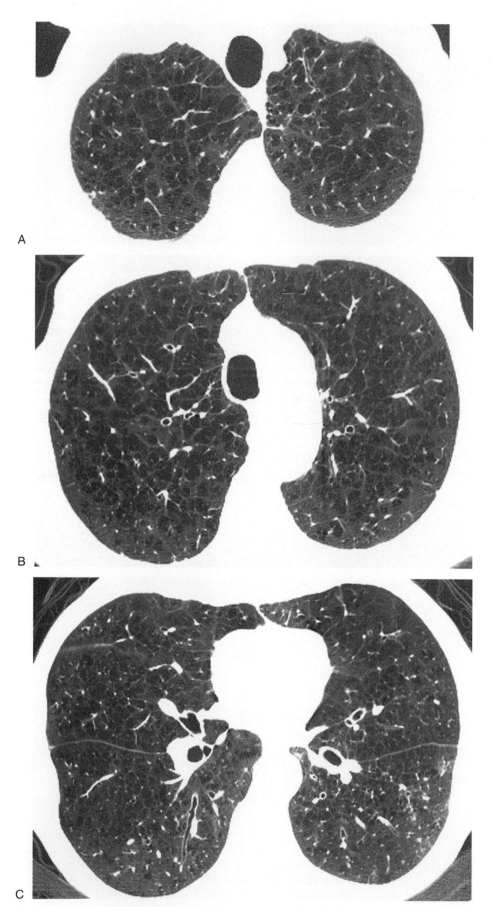

FIG. 3-123. A–C: Centrilobular emphysema on HRCT showing an upper lobe predominance. Spotty areas of lucency predominate in the upper lobes **(A)**, and some are centrilobular in location, surrounding small vessels. At lower levels **(B** and **C)**, lucencies are smaller in size and more normal lung is visible.

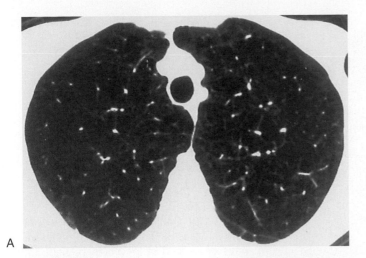

A

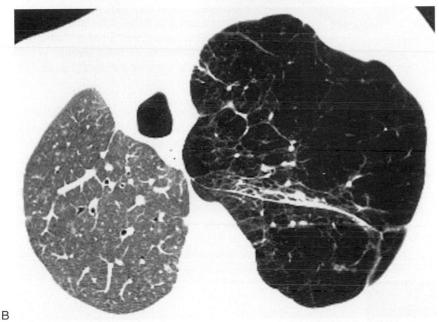

B

FIG. 3-124. Panlobular emphysema in two patients. **A:** On HRCT, lung volumes are increased, the lungs appear lucent, and the size of pulmonary vessels is diminished. Focal lucencies, as seen in patients with centrilobular emphysema, are not visible. **B:** Panlobular emphysema in a patient who has had a right lung transplantation. The right lung is normal in appearance and attenuation. The emphysematous left lung is abnormally lucent, increased in volume, and contains fewer and smaller visible vessels.

Cavitary Nodules

Cavitary nodules have thicker and more irregular walls than lung cysts, but there is some overlap between these appearances (Figs. 3-133 and 3-134). In patients with diffuse lung diseases, such nodules have been reported in Langerhans histiocytosis [92,93], tuberculosis [65], fungal infections, and sarcoidosis [97], but they could also be seen in patients with such disorders as rheumatoid lung disease, septic embolism, pneumonia, metastatic tumor, tracheobronchial papillomatosis (Fig. 3-134), and Wegener's granulomatosis. Also, some nodular opacities that have central lucencies may represent dilated bronchioles surrounded by areas of consolidation or interstitial thickening [92].

Bronchiectasis

Bronchiectasis is generally defined as localized, irreversible bronchial dilatation, often with thickening of the bronchial wall [6,234]. Generally speaking, a bronchus is considered to be dilated if its internal diameter is greater than that of its accompanying artery (Figs. 3-7, 3-109, and 3-135). However, this appearance is sometimes seen in normals [235]. Also, a bronchus may normally appear larger than its adjacent artery if the scan traverses an undivided bronchus near its branch point, and its accompanying artery has already branched. In this situation, two artery branches may be seen to lie adjacent to the "dilated" bronchus (Fig. 3-135). The presence of bronchial wall thickening in addition to an increase in bronchial diameter can be helpful in diagnosing true bronchiectasis.

Although bronchiectasis usually results from chronic infection, airway obstruction by tumor, stricture, impacted material, or inherited abnormalities can also play a significant role. Bronchiectasis has been classified into three types, depending on the morphology of the abnormal bronchi, although these distinctions are of little clinical value [216]. The HRCT diagnosis of bronchiectasis is described in detail in Chapter 8.

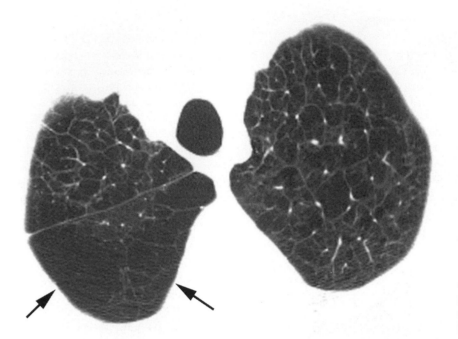

FIG. 3-125. Confluent centrilobular emphysema. Areas of centrilobular emphysema have coalesced in the posterior right lung (*arrows*), resulting in an area of very low attenuation that mimics the appearance of panlobular emphysema. Mild interlobular septal thickening is also visible, usually indicative of some associated fibrosis.

Cylindrical bronchiectasis, the mildest form of this disease, is characterized on HRCT by the presence of thick-walled bronchi that extend into the lung periphery and fail to show normal tapering. On HRCT, bronchi are not normally visible in the peripheral 1 cm of lung, but in patients with bronchiectasis, bronchial wall thickening, peribronchial fibrosis, and dilatation of the bronchial lumen, they can be seen in the lung periphery (Figs. 3-7, 3-109, 3-135, and 3-136) [236,237]. Depending on their orientation relative to the scan plane they can simulate tram tracks or can show the signet ring sign, in which the dilated, thick-walled bronchus and its accompanying pulmonary artery branch are seen adjacent to each other [34]. Ectatic bronchi containing fluid or mucus appear as tubular opacities.

Varicose bronchiectasis is similar in appearance to cylindrical bronchiectasis; however, with varicose bronchiectasis the bronchial walls are more irregular and can assume a beaded appearance (Figs. 3-109, 3-137, and 3-138). The term *string of pearls* has been used to describe varicose bronchiectasis. Traction bronchiectasis often appears varicose.

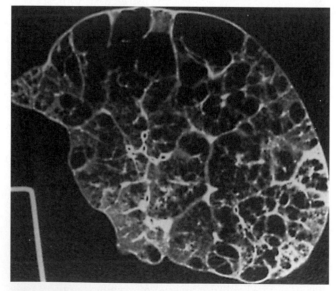

FIG. 3-126. Confluent centrilobular emphysema in an isolated lung. On HRCT, areas of centrilobular emphysema have coalesced to form peripheral bulla. These are marginated by residual normal septa. Because of its peripheral location, this may be termed *paraseptal emphysema.*

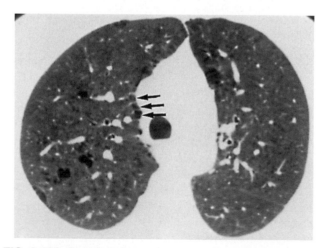

FIG. 3-127. Centrilobular and paraseptal emphysema. Small isolated areas of destruction are present within the central upper lobes and adjacent to the mediastinal pleura. Some of the paramediastinal cysts (*arrows*) have visible walls, as is characteristic of paraseptal emphysema.

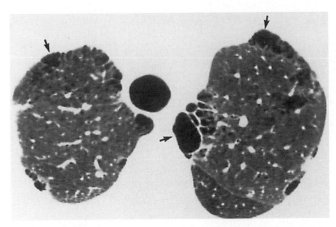

FIG. 3-128. HRCT in a patient with paraseptal and centrilobular emphysema. The larger areas of subpleural emphysema (*arrows*) are most appropriately termed *bullae*.

Cystic bronchiectasis most often appears as a group or cluster of air-filled cysts, but cysts can also be fluid-filled, giving the appearance of a cluster of grapes. Cystic bronchiectasis is often patchy in distribution, allowing it to be distinguished from a cystic lung disease such as LAM (Figs. 3-109 and 3-139). Also, air-fluid levels, which may be present in the dependent portions of the cystic dilated bronchi, are a very specific sign of bronchiectasis and are not usually seen in patients with lung cysts.

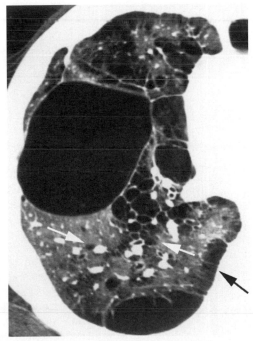

FIG. 3-129. HRCT in a patient with paraseptal and centrilobular emphysema associated with large bullae. Small lucencies lacking walls in the central lung (*white arrows*) represent centrilobular emphysema. Subpleural lucencies (*black arrow*) reflect associated paraseptal emphysema. Large bullae are also subpleural in location.

Traction Bronchiectasis

In patients with lung fibrosis and distortion of lung architecture, traction bronchiectasis is commonly present (Figs. 3-28, 3-29, 3-82, and 3-140). In this condition, traction by fibrous tissue on the walls of bronchi results in irregular bronchial dilatation, or bronchiectasis, which is typically varicose in appearance [31,32]. Traction bronchiectasis usually involves the segmental and subsegmental bronchi and can also affect small peripheral bronchi or bronchioles. Dilatation of intralobular bronchioles because of surrounding fibrosis is termed *traction bronchiolectasis*. In patients with honeycombing, bronchiolar dilatation contributes to the cystic appearance seen on HRCT [8].

The increased transpulmonary pressure and elastic recoil associated with advanced pulmonary fibrosis, along with local distortion of airways by fibrotic tissue, contribute to the varicose dilatation of airways seen in these conditions. Because of peribronchial interstitial thickening, bronchial walls can appear to measure up to several millimeters in thickness. Traction bronchiectasis is usually most marked in areas of lung that show the most severe fibrosis. It is commonly seen in association with honeycombing, as is bronchiolectasis. Mucoid impaction or air-fluid levels are characteristically absent.

Mosaic Perfusion

Lung density and attenuation are partially determined by the amount of blood present in lung tissue. On HRCT, inhomogeneous lung opacity can result from regional differences in lung perfusion in patients with airways disease or pulmonary vascular disease [124,125,238]. Because this phenomenon is often patchy or mosaic in distribution, with adjacent areas of lung being of differing attenuation, it has been termed *mosaic perfusion* [5] or *mosaic oligemia* [239], although the former term is most appropriate [6]. Areas of relatively decreased lung opacity seen on HRCT can be of varying sizes and sometimes appear to correspond to lobules, segments, lobes, or an entire lung (Figs. 3-63, 3-109, 3-138, and 3-141 through 3-145). In almost all cases, mosaic perfusion is seen in association with diseases causing regional decreases in lung perfusion. However, differences in attenuation between normal and abnormal lung regions recognizable on HRCT are accentuated by compensatory increased perfusion of normal or relatively normal lung areas.

Mosaic perfusion is most frequent in patients with airways diseases that result in focal air-trapping or poor ventilation of lung parenchyma (Figs. 3-141 through 3-144) [124,125,238]; in these patients, areas of poorly ventilated lung are poorly perfused because of reflex vasoconstriction or because of a permanent reduction in the pulmonary capillary bed. In our experience, this finding has been most common in patients with bronchiolitis obliterans (constrictive bronchiolitis) (Figs. 3-142 through 3-144) or other diseases associated with small airways obstruction such as cystic fibrosis or bronchiectasis of any cause

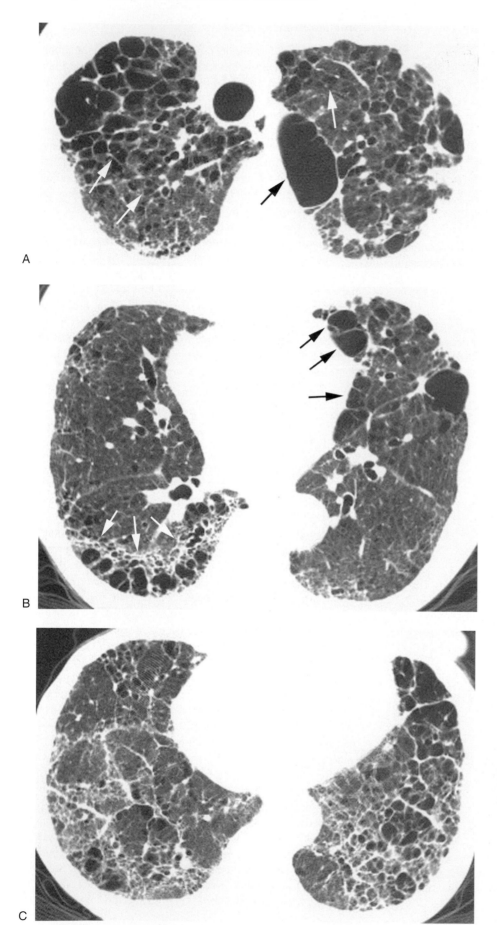

A

B

C

FIG. 3-130. HRCT at three levels in a patient with combined honeycombing and centrilobular and paraseptal emphysema. **A:** In the upper lobes, clear-cut areas of centrilobular emphysema (*white arrows*) can be seen, with subpleural bullae due to paraseptal emphysema (*black arrow*). **B:** At a lower level, findings of both emphysema and fibrosis are visible. Areas of paraseptal emphysema are visible anteriorly (*black arrows*) whereas honeycombing and traction bronchiectasis are visible in the posterior lung (*white arrows*). Paraseptal emphysema occurs in a single layer whereas honeycomb cysts occur in multiple layers. **C:** Near the lung bases, findings of honeycombing and fibrosis predominate.

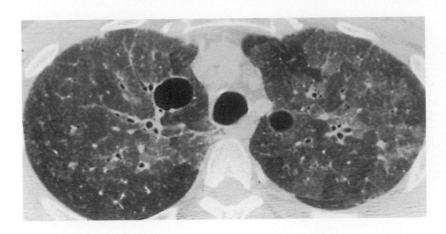

FIG. 3-131. HRCT in a patient with *Pneumocystis carinii* pneumonia shows ground-glass opacity and focal lung cysts representing pneumatoceles.

(Figs. 3-63 and 3-141), but it can also be seen as a result of large bronchial obstruction [240–242]. Mosaic perfusion has also been reported in association with pulmonary vascular obstruction such as that caused by chronic pulmonary embolism [239,243,244].

Regardless of its cause, when mosaic perfusion is present, pulmonary vessels in the areas of decreased opacity often appear smaller than vessels in relatively dense areas of lung [125,244] (Figs. 3-141 through 3-145). This discrepancy reflects differences in regional blood flow and can be quite

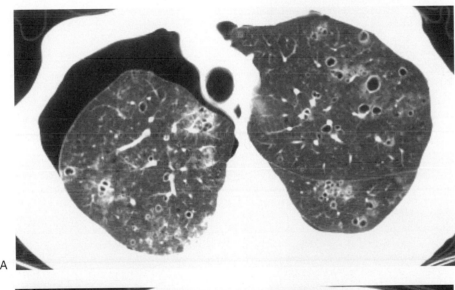

A

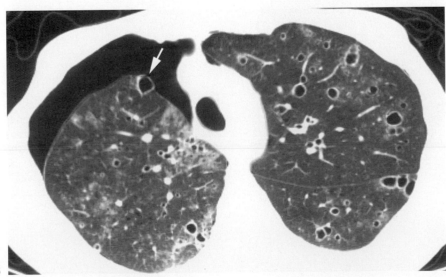

B

FIG. 3-132. HRCT at two levels in an acquired immunodeficiency syndrome patient with recurrent *Pneumocystis carinii* pneumonia associated with pneumatoceles and pneumothorax. **A:** Patchy areas of ground-glass opacity are associated with a number of small cystic spaces representing pneumatoceles. A moderate pneumothorax is present on the right, and a small pneumothorax is visible on the left. **B:** At a lower level, one of the cystic lesions (*arrow*) in the right lung is visible protruding into the air-filled pleural space. The rupture of such a lesion likely accounts for the pneumothorax.

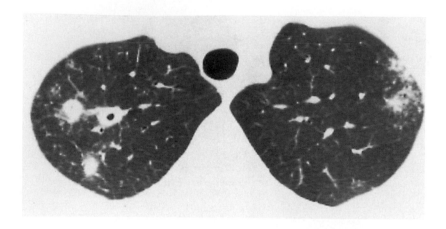

FIG. 3-133. Cavitary nodules in an acquired immunodeficiency syndrome patient with a fungal pneumonia. Nodules appear both solid and cavitary. The cavitated nodule in the right upper lobe is thick-walled.

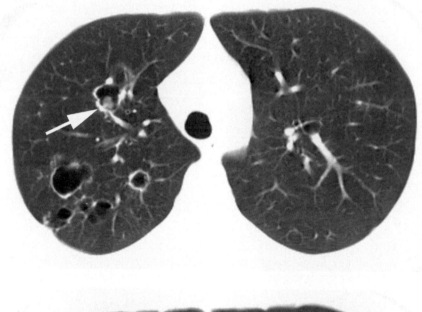

A

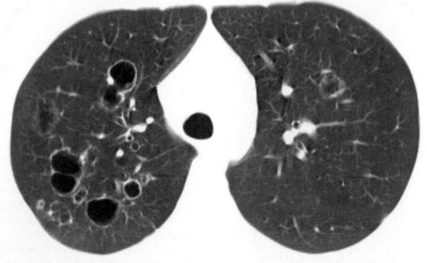

B

FIG. 3-134. A–C: Cavitary nodules or cysts in a patient with tracheobronchial papillomatosis. Thin-walled cystic lesions are visible, with a predominance in the right lung. Associated nodules may be seen within cysts (*arrow*, **A**) or within lung parenchyma (*arrow*, **C**). *Continued*

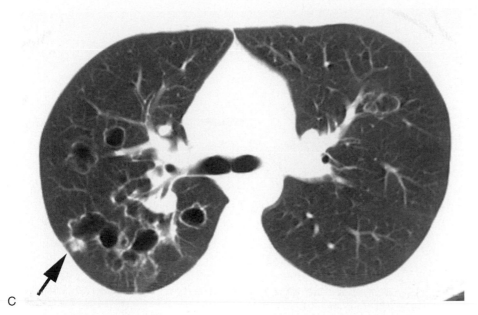

C

FIG. 3 134. *Continued*

helpful in distinguishing mosaic perfusion from ground-glass opacity, which can otherwise have a similar patchy appearance. In patients with ground-glass opacity, vessels usually appear equal in size throughout the lung. For example, in a series of 48 patients with mosaic perfusion primarily due to airways disease, Im et al. [245] observed smaller vessels in areas of low attenuation in 93.8% of cases. It must be pointed out, however, that decreased vessel size may be subtle and difficult to observe in some patients with mosaic perfusion. In a blinded study by Arakawa et al. [246] of patients with inhomogeneous lung opacity of various causes, only 68% of patients with airways or vascular disease were thought to show small vessels in areas of low attenuation.

Mosaic Perfusion Due to Airways Disease

In patients with mosaic perfusion resulting from airways disease, abnormal dilated or thick-walled airways (i.e., bronchiectasis) may be visible in the relatively lucent lung regions, thus suggesting the proper diagnosis [125,242,246]. In one study [247], abnormal airways were seen in 70% of patients with airways disease and mosaic lung attenuation (Figs. 3-141, 3-142, and 3-144). Mosaic perfusion can be seen in a variety of airways diseases including bronchiectasis, cystic fibrosis, and constrictive bronchiolitis. In patients with mosaic perfusion secondary to airways disease, lobular areas of low attenuation are common. Air-trapping on expi-

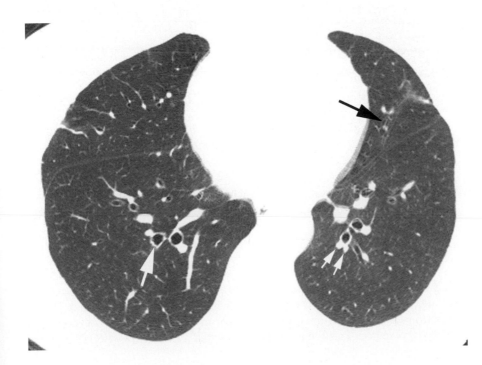

FIG. 3-135. Bronchiectasis and pseudobronchiectasis. Bronchiectasis is considered to be present if the internal diameter of a bronchus is greater than that of its accompanying artery (i.e., the signet ring sign) (*large white arrow*). In the left lower lobe, a bronchus appears to be dilated because its adjacent artery has divided into two branches (*small white arrows*). In the left upper lobe (*black arrow*), a cardiac pulsation or "doubling" artifact results in the appearance of bronchiectasis.

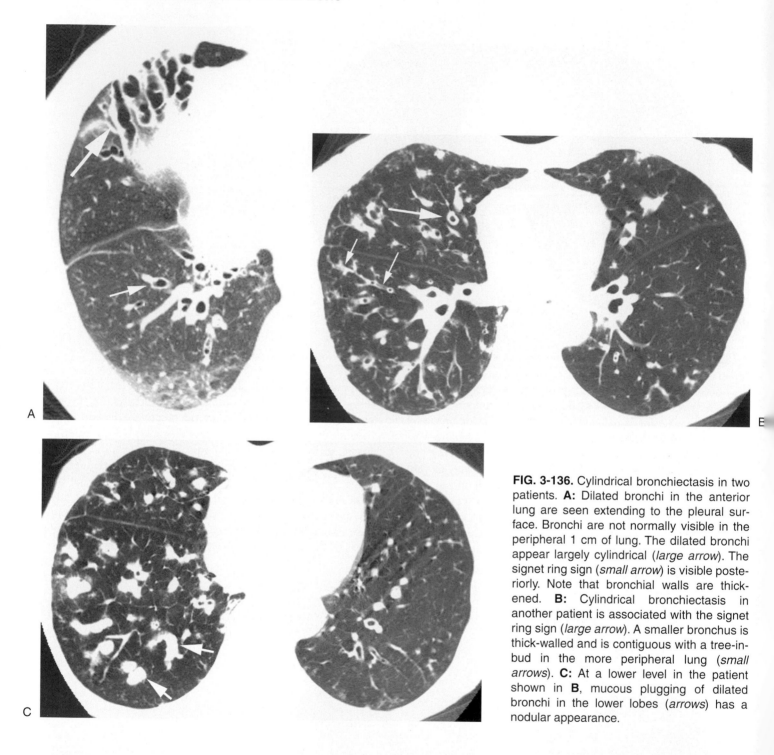

A

C

B

FIG. 3-136. Cylindrical bronchiectasis in two patients. **A:** Dilated bronchi in the anterior lung are seen extending to the pleural surface. Bronchi are not normally visible in the peripheral 1 cm of lung. The dilated bronchi appear largely cylindrical (*large arrow*). The signet ring sign (*small arrow*) is visible posteriorly. Note that bronchial walls are thickened. **B:** Cylindrical bronchiectasis in another patient is associated with the signet ring sign (*large arrow*). A smaller bronchus is thick-walled and is contiguous with a tree-in-bud in the more peripheral lung (*small arrows*). **C:** At a lower level in the patient shown in **B**, mucous plugging of dilated bronchi in the lower lobes (*arrows*) has a nodular appearance.

ratory scans, described in the section below, is often helpful in confirming the diagnosis.

Mosaic Perfusion Due to Vascular Disease

Inhomogeneous lung attenuation is common in patients with chronic pulmonary embolism (CPE), and decreased vessel size in less opaque regions is often visible (Fig. 3-145). In a study of pulmonary parenchymal abnormalities in 75 patients with CPE, 58 patients (77.3%) showed

mosaic perfusion with normal or dilated arteries in areas of hyperattenuation [244]; areas of relatively increased attenuation averaged –727 HU, whereas areas of decreased attenuation averaged –868 HU. In another study of patients with pulmonary hypertension due to CPE, pulmonary hypertension of other causes, and a variety of other pulmonary diseases, HRCT was thought to show mosaic perfusion in all patients with CPE [248]. Considerably more variation in vessel size in different lung regions was also visible in the patients with CPE. Overall, HRCT had a sen-

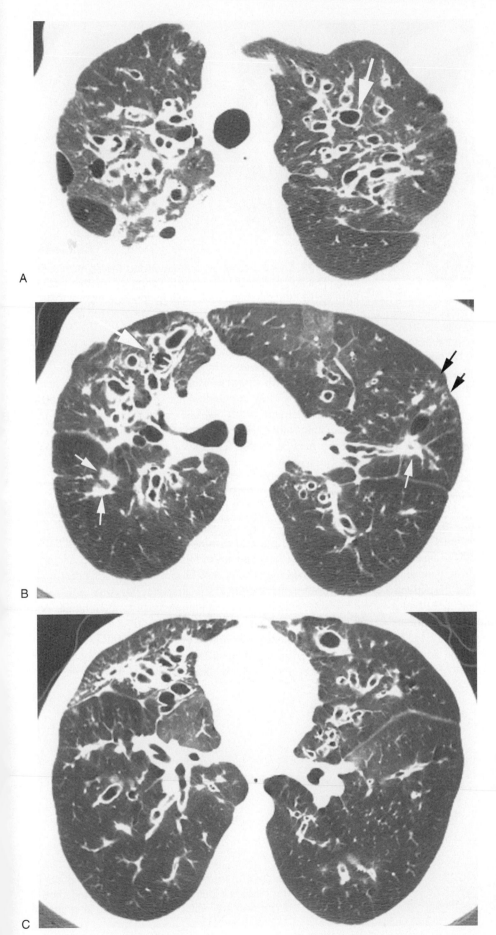

FIG. 3-137. Bronchiectasis in a patient with cystic fibrosis. **A:** In the upper lung, multiple dilated thick-walled bronchi are present. The signet ring sign is visible (*arrow*). **B:** Irregular or varicose bronchiectasis is visible in the anterior right lung (*large white arrow*). Mucous plugging of bronchi is also visible (*small white arrows*), as is tree-in-bud (*black arrows*). **C:** Multiple dilated bronchi with examples of the signet ring sign are also visible at the lung bases.

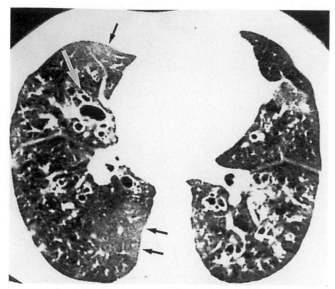

FIG. 3-138. HRCT in a patient with varicose bronchiectasis resulting from allergic bronchopulmonary aspergillosis. Irregular bronchial dilatation (*white arrow*) is visible in the anterior right lung. Dilatation of small bronchioles in the peripheral lung is visible, as is tree-in-bud. Patchy lung opacity, with focal regions of decreased and increased attenuation (*black arrows*), reflects mosaic perfusion.

sitivity of 94% to 100% and a specificity of 96% to 98% in diagnosing CPE [248].

The frequency with which a mosaic pattern of lung opacity is seen on CT in patients with various causes of pulmonary artery hypertension (PAH) has also been studied [249]. Twenty-one patients had PAH caused by lung disease; 17 patients, caused by cardiac disease; and 23 patients, caused by vascular disease. Of the 23 patients with PAH caused by vascular disease, 17 patients (74%) had a mosaic pattern of lung attenuation; 12 of these had CPE. Of the 21 patients with PAH caused by lung disease, one patient (5%) had a mosaic pattern of lung attenuation. Among the 17 patients with PAH caused by cardiac disease, two patients (12%) had a mosaic pattern of lung attenuation [249]. Thus, a mosaic pattern of lung attenuation was seen significantly more often

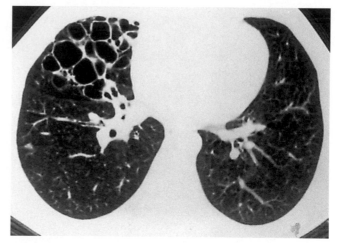

FIG. 3-139. Cystic bronchiectasis involving the right middle lobe. The focal distribution allows distinction of this entity from cystic lung disease, such as in lymphangiomyomatosis.

in patients with PAH caused by vascular disease than in patients with PAH caused by cardiac or lung disease.

In patients with vascular disease as a cause of mosaic perfusion, areas of low attenuation are usually larger than lobules. In patients with mosaic perfusion occurring in association with CPE, enlargement of the main pulmonary arteries may be visible because of pulmonary hypertension (see Chapter 9).

Algorithmic Approach to the Diagnosis of Decreased Lung Opacity

The following series of algorithms may be used to help conceptualize the diagnosis of focal or diffuse lung lucencies.

Decreased lung opacity may be caused by (i) lung destruction, resulting in discrete cystic airspaces not containing recognizable vessels, or (ii) reduction in lung attenuation, or inhomogeneous lung attenuation, without the presence of discrete air-filled spaces or loss of visible vessels (Algorithm 7A). The presence of air-filled cystic spaces or focal lung destruction may indicate the presence of honeycombing,

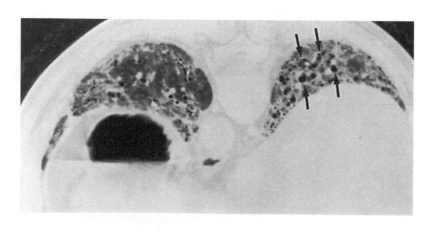

FIG. 3-140. Traction bronchiectasis in a patient with idiopathic pulmonary fibrosis. Dilated bronchi (*arrows*) are visible in the posterior lung base.

emphysema, cystic bronchiectasis, lung cysts, or pneumatoceles. A reduction in lung attenuation or patchy inhomogeneous lung attenuation may be seen in patients with panlobular emphysema, airways disease, vascular disease, or mixed airway and infiltrative disease.

Air-filled cystic spaces first may be classified as subpleural or intraparenchymal for the purposes of differential diagnosis (Algorithm 7B). Air-filled cystic spaces in the subpleural regions may represent paraseptal emphysema or honeycomb-

ing. Both have distinct walls. Paraseptal emphysema is usually distinguishable from honeycombing because the cystic spaces occur in a single layer, whereas honeycomb cysts usually occur in multiple layers. Areas of paraseptal emphysema also can be larger (bullae) than typical honeycomb cysts. Paraseptal emphysema tends to have an upper lobe predominance and may be associated with centrilobular emphysema, whereas honeycombing usually has a lower lobe predominance and is associated with findings of fibrosis.

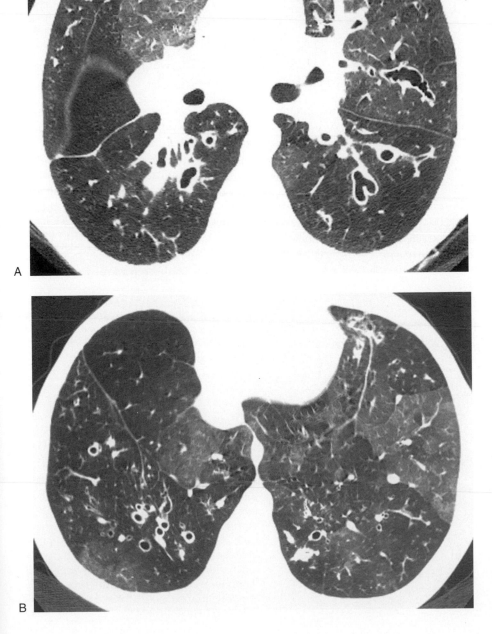

FIG. 3-141. A–C: Mosaic perfusion in three patients with cystic fibrosis. In each patient, vessels appear larger in relatively dense lung regions, a finding of great value in making the diagnosis of mosaic perfusion. The relatively dense lung regions are normally perfused or overperfused because of shunting of blood away from the abnormal areas. Also note that abnormal airways (i.e., bronchiectasis, bronchial wall thickening, tree-in-bud) are often visible in relatively lucent lung regions. These areas are poorly ventilated and poorly perfused. *Continued*

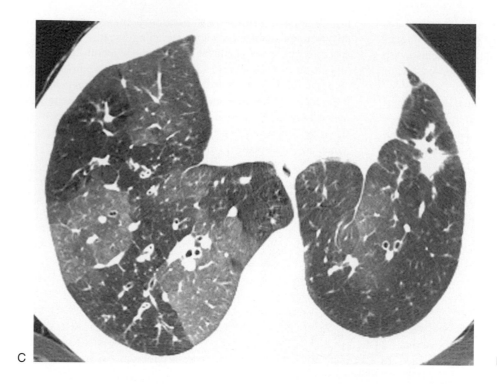

C

FIG. 3-141. *Continued*

Intraparenchymal cystic airspaces (i.e., those not occurring primarily at the pleural surface) can represent centrilobular emphysema, lung cysts, dilated bronchi, or pneumatoceles (Algorithm 7C). In patients with centrilobular emphysema, areas of lucency do not usually have recognizable walls, have an upper lobe distribution in most patients, are relatively small (less than 1 cm in diameter), have a spotty distribution, and may sometimes be seen surrounding a centrilobular artery. Cystic bronchiectasis may result in clustered or scattered thin-walled cystic airspaces. The correct diagnosis may be suggested if air-fluid levels or other findings of bronchiectasis are visible. The term *lung cyst* is used to describe a thin-walled, well-defined and circumscribed air-containing lesion that is 1 cm or larger in diameter. Langerhans histiocytosis and LAM result in multiple lung cysts [92,93,220–224]. The cysts have a thin but easily discernible wall, ranging up to a few millimeters in thickness. Associated findings of fibrosis are usually absent or much less conspicuous than they are in patients with honeycombing. In these diseases, the cysts are usually interspersed within areas of normal-appearing lung. In patients with histiocytosis, the cysts can have bizarre shapes, typi-

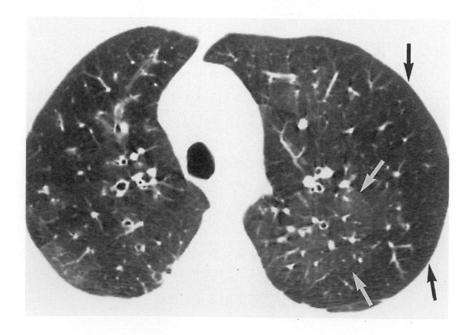

FIG. 3-142. HRCT in a patient with bronchiolitis obliterans related to rheumatoid arthritis. Bronchiectasis is visible, along with patchy lung attenuation, a finding that reflects mosaic perfusion. Note that the pulmonary vessels in the lucent-appearing peripheral left lung (*black arrows*) are smaller than vessels in the denser medial left lung (*white arrows*).

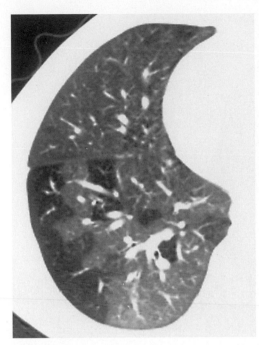

FIG. 3-143. HRCT in a 9-year-old boy with postinfectious bronchiolitis obliterans. Patchy areas of mosaic perfusion are visible, with decreased vascular size within the lucent regions.

cally have an upper lobe predominance, and may occur in men. LAM is associated with rounder and more uniformly shaped cysts, is diffusely distributed from apex to base, and exclusively occurs in women. Cysts are rarely seen in patients with LIP associated with Sjögren's syndrome, AIDS, or other systemic diseases; cystic airspaces in LIP have thin walls, measure 1 to 30 mm in diameter, and are typically less numerous than with histiocytosis and LAM [17,225,250]. Cysts representing pneumatoceles can be seen in patients with infection, particularly *P. carinii* pneumonia; pneumatoceles are often scattered and patchy in distribution and limited in number, and findings of pneumonia or a history of pneumonia may be present.

Decreased lung attenuation in the absence of cystic airspaces, when diffuse, can reflect panlobular emphysema or diffuse airways disease with air-trapping (Algorithm 7D). [124,238]. Patchy, decreased lung opacity often reflects "mosaic perfusion" [239]; it most often is caused by airway and obstructive diseases, such as cystic fibrosis or bronchiolitis obliterans, but can also be seen with vascular diseases such as CPE. Mosaic perfusion may be recognized by the presence of decreased vessel size in areas of lucency. The presence of vascular disease as a cause may be suggested if findings of pulmonary hypertension or cronic pulmonary embolism is present. Similarly, if large or small airway abnormalities are visible, then obstructive disease is the likely cause (Algorithm 7D). Because inhomogeneous lung attenuation resulting from subtle ground-glass opacity may also mimic mosaic perfusion, the presence of infiltrative disease must also be considered in patients with an appearance suggesting mosaic perfusion.

Inhomogeneous Lung Opacity: Differentiation of Mosaic Perfusion from Ground-Glass Opacity

The presence of inhomogeneous lung attenuation on HRCT is a common finding; in one study, inhomogeneous lung opacity was the predominant HRCT abnormality in 19% of scans reviewed [246]. This appearance can be a diagnostic dilemma,

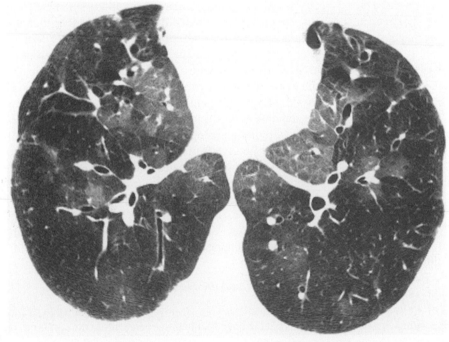

A

FIG. 3-144. A,B: HRCT in a bone marrow transplant recipient with bronchiolitis obliterans. Patchy areas of mosaic perfusion are visible, associated with findings of bronchiectasis. In patients with bronchiolitis obliterans, bronchiectasis is commonly visible. *Continued*

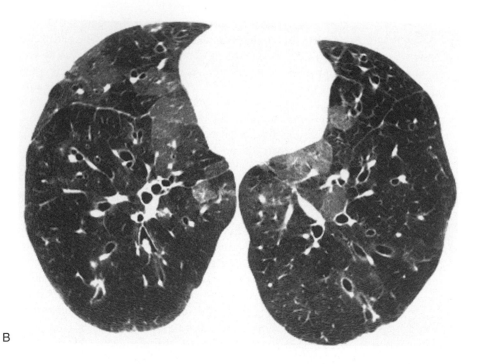

B

FIG. 3-144. *Continued*

resulting from (i) ground-glass opacity, (ii) mosaic perfusion resulting from airways obstruction and reflex vasoconstriction, (iii) mosaic perfusion resulting from vascular obstruction, or (iv) a combination of these (i.e., mixed disease). Because the finding of inhomogeneous lung opacity may be nonspecific, it has been referred to as the *mosaic pattern* [251]. However, most cases of inhomogeneous opacity can be correctly classified as one of these based on HRCT findings [246,247].

On inspiratory scans, it is often possible to distinguish among ground-glass opacity, mosaic perfusion caused by airways disease, and mosaic perfusion caused by vascular disease (Algorithm 8). In two studies [246,247], an accurate distinction was possible in more than 80% of cases based on HRCT findings. The use of expiratory scanning, described in the next section, can also be very helpful in the diagnosis of inhomogeneous lung opacity.

The most important finding in making the diagnosis of mosaic perfusion is that of reduced vessel size in lucent lung regions. If reduced vessel size is visible, a confident diagnosis of mosaic perfusion can usually be made. Also, in patients with mosaic perfusion, some lung regions may appear too lucent to be normal, but this is somewhat subjective and based on experience with the window settings used for scan viewing.

In patients with mosaic perfusion resulting from airways disease, abnormal dilated or thick-walled airways (i.e., bronchiectasis) may be visible in the relatively lucent lung regions, suggesting the proper diagnosis; this is visible in approximately 70% of cases and is very helpful in suggesting the correct diagnosis [241,252–255]. Furthermore, lobular areas of lucency are common in patients with airways disease. In a study by Im et al. [245] of 48 consecutive patients with lobular areas of low attenuation seen on

HRCT, 46 (95%) had symptoms related to respiratory disease, such as productive cough (n = 25) and hemoptysis (n = 18). Only two patients with this appearance, one with chronic pulmonary embolism and one with Takayasu's arteritis combined with bronchiectasis, had pulmonary vascular disease.

In patients with vascular obstruction (e.g., cronic pulmonary embolism) as a cause of mosaic perfusion, dilatation of central pulmonary arteries may be present as a result of pulmonary hypertension, lobular areas of lucency are typically absent, and larger areas of low attenuation are usually visible.

Ground-glass opacity may be accurately diagnosed as the cause of inhomogeneous lung opacity if it is associated with other findings of infiltrative disease such as consolidation, reticular opacities (i.e., the crazy-paving pattern), or nodules. Also, a pattern in which the areas of higher attenuation are centrilobular almost always represents ground-glass opacity with a centrilobular distribution. This pattern is not seen with mosaic perfusion resulting from airways disease; it is uncommonly the result of vascular disease with mosaic perfusion. Ground-glass opacity may also result in very ill-defined and poorly marginated areas of increased opacity, lacking the sharply marginated and geographic appearance sometimes seen in patients with mosaic perfusion. Ground-glass opacity can often be diagnosed simply because lung looks too dense, although this is quite subjective and depends on using consistent window settings and being familiar with the appearance of normal lung parenchyma.

Mixed Disease and the Head-Cheese Sign

In occasional patients, inspiratory scans show a patchy pattern of variable lung attenuation, representing the combination

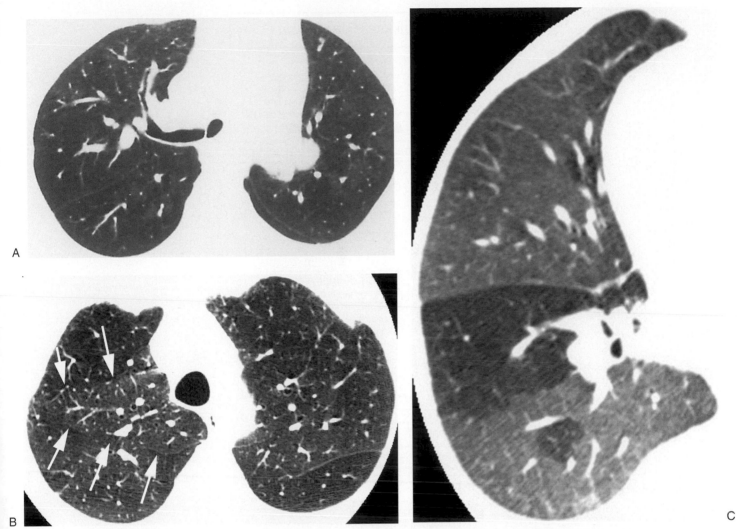

FIG. 3-145. Mosaic perfusion with patchy lung attenuation in three patients with pulmonary embolism.
A: In a patient with chronic pulmonary embolism, peripheral pulmonary vessels are largest in the relatively dense anterior right upper lobe. The main pulmonary artery appears enlarged. **B:** In a patient with acute pulmonary embolism, vessels appear larger in a wedge-shaped area of the relatively dense right upper lobe (*arrows*). **C:** Multidetector-row HRCT through the right lower lobe in a patient with chronic pulmonary thromboembolism shows areas of reduced attenuation caused by vascular obstruction.

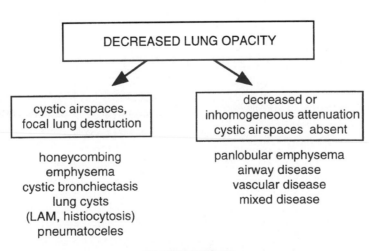

ALGORITHM 7A

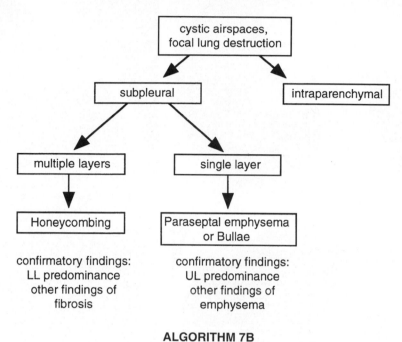

DECREASED LUNG OPACITY

cystic airspaces,
focal lung destruction

↙ subpleural ↘ intraparenchymal

subpleural
↙ multiple layers ↘ single layer

multiple layers
↓
Honeycombing

confirmatory findings:
LL predominance
other findings of
fibrosis

single layer
↓
Paraseptal emphysema
or Bullae

confirmatory findings:
UL predominance
other findings of
emphysema

ALGORITHM 7B

DECREASED LUNG OPACITY

cystic airspaces,
focal lung destruction

↙ subpleural ↓ intraparenchymal

intraparenchymal
↙ no visible walls ↘ visible walls

no visible walls
↓
spotty,
holes small,
UL predominant
↓
Centrilobular
Emphysema

visible walls
↙ patchy or central, signet ring sign ↓ numerous, symmetrical, intervening lung normal ↘ few and scattered, pneumonia

patchy or
central,
signet ring sign
↓
Cystic
Bronchiectasis

numerous,
symmetrical,
intervening lung
normal
↓
Lung Cysts

few and scattered,
pneumonia
↓
Pneumatoceles
e.g., PCP

Lung Cysts
↙ UL predominant irregular shapes ↓ woman uniform distribution cysts round ↘ Sjögrens syn, AIDS limited lung involvement

UL predominant
irregular shapes
↓
Histiocytosis

woman
uniform distribution
cysts round
↓
LAM

Sjögrens syn, AIDS
limited lung involvement
↓
LIP

ALGORITHM 7C

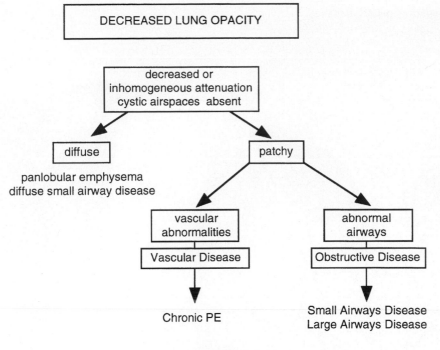

ALGORITHM 7D

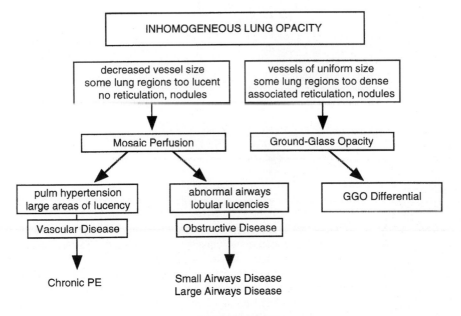

ALGORITHM 8

of ground-glass opacity (or consolidation), normal lung, and reduced lung attenuation as a result of mosaic perfusion. This combination of mixed densities, including the presence of mosaic perfusion, often gives the lung a geographic appearance and has been termed the *head-cheese sign* because of its resemblance to the variegated appearance of a sausage made from parts of the head of a hog (Fig. 3-146) [256]. If you can be sure that both ground-glass opacity or consolidation and mosaic perfusion are visible (rather than one or the other), the head-cheese sign is present. Air-trapping is commonly visible on expiratory scans (Fig. 3-158).

The head-cheese sign is usually indicative of mixed infiltrative and obstructive disease, usually associated with bronchiolitis. In patients with this appearance, the presence of ground-glass opacity or consolidation is caused by lung infiltration, whereas the presence of mosaic perfusion with decreased vessel size is usually caused by small airway obstruction.

The most common causes of this pattern are hypersensitivity pneumonitis, sarcoidosis, and, in our experience, atypical infections with associated bronchiolitis. Each of these diseases results in infiltrative abnormalities and may be associated with airway abnormalities.

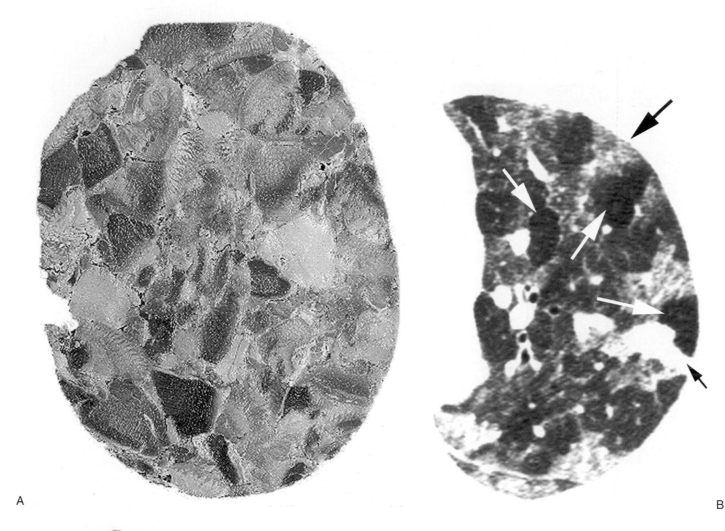

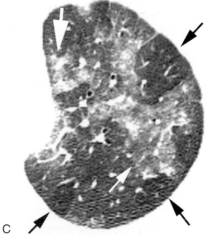

FIG. 3-146. Head cheese and the head-cheese sign. **A:** A slice of head cheese shows a variegated appearance, consisting of chunks of different meats from the head of a hog. Some appear dark, some appear light, and some are gray. **B:** In a patient with *Mycoplasma* pneumonia associated with lung infiltration and bronchiolitis, the head-cheese sign is associated with consolidation (*small black arrow*), ground-glass opacity (*large black arrow*), and lobular areas of mosaic perfusion (*white arrows*). Note the pulmonary arteries are small or invisible in the regions of mosaic perfusion. **C:** In a patient with hypersensitivity pneumonitis showing the head-cheese sign, areas of varying attenuation are visible, including consolidation (*large white arrow*), ground-glass opacity (*small white arrow*), normal lung, and areas of reduced attenuation due to mosaic perfusion (*black arrows*).

EXPIRATORY HIGH-RESOLUTION COMPUTED TOMOGRAPHY

Obtaining HRCT scans at selected levels after expiration may be useful in (i) the diagnosis of air-trapping in patients with obstructive lung disease [246,254,255], (ii) the diagnosis of airways disease unassociated with distinct morphologic abnormalities on inspiratory images [257], (iii) distinguishing mosaic perfusion from ground-glass opacity [246,247], and (iv) allowing the diagnosis of mixed infiltrative and obstructive diseases [246,258,259].

Diagnosis of Air-Trapping in Obstructive Lung Disease

Expiratory HRCT scans have proved useful in the evaluation of patients with a variety of lung diseases characterized by

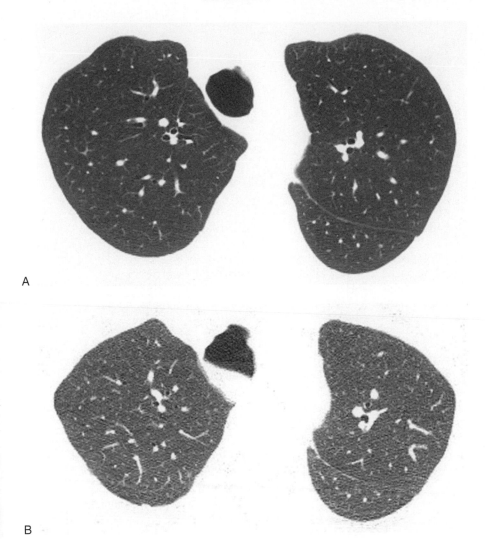

FIG. 3-147. Normal postexpiratory HRCT. Inspiratory image **(A)** shows homogeneous lung attenuation. **B:** After expiration, there has been a significant reduction in lung volume associated with an increase in lung attenuation. Lung attenuation remains homogeneous. Note flattening of the posterior tracheal membrane.

obstruction of airflow [241,242]. Air-trapping visible using expiratory or postexpiratory HRCT techniques has been recognized in patients with emphysema [253,260,261], chronic airways disease [255], asthma [262–264], bronchiolitis obliterans [238,253,257,265–271], the cystic lung diseases associated with Langerhans histiocytosis and tuberous sclerosis [272], bronchiectasis [253,273], and airways disease related to AIDS [274]. Expiratory HRCT also has proved valuable in demonstrating the presence of bronchiolitis in patients with primarily infiltrative diseases such as hypersensitivity pneumonitis [259,275], sarcoidosis [258,276], and pneumonia.

It must be recognized that limited air-trapping can be seen in normal subjects, particularly in the superior segments of the lower lobes or in isolated secondary lobules. Abnormal air-trapping differs from this occurrence to an extent. Expiratory CT techniques and normal findings are described in Chapters 1 and 2.

Lung Attenuation Abnormalities

In normal subjects, lung increases significantly in attenuation during expiration (see Fig. 2-19 through 2-21; Fig. 3-147).

In the presence of airway obstruction and air-trapping, lung remains lucent on expiration and shows little change in a cross-sectional area. Areas of air-trapping are seen as relatively low in attenuation on expiratory scans.

On expiratory HRCT, the diagnosis of air-trapping is easiest to make when the abnormality is patchy in distribution, and normal lung regions can be contrasted with abnormal, lucent lung regions (Figs. 3-148 through 3-153) [125,242]. Areas of air-trapping can be patchy and nonanatomic, can correspond to individual secondary pulmonary lobules, segments, and lobes, or may involve an entire lung [252,277]. Air-trapping in a lobe or lung is usually associated with large airway or generalized small airway abnormalities, whereas lobular or segmental air-trapping is associated with diseases that produce small airway abnormalities [252]. Pulmonary vessels within the low-attenuation areas of air-trapping often appear small relative to vessels in the more opaque normal lung regions [252].

In patients with airways disease or emphysema who have a diffuse abnormality, expiratory inhomogeneities in lung attenuation may not be visible, but air-trapping can be detected by measuring the lung attenuation change occurring

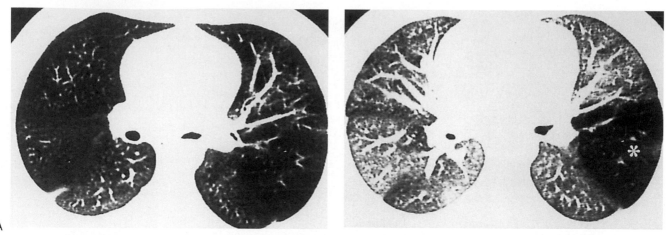

A   B

FIG. 3-148. Dynamic inspiratory **(A)** and expiratory **(B)** HRCT in a patient with postinfectious bronchiolitis obliterans. On expiration, marked inhomogeneity in lung attenuation is noted, with focal air-trapping in the left upper lobe (*asterisk*). Note the relatively small size of pulmonary vessels in the region of air-trapping. A region of interest placed in the area of air-trapping shows a paradoxical decrease in lung attenuation of 30 HU during expiration.

with expiration [241,252–255]. Areas of air-trapping show significantly less attenuation increase than seen in normal lung [269]. The normal mean attenuation difference between full inspiration and expiration usually ranges from 80 to 300 HU. On dynamic scans, a lung attenuation change of less than 70 or 80 HU between full inspiration and full exhalation may be regarded as abnormal (Fig. 3-153). On simple post-expiratory scans, a lung attenuation change of less than 70 HU sometimes may be seen. Lung attenuation change is most simply measured using small (1 to 2 cm) regions of interest on both inspiratory and expiratory scans [254]. Measuring the change in overall lung attenuation from inspiration to expiration may be used in patients with diffuse air-trapping [254] but is clearly less sensitive in patients with patchy disease.

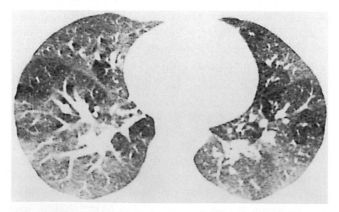

FIG. 3-149. Dynamic expiratory HRCT in a patient with asthma. On expiration, marked inhomogeneity in lung attenuation is noted, with multifocal regions of air-trapping. (From Webb WR. High-resolution computed tomography of obstructive lung disease. *Radiol Clin North Am* 1994;32:745, with permission.)

A second method is to compare equivalent areas in each lung on expiratory scans. In healthy subjects, the mean difference in attenuation change between symmetric regions of the right and left lungs during exhalation was measured as 36 HU ± 14 [278]. From this, a right-left difference in attenuation increase during exhalation exceeding 78 HU [more than three standard deviations greater than the mean] can be considered abnormal. This method is especially useful when air-trapping is unilateral.

Occasionally, lung attenuation decreases during expiration in regions of air-trapping; a decrease of attenuation by as much as –258 HU has been reported during dynamic expiration [253]. Although there is no definite explanation for this phenomenon, several suggestions have been made [253]. The most likely is that during exhalation, lung units trapping air compress small pulmonary vessels, squeezing blood out of the lung and decreasing lung perfusion. Another possible explanation is so-called pendelluft, in which air may pass from a normally ventilated lung unit to a partially obstructed lung unit during rapid expiration, resulting in an increased gas volume [252].

Although measurement of lung attenuation can be used to diagnose air-trapping except in patients with diffuse air-trapping (e.g., emphysema, large bronchial obstruction), the extent of air-trapping rather than overall lung attenuation better predicts pulmonary function test findings of obstruction [252,253].

Pixel Index

The *pixel index* (PI) is defined as the percentage of pixels in both lungs on a single scan that show an attenuation lower than a predetermined threshold value (usually –900 HU to –950 HU) (Fig. 3-154) [260,262,279]. Although the inspiratory PI has wide normal range, the expiratory PI is relatively constant. The normal PI at full inspiration ranges from 0.6 to as much as 58.0 when the threshold is –900 HU [280],

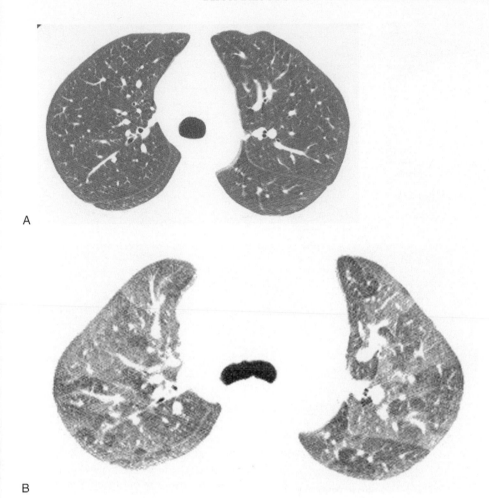

A

B

FIG. 3-150. Expiratory air-trapping in a patient with bronchiolitis obliterans. **A:** Inspiratory scan is normal. **B:** Post-expiratory scan shows patchy lung attenuation with the relatively lucent regions representing regions of air-trapping. Normally ventilated areas increase significantly in attenuation on expiration.

although the mean value ranges from 10 to 25 depending on the level scanned and on the CT scan collimation (Fig. 3-154) [262]. In a study of 42 healthy subjects (21 men, 21 women) aged 23 to 71 years, the inspiratory PI measured using –950 HU ranged from 1.2 to 22.3 (mean, 7.8) [279]. At full expiration, with a threshold value of –900 HU, the normal range of PI is rather small with a mean of less than 1.04 (SD, 1.3) [262]. Thus, in normals, the area of lung having an attenuation of less than –900 HU at full expiration in normals can generally be regarded as less than a few percent.

The expiratory PI can be used to quantitatively assess the area of low attenuation lung in patients with air-trapping or emphysema (Fig. 3-155). For example, in one study [260], 64 patients underwent both inspiratory and expiratory CT correlated with pulmonary physiology. There were 28 patients with an inspiratory PI of more than 40, and 14 of these had an expiratory PI of more than 15. This group showed markedly abnormal pulmonary function test values suggestive of emphysema, whereas other patients showed preserved lung function. Also, an expiratory PI over 15 accurately reflected and quantitated the degree of emphysema estimated by various pulmonary function tests.

The expiratory PI has also been used to quantitatively discriminate asthmatic patients from normal subjects. In one

study of both asthmatic and normal subjects [262], both inspiratory and expiratory PI were obtained at two levels (at the transverse aorta and just superior to the diaphragm) and compared with pulmonary function tests. Using collimations of 10 mm and 1.5 mm, the expiratory PI at a level immediately superior to the diaphragm was significantly higher in asthmatic subjects (4.45 and 10.03 for the two collimations, respectively) than in normal subjects (0.16 and 1.04, respectively) and provided the best separation between the groups [262].

Air-Trapping Score

The extent of air-trapping present on expiratory scans can be measured using a semiquantitative scoring system, which estimates the percentage of lung that appears abnormal on each scan [253–255,273,278,281,282]. Such systems have the advantage of being simple, quick, and easy to perform at the time of image interpretation. Furthermore, in one study [281], a simple 5-point scoring system was found to be associated with better interobserver agreement than a more detailed scoring system.

For example, in the scoring system proposed by Webb et al. [278] and Stern et al. [253], estimates of air-trapping are made at three levels scanned using expiratory technique (at

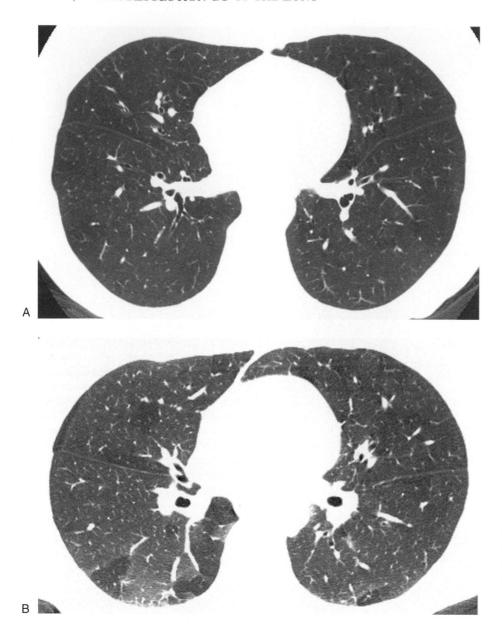

FIG. 3-151. Postexpiratory air-trapping in a patient with asthma. **A:** An inspiratory scan is normal. **B:** Routine postexpiratory scan obtained during suspended respiration after a forced exhalation scan shows patchy air-trapping.

the aortic arch, carina, and 5 cm below the carina). At each level and for each lung, a 5-point scale is used to estimate the extent of air-trapping visible subjectively: 0 = no air-trapping; 1 = 1% to 25% of cross-sectional area of lung affected; 2 = 26% to 50% of affected lung; 3 = 51% to 75% of affected lung; 4 = 76% to 100% of affected lung. The air-trapping score is the sum of these numbers for the three levels studied and ranges from 0 to 24. In several studies using this method, significant differences were found in the extent of air-trapping in normal patients and those with airway obstruction [254], and significant correlations were found between the extent of air-trapping and pulmonary function test measures of airway obstruction [246,253,254].

Other methods of visually scoring the extent of air-trapping on expiratory scans have been used and validated [255,273]. Lucidarme et al. [255] and Lee et al. [282] used a grid superimposed on the expiratory HRCT image and

counted the number of squares containing lucent lung and the number encompassing the entire lung. The air-trapping score represented the ratio of air-trapping squares to the total number of squares overlying lung and approximated the cross-sectional percent of abnormal lung. Excellent interobserver agreement was achieved using this method [255].

In patients studied using postexpiratory HRCT, correlations between the air-trapping score and various pulmonary function test findings of obstruction range from approximately $r = -0.4$ to $r = -0.6$ [246,254,282]; correlations are generally best when normal and abnormal patients are grouped together and when patients with emphysema are included among those with airway obstruction [254]. Thus, in a study by Chen et al. [254], considering only patients with obstructive disease, air-trapping score correlated significantly with forced expiratory volume in 1 second (FEV_1) ($r = -0.78$), FEV_1/forced vital capacity (FVC) ($r = -0.64$), FVC ($r = -0.61$),

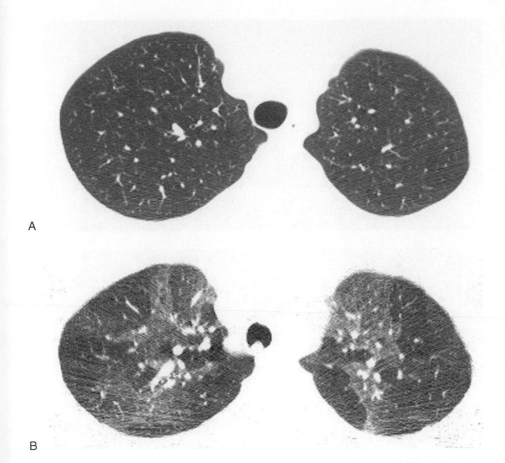

A

B

FIG. 3-152. Postexpiratory air-trapping in a patient with bronchiolitis obliterans related to smoke inhalation. **A:** An inspiratory scan is normal. **B:** A low-dose dynamic expiratory scan shows patchy air-trapping. Note anterior bowing of the posterior tracheal membrane, a good indication of forceful exhalation.

and forced expiratory flow (FEF) at 25% to 75% of vital capacity ($r = -0.65$); when both normal and abnormal patients were considered together, correlations were higher, with r values measuring -0.89, -0.74, -0.77, and -0.81, respectively. In a study by Lucidarme et al. [255] of 74 patients with suspected chronic airway disease, expiratory air-trapping was seen in 18 of 35 (51%) patients with severe airway obstruction (FEV$_1$/FVC <80%), in 21 of 29 (72%) patients with predominantly small airway obstruction (abnormal flow-volume curve and FEV$_1$/FVC ≥80%), and in four of ten (40%) patients with normal PFT results. Air-trapping scores were 27%, 12%, and 8% for these groups, respectively, with significant negative correlations with FEV$_1$ ($r = -0.45$), FEV$_1$/FVC ($r = -0.31$), and FEF at 25% of vital capacity ($r = -0.57$). Lee et al. [282] studied 47 asymptomatic subjects using PFT and expiratory HRCT; in all, PFT were considered to be normal. In this study, the air-trapping grade correlated with FEV$_1$/FVC ($r = -0.44$) In a study of 70 patients with chronic purulent sputum production [273], the air-trapping score defined at a lobular level significantly correlated with values of FEV$_1$ and FEV$_1$/FVC.

Air-trapping can also be seen in normal subjects, although its extent is limited. Air-trapping in one or more secondary pulmonary lobules is not uncommon. Also, focal areas of relative lucency can be seen in normal subjects on expiratory scans in the superior segments of the lower lobes and in the lingula or middle lobe [252,278]. It is postulated that the slender segments may be less well ventilated than adjacent lung, having a tendency to trap air during exhalation [252]. In their study of ten young normal subjects, Webb et al. [278] found that, although air-trapping was present in four patients, the air-trapping score never exceeded a total of 2 (i.e., 25%) at any one level. In subsequent experience with patients having normal PFT, an air-trapping score of up to 6/24 (i.e., 25%) has been found when the superior segments are included in analysis [254]. In a study by Lucidarme et al. [255] of ten normal nonsmokers, excluding the superior segments of the lower lobes and isolated pulmonary lobules, no air-trapping was visible. In a study by Lee et al. [282], an air-trapping score equivalent to less than 5% of lung was seen in 32% of asymptomatic patients, and an air-trapping score of between 5% and 25% was seen in an additional 20%. In this study, although all patients were considered normal, an air-trapping extent between 5% and 25% was more frequent in smokers (33%) than nonsmokers (14%) [282].

Lung Area Changes

Robinson and Kreel have shown that a significant correlation exists between changes in cross-sectional lung area measured using CT and lung volume ($r = 0.569$) [283]. The percentage decrease in lung cross-sectional area that occurred during exhalation also correlates with the attenuation increase [278,283]. In a study using dynamic ultrafast

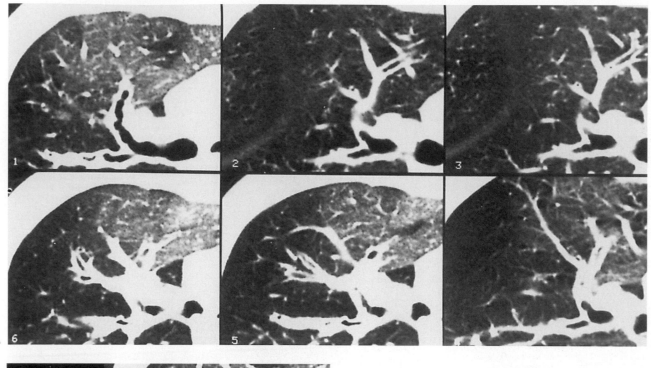

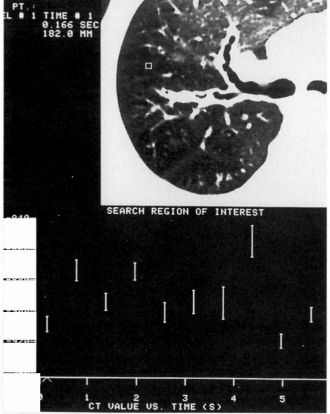

FIG. 3-153. Dynamic expiratory HRCT in a patient with cystic fibrosis obtained using an electron-beam scanner. **A:** Six dynamic images from a sequence of ten, through the right upper lobe region, shown sequentially in a clockwise fashion from the upper left to lower left. On inspiration (*top middle*), lung opacity appears homogeneous. On expiration (*lower left corner*), a part of the anterior segment shows a normal increase in opacity, whereas the remainder of the upper lobe remains lucent. **B:** Time-attenuation curve measured in a lucent region of the upper lobe shows little change in attenuation during expiration.

HRCT [278], a significant correlation between cross-sectional lung area and lung attenuation was found for each of three lung regions evaluated (upper lung: $r = 0.51$, $p = .03$, midlung: $r = 0.58$, $p = .01$; lower lung: $r = 0.51$, $p = .05$).

Usually, areas of air-trapping show little or no area and volume change during exhalation and can help to identify areas of air-trapping. In one study of nine cases of Swyer-James syndrome [238], expiratory CT scans in areas of

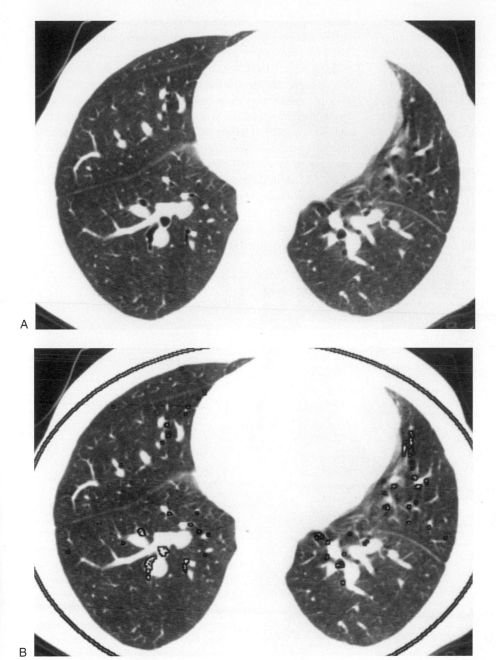

FIG. 3-154. Pixel index measured in a patient with bilateral lung transplantation and normal lung function. An expiratory scan **(A)** and scan with pixels measuring less than –900 HU (highlighted) **(B)** are shown. The low attenuation pixels shown in **B** represent 0.6% of lung area (pixel index, 0.6). This is normal. (From Arakawa H, Webb WR. Expiratory HRCT scan. *Radiol Clin North Am* 1998;36:189, with permission.)

abnormal lung showed no significant lung volume change, and mediastinal shift toward the normal lung was also seen.

In a study by Lucidarme et al. [255] of 74 patients with suspected chronic airway disease and ten normal subjects, an area-reduction score was measured, representing the reduction in cross-sectional lung area from inspiration to expiration. Area-reduction scores were 18%, 30%, and 35%, respectively, for groups of patients with severe airway obstruction ($FEV_1/FVC <80\%$), predominantly small airways obstruction (abnormal flow-volume curve and $FEV_1/FVC \geq 80\%$), and normal PFT results. In the normal subjects, the area-reduction score was 43%. Area-reduction score correlated significantly with all PFT indexes ($r = 0.35$ to 0.66) except total lung capacity.

Diagnosis of Air-Trapping in Patients with Normal Inspiratory Scans

In some patients, inhomogeneous lung attenuation is visible on expiratory scans in the presence of normal inspiratory scans, indicating the presence of obstructive disease (Figs. 3-149 through 3-152). In one study [257], HRCT in 273 consecutive patients with suspected diffuse lung disease was reviewed. Forty-five patients showed air-trapping on expiratory HRCT scans. Of these 45 patients, inspiratory HRCT scans showed abnormal findings in 36 (bronchiectasis, bronchiolitis obliterans, asthma, chronic bronchitis, and cystic fibrosis). In the remaining nine patients, inspiratory HRCT showed normal findings; conditions in these nine patients included bronchiolitis obliterans (n = 5), asthma (n = 3), and chronic bronchitis (n = 1). Results of pulmonary function tests in patients with air-trapping and normal findings on inspiratory scans were intermediate, falling between those of patients with normal findings on inspiratory and expiratory HRCT scans and those of patients with air-trapping and abnormal findings on inspiratory scans. This appearance can also be seen in patients with hypersensitivity pneumonitis.

Inhomogeneous Lung Opacity: Differentiation of Mosaic Perfusion from Ground-Glass Opacity

As indicated above, the presence of inhomogeneous lung attenuation on inspiratory scans is a common finding [246]. This appearance may result from ground-glass opacity,

mosaic perfusion resulting from airways obstruction and reflex vasoconstriction, mosaic perfusion resulting from vascular obstruction, or a combination of these.

Expiratory HRCT scans may be useful in the diagnosis of inhomogeneous opacity and can usually allow the differentiation of mosaic perfusion resulting from airways obstruction from other abnormalities when the inspiratory scans are inconclusive (Algorithm 9). In patients with ground-glass opacity, expiratory HRCT typically shows a proportional increase in attenuation in areas of both increased and decreased opacity (Fig. 3-156). In patients with mosaic perfusion resulting from airways disease, attenuation differences are accentuated on expiration (Fig. 3-157); relatively dense areas increase in attenuation, whereas lower attenuation regions remain lucent (i.e., air-trapping is present) [125,252,272,278].

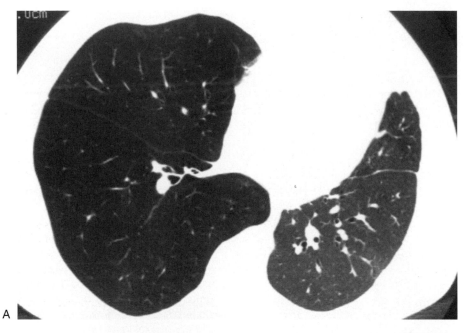

A

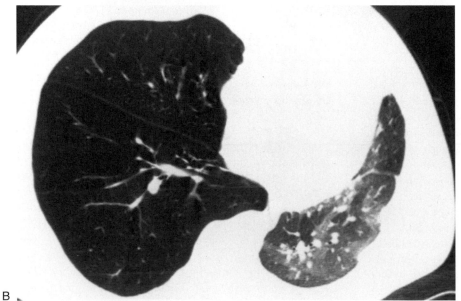

B

FIG. 3-155. Inspiratory and postexpiratory images in a patient with left lung transplantation for panlobular emphysema. **A:** Inspiratory HRCT shows extensive right-sided emphysema. **B:** On a postexpiratory HRCT, measured using a region of interest, there was little or no attenuation increase in the right lung. As compared to the inspiratory image, patchy air-trapping on the left is visible as inhomogeneous opacity. This finding suggests small airway obstruction and is consistent with constrictive bronchiolitis. This was confirmed on transbronchoscopic biopsy. **C:** Pixels having a value of less than −900 HU in the post–expiratory image have been highlighted. The pixel index for the emphysematous right lung measures 72 and is markedly abnormal. The pixel index for the left lung measures 0.7, and is within normal limits. (From Arakawa H, Webb WR. Expiratory HRCT scan. *Radiol Clin North Am* 1998;36:189, with permission.) *Continued*

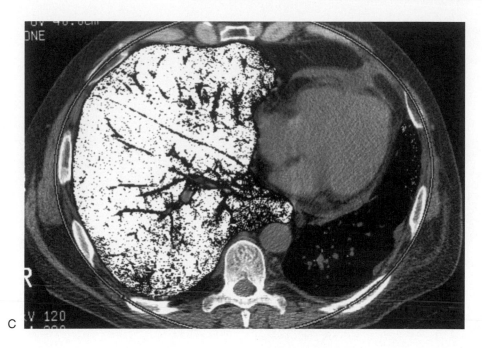

C

FIG. 3-155. *Continued*

In a study by Arakawa et al. [246] of patients showing inhomogeneous opacity as their predominant HRCT abnormality, the accuracy of HRCT in correctly diagnosing the type of disease present increased from 81% to 89% in patients with ground-glass opacity and from 84% to 100% in diagnosing airways disease when expiratory scans were included in the analysis [246]. Some patients who appear to show ground-glass opacity on inspiratory scans and show air-trapping on expiratory scans thus may be correctly diagnosed as having obstructive disease (Algorithm 9).

In patients with mosaic perfusion resulting from vascular disease, expiratory HRCT findings mimic those seen in patients with ground-glass opacity; both low-attenuation and high-attenuation regions increase in attenuation on expiration. In patients with mosaic perfusion due to vascular disease, air-trapping is not usually seen. However, in a study of

patients with inhomogeneous lung attenuation of various causes [247], air-trapping was thought to be present on expiratory scans in some patients with vascular disease when scans were viewed blindly.

Mixed Disease

In patients with mixed infiltrative and airways disease, inspiratory scans may show a patchy pattern of variable lung attenuation, representing the combination of ground-glass opacity (or consolidation), normal lung, and reduced lung attenuation as a result of mosaic perfusion. This combination of mixed densities has been termed the head-cheese sign (Fig. 3-146) [256] and is most typical of hypersensitivity pneumonitis (Fig. 3-158), sarcoidosis, and atypical infections with associated bronchiolitis (Fig. 3-159).

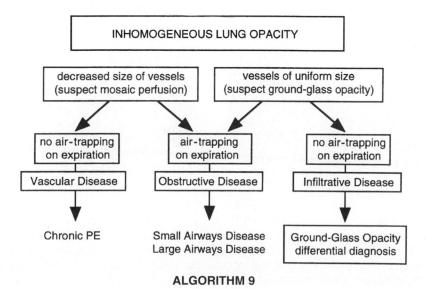

ALGORITHM 9

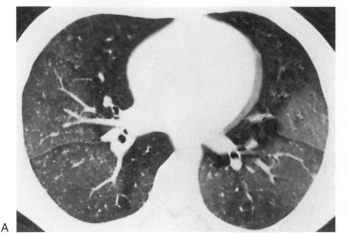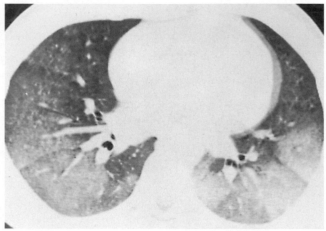

A B

FIG. 3-156. Inspiratory and postexpiratory HRCT in a patient with pulmonary hemorrhage and ground-glass opacity. **A:** Patchy differences in lung opacity are visible on the inspiratory scan. This appearance mimics mosaic perfusion. **B:** On a postexpiratory scan, proportional increases in lung opacity are seen throughout the lungs. Lung attenuation increased by 150 to 200 HU on the expiratory scan in all lung regions.

In some patients with mixed infiltrative and obstructive diseases, ground-glass opacity may be seen on the inspiratory scans without clear-cut findings of mosaic perfusion. However, in such cases, the presence of air-trapping on expiratory images may allow the correct diagnosis of mixed infiltrative and obstructive disease [246]. The combination of ground-glass opacity or consolidation on inspiratory scans and air-trapping on expiratory scans should also be considered indicative of a mixed abnormality (Fig. 3-158) [246].

In a study by Chung et al. [256], 14 of 400 consecutive patients having HRCT with routine expiratory images showed findings of infiltrative lung disease on inspiratory scans and significant air-trapping on expiratory scans. These 14 patients included six with hypersensitivity pneumonitis, five with sarcoidosis, two with atypical infections, and one with pulmonary edema. Ten patients showed ground-glass opacity on inspiratory scans, whereas four patients with sarcoidosis showed nodules. Mosaic perfusion was seen in ten patients. Pulmonary function tests demonstrated a mixed pattern in five patients, an obstructive pattern in four patients, and a restrictive pattern in three patients. FEV_1/FVC correlated significantly with the extent of air-trapping score ($r = 0.58$, $p = .05$). The extent of infiltrative abnormalities correlated significantly with

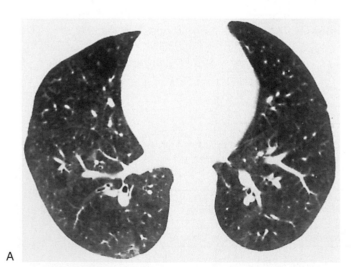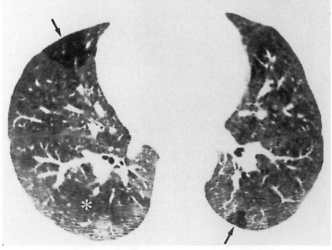

A B

FIG. 3-157. Inspiratory and postexpiratory HRCT in a patient with bronchiolitis obliterans. **A:** Inspiratory scan shows subtle differences in opacity in different lung regions, representing mosaic perfusion. **B:** Postexpiratory HRCT shows a marked accentuation in attenuation inhomogeneities due to air-trapping. Regions of lucency increased in attenuation by approximately 50 HU on expiration. Although some areas of air-trapping appear patchy and nonanatomic (*asterisk*), others appear subsegmental or lobular (*arrows*).

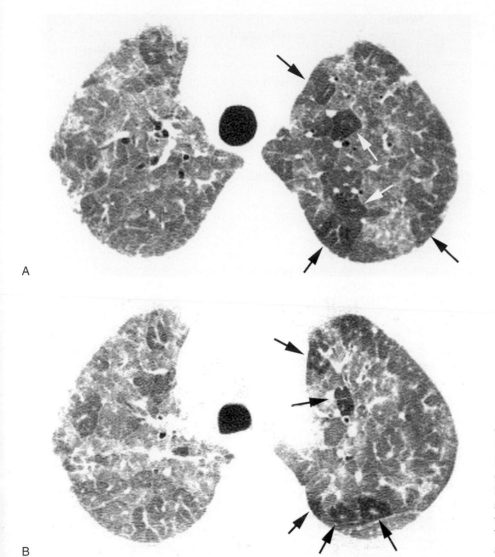

FIG. 3-158. Hypersensitivity pneumonitis with the head-cheese sign. **A:** An inspiratory scan shows inhomogeneous lung attenuation consisting of ground-glass opacity and lobular areas of lucency (*arrows*) due to mosaic perfusion. **B:** Expiratory scan shows air-trapping in the lucent regions (*arrows*). These areas show little or no change in attenuation on the expiratory scans.

FVC ($r = -0.77$, $p = .003$) and diffusing capacity (DLCO) ($r = -0.75$, $p = .01$).

Air-trapping in association with ground-glass opacity is a common HRCT finding in both the subacute and chronic stages of hypersensitivity pneumonitis [259]. In a series of 22 patients with hypersensitivity pneumonitis, HRCT scans with a limited number of expiratory images were correlated with pulmonary function tests [259]. Areas of decreased attenuation, mosaic perfusion, and air-trapping were seen in 19 patients and were the most frequent findings. In addition, the extent of decreased attenuation correlated well with severity of functional index of air-trapping as indicated by increased residual volume ($r = 0.58$, $p < .01$).

In patients with sarcoidosis, HRCT commonly shows findings of mosaic perfusion and air-trapping in addition to findings of infiltrative disease [258,276]. Hansell et al. [258] attempted to determine the relationship between the obstructive defects of pulmonary sarcoidosis and HRCT patterns of disease in 45 patients. The most prevalent CT patterns were decreased lung attenuation on expiratory scans ($n = 40$), a reticular pattern ($n = 37$), and a nodular pattern ($n = 36$). A reticular pattern was the main determinant of functional impairment, particularly airflow obstruction, as shown by inverse relationships with FEV_1 and FEV_1/FVC, among others. Decreased attenuation on expiratory scans was also significantly related to measures of airway obstruction, although correlations were weaker.

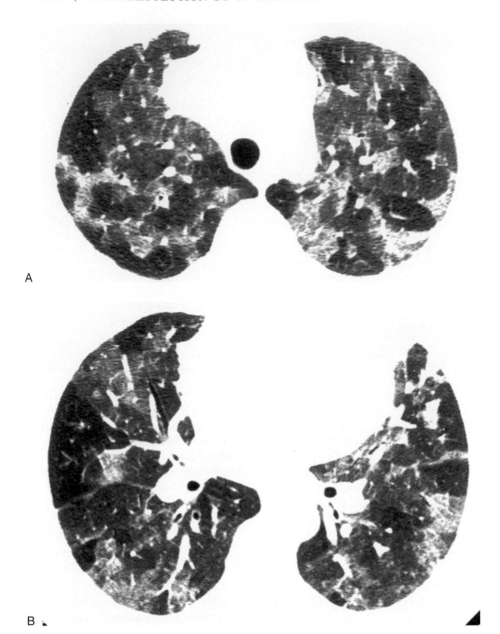

A

B

FIG. 3-159. A,B: *Mycoplasma* pneumonia with the head-cheese sign. Inspiratory images show inhomogeneous lung attenuation consisting of ground-glass opacity and multiple lobular areas of lucency due to mosaic perfusion, and secondary to bronchiolitis. Air-trapping was present on expiratory scans.

DISTRIBUTION OF PARENCHYMAL ABNORMALITIES IN THE DIAGNOSIS OF LUNG DISEASE

When attempting to reach a diagnosis or differential diagnosis of lung disease using HRCT, the overall distribution of pulmonary abnormalities should be considered along with their morphology, HRCT appearance, and distribution relative to lobular structures [41,60,76,101]. Many lung diseases show specific regional distributions or preferences, a fact that is likely related to their underlying pathogenesis and pathophysiology [284].

Preferential or predominant involvement of one or more lung regions is commonly seen on HRCT, even in patients with chest radiographs showing a diffuse abnormality. For the purposes of interpreting HRCT, the regional distribution of lung abnormalities can be categorized in several ways: central lung versus peripheral lung, upper lung versus lower lung, anterior lung versus posterior lung, or unilateral versus bilateral.

An important caveat to keep in mind when reading the following section is that significant variations in classical patterns of lung involvement can be seen in individual patients. A specific diagnosis should not be excluded because of an atypical distribution of abnormalities.

Central Lung versus Peripheral Lung

Some diseases have a central, perihilar, bronchocentric, or bronchovascular distribution [9,60], whereas others favor the peripheral or subpleural parenchyma, or lung cortex (Table 3-13). Diseases that can have a central or perihilar predominance include sarcoidosis (Fig. 3-81),

TABLE 3-13. *Predominance of lung disease on HRCT: central lung versus peripheral lung*

Lung disease	Findings
Central lung	
Sarcoidosis	Peribronchovascular nodules; conglomerate fibrosis with traction bronchiectasis
Silicosis	Conglomerate masses of fibrosis
Talcosis	Conglomerate masses of fibrosis
Lymphangitic spread of carcinoma	Peribronchovascular interstitial thickening or nodules
Large airways diseases	Bronchiectasis (e.g., cystic fibrosis)
Peripheral lung	
Usual interstitial pneumonitis—idiopathic pulmonary fibrosis; collagen diseases; asbestosis	Subpleural fibrosis; honeycombing; sometimes ground-glass opacity
Nonspecific interstitial pneumonia	Subpleural ground-glass opacity; reticulation
Chronic eosinophilic pneumonia	Subpleural consolidation or ground-glass opacity
Bronchiolitis obliterans organizing pneumonia	Subpleural consolidation or ground-glass opacity
Acute interstitial pneumonia	Peripheral consolidation; ground-glass opacity
Desquamative interstitial pneumonia	Peripheral ground-glass opacity in some
Hypersensitivity pneumonitis	Peripheral ground-glass opacity in some
Hematogenous metastases	Peripheral predominance of nodules common

silicosis (Fig. 3-83), lymphangitic spread of carcinoma [285], and large airways diseases, such as bronchiectasis, cystic fibrosis, and allergic bronchopulmonary aspergillosis (Fig. 3-138) [11,12,41,56,76,90,101]. In a study by Grenier et al. [285], a predominantly central distribution of abnormalities was visible in 16% of patients with sarcoidosis, 31% of patients with silicosis, and 8% of those with lymphangitic spread of carcinoma. In another study [76], a central or peribronchovascular predominance was seen in 70% of patients with sarcoidosis and 60% of patients with lymphangitic spread of carcinoma.

A peripheral, cortical, or subpleural predominance of abnormalities has been reported in nearly all patients with eosinophilic pneumonia (Figs. 3-103 and 3-104) [204] and asbestosis [62], 81% to 94% of patients with IPF (Figs. 3-25 and 3-95) [62,76,77], and a similar high percentage of patients with scleroderma, rheumatoid lung disease (Figs. 3-17 and 3-36), or interstitial pneumonia of other causes [143,285]. Peripheral predominance of abnormalities is somewhat less common, visible in approximately half of patients with BOOP (Fig. 3-102) and DIP [62,76,134,193]. It is occasionally present in patients with hypersensitivity pneumonitis and sarcoidosis, ranging from a few percent to 18% in different studies, and in patients with AIP [185]. In patients with hematogenous metastases, nodules may have a peripheral predominance. A subpleural predominance is also typical of amyloidosis, although this disease is quite rare.

Upper Lung versus Lower Lung

The relative extent and severity of abnormalities in the upper lungs and midlungs and at the lung bases can be deter-

mined on HRCT if scans have been obtained at several levels and if one level is compared to the others. Some diseases tend to predominate in the upper lobes, whereas others predominate in the lower lobes (Table 3-14) [286].

Diseases that have been recognized to have an upper lobe predominance on HRCT include sarcoidosis (Figs. 3-5, 3-6, and 3-81), Langerhans histiocytosis (Figs. 3-113 through 3-115), CWP and silicosis (Fig. 3-49), and centrilobular emphysema (Fig. 3-123) [21,58,76,77,90,92,93,101,285]. An upper lobe predominance of abnormalities is present in nearly equal percentages of patients with sarcoidosis (47% to 50%), Langerhans histiocytosis (57% to 62%), and silicosis (55% to 69%), whereas a lower lobe predominance is present in less than 10% of patients with these diseases [77,285]. An upper lobe predominance may be present in patients with respiratory bronchiolitis [109].

A basal distribution is most typical of lymphangitic metastasis (46%), hematogenous metastases, IPF (68%) (Fig. 3-30), collagen-vascular diseases such as rheumatoid lung disease and scleroderma (80%), and asbestosis [39,41,42,62,63,76,77,143,285]. Pulmonary fibrosis of any cause has a basal predominance in approximately 60% of cases [76,77]. Although hypersensitivity pneumonitis is believed to have an upper lobe predominance, it more often appears to be diffuse or preponderant in the mid [23,62] or lower lung zones (30%) [285].

Anterior versus Posterior

Some diseases produce their initial or most extensive abnormalities in the posterior lung (Table 3-15). The distinction between anterior and posterior, of course, is easily made

TABLE 3-14. *Predominance of lung disease on HRCT: upper lung versus lower lung*

Lung disease	Findings
Upper lung	
Sarcoidosis	Nodules; fibrosis; conglomerate masses
Langerhans histiocytosis	Nodules; cysts
Silicosis	Nodules; conglomerate masses
Talcosis	Conglomerate masses of fibrosis
Tuberculosis	Consolidation; nodules; cavities; scarring
Cystic fibrosis	Bronchiectasis; emphysema
Centrilobular emphysema	Focal lucencies
Respiratory bronchiolitis	Ground-glass opacity
Lower lung	
Usual interstitial pneumonitis—idiopathic pulmonary fibrosis; collagen diseases; asbestosis	Subpleural fibrosis; honeycombing; sometimes ground-glass opacity
Nonspecific interstitial pneumonia	Subpleural ground-glass opacity; reticulation
Lipoid pneumonia	Consolidation; ground-glass opacity
Bronchiolitis obliterans organizing pneumonia	Subpleural consolidation or ground-glass opacity
Hematogenous or lymphangitic metastases	Nodules; septal thickening

on HRCT. However, it is important to recognize the value of using both prone and supine scans in this regard. Areas of increased attenuation that are limited to the posterior lung on scans obtained in the supine position can reflect normal dependent volume loss; prone scans are essential in making a confident diagnosis of early posterior lung disease. Although the percentages vary in different series, a posterior preponderance of disease is particularly common in scleroderma (60%), sarcoidosis (32% to 36%) (Fig. 3-82), silicosis (31% to 38%) (Fig. 3-49), hypersensitivity pneumonitis (23%), IPF (9% to 21%), and other causes of UIP (Figs. 3-31 and 3-36) [58,76,77,90,285]. A posterior predominance of abnormalities is also common in patients with asbestosis,

lymphangitic carcinomatosis, and pulmonary edema [39,41,63,76,77,90,143,285]. In patients with pulmonary edema, the predominant abnormality is more appropriately referred to as *dependent* (Fig. 3-10) rather than *posterior*.

An anterior predominance of lung disease is unusual but has been reported in adult survivors of ARDS [71]. In this study, HRCT was obtained during the acute illness and at follow-up in 27 patients with ARDS. At follow-up CT, a reticular pattern was the most prevalent abnormality (85%), with a striking anterior distribution (see Fig. 6-76). This finding was related to the duration of mechanical ventilation and was inversely correlated with the extent of parenchymal opacification on scans obtained during the acute illness.

TABLE 3-15. *Predominance of lung disease on HRCT: posterior lung versus anterior lung*

Lung disease	Findings
Posterior lung	
Usual interstitial pneumonia; Nonspecific interstitial pneumonia	Fibrosis; ground-glass opacity
Asbestosis	Fibrosis
Scleroderma	Fibrosis; ground-glass opacity
Silicosis	Nodules; conglomerate masses
Sarcoidosis	Nodules; conglomerate masses
Pulmonary edema	Septal thickening; ground-glass opacity; consolidation
Adult respiratory distress syndrome (ARDS)	Ground-glass opacity; consolidation
Hypersensitivity pneumonitis	Ground-glass opacity; nodules; fibrosis
Lipoid pneumonia	Consolidation; ground-glass opacity
Anterior lung	
Post-ARDS fibrosis	Subpleural fibrosis; honeycombing; traction bronchiectasis

TABLE 3-16. *Predominance of lung disease on HRCT: unilateral or markedly asymmetric disease*

Disease	Findings
Pneumonia	Variable
Lymphangitic spread of carcinoma	Peribronchovascular interstitial thickening; nodules; septal thickening
Sarcoidosis	Peribronchovascular; subpleural; septal nodules
Bronchiectasis	Findings of bronchiectasis

Unilateral versus Bilateral

A unilateral predominance of abnormalities is most typical of lymphangitic spread of carcinoma, which is often asymmetric in distribution (Table 3-16); this was seen in nearly 40% of patients with lymphangitic spread of carcinoma in one series (Figs. 3-4 and 3-9) [76]. Asymmetry or unilateral predominance of findings is also common in patients with sarcoidosis, ranging from 9% to 21%. It is somewhat less frequent in association with silicosis (2% to 21%), pulmonary fibrosis (3% to 14%), Langerhans histiocytosis (12%), and hypersensitivity pneumonitis (5%) [76,77].

Diffuse Lung Involvement

Some diseases that appear diffuse on chest films are in fact diffuse and involve the lung uniformly from apex to base, from anterior to posterior, and from central to peripheral (Table 3-17) [76,101]. This is not to say that the disease may not be patchy in distribution with some areas much more abnormal than others, but rather that there is no consistent pattern to the disease. Many of the diseases that are described in the previous section as showing a particular distribution can also be diffuse; these include lymphangitic spread of car-

cinoma, sarcoidosis, and silicosis. One disease that typically shows this uniform distribution is hypersensitivity pneumonitis [76,101,130]. LAM tends to be diffuse, whereas Langerhans histiocytosis does not [224].

TABLE 3-17. *Diffuse lung disease*

Disease	Findings
Diffuse pneumonia	Ground-glass opacity; consolidation
Lymphangitic spread of carcinoma	Peribronchovascular interstitial thickening; nodules; septal thickening
Hematogenous metastases	Nodules
Sarcoidosis	Peribronchovascular; subpleural; septal nodules
Hypersensitivity pneumonitis	Ground-glass opacity; nodules; fibrosis
Lymphangiomyomatosis	Lung cysts
Bronchiectasis	Findings of bronchiectasis

REFERENCES

1. Müller NL, Miller RR. Computed tomography of chronic diffuse infiltrative lung disease: part 1. *Am Rev Respir Dis* 1990;142:1206–1215.
2. Müller NL, Miller RR. Computed tomography of chronic diffuse infiltrative lung disease: part 2. *Am Rev Respir Dis* 1990;142:1440–1448.
3. Webb WR. High-resolution CT of the lung parenchyma. *Radiol Clin North Am* 1989;27:1085–1097.
4. Zerhouni E. Computed tomography of the pulmonary parenchyma: an overview. *Chest* 1989;95:901–907.
5. Webb WR, Müller NL, Naidich DP. Standardized terms for high-resolution computed tomography of the lung: a proposed glossary. *J Thorac Imag* 1993;8:167–185.
6. Austin JH, Müller NL, Friedman PJ, et al. Glossary of terms for CT of the lungs: recommendations of the Nomenclature Committee of the Fleischner Society. *Radiology* 1996;200:327–331.
7. Zerhouni EA, Naidich DP, Stitik FP, et al. Computed tomography of the pulmonary parenchyma: part 2. Interstitial disease. *J Thorac Imaging* 1985;1:54–64.
8. Nishimura K, Kitaichi M, Izumi T, et al. Usual interstitial pneumonia: histologic correlation with high-resolution CT. *Radiology* 1992;182:337–342.
9. Murata K, Takahashi M, Mori M, et al. Peribronchovascular interstitium of the pulmonary hilum: normal and abnormal findings on thin-section electron-beam CT. *AJR Am J Roentgenol* 1996;166:309–312.
10. Weibel ER. Looking into the lung: what can it tell us? *AJR Am J Roentgenol* 1979;133:1021–1031.
11. Munk PL, Müller NL, Miller RR, et al. Pulmonary lymphangitic carcinomatosis: CT and pathologic findings. *Radiology* 1988;166:705–709.
12. Stein MG, Mayo J, Müller N, et al. Pulmonary lymphangitic spread of carcinoma: appearance on CT scans. *Radiology* 1987;162:371–375.
13. Bergin CJ, Müller NL. CT in the diagnosis of interstitial lung disease. *AJR Am J Roentgenol* 1985;145:505–510.
14. Johkoh T, Ikezoe J, Tomiyama N, et al. CT findings in lymphangitic carcinomatosis of the lung: correlation with histologic findings and pulmonary function tests. *AJR Am J Roentgenol* 1992;158:1217–1222.
15. Lee KS, Kim Y, Primack SL. Imaging of pulmonary lymphomas. *AJR Am J Roentgenol* 1997;168:339–345.
16. Heyneman LE, Johkoh T, Ward S, et al. Pulmonary leukemic infiltrates: high-resolution CT findings in 10 patients. *AJR Am J Roentgenol* 2000;174:517–521.
17. Johkoh T, Müller NL, Pickford HA, et al. Lymphocytic interstitial pneumonia: thin-section CT findings in 22 patients. *Radiology* 1999;212:567–572.
18. Ichikawa Y, Kinoshita M, Koga T, et al. Lung cyst formation in lymphocytic interstitial pneumonia: CT features. *J Comput Assist Tomogr* 1994;18:745–748.
19. McGuinness G, Scholes JV, Jagirdar JS, et al. Unusual lymphoproliferative disorders in nine adults with HIV or AIDS: CT and pathologic findings. *Radiology* 1995;197:59–65.
20. Traill ZC, Maskell GF, Gleeson FV. High-resolution CT findings of pulmonary sarcoidosis. *AJR Am J Roentgenol* 1997;168:1557–1660.
21. Müller NL, Kullnig P, Miller RR. The CT findings of pulmonary sarcoidosis: analysis of 25 patients. *AJR Am J Roentgenol* 1989;152:1179–1182.
22. Kim TS, Lee KS, Chung MP, et al. Nonspecific interstitial pneumonia with fibrosis: high-resolution CT and pathologic findings. *AJR Am J Roentgenol* 1998;171:1645–1650.
23. Adler BD, Padley SP, Müller NL, et al. Chronic hypersensitivity pneumonitis: high-resolution CT and radiographic features in 16 patients. *Radiology* 1992;185:91–95.
24. Wintermark M, Wicky S, Schnyder P, et al. Blunt traumatic pneumomediastinum: using CT to reveal the Macklin effect. *AJR Am J Roentgenol* 1999;172:129–130.

25. Kemper AC, Steinberg KP, Stern EJ. Pulmonary interstitial emphysema: CT findings. *AJR Am J Roentgenol* 1999;172:1642.

26. Satoh K, Kobayashi T, Kawase Y, et al. CT appearance of interstitial pulmonary emphysema. *J Thorac Imaging* 1996;11:153–154.

27. Bessis L, Callard P, Gotheil C, et al. High-resolution CT of parenchymal lung disease: precise correlation with histologic findings. *Radiographics* 1992;12:45–58.

28. Storto ML, Kee ST, Golden JA, et al. Hydrostatic pulmonary edema: high-resolution CT findings. *AJR Am J Roentgenol* 1995;165:817–820.

29. Weibel ER, Taylor CR. Design and structure of the human lung. In: Fishman AP, ed. *Pulmonary diseases and disorders*. New York: McGraw-Hill, 1988:11–60.

30. Bankier AA, Fleischmann D, De Maertelaer V, et al. Subjective differentiation of normal and pathological bronchi on thin-section CT: impact of observer training. *Eur Respir J* 1999;13:781–786.

31. Westcott JL, Cole SR. Traction bronchiectasis in end-stage pulmonary fibrosis. *Radiology* 1986;161:665–669.

32. Webb WR, Stein MG, Finkbeiner WE, et al. Normal and diseased isolated lungs: high-resolution CT. *Radiology* 1988;166:81–87.

33. Logan PM. Thoracic manifestations of external beam radiotherapy. *AJR Am J Roentgenol* 1998;171:569–577.

34. Naidich DP, McCauley DI, Khouri NF, et al. Computed tomography of bronchiectasis. *J Comput Assist Tomogr* 1982;6:437–444.

35. Grenier P, Maurice F, Musset D, et al. Bronchiectasis: assessment by thin-section CT. *Radiology* 1986;161:95–99.

36. Munro NC, Cooke JC, Currie DC, et al. Comparison of thin section computed tomography with bronchography for identifying bronchiectatic segments in patients with chronic sputum production. *Thorax* 1990;45:135–139.

37. Grenier P, Lenoir S, Brauner M. Computed tomographic assessment of bronchiectasis. *Semin Ultrasound CT MR* 1990;11:430–441.

38. Neeld DA, Goodman LR, Gurney JW, et al. Computerized tomography in the evaluation of allergic bronchopulmonary aspergillosis. *Am Rev Respir Dis* 1990;142:1200–1206.

39. Aberle DR, Gamsu G, Ray CS, et al. Asbestos-related pleural and parenchymal fibrosis: detection with high-resolution CT. *Radiology* 1988;166:729–734.

40. Todo G, Herman PG. High-resolution computed tomography of the pig lung. *Invest Radiol* 1986;21:689–696.

41. Swensen SJ, Aughenbaugh GL, Brown LR. High-resolution computed tomography of the lung. *Mayo Clin Proc* 1989;64:1284–1294.

42. Müller NL, Miller RR, Webb WR, et al. Fibrosing alveolitis: CT-pathologic correlation. *Radiology* 1986;160:585–588.

43. Murata K, Itoh H, Todo G, et al. Centrilobular lesions of the lung: demonstration by high-resolution CT and pathologic correlation. *Radiology* 1986;161:641–645.

44. Akira M, Yamamoto S, Yokoyama K, et al. Asbestosis: high-resolution CT-pathologic correlation. *Radiology* 1990;176:389–394.

45. Bergin CJ, Coblentz CL, Chiles C, et al. Chronic lung diseases: specific diagnosis using CT. *AJR Am J Roentgenol* 1989;152:1183–1188.

46. Kang EY, Grenier P, Laurent F, et al. Interlobular septal thickening: patterns at high-resolution computed tomography. *J Thoracic Imaging* 1996;11:260–264.

47. Cassart M, Genevois PA, Kramer M, et al. Pulmonary venoocclusive disease: CT findings before and after single-lung transplantation. *AJR Am J Roentgenol* 1993;160:759–760.

48. Swensen SJ, Tashjian JH, Myers JL, et al. Pulmonary venoocclusive disease: CT findings in eight patients. *AJR Am J Roentgenol* 1996;167:937–940.

49. Ren H, Hruban RH, Kuhlman JE, et al. Computed tomography of inflation-fixed lungs: the beaded septum sign of pulmonary metastases. *J Comput Assist Tomogr* 1989;13:411–416.

50. Graham CM, Stern EJ, Finkbeiner WE, et al. High-resolution CT appearance of diffuse alveolar septal amyloidosis. *AJR Am J Roentgenol* 1992;158:265–267.

51. Murch CR, Carr DH. Computed tomography appearances of pulmonary alveolar proteinosis. *Clin Radiol* 1989;40:240–243.

52. Godwin JD, Müller NL, Takasugi JE. Pulmonary alveolar proteinosis: CT findings. *Radiology* 1988;169:609–613.

53. Lee KN, Levin DL, Webb WR, et al. Pulmonary alveolar proteinosis: high-resolution CT, chest radiographic, and functional correlations. *Chest* 1997;111:989–995.

54. Murayama S, Murakami J, Yabuuchi H, et al. "Crazy-paving appearance" on high resolution CT in various diseases. *J Comput Assist Tomogr* 1999;23:749–752.

55. Johkoh T, Itoh H, Müller NL, et al. Crazy-paving appearance at thin-section CT: spectrum of disease and pathologic findings. *Radiology* 1999;211:155–160.

56. Lynch DA, Webb WR, Gamsu G, et al. Computed tomography in pulmonary sarcoidosis. *J Comput Assist Tomogr* 1989;13:405–410.

57. Remy-Jardin M, Beuscart R, Sault MC, et al. Subpleural micronodules in diffuse infiltrative lung diseases: evaluation with thin-section CT scans. *Radiology* 1990;177:133–139.

58. Remy-Jardin M, Degreef JM, Beuscart R, et al. Coal worker's pneumoconiosis: CT assessment in exposed workers and correlation with radiographic findings. *Radiology* 1990;177:363–371.

59. Pickford HA, Swensen SJ, Utz JP. Thoracic cross-sectional imaging of amyloidosis. *AJR Am J Roentgenol* 1997;168:351–355.

60. Murata K, Khan A, Herman PG. Pulmonary parenchymal disease: evaluation with high-resolution CT. *Radiology* 1989;170:629–635.

61. Johkoh T, Müller NL, Ichikado K, et al. Perilobular pulmonary opacities: high-resolution CT findings and pathologic correlation. *J Thorac Imaging* 1999;14:172–177.

62. Primack SL, Hartman TE, Hansell DM, et al. End-stage lung disease: CT findings in 61 patients. *Radiology* 1993;189:681–686.

63. Aberle DR, Gamsu G, Ray CS. High-resolution CT of benign asbestos-related diseases: clinical and radiographic correlation. *AJR Am J Roentgenol* 1988;151:883–891.

64. Lynch DA, Gamsu G, Ray CS, et al. Asbestos-related focal lung masses: manifestations on conventional and high-resolution CT scans. *Radiology* 1988;169:603–607.

65. Im JG, Itoh H, Shim YS, et al. Pulmonary tuberculosis: CT findings—early active disease and sequential change with antituberculous therapy. *Radiology* 1993;186:653–660.

66. Colby TV, Swensen SJ. Anatomic distribution and histopathologic patterns in diffuse lung disease: correlation with HRCT. *J Thorac Imag* 1996;11:1–26.

67. Johkoh T, Müller NL, Cartier Y, et al. Idiopathic interstitial pneumonias: diagnostic accuracy of thin-section CT in 129 patients. *Radiology* 1999;211:555–560.

68. Park JS, Lee KS, Kim JS, et al. Nonspecific interstitial pneumonia with fibrosis: radiographic and CT findings in seven patients. *Radiology* 1995;195:645–648.

69. Kim EY, Lee KS, Chung MP, et al. Nonspecific interstitial pneumonia with fibrosis: serial high-resolution CT findings with functional correlation. *AJR Am J Roentgenol* 1999;173:949–953.

70. Genereux GP. The end-stage lung: pathogenesis, pathology, and radiology. *Radiology* 1975;116:279–289.

71. Desai SR, Wells AU, Rubens MB, et al. Acute respiratory distress syndrome: CT abnormalities at long-term follow-up. *Radiology* 1999;210:29–35.

72. Remy-Jardin M, Giraud F, Remy J, et al. Importance of ground-glass attenuation in chronic diffuse infiltrative lung disease: pathologic-CT correlation. *Radiology* 1993;189:693–698.

73. Wells AU, Hansell DM, Rubens MB, et al. The predictive value of appearances of thin-section computed tomography in fibrosing alveolitis. *Am Rev Respir Dis* 1993;148:1076–1082.

74. Tung KT, Wells AU, Rubens MB, et al. Accuracy of the typical computed tomographic appearances of fibrosing alveolitis. *Thorax* 1993;48:334–338.

75. Al-Jarad N, Strickland B, Pearson MC, et al. High-resolution computed tomographic assessment of asbestosis and cryptogenic fibrosing alveolitis: a comparative study. *Thorax* 1992;47:645–650.

76. Mathieson JR, Mayo JR, Staples CA, et al. Chronic diffuse infiltrative lung disease: comparison of diagnostic accuracy of CT and chest radiography. *Radiology* 1989;171:111–116.

77. Grenier P, Valeyre D, Cluzel P, et al. Chronic diffuse interstitial lung disease: diagnostic value of chest radiography and high-resolution CT. *Radiology* 1991;179:123–132.

78. Padley SPG, Hansell DM, Flower CDR, et al. Comparative accuracy of high resolution computed tomography and chest radiography in the diagnosis of chronic diffuse infiltrative lung disease. *Clin Radiol* 1991;44:222–226.

79. Nishimura K, Izumi T, Kitaichi M, et al. The diagnostic accuracy of high-resolution computed tomography in diffuse infiltrative lung diseases. *Chest* 1993;104:1149–1155.

80. Swensen SJ, Aughenbaugh GL, Myers JL. Diffuse lung disease: diagnostic accuracy of CT in patients undergoing surgical biopsy of the lung. *Radiology* 1997;205:229–234.

81. Yoshimura H, Hatakeyama M, Otsuji H, et al. Pulmonary asbestosis: CT study of subpleural curvilinear shadow. Work in progress. *Radiology* 1986;158:653–658.

82. Schurawitzki H, Stiglbauer R, Graninger W, et al. Interstitial lung disease in progressive systemic sclerosis: high-resolution CT versus radiography. *Radiology* 1990;176:755–759.

83. Swensen SJ, Aughenbaugh GL, Douglas WW, et al. High-resolution CT of the lungs: findings in various pulmonary diseases. *AJR Am J Roentgenol* 1992;158:971–979.

84. Morimoto S, Takeuchi N, Imanaka H, et al. Gravity dependent atelectasis: radiologic, physiologic and pathologic correlation in rabbits on high-frequency ventilation. *Invest Radiol* 1989;24:522–530.

85. Kubota H, Hosoya T, Kato M, et al. Plate-like atelectasis at the corticomedullary junction of the lung: CT observation and hypothesis. *Radiat Med* 1983;1:305–310.

86. Remy-Jardin M, Remy J, Deffontaines C, et al. Assessment of diffuse infiltrative lung disease: comparison of conventional CT and high-resolution CT. *Radiology* 1991;181:157–162.

87. Lee KS, Im JG. CT in adults with tuberculosis of the chest: characteristic findings and role in management. *AJR Am J Roentgenol* 1995;164:1361–1367.

88. Im JG, Itoh H, Han MC. CT of pulmonary tuberculosis *Semin Ultrasound CT MR* 1995;16:420–434.

89. Hong SH, Im JG, Lee JS, et al. High resolution CT findings of miliary tuberculosis. *J Comput Assist Tomogr* 1998;22:220–224.

90. Brauner MW, Grenier P, Mompoint D, et al. Pulmonary sarcoidosis: evaluation with high-resolution CT. *Radiology* 1989;172:467–471.

91. Nakata H, Kimoto T, Nakayama T, et al. Diffuse peripheral lung disease: evaluation by high-resolution computed tomography. *Radiology* 1985;157:181–185.

92. Brauner MW, Grenier P, Mouelhi MM, et al. Pulmonary histiocytosis X: evaluation with high resolution CT. *Radiology* 1989;172:255–258.

93. Moore AD, Godwin JD, Müller NL, et al. Pulmonary histiocytosis X: comparison of radiographic and CT findings. *Radiology* 1989;172:249–254.

94. Bergin CJ, Müller NL, Vedal S, et al. CT in silicosis: correlation with plain films and pulmonary function tests. *AJR Am J Roentgenol* 1986;146:477–483.

95. Akira M, Higashihara T, Yokoyama K, et al. Radiographic type p pneumoconiosis: high-resolution CT. *Radiology* 1989;171:117–123.

96. Hruban RH, Meziane MA, Zerhouni EA, et al. High resolution computed tomography of inflation fixed lungs: pathologic-radiologic correlation of centrilobular emphysema. *Am Rev Respir Dis* 1987;136:935–940.

97. Nishimura K, Itoh H, Kitaichi M, et al. Pulmonary sarcoidosis: correlation of CT and histopathologic findings. *Radiology* 1993;189:105–109.

98. Brauner MW, Lenoir S, Grenier P, et al. Pulmonary sarcoidosis: CT assessment of lesion reversibility. *Radiology* 1992;182:349–354.

99. Bergin CJ, Bell DY, Coblentz CL, et al. Sarcoidosis: correlation of pulmonary parenchymal pattern at CT with results of pulmonary function tests. *Radiology* 1989;171:619–624.

100. Bégin R, Bergeron D, Samson L, et al. CT assessment of silicosis in exposed workers. *AJR Am J Roentgenol* 1987;148:509–514.

101. Bergin CJ, Müller NL. CT of interstitial lung disease: a diagnostic approach. *AJR Am J Roentgenol* 1987;148:9–15.

102. Naidich DP, Zerhouni EA, Hutchins GM, et al. Computed tomography of the pulmonary parenchyma: part 1. Distal airspace disease. *J Thorac Imaging* 1985;1:39–53.

103. Itoh H, Tokunaga S, Asamoto H, et al. Radiologic-pathologic correlations of small lung nodules with special reference to peribronchiolar nodules. *AJR Am J Roentgenol* 1978;130:223–231.

104. Murata K, Herman PG, Khan A, et al. Intralobular distribution of oleic acid-induced pulmonary edema in the pig: evaluation by high-resolution CT. *Invest Radiol* 1989;24:647–653.

105. Gruden JF, Webb WR, Naidich DP, et al. Multinodular disease: anatomic localization at thin-section CT: multireader evaluation of a simple algorithm. *Radiology* 1999;210:711–720.

106. Lee KS, Kim TS, Han J, et al. Diffuse micronodular lung disease: HRCT and pathologic findings. *J Comput Assist Tomogr* 1999;23:99–106.

107. Gruden JF, Webb WR, Warnock M. Centrilobular opacities in the lung on high-resolution CT: diagnostic considerations and pathologic correlation. *AJR Am J Roentgenol* 1994;162:569–574.

108. Remy-Jardin M, Remy J, Boulenguez C, et al. Morphologic effects of cigarette smoking on airways and pulmonary parenchyma in healthy adult volunteers: CT evaluation and correlation with pulmonary function tests. *Radiology* 1993;186:107–115.

109. Remy-Jardin M, Remy J, Gosselin B, et al. Lung parenchymal changes secondary to cigarette smoking: pathologic-CT correlations. *Radiology* 1993;186:643–651.

110. Liebow AA, Carrington CB. Diffuse pulmonary lymphoreticular infiltration associated with dysproteinemia. *Med Clin North Am* 1973;57:809–843.

111. Steimlam CV, Rosenow EC, Divertie MB, et al. Pulmonary manifestations of Sjögren's syndrome. *Chest* 1976;70:354–361.

112. Joshi VV, Oleske JM, Minnefor AB, et al. Pathologic pulmonary findings in children with the acquired immunodeficiency syndrome. *Hum Pathol* 1985;16:241–246.

113. Grieco MH, Chinoy-Acharya P. Lymphoid interstitial pneumonia associated with the acquired immune deficiency syndrome. *Am Rev Respir Dis* 1985;131:952–955.

114. Honda O, Johkoh T, Ichikado K, et al. Differential diagnosis of lymphocytic interstitial pneumonia and malignant lymphoma on high-resolution CT. *AJR Am J Roentgenol* 1999;173:71–74.

115. Murata K, Takahashi M, Mori M, et al. Pulmonary metastatic nodules: CT-pathologic correlation. *Radiology* 1992;182:331–335.

116. Kim JS, Ryu CW, Lee SI, et al. High-resolution CT findings of varicella-zoster pneumonia. *AJR Am J Roentgenol* 1999;172:113–116.

117. Lee KS, Kim YH, Kim WS, et al. Endobronchial tuberculosis: CT features. *J Comput Assist Tomogr* 1991;15:424–428.

118. Hartman TE, Swensen SJ, Williams DE. Mycobacterium avium-intracellulare complex: evaluation with CT. *Radiology* 1993;187:23–26.

119. Swensen SJ, Hartman TE, Williams DE. Computed tomography in diagnosis of Mycobacterium avium-intracellulare complex in patients with bronchiectasis. *Chest* 1994;105:49–52.

120. McGuinness G, Gruden JF, Bhalla M, et al. AIDS-related airway disease. *AJR Am J Roentgenol* 1997;168:67–77.

121. Seely JM, Effmann EL, Müller NL. High-resolution CT of pediatric lung disease: imaging findings. *AJR Am J Roentgenol* 1997;168:1269–1275.

122. Logan PM, Primack SL, Miller RR, et al. Invasive aspergillosis of the airways: radiographic, CT, and pathologic findings. *Radiology* 1994;193:383–388.

123. Müller NL, Miller RR. Diseases of the bronchioles: CT and histopathologic findings. *Radiology* 1995;196:3–12.

124. Lynch DA, Brasch RC, Hardy KA, et al. Pediatric pulmonary disease: assessment with high-resolution ultrafast CT. *Radiology* 1990;176:243–248.

125. Webb WR. High-resolution computed tomography of obstructive lung disease. *Rad Clin N Am* 1994;32:745–757.

126. Akira M, Kitatani F, Lee Y-S, et al. Diffuse panbronchiolitis: evaluation with high-resolution CT. *Radiology* 1988;168:433–438.

127. Nishimura K, Kitaichi M, Izumi T, et al. Diffuse panbronchiolitis: correlation of high-resolution CT and pathologic findings. *Radiology* 1992;184:779–785.

128. Akira M, Higashihara T, Sakatani M, et al. Diffuse panbronchiolitis: follow-up CT examination. *Radiology* 1993;189:559–562.

129. Ward S, Heyneman L, Lee MJ, et al. Accuracy of CT in the diagnosis of allergic bronchopulmonary aspergillosis in asthmatic patients. *AJR Am J Roentgenol* 1999;173:937–942.

130. Silver SF, Müller NL, Miller RR, et al. Hypersensitivity pneumonitis: evaluation with CT. *Radiology* 1989;173:441–445.

131. Lynch DA, Rose CS, Way D, et al. Hypersensitivity pneumonitis: sensitivity of high-resolution CT in a population-based study. *AJR Am J Roentgenol* 1992;159:469–472.

132. Akira M, Kita N, Higashihara T, et al. Summer-type hypersensitivity pneumonitis: comparison of high-resolution CT and plain radiographic findings. *AJR Am J Roentgenol* 1992;158:1223–1228.

133. Remy-Jardin M, Remy J, Wallaert B, et al. Subacute and chronic bird breeder hypersensitivity pneumonitis: sequential evaluation with CT and correlation with lung function tests and bronchoalveolar lavage. *Radiology* 1993;198:111–118.

134. Müller NL, Staples CA, Miller RR. Bronchiolitis obliterans organizing pneumonia: CT features in 14 patients. *AJR Am J Roentgenol* 1990;154:983–987.

135. Leung AN, Miller RR, Müller NL. Parenchymal opacification in chronic infiltrative lung diseases: CT-pathologic correlation. *Radiology* 1993;188:209–214.

136. Collins J, Blankenbaker D, Stern EJ. CT patterns of bronchiolar disease: what is tree-in-bud? *AJR Am J Roentgenol* 1998;171:365–370.

137. Aquino SL, Gamsu G, Webb WR, et al. Tree-in-bud pattern: frequency and significance on thin section CT. *J Comput Assist Tomogr* 1996;20:594–599.

138. Gruden JF, Webb WR. CT findings in a proved case of respiratory bronchiolitis. *AJR Am J Roentgenol* 1993;161:44–46.

139. Holt RM, Schmidt RA, Godwin JD, et al. High resolution CT in respiratory bronchiolitis-associated interstitial lung disease. *J Comput Assist Tomogr* 1993;17:46–50.

140. Heyneman LE, Ward S, Lynch DA, et al. Respiratory bronchiolitis, respiratory bronchiolitis-associated interstitial pneumonia: different entities or part of the spectrum of the same disease process? *AJR Am J Roentgenol* 1999;173:1617–1622.

141. Akira M, Yokoyama K, Yamamoto S, et al. Early asbestosis: evaluation with high-resolution CT. *Radiology* 1991;178:409–416.

142. Howling SJ, Hansell DM, Wells AU, et al. Follicular bronchiolitis: thin-section CT and histologic findings. *Radiology* 1999;212:637–642.

143. Remy-Jardin M, Remy J, Wallaert B, et al. Pulmonary involvement in progressive systemic sclerosis: sequential evaluation with CT, pulmonary function tests, and bronchoalveolar lavage. *Radiology* 1993;188:499–506.

144. Remy-Jardin M, Remy J, Cortet B, et al. Lung changes in rheumatoid arthritis: CT findings. *Radiology* 1994;193:375–382.

145. Gruden JF, Webb WR, Sides DM. Adult-onset disseminated tracheobronchial papillomatosis: CT features. *J Comput Assist Tomogr* 1994;18:640–642.

146. Akira M, Atagi S, Kawahara M, et al. High-resolution CT findings of diffuse bronchioloalveolar carcinoma in 38 patients. *AJR Am J Roentgenol* 1999;173:1623–1629.

147. Padley SPG, Adler BD, Staples CA, et al. Pulmonary talcosis: CT findings in three cases. *Radiology* 1993;186:125–127.

148. Connolly B, Manson D, Eberhard A, et al. CT appearance of pulmonary vasculitis in children. *AJR Am J Roentgenol* 1996;167:901–904.

149. Primack SL, Miller RR, Müller NL. Diffuse pulmonary hemorrhage: clinical, pathologic, and imaging features. *AJR Am J Roentgenol* 1995;164:295–300.

150. Johkoh T, Ikezoe J, Nagareda T, et al. Metastatic pulmonary calcification: early detection by high-resolution CT. *J Comput Assist Tomogr* 1993;17:471–473.

151. Hartman TE, Müller NL, Primack SL, et al. Metastatic pulmonary calcification in patients with hypercalcemia: findings on chest radiographs and CT scans. *AJR Am J Roentgenol* 1994;162:799–802.

152. Nolan RL, McAdams HP, Sporn TA, et al. Pulmonary cholesterol granulomas in patients with pulmonary artery hypertension: chest radiographic and CT findings. *AJR Am J Roentgenol* 1999;172:1317–1319.

153. Dufour B, Maitre S, Humbert M, et al. High-resolution CT of the chest in four patients with pulmonary capillary hemangiomatosis or pulmonary venoocclusive disease. *AJR Am J Roentgenol* 1998;171:1321–1324.

154. Gruden JF, Webb WR. Identification and evaluation of centrilobular opacities on high-resolution CT. *Semin Ultrasound CT MR* 1995;16:435–449.

155. Reid L, Simon G. The peripheral pattern in the normal bronchogram and its relation to peripheral pulmonary anatomy. *Thorax* 1958;13:103–109.

156. Gruden JF, Huang L, Turner J, et al. High-resolution CT in the evaluation of clinically suspected *Pneumocystis carinii* pneumonia in AIDS patients with normal, equivocal, or nonspecific radiographic findings. *AJR Am J Roentgenol* 1997;169:967–975.

157. Tuddenham WJ. Glossary of terms for thoracic radiology: recommendations of the Nomenclature Committee of the Fleischner Society. *AJR Am J Roentgenol* 1984;143:509–517.

158. Davis SD. CT evaluation for pulmonary metastases in patients with extrathoracic malignancy. *Radiology* 1991;180:1–12.

159. Diederich S, Semik M, Lentschig MG, et al. Helical CT of pulmonary nodules in patients with extrathoracic malignancy: CT-surgical correlation. *AJR Am J Roentgenol* 1999;172:353–360.

160. McCulloch GL, Sinnatamby R, Stewart S, et al. High-resolution computed tomographic appearance of MALToma of the lung. *Eur Radiol* 1998;8:1669–1673.

161. Lewis ER, Caskey CI, Fishman EK. Lymphoma of the lung: CT findings in 31 patients. *AJR Am J Roentgenol* 1991;156:711–714.

162. Collins J, Müller NL, Leung AN, et al. Epstein-Barr-virus-associated lymphoproliferative disease of the lung: CT and histologic findings. *Radiology* 1998;208:749–759.

163. Rappaport DC, Chamberlain DW, Shepherd FA, Hutcheon MA. Lymphoproliferative disorders after lung transplantation: imaging features. *Radiology* 1998;206:519–524.

164. Akira M, Yamamoto S, Sakatani M. Bronchiolitis obliterans organizing pneumonia manifesting as multiple large nodules or masses. *AJR Am J Roentgenol* 1998;170:291–295.

165. Hoffman GS, Kerr GS, Leavitt RY, et al. Wegener granulomatosis: an analysis of 158 patients. *Ann Intern Med* 1992;116:488–498.

166. Aberle DR, Gamsu G, Lynch D. Thoracic manifestations of Wegener granulomatosis: diagnosis and course. *Radiology* 1990;174:703–709.

167. Weir IH, Müller NL, Chiles C, et al. Wegener's granulomatosis: findings from computed tomography of the chest in 10 patients. *Can Assoc Radiol J* 1992;43:31–34.

168. Foo SS, Weisbrod GL, Herman SJ, et al. Wegener granulomatosis presenting on CT with atypical bronchovasocentric distribution. *J Comput Assist Tomogr* 1990;14:1004–1006.

169. Worthy SA, Müller NL, Hansell DM, et al. Churg-Strauss syndrome: the spectrum of pulmonary CT findings in 17 patients. *AJR Am J Roentgenol* 1998;170:297–300.

170. Utz JP, Swensen SJ, Gertz MA. Pulmonary amyloidosis. The Mayo Clinic experience from 1980 to 1993. *Ann Intern Med* 1996;124:407–413.

171. Mori M, Galvin JR, Barloon TJ, et al. Fungal pulmonary infections after bone marrow transplantation: evaluation with radiography and CT. *Radiology* 1991;178:721–726.

172. Kuhlman JE, Fishman EK, Burch PA, et al. Invasive pulmonary aspergillosis in acute leukemia: the contribution of CT to early diagnosis and aggressive management. *Chest* 1987;92:95–99.

173. Gaeta M, Volta S, Stroscio S, et al. CT "halo sign" in pulmonary tuberculoma. *J Comput Assist Tomogr* 1992;16:827–828.

174. Primack SL, Hartman TE, Lee KS, et al. Pulmonary nodules and the CT halo sign. *Radiology* 1994;190:513–515.

175. Won HJ, Lee KS, Cheon JE, et al. Invasive pulmonary aspergillosis: prediction at thin-section CT in patients with neutropenia: a prospective study. *Radiology* 1998;208:777–782.

176. Doyle TC, Lawler GA. CT features of rounded atelectasis of the lung. *AJR Am J Roentgenol* 1984;143:225–228.

177. Ren H, Hruban RH, Kuhlman JE, et al. Computed tomography of rounded atelectasis. *J Comput Assist Tomogr* 1988;12:1031–1034.

178. McHugh K, Blaquiere RM. CT features of rounded atelectasis. *AJR Am J Roentgenol* 1989;153:257–260.

179. Müller NL, Staples CA, Miller RR, et al. Disease activity in idiopathic pulmonary fibrosis: CT and pathologic correlation. *Radiology* 1987;165:731–734.

180. Engeler CE, Tashjian JH, Trenkner SW, et al. Ground-glass opacity of the lung parenchyma: a guide to analysis with high-resolution CT. *AJR Am J Roentgenol* 1993;160:249–251.

181. Remy-Jardin M, Remy J, Giraud F, et al. Computed tomography assessment of ground-glass opacity: semiology and significance. *J Thorac Imag* 1993;8:249–264.

182. Wells AU, Hansell DM, Corrin B, et al. High resolution computed tomography as a predictor of lung histology in systemic sclerosis. *Thorax* 1992;47:508–512.

183. Wells AU, Rubens MB, du Bois RM, et al. Serial CT in fibrosing alveolitis: prognostic significance of the initial pattern. *AJR Am J Roentgenol* 1993;161:1159–1165.

184. Ikezoe J, Takashima S, Morimoto S, et al. CT appearance of acute radiation-induced injury in the lung. *AJR Am J Roentgenol* 1988;150:765–770.

185. Primack SL, Hartman TE, Ikezoe J, et al. Acute interstitial pneumonia: radiographic and CT findings in nine patients. *Radiology* 1993;188:817–820.

186. Bergin CJ, Wirth RL, Berry GJ, et al. *Pneumocystis carinii* pneumonia: CT and HRCT observations. *J Comput Assist Tomogr* 1990;14:756–759.

187. Moskovic E, Miller R, Pearson M. High resolution computed tomography of *Pneumocystis carinii* pneumonia in AIDS. *Clin Radiol* 1990;42:239–243.

188. Graham NJ, Müller NL, Miller RR, et al. Intrathoracic complications following allogeneic bone marrow transplantation: CT findings. *Radiology* 1991;181:153–156.

189. McGuinness G, Scholes JV, Garay SM, et al. Cytomegalovirus pneumonitis: spectrum of parenchymal CT findings with pathologic correlation in 21 AIDS patients. *Radiology* 1994;192:451–459.

190. Reittner P, Müller NL, Heyneman L, et al. Mycoplasma pneumoniae pneumonia: radiographic and high-resolution CT features in 28 patients. *AJR Am J Roentgenol* 1999;174:37–41.

191. Cheon JE, Lee KS, Jung GS, et al. Acute eosinophilic pneumonia: radiographic and CT findings in six patients. *AJR Am J Roentgenol* 1996;167:1195–1199.

192. Ikezoe J, Morimoto S, Takashima S, et al. Acute radiation-induced pulmonary injury: computed tomographic evaluation. *Semin Ultrasound CT MR* 1990;11:409–416.

193. Hartman TE, Primack SL, Swensen SJ, et al. Desquamative interstitial pneumonia: thin-section CT findings in 22 patients. *Radiology* 1993;187:787–790.

194. Franquet T, Giménez A, Bordes R, et al. The crazy-paving pattern in exogenous lipoid pneumonia: CT-pathologic correlation. *AJR Am J Roentgenol* 1998;170:315–317.

195. Tan RT, Kuzo RS. High-resolution CT findings of mucinous bronchioloalveolar carcinoma: a case of pseudopulmonary alveolar proteinosis. *AJR Am J Roentgenol* 1997;168:99–100.

196. Murdoch J, Müller NL. Pulmonary sarcoidosis: changes on follow-up CT examinations. *AJR Am J Roentgenol* 1992;159:473–477.

197. Hommeyer SH, Godwin JD, Takasugi JE. Computed tomography of airspace disease. *Radiol Clin North Am* 1991;29:1065–1084.

198. Nishimura K, Itoh H. High-resolution computed tomographic features of bronchiolitis obliterans organizing pneumonia. *Chest* 1992;102:26S–31S.

199. Müller NL, Miller RR. Ground-glass attenuation, nodules, alveolitis, and sarcoid granulomas (editorial). *Radiology* 1993;189:31–32.

200. Lee JS, Im JG, Ahn JM, et al. Fibrosing alveolitis: prognostic implication of ground-glass attenuation at high-resolution CT. *Radiology* 1992;184:415–454.

201. Akira M, Sakatani M, Ueda E. Idiopathic pulmonary fibrosis: progression of honeycombing at thin-section CT. *Radiology* 1993;189:687–691.

202. Terriff BA, Kwan SY, Chan-Yeung MM, et al. Fibrosing alveolitis: chest radiography and CT as predictors of clinical and functional impairment at follow-up in 26 patients. *Radiology* 1992;184:445–449.

203. Bouchardy LM, Kuhlman JE, Ball WC, et al. CT findings in bronchiolitis obliterans organizing pneumonia (BOOP) with radiographic, clinical, and histologic correlation. *J Comput Assist Tomogr* 1993;17:352–357.

204. Mayo JR, Müller NL, Road J, et al. Chronic eosinophilic pneumonia: CT findings in six cases. *AJR Am J Roentgenol* 1989;153:727–730.

205. Bourgouin P, Cousineau G, Lemire P, et al. Differentiation of radiation-induced fibrosis from recurrent pulmonary neoplasm by CT. *Can Assoc Radiol J* 1987;38:23–26.

206. Libshitz HI, Shuman LS. Radiation-induced pulmonary change: CT findings. *J Comput Assist Tomogr* 1984;8:15–19.

207. Kuhlman JE. The role of chest computed tomography in the diagnosis of drug-related reactions. *J Thorac Imaging* 1991;6(1):52–61.

208. Hamrick-Turner J, Abbitt PL, et al. Diffuse lung calcification following fat emboli and adult respiratory distress syndromes: CT findings. *J Thorac Imag* 1994;9:47–50.

209. Gevenois PA, Abehsera M, Knoop C, et al. Disseminated pulmonary ossification in end-stage pulmonary fibrosis: CT demonstration. *AJR Am J Roentgenol* 1994;162:1303–1304.

210. Kuhlman JE, Ren H, Hutchins GM, Fishman EK. Fulminant pulmonary calcification complicating renal transplantation: CT demonstration. *Radiology* 1989;173:459–460.

211. Cluzel P, Grenier P, Bernadac P, et al. Pulmonary alveolar microlithiasis: CT findings. *J Comput Assist Tomogr* 1991;15:938–942.

212. Korn MA, Schurawitzki H, Klepetko W, et al. Pulmonary alveolar microlithiasis: findings on high-resolution CT. *AJR Am J Roentgenol* 1992;158:981–982.

213. Helbich TH, Wojnarovsky C, Wunderbaldinger P, et al. Pulmonary alveolar microlithiasis in children: radiographic and high-resolution CT findings. *AJR Am J Roentgenol* 1997;168:63–65.

214. Kuhlman JE, Teigen C, Ren H, et al. Amiodarone pulmonary toxicity: CT findings in symptomatic patients. *Radiology* 1990;177:121–125.

215. Akira M. Uncommon pneumoconioses: CT and pathologic findings. *Radiology* 1995;197:403–409.

216. Naidich DP. High-resolution computed tomography of cystic lung disease. *Semin Roentgenol* 1991;26:151–174.

217. Hogg JC. Benjamin Felson lecture. Chronic interstitial lung disease of unknown cause: a new classification based on pathogenesis. *AJR Am J Roentgenol* 1991;156:225–233.

218. Aquino SL, Webb WR, Zaloudek CJ, et al. Lung cysts associated with honeycombing: change in size on expiratory CT scans. *AJR Am J Roentgenol* 1994;162:583–584.

219. Worthy SA, Brown MJ, Müller NL. Technical report: Cystic airspaces in the lung: change in size on expiratory high-resolution CT in 23 patients. *Clin Radiol* 1998;53:515–519.

220. Lenoir S, Grenier P, Brauner MW, et al. Pulmonary lymphangiomyomatosis and tuberous sclerosis: comparison of radiographic and thin-section CT findings. *Radiology* 1990;175:329–334.

221. Templeton PA, McLoud TC, Müller NL, et al. Pulmonary lymphangioleiomyomatosis: CT and pathologic findings. *J Comput Assist Tomogr* 1989;13:54–57.

222. Sherrier RH, Chiles C, Roggli V. Pulmonary lymphangioleiomyomatosis: CT findings. *AJR Am J Roentgenol* 1989;153:937–940.

223. Rappaport DC, Weisbrod GL, Herman SJ, et al. Pulmonary lymphangiolciomyomatosis: high resolution CT findings in four cases. *AJR Am J Roentgenol* 1989;152:961–964.

224. Müller NL, Chiles C, Kullnig P. Pulmonary lymphangiomyomatosis: correlation of CT with radiographic and functional findings. *Radiology* 1990;175:335–339.

225. Desai SR, Nicholson AG, Stewart S, et al. Benign pulmonary lymphocytic infiltration and amyloidosis: computed tomographic and pathologic features in three cases. *J Thorac Imaging* 1997;12:215–220.

226. Sanders C, Nath PH, Bailey WC. Detection of emphysema with computed tomography: correlation with pulmonary function tests and chest radiography. *Invest Radiol* 1988;23:262–266.

227. Müller NL, Staples CA, Miller RR, et al. "Density mask": an objective method to quantitate emphysema using computed tomography. *Chest* 1988;94:782–787.

228. Miller RR, Müller NL, Vedal S, et al. Limitations of computed tomography in the assessment of emphysema. *Am Rev Respir Dis* 1989;139:980 983.

229. Kinsella N, Müller NL, Vedal S, et al. Emphysema in silicosis: a comparison of smokers with nonsmokers using pulmonary function testing and computed tomography. *Am Rev Respir Dis* 1990;141:1497–1500.

230. Stern EJ, Webb WR, Weinacker A, et al. Idiopathic giant bullous emphysema (vanishing lung syndrome): imaging findings in nine patients. *AJR Am J Roentgenol* 1994;162:279–282.

231. Feuerstein I, Archer A, Pluda JM, et al. Thin-walled cavities, cysts, and pneumothorax in *Pneumocystis carinii* pneumonia: further observations with histopathologic correlation. *Radiology* 1990;174:697–702.

232. Panicek DM. Cystic pulmonary lesions in patients with AIDS [editorial]. *Radiology* 1989;173:12–14.

233. Gurney JW, Bates FT. Pulmonary cystic disease: comparison of *Pneumocystis carinii* pneumatoceles and bullous emphysema due to intravenous drug abuse. *Radiology* 1989;173:27–31.

234. Grenier P, Cordeau MP, Beigelman C. High-resolution computed tomography of the airways. *J Thorac Imag* 1993;8:213–229.

235. Lynch DA, Newell JD, Tschomper BA, et al. Uncomplicated asthma in adults: comparison of CT appearance of the lungs in asthmatic and healthy subjects. *Radiology* 1993;188:829–833.

236. Kim JS, Müller NL, Park CS, et al. Cylindrical bronchiectasis: diagnostic findings on thin-section CT. *AJR Am J Roentgenol* 1997;168:751–754.

237. Kang EY, Miller RR, Müller NL. Bronchiectasis: comparison of preoperative thin-section CT and pathologic findings in resected specimens. *Radiology* 1995;195:649–654.

238. Marti-Bonmati L, Ruiz PF, Catala F, et al. CT findings in Swyer-James syndrome. *Radiology* 1989;172:477–480.

239. Martin KW, Sagel SS, Siegel BA. Mosaic oligemia simulating pulmonary infiltrates on CT. *AJR Am J Roentgenol* 1986;147:670–673.

240. Worthy SA, Park CS, Kim JS, et al. Bronchiolitis obliterans after lung transplantation: high resolution CT findings in 15 patients. *AJR Am J Roentgenol* 1997;169:673–677.

241. Arakawa H, Webb WR. Expiratory high-resolution CT scan. *Radiol Clin North Am* 1998;36:189–209.
242. Webb WR. Radiology of obstructive pulmonary disease. *AJR Am J Roentgenol* 1997;169:637–647.
243. King MA, Bergin CJ, Yeung DWC, et al. Chronic pulmonary thromboembolism: detection of regional hypoperfusion with CT. *Radiology* 1994;191:359–363.
244. Schwickert HC, Schweden F, Schild HH, et al. Pulmonary arteries and lung parenchyma in chronic pulmonary embolism: preoperative and postoperative CT findings. *Radiology* 1994;191:351–357.
245. Im JG, Kim SH, Chung MJ, et al. Lobular low attenuation of the lung parenchyma on CT: evaluation of forty-eight patients. *J Comput Assist Tomogr* 1996;20:756–762.
246. Arakawa H, Webb WR, McCowin M, et al. Inhomogeneous lung attenuation at thin-section CT: diagnostic value of expiratory scans. *Radiology* 1998;206:89–94.
247. Worthy SA, Müller NL, Hartman TE, et al. Mosaic attenuation pattern on thin-section CT scans of the lung: differentiation among infiltrative lung, airway, and vascular diseases as a cause. *Radiology* 1997;205:465–470.
248. Bergin CJ, Rios G, King MA, et al. Accuracy of high-resolution CT in identifying chronic pulmonary thromboembolic disease. *AJR Am J Roentgenol* 1996;166:1371–1377.
249. Sherrick AD, Swensen SJ, Hartman TE. Mosaic pattern of lung attenuation on CT scans: frequency among patients with pulmonary artery hypertension of different causes. *AJR Am J Roentgenol* 1997;169:79–82.
250. Franquet T, Giménez A, Monill JM, et al. Primary Sjögren's syndrome and associated lung disease: CT findings in 50 patients. *AJR Am J Roentgenol* 1997;169:655–658.
251. Stern EJ, Swensen SJ, Hartman TE, et al. CT mosaic pattern of lung attenuation: distinguishing different causes. *AJR Am J Roentgenol* 1995;165:813–816.
252. Stern EJ, Webb WR. Dynamic imaging of lung morphology with ultrafast high-resolution computed tomography. *J Thorac Imag* 1993;8:273–282.
253. Stern EJ, Webb WR, Gamsu G. Dynamic quantitative computed tomography: a predictor of pulmonary function in obstructive lung diseases. *Invest Radiol* 1994;29:564–569.
254. Chen D, Webb WR, Storto ML, et al. Assessment of air trapping using postexpiratory high-resolution computed tomography. *J Thorac Imaging* 1998;13:135–143.
255. Lucidarme O, Coche E, Cluzel P, et al. Expiratory CT scans for chronic airway disease: correlation with pulmonary function test results. *AJR Am J Roentgenol* 1998;170:301–307.
256. Chung MH, Edinburgh KJ, Webb EM, et al. Mixed infiltrative and obstructive disease on high-resolution CT: differential diagnosis and functional correlates in a consecutive series. *Society of Thoracic Radiology*, 1998.
257. Arakawa H, Webb WR. Air trapping on expiratory high-resolution CT scans in the absence of inspiratory scan abnormalities: correlation with pulmonary function tests and differential diagnosis. *AJR Am J Roentgenol* 1998;170:1349–1353.
258. Hansell DM, Milne DG, Wilsher ML, et al. Pulmonary sarcoidosis: morphologic associations of airflow obstruction at thin-section CT. *Radiology* 1998;209:697–704.
259. Hansell DM, Wells AU, Padley SP, et al. Hypersensitivity pneumonitis: correlation of individual CT patterns with functional abnormalities. *Radiology* 1996;199:123–128.
260. Knudson RJ, Standen JR, Kaltenborn WT, et al. Expiratory computed tomography for assessment of suspected pulmonary emphysema. *Chest* 1991;99:1357–1366.
261. Kitahara Y, Takamoto M, Maruyama M, et al. Differential diagnosis of pulmonary emphysema using the CT index: LL% (in Japanese). *Nippon Kyobu Shikkan Gakkai Zasshi* 1989;27:689–695.
262. Newman KB, Lynch DA, Newman LS, et al. Quantitative computed tomography detects air trapping due to asthma. *Chest* 1994;106:105–109.
263. Park CS, Müller NL, Worthy SA, et al. Airway obstruction in asthmatic and healthy individuals: inspiratory and expiratory thin-section CT findings. *Radiology* 1997;203:361–367.
264. Lynch DA. Imaging of asthma and allergic bronchopulmonary mycosis. *Rad Clin N Amer* 1998;36:129–142.
265. Garg K, Newell JD, King TE, et al. Proliferative and constrictive bronchiolitis: classification and radiologic features. *AJR Am J Roentgenol* 1994;162:803–808.
266. Padley SPG, Adler BD, Hansell DM, et al. Bronchiolitis obliterans: high-resolution CT findings and correlation with pulmonary function tests. *Clin Radiol* 1993;47:236–240.
267. Moore ADA, Godwin JD, Dietrich PA, et al. Swyer-James syndrome: CT findings in eight patients. *AJR Am J Roentgenol* 1992;158:1211–1215.
268. Sweatman MC, Millar AB, Strickland B, et al. Computed tomography in adult obliterative bronchiolitis. *Clin Radiol* 1990;41:116–119.
269. Aquino SL, Webb WR, Golden J. Bronchiolitis obliterans associated with rheumatoid arthritis: findings on HRCT and dynamic expiratory CT. *J Comput Assist Tomogr* 1994;18:555–558.
270. Leung AN, Fisher K, Valentine V, et al. Bronchiolitis obliterans after lung transplantation: detection using expiratory HRCT. *Chest* 1998;113:365–370.
271. Yang CF, Wu MT, Chiang AA, et al. Correlation of high-resolution CT and pulmonary function in bronchiolitis obliterans: a study based on 24 patients associated with consumption of *Sauropus Androgynus*. *AJR Am J Roentgenol* 1997;168:1045–1050.
272. Stern EJ, Webb WR, Golden JA, et al. Cystic lung disease associated with eosinophilic granuloma and tuberous sclerosis: air trapping at dynamic ultrafast high-resolution CT. *Radiology* 1992;182:325–329.
273. Hansell DM, Wells AU, Rubens MB, et al. Bronchiectasis: functional significance of areas of decreased attenuation at expiratory CT. *Radiology* 1994;193:369–374.
274. Gelman M, King MA, Neal DE, et al. Focal air trapping in patients with HIV infection: CT evaluation and correlation with pulmonary function test results. *AJR Am J Roentgenol* 1999;172:1033–1038.
275. Small JH, Flower CD, Traill ZC, et al. Air-trapping in extrinsic allergic alveolitis on computed tomography. *Clin Radiol* 1996;51:684–688.
276. Gleeson FV, Traill ZC, Hansell DM. Evidence of expiratory CT scans of small-airway obstruction in sarcoidosis. *AJR Am J Roentgenol* 1996;166:1052–1054.
277. Ringertz HG, Brasch RC, Gooding CA, et al. Quantitative density-time measurements in the lungs of children with suspected airway obstruction using ultrafast CT. *Pediatr Radiol* 1989;19:366–370.
278. Webb WR, Stern EJ, Kanth N, et al. Dynamic pulmonary CT: findings in normal adult men. *Radiology* 1993;186:117–124.
279. Gevenois PA, Scillia P, de Maertelaer V, et al. The effects of age, sex, lung size, and hyperinflation on CT lung densitometry. *AJR Am J Roentgenol* 1996;167:1169–1173.
280. Adams H, Bernard MS, McConnochie K. An appraisal of CT pulmonary density mapping in normal subjects. *Clin Radiol* 1991;43:238–242.
281. Ng CS, Desai SR, Rubens MB, et al. Visual quantitation and observer variation of signs of small airways disease at inspiratory and expiratory CT. *J Thorac Imaging* 1999;14:279–285.
282. Lee KW, Chung SY, Yang I, et al. Correlation of aging and smoking with air trapping at thin-section CT of the lung in asymptomatic subjects. *Radiology* 2000;214:831–836.
283. Robinson PJ, Kreel L. Pulmonary tissue attenuation with computed tomography: comparison of inspiration and expiration scans. *J Comput Assist Tomogr* 1979;3:740–748.
284. Gurney JW. Cross-sectional physiology of the lung. *Radiology* 1991;178:1–10.
285. Grenier P, Chevret S, Beigelman C, et al. Chronic diffuse infiltrative lung disease: determination of the diagnostic value of clinical data, chest radiography, and CT with Bayesian analysis. *Radiology* 1994;191:383–390.
286. Gurney JW, Schroeder BA. Upper lobe disease: physiological correlates. *Radiology* 1988;167:359–366.

CHAPTER 4

Diseases Characterized Primarily by Linear and Reticular Opacities

The diseases discussed in this chapter are those primarily characterized by the presence of fibrosis and linear or reticular abnormalities on high-resolution computed tomography (HRCT). These notably may include the idiopathic interstitial pneumonias [usual interstitial pneumonia (UIP), desquamative interstitial pneumonia (DIP), acute interstitial pneumonia (AIP), and nonspecific interstitial pneumonia (NSIP)], idiopathic pulmonary fibrosis (IPF), collagen-vascular diseases, and asbestosis. Also reviewed in this chapter are drug-induced lung diseases and radiation fibrosis. It should be recognized, however, that many of the other lung diseases discussed in this book result in pulmonary fibrosis and may produce similar HRCT abnormalities; the differential diagnosis of reticular abnormalities should not be limited to the diseases reviewed in this chapter.

Furthermore, although the diseases discussed in this chapter are primarily reticular, they commonly show other HRCT findings as well. In this and the following three chapters, lung diseases have been classified according to their most common and most diagnostic appearances. In the discussion of individual diseases, however, the entire spectrum of abnormalities seen with each is also reviewed.

IDIOPATHIC INTERSTITIAL PNEUMONIAS

The idiopathic interstitial pneumonias are a heterogeneous group of interstitial inflammatory and fibrosing lesions that

TABLE 4-1. *Clinical and pathologic features of the idiopathic interstitial pneumonias*

	Usual interstitial pneumonia	Desquamative interstitial pneumonia	Respiratory bronchiolitis-interstitial lung disease	Acute interstitial pneumonia	Nonspecific interstitial pneumonia
Clinical findings					
Mean age (yr)	57	42	36	49	49
Onset	Insidious	Insidious	Insidious	Acute	Subacute, insidious
Mortality rate	68%	27%	0%	62%	11%
Mean survival	5–6 yr	12 yr	—	1–2 mo	17 mo
Steroid response	Poor	Good	Good	Poor	Good
Complete recovery	No	Possible	Possible	Possible	Possible
Pathologic findings					
Temporal appearance	Heterogeneous	Uniform	Uniform	Uniform	Uniform
Interstitial inflammation	Scant	Scant	Scant	Scant	Usually prominent
Collagen fibrosis	Yes, patchy	Variable, diffuse	Mild, focal	No	Variable, diffuse
Fibroblastic proliferation	Foci prominent	No	No	Diffuse	Occasional
Microscopic honeycombing	Yes	No	No	No	Rare
Intraalveolar macrophages	Occasional	Diffuse	Focal	No	Occasional
Bronchiolitis obliterans organizing pneumonia	No	No	No	No	Occasional, focal
HRCT findings		See Chapter 6	See Chapter 6	See Chapter 6	See Chapter 6
Honeycombing	+++	—	—	++ (late stage)	+
Reticulation	+++	+	—	++ (late stage)	++
Ground-glass opacity	+	+++ (diffuse)	+++ (centrilobular)	+++ (acute stage)	+++
Consolidation	+	—	—	+++ (acute stage)	++

+, uncommon; ++, common; +++, typical.
Modified from Katzenstein AL, Myers JL. Idiopathic pulmonary fibrosis: clinical relevance of pathologic classification. *Am J Respir Crit Care Med* 1998;157:1301.

occur without any known cause. Based on their histologic appearance, they are currently classified into four types: UIP, DIP, AIP, and NSIP (Table 4-1) [1–4].

There has been considerable controversy regarding the nomenclature of the idiopathic interstitial pneumonias and confusion between histologic and clinical terminology. The American Thoracic Society and European Respiratory Society established an international multidisciplinary consensus group with the aim of standardizing the classification of the idiopathic interstitial pneumonias. The classification presented in this book follows the guidelines of this International Consensus Classification of Idiopathic Interstitial Pneumonias panel [3].

UIP, as the name implies, is the most common type of idiopathic interstitial pneumonia [1–4]. Histologically, UIP is characterized by a patchy heterogeneous pattern with foci of normal lung, interstitial inflammation, fibroblastic prolifera-

tion, interstitial fibrosis, and honeycombing, a heterogeneity that is best seen at low-power magnification (Table 4-1) [2,4,5]. Histologic abnormalities appear to represent different stages in the evolution of fibrosis, a combination of old and active lesions; this is termed *temporal heterogeneity* and is characteristic of UIP [4]. The fibrosis and honeycombing predominantly involve the subpleural and paraseptal lung regions (Fig. 4-1) [6,7]. Lack of subpleural honeycombing on open-lung biopsy should suggest an alternative diagnosis [2].

It should be clearly understood that, like the other interstitial pneumonias, UIP is a histologic diagnosis and a lung reaction pattern to injury. It may occur secondary to exposure to dusts (e.g., asbestos), drugs (e.g., bleomycin), or radiation, or be seen in association with collagen-vascular diseases [7]. When, after careful clinical evaluation, no etiology is found, it is classified as an idiopathic interstitial pneumonia, and in

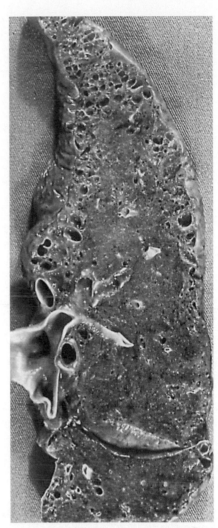

FIG. 4-1. Usual interstitial pneumonia (UIP). Gross pathologic specimen of a patient with idiopathic pulmonary fibrosis and UIP, which has been cut in the transverse plane. Fibrosis and honeycombing that almost exclusively involve the lung periphery are typical.

this context it is now considered synonymous with IPF [2,3]. In this book, we use the term *UIP* only to refer to the histologic abnormality; we use the term *IPF* to describe the disease that so commonly results in this histologic finding.

DIP is an uncommon condition characterized histologically by a relatively uniform pattern that consists predominantly of accumulation of macrophages within the alveoli (Table 4-1) [2,8]. Although DIP is classified as an idiopathic interstitial pneumonia, the majority of patients who have DIP are smokers [4,9]; therefore, it is likely that in many cases it represents a reaction to cigarette smoke. A histologic pattern of DIP can also be seen after exposure to various dusts such as asbestos, aluminum, silica, and hard metals [7]. The term *alveolar macrophage pneumonia* has been suggested by the American Thoracic Society/European Respiratory Society

International Multidisciplinary Consensus Committee for classification of idiopathic interstitial pneumonias as an alternative to or replacement for DIP [3].

Because there is considerable overlap between the histologic findings of DIP and those of respiratory bronchiolitis-interstitial lung disease (RB-ILD), a condition seen exclusively in smokers, it has been suggested that the term *DIP* be discarded and replaced with *RB-ILD* [4]. However, histologically RB-ILD has a predominantly bronchiolocentric distribution whereas DIP is diffuse [3]. Therefore, although RB-ILD and DIP may represent different parts of the spectrum of the same disease process [4], they are currently considered separate entities [3].

AIP is a clinicopathologic entity characterized by the presence of organizing diffuse alveolar damage (DAD) in patients who present with respiratory failure developing over days or weeks and in whom no etiologic agent is identified [2,10,11]. It is characterized histologically by the presence of hyaline membranes within the alveoli and diffuse, active interstitial fibrosis (Table 4-1) [4,10].

NSIP is characterized histologically by the presence of varying proportions of interstitial inflammation and fibrosis but without any specific features that would allow a diagnosis of UIP, DIP, or AIP (Table 4-1) [4,12]. It is therefore largely a diagnosis of exclusion. NSIP may be idiopathic or represent a reaction pattern seen in patients who have collagenvascular diseases or hypersensitivity pneumonitis [4,12].

In the majority of patients who have DIP, RB-ILD, AIP, and NSIP, the predominant abnormality on HRCT is parenchymal opacification. Therefore, these conditions are discussed in detail in Chapter 6.

IDIOPATHIC PULMONARY FIBROSIS

IPF occurs most commonly in patients between 40 and 70 years of age [4,9,13]. Patients who have IPF typically present with progressive shortness of breath and a dry cough. On physical examination, finger clubbing is seen in 25% to 50% of cases, and on auscultation, late inspiratory crackles (socalled Velcro rales) are characteristic. Pulmonary function tests show a restrictive pattern with reduced lung volumes and impairment in gas exchange [9,14]. IPF has a poor prognosis, with a mean survival of approximately 4 years from the onset of symptoms [15,16].

The diagnosis of IPF is limited to patients who have histologic findings of UIP [2,3]. Patients who have histologic findings of DIP, AIP, or NSIP and in whom no etiology is found are considered to have idiopathic DIP, AIP, or NSIP and not IPF. The earliest histologic abnormality in IPF is alveolitis with increased cellularity of the alveolar walls [7,17]. This inflammatory process can lead to progressive fibrosis [18]. Alveolar wall inflammation and intraalveolar macrophages in IPF indicate disease activity and are potentially reversible [19,20]. Fibrosis and honeycombing are considered irreversible.

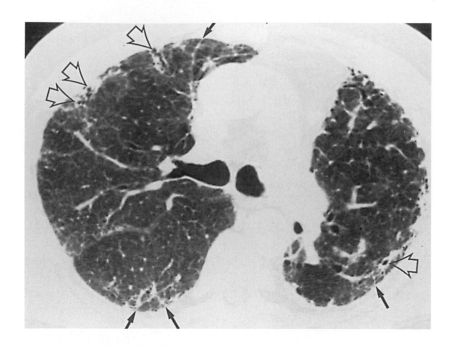

FIG. 4-2. Reticular opacities in a 69-year-old man with mild idiopathic pulmonary fibrosis. HRCT at the level of the right upper-lobe bronchus demonstrates irregular reticular opacities bilaterally in the subpleural lung regions. In several areas, irregular septal thickening (*small arrows*) and traction bronchiolectasis (*open arrows*) are visible. Irregular interfaces are present along the mediastinal and costal lung surfaces.

Recently it has been proposed in a Joint Statement of the American Thoracic Society (ATS) and the European Respiratory Society (ERS) [20a], that, in the absence of open-lung biopsy confirmation of UIP, a diagnosis of IPF may be considered likely in the presence of four major criteria and three of four minor criteria. Major criteria include (i) exclusion of known causes of infiltrative lung disease such as exposures, drugs, and connective tissue disease, (ii) abnormal pulmonary function tests with evidence of restriction and impaired gas exchange, (iii) HRCT findings of bibasilar reticulation with minimal ground-glass opacity, and (iv) transbronchial lung biopsy or bronchoalveolar lavage showing no evidence of another disease. Minor criteria for diagnosis are (i) age older than 50 years, (ii) insidious onset of dyspnea on exertion, (iii) duration of illness of 3 months or more, and (iv) bibasilar inspiratory crackles [20a].

One of the most characteristic features of IPF histologically is its heterogeneity. Areas of normal lung, active inflammation or alveolitis, and end-stage fibrosis are often present within the same open-lung biopsy specimen [2,4,7]. Regardless of the severity of disease, the predominant abnormalities are located in the subpleural lung regions and in the interstitium adjacent to the interlobular septa [6,7,13,21].

The most common radiographic finding in IPF, described in approximately 80% of patients who have biopsy-proven disease, consists of bilateral irregular linear opacities causing a reticular pattern [9,22,23]. Although these opacities may be diffuse throughout both lungs, in 50% to 80% of cases they involve predominantly or exclusively the lower lung zones [24]. As fibrosis develops, a fine reticular pattern appears that may be diffuse but is often first seen and more severe in the lower lung zones. As fibrosis progresses, the reticular pattern becomes coarser, and there is progressive loss of lung volume. In the end stage there is diffuse honeycombing. It is

well known, however, that the plain radiographic appearance of IPF is nonspecific, being similar to that seen in many other interstitial diseases. Furthermore, it has been repeatedly demonstrated that the severity of interstitial disease assessed on the chest radiograph correlates poorly with the clinical and functional impairment [13,25,26]. Patients may have severe dyspnea and a normal chest radiograph, or they may have extensive changes on the radiograph and minimal symptomatology.

High-Resolution Computed Tomography Findings

On HRCT, IPF is characterized by the presence of reticular opacities that correspond to areas of irregular fibrosis (Figs. 4-2 and 4-3) and reflect the typical pathologic features of UIP (Table 4-2) [1,2,21]. The predominant HRCT features of IPF include honeycombing and intralobular interstitial thickening; irregular interlobular septal thickening and ground-glass opacity may also be present but are usually less conspicuous findings.

Intralobular interstitial thickening is often visible on HRCT in patients who have IPF (Figs. 4-4 through 4-7), resulting in a fine reticular pattern that may predominate in patients who have this disease [27]. Nishimura et al. [13] reported the presence of a fine reticulation or ill-defined increased lung attenuation in 96% of cases, associated with visibility of centrilobular bronchioles (i.e., traction bronchiolectasis). Thickening of the intralobular interstitium also results in the presence of irregular interfaces between the lung and pulmonary vessels, bronchi, and pleural surfaces (Fig. 4-5) [13,28]. In areas of severe fibrosis, the segmental and subsegmental bronchi become dilated and tortuous, a finding referred to as *traction bronchiectasis* (Figs. 4-5 and 4-7) [29]. Subpleural lines can also be seen, usually indicating fibrosis (Fig. 4-4).

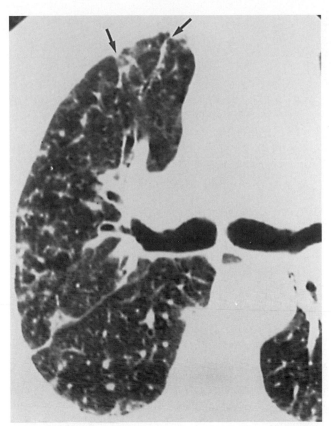

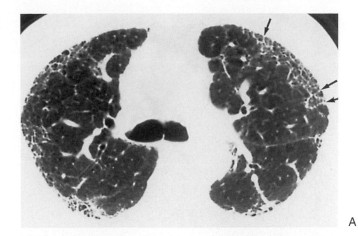

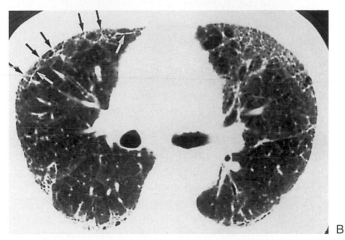

FIG. 4-3. Irregular reticular opacities in a 58-year-old woman with idiopathic pulmonary fibrosis. HRCT is targeted to the right lung. Reticular opacities are slightly more prominent in the subpleural regions. Irregular septal thickening (*small arrows*) is visible in several locations.

FIG. 4-4. Reticular opacities in a patient with idiopathic pulmonary fibrosis. Scans at two levels **(A,B)** show a peripheral predominance of abnormalities indicative of fibrosis, including irregular interlobular septal thickening (*black arrows*) and subpleural lines (*white arrows*). However, the predominant pattern is that of intralobular interstitial thickening with areas of honeycombing.

In many cases of IPF, findings of honeycombing predominate [21,27]. In such cases, there is gross distortion of lung architecture, and individual lobules are no longer visible (Figs. 4-8 through 4-11). Honeycomb cysts usually range from 2 to 20 mm in diameter, but they can be larger (Figs. 4-8 through 4-11) [21,27,30]. They typically appear to share walls on HRCT and usually occur in several layers in the subpleural lung. Honeycomb cysts have been reported on HRCT in 24%

TABLE 4-2. *HRCT findings in idiopathic pulmonary fibrosis*

Findings of fibrosis (i.e., honeycombing, traction bronchiectasis and bronchiolectasis, intralobular interstitial thickening, irregular interlobular septal thickening, irregular interfaces)[a]

Ground-glass opacity (usually in areas showing fibrosis)[a]

Peripheral and subpleural predominance of abnormalities[a,b]

Lower lung zone and posterior predominance[a,b]

[a]Most common finding(s).
[b]Finding(s) most helpful in differential diagnosis.

---

to 90% of patients who have IPF [13,26], and the frequency of this finding varies with the severity or stage of the disease. Findings of honeycombing and fibrosis are most often symmetric, but asymmetry may be present.

Interlobular septal thickening is sometimes seen on HRCT in patients who have IPF, but it is a less conspicuous finding than intralobular interstitial thickening or honeycombing (Figs. 4-2 through 4-4 and 4-12). In patients who have honeycombing, findings of septal thickening are usually visible only in less abnormal lung regions. When visible, septal thickening is characteristically irregular in contour (Figs. 4-2 through 4-4 and 4-12) [27,31], and septa marginate pulmonary lobules that can appear irregular in shape or distorted. Abnormal prominence of the centrilobular vessel, which normally appears as a dot- or Y-shaped branching opacity in the lobular core, is often present in patients who show septal thickening, but is not a conspicuous finding in most [27]. In addition, the centrilobular

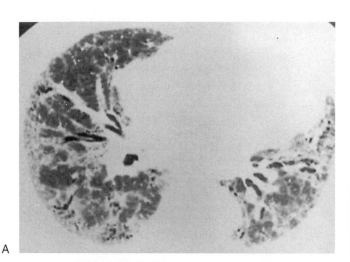

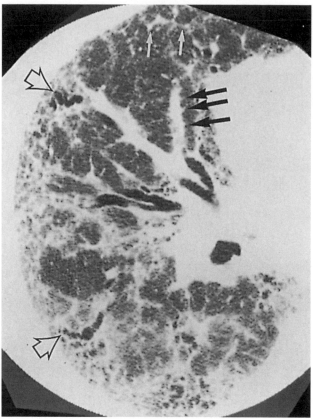

FIG. 4-5. HRCT findings of idiopathic pulmonary fibrosis: fibrosis and a peripheral, subpleural predominance. **A:** A 1.5-mm collimation scan using the standard reconstruction algorithm demonstrates a patchy distribution of reticular opacities in the peripheral aspects of both lungs. **B:** The distinction between normal and abnormal lung parenchyma is more readily made on this image targeted to the right lung and reconstructed using the bone algorithm; the patchy distribution of abnormalities is clearly seen. The fine reticular pattern visible largely reflects intralobular interstitial thickening, but irregular septal thickening (*white arrows*) is visible anteriorly in areas that are less abnormal. Irregular interfaces (*black arrows*) are visible throughout the lung at the margins of vessels and bronchi. Traction bronchiectasis and bronchiolectasis are seen within the peripheral lung regions (*open arrows*). Ground-glass opacity is visible in the right lower lobe, but the right middle lobe appears spared. (From Müller NL, Staples CA, et al. Disease activity in idiopathic pulmonary fibrosis: CT and pathologic correlation. *Radiology* 1987;165:731, with permission.)

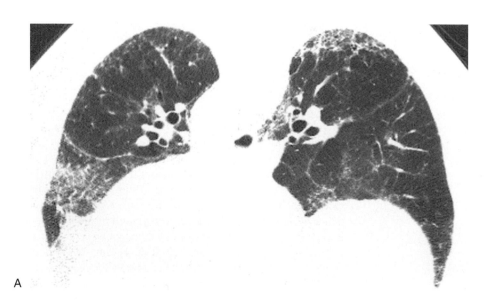

FIG. 4-6. A–C: Prone HRCT in a 71-year-old man with idiopathic pulmonary fibrosis and progressive shortness of breath. Abnormalities predominate in the posterior, subpleural lower lobes and are characterized by intralobular interstitial thickening (*arrows*, **B**) and interlobular septal thickening (*arrow*, **C**). Although ground-glass opacity is superimposed on the abnormal reticulation, this was found to represent end-stage fibrosis on biopsy. *Continued*

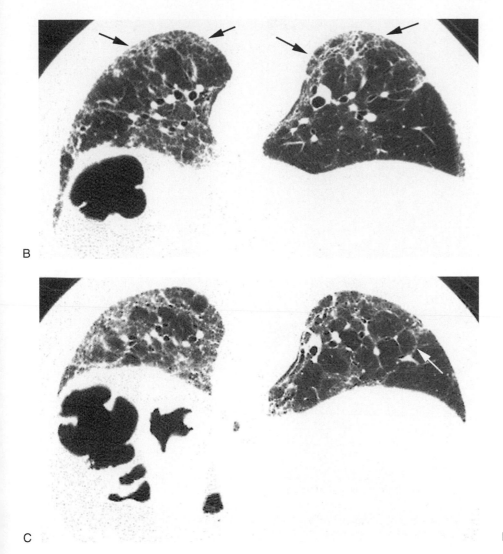

B

C

FIG. 4-6. *Continued*

bronchiole, which is not normally seen, is sometimes visible because of a combination of dilatation (i.e., traction bronchiolectasis), thickening of the peribronchiolar interstitium, and increased opacity of surrounding lung (Figs. 4-2 and 4-5) [27].

Ground-glass opacity may be visible on HRCT in patients who have IPF. It may indicate the presence of active inflammation and potentially treatable disease (Figs. 4-13 through 4-15) [32] or the presence of fibrosis below the resolution of HRCT. Ground-glass opacity should be considered to represent an active process only when there are no associated HRCT findings of fibrosis. Findings of fibrosis in association with ground-glass opacity, thus suggesting an irreversible process, include intralobular interstitial thickening, honeycombing, and traction bronchiectasis and bronchiolectasis (Fig. 4-6) [33].

Patients who have predominantly ground-glass opacity on HRCT are more likely to respond to treatment than patients who predominantly have reticulation [34–36]. It should be emphasized, however, that most patients who have IPF present with HRCT findings of reticulation and have progressive disease and a poor prognosis. IPF presenting with ground-glass

opacity as a predominant finding is distinctly uncommon. In some patients, areas of ground-glass opacity frequently can be seen to progress to fibrosis and honeycombing [34,37].

Another hallmark of IPF on HRCT is its patchy distribution (Fig. 4-16). Areas of mild and severe fibrosis, mild and marked inflammatory activity, and normal lung are often present in the same patient, in the same lung, and in the same lobe. Also, and most important diagnostically, findings of IPF often predominate in the peripheral and subpleural regions (Figs. 4-1, 4-2, 4-4, and 4-5) and in the lung bases [21]. Concentric subpleural honeycombing is characteristic of IPF (Figs. 4-1 and 4-8 through 4-11). This subpleural predominance is evident on HRCT in 80% to 95% of patients [13,21,38]. In approximately 70% of patients, the fibrosis is most severe in the lower lung zones; in approximately 20%, all zones are involved to a similar degree; and in approximately 10%, mainly the middle or upper lung zones are involved [34,38].

A common finding on HRCT in patients who have IPF is the presence of mediastinal lymphadenopathy [39–41]. This usually involves only one or two nodal stations, and the nodes usually measure less than 15 mm in short axis diame-

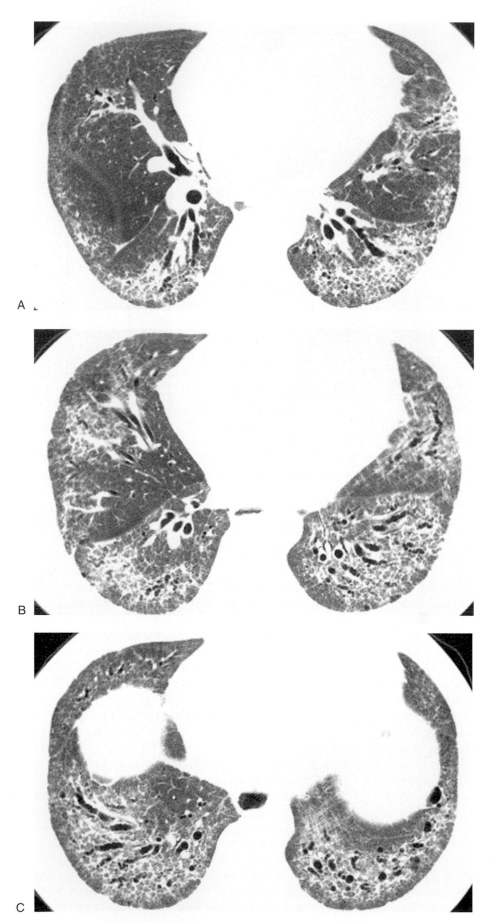

FIG. 4-7. A–C: HRCT in a 34-year-old man with progressive shortness of breath and idiopathic pulmonary fibrosis (IPF) diagnosed on lung biopsy. The predominant abnormalities are intralobular interstitial thickening and traction bronchiectasis. A posterior, subpleural, and basal predominance is also visible and typical of IPF.

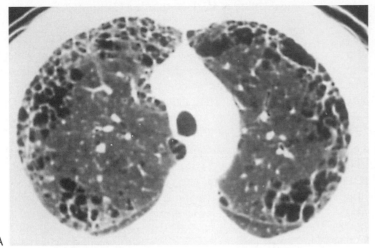

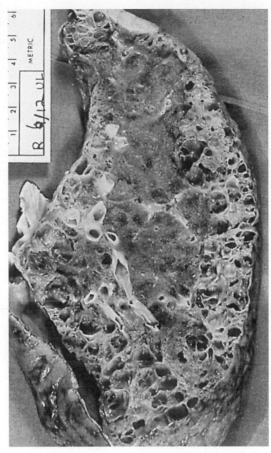

A

FIG. 4-8. Peripheral honeycombing in a 60-year-old patient with idiopathic pulmonary fibrosis. **A:** A 1.5-mm collimation scan (reconstructed with the standard algorithm) at the level of the aortic arch shows honeycombing that is almost exclusively in the subpleural lung regions. **B:** The macroscopic pathologic specimen of the right upper lobe, cut in the same plane and at the same level as the HRCT, mirrors the appearance of the HRCT image. Honeycomb cysts measuring 2 to 10 mm in diameter are present in the subpleural lung regions; the remaining parenchyma is normal. (From Müller NL, Miller RR, et al. Fibrosing alveolitis: CT-pathologic correlation. *Radiology* 1986,160:585, with permission.)

B

ter [40]. Enlarged mediastinal nodes have been reported in 48% to 90% of patients who have IPF [39–41]. The likelihood of lymphadenopathy increases with the extent of parenchymal involvement and decreases in the presence of recent steroid treatment. In a study by Franquet et al. [41], the prev-

alence of enlarged nodes was 14% in patients who had recently received oral steroids, and 71% in patients who had not taken steroids for at least 6 months.

In the majority of patients who have IPF, serial HRCT scans show an increase in the extent of reticulation and hon-

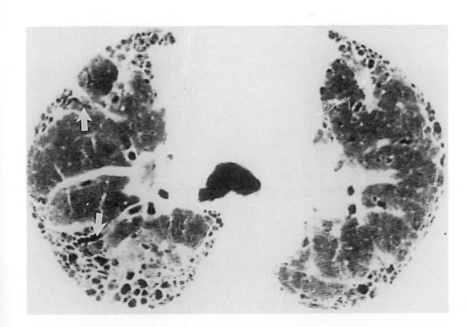

FIG. 4-9. End-stage idiopathic pulmonary fibrosis. Typical honeycomb cysts are present mainly in the subpleural lung regions. Also noted is traction bronchiectasis (*arrows*).

eycombing (Fig. 4-17) [37,42,43]. This progression usually occurs gradually over several months or years (Fig. 4-18). Occasionally, patients develop a fulminant and often fatal acute exacerbation [44,45]. The clinical diagnosis is based on rapid deterioration in the absence of demonstrable infection or congestive heart failure. The HRCT findings consist of extensive multifocal, peripheral, or diffuse ground-glass opacification superimposed on a background of interstitial fibrosis (Figs. 4-19 and 4-20) [46,47]. This appearance correlates with the presence of diffuse alveolar damage on lung biopsy [46,47]. Patients who have an acute exacerbation and peripheral or multifocal ground-glass opacities on HRCT often show at least partial improvement after corticosteroid therapy. Patients who have diffuse ground-glass opacification on HRCT usually die within 3 months of presentation [46].

Clinical Utility of High-Resolution Computed Tomography

Several studies have shown that CT and HRCT are superior to plain chest radiographs in the assessment of patients who have IPF. For example, honeycombing is seen in up to 90% of CT studies, as compared to 30% of cases on plain radiographs [26]. HRCT findings have been shown to correlate with symptoms and pulmonary function abnormalities in patients who have IPF. Staples et al. [26] compared CT with clinical, functional, and radiologic findings in 23 patients who had IPF. The CT scans provided a better estimate of the pattern, distribution, and extent of pulmonary fibrosis and showed more extensive honeycombing than did radiographs. In this study, there was also good correlation between the extent of disease, assessed by the percentage of lung showing

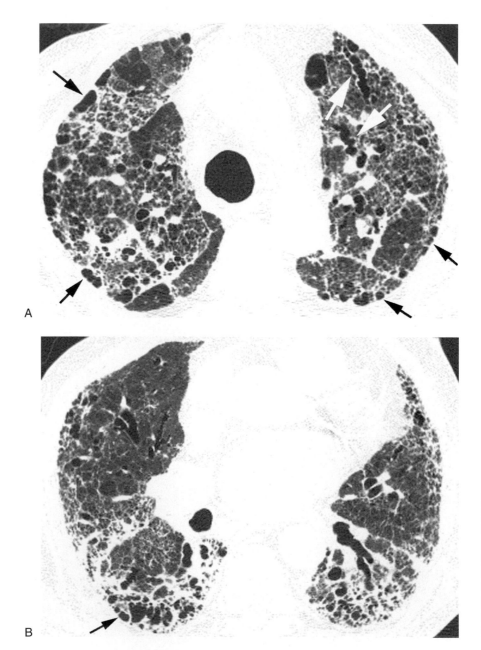

A

B

FIG. 4-10. A–C: HRCT at three levels in a 54-year-old man with idiopathic pulmonary fibrosis. Abnormalities include intralobular interstitial thickening and traction bronchiectasis (*white arrows*, **A**). Honeycombing characterized by subpleural cystic lucencies is also present (*black arrows*). At the lung bases **(C)**, some overlap between the appearances of honeycombing and traction bronchiolectasis is visible. *Continued*

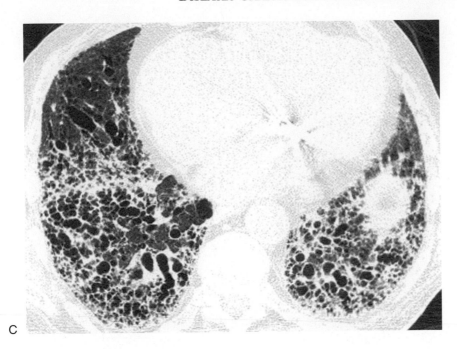

C

FIG. 4-10. *Continued*

evidence of fibrosis on CT, and the severity of dyspnea ($r = 0.64$; $p < .001$). A significant correlation between the extent of ground-glass opacities seen on CT or HRCT and the severity of dyspnea and reduction in total lung capacity (TLC) and carbon monoxide diffusing capacity (DLCO) ($p < .01$) has also been found [37].

Both the long-term survival in IPF and its response to treatment with corticosteroids correlate with the histologic findings at biopsy. The best response to steroids is observed in patients who have marked disease activity and little fibrosis [19,20,36]. Although open-lung biopsy provides the gold standard for evaluating patients who have IPF, it has limitations. Most important, it is invasive and usually assesses only a small part of the lung. Thus, the region sampled may not be representative of the lung as a whole, and the presence of inflammation may be missed.

Several studies have demonstrated that HRCT allows a distinction of active, potentially reversible alveolitis from irreversible fibrosis in the majority of patients who have IPF without the need for lung biopsy [32,35,36,48]. Several investigators routinely use HRCT to assess disease activity in patients who have IPF, with HRCT findings governing treatment. In some patients who have IPF, definite diagnoses of end-stage lung (honeycombing without ground-glass opacity) or active alveolitis (ground-glass opacity) can be made on the basis of HRCT findings.

Müller et al. [48] reported 12 patients who have IPF in whom disease activity assessed by CT was correlated with the open-lung biopsy findings. In this study, the CT finding of airspace opacification (ground-glass opacity) was used to diagnose alveolitis and activity. Two independent

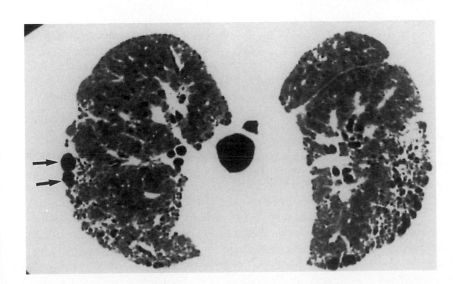

FIG. 4-11. End-stage idiopathic pulmonary fibrosis with honeycombing. A prone scan shows subpleural cysts typical of honeycombing. Some cysts (*arrows*) can be large. Honeycomb cysts typically share walls on HRCT and occur in several layers in the subpleural lung.

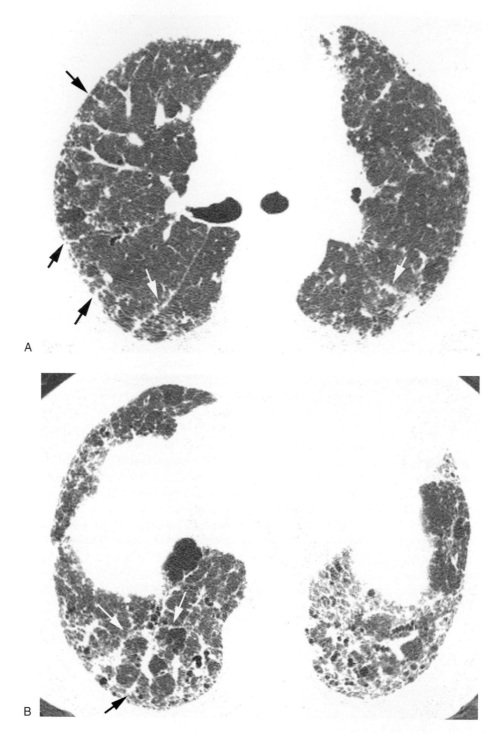

FIG. 4-12. A,B: HRCT in a 60-year-old woman with idiopathic pulmonary fibrosis. **A:** Irregular interlobular septal thickening (*black arrows*), irregular thickening of the major fissures (*white arrows*), and irregular reticular opacities are visible in the peripheral lung. **B:** Abnormalities are more extensive at the lung bases, characterized by intralobular interstitial thickening, traction bronchiectasis, and irregular interlobular septal thickening (*arrows*).

observers correctly identified the five patients who had marked-disease activity and five out of seven patients who had low-disease activity. In another study, of 14 patients who had IPF who showed ground-glass opacity on HRCT, 12 (86%) had inflammation on biopsy that indicated the presence of active disease [32].

Lee et al. [49] correlated the extent of ground-glass opacity at presentation with the improvement in pulmonary function after treatment with corticosteroids in 19 patients who had IPF. The extent of ground-glass opacity on CT correlated significantly with the improvement in the forced vital capacity ($r = 0.7$; $p < .001$) and in gas transfer as assessed by the DLCO ($r = 0.67$; $p < .002$) after treatment. Wells et al. [35] assessed whether CT could predict response to treatment and prognosis in 76 patients who had IPF. The CT abnormalities were categorized as consisting predominantly of ground-glass opacity (n = 8), a mixed pattern (n = 18), or a predominantly reticular pattern (n = 50). Response to treatment was seen in approximately 80% of patients who had ground-glass opacity as the predominant abnormality compared to only

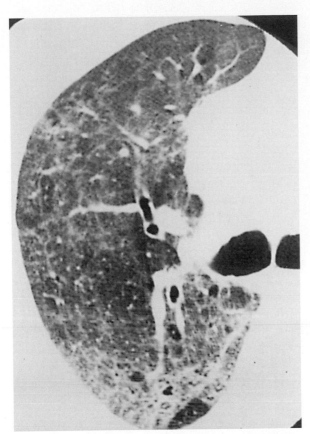

FIG. 4-13. Ground-glass opacity in a 65-year-old man with idiopathic pulmonary fibrosis. HRCT at the level of the right upper lobe shows a ground-glass increase in lung opacity involving most of the right lung. This ground-glass pattern reflects the presence of active disease. Reticular abnormalities indicating fibrosis are few, but some septal thickening is visible.

20% of patients who had a mixed pattern and 4% of patients who had a predominant reticular pattern. Overall the prognosis in the patients was poor with a 50% 4-year survival. All eight patients who had predominant ground-glass opacity at presentation were alive after 4 years, compared to only 40%

of patients who had mixed pattern and 20% of patients who had a predominant reticular pattern at presentation [35].

Wells et al. [34] also performed serial CT scans in 21 patients who had IPF. They demonstrated that improvement with treatment was associated with a decrease in the extent of ground-glass opacity. Deterioration on follow-up was associated with an increase in the extent of ground-glass opacity or an increase in the extent of reticular abnormalities [34].

Gay et al. compared pretreatment clinical, HRCT, and open-lung biopsy features with likelihood of response to treatment in 38 patients who had biopsy-proven IPF [36]. Responders to treatment had a lower age, greater extent of ground-glass opacity, less fibrosis on HRCT, and greater cellular infiltration scores (disease activity) on lung biopsy specimens than nonresponders [36]. The only parameters that were helpful in predicting death during follow-up were the extent of fibrosis on HRCT or open-lung biopsy specimens [36]. No clinical or pulmonary function parameter was helpful in predicting long-term survival.

It should be emphasized that the majority of patients who have IPF have a predominantly reticular pattern at presentation; such patients do not respond well to treatment [34,35,37,42]. Furthermore, although patients who have areas of ground-glass opacity are more likely to respond to treatment, it has been shown that in patients who do not respond to treatment, areas of ground-glass opacity visible on HRCT precede and predict development of a reticular pattern or honeycombing in the same location [37,42] (Fig. 4-15).

In summary, HRCT can be helpful in predicting potential response to treatment and long-term prognosis in patients who have IPF [35,36]. In patients who do not respond to treatment, the progression of fibrosis and honeycombing is faster in patients who have active inflammation and ground-glass opacities than in patients who did not have ground-glass opacity [50]. CT is also helpful in determining the optimal site for lung biopsy, if this procedure is considered necessary. As pointed out by Carrington and Gaensler [9], at the time of open-lung biopsy, the surgeon must attempt to obtain diagnostic tissue by avoiding areas of extensive honeycombing.

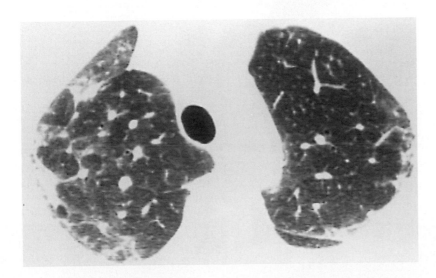

FIG. 4-14. Active idiopathic pulmonary fibrosis in a 63-year-old woman. HRCT shows ground-glass opacities in the subpleural lung regions, particularly on the right.

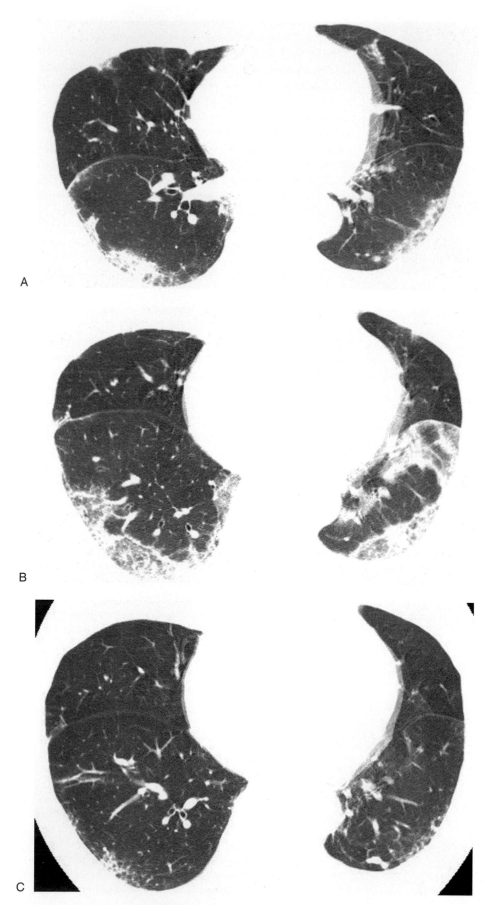

FIG. 4-15. Active idiopathic pulmonary fibrosis (IPF) in a 59-year-old woman with a history of nonproductive cough and progressive shortness of breath over a period of several months. HRCT at two levels (**A** and **B**) shows ground-glass opacity and consolidation to be predominant findings. Open-lung biopsy showed findings of active IPF. **C:** After treatment, there has been significant resolution of the ground-glass opacities, although some intralobular interstitial thickening persists.

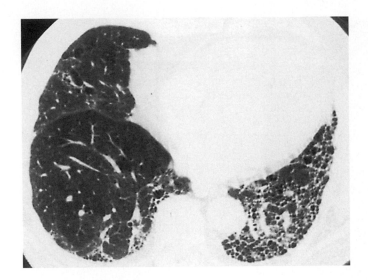

FIG. 4-16. A 73-year-old man with idiopathic pulmonary fibrosis. HRCT through the lung bases shows a patchy distribution of abnormalities, with mild honeycombing in the right lower lobe and extensive honeycombing and marked loss of lung volume in the left lower lobe.

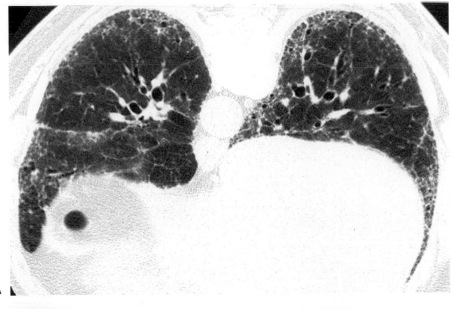

A

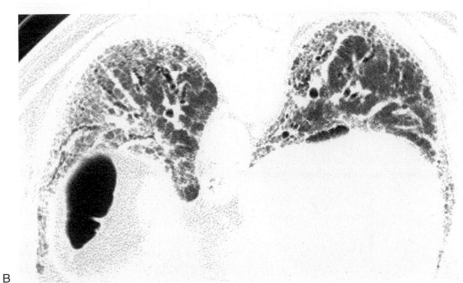

B

FIG. 4-17. Progression of idiopathic pulmonary fibrosis. A: The initial HRCT shows mild subpleural reticulation. B: Five months later, despite treatment, there has been progression of pulmonary fibrosis with intralobular interstitial thickening, traction bronchiectasis, and more extensive lung involvement. The presence of ground-glass opacity superimposed on reticulation likely represents fibrosis.

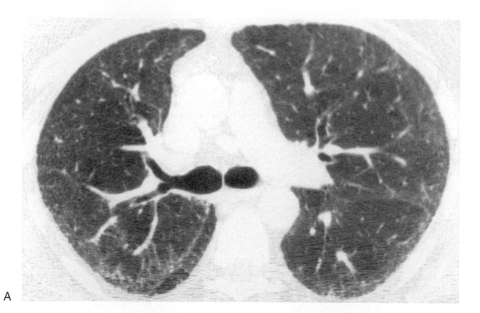

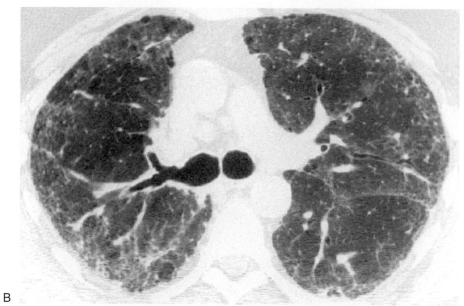

FIG. 4-18. Idiopathic pulmonary fibrosis with progression over 3 years. **A:** HRCT at presentation demonstrates patchy ground-glass opacities and mild reticular pattern involving mainly the subpleural lung regions. **B:** HRCT 3 years later demonstrates more extensive reticular changes and mild subpleural honeycombing.

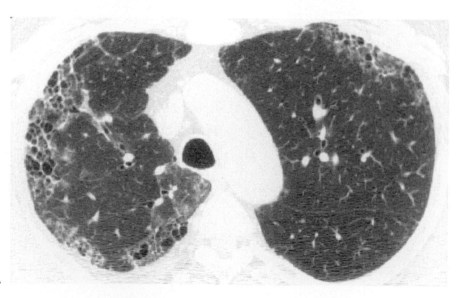

FIG. 4-19. Acute exacerbation of idiopathic pulmonary fibrosis. **A:** HRCT shows irregular linear opacities, small foci of ground-glass attenuation, and honeycombing in a patchy distribution predominantly in the subpleural lung regions. *Continued*

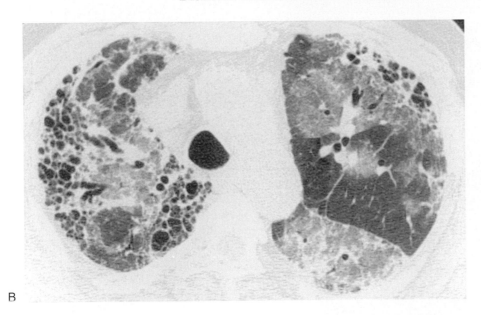

FIG. 4-19. *Continued* B: HRCT performed when the patient presented with acute exacerbation of clinical symptoms and rapid development of severe hypoxemia demonstrates extensive bilateral areas of ground-glass attenuation. Also noted is slight progression of the honeycombing.

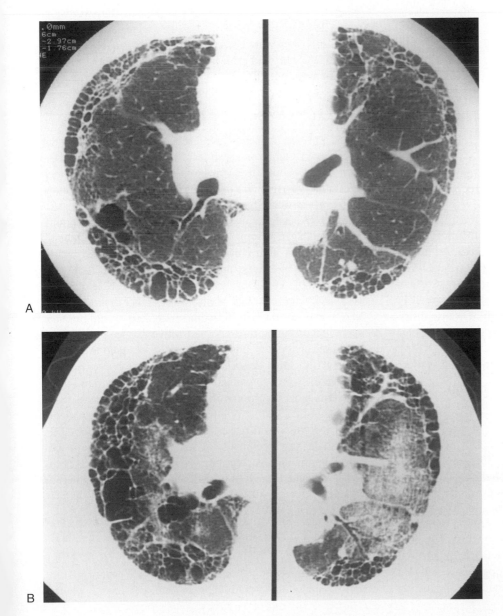

FIG. 4-20. HRCT in a 64-year-old man with acute exacerbation of idiopathic pulmonary fibrosis. **A:** HRCT obtained 6 months before clinical deterioration shows bilateral subpleural honeycombing. **B:** HRCT obtained during acute exacerbation shows areas of ground-glass opacity superimposed on peripheral honeycombing. *Continued*

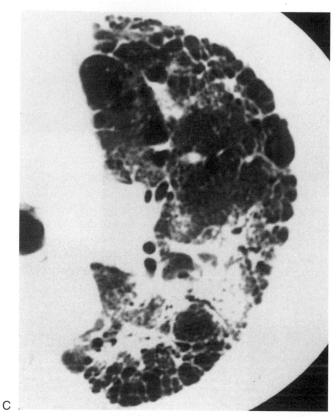

C

FIG. 4-20. *Continued* C: HRCT obtained 14 days after that shown in **(B)** shows evolution of ground-glass opacity into dense consolidation. At autopsy, this represented dense fibrosis. (From Akira M. Computed tomography and pathologic findings in fulminant forms of idiopathic interstitial pneumonia. *J Thorac Imag* 1999;14:76, with permission.)

This can be difficult in cases of IPF, because the most severe honeycombing is typically subpleural in location. An important role for CT in the assessment of patients who have IPF is to help the surgeon choose the best area for biopsy. Areas of honeycombing can be avoided, and less abnormal areas, or areas of ground-glass opacity, can be sought. Disease distribution cannot be adequately assessed from the conventional radiographs, but it can be easily determined using CT [51]; CT scans may demonstrate areas of abnormal lung that are not apparent on chest radiographs [52].

Accuracy in Diagnosis

HRCT findings have been shown to be highly accurate in making a diagnosis of UIP and IPF [53–55]. As shown by Tung et al., in a study of 86 patients, including 41 with IPF and 45 with various other diffuse lung diseases, HRCT accurately identified 88% of patients who had IPF. Even more important, in the majority of patients who present with clinical features of IPF, the presence of predominantly subpleural and basal distribution of fibrosis on HRCT can be sufficiently characteristic to obviate biopsy, especially in those patients in whom HRCT shows no evidence suggesting

disease activity [33,35]. Generally speaking, biopsy should be avoided in patients who have typical basal honeycombing; if atypical findings are present, biopsy is warranted.

Several other studies have assessed the accuracy of HRCT in the diagnosis of UIP. However, in these studies, because biopsy proof was required for participation, there may be a bias toward exclusion of cases with typical HRCT findings. In a study of 85 patients having one of 16 different diseases proven by surgical biopsy [56], 18 patients were proven to have UIP. Among the 85 patients, 14 were diagnosed as having UIP with a high degree of confidence; 12 had UIP, and two had other interstitial pneumonias. In a study of 129 patients who had proven idiopathic interstitial pneumonia [57], UIP was correctly diagnosed in 71% of cases overall, and in 76% when readers were confident. In a yet-unpublished study of 91 patients suspected of having UIP and IPF (Lynch et al., Society of Thoracic Radiology, March 1999), 54 were proven to have IPF pathologically. Four radiologists were certain of the presence or absence of IPF in 52 cases. When they were certain that IPF was present, they were correct in 26 of 27 cases (96%); when they were certain that IPF was absent, they were correct in 21 of 25 (84%). However, in 28 patients who had pathologic IPF, a confident diagnosis was not made on HRCT.

COLLAGEN-VASCULAR DISEASES

Each of the collagen-vascular diseases can involve the respiratory system and cause focal or diffuse pulmonary disease; however, the frequency of lung abnormalities varies among the different diseases [58,59]. The two most common conditions associated with interstitial fibrosis are rheumatoid arthritis (RA) and progressive systemic sclerosis (scleroderma).

Most collagen-vascular diseases can cause chronic interstitial pneumonia with clinical, radiologic, HRCT, and pathologic features indistinguishable from those of IPF (Table 4-2) [25,26,58,60]. However, collagen-vascular disease may be associated with histologic abnormalities other than UIP (e.g., NSIP), and several HRCT findings may help to differentiate interstitial pneumonitis associated with collagen disease from IPF in selected cases. First, collagen diseases tend to be associated with a finer reticular pattern and less honeycombing than typically seen in patients who have IPF, and ground-glass opacity is more common as a predominant abnormality. Second, pleural thickening or effusion may be present in patients who have collagen diseases, but neither is a feature of IPF. Also, collagen-vascular disease may be associated with specific abnormalities, such as bronchiectasis, bronchiolitis obliterans, follicular bronchiolitis, LIP, and bronchiolitis obliterans organizing pneumonia (BOOP), not seen in patients who have IPF and having distinct HRCT appearances.

Rheumatoid Arthritis

RA is commonly associated with thoracic abnormalities [61,62], including interstitial pneumonia and fibrosis, pleural

TABLE 4-3. *HRCT findings in rheumatoid arthritis*

Bronchiectasis without fibrosis[a]

Findings of fibrosis (i.e., traction bronchiectasis and bronchiolectasis, intralobular interstitial thickening, irregular interlobular septal thickening, irregular interfaces)[a]

Honeycombing (less common than in idiopathic pulmonary fibrosis)

Ground-glass opacity[a]

Peripheral and subpleural predominance of fibrosis or ground-glass opacity[a,b]

Lower lung zone and posterior predominance[a,b]

Pleural thickening or effusion[a,b]

Small centrilobular nodules (follicular bronchiolitis)

Large (rheumatoid) nodules

Findings of bronchiolitis obliterans (i.e., air-trapping, mosaic perfusion)

[a]Most common finding(s).
[b]Finding(s) most helpful in differential diagnosis.

effusion or pleural thickening, necrobiotic nodules, BOOP, bronchiectasis, and bronchiolitis obliterans [63,64].

Pulmonary function abnormalities consistent with interstitial pneumonia have been reported in as many as 40% of patients who have RA [65,66], but in more than half of these patients, the chest radiograph is normal [61,66]. The prevalence of radiologically detectable interstitial disease in patients who have RA is probably around 10% [61,65,66]. Clinical evidence of arthritis precedes the development of pulmonary fibrosis in approximately 90% of patients, and 90% have a positive serum rheumatoid factor. Whereas the

majority of patients who have interstitial fibrosis associated with RA have UIP, a small percentage have histologic findings of NSIP [12]. The HRCT findings of NSIP are discussed in Chapter 6.

High-Resolution Computed Tomography Findings

Radiologically and on HRCT, the appearance of RA with interstitial fibrosis is usually indistinguishable from that of IPF (see Figs. 3-17, 3-33, 3-36, and Figs. 4-21 through 4-23) [26,62,63]. In one study, HRCT findings of pulmonary fibrosis, with or without honeycombing, were seen in 10% of patients, and ground-glass opacity was present in 14% [63]. However, patients who have rheumatoid disease may show other abnormalities not typical of IPF. HRCT findings also reported in patients who have RA include bronchial abnormalities and bronchiectasis (21%), consolidation (6%), enlarged lymph nodes (9%), pleural abnormalities (16%), and nodules 3 mm to 3 cm in diameter that are predominantly subpleural in location (22%) (Table 4-3) [63].

Bronchiectasis and airways disease are common in RA and can be associated with chronic infection, which has an increased incidence in rheumatoid patients, or bronchiolitis obliterans [64,67] (see Fig. 3-142). For example, in a study of 20 nonsmoking RA patients who had normal chest radiographs, five (25%) were found to have unsuspected basal bronchiectasis on HRCT [68]. Perez et al. [64] reviewed the prevalence and characteristics of airways involvement in 50 RA patients who did not have ILD. They found HRCT to be more sensitive in detecting airway abnormalities than were pulmonary function tests. HRCT demonstrated bronchial or lung abnormalities, or both, in 35 cases (70%), consisting of air-trapping (n = 16; 32%), cylindrical bronchiectasis (n = 15; 30%), and mild

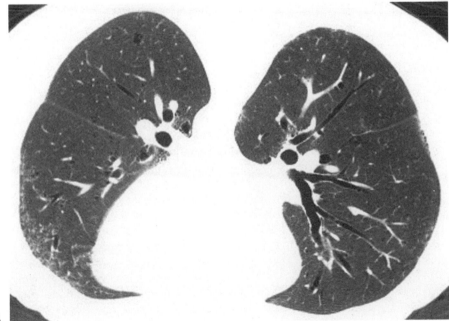

FIG. 4-21. A–C: Prone HRCT at three levels in a patient with rheumatoid arthritis and lung disease. Subpleural opacities in the midlung (**A** and **B**) have a small nodular or branching appearance, consistent with that of follicular bronchiolitis. At a lower level (**C**), findings of intralobular interstitial thickening and traction bronchiectasis are typical of fibrosis. *Continued*

A

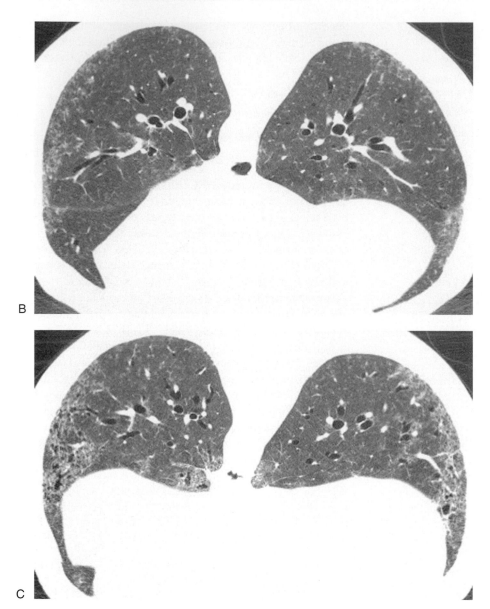

B

C

FIG. 4-21. *Continued*

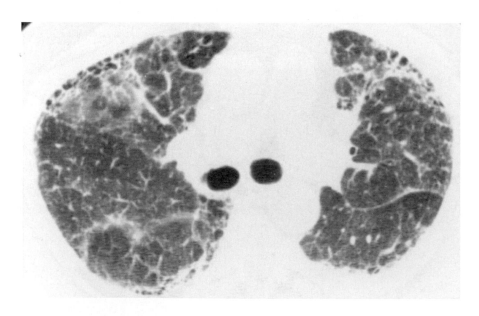

FIG. 4-22. Usual interstitial pneumonia in rheumatoid arthritis. HRCT shows a reticular pattern and mild honeycombing predominantly in the subpleural lung regions. Also noted are patchy areas of ground-glass attenuation consistent with active alveolitis.

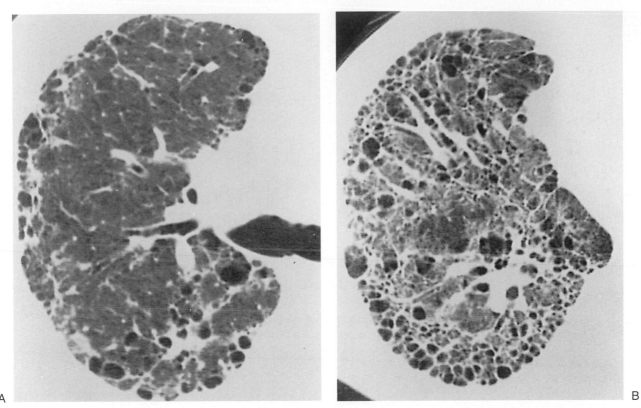

FIG. 4-23. Rheumatoid arthritis and end-stage usual interstitial pneumonia with honeycombing in a 60-year-old man. **A:** HRCT at the level of the tracheal carina shows subpleural honeycombing and interlobular septal thickening indistinguishable from idiopathic pulmonary fibrosis. **B:** HRCT through the right lung base shows diffuse honeycombing and septal thickening.

heterogeneity in lung attenuation (i.e., mosaic perfusion) (n = 10; 20%). On the other hand, pulmonary function tests demonstrated airway obstruction [i.e., reduced forced expiratory volume in 1 second (FEV$_1$)/forced vital capacity (FVC)] in only nine patients (18%) and evidence of small airways disease in only four (8%). Pulmonary function test findings of airway obstruction and small airways disease correlated with the presence of bronchiectasis and bronchial-wall thickening ($p = .003$) [64]. The occurrence of bronchiolitis obliterans in patients who have RA is discussed in Chapter 8.

An uncommon abnormality seen in patients who have RA or other collagen-vascular diseases is follicular bronchiolitis [69,70]. This is a benign condition characterized by prominent hyperplasia of lymphoid follicles around the bronchioles and, to a lesser extent, bronchi [70]. HRCT findings of follicular bronchiolitis consist of multiple small nodules in a predominantly centrilobular, subpleural, and peribronchial distribution (Fig. 4-21) [70,71]. The nodules usually measure 1 to 4 mm in diameter but may occasionally be 1 cm or more in diameter [71]. Large nodules seen in patients who have RA probably represent necrobiotic (rheumatoid) nodules.

Pleural disease, either pleural effusion or pleural thickening, is common in patients who have RA, being seen in up to 40% of patients at autopsy. However, symptomatic pleural disease is less common, and radiographic evidence of pleural thickening or pleural effusion is present in only 5% to 20% of patients [59,61]. In a study by Fujii et al. [72], pleural thickening was visible on HRCT in 33% of the 91 patients studied and in 44% of the patients who had HRCT findings of interstitial pneumonia.

Utility of High-Resolution Computed Tomography

HRCT is more sensitive than chest radiographs in the diagnosis of lung disease in patients who have RA. Fujii et al. [72] reviewed the chest radiographic and HRCT findings of 91 patients who had RA. On HRCT, 43 patients had findings of UIP with fibrosis, five had findings consistent with bronchiolitis obliterans, and 43 had a normal HRCT. In approximately half of these 91 patients, chest radiographic findings were similar to those shown on HRCT. However, 17 of 46 (37%) patients thought to have normal chest radiographs had HRCT abnormalities consistent with rheumatoid lung disease. Furthermore, 14 of 43 (33%) patients thought to have abnormal chest radiographs had no evidence of significant lung disease on HRCT. Also, HRCT can be useful in demonstrating lung disease in RA patients who have normal chest radiographs but have pulmonary function abnormalities [59,73]. Some HRCT findings are more frequent in symptomatic patients who have rheumatoid lung disease [63].

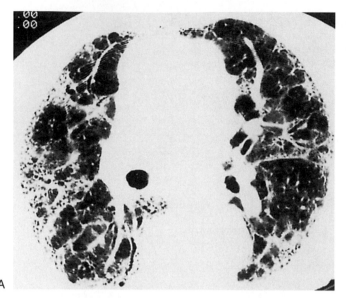
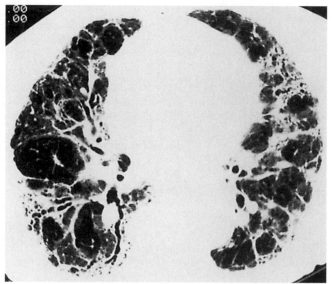

FIG. 4-24. A,B: Findings of fibrosis in a patient with scleroderma. Subpleural honeycombing, traction bronchiectasis, and some irregular interlobular septal thickening are the predominant features. These abnormalities closely mimic the appearance of idiopathic pulmonary fibrosis.

These include honeycombing, bronchiectasis, nodules, and ground-glass opacity.

Progressive Systemic Sclerosis (Scleroderma)

Progressive systemic sclerosis (PSS) leads to some degree of interstitial fibrosis in nearly all cases [74,75]. As many as 75% of patients who have PSS have evidence of lung disease at autopsy, although only 1% present with symptoms of pulmonary dysfunction [75]. As with RA, chest radiographs may appear normal despite abnormal pulmonary function tests. The incidence of radiographically recognizable interstitial disease is probably around 25%, although various studies quote an incidence ranging from 10% to 80% [74,75]. In addition to UIP, PSS is commonly associated with pulmonary vasculitis and pulmonary hypertension. Recently, it has been shown that at least some of the patients who have PSS and interstitial fibrosis have NSIP rather than UIP [4,12]. The prevalence of NSIP in patients who have PSS is not known.

High-Resolution Computed Tomography Findings

The HRCT findings of interstitial fibrosis in PSS are similar to those of IPF, including honeycombing, irregular reticulation, subpleural lines, ground-glass opacity, consolidation, and a subpleural distribution (Figs. 4-24 through 4-27) (Table 4-4) [23,76]. Chan et al. compared the HRCT findings in 52 patients who had interstitial fibrosis associated with PSS with those of 55 patients who had IPF [77]. In both groups of patients, the fibrosis had a predominantly subpleural and basal distribution. Increasingly extensive disease on HRCT was associated with a coarser reticular

pattern and increasing upper lung zone involvement. The only differences between the two groups were that patients who had PSS tended to have a finer reticular pattern and less upper lung zone involvement for the same extent of disease than did patients who had IPF [77].

Schurawitzki et al. [76] studied 23 patients who had PSS. HRCT findings in their patients included subpleural lines (74%), septal thickening or parenchymal bands (43%), and honeycombing (43%). Honeycombing had a uniform or peripheral distribution. Parenchymal abnormalities had upper lung to middle lung to lower lung distribution ratios of 1:2.4:3.8, confirming the typical lower lung zone predominance of abnormalities in this disease.

Remy-Jardin et al. [78] reviewed the HRCT, pulmonary function test, and bronchoalveolar lavage (BAL) results of 53 patients who had PSS, emphasizing the frequency of honeycombing and ground-glass opacity in these subjects. Among the 32 patients who had abnormal HRCT findings, 26 (81%) had ground-glass opacities and 19 (59%) had honeycombing. Honeycombing in PSS is usually characterized by the presence of small irregular cysts, often associated with areas of ground-glass opacity. In the study by Remy-Jardin et al., all patients who had honeycombing also showed ground-glass opacity [78]. These abnormalities had a distinct basal, posterior, and peripheral predominance. Small nodules with or without associated honeycombing have also been reported in patients who have PSS and are presumed to represent focal lymphoid hyperplasia (follicular bronchiolitis), a common finding in PSS [78,79]. However, nodules are not a prominent feature of this disease. In patients who have PSS, HRCT findings of ground-glass opacity are often associated with a reduction in diffusing capacity, whereas honeycombing generally indicates a reduction in lung volumes and diffusing capacity [78].

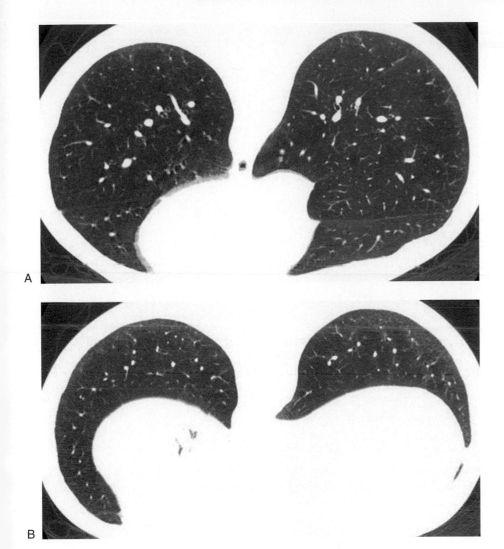

FIG. 4-25. A,B: Subpleural ground-glass opacity in a young patient with scleroderma. A subtle but distinct increase in opacity is visible in the posterior lungs on prone scans.

Other findings on CT in patients who have PSS include diffuse pleural thickening, seen in one-third of cases [78]; asymptomatic esophageal dilatation, present in 40% to 80% of cases (Fig. 4-27) [23,80]; and enlarged mediastinal nodes, seen in approximately 60% of cases [80]. The presence of esophageal dilatation may be helpful in the differential diagnosis of PSS from other diffuse ILDs. The coronal luminal diameter of the esophagus in patients who have PSS, as shown on CT, has been reported to range from 12 to 40 mm (mean, 23 mm), a finding that was not seen in a control group of 13 patients who have a variety of other parenchymal and airway abnormalities [80].

Seely et al. assessed the radiographic and HRCT findings in 11 children (mean age, 11 years) with PSS [81]. ILD was evident on the radiograph in two patients and on HRCT in eight. The HRCT findings consisted of ground-glass opacity, seen in all eight patients; linear opacities, seen in six; honeycombing, seen in five; and small subpleural nodules, seen in seven [81]. There was no correlation between duration of PSS and severity of ILD. Overall the pattern and distribution of abnormalities were similar to those seen in adults. How-

ever, whereas in adults honeycombing predominates in the lower lung zones, in children the honeycombing was most severe in the upper lung zones [81].

Utility of High-Resolution Computed Tomography

Schurawitzki et al. [76] studied 23 patients who had PSS using plain radiographs and HRCT. Chest radiographs were abnormal in only 15 (65%), but HRCT showed evidence of ILD in 21 (91%); the authors concluded that HRCT was clearly superior to chest radiographs for detecting minimal lung disease.

Wells et al. [82] assessed the potential role of HRCT as a predictor of lung histology on open-lung biopsy specimens in patients who had PSS. In this study, CT discriminated correctly between inflammatory and fibrotic histologic appearances in 16 of 20 (80%) biopsy specimens. Predominant ground-glass opacities often correlated with the presence of inflammation; the presence of a predominantly reticular pattern on HRCT correlated closely with the presence of fibrosis on the pathologic specimens [82]. Although Remy-Jardin

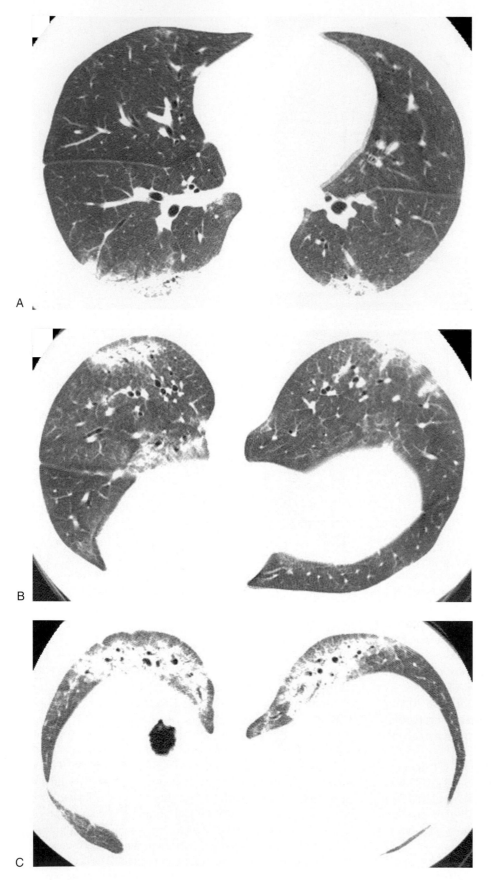

FIG. 4-26. Subpleural ground-glass opacity and consolidation in a patient with scleroderma. Before treatment **(A–C)**, subpleural opacities are the predominant abnormality. Traction bronchiectasis **(C)** seen within areas of opacity in the posterior costophrenic sulcus indicates some evidence of fibrosis. *Continued*

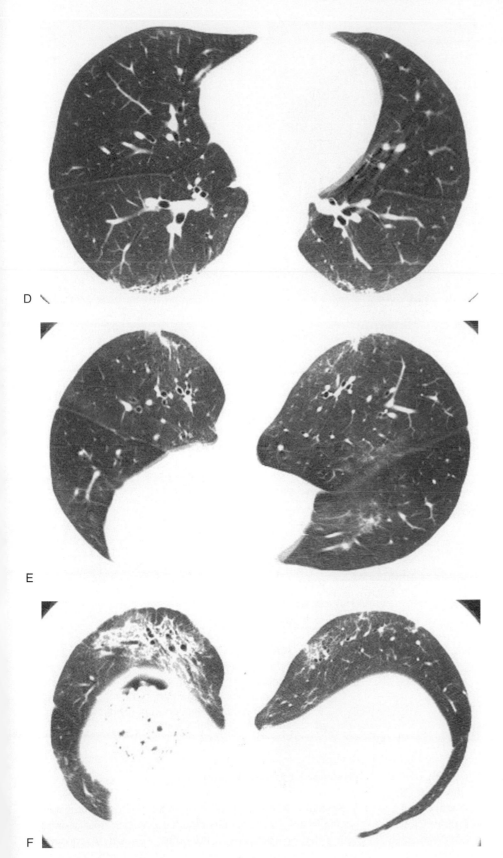

FIG. 4-26. *Continued* After treatment, scans at similar levels **(D–F)** show considerable reduction in opacity. Persistent abnormalities in the posterior lungs and at the lung bases, including irregular reticulation and traction bronchiectasis, likely represent fibrosis.

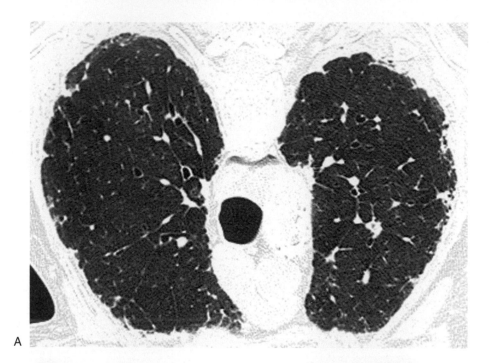

A

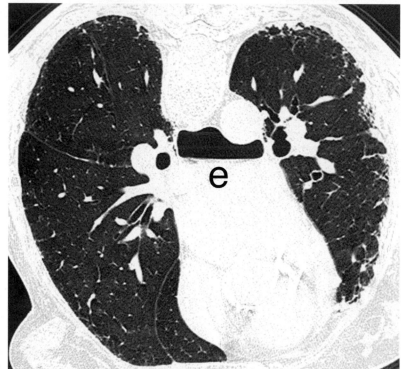

B

FIG. 4-27. A,B: Prone HRCT in a patient with scleroderma with mild interstitial fibrosis and esophageal dilatation. Irregular reticular opacities are visible in the peripheral lung, consistent with fibrosis. The esophagus (e) is dilatated and contains an air-fluid level.

et al. [78] did not find a strong correlation between HRCT findings and the results of BAL in patients who have PSS, BAL is less valid than biopsy as a predictor of activity.

UIP associated with PSS follows a less progressive course and has a better long-term prognosis than UIP associated with IPF [35,82]. Improvement after treatment similar to that seen in patients who have IPF is more frequent in patients who have a prominent ground-glass component than in those with predominant reticular abnormalities (Fig. 4-26) [35].

Systemic Lupus Erythematosus

Systemic lupus erythematosus (SLE) is a multisystem autoimmune disease usually associated with increased circulating serum antinuclear antibodies. Clinical diagnosis is based on the presence of at least four of the following ten features: rash, discoid lupus, photosensitivity, oral ulcers, arthritis, serositis, renal disorders, neurologic disorders, hematologic disorders, and immunologic disorders [83].

TABLE 4-4. *HRCT findings in progressive systemic sclerosis (scleroderma)*

Ground-glass opacity or consolidation[a]

Findings of fibrosis (i.e., honeycombing, traction bronchiectasis and bronchiolectasis, intralobular interstitial thickening, irregular interlobular septal thickening, irregular interfaces)[a]

Peripheral and subpleural predominance of fibrosis or ground-glass opacity[a,b]

Lower lung zone and posterior predominance[a,b]

Pleural thickening or effusion[a,b]

Small centrilobular nodules (follicular bronchiolitis)

Esophageal dilatation[a,b]

[a]Most common finding(s).
[b]Finding(s) most helpful in differential diagnosis.

SLE is commonly associated with pleural and pulmonary abnormalities. Pleuritis or pleural fibrosis is present in up to 85% of cases at autopsy, and pleural effusion is often visible on chest radiographs in patients who have SLE [84]. More than 50% of patients who have SLE have lung disease at some time [59].

The most common pulmonary complications of SLE are pneumonia (usually of bacterial etiology), lupus pneumonitis, and pulmonary hemorrhage [62,85]. BOOP is seen with increased frequency in patients who have SLE [86]. Pulmonary fibrosis is evident on the chest radiograph in approximately 3% of patients who have SLE [62,87], although the incidence of fibrosis is higher [88–90].

High-Resolution Computed Tomography Findings

HRCT findings in patients who have SLE include (i) findings of fibrosis, although they are less common than in patients who have IPF, RA, or scleroderma; (ii) ground-glass opacity; (iii) small nodules; (iv) bronchial wall thickening or bronchiectasis; and (v) pleural thickening or effusion (Table 4-5).

TABLE 4-5. *HRCT findings in systemic lupus erythematosus*

Findings of fibrosis (i.e., intralobular interstitial thickening, irregular interlobular septal thickening, irregular interfaces, bronchiectasis and bronchiolectasis)[a]

Honeycombing (less common than with idiopathic pulmonary fibrosis)

Ground-glass opacity

Peripheral and subpleural predominance of fibrosis or ground-glass opacity[a,b]

Lower lung zone and posterior predominance[a,b]

Bronchiectasis

Pleural thickening or effusion[a,b]

[a]Most common finding(s).
[b]Finding(s) most helpful in differential diagnosis.

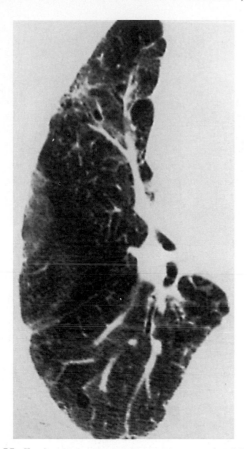

FIG. 4-28. Systemic lupus erythematosus and mild pulmonary fibrosis in a 65-year-old woman. HRCT through the right lung base shows patchy distribution of reticular and ground-glass opacities.

Pulmonary fibrosis resembling IPF is seen on HRCT in 30% to 35% of patients who have SLE (Figs. 4-28 and 4-29) [62,88,89,91]. It may be manifested by such findings as interlobular septal thickening (33%), intralobular interstitial thickening (33%), or architectural distortion (22%) [88]. Honeycombing is uncommon.

Ground-glass opacity, seen in 13% of patients who had SLE studied by Bankier et al. [88], and consolidation, seen in 7%, may be associated with pneumonia, lupus pneumonitis (Fig. 4-30), or pulmonary hemorrhage (Fig. 4-31) [62]. Occasionally similar findings may be due to BOOP, which occurs in some patients who have SLE. As in patients who have other collagen-vascular diseases, hazy or fluffy centrilobular perivascular opacities may be seen, likely related to vasculitis [92].

Findings of airways disease such as bronchial wall thickening and bronchiectasis have been seen in 18% to 20% of patients who have SLE [88,89]. Pleuropericardial abnormalities were seen in 15% to 17% of cases in two studies [89,91].

Utility of High-Resolution Computed Tomography

Several studies have shown that interstitial fibrosis is seen more frequently on HRCT than on chest radiographs

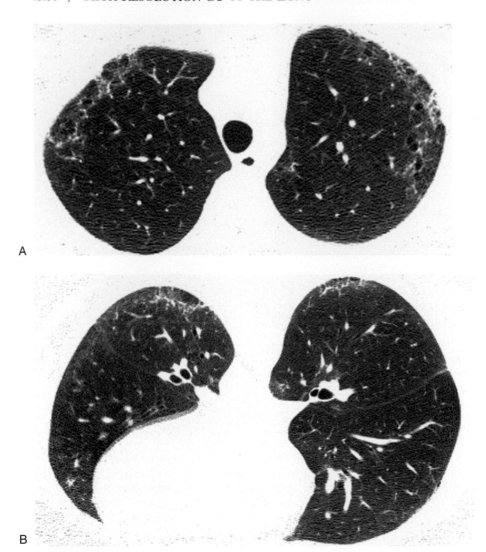

A

B

FIG. 4-29. Supine **(A)** and prone **(B)** HRCT in a 34-year-old woman with systemic lupus erythematosus, interstitial lung disease, and progression of pulmonary function test abnormalities. Reticular opacities in the peripheral lung are consistent with fibrosis. The appearance is indistinguishable from that of idiopathic pulmonary fibrosis, although the abnormalities are more limited in extent.

[88–90]. Bankier et al. [88] performed a prospective study in 48 patients who had SLE and no prior clinical evidence of lung involvement. Three (6%) of patients had evidence of fibrosis on radiographs. Of the 45 patients who had normal chest radiographs, 17 (38%) had abnormalities evident on HRCT. These consisted of interlobular septal thickening in 15 patients (33%), intralobular interstitial thickening in 15 (33%), architectural distortion in ten (22%), small nodules in ten (22%), bronchial wall thickening in nine (20%), bronchial dilatation in eight (18%), areas of ground-glass

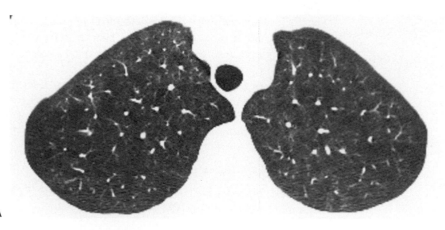

A

FIG. 4-30. HRCT in a 29-year-old woman with systemic lupus erythematosus and shortness of breath. **A:** Patchy ground-glass opacities are visible. *Continued*

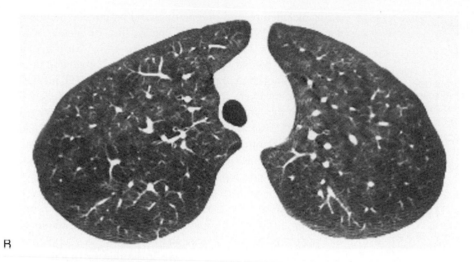

FIG. 4-30. ***Continued*** **B:** Four months later, there has been progression of the abnormalities. Lung biopsy revealed lupus pneumonitis.

opacity in six (13%), and areas of airspace consolidation in three (7%) [88].

Fenlon et al. assessed the radiographic and HRCT findings in 34 patients who had SLE [89]. Abnormalities were identified on chest radiographs in eight (24%) patients and on HRCT in 24 (70%). The most common findings on HRCT were interstitial fibrosis seen in 11 (32%) patients, bronchiectasis in seven (20%), mediastinal or axillary lymphadenopathy in six (18%), and pleuropericardial abnormalities in five (15%) [89]. In another study of 29 patients who had SLE, the chest radiograph was abnormal in ten (34%) and the HRCT in 20 (72%) patients. The most frequently detected

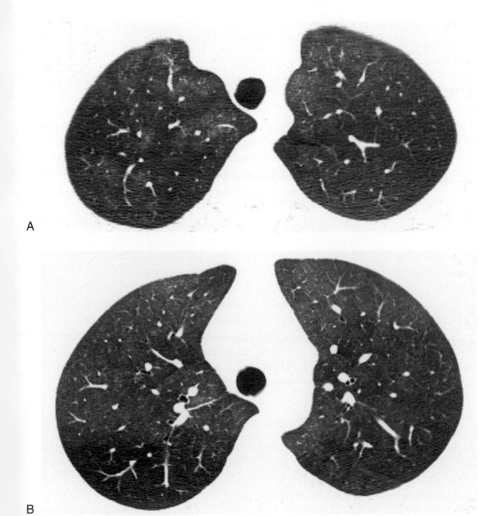

FIG. 4-31. A,B: HRCT in a 19-year-old woman with newly diagnosed systemic lupus erythematosus and pulmonary hemorrhage. Patchy areas of ground-glass opacity, which appear centrilobular and lobular, are visible.

TABLE 4-6. *HRCT findings in polymyositis/dermatomyositis*

Ground-glass opacity[a]

Findings of fibrosis (i.e., traction bronchiectasis and bronchiolectasis, intralobular interstitial thickening, irregular interlobular septal thickening, irregular interfaces)[a]

Honeycombing (less common than with idiopathic pulmonary fibrosis)

Consolidation (secondary to bronchiolitis obliterans organizing pneumonia)[a,b]

Peripheral and subpleural predominance of fibrosis or ground-glass opacity[a,b]

Lower lung zone and posterior predominance[a,b]

[a]Most common finding(s).
[b]Finding(s) most helpful in differential diagnosis.

abnormality on HRCT was ILD, which was seen in 11 (38%) patients. Of 15 patients who had normal clinical examination, normal pulmonary function tests, and normal chest radiographs, four (26%) had HRCT features of ILD [91].

Polymyositis-Dermatomyositis

Polymyositis-dermatomyositis (PM-DM) is a disorder characterized by weakness in the proximal limb muscles. Approximately 50% of patients have a characteristic skin rash, which enables distinction of dermatomyositis from polymyositis. PM-DM is less commonly associated with pulmonary involvement than with other connective tissue diseases. The reported incidence of pulmonary function abnormalities is approximately 30%, whereas approximately 5% of patients show chest radiographic abnormalities [59,93,94]. The pattern of involvement is typically that of UIP or BOOP [95].

High-Resolution Computed Tomography Findings

HRCT findings of PM-DM include (i) ground-glass opacity; (ii) findings of fibrosis, although honeycombing is uncommon; and (iii) consolidation (Table 4-6). Ikezoe et al. [96] reviewed the HRCT findings in 25 patients who had PM-DM; 23 had abnormal HRCT scans. The most common findings seen in these 23 patients included ground-glass opacities (92%), linear opacities (92%), irregular interfaces (88%), airspace consolidation (52%), parenchymal micronodules (28%), and honeycombing (16%). A relatively high prevalence of airspace consolidation (52%) and a low prevalence of honeycombing (16%) were observed. Correlation of HRCT with pathologic findings showed that two patients who had extensive consolidation had diffuse alveolar damage; eight patients who had subpleural bandlike opacities or airspace consolidation, or both, had BOOP, and four patients who had honeycombing had UIP. Mino et al. assessed the HRCT findings before and after treatment with corticosteroids and immunosuppressants in 19 patients who had PM-DM [97]. Findings on the initial HRCT

scans included pleural irregularities and prominent interlobular septa (n = 19), ground-glass opacity (n = 19), patchy consolidation (n = 19), parenchymal bands (n = 15), irregular peribronchovascular thickening (n = 15), and subpleural lines (n = 7). Honeycombing was not detected on any CT images. These findings were more severe in the basal and subpleural regions of the lungs. In 16 of the 17 patients who underwent sequential CT, areas of consolidation, parenchymal bands, and irregular peribronchovascular thickening improved, becoming pleural irregularities and prominent interlobular septa, ground-glass opacity, and subpleural lines on follow-up CT scans [97].

Akira et al. performed sequential HRCT scans in seven patients who had PM-DM, five of whom had histologic confirmation of pulmonary involvement [98]. The predominant finding on the initial CT scans in four patients was subpleural consolidation, which was shown to be due to BOOP. One patient with bilateral patchy areas of ground-glass opacity and consolidation was shown to have diffuse alveolar damage. In most cases, consolidation improved with use of corticosteroid or immunosuppressive therapy, or both; in two patients, however, consolidation evolved into honeycombing. In one patient with subpleural linear opacities, parenchymal abnormalities slowly progressed, and linear opacities had evolved into honeycombing at the patient's 8-year follow-up.

Mixed Connective Tissue Disease

Mixed connective tissue disease (MCTD) is associated with clinical and laboratory findings overlapping those of PSS, SLE, and PM-DM. A prerequisite for diagnosis is the presence of high titers of circulating antibodies against small nuclear ribonucleoprotein [99]. MCTD is commonly associated with radiologic and functional evidence of ILD or pleural effusion, or both; several studies indicate a prevalence of up to 80% [59,93,100]. Pulmonary vasculitis with pulmonary hypertension and pulmonary hemorrhage are also associated with MCTD.

More than two-thirds of patients who have MCTD have abnormal pulmonary function tests, but chest radiographic abnormalities are less frequent, visible in approximately 20% [99,100]. The ILD of MCTD appears identical to that of IPF on histologic examination and radiographs and in the few cases in which HRCT findings have been reported, although there is a tendency for the reticular abnormalities to be less severe than in IPF (Figs. 4-32 through 4-35) [73,100]. Hazy or fluffy centrilobular perivascular opacities may also be seen, likely related to vasculitis [92]. Pleural effusion or pleural thickening is present in fewer than 10% of cases of MCTD [100].

Sjögren's Syndrome

Sjögren's syndrome consists of the clinical triad of keratoconjunctivitis sicca, xerostomia, and recurrent swelling of the parotid gland. Although Sjögren's syndrome can occur in isolation, the majority of patients have coexistent collagenvascular disease, most commonly RA [101]. Pleuropulmonary

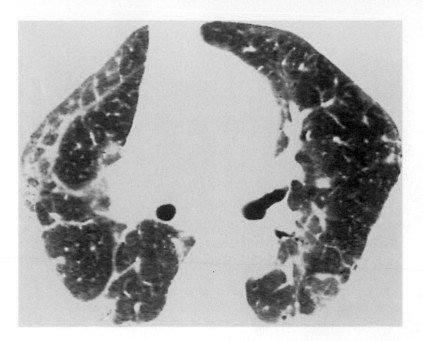

FIG. 4-32. Ground-glass opacity in a 63-year-old woman with mixed connective tissue disease and pulmonary fibrosis. HRCT shows bilateral asymmetric areas of ground-glass opacity and interlobular septal thickening, which have a predominantly subpleural distribution. Areas of ground-glass opacity are characteristic of active disease. The combination of disease activity and mild fibrosis suggests that the patient has early disease.

manifestations are relatively common and include lymphocytic interstitial pneumonia (LIP), UIP, BOOP, follicular bronchiolitis [71], tracheobronchial gland inflammation, and pleuritis with or without effusion [5].

The frequency of reported radiographic abnormalities ranges from 2% to 34% [101]. The most common radiographic finding consists of a reticular or reticulonodular pattern, usually with a basal predominance [5,101]. This pattern may be caused by LIP, interstitial fibrosis, or, occasionally, lymphoma [5,102].

High-Resolution Computed Tomography Findings

Common HRCT findings in Sjögren's syndrome include (i) ground-glass opacity, (ii) findings of fibrosis, (iii) centrilobular nodular opacities, and (iv) lung cysts (Table 4-7). Franquet et al. assessed the HRCT findings in 50 patients who had Sjögren's syndrome for a mean of 12 years (range, 2 to 37 years) after the onset of disease [101]. Abnormalities were detected in 17 patients (34%) on HRCT compared with

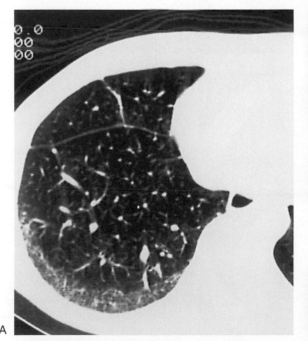

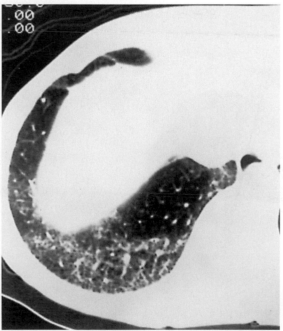

A   B

FIG. 4-33. Mixed connective tissue disease with pulmonary fibrosis. **A,B:** HRCT at two levels shows a fine reticular pattern posteriorly, which reflects septal thickening and intralobular interstitial fibrosis.

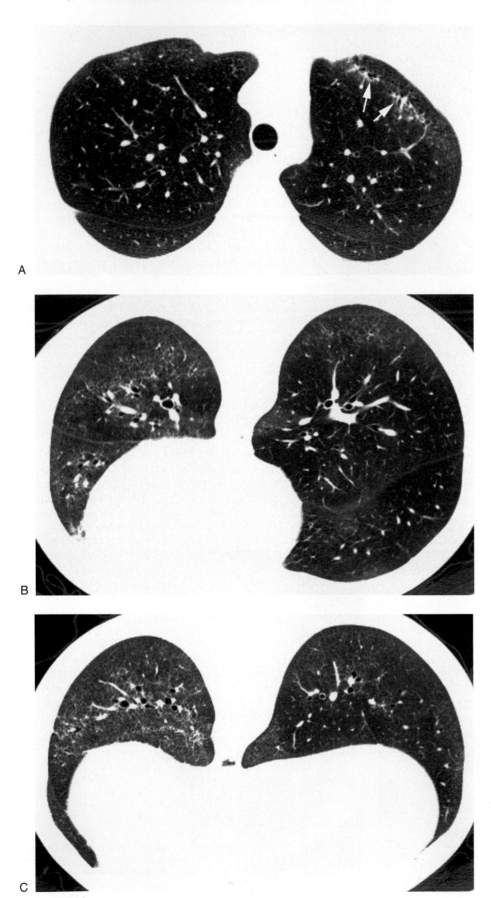

A

B

C

FIG. 4-34. A–C: HRCT in a 26-year-old woman with mixed connective tissue disease, basilar crackles on physical examination, and restrictive disease on pulmonary function tests. Intralobular interstitial thickening results in a very fine reticular pattern in the subpleural lung and lower lobes. Traction bronchiectasis (*arrows*, **A**) is also visible.

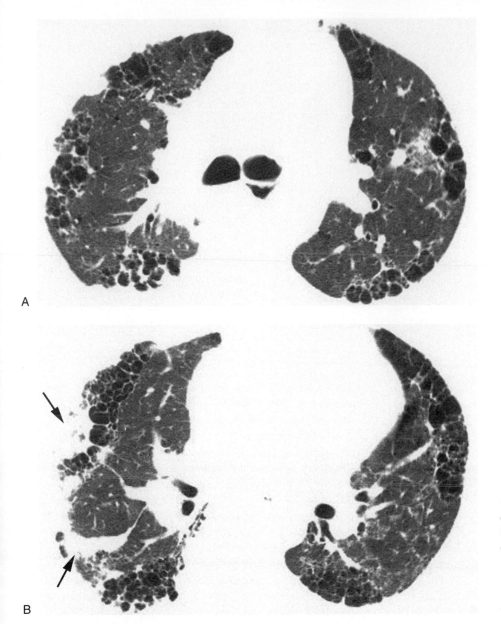

A

B

FIG. 4-35. HRCT in a patient with mixed connective tissue disease, findings of honeycombing, and associated lung carcinoma. **A:** Honeycombing is visible in the peripheral subpleural lung (**A** and **B**). A peripheral adenocarcinoma with infiltration of the pleura (*arrows*, **B**) is also present.

TABLE 4-7. *HRCT findings in Sjögren's syndrome*

Ground-glass opacity

Findings of fibrosis (i.e., traction bronchiectasis or bronchiolectasis, intralobular interstitial thickening, irregular interlobular septal thickening, irregular interfaces)

Honeycombing (less common than in idiopathic pulmonary fibrosis)

Peripheral and subpleural predominance of fibrosis or ground-glass opacity

Lower lung zone and posterior predominance

Small centrilobular nodules (follicular bronchiolitis)

Cysts or small subpleural nodules (lymphocytic interstitial pneumonia)[a,b]

---
[a]Most common finding(s).
[b]Finding(s) most helpful in differential diagnosis.

---

seven (14%) on chest radiographs. The most common findings consisted of bronchiolectasis and poorly defined centrilobular nodular or branching linear opacities (seen in 11 patients), areas of ground-glass opacity (in seven), and honeycombing (in four). The latter was bilateral, asymmetric, and present almost exclusively in the periphery of the lower lobes [101]. A tree-in-bud appearance related to infection or follicular bronchiolitis was visible in three.

Salaffi et al. performed chest radiographs, HRCT scans, and BAL 2 years after documented and treated alveolitis in 18 nonsmoking women with primary Sjögren's syndrome [103]. Five patients had abnormal HRCT scans and only one had an abnormal chest radiograph. The HRCT abnormalities consisted of isolated septal lines in three patients, ground-glass opacities with irregular pleural margins in one patient, and ground-glass opacities associated with septal lines in another.

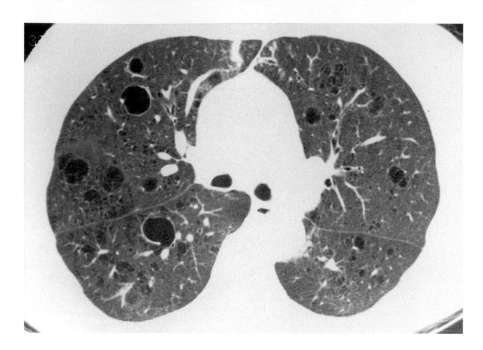

FIG. 4-36. Lymphocytic interstitial pneumonia in Sjögren's syndrome. HRCT scan demonstrates bilateral thin-walled cystic lesions in a random distribution. Also noted are small foci of ground-glass attenuation and a few linear opacities. More extensive areas of ground-glass attenuation were present in the lower lung zones. (Courtesy of Dr. Jim Barrie, University of Alberta Medical Centre, Edmonton, Alberta.)

All of these patients had abnormal BAL results with an increased proportion of neutrophils and lymphocytes [103].

The HRCT manifestations of LIP in Sjögren's syndrome are similar to those seen in LIP associated with other conditions (see Chapter 5) [104,105]. The predominant findings consist of extensive areas of ground-glass opacity and randomly distributed thin-walled cysts (Fig. 4-36) [104,105] The presence of cystic lesions and focal regions of air-trapping on expiratory HRCT have been associated with follicular bronchiolitis in a patient with this disease [106]. Other common findings in LIP include interlobular septal thickening, intralobular linear opacities, areas of consolidation, centrilobular nodules, and subpleural nodules [105]. Amyloidosis occurring in relation to Sjögren's syndrome may appear as multiple nodules, cystic lesions, or a combination of both [107]. Lymphoma in patients who have Sjögren's syndrome may result in diffuse interstitial infiltration or multiple nodules.

Ankylosing Spondylitis

Extensive upper-zonal pulmonary fibrosis may appear in patients who have ankylosing spondylitis, usually 10 years or more after the onset of the disease [59,102]. The precise frequency of pulmonary involvement is not known, and a range of 0% to 30% has been reported. The largest single series indicates a frequency of approximately 1% [108]. Radiologically, the process begins as apical pleural involvement, and then an apical infiltrate develops and progresses to cyst formation. Generally, the disease begins unilaterally and becomes bilateral. The chest radiographic findings may closely mimic those of tuberculosis. Symptoms are usually absent, but the cavities become secondarily infected, most commonly by *Aspergillus fumigatus*, although a variety of other organisms may also be involved.

The histologic lesions consist of nonspecific inflammation and fibrosis. Bronchiolitis obliterans, together with a distal lipid pneumonia, is commonly present.

Limited information is available about the HRCT findings of ankylosing spondylitis [62,109,110]. Fenlon et al. prospectively assessed the chest radiographic and HRCT findings in 26 patients who had ankylosing spondylitis [109]. Abnormalities were evident on the radiograph in four (15%) patients and on HRCT in 18 (69%). The most common findings on HRCT consisted of ILD seen in four patients; bronchiectasis, seen in six; mediastinal lymphadenopathy, seen in three; paraseptal emphysema, seen in three; tracheal dilatation, seen in two; and apical fibrosis, seen in two [109]. Plain chest radiography failed to identify any of the patients who had ILD. Apical fibrosis in ankylosing spondylitis is frequently associated with apical bullae and cavities [62].

DRUG-INDUCED LUNG DISEASE

Many drugs can be associated with lung disease, but the highest incidence of adverse effects occurs with cytotoxic agents [111,112]. Up to 10% of patients receiving cytotoxic chemotherapeutic agents develop an adverse reaction [113]. Drugs can result in a variety of pathologic reactions in the lung parenchyma, including noncardiogenic pulmonary edema, diffuse alveolar damage (DAD), and adult respiratory distress syndrome (ARDS), chronic interstitial pneumonitis with fibrosis, eosinophilic pneumonia, hypersensitivity pneumonitis, BOOP, pulmonary hemorrhage, a lupuslike syndrome, pulmonary vasculitis or arteriopathy, and granulomatous lesions [111,112,114]. Prompt recognition of pulmonary drug complications is important, because early abnormalities may resolve completely when treatment with the drug is discontinued [115,116].

TABLE 4-8. *HRCT findings in drug-induced lung disease associated with chronic pneumonitis and fibrosis*

Findings of fibrosis (i.e., honeycombing, traction bronchiectasis and bronchiolectasis, intralobular interstitial thickening, irregular interlobular septal thickening, irregular interfaces)[a]

Ground-glass opacity; consolidation

Peripheral and subpleural predominance of abnormalities[a]

Lower and posterior lung zone predominance[a]

[a]Most common finding(s).

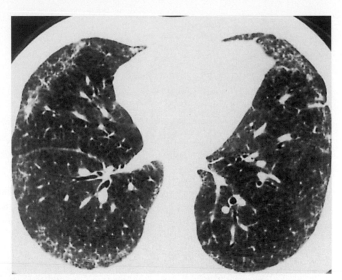

FIG. 4-37. A 61-year-old man with chronic lymphocytic leukemia developed shortness of breath after 5 months of treatment with chlorambucil. HRCT at the level of the inferior pulmonary veins demonstrates bilateral irregular reticular opacities involving predominantly the subpleural lung regions. The findings are similar to those seen in usual interstitial pneumonia.

CT has been shown to be superior to chest radiography in the detection of abnormalities associated with pulmonary drug toxicity. Padley et al. [117] reviewed the chest radiographs and HRCT scans of 23 patients and five normal controls. Two independent observers detected abnormal findings on chest radiographs consistent with drug-induced lung disease in 17 (74%) of the 23 patients, whereas all 23 patients were considered to have abnormal HRCT studies. Bellamy et al. [115] reviewed the chest radiographs and CT scans in 100 patients receiving bleomycin. Pulmonary abnormalities due to bleomycin were detected on 15% of the chest radiographs and 38% of CT scans. These authors also demonstrated significant correlation between the extent of abnormalities on CT and changes in lung volume ($p > .01$).

Five primary patterns of drug-related lung injury have been described. These are (i) chronic pneumonitis and fibrosis, (ii) BOOP, (iii) hypersensitivity lung disease and eosinophilic pneumonia, (iv) noncardiogenic pulmonary edema and DAD with ARDS, and (v) bronchiolitis obliterans [111,112,118]. Each of these five patterns is characteristically associated with a different group of drugs, although many drugs can result in more than one type of lung reaction. HRCT findings associated with these patterns have been reported [117], but it should be pointed out that in most cases, the HRCT appearances of a drug-related lung disease are nonspecific and the diagnosis must be based on a temporal relationship between the administration of a drug and the development of pulmonary abnormalities.

Chronic Pneumonitis and Fibrosis

Both UIP and NSIP have been associated with drug injury. The clinical and radiographic presentations are often identical to those of IPF [119]. A long list of drugs has been implicated in the development of chronic pneumonitis [111,112,116], but this pattern is most commonly the result of cytotoxic chemotherapeutic agents such as bleomycin, busulfan, vincristine, methotrexate, doxorubicin hydrochloride (Adriamycin), and carmustine (BCNU). Nitrofurantoin, amiodarone, gold, and penicillamine are noncytotoxic drugs that can also result in this type of reaction. Plain radiographs in patients who have chronic pneumonitis and fibrosis typically show a mixture of reticulation and consolidation.

In a study by Padley et al. [117], the most common pattern seen on HRCT in patients who have drug-induced lung injury was that of fibrosis, with or without associated consolidation (Table 4-8) [117]. This pattern was visible in 12 of the 23 patients. The fibrosis was characterized by the presence of irregular reticular opacities, honeycombing, architectural distortion, and traction bronchiectasis. Of the 12 examples of this pattern, four were the result of bleomycin, four resulted from nitrofurantoin toxicity, and the remaining cases were caused by amiodarone, busulfan, and gold. HRCT findings of fibrosis were similar to those seen in UIP (Fig. 4-37) [111,112, 115,117,120–122].

HRCT abnormalities (Figs. 4-37 and 4-38) were usually bilateral and symmetric, with predominant lower-lung zone involvement [118]. A peripheral and subpleural distribution of abnormalities was common, particularly in patients who had bleomycin toxicity. In some patients, findings of fibrosis were patchy in distribution and predominantly peribronchovascular; this pattern was most common in patients receiving nitrofurantoin [118]. The extent of abnormalities depends on the severity of lung damage. Mild damage is often limited to the posterior subpleural lung regions of the lower lung zones. In patients who have more severe abnormalities, there is greater involvement of the remaining lung parenchyma [115].

Bronchiolitis Obliterans Organizing Pneumonia

An interstitial pneumonitis that has characteristics of BOOP has been reported with several of the drugs described previously, including methotrexate, gold, penicillamine, nitrofurantoin, amiodarone, bleomycin, and busulfan [123].

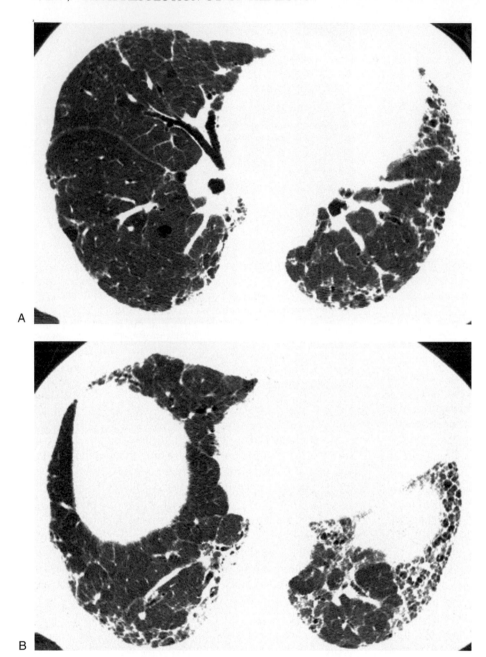

A

B

FIG. 4-38. A,B: HRCT at two levels in a 86-year-old man with chronic myelogenous leukemia treated using methotrexate who now complains of increased shortness of breath. Subpleural reticulation and honeycombing are present, indicative of fibrosis.

Like other causes of BOOP, this reaction is characterized by the presence of consolidation that may have a patchy or nodular distribution or may be predominantly peribronchial or subpleural in location [123].

Hypersensitivity Lung Disease and Eosinophilic Pneumonia

Hypersensitivity lung disease can be attributed to a large number of drugs but is most commonly due to methotrexate, nitrofurantoin, bleomycin, procarbazine, BCNU, cyclophosphamide, nonsteroidal antiinflammatory drugs, and sulfonamides [111,112,117,124]. Cough and dyspnea, with or without fever, can be acute in onset or progress over a period of several months after institution of treatment and is unre-

lated to the cumulative drug dose. A peripheral eosinophilia is present in up to 40% of patients [111,112]. This reaction is characterized on HRCT by the presence of patchy areas of ground-glass opacity, sometimes associated with small areas of consolidation [117]. This pattern is similar to that seen with eosinophilic pneumonia or hypersensitivity pneumonitis, described in detail in Chapter 6. In the study by Padley [117], this pattern was visible in seven of the 23 patients and was due to methotrexate, nitrofurantoin, bleomycin, BCNU, and cyclophosphamide.

Pulmonary Edema or Diffuse Alveolar Damage

Pulmonary edema or DAD with ARDS can be caused by a variety of drugs, most typically cytotoxic agents such as bleomycin, aspirin, and narcotics [111,112]. Although the mechanism of lung injury is unclear, it is likely due to increased capillary permeability. Onset is usually sudden and within a few days of the onset of chemotherapy [111,112,117,118]. The HRCT appearance of pulmonary edema occurring as a result of a drug reaction is partially determined by the presence or absence of DAD. If DAD is present, HRCT typically shows extensive bilateral parenchymal consolidation that may be more marked in the dependent lung regions (see Fig. 6-15) [117]. Other than a temporal relationship to chemotherapy, there are no clinical or HRCT findings that allow this appearance to be distinguished from other causes or ARDS. Pulmonary edema may occur without accompanying DAD in patients who have a drug reaction; a good example is treatment with interleukin-2 [125,126]. In such cases, interlobular septal thickening may be the predominant HRCT finding, with ground-glass opacity or consolidation being less conspicuous. The prognosis of drug-related pulmonary edema is related to the severity of the lung injury. Two patients in the study by Padley et al. [117] developed ARDS as a result of mitomycin-C and busulfan therapy; both of these patients died.

Bronchiolitis Obliterans

The least common lung reaction to drugs is bronchiolitis obliterans, a finding that has been described primarily in association with penicillamine therapy for RA (see Fig. 8-59) [111,112,127]. However, the role of penicillamine is controversial, as bronchiolitis obliterans can be seen in patients who have RA who have not been treated using this drug [67]. Bronchiolitis obliterans has also been seen in patients treated with sulfasalazine [111]. The abnormalities seen on HRCT in these patients consist of bronchial wall thickening and a pattern of mosaic perfusion, similar to that seen with other causes of bronchiolitis obliterans (see Table 8-10) [117,128].

Reactions to Specific Drugs

Drug reactions may occur during treatment with a wide variety of agents [116]. Some of the more common drugs that result in significant pulmonary disease are described below.

Bleomycin

Bleomycin is a cytotoxic drug used in the treatment of lymphomas and some carcinomas [112,116,129]. Bleomycin pulmonary toxicity is the most common pulmonary disease related to chemotherapy [130], with an incidence of approximately 4%. It is most likely with cumulative doses above 450 units [112]. Associated risk factors for development of lung disease include recent radiation, oxygen therapy, or old age [116]. A wide variety of reactions to bleomycin have been reported including DAD

with respiratory failure, chronic pneumonitis with fibrosis, BOOP, and hypersensitivity lung disease. Reported CT and HRCT appearances have varied accordingly, including reticulation, consolidation, and ground-glass opacity with predominant subpleural and lower lobe predominance when mild [115,117,121]. When severe or extensive, more diffuse involvement of the lower, middle, and upper lungs is typically visible. A unique manifestation of bleomycin-related lung toxicity is the presence of multiple pulmonary nodules that mimic the appearance of metastases and have histologic characteristics of BOOP [131–133]. Resolution of some abnormalities after cessation of treatment may occur [115].

Busulfan

Busulfan is an alkylating agent used in treating chronic myeloproliferative diseases, and clinically recognized lung toxicity occurs in approximately 5% of cases [113]. Its use may result in findings of chronic pneumonitis and fibrosis, BOOP, or DAD. HRCT findings include patchy or diffuse consolidation or reticulation.

Cyclophosphamide

Cyclophosphamide is an alkylating agent used in the treatment of a variety of malignancies and autoimmune diseases; it is commonly used in combination with other therapeutic agents [113]. Histologic findings associated with lung injury are similar to those seen in patients who have bleomycin toxicity and include chronic pneumonitis and fibrosis, BOOP, DAD, pulmonary edema, and hypersensitivity reactions. HRCT appearances vary accordingly [117].

Methotrexate

Methotrexate is a folate antagonist used in the treatment of malignancies and inflammatory diseases [116]. Pulmonary toxicity occurs in 5% to 10% of cases and is unrelated to toxicity and duration of treatment or cumulative dose. In contrast to many other cytotoxic agents, methotrexate often results in reversible abnormalities. In most cases, the histologic appearance resembles hypersensitivity pneumonitis or less often BOOP or DAD; peripheral eosinophilia may be present. HRCT has shown ground-glass opacities as the predominant abnormality [117].

Amiodarone

Although the majority of drug reactions have a somewhat nonspecific appearance on CT, amiodarone-related lung toxicity often can be readily recognized by the presence of lung attenuation greater than that of soft tissue due to the tissue accumulation of this iodinated compound [117,120] (see Fig. 3-108; Figs. 4-39 and 4-40). Amiodarone is used in the treatment of refractory cardiac tach-

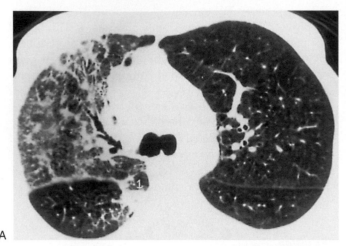
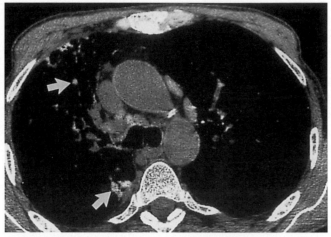

FIG. 4-39. A 61-year-old man with amiodarone lung. **A:** HRCT at the level of the tracheal carina demonstrates irregular linear opacities in the right upper lobe with associated traction bronchiectasis and architectural distortion as well as areas of ground-glass opacity. A localized area of consolidation is present in the right lower lobe. **B:** Corresponding soft-tissue windows demonstrate increased attenuation of the lung parenchyma (*arrows*). The attenuation of the area of consolidation in the right lower lobe measured 135 HU compared to 23 HU for the soft tissues of the chest wall. Also note increased attenuation of the mediastinal lymph nodes.

yarrhythmias. It accumulates in the liver and lung, where it becomes entrapped in macrophage lysosomes. Patients who have amiodarone pulmonary toxicity almost always show increased liver attenuation on CT, although this finding is also present in patients treated with amiodarone in the absence of drug toxicity [117,120,122] (Fig. 4-40). The patterns of pulmonary reaction to amiodarone include focal or diffuse areas of consolidation, reticular opacities and, less commonly, conglomerate masses (see Fig. 3-108; Figs. 4-39 through 4-41) [117,120,122].

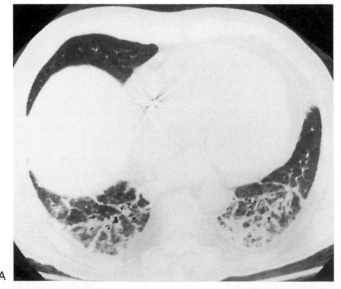
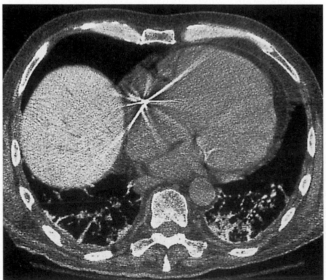

FIG. 4-40. A 68-year-old man with amiodarone lung. **A:** HRCT through the lung bases demonstrates a reticular pattern with associated traction bronchiectasis and ground-glass opacity. **B:** Corresponding mediastinal windows demonstrate increased attenuation of the lung parenchyma and of the liver. Also note cardiomegaly and presence of a pacemaker.

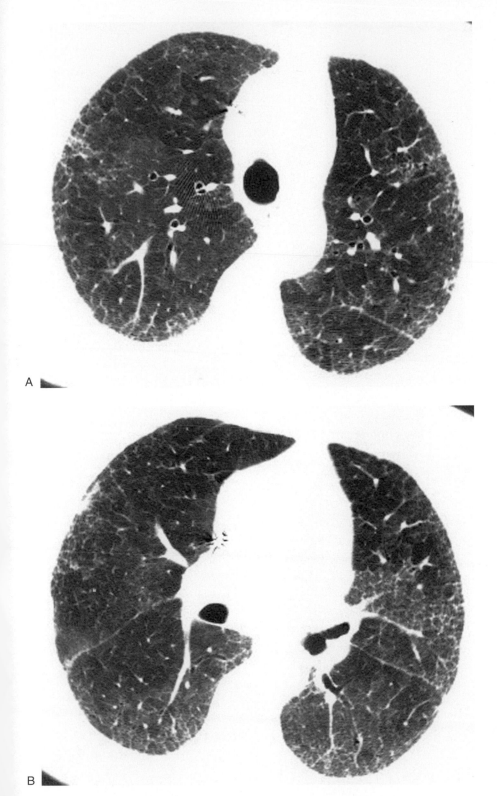

FIG. 4-41. HRCT in a patient with amiodarone lung toxicity and progressive fibrosis. Initial HRCT at three levels **(A–C)** shows peripheral reticulation characterized by intralobular interstitial thickening and ground-glass opacity **(C)**. Six months later **(D–F)**, there has been progression of abnormalities with increase in reticulation at the lung bases **(F)**. *Continued*

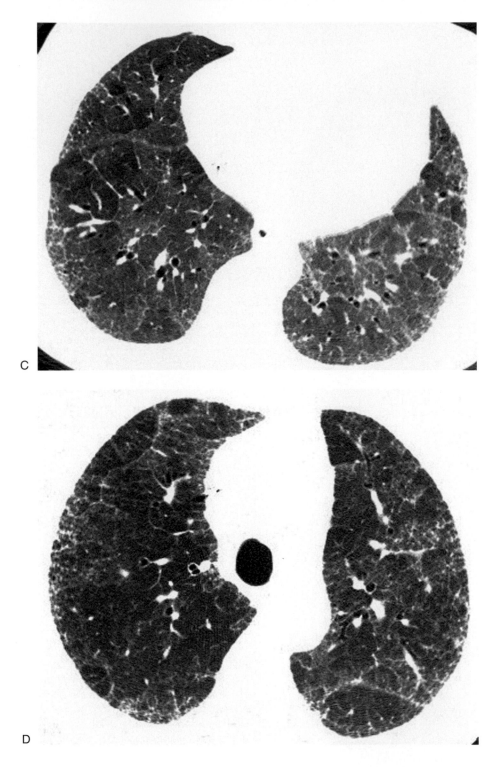

C

D

FIG. 4-41. *Continued*

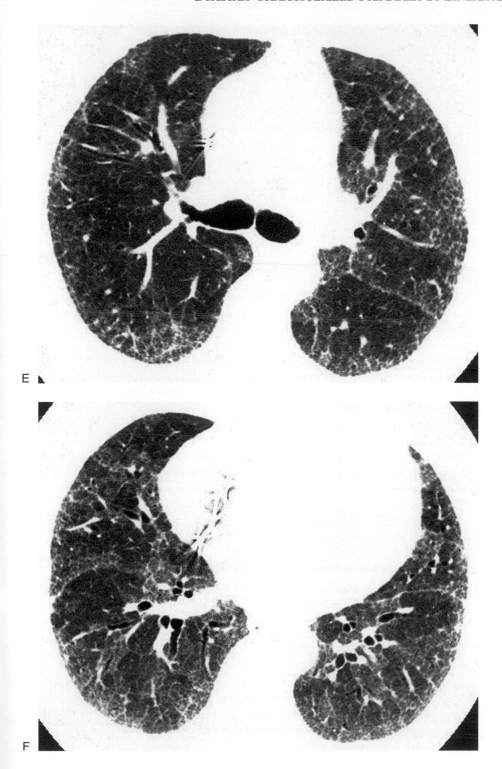

E

F

FIG. 4-41. *Continued*

RADIATION PNEUMONITIS AND FIBROSIS

After external beam radiotherapy of the thorax, approximately 40% of patients develop radiographic abnormalities and 7% develop symptomatic radiation pneumonitis [134–136]. The development and appearance of radiation lung injury depend on a number of factors, including (i) volume of lung irradiated, (ii) shape of the radiation fields, (iii) radiation dose, (iv) number of fractions of radiation given, (v) time period over which the radiation is delivered, (vi) prior irradiation, (vii) whether chemotherapy is also used, (viii) corticosteroid therapy withdrawal, (ix) preexisting lung disease, (x) type of radiation used, and (xi) individual susceptibility [134,136–138]. Generally, radiation is best tolerated by the patient if given in smaller doses, over a long period of time, and to a single lung or a small lung region. For unilateral radiation with fractionated doses, radiographic findings of radiation pneumonitis are seldom detected with doses below 3,000 cGy, are variably present with doses between 3,000 and 4,000 cGy, and are nearly always visible at doses of 4,000 cGy [138]. Radiographic findings of radiation pneumonitis are usually unassociated with symptoms, although low-grade fever, cough, and dyspnea may be present in some patients.

Pulmonary abnormalities related to radiation injury have been divided into early and late manifestations [135]. The early stage of radiation lung injury, referred to as *radiation pneumonitis*, occurs 1 to 3 months after radiation therapy is completed and is most severe 3 to 4 months after treatment [135,137–139]. Radiation pneumonitis is not generally apparent after doses of less than 20 Gy; its likelihood is increased by a second course of radiation, the withdrawal of corticosteroid treatment, and the use of concomitant chemotherapy. Radiation pneumonitis is associated with histologic findings of DAD, intraalveolar proteinaceous exudates, and hyaline membranes. Depending on the severity of lung injury, these abnormalities may resolve completely, but they more often undergo progressive organization and eventually lead to fibrosis [137].

The late stage of radiation-induced lung injury, termed *radiation fibrosis,* develops gradually in patients who have radiation pneumonitis when complete resolution does not occur [137]. Radiation fibrosis evolves in the previously irradiated field, 6 to 12 months after radiation therapy, and usually becomes stable within 2 years of treatment [134,140]. Histologically, dense fibrosis with obliteration of lung architecture and bronchiectasis are present. Patients can present with radiation fibrosis without a history of acute pneumonitis [134].

Computed Tomography and High-Resolution Computed Tomography Findings

The hallmark of radiation pneumonitis on CT is the presence of increased lung attenuation corresponding closely to the location of the radiation ports (Table 4-9) [135]. On CT, radiation pneumonitis can be associated with three patterns. These are (i) homogeneous ground-glass opacity that uniformly involves the irradiated portions of lung (Fig. 4-42),

TABLE 4-9. *HRCT findings in radiation pneumonitis*

Early (radiation pneumonitis)
Patchy or dense consolidation[a]
Ground-glass opacity[a]
Abnormalities largely limited to radiation port[a,b]
Late (radiation fibrosis)
Streaky opacities[a]
Dense consolidation with volume loss[a]
Traction bronchiectasis in abnormal regions[a]
Abnormalities largely limited to radiation port[a,b]

[a]Most common finding(s).
[b]Finding(s) most helpful in differential diagnosis.

(ii) patchy consolidation that is contained within the irradiated lung but does not conform to the shape of the radiation ports, and (iii) discrete consolidation that conforms to the shape of the radiation ports but does not uniformly involve the irradiated lung parenchyma [141,142].

The first two patterns likely represent the presence of diffuse or patchy radiation pneumonitis, whereas the third pattern is thought to indicate the presence of progressive organization and early fibrosis [137,138,141]. Abnormalities are typically nonanatomic and do not tend to respect normal lung boundaries, such as interlobar fissures or lung segments (Fig. 4-42). Volume loss or pleural thickening can be seen in some cases [143]; this is due to obstruction of bronchioles by inflammatory exudate, loss of surfactant, or both [135]. On CT, these abnormalities can be seen as early as 4 weeks after treatment [138,141]. Large airways are patent, and air bronchograms are commonly visible [135].

Although findings of radiation pneumonitis are characteristically confined to areas of irradiated lung, relatively mild abnormalities may be detected outside of the radiation portal in as many as 20% of cases, perhaps related to a hypersensitivity reaction (Fig. 4-42) [135,142,143]. In a prospective study of CT findings in 54 irradiated patients, Mah et al. [143] demonstrated that two patients had minor extension of radiation injury beyond the boundaries of the radiation field. Ikezoe et al. [142] demonstrated CT findings of radiation pneumonitis beyond the radiation portals in four of 17 patients. The abnormalities seen in these four patients consisted of subtle areas of ground-glass opacity or patchy or homogeneous consolidation. The severity of the abnormalities seen outside the radiation ports in these patients was less severe than that seen within the radiation ports [142]. Rarely, areas of consolidation initially limited to the radiation field may migrate within both lungs [144,145]. This pattern has been shown to be due to BOOP triggered by lung irradiation [144,145].

Progression of CT abnormalities more than 9 months after treatment likely indicates fibrosis [137]. The development of radiation fibrosis can be recognized on CT by the appearance of streaky opacities, progressive volume loss, progressive

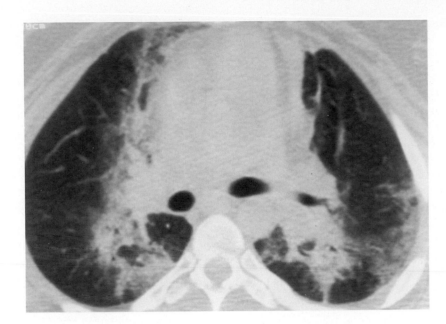

FIG. 4-42. Radiation pneumonitis in a patient who had mediastinal and hilar radiation. Bilateral ill-defined regions of consolidation and ground-glass opacity correspond closely to the radiation ports, although increased opacity is also visible in the peripheral nonirradiated lung. (Courtesy of Joseph Cherian, M.D., Al-Sabah Hospital, Kuwait.)

dense consolidation, traction bronchiectasis, or pleural thickening within the irradiated lung [135,137] (Fig. 4-43). Fibrosis and volume loss typically result in a sharper demarcation between normal and irradiated lung regions than is seen in patients who have radiation pneumonitis. This gives the abnormal lung regions a characteristically straight and sharply defined edge [137] (Table 4-9) (Fig. 4-44). The adjacent lung is frequently hyperinflated and may show extensive bullous changes [135]. Libshitz [138,141] has reported that patients who have radiation fibrosis generally show dense consolidation, conforming to and totally involving the irradiated portions of lung and containing ectatic air bronchograms. However, linear opacities at the margins of the radiation port,

reticular opacities similar to those seen in patients who have UIP, or discrete consolidation that conforms to the shape of the radiation portals but does not uniformly involve the irradiated lung can be seen in some patients.

Pleural effusions are uncommon as a result of radiation, but they may occur. Development within 6 months of treatment in conjunction with radiation pneumonitis and spontaneous resolution is suggestive [135]. On the other hand, rapid accumulation suggests malignant effusion. Pleural thickening is common as a manifestation of radiation.

Mediastinal lymph node calcification, particularly after radiation of lymphomas, and the development of thymic cysts, pericarditis, and cardiomyopathy may also be seen [135].

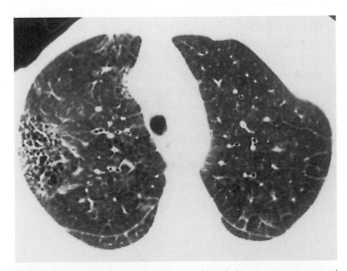

FIG. 4-43. A 78-year-old woman after right mastectomy and tangential beam radiation for breast carcinoma. HRCT 2 years later demonstrates marked fibrosis with honeycombing and traction bronchiectasis involving predominantly the axillary region of the right lung.

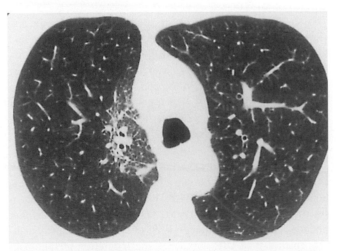

FIG. 4-44. A 67-year-old man after undergoing radiation therapy for carcinoma of the lung. HRCT scan performed 1 year later demonstrates reticular pattern and ground-glass opacity in the medial aspect of the right upper lobe. Note traction bronchiectasis due to fibrosis and sharp demarcation between normal and irradiated lung.

Utility of Computed Tomography and High-Resolution Computed Tomography

CT is more sensitive than radiographs in the detection and assessment of radiation-induced lung injury [135,142,146], and HRCT is superior to conventional CT [142,147]. Ikezoe et al. [142] performed serial CT scans in 17 patients and detected abnormalities on CT in 15 cases, most of which were present within 4 weeks of radiation therapy. In three of their patients, abnormalities were detected on CT but not on chest radiographs. In three other patients, radiation pneumonitis was detected earlier on CT than on the radiographs. Similarly, Bell et al. [146] demonstrated that CT allowed detection of radiation pneumonitis in patients who had normal chest radiographs. CT can also be extremely helpful in detecting tumor recurrence within the irradiated field [138]. Evidence of a mass or increased opacity developing within the irradiated field, particularly if it does not contain air-bronchograms, should suggest tumor recurrence [135,138,148].

ASBESTOSIS AND ASBESTOS-RELATED DISEASE

Asbestos exposure in the workplace, and to a lesser degree in the general population, is a major public health concern in the United States. Inhalation of asbestos fibers has been known to cause pulmonary and pleural fibrosis for more than 80 years. Asbestos-related abnormalities include asbestosis, asbestos-related rounded atelectasis, and asbestos-related pleural disease.

Asbestosis

The lung disease associated with asbestos fiber inhalation is known as *asbestosis* [149,150]. Asbestosis is defined in pathologic terms, quite simply, as interstitial pulmonary fibrosis associated with the presence of intrapulmonary asbestos bodies or asbestos fibers [151,152].

After inhalation, asbestos fibers are first deposited in the respiratory bronchioles and alveolar ducts, but with longer and more extensive exposure they also accumulate in a subpleural location [151–154]. In patients who have asbestosis, the earliest changes of fibrosis occur in the peribronchiolar region of the lobular core [153–155]. As the fibrosis progresses, it involves the alveolar walls throughout the lobule and, eventually, the interlobular septa. Honeycombing can be seen in advanced cases. Visceral pleural thickening often overlies areas of parenchymal fibrosis. In asbestosis, abnormalities are usually most severe in the lower and posterior lungs and in a subpleural location [154]. Yamamoto et al. [156] have classified the lung fibrosis of asbestosis as two types: honeycombing predominant fibrosis, seen in approximately 40% of cases and indistinguishable from that of UIP, and atelectatic induration predominant fibrosis, seen in the remainder and unlike that seen in UIP.

It is uncommon, in clinical practice, to obtain histologic proof of asbestosis; this diagnosis is usually presumptive and based on indirect evidence [151,157–159]. The expression "clinical diagnosis of asbestosis" has been adopted by the

---

TABLE 4-10. *Criteria for a clinical diagnosis of asbestosis*

Reliable history of exposure to asbestos

Appropriate time interval between exposure and detection

Chest radiographic evidence of International Labor Organization type s, t, or u (small irregular) opacities with a profusion (severity) of 1/1 or greater

Restrictive lung impairment with a forced vital capacity below the lower limit of normal

Diffusing capacity below the lower limit of normal

Bilateral late or paninspiratory crackles at the posterior lung base, not cleared by coughing

Modified from Schwartz A, Rockoff SD, et al. A clinical diagnostic model for the assessment of asbestosis: a new algorithmic approach. *J Thorac Imag* 1988;3:29; McLoud TC. The use of CT in the examination of asbestos-exposed persons [Editorial]. *Radiology* 1988;169:862; and American Thoracic Society. The diagnosis of nonmalignant diseases related to asbestos. *Am Rev Respir Dis* 1986;134:363.

American Thoracic Society to refer to a diagnosis based on a combination of chest radiographic abnormalities, restrictive abnormalities on pulmonary function tests, appropriate physical findings, and known exposure to asbestos (Table 4-10) [158–160]. Although none of these clinical or radiographic criteria is specific, the presence of multiple abnormal findings in an individual with significant asbestos exposure is taken as presumptive evidence of asbestosis. A diagnosis of asbestosis is difficult to make and is probably inappropriate when only a few physical or functional abnormalities are present. Limitations in the accuracy of these criteria have been pointed out, and interstitial fibrosis in asbestos-exposed patients does not always reflect asbestosis; in one study, 5% of patients who had biopsy-proven ILD and asbestos exposure had a disease other than asbestosis on lung biopsy [161].

Symptoms and physical findings are present in only a small minority of patients who have asbestosis, unless the disease is relatively advanced [149,151,158]. Similarly, reductions in lung volumes and diffusing capacity, which are typical of restrictive lung disease, are insensitive for detecting early or mild degrees of dysfunction in patients who have asbestosis. The chest radiograph is often relied on to help in diagnosis, but it is quite limited in its ability to detect early disease. Clinical symptoms and radiographic findings of asbestosis are not usually detected until 10 years after exposure, and this latent period is sometimes as long as 40 years [151,158,160]. Gallium scintigraphy can be of value in patients who have early disease [155,162].

Plain Radiographs in Diagnosing Asbestosis

The International Labor Organization (ILO) classification of pneumoconiosis radiographs provides a method for objectively recording and quantitating the parenchymal and pleural abnormalities seen in patients who have asbestos-related diseases [158,159,163,164]. Although certain ILO abnor-

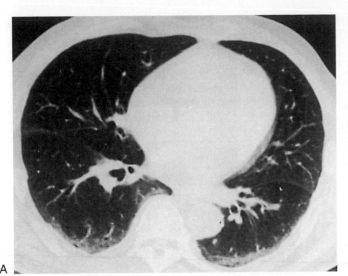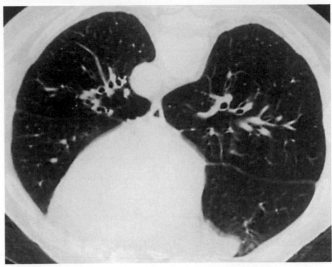

A

B

FIG. 4-45. Dependent lung opacity (atelectasis) in a patient with asbestos exposure. **A:** In the supine position, ill-defined areas of increased opacity are visible posteriorly. Irregularity of the costal pleural surfaces reflects pleural thickening and plaques. **B:** In the prone position, the lungs are normal in appearance. There is no evidence of septal thickening or fibrosis. The pleural irregularity, particularly within the posterior lung, remains visible.

malities (Table 4-10) are often assumed to be diagnostic of asbestosis in patients who have been exposed to asbestos, numerous authors have stressed the limitations of chest radiographs in detecting or making a confident diagnosis of this disease [151,158,159,163–167].

Chest radiographs are relatively insensitive in detecting the presence of asbestosis. In a study performed by Epler and associates [168] of 58 patients who had asbestosis diagnosed on lung biopsy, six (10%) had normal chest radiographs according to ILO standards. Kipen and coworkers [166] found that 25 (18%) of 138 asbestos-exposed patients who had histologic proof of pulmonary fibrosis had no radiographic findings of this disease. Furthermore, 80% of the cases that were graded as less than 1/0 according to ILO standards had moderate or severe histologic grades of fibrosis.

It is also clear that the ILO classification of radiographs lacks specificity for diagnosing asbestosis [163,164]; there are no plain radiographic findings that are pathognomonic of this disease. Epstein and associates [169] found that 36 (18%) of 200 screening chest radiographs showed small opacities that were consistent with pneumoconiosis using the ILO classification system; of these, 22 (61%) had no known occupational exposure to asbestos. In other studies, it has been suggested that cigarette smoking results in radiographic abnormalities indistinguishable from those produced by asbestosis, but this is controversial [159,163,170].

High-Resolution Computed Tomography Techniques in Asbestos-Exposed Subjects

In patients who have asbestos exposure, it has been recommended that scans should be obtained both supine and prone

at each level [151,157,171] or in the prone position only [150,172]. It is particularly important to scan asbestos-exposed individuals in the prone position, because the posterior lung is typically involved earlier and to a greater degree than the anterior lung [150]. Unless prone scans are obtained, it may be impossible to distinguish normal dependent atelectasis from fibrosis in the posterior lung (Fig. 4-45).

In evaluating patients who have asbestos exposure, several authors have indicated that a limited number of scans should be sufficient for the diagnosis of lung disease [150,151, 157,167,171,172]. Because of the typical basal distribution of asbestosis, obtaining four or five scans near the lung bases, with the most cephalad scan obtained at the level of the carina, should be sufficient for detection of an abnormality. Indeed, this approach has proven to have good sensitivity in patients who have suspected asbestosis and would be appropriate for screening groups of asbestos-exposed individuals [173]. In an individual patient with asbestos exposure and suspected lung disease, however, the most appropriate protocol is to obtain HRCT at 2-cm intervals, both prone and supine. This technique allows a more complete assessment of abnormal findings, including lung masses, emphysema, and pleural abnormalities [150]; allows a more accurate diagnosis of the type of lung disease present; and is more accurate in distinguishing fibrotic lung disease from emphysema, which can have similar symptoms.

High-Resolution Computed Tomography Findings of Asbestosis

On HRCT, asbestosis can result in a variety of findings, depending on the severity of the disease [150,151,153,157,159,

TABLE 4-11. *HRCT findings in asbestosis*

Findings of fibrosis (i.e., traction bronchiectasis or bronchiolectasis, intralobular interstitial thickening, irregular interlobular septal thickening, irregular interfaces)[a]

Honeycombing in advanced disease

Subpleural dotlike opacities in early disease (peribronchiolar fibrosis)[a]

Subpleural lines[a]

Parietal pleural thickening or plaques[a,b]

Parenchymal bands particularly in association with pleural thickening[a,b]

Earliest abnormalities posterior and basal

Ground-glass opacity

[a]Most common finding(s).
[b]Finding(s) most helpful in differential diagnosis.

167,171,174,175]. In general, HRCT findings reflect the presence of interstitial fibrosis and are similar to those seen in patients who have IPF. Although none of these findings is specific for asbestosis, the presence of parietal pleural thickening in association with lung fibrosis is highly suggestive (Table 4-11).

The earliest abnormal findings recognizable on HRCT in patients who have asbestosis reflect the presence of centrilobular, peribronchiolar fibrosis (Table 4-11) [153,175]. In one study [153], dotlike opacities were visible in the subpleural lung in patients who had early asbestosis, forming clusters and subpleural curvilinear opacities when confluent; these correlated with the presence of peribronchiolar fibrosis extending

to involve the contiguous airspaces and alveolar interstitium (Fig. 4-46). In a subsequent study [175], subpleural nodular opacities or "dots" were visible in 21 of 23 patients who had early asbestosis, reflecting peribronchiolar fibrosis. These nodules are typically visible several millimeters from the pleural surface (Figs. 4-46 and 4-47). The presence of peribronchiolar fibrosis can also result in an abnormal prominence of the centrilobular arteries, giving rise to an increased reticulation in the peripheral lung [153,157].

As pulmonary fibrosis extends from the peribronchiolar regions to involve the remainder of the pulmonary lobule, other findings of fibrosis can be recognized. Thickening of interlobular septa, intralobular interstitial thickening, traction bronchiectasis, architectural distortion, and findings of honeycombing can all be seen in patients who have asbestosis, depending on the severity of their disease (Figs. 4-48 through 4-51) [151,153,157,167]. Interlobular septal thickening is common in early disease (Fig. 4-52) [151,171,176] but is less frequent in patients who have severe disease because of superimposed honeycombing [54]. Honeycombing typically predominates in the peripheral and posterior lung and is common in advanced asbestosis. In a study of patients who had end-stage lung disease [54], subpleural honeycombing was present in 100% of patients who had asbestosis. This appearance, however, is seen in a minority of patients who have asbestosis.

Parenchymal bands are common in patients who have asbestosis (Figs. 4-52 through 4-54) [151,153,157,172,176], and may reflect thickening of interlobular septa, fibrosis along the bronchovascular sheaths [153], coarse scars, or areas of atelectasis adjacent to pleural plaques or areas of visceral pleural thickening [177] (Figs. 4-52 through 4-54). Often in

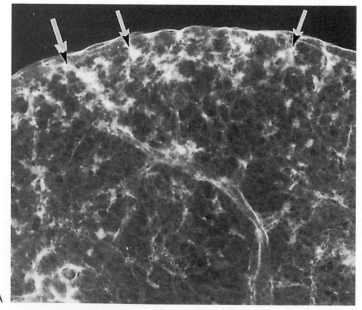
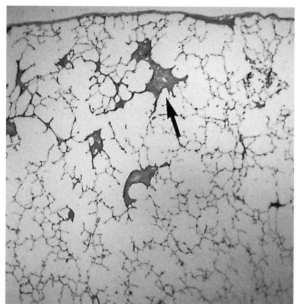

A   B

FIG. 4-46. Subpleural dotlike opacities in asbestosis. Radiograph **(A)** and histologic section **(B)** of an inflation-fixed lung obtained from a patient with early asbestosis. Small nodular opacities (*arrows*) are visible in the subpleural lung regions, representing peribronchiolar fibrosis. (From Akira M, Yokoyama K, et al. Early asbestosis: evaluation with high-resolution CT. *Radiology* 1991;178:409, with permission.)

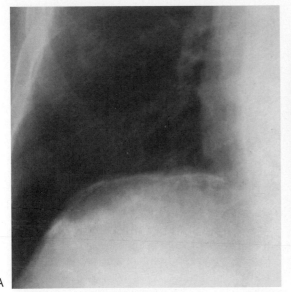

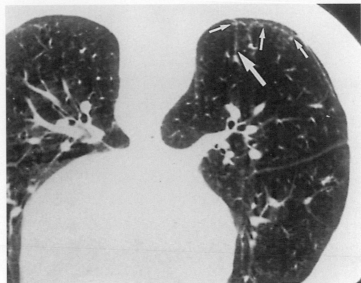

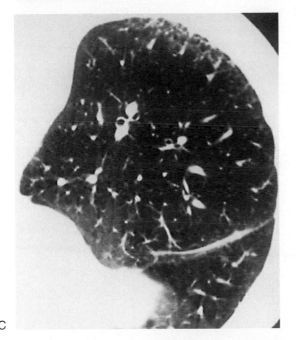

FIG. 4-47. Early fibrosis in asbestosis with dotlike opacities and a subpleural line. **A:** Plain radiograph shows calcified pleural plaques but no evidence of pulmonary fibrosis. **B:** Prone HRCT shows an irregular subpleural line in the posterior right lung (*small arrows*) and a parenchymal band (*long arrow*). The posterior left lung is only minimally abnormal. **C:** A targeted image of the posterior right lung shows a number of small dotlike opacities in the peripheral lung. These are quite similar to the subpleural opacities, reported by Akira et al. (175), and reflect the presence of peribronchiolar fibrosis.

patients who have asbestos-related disease, parenchymal bands are associated with areas of thickened pleura and have a basal predominance [151,178]. In one study, they were found to be unilateral in 69% of cases [177], and several bands occurring in the same location may give the appearance of crow's feet. Gevenois et al. [177] consider parenchymal bands to be related to visceral pleural fibrosis and to be distinct from findings of pulmonary fibrosis—namely septal lines, intralobular lines, and honeycombing. Parenchymal bands can be seen in a number of fibrotic diseases but are particularly common in patients who have asbestosis. In one study, multiple parenchymal bands were seen in 66% of asbestos-exposed patients, whereas parenchymal bands were much less frequent in a control group of patients who did not have asbestos exposure [151]. In another study, it was found that parenchymal bands

were present in 79% of patients who had asbestosis, as compared to only 11% of patients who had IPF [55]. In a study of patients who had histologically proven asbestosis [176], parenchymal bands were visible on HRCT in 76%.

Subpleural lines can reflect early fibrosis occurring in patients who have asbestosis (Fig. 4-47) [153,179]; this finding has been associated with the presence of peribronchiolar fibrosis and associated lung fibrosis, resulting in collapse and flattening of alveoli [153]. In patients who have more severe fibrosis, a subpleural line can reflect honeycombing (Fig. 4-51) [179]. Subpleural lines can also reflect atelectasis; in asbestos-exposed individuals, subpleural lines representing atelectasis have a propensity to occur adjacent to plaques [172].

Ground-glass opacity is uncommon in patients who have asbestosis [55], but when present, it correlates with the pres-

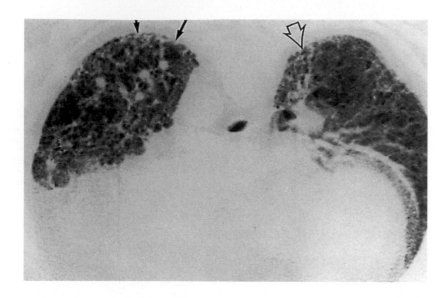

FIG. 4-48. Fibrosis in asbestosis. On a prone scan, an irregular subpleural line is present on the left (*arrows*). Subpleural dotlike opacities are visible bilaterally. Irregular septal thickening is also seen. Some subpleural lucencies (*open arrow*) may represent traction bronchiolectasis.

ence of mild alveolar wall and interlobular septal fibrosis or edema [153]. This finding is much more frequent in association with IPF or other causes of interstitial pneumonia than it is in patients who have asbestosis [55].

Scoring systems for use with HRCT analogous to the ILO system have been proposed by Al-Jarad et al. and Kraus et al., one of which involves the use of 28 additional symbols [180–182]. In a study by Al-Jarad et al. [180], the HRCT scoring system was found to have better interobserver repeatability than the ILO system, although both HRCT and the ILO system scores correlated to a similar degree with impairment of lung function. Krause et al. [181,182] have found their system practical and reproducible. Gamsu et al. [176] assessed the relative accuracy of a subjective semi-quantitative scoring system for HRCT and a relatively simple method of scoring based on the cumulative number of HRCT findings present in patients who have proven asbestosis; similar results were found for both scoring systems.

It should be kept in mind that patients who have asbestosis usually show a number of HRCT findings indicative of lung fibrosis, and the abnormalities are usually bilateral and often somewhat symmetric [177]. The presence of focal or unilateral HRCT abnormalities should not be considered sufficient for making this diagnosis. In fact, in one study, three abnormal findings indicative of interstitial disease were required before a definite diagnosis could be made [176]. Furthermore, although asbestosis can be present in the absence of visible pleural plaques, a diagnosis of asbestosis should be considered questionable unless pleural thickening is visible on HRCT.

Utility of High-Resolution Computed Tomography in the Diagnosis of Asbestosis

In patients who have significant asbestos exposure but no evidence of asbestosis on chest radiographs, it has been reported that as many as 20% to 30% will have some abnormal HRCT findings consistent with this disease (i.e., find-

ings of pulmonary fibrosis) [157,165]. However, other studies report the percentage of asbestos-exposed patients who have normal chest radiographs and abnormal HRCT studies to be as low as 5% [172,183]. Although the precise figures may vary depending on the population studied, it is

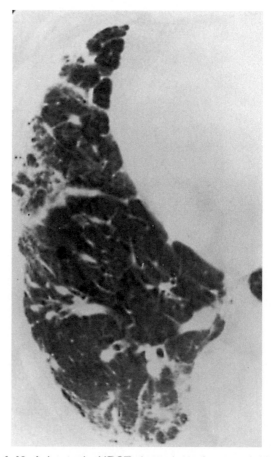

FIG. 4-49. Asbestosis. HRCT shows irregular septal thickening and early honeycombing.

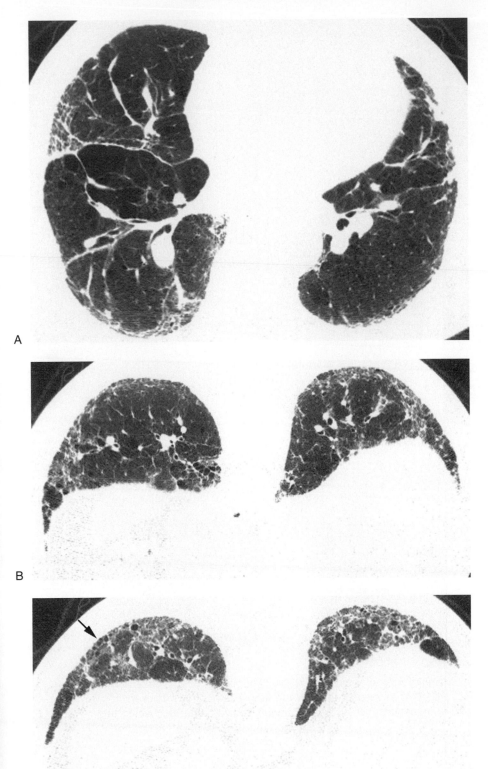

FIG. 4-50. A–C: Supine and prone HRCT in 81-year-old man with significant occupational exposure to asbestos, dyspnea, and abnormal chest radiograph. Images show subpleural reticulation predominantly representing intralobular interstitial thickening. Early honeycombing (*arrow*, **C**) is visible at the lung base.

universally conceded that HRCT is more sensitive than chest radiographs in detecting this disease. As stated previously, 10% to 20% of patients who have asbestosis diagnosed histologically have normal chest radiographs [166,168].

Certainly, chest films underestimate the presence of histologic asbestosis [166,168], but what is the significance of

HRCT abnormalities in asbestos-exposed patients who have normal or near-normal chest radiographs?

This question was addressed in a study of 169 asbestos-exposed workers with normal chest radiographs (ILO, 0/0 or 0/1) who also had HRCT (109). In this group, HRCT scans were read as normal or nearly normal in 76 (45%), abnormal

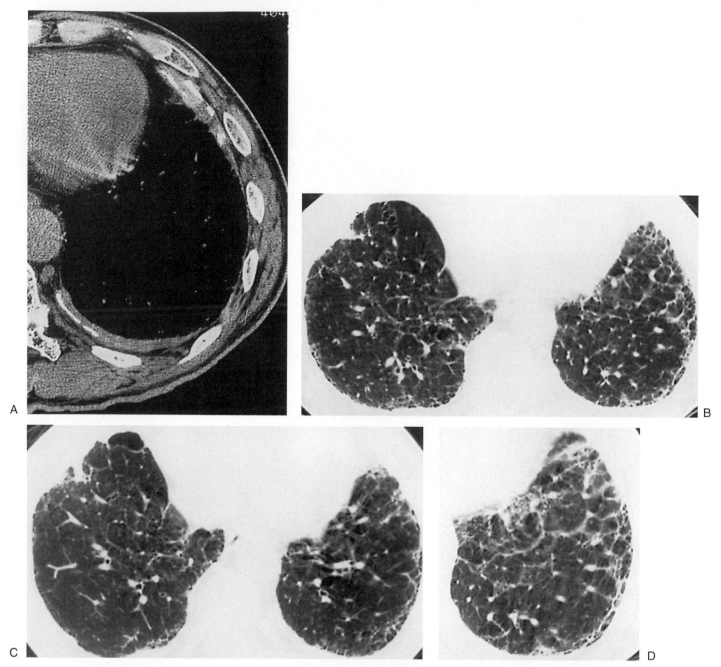

FIG. 4-51. Asbestosis with honeycombing in a 66-year-old man. **A:** Calcified pleural plaques are visible, typical of asbestos exposure. **B,C:** HRCT at two levels through the lung bases shows thickening of interlobular septa and the intralobular interstitium. **D:** A targeted image shows septal thickening and early subpleural honeycombing.

and suggestive of asbestosis in 57 (34%), or abnormal but not suggestive of pulmonary fibrosis in 36 (21%). Comparing the two groups in whom HRCT was interpreted as normal or suggestive of asbestosis, the group considered to be abnormal on HRCT had significantly lower vital capacity (percent predicted) and diffusing capacity (percent predicted) than did the normal group; these are functional findings typically associated with asbestosis [165]. On the other hand, there was no difference between the groups in a num-

ber of other clinical and functional parameters, including smoking history and measures of airway obstruction. Thus, based on this study, it appears as if HRCT is able to discriminate between groups of patients who have normal and abnormal lung function and indicates the significance of the abnormalities identified on HRCT. In another study, HRCT findings were found to correlate better with pulmonary function abnormalities in patients who had early asbestosis than did chest radiographs (126).

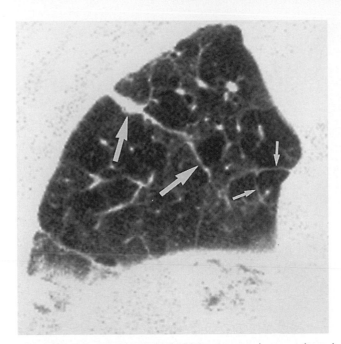

FIG. 4-52. Interlobular septal thickening and parenchymal bands in a patient with early asbestosis. View of the posterior lower lobe on a prone scan shows interlobular septal thickening (*small arrows*) and a thicker parenchymal band (*large arrows*).

In another study, Harkin et al. [184] studied 37 asbestos-exposed individuals having normal or near-normal chest radiographs using HRCT, pulmonary function tests, and bronchoalveolar lavage (BAL). A normal HRCT proved to be an excellent predictor of normality, with pulmonary function test values close to 100% predicted for FVC, FEV_1, TLC, DLco, and normal BAL. On the other hand, HRCT abnormalities were associated with reduced FEV_1/FVC ratio, reduced diffusing capacity, and alveolitis consistent with a definition of asbestosis.

Bergin et al. [185] have emphasized the nonspecific nature of the HRCT findings used to diagnose mild degrees of asbestosis. In a study of 157 patients who did not have evidence of asbestos exposure [185], HRCT showed dependent subpleural lines in 32 (20%), nondependent subpleural lines in 19 (12%), parenchymal bands in 47 (30%), thickened septal lines in dependent areas in 93 (59%), septal lines in nondependent areas in 67 (43%), and honeycomb lung in five (3%). Gamsu et al. [176] studied 30 asbestos-exposed patients who had HRCT and histologic assessment of lung tissue; 25 had findings of asbestosis on pathologic examination. Considering those 14 with normal or near normal chest radiographs (ILO, 0/0 or 0/1), five of ten with asbestosis showed two or more abnormal HRCT findings (i.e., interstitial lines, parenchymal bands, architectural distortion),

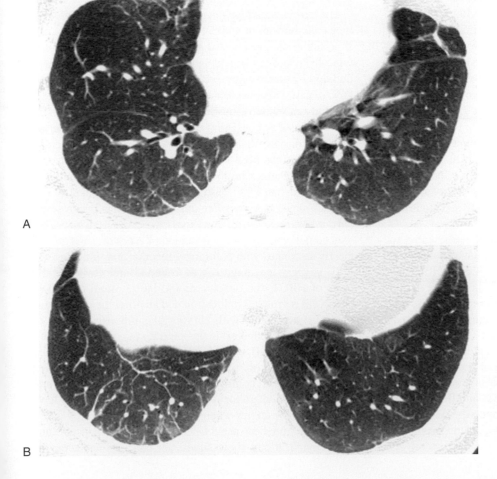

A

B

FIG. 4-53. A,B: HRCT in a 58-year-old man with a history of asbestos exposure and pleural thickening. Parenchymal bands and interlobular septal thickening are associated with pleural thickening. This finding does not necessarily indicate the presence of asbestosis but may reflect atelectasis or coarse scars.

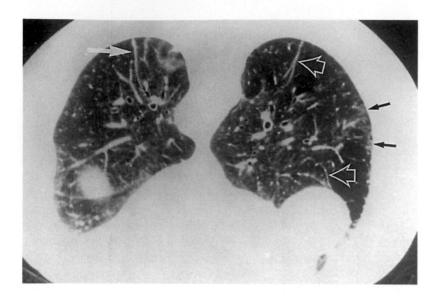

FIG. 4-54. Parenchymal bands in asbestosis. On a prone scan, areas of peripheral lung fibrosis are evident, particularly in the right lung (*small arrows*). Parenchymal bands are visible posteriorly on both sides. One of these bands (*large arrow*) is associated with a bronchus, perhaps representing fibrosis along the bronchovascular sheath associated with atelectasis or coarse scarring. Other bands (*open arrows*) appear to represent thickened interlobular septa.

whereas this was seen in one of four patients who did not have asbestosis [176]. Overall, one or two abnormal findings were seen in 40% of normals and 88% of patients who had asbestosis.

HRCT can also be valuable for eliminating the diagnosis of asbestosis in patients who have chest radiographic findings that suggest this disease, but who have some other abnormality. Friedman et al. [172] reported that approximately 20% of patients suspected of having interstitial disease on the basis of plain radiographs were shown by HRCT to have emphysema, prominent vessels, pleural disease, or bronchiectasis as the cause of their abnormal plain film findings. Many asbestos-exposed patients who have respiratory disability are smokers who have emphysema; HRCT can allow some estimation of the relative contribution of emphysema and fibrosis to the patient's respiratory difficulties.

On the other hand, a normal HRCT cannot exclude the presence of asbestosis. In a study by Gamsu et al. [176] of 25 cases of histologically proven asbestosis, five had normal HRCT and four had abnormalities thought unlikely to represent asbestosis. Thus, in this group, only 64% had scans suggestive of this diagnosis.

HRCT need not be performed in all patients who have asbestos exposure; if significant chest film abnormalities are present in the appropriate clinical setting (Table 4-10), CT is not necessary [162]. It would seem most appropriate to limit the use of HRCT in asbestos-exposed patients to those who have (i) equivocal chest radiographic findings of asbestosis, (ii) pulmonary function abnormalities or symptoms and normal chest radiographs, and (iii) extensive pleural abnormalities in whom the differentiation of pleural and parenchymal abnormalities may be difficult. In each of these three settings, the absence of findings of fibrosis on HRCT can be taken to mean that clinically significant asbestosis is not present, whereas the presence of fibrosis can lend strong support to the diagnosis.

Rounded Atelectasis and Focal Fibrotic Masses

Focal mass–like lung opacities can be seen in patients who have asbestos exposure, reflecting the presence of rounded atelectasis or focal subpleural fibrosis (Fig. 4-55) [172,178]. In one study [178], such masses were visible in approximately 10% of patients. It is important to distinguish these masses from lung cancer, which has an increased incidence in asbestos-exposed individuals.

The term *rounded atelectasis* refers to the presence of focal lung collapse with or without folding of the lung parenchyma. It occurs in the presence of a variety of abnormalities, but is typically associated with pleural disease, and thus is a common finding in patients who have asbestos exposure; in one study, 86% of cases were associated with asbestos [186]. In patients who have asbestos exposure, rounded atelectasis can represent the sequela of a preexisting exudative effusion or can be the result of adjacent pleural fibrosis or diffuse pleural thickening [177,186]. It has been suggested that rounded atelectasis in patients who have asbestos exposure may reflect evolution of parenchymal bands [177]. In a study by Gevenois et al. [177], rounded atelectasis was often unilateral. In some patients who have asbestos exposure, these masses are largely fibrotic, but they do not represent a manifestation of asbestosis and are not clearly associated with pulmonary function abnormalities.

To suggest the diagnosis of rounded atelectasis on the basis of HRCT, the opacity should be (i) round or oval in shape, (ii) peripheral in location and abutting the pleural surface, (iii) associated with curving of pulmonary vessels or bronchi into the edge of the lesion (i.e., the comet-tail sign), and (iv) associated with an ipsilateral pleural abnormality, either effusion or pleural thickening [187]. Rounded atelectasis is most common in the posterior lower lobes, and is sometimes bilateral or symmetrical [186,187]. It may have acute or obtuse angles where it contacts the pleura.

Because rounded atelectasis represents collapsed lung parenchyma, it can show significant enhancement after the

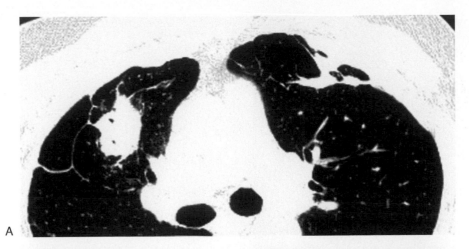

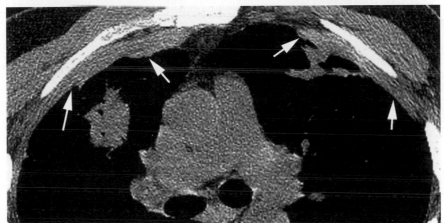

FIG. 4 55. A,B: Rounded atelectasis or focal fibrotic masses in a patient with asbestos exposure and pleural thickening. **A:** Irregular masses are visible bilaterally in the anterior lung. **B:** A tissue window scan shows that these opacities are adjacent to areas of pleural thickening (*arrows*). Although this appearance is common in patients with asbestos exposure and focal fibrotic masses, a definite diagnosis of this entity cannot be made based on their appearance, and carcinoma must be considered. However, repeated negative biopsy and follow-up has indicated their benign nature.

intravenous injection of contrast agents [188]. In a study of dynamic CT after contrast infusion, a significant increase in attenuation of rounded atelectasis was consistently found, with a minimum attenuation increase of 200% [189]. Although lung cancers opacify to some degree after contrast injection [190,191], dense opacification as seen in these patients has not been reported as a characteristic of lung cancer.

If the criteria for rounded atelectasis listed above are met, a confident diagnosis can usually be made. However, atypical cases are frequently encountered in patients who have asbestos exposure with appearances best described as lenticular, wedge-shaped, or irregular (Fig. 4-55) [178]. Furthermore, they may not be associated with curving of adjacent vessels, particularly if small in size, and they may not have significant contact with the pleural surface. If these lesions can be shown to be unchanged in size for longer than 1 year, they are likely benign; if not, needle biopsy may be necessary.

Asbestos-Related Pleural Disease

Benign exudative pleural effusion can be an early manifestation of asbestos exposure, as it is the only finding present in the first 10 years after exposure and the most common finding present in the first 20 years after exposure [192].

Asbestos-related pleural effusions can be unilateral or bilateral and may be persistent or recurrent [150]. CT in such patients sometimes shows the presence of pleural thickening or plaques invisible on chest radiographs, typical of asbestos exposure. However, the diagnosis of benign asbestos-related effusion is by exclusion; malignant mesothelioma must be considered in the differential diagnosis.

Parietal pleural thickening occurs commonly in patients who have occupational asbestos exposure [151,157,159, 167,172,192]. In fact, the combination of pleural thickening and ILD is most frequent in patients who have asbestos exposure. Parietal pleural plaques are the most common manifestation and the most characteristic radiographic feature of asbestos exposure. They represent focal and discrete regions of pleural thickening and predominate along the posterolateral costal pleural and diaphragmatic surfaces, but they typically spare the apices and costophrenic sulci.

High-Resolution Computed Tomography Findings of Pleural Thickening

On HRCT, parietal pleural thickening is easiest to see internal to visible rib segments; only the pleura, extrapleural fat, and endothoracic fascia pass internal to ribs (see

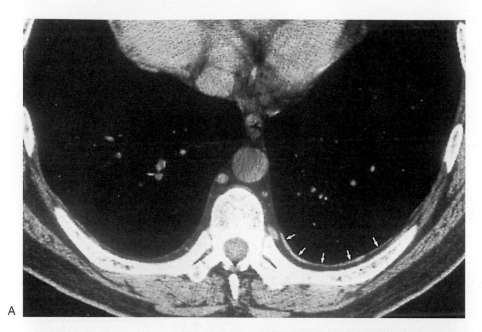

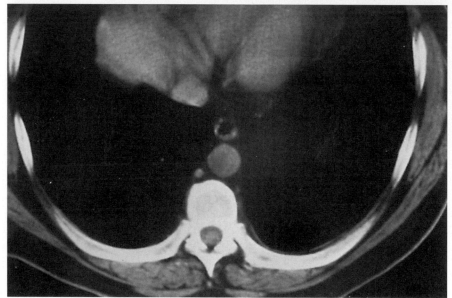

FIG. 4-56. Pleural thickening internal to a rib in asbestos exposure. **A:** HRCT shows a distinct white line (*arrows*) internal to a left posterior rib, representing pleural thickening. Extrapleural fat separates the thickened parietal pleura from the rib. Minimal pleural thickening is present on the right. The paravertebral line is normal. **B:** This finding is much more difficult to appreciate with 1-cm collimation and conventional CT technique.

Fig. 2-16), and in most normal patients these are too thin to recognize on HRCT. Thickened pleura measuring as little as 1 to 2 mm can be readily diagnosed in this location (Fig. 4-56). Although the normal innermost intercostal muscle is visible on HRCT as a 1- to 2-mm thick opaque stripe between adjacent rib segments (see Fig. 2-17), it does not pass internal to them and should not be confused with pleural thickening. Pleural thickening is also easy to recognize in the paravertebral regions. In the paravertebral regions, the intercostal muscles are anatomically absent (see Fig. 2-18), and any distinct stripe of density indicates pleural thickening (Figs. 4-57 and 4-58).

The HRCT diagnosis of pleural thickening is made easier in many locations by the presence of a distinct layer of extrapleural fat, usually measuring from 1 to 4 mm in thickness,

that separates the thickened pleura from adjacent structures of the chest wall, such as rib, innermost intercostal muscle, intercostal vein, or subcostalis muscle (Figs. 4-56, 4-58, and 4-59) [193]. This layer of extrapleural fat represents the normal fatty connective tissue present external to the parietal pleura and is likely thickened in patients who have asbestos exposure as a result of pleural inflammation. Extrapleural fat allows the thickened pleura to be seen on HRCT as a discrete linear opacity, even when the pleural thickening is minimal.

Asbestos-related pleural thickening has a typical appearance on HRCT [151,157,167,193]. The pleural thickening appears smooth and sharply defined and can be recognized when measuring only 1 or 2 mm in thickness (Figs. 4-56 through 4-59) [193]. Early pleural thickening is discontinuous, and abnormal areas can be easily contrasted with adja-

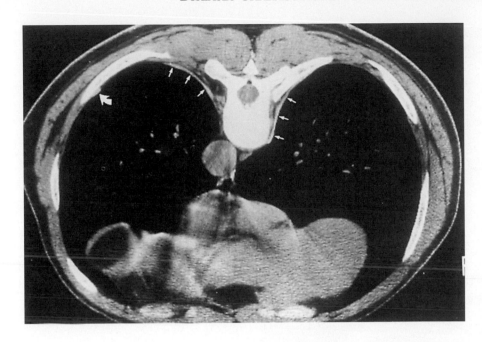

FIG. 4-57. Paravertebral pleural thickening in asbestos exposure. Prone HRCT shows 2- to 3-mm-thick lines (*arrows*) in both paravertebral regions, representing parietal pleural thickening. A small focus of pleural thickening internal to a rib (*large arrow*) is also seen.

cent normal regions. Areas of pleural thickening or plaques of thickened pleura are commonly visible adjacent to the inner surfaces of ribs or vertebral bodies (Figs 4-56 and 4-57). Plaques are usually bilateral, although they may appear unilateral in up to one-third of cases [177]. The presence of bilateral pleural plaques or focal pleural thickening is strongly suggestive of asbestos exposure, particularly when calcification is also visible (Fig. 4-60). Pleural calcification is visible on HRCT in approximately 15% of patients (Fig. 4-60) [171,172]. In one study [157], calcification was identified with HRCT in 20% of 100 subjects but was seen in only 16% with conventional CT and in 13% with chest radiographs. Often, even when not grossly calcified, asbestos-related areas of pleural thickening appear slightly denser than adjacent intercostal muscles (Figs. 4-57 and 4-59).

The diaphragmatic pleura is commonly involved in patients who have asbestos-related pleural disease (Fig. 4-60). However, the diaphragm lies roughly in the plane of the scan, and the detection of uncalcified pleural plaques on the diaphragmatic surface can be difficult with HRCT. In some patients, however, diaphragmatic pleural plaques are visible deep in the posterior costophrenic angle below the lung base; in this location, the pleural disease can be localized with certainty to the parietal pleura because only parietal pleura is present below the lung base.

Pleural plaques along the mediastinum have been considered unusual in patients who have asbestos-related pleural disease but are visible on CT scans in approximately 40% of patients [151,157,167,192,193]. Paravertebral pleural thickening is commonly seen on HRCT [193]. Although it is unusual, pleural thickening can involve a fissure and result in a localized intrapulmonary pleural plaque. These may simulate a lung nodule on CT, unless the plane of the fissure is identified. In patients who also have pulmonary fibrosis, vis-

ceral pleural thickening with irregularity of the pleural surface can also be seen at soft-tissue window settings.

Diffuse pleural thickening (DPT) is another common manifestation of asbestos exposure [192]. DPT represents a synthesis and fusion of thickened visceral and parietal pleural layers and is usually related to the presence of prior asbestos-related benign pleural effusion. On CT, DPT is defined by the presence of a sheet of thickened pleura at least 5 cm in lateral dimension and 8 cm in craniocaudal dimension [157]. DPT was found by Aberle and coworkers [157] in seven of 100 exposed individuals. Because of visceral pleural thickening or associated lung fibrosis, the thickened pleura may appear ill defined or irregular. Extensive calcification is uncommon.

DPT is associated with significant impairment of pulmonary function; pulmonary function in patients who have pleural plaques is normal or slightly reduced [194,195]. Kee et al. [196] studied the relationship between DPT and pulmonary function in 84 asbestos-exposed subjects with DPT detected using HRCT and 53 patients matched for age, smoking history, length of asbestos exposure, and latency. Individuals with DPT demonstrated significantly reduced FVC ($p = .002$) and DLCO ($p = .002$) as compared to the matched controls.

There is a significant correlation between the presence and severity of pleural disease and the presence and severity of asbestosis [151]. In one study, HRCT findings of parenchymal fibrosis were visible in 14% of exposed patients who did not have evidence of pleural thickening, in 56% of those with focal plaques, and in 88% of those with DPT [195]. It is important to note, however, that pleural thickening and plaques commonly occur in the absence of pulmonary fibrosis [197], and asbestosis can sometimes be seen in the absence of visible pleural plaques [195], although this is more unusual.

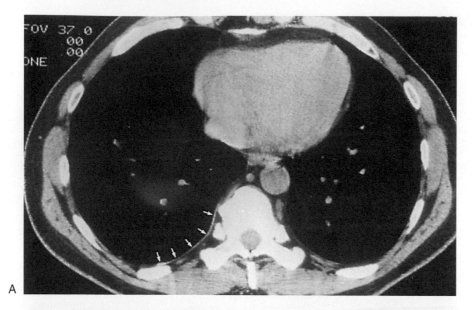

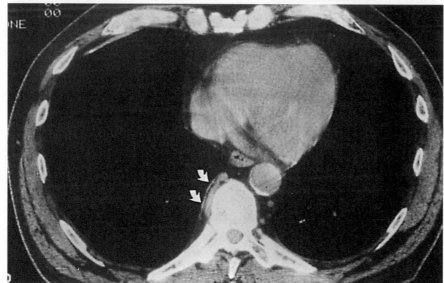

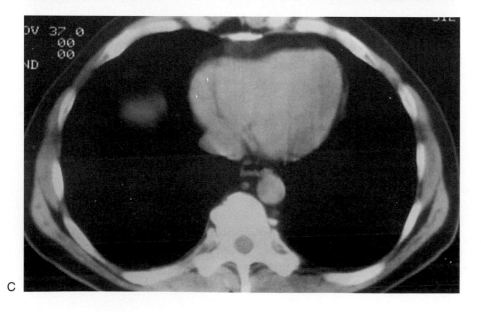

FIG. 4-58. Paravertebral pleural thickening in asbestos exposure. **A,B:** HRCT at two levels shows thickening of the right paravertebral line (*small arrows*). At one level, the thickened pleura (*large arrows*, **B**) is separated from the adjacent intercostal vein by fat. **C:** With 1-cm collimation and conventional CT technique these findings are difficult to see.

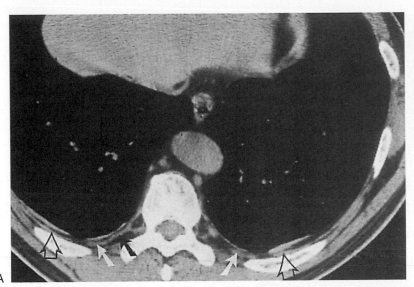 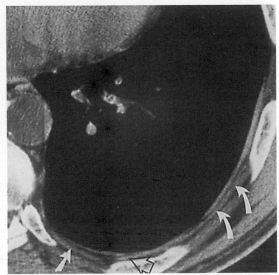

FIG. 4-59. Pleural thickening in asbestos exposure. **A,B:** HRCT in two different patients shows thickened pleura separated from intercostal vein (*arrows*), subcostalis muscle (*open arrows*), and intercostal muscle (*curved arrows*, **B**) by a layer of fat.

Utility of High-Resolution Computed Tomography in Diagnosing Asbestos-Related Pleural Disease

Pleural thickening is frequently seen on plain radiographs in patients who have asbestos exposure (Fig. 4-47), but CT and, particularly, HRCT are much more sensitive in detecting pleural disease [151,157,167]. Aberle and colleagues [157] studied the detection of pleural plaques and calcification with conventional radiographs, conventional CT, and HRCT in 100 subjects occupationally exposed to asbestos. Although HRCT was obtained only at selected levels, it was more sensitive in detecting plaques than were the other two modalities (Figs. 4-56 and 4-58). Plaques were identified in 64 persons with HRCT, in 56 with conventional CT, and in 49 with chest radiographs. In another study [193] of 13 patients who had evidence of asbestos-related pleural disease visible on HRCT, conventional CT showed some evidence of pleural abnormality in only 11; however, in all 13, some abnormal areas visible on HRCT were not seen with conventional CT. Similar results have been reported by others [167,198].

Furthermore, HRCT is much more accurate than plain films or conventional CT in distinguishing true pleural disease from extrapleural fat pads that can closely mimic the appearance of pleural thickening (Fig. 4-61). In one study of patients with low levels of asbestos exposure, posteroanterior and right anterior oblique radiographs were thought to show pleural thickening in all, whereas HRCT showed true pleural plaques in only 13% to 26% [199]; most of the false-positive interpretations on chest radiographs were due to the presence of extrapleural fat.

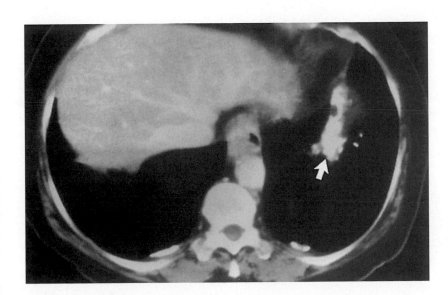

FIG. 4-60. Pleural plaques in a patient with asbestos exposure. CT shows calcified plaques posteriorly, and on the dome of the left hemidiaphragm (*arrow*).

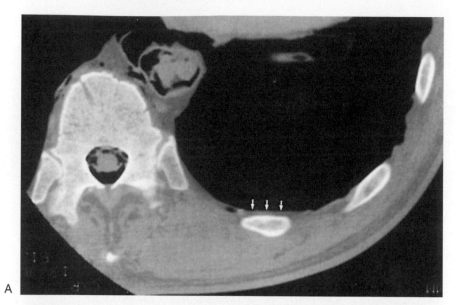

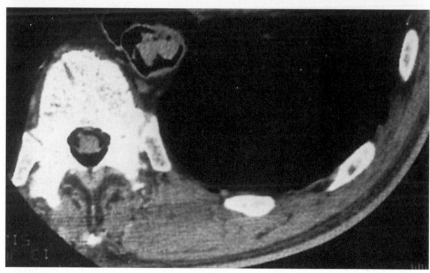

FIG. 4-61. Normal extrapleural fat pad in a cadaver. **A:** With a wide-window setting, soft tissue (*arrows*) is visible internal to the posterior rib segment. This appearance mimics pleural thickening. **B:** At a soft-tissue window setting, the low density of the fat is apparent. (From Im JG, Webb WR, et al. Costal pleura: appearances at high-resolution CT. *Radiology* 1989;171:125, with permission.)

Differential Diagnosis and Mimics of Parietal Pleural Thickening

Parietal pleural thickening or pleural effusion in association with lung disease can also be seen in patients who have RA [200], lymphangiomyomatosis (LAM) [201,202], coal worker's pneumoconiosis [203], tuberculosis [204], nontuberculous mycobacteria, and lymphangitic spread of carcinoma [23].

Normal extrapleural fat can be seen on HRCT internal to ribs in several locations and can mimic pleural thickening (Fig. 4-61) [172]. The normal layer of extrapleural fat between the parietal pleura and the endothoracic fascia is notably thicker adjacent to the lateral ribs than in other sites [193,205,206]. It is most abundant over the posterolateral fourth to eighth ribs and can result in fat pads several millimeters thick that extend into the intercostal spaces [205,206]. In normal subjects, these costal fat pads can be difficult to distinguish from pleural thickening or plaques when extended window settings [width 2,000 Hounsfield units (HU)] are used, but are very low in attenuation and difficult to see with soft-tissue window settings [193].

The transversus thoracis and subcostalis muscles can also mimic pleural thickening in some patients. Anteriorly, at the level of the heart and adjacent to the lower sternum or xiphoid process, the transversus thoracis muscles are nearly always visible internal to the anterior ends of ribs or costal cartilages (Fig. 4-62) [193]. Posteriorly, at the same level, a 1- to 2-mm-thick line is sometimes seen internal to one or more ribs, representing the subcostalis muscle; this muscle is present in only a small percentage of patients (Fig. 4-61) [193]. In contrast to pleural thickening, these muscles are smooth, uniform in thickness, and symmetric bilaterally.

Segments of intercostal veins are commonly visible in the paravertebral regions and can mimic focal pleural thickening (Fig. 4-62). Continuity of these opacities with the azygos or hemizygos veins can sometimes allow them to be correctly identified [193]. Furthermore, when viewed using

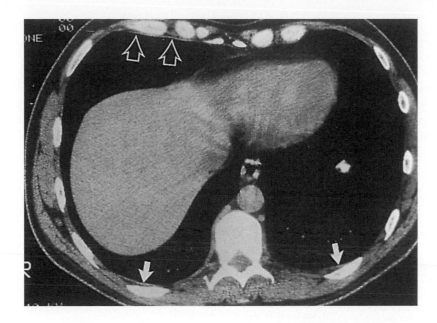

FIG. 4-62. Normal transversus thoracis and subcostalis muscles. HRCT in a normal subject shows the right transversus thoracis muscle internal to the anterior rib and costal cartilage (*open arrows*). Posteriorly, the subcostalis muscles (*solid arrows*) are visible bilaterally, anterior to ribs. Prominent intercostal veins are visible in the paravertebral regions.

lung window settings, intercostal vein segments do not indent the lung surface; pleural plaques of the same thickness certainly would.

Visceral pleural thickening (i.e., thickening of the subpleural interstitium) can be seen on HRCT in a number of lung diseases that produce pulmonary fibrosis. However, visceral pleural thickening can usually be distinguished from parietal pleural thickening by its irregular appearance; visceral pleural thickening usually appears very irregular at soft-tissue or wide-window settings (Fig. 4-63) because of abnormal lung reticulation and the interface sign. Because

its presence reflects an interstitial abnormality, visceral pleural thickening is usually localized to areas in which the underlying lung is abnormal; this is not true of asbestos-related parietal pleural thickening.

Confluent subpleural nodules, so-called pseudoplaques [203,207], can be seen in patients who have silicosis, coal worker's pneumoconiosis, or sarcoidosis (see Fig. 3-46). These can mimic the appearance of parietal pleural plaques that occur in patients who have asbestos exposure, but they are associated with lung nodules rather than findings of fibrosis.

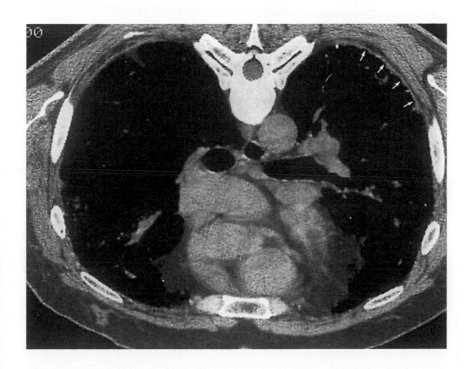

FIG. 4-63. Visceral pleural thickening in a patient with pulmonary fibrosis and no history of asbestos exposure. The pleural opacity (*arrows*) visible on prone HRCT appears very irregular.

ALUMINUM DUST PNEUMOCONIOSIS

Inhalation of dusts containing metallic or oxidized aluminum have been associated with pulmonary fibrosis, granuloma formation, DIP, and alveolar proteinosis, but pneumoconiosis related to aluminum dust is rare. HRCT findings in six reported cases include subpleural or diffuse honeycombing resembling the appearance of IPF, centrilobular nodules resembling those seen in silicosis, or irregular reticulation [208]. In five of the six cases, abnormalities had an upper lobe predominance.

HARD-METAL PNEUMOCONIOSIS

Hard metal is an alloy of tungsten carbide and cobalt, sometimes mixed with other metals. Of these, at least cobalt is toxic to the lung. Exposure to hard metal results in interstitial inflammation with fibrosis and lung destruction, which may develop within a few years of exposure. HRCT findings in two reported patients [208] include coarse reticular opacities, consolidation, architectural distortion, traction bronchiectasis and bronchiolectasis, and subpleural bullae (Fig. 4-64). The distribution may be patchy or with a lower lobe predominance.

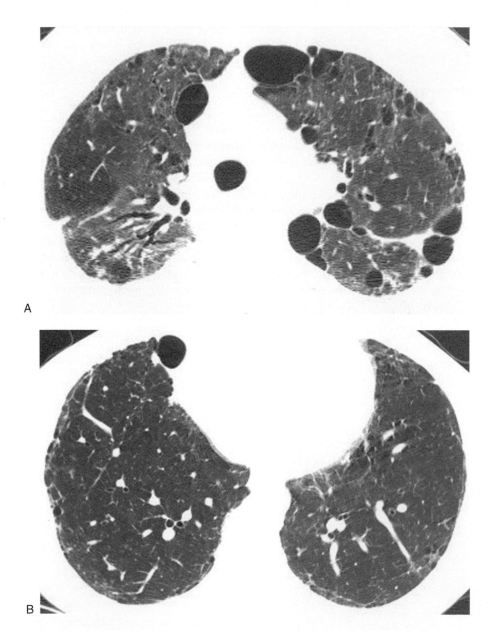

A

B

FIG. 4-64. A,B: Hard metal pneumoconiosis. HRCT in a patient with hard metal pneumoconiosis shows subpleural bullae in the upper lobes, posterior lung fibrosis, and subpleural reticular opacities.

END-STAGE LUNG

So-called end-stage lung represents the final common pathway of a number of chronic infiltrative lung diseases and is characterized by acute and chronic inflammation, the presence of fibrosis, alveolar dissolution, bronchiolectasis, and disruption of normal lung architecture. Generally speaking, end-stage lung is considered to be present in patients who have morphologic evidence of honeycombing, extensive cystic changes, or conglomerate fibrosis [209–212].

Based on the analysis of chest radiographs and fragmentary lung histology obtained at open-lung biopsy, it had been assumed that the morphologic appearance of end-stage lung lacked specificity, with the observed findings being similar regardless of etiology [54,210]. Although significant overlap can occur between the HRCT appearances of different fibrotic diseases, Primack et al. [54] demonstrated that the pattern and distribution of abnormalities seen on HRCT in patients who have end-stage lung are determined at least in part by the underlying disease, and that in most cases a specific diagnosis can be made on HRCT.

Primack et al. [54] reviewed the HRCT scans of 61 consecutive patients who had end-stage lung. Two independent observers, without knowledge of the clinical or pathologic data, listed the three most likely diagnoses and recorded the degree of confidence in their first-choice diagnosis on a three-point scale. On the average, the two observers made a correct first-choice diagnosis in 87% of cases. A correct first-choice diagnosis was made most often in silicosis (100%), Langerhans histiocytosis (100%), asbestosis (90%), UIP (88%), hypersensitivity pneumonitis (87%), and sarcoidosis (83%). The observers had a high degree of confidence in their first-choice diagnosis in 62% of the interpretations, and when they were confident in their diagnosis, they were correct in 100% of the cases. The most common conditions leading to end-stage lung disease in the study by Primack et al. [54] included UIP (43%), sarcoidosis (15%), Langerhans histiocytosis (13%), asbestosis (8%), and hypersensitivity pneumonitis (extrinsic allergic alveolitis) (6%).

UIP was characterized by predominant involvement of the lower lung zones and subpleural regions, with peripheral honeycombing being the most common finding (Figs. 4-2 through 4-10). The abnormalities in patients who had sarcoidosis involved mainly the upper lung zones and had a peribronchovascular distribution (see Figs. 3-82, 5-44 through 5-48). End-stage fibrosis in sarcoidosis was associated with three different patterns: (i) subpleural honeycombing, (ii) central cystic changes due to markedly ectatic bronchi, and (iii) conglomerate fibrosis. In the six patients who had sarcoidosis and conglomerate fibrosis, bronchi could be seen within the areas of fibrosis. Langerhans histiocytosis was characterized in all cases by an upper-lung zone predominance of randomly distributed cystic spaces with relative sparing of the lung bases (see Figs. 7-2 and 7-3). Asbestosis had an appearance identical to that of UIP, except that all five patients who had asbestosis also had pleural plaques or

DPT (Figs. 4-46 through 4-51). Parenchymal bands are also much more common in patients who have asbestosis (Fig. 4-52) [180]. The abnormalities in end-stage hypersensitivity pneumonitis involved all lung zones to a similar degree in three patients and had an upper-lung zone predominance in one. Honeycombing was predominantly subpleural in three cases, but unlike UIP, in chronic hypersensitivity pneumonitis there was relative sparing of the lung bases (see Figs. 6-14 and 6-15). All patients who had hypersensitivity pneumonitis had associated extensive areas of ground-glass opacity in a random distribution.

The ability to make a confident correct specific diagnosis on HRCT in the majority of patients who have end-stage lung may be of significant clinical utility, as open-lung biopsy is not usually diagnostic in patients who have this pattern of abnormalities, and its use is not recommended [213]. Gaensler and Carrington [213] reviewed their experience with open-lung biopsy in 502 patients who had chronic diffuse infiltrative lung disease. Nonspecific honeycombing, or end-stage lung, was the only diagnosis possible in 3.4% of patients. Based on their experience, they did not consider it advisable to perform lung biopsy in patients who have radiographic evidence of extensive honeycombing, because in such patients, biopsy has made no contribution from either the diagnostic or the therapeutic standpoint [213]. Overall, the diagnostic yield in this study [213] was 92%, with a mortality rate of 0.3% and a 2.5% rate of significant complications, such as emphysema, respiratory insufficiency, and myocardial ischemia. If end-stage lung disease is the only abnormality seen on CT, open-lung biopsy is not likely warranted. The diagnosis in those patients can be based on clinical history and the pattern and distribution of findings on HRCT.

REFERENCES

1. McAdams HP, Rosado-de-Christenson ML, Wehunt WD, et al. The alphabet soup revisited: the chronic interstitial pneumonias in the 1990s. *Radiographics* 1996;16:1009–1034.
2. Müller NL, Colby TV. Idiopathic interstitial pneumonias: high-resolution CT and histologic findings. *Radiographics* 1997;17:1016–1022.
3. ATS/ERS International Multidisciplinary Consensus Classification of Idiopathic Interstitial Pneumonias: General Principles and Guidelines. American Thoracic Society, Toronto, May 2000.
4. Katzenstein AL, Myers JL. Idiopathic pulmonary fibrosis: clinical relevance of pathologic classification. *Am J Respir Crit Care Med* 1998;157:1301–1315.
5. Kadota J, Kusano S, Kawakami K, et al. Usual interstitial pneumonia associated with primary Sjögren's syndrome. *Chest* 1995;108:1756–1758.
6. Müller NL, Miller RR. Computed tomography of chronic diffuse infiltrative lung disease: part 1. *Am Rev Respir Dis* 1990;142:1206–1215.
7. Colby T, Carrington C. Interstitial Lung Disease. In: Thurlbeck WM, Churg AM, eds. *Pathology of the lung.* New York: Thieme, 1995:589–737.
8. Muhm JR, Miller WE, Fontana RS, et al. Lung cancer detected during a screening program using four-month chest radiographs. *Radiology* 1983;148:609–615.
9. Carrington CB, Gaensler EA, Coute RE, et al. Natural history and treated course of usual and desquamative interstitial pneumonia. *N Engl J Med* 1978;298:801–809.
10. Katzenstein ALA, Myers JL, Mazur MT. Acute interstitial pneumonia: a clinicopathologic, ultrastructural, and cell kinetic study. *Am J Surg Pathol* 1986;10:256–267.

11. Ichikado K, Johkoh T, Ikezoe J, et al. Acute interstitial pneumonia: high-resolution CT findings correlated with pathology. *AJR Am J Roentgenol* 1997;168:333–338.
12. Katzenstein AL, Fiorelli RF. Nonspecific interstitial pneumonia/fibrosis: histologic features and clinical significance. *Am J Surg Pathol* 1994;18:136–147.
13. Nishimura K, Kitaichi M, Izumi T, et al. Usual interstitial pneumonia: histologic correlation with high-resolution CT. *Radiology* 1992; 182:337–342.
14. Crystal RG, Bitterman PB, Rennard SI, et al. Interstitial lung diseases of unknown cause: disorders characterized by chronic inflammation of the lower respiratory tract. *N Engl J Med* 1984;310:154–166.
15. Stack BHR, Choo-King YF, Heard BE. The prognosis of cryptogenic fibrosing alveolitis. *Thorax* 1972;27:535–542.
16. Bjoraker JA, Ryu JH, Edwin MK, et al. Prognostic significance of histopathologic subsets in idiopathic pulmonary fibrosis. *Am J Respir Crit Care Med* 1998;157:199–203.
17. Hansell DM, Wells AU. CT evaluation of fibrosing alveolitis—applications and insights. *J Thorac Imaging* 1996;11:231–249.
18. Scadding JG, Hinson KFW. Diffuse fibrosing alveolitis (diffuse interstitial fibrosis of the lungs): correlation of histology at biopsy with prognosis. *Thorax* 1967;22:291–304.
19. Watters LC, King TE, Schwarz MI, et al. A clinical, radiographic and physiologic scoring system for the longitudinal assessment of patients who have idiopathic pulmonary fibrosis. *Am Rev Respir Dis* 1986;133:97–103.
20. Wright PH, Heard BE, Steel SJ, et al. Cryptogenic fibrosing alveolitis: assessment by graded trephine lung biopsy histology compared with clinical, radiographic and physiologic features. *Br J Dis Chest* 1981;75:61–70.
20a. Idiopathic pulmonary fibrosis: diagnosis and treatment. International consensus statement. *Am J Respir Crit Care Med* 2000;161:646–664.
21. Müller NL, Miller RR, Webb WR, et al. Fibrosing alveolitis: CT-pathologic correlation. *Radiology* 1986;160:585–588.
22. McLoud TC, Carrington CB, Gaensler EA. Diffuse infiltrative lung disease: a new scheme for description. *Radiology* 1983;149:353–363.
23. Grenier P, Chevret S, Beigelman C, et al. Chronic diffuse infiltrative lung disease: determination of the diagnostic value of clinical data, chest radiography, and CT with Bayesian analysis. *Radiology* 1994;191:383–390.
24. Müller NL, Guerry-Force ML, Staples CA, et al. Differential diagnosis of bronchiolitis obliterans with organizing pneumonia and usual interstitial pneumonia: clinical, functional, and radiologic findings. *Radiology* 1987;162:151–156.
25. Crystal RG, Fulmer JD, Roberts WC, et al. Idiopathic pulmonary fibrosis: clinical, histologic, radiographic, physiologic, scintigraphic, cytologic, and biochemical aspects. *Ann Intern Med* 1976;85:769–788.
26. Staples CA, Müller NL, Vedal S, et al. Usual interstitial pneumonia: correlation of CT with clinical, functional, and radiologic findings. *Radiology* 1987;162:377–381.
27. Webb WR, Stein MG, Finkbeiner WE, et al. Normal and diseased isolated lungs: high-resolution CT. *Radiology* 1988;166:81–87.
28. Zerhouni EA, Naidich DP, Stitik FP, et al. Computed tomography of the pulmonary parenchyma: part 2. interstitial disease. *J Thorac Imaging* 1985;1:54–64.
29. Westcott JL, Cole SR. Traction bronchiectasis in end-stage pulmonary fibrosis. *Radiology* 1986;161:665–669.
30. Aquino SL, Webb WR, Zaloudek CJ, et al. Lung cysts associated with honeycombing: change in size on expiratory CT scans. *AJR Am J Roentgenol* 1994;162:583–584.
31. Kang EY, Grenier P, Laurent F, et al. Interlobular septal thickening: patterns at high-resolution computed tomography. *J Thorac Imaging* 1996;11:260–264.
32. Leung AN, Miller RR, Müller NL. Parenchymal opacification in chronic infiltrative lung diseases: CT-pathologic correlation. *Radiology* 1993;188:209–214.
33. Remy-Jardin M, Giraud F, Remy J, et al. Importance of ground glass attenuation in chronic diffuse infiltrative lung disease: pathologic-CT correlation. *Radiology* 1993;189:693–698.
34. Wells AU, Rubens MB, du Bois RM, et al. Serial CT in fibrosing alveolitis: prognostic significance of the initial pattern. *AJR Am J Roentgenol* 1993;161:1159–1165.
35. Wells AU, Hansell DM, Rubens MB, et al. The predictive value of appearances of thin-section computed tomography in fibrosing alveolitis. *Am Rev Respir Dis* 1993;148:1076–1082.
36. Gay SE, Kazerooni EA, Toews GB, et al. Idiopathic pulmonary fibrosis: predicting response to therapy and survival. *Am J Respir Crit Care Med* 1998;157:1063–1072.
37. Terriff BA, Kwan SY, Chan-Yeung MM, et al. Fibrosing alveolitis: chest radiography and CT as predictors of clinical and functional impairment at follow-up in 26 patients. *Radiology* 1992;184:445–449.
38. Mathieson JR, Mayo JR, Staples CA, et al. Chronic diffuse infiltrative lung disease: comparison of diagnostic accuracy of CT and chest radiography. *Radiology* 1989;171:111–116.
39. Bergin C, Castellino RA. Mediastinal lymph node enlargement on CT scans in patients who have unusual interstitial pneumonitis. *AJR Am J Roentgenol* 1990;154:251–254.
40. Niimi H, Kang EY, Kwong JS, et al. CT of chronic infiltrative lung disease: prevalence of mediastinal lymphadenopathy. *J Comput Assist Tomogr* 1996;20:305–308.
41. Franquet T, Gimenez A, Alegret X, et al. Mediastinal lymphadenopathy in cryptogenic fibrosing alveolitis: the effect of steroid therapy on the prevalence of nodal enlargement. *Clin Radiol* 1998; 53:435–438.
42. Akira M, Sakatani M, Ueda E. Idiopathic pulmonary fibrosis: progression of honeycombing at thin-section CT. *Radiology* 1993;189:687–691.
43. Hartman TE, Primack SL, Kang EY, et al. Disease progression in usual interstitial pneumonia compared with desquamative interstitial pneumonia: assessment with serial CT. *Chest* 1996;110:378–382.
44. Colby T. Interstitial diseases. In: Colby TV, Lombard C, Yousem SA, et al., eds. *Atlas of pulmonary surgical pathology.* Philadelphia: WB Saunders, 1991:227–306.
45. Kondoh Y, Taniguchi H, Kawabata Y, et al. Acute exacerbation in idiopathic pulmonary fibrosis: analysis of clinical and pathologic findings in three cases. *Chest* 1993;103:1808–1812.
46. Akira M, Hamada H, Sakatani M, et al. CT findings during phase of accelerated deterioration in patients who have idiopathic pulmonary fibrosis. *AJR Am J Roentgenol* 1997;168:79–83.
47. Akira M. Computed tomography and pathologic findings in fulminant forms of idiopathic interstitial pneumonia. *J Thorac Imag* 1999;14:76–84.
48. Müller NL, Staples CA, Miller RR, et al. Disease activity in idiopathic pulmonary fibrosis: CT and pathologic correlation. *Radiology* 1987;165:731–734.
49. Lee JS, Im JG, Ahn JM, et al. Fibrosing alveolitis: prognostic implication of ground glass attenuation at high-resolution CT. *Radiology* 1992;184:415–454.
50. Lee JS, Gong G, Song KS, et al. Usual interstitial pneumonia: relationship between disease activity and the progression of honeycombing at thin-section computed tomography. *J Thorac Imag* 1998; 13:199–203.
51. Miller RR, Nelems B, Müller NL, et al. Lingular and right middle lobe biopsy in the assessment of diffuse lung disease. *Ann Thorac Surg* 1987;44:269–273.
52. Vedal S, Welsh EV, Miller RR, et al. Desquamative interstitial pneumonia: computed tomographic findings before and after treatment with corticosteroids. *Chest* 1988;93:215–217.
53. Tung KT, Wells AU, Rubens MB, et al. Accuracy of the typical computed tomographic appearances of fibrosing alveolitis. *Thorax* 1993;48:334–338.
54. Primack SL, Hartman TE, Hansell DM, et al. End-stage lung disease: CT findings in 61 patients. *Radiology* 1993;189:681–686.
55. Al-Jarad N, Strickland B, Pearson MC, et al. High-resolution computed tomographic assessment of asbestosis and cryptogenic fibrosing alveolitis: a comparative study. *Thorax* 1992;47:645–650.
56. Swensen SJ, Aughenbaugh GL, Myers JL. Diffuse lung disease: diagnostic accuracy of CT in patients undergoing surgical biopsy of the lung. *Radiology* 1997;205:229–234.
57. Johkoh T, Müller NL, Cartier Y, et al. Idiopathic interstitial pneumonias: diagnostic accuracy of thin-section CT in 129 patients. *Radiology* 1999;211:555–560.
58. Colby TV, Carrington CB. Infiltrative lung disease. In: Thurlbeck WM, Churg AM, eds. *Pathology of the lung.* Stuttgart: Thieme, 1988:425–518.

59. Gamsu G. Radiographic manifestations of thoracic involvement by collagen-vascular diseases. *J Thorac Imag* 1992;7(3):1–12.

60. Turner-Warwick M, Burrows B, Johnson A. Cryptogenic fibrosing alveolitis: clinical features and their influence on survival. *Thorax* 1980;35:171–180.

61. Shannon TM, Gale ME. Noncardiac manifestations of rheumatoid arthritis in the thorax. *J Thorac Imag* 1992;7(2):19–29.

62. Primack SL, Müller NL. Radiologic manifestations of the systemic autoimmune diseases. *Clin Chest Med* 1998;19:573–586.

63. Remy-Jardin M, Remy J, Cortet B, et al. Lung changes in rheumatoid arthritis: CT findings. *Radiology* 1994;193:375–382.

64. Perez T, Remy-Jardin M, Cortet B. Airways involvement in rheumatoid arthritis: clinical, functional, and HRCT findings. *Am J Respir Crit Care Med* 1998;157:1658–1665.

65. Laitinen O, Nissila M, Salorinne Y, et al. Pulmonary involvement in patients who have rheumatoid arthritis. *Scand J Respir Dis* 1975;56:297.

66. Frank ST, Weg JG, Harkleroad LE, et al. Pulmonary dysfunction in rheumatoid disease. *Chest* 1973;63:27–34.

67. Aquino SL, Webb WR, Golden J. Bronchiolitis obliterans associated with rheumatoid arthritis: findings on HRCT and dynamic expiratory CT. *J Comput Assist Tomogr* 1994;18:555–558.

68. Hassan WU, Keaney NP, Holland CD, et al. High resolution computed tomography of the lung in lifelong non-smoking patients who have rheumatoid arthritis. *Ann Rheum Dis* 1995;54:308–310.

69. Kinoshita M, Higashi T, Tanaka C, et al. Follicular bronchiolitis associated with rheumatoid arthritis. *Intern Med* 1992;31:674–677.

70. Hayakawa H, Sato A, Imokawa S, et al. Bronchiolar disease in rheumatoid arthritis. *Am J Respir Crit Care Med* 1996;154:1531–1536.

71. Howling SJ, Hansell DM, Wells AU, et al. Follicular bronchiolitis: thin-section CT and histologic findings. *Radiology* 1999;212:637–642.

72. Fujii M, Adachi S, Shimizu T, et al. Interstitial lung disease in rheumatoid arthritis: assessment with high-resolution computed tomography. *J Thorac Imag* 1993;8:54–62.

73. Meziane MA. High-resolution computed tomography scanning in the assessment of interstitial lung diseases. *J Thorac Imag* 1992;7(3):13–25.

74. Taormina VJ, Miller WT, Gefter WB, et al. Progressive systemic sclerosis subgroups: variable pulmonary features. *AJR Am J Roentgenol* 1981;137:277–285.

75. Arroliga AC, Podell DN, Matthay RA. Pulmonary manifestations of scleroderma. *J Thorac Imag* 1992;7(2):30–45.

76. Schurawitzki H, Stiglbauer R, Graninger W, et al. Interstitial lung disease in progressive systemic sclerosis: high-resolution CT versus radiography. *Radiology* 1990;176:755–759.

77. Chan TY, Hansell DM, Rubens MB, et al. Cryptogenic fibrosing alveolitis and the fibrosing alveolitis of systemic sclerosis: morphological differences on computed tomographic scans. *Thorax* 1997;52:265–270.

78. Remy-Jardin M, Remy J, Wallaert B, et al. Pulmonary involvement in progressive systemic sclerosis: sequential evaluation with CT, pulmonary function tests, and bronchoalveolar lavage. *Radiology* 1993;188:499–506.

79. Harrison NK, Myers AR, Corrin B, et al. Structural features of interstitial lung disease in systemic sclerosis. *Am Rev Respir Dis* 1991;144:706–713.

80. Bhalla M, Silver RM, Shepard JO, et al. Chest CT in patients who have scleroderma: prevalence of asymptomatic esophageal dilatation and mediastinal lymphadenopathy. *AJR Am J Roentgenol* 1993;161:269–272.

81. Seely JM, Jones LT, Wallace C, et al. Systemic sclerosis: using high-resolution CT to detect lung disease in children. *AJR Am J Roentgenol* 1998;170:691–697.

82. Wells AU, Hansell DM, Corrin B, et al. High resolution computed tomography as a predictor of lung histology in systemic sclerosis. *Thorax* 1992;47:508–512.

83. Panush RS, Greer JM, Morshedian KK. What is lupus? What is not lupus? *Rheum Dis Clin North Am* 1993;19:223–234.

84. Wiedemann HP, Matthay RA. Pulmonary manifestations of systemic lupus erythematosus. *J Thorac Imag* 1992;7(2):1–18.

85. Kim JS, Lee KS, Koh EM, et al. Thoracic involvement of systemic lupus erythematosus: clinical, pathologic, and radiologic findings. *J Comput Assist Tomogr* 2000;24:9–18.

86. Gammon RB, Bridges TA, al-Nezir H, et al. Bronchiolitis obliterans organizing pneumonia associated with systemic lupus erythematosus. *Chest* 1992;102:1171–1174.

87. Eisenberg H, Dubois EL, Sherwin RP, et al. Diffuse interstitial lung disease in systemic lupus erythematosus. *Ann Intern Med* 1973;79:37–45.

88. Bankier AA, Kiener HP, Wiesmayr MN, et al. Discrete lung involvement in systemic lupus erythematosus: CT assessment. *Radiology* 1995;196:835–840.

89. Fenlon HM, Doran M, Sant SM, et al. High-resolution chest CT in systemic lupus erythematosus. *AJR Am J Roentgenol* 1996;166:301–307.

90. Ooi GC, Ngan H, Peh WC, et al. Systemic lupus erythematosus patients who have respiratory symptoms: the value of HRCT. *Clin Radiol* 1997;52:775–781.

91. Sant SM, Doran M, Fenelon HM, et al. Pleuropulmonary abnormalities in patients who have systemic lupus erythematosus: assessment with high resolution computed tomography, chest radiography and pulmonary function tests. *Clin Exp Rheumatol* 1997;15:507–513.

92. Connolly B, Manson D, Eberhard A, et al. CT appearance of pulmonary vasculitis in children. *AJR Am J Roentgenol* 1996;167:901–904.

93. Hunninghake GW, Fauci AS. Pulmonary involvement in the collagen-vascular diseases. *Am Rev Respir Dis* 1979;119:471–503.

94. Schwarz MI. Pulmonary and cardiac manifestations of polymyositis-dermatomyositis. *J Thorac Imag* 1992;7(2):46–54.

95. Tazelaar HD, Viggiano RW, Pickersgill J, et al. Interstitial lung disease in polymyositis and dermatomyositis: clinical features and prognosis as correlated with histologic findings. *Am Rev Respir Dis* 1990;141:727–733.

96. Ikezoe J, Johkoh T, Kohno N, et al. High-resolution CT findings of lung disease in patients who have polymyositis and dermatomyositis. *J Thorac Imag* 1996;11:250–259.

97. Mino M, Noma S, Taguchi Y, et al. Pulmonary involvement in polymyositis and dermatomyositis: sequential evaluation with CT. *AJR Am J Roentgenol* 1997;169:83–87.

98. Akira M, Hara H, Sakatani M. Interstitial lung disease in association with polymyositis-dermatomyositis: long-term follow-up CT evaluation in seven patients. *Radiology* 1999;210:333–338.

99. Prakash UB. Respiratory complications in mixed connective tissue disease. *Clin Chest Med* 1998;19:733–746, ix.

100. Prakash UB. Lungs in mixed connective tissue disease. *J Thorac Imag* 1992;7(2):55–61.

101. Franquet T, Giménez A, Monill JM, et al. Primary Sjögren's syndrome and associated lung disease: CT findings in 50 patients. *AJR Am J Roentgenol* 1997;169:655–658.

102. Tanoue LT. Pulmonary involvement in collage vascular disease: a review of the pulmonary manifestations of the Marfan syndrome, ankylosing spondylitis, Sjögren's syndrome, and relapsing polychondritis. *J Thorac Imag* 1992;7(2):62–77.

103. Salaffi F, Manganelli P, Carotti M, et al. A longitudinal study of pulmonary involvement in primary Sjögren's syndrome: relationship between alveolitis and subsequent lung changes on high-resolution computed tomography. *Br J Rheumatol* 1998;37:263–269.

104. Carignan S, Staples CA, Müller NL. Intrathoracic lymphoproliferative disorders in the immunocompromised patient: CT findings. *Radiology* 1995;197:53–58.

105. Johkoh T, Müller NL, Pickford HA, et al. Lymphocytic interstitial pneumonia: thin-section CT findings in 22 patients. *Radiology* 1999;212:567–572.

106. Meyer CA, Pina JS, Taillon D, et al. Inspiratory and expiratory high-resolution CT findings in a patient with Sjögren's syndrome and cystic lung disease. *AJR Am J Roentgenol* 1997;168:101–103.

107. Desai SR, Nicholson AG, Stewart S, et al. Benign pulmonary lymphocytic infiltration and amyloidosis: computed tomographic and pathologic features in three cases. *J Thorac Imag* 1997;12:215–220.

108. Rosenow EC, Strimlan CV, Muhm JR, et al. Pleuropulmonary manifestations of ankylosing spondylitis. *Mayo Clin Proc* 1977;52:641–649.

109. Fenlon HM, Casserly I, Sant SM, et al. Plain radiographs and thoracic high-resolution CT in patients who have ankylosing spondylitis. *AJR Am J Roentgenol* 1997;168:1067–1072.

110. Casserly IP, Fenlon HM, Breatnach E, et al. Lung findings on high-resolution computed tomography in idiopathic ankylosing spondylitis—correlation with clinical findings, pulmonary function testing and plain radiography. *Br J Rheumatol* 1997;36:677–682.

111. Cooper JAD, White DA, Matthay RA. Drug induced pulmonary disease: part 2. Noncytotoxic drugs. *Am Rev Respir Dis* 1986;133:488–503.

112. Cooper JAD, White DA, Matthay RA. Drug induced pulmonary disease: part 1. Cytotoxic drugs. *Am Rev Respir Dis* 1986;133:321–340.
113. Rosenow EC III, Limper AH. Drug-induced pulmonary disease. *Semin Respir Infect* 1995;10:86–95.
114. Colby TV. Anatomic distribution and histopathologic patterns in interstitial lung disease. In: Schwarz MI, King TE Jr, eds. *Interstitial lung disease.* St. Louis: Mosby–Year Book, 1993:59–77.
115. Bellamy EA, Husband JE, Blaquiere RM, et al. Bleomycin-related lung damage: CT evidence. *Radiology* 1985;156:155–158.
116. Aronchick JM, Gefter WB. Drug-induced pulmonary disorders. *Semin Roentgenol* 1995;30:18–34.
117. Padley SPG, Adler B, Hansell DM, et al. High-resolution computed tomography of drug-induced lung disease. *Clin Radiol* 1992;46:232–236.
118. Pietra GG. Pathologic mechanisms of drug-induced lung disorders. *J Thorac Imag* 1991;6(1):1–7.
119. Cooper JJ. Drug-induced lung disease. *Adv Intern Med* 1997;42:231–268.
120. Kuhlman JE, Teigen C, Ren H, et al. Amiodarone pulmonary toxicity: CT findings in symptomatic patients. *Radiology* 1990;177:121–125.
121. Rimmer MJ, Dixon AK, Flower CD, et al. Bleomycin lung: computed tomographic observations. *Br J Radiol* 1985;58:1041–1045.
122. Kuhlman JE. The role of chest computed tomography in the diagnosis of drug-related reactions. *J Thorac Imaging* 1991;6(1):52–61.
123. Rosenow EC, Myers JL, Swensen SJ, et al. Drug-induced pulmonary disease: an update. *Chest* 1992;102:239–250.
124. Searles G, McKendry RJR. Methotrexate pneumonitis in rheumatoid arthritis: potential risk factors. Four case reports and a review of the literature. *J Rheumatol* 1987;14:1164–1171.
125. Saxon RR, Klein JS, Bar MH, et al. Pathogenesis of pulmonary edema during interleukin-2 therapy: correlation of chest radiographic and clinical findings in 54 patients. *AJR Am J Roentgenol* 1991;156:281–285.
126. Ketai LH, Godwin JD. A new view of pulmonary edema and acute respiratory distress syndrome. *J Thorac Imaging* 1998;13:147–171.
127. Geddes DM, Corrin B, Brewerton DA, et al. Progressive airway obliteration in adults and its association with rheumatoid disease. *Q J Med* 1977;46:427–444.
128. Morrish WF, Herman SJ, Weisbrod GL, et al. Bronchiolitis obliterans after lung transplantation: findings at chest radiography and high-resolution CT. *Radiology* 1991;179:487–490.
129. Bellamy EA, Nicholas D, Husband JE. Quantitative assessment of lung damage due to bleomycin using computed tomography. *Br J Radiol* 1987;60:1205–1209.
130. Jules-Elysee K, White DA. Bleomycin-induced pulmonary toxicity. *Clin Chest Med* 1990;11:1–20.
131. Glasier CM, Siegel MJ. Multiple pulmonary nodules: unusual manifestation of bleomycin toxicity. *AJR Am J Roentgenol* 1981;137:155–156.
132. Cohen MB, Austin JH, Smith-Vaniz A, et al. Nodular bleomycin toxicity. *Am J Clin Pathol* 1989;92:101–104.
133. Santrach PJ, Askin FB, Wells RJ, et al. Nodular form of bleomycin-related pulmonary injury in patients who have osteogenic sarcoma. *Cancer* 1989;64:806–811.
134. Movsas B, Raffin TA, Epstein AH, et al. Pulmonary radiation injury. *Chest* 1997;111:1061–1076.
135. Logan PM. Thoracic manifestations of external beam radiotherapy. *AJR Am J Roentgenol* 1998;171:569–577.
136. Bush DA, Dunbar RD, Bonnet R, et al. Pulmonary injury from proton and conventional radiotherapy as revealed by CT. *AJR Am J Roentgenol* 1999;172:735–739.
137. Davis SD, Yankelevitz DF, Henschke CI. Radiation effects on the lung: clinical features, pathology, and imaging findings. *AJR Am J Roentgenol* 1992;159:1157–1164.
138. Libshitz HI. Radiation changes in the lung. *Semin Roentgenol* 1993;28:303–320.
139. Maasilta P. Radiation-induced lung injury: from the chest physician's point of view. *Lung Cancer* 1991;7:367–384.
140. Gross NJ. The pathogenesis of radiation-induced lung damage. *Lung* 1981;159:115–125.
141. Libshitz HI, Shuman LS. Radiation-induced pulmonary change: CT findings. *J Comput Assist Tomogr* 1984;8:15–19.
142. Ikezoe J, Takashima S, Morimoto S, et al. CT appearance of acute radiation-induced injury in the lung. *AJR Am J Roentgenol* 1988;150:765–770.
143. Mah K, Poon PY, Van DJ, et al. Assessment of acute radiation-induced pulmonary changes using computed tomography. *J Comput Assist Tomogr* 1986;10:736–743.
144. Crestani B, Kambouchner M, Soler P, et al. Migratory bronchiolitis obliterans organizing pneumonia after unilateral radiation therapy for breast carcinoma. *Eur Respir J* 1995;8:318–321.
145. Bayle JY, Nesme P, Bejui-Thivolet F, et al. Migratory organizing pneumonitis "primed" by radiation therapy. *Eur Respir J* 1995;8:322–326.
146. Bell J, McGivern D, Bullimore J, et al. Diagnostic imaging of post-irradiation changes in the chest. *Clin Radiol* 1988;39:109–119.
147. Ikezoe J, Morimoto S, Takashima S, et al. Acute radiation-induced pulmonary injury: computed tomographic evaluation. *Semin Ultrasound CT MR* 1990;11:409–416.
148. Bourgouin P, Cousineau G, Lemire P, et al. Differentiation of radiation-induced fibrosis from recurrent pulmonary neoplasm by CT. *Can Assoc Radiol J* 1987;38:23–26.
149. Becklake MR. Asbestos-related diseases of the lungs and pleura: current clinical issues. *Am Rev Respir Dis* 1982;126:187–194.
150. Staples CA. Computed tomography in the evaluation of benign asbestos-related disorders. *Radiol Clin North Am* 1992;30:1191–1207.
151. Aberle DR, Gamsu G, Ray CS, et al. Asbestos-related pleural and parenchymal fibrosis: detection with high-resolution CT. *Radiology* 1988;166:729–734.
152. Kagan E. Current issues regarding the pathobiology of asbestosis: a chronologic perspective. *J Thorac Imaging* 1988;3(4):1–9.
153. Akira M, Yamamoto S, Yokoyama K, et al. Asbestosis: high-resolution CT-pathologic correlation. *Radiology* 1990;176:389–394.
154. Craighead JE, Abraham JL, Churg A, et al. The pathology of asbestos-associated disease of the lungs and pleural cavities: diagnostic criteria and proposed grading schema. *Arch Pathol Lab Med* 1982;106:544–596.
155. Bégin R, Ostiguy G, Filion R, et al. Recent advances in the early diagnosis of asbestosis. *Semin Roentgenol* 1992;27:121–139.
156. Yamamoto S. Histopathological features of pulmonary asbestosis with particular emphasis on the comparison with those of usual interstitial pneumonia. *Osaka City Medical Journal* 1997;43:225–242.
157. Aberle DR, Gamsu G, Ray CS. High-resolution CT of benign asbestos-related diseases: clinical and radiographic correlation. *AJR Am J Roentgenol* 1988;151:883–891.
158. Schwartz A, Rockoff SD, Christiani D, et al. A clinical diagnostic model for the assessment of asbestosis: a new algorithmic approach. *J Thorac Imaging* 1988;3:29–35.
159. McLoud TC. The use of CT in the examination of asbestos-exposed persons [Editorial]. *Radiology* 1988;169:862–863.
160. American Thoracic Society. The diagnosis of nonmalignant diseases related to asbestos. *Am Rev Respir Dis* 1986;134:363–368.
161. Gaensler EA, Jederlinic PJ, Churg A. Idiopathic pulmonary fibrosis in asbestos-exposed workers. *Am Rev Respir Dis* 1991;144:477–478.
162. Klaas VE. A diagnostic approach to asbestosis, utilizing clinical criteria, high resolution computed tomography, and gallium scanning. *Am J Ind Med* 1993;23:801–809.
163. Gefter WB, Conant EF. Issues and controversies in the plain-film diagnosis of asbestos-related disorders in the chest. *J Thorac Imag* 1988;3:11–28.
164. Rockoff SD, Schwartz A. Roentgenographic underestimation of early asbestosis by International Labor Organization classification: analysis of data and probabilities. *Chest* 1988;93:1088–1091.
165. Staples CA, Gamsu G, Ray CS, et al. High resolution computed tomography and lung function in asbestos-exposed workers with normal chest radiographs. *Am Rev Respir Dis* 1989;139:1502–1508.
166. Kipen HM, Lilis R, Suzuki Y, et al. Pulmonary fibrosis in asbestos insulation workers with lung cancer: a radiological and histopathological evaluation. *Br J Indust Med* 1987;44:96–100.
167. Friedman AC, Fiel SB, Fisher MS, et al. Asbestos-related pleural disease and asbestosis: a comparison of CT and chest radiography. *AJR Am J Roentgenol* 1988;150:268–275.
168. Epler GR, McLoud TC, Gaensler EA, et al. Normal chest roentgenograms in chronic diffuse infiltrative lung disease. *N Engl J Med* 1978;298:801–809.
169. Epstein DM, Miller WT, Bresnitz EA, et al. Application of ILO classification to a population without industrial exposure: findings to be differentiated from pneumoconiosis. *AJR Am J Roentgenol* 1984;142:53–58.

170. Blanc PD, Gamsu G. The effect of cigarette smoking on the detection of small radiographic opacities in inorganic dust diseases. *J Thorac Imag* 1988;3:51–56.

171. Gamsu G, Aberle DR, Lynch D. Computed tomography in the diagnosis of asbestos-related thoracic disease. *J Thorac Imag* 1989;4:61–67.

172. Friedman AC, Fiel SB, Radecki PD, et al. Computed tomography of benign pleural and pulmonary parenchymal abnormalities related to asbestos exposure. *Semin Ultrasound CT MR* 1990;11:393–408.

173. Murray K, Gamsu G, Webb WR, et al. High-resolution CT sampling for detection of asbestos-related lung disease. *Acad Radiol* 1995;2:111–115.

174. Aberle DR, Balmes JR. Computed tomography of asbestos-related pulmonary parenchymal and pleural diseases. *Clin Chest Med* 1991;12:115–131.

175. Akira M, Yokoyama K, Yamamoto S, et al. Early asbestosis: evaluation with high-resolution CT. *Radiology* 1991;178:409–416.

176. Gamsu G, Salmon CJ, Warnock ML, et al. CT quantification of interstitial fibrosis in patients who have asbestosis: a comparison of two methods. *Am J Roentgenol* 1995;164:63–68.

177. Gevenois PA, de Maertelaer V, Madani A, et al. Asbestosis, pleural plaques and diffuse pleural thickening: three distinct benign responses to asbestos exposure. *Eur Respir J* 1998;11:1021–1027.

178. Lynch DA, Gamsu G, Ray CS, et al. Asbestos-related focal lung masses: manifestations on conventional and high-resolution CT scans. *Radiology* 1988;169:603–607.

179. Yoshimura H, Hatakeyama M, Otsuji H, et al. Pulmonary asbestosis: CT study of subpleural curvilinear shadow. work in progress. *Radiology* 1986;158:653–658.

180. Al-Jarad N, Wilkinson P, Pearson MC, et al. A new high resolution computed tomography scoring system for pulmonary fibrosis, pleural disease, and emphysema in patients who have asbestos related disease. *Br J Ind Med* 1992;49:73–84.

181. Kraus T, Raithel HJ, Lehnert G. Computer-assisted classification system for chest X-ray and computed tomography findings in occupational lung disease. *Int Arch Occup Environ Health* 1997;69: 482–486.

182. Kraus T, Raithel HJ, Hering KG. Evaluation and classification of high-resolution computed tomographic findings in patients who have pneumoconiosis. *Int Arch Occup Environ Health* 1996;68:249–254.

183. Friedman PJ. Lung cancer: update on staging classifications. *AJR Am J Roentgenol* 1988;150:261–264.

184. Harkin TJ, McGuinness G, Goldring R, et al. Differentiation of the ILO boundary chest roentgenograph (0/1 to 1/0) in asbestosis by high-resolution computed tomography scan, alveolitis, and respiratory impairment. *J Occup Environ Med* 1996;38:46–52.

185. Bergin CJ, Castellino RA, Blank N, et al. Specificity of high-resolution CT findings in pulmonary asbestosis: do patients scanned for other indications have similar findings? *AJR Am J Roentgenol* 1994;163:551–555.

186. Hillerdal G. Rounded atelectasis: clinical experience with 74 patients. *Chest* 1989;95:836–941.

187. McHugh K, Blaquiere RM. CT features of rounded atelectasis. *AJR Am J Roentgenol* 1989;153:257–260.

188. Taylor PM. Dynamic contrast enhancement of asbestos-related pulmonary pseudotumours. *Br J Radiol* 1988;61:1070–1072.

189. Westcott JL, Hallisey MJ, Volpe JP. Dynamic CT of round atelectasis. *Radiology* 1991;181(P):182.

190. Swensen SJ. Lung nodule enhancement at CT—Response. *Radiology* 1997;204:283.

191. Swensen SJ, Brown LR, Colby TV, et al. Lung nodule enhancement at CT: prospective findings. *Radiology* 1996;201:447–455.

192. McLoud TC, Woods BO, Carrington CB, et al. Diffuse pleural thickening in an asbestos-exposed population: prevalence and causes. *AJR Am J Roentgenol* 1985;144:9–18.

193. Im JG, Webb WR, Rosen A, et al. Costal pleura: appearances at high-resolution CT. *Radiology* 1989;171:125–131.

194. Hillerdal G, Malmberg P, Hemmingsson A. Asbestos-related lesions of the pleura: parietal plaques compared to diffuse thickening studied with chest roentgenography, computed tomography, lung function, and gas exchange. *Am J Ind Med* 1990;18:627–639.

195. Schwartz DA, Galvin JR, Dayton CS, et al. Determinants of restrictive lung function in asbestos-induced pleural fibrosis. *J Appl Physiol* 1990;68:1932–1937.

196. Kee ST, Gamsu G, Blanc P. Causes of pulmonary impairment in asbestos-exposed individuals with diffuse pleural thickening. *Am J Respir Crit Care Med* 1996;154:789–793.

197. Ren H, Lee DR, Hruban RH, et al. Pleural plaques do not predict asbestosis: high-resolution computed tomography and pathology study. *Mod Pathol* 1991;4:201–209.

198. Al Jarad N, Poulakis N, Pearson MC, et al. Assessment of asbestos-induced pleural disease by computed tomography—correlation with chest radiograph and lung function. *Respir Med* 1991;85:203–208.

199. Ameille J, Brochard P, Brechot JM, et al. Pleural thickening: a comparison of oblique chest radiographs and high-resolution computed tomography in subjects exposed to low levels of asbestos pollution. *Int Arch Occup Environ Health* 1993;64:545–548.

200. Steinberg DL, Webb WR. CT appearances of rheumatoid lung disease. *J Comput Assist Tomogr* 1984;8:881–884.

201. Rappaport DC, Weisbrod GL, Herman SJ, et al. Pulmonary lymphangioleiomyomatosis: high-resolution CT findings in four cases. *AJR Am J Roentgenol* 1989;152:961–964.

202. Sherrier RH, Chiles C, Roggli V. Pulmonary lymphangioleiomyomatosis: CT findings. *AJR Am J Roentgenol* 1989;153:937–940.

203. Remy-Jardin M, Degreef JM, Beuscart R, et al. Coal worker's pneumoconiosis: CT assessment in exposed workers and correlation with radiographic findings. *Radiology* 1990;177:363–371.

204. Im JG, Webb WR, Han MC, et al. Apical opacity associated with pulmonary tuberculosis: high-resolution CT findings. *Radiology* 1991;178:727–731.

205. Vix VA. Extrapleural costal fat. *Radiology* 1974;112:563–565.

206. Sargent EN, Boswell WD, Ralls PW, et al. Subpleural fat pads in patients exposed to asbestos: distinction from non-calcified pleural plaques. *Radiology* 1984;152:273–277.

207. Remy-Jardin M, Beuscart R, Sault MC, et al. Subpleural micronodules in diffuse infiltrative lung diseases: evaluation with thin-section CT scans. *Radiology* 1990;177:133–139.

208. Akira M. Uncommon pneumoconioses: CT and pathologic findings. *Radiology* 1995;197:403–409.

209. Hogg JC. Benjamin Felson lecture. Chronic interstitial lung disease of unknown cause: a new classification based on pathogenesis. *AJR Am J Roentgenol* 1991;156:225–233.

210. Genereux GP. The end-stage lung: pathogenesis, pathology, and radiology. *Radiology* 1975;116:279–289.

211. Snider GL. Interstitial pulmonary fibrosis. *Chest* 1986; 89[Suppl]: 115–121.

212. Fulmer JD, Crystal RG. Interstitial lung disease. *Curr Pulmonol* 1979;1:1–65.

213. Gaensler EA, Carrington CB. Open biopsy for chronic diffuse infiltrative lung disease: clinical, roentgenographic, and physiologic correlations in 502 patients. *Ann Thorac Surg* 1980;30:411–426.

CHAPTER 5

Diseases Characterized Primarily by Nodular or Reticulonodular Opacities

Because the presence of pulmonary nodules can be of great value in differential diagnosis, it is important to distinguish between true nodular disease and disease that merely appears nodular on chest radiographs. On plain radiographs, the finding of reticulonodular opacities is quite nonspecific, and its correlation with histology is often poor [1]. This radiographic pattern can reflect the presence of true nodules occurring in association with reticular interstitial thickening or the radiographic summation of purely nodular or reticular opacities [2–4]. On high-resolution computed tomography (HRCT), the presence of small nodules can be accurately diagnosed, even in patients who have extensive associated reticular opacities. Thus, the presence of nodular or reticulonodular interstitial disease can be much more precisely defined using HRCT than is possible on plain films. Furthermore, because of the absence of summation artifacts, the presence, size, number, and distribution of small nodular opacities can more accurately be assessed using HRCT than chest radiographs [5–9].

Diseases in which HRCT can identify the presence of small nodules include neoplastic processes such as lymphangitic spread of carcinoma, hematogenous metastases, bronchioloalveolar carcinoma (BAC), Kaposi's sarcoma (KS), lymphoproliferative diseases, lymphoma, and leukemia; sarcoidosis; silicosis and coal worker's pneumoconiosis (CWP); talcosis; amyloidosis; and mycobacterial and fungal infections. In patients who have lymphangitic spread of carcinoma, other neoplasms, sarcoidosis, and amyloidosis, nodules are often associated with reticular opacities, whereas nodules usually predominate with the other entities.

PULMONARY LYMPHANGITIC CARCINOMATOSIS

Pulmonary lymphangitic carcinomatosis (PLC) is a term that refers to tumor growth in the lymphatic system of the lungs. It occurs most commonly in patients who have carcinomas of the breast, lung, stomach, pancreas, prostate, cervix, or thyroid, and in patients who have metastatic adenocarcinoma from an unknown primary site [10,11]. PLC usually results from a hematogenous spread to lung, with subsequent interstitial and lymphatic invasion, but can also occur because of direct lymphatic spread of tumor from mediastinal and hilar lymph nodes [11]. Symptoms of shortness of breath are common and can predate radiographic abnormalities.

The radiographic manifestations of PLC include reticular or reticulonodular opacities, septal lines, hilar and mediastinal lymphadenopathy, and pleural effusion [12,13]. However, these findings are nonspecific. In one study, an accurate chest radiographic diagnosis was made in only 20 of 87 (23%) patients who had PLC [13]. Furthermore, the chest radiograph is normal in approximately 50% of cases of pathologically proven PLC [13,14].

The pulmonary lymphatics involved in patients who have PLC are located in the axial interstitial compartment (the peribronchovascular and centrilobular interstitium) and in the peripheral interstitial compartment (within the interlobular septa and in the subpleural regions) [1]. Tumor growth in the lymphatics located within these compartments and associated edema result in the characteristic HRCT findings of PLC [15,16]. As discussed in Chapter 3, this distribution of abnormalities has been termed *lymphatic* or *perilymphatic* [17,18].

High-Resolution Computed Tomography Findings

PLC is characterized on HRCT by reticular opacities, sometimes associated with nodules (see Figs. 3-12, 3-51, and 3-52; Figs. 5-1 and 5-2). Specific findings include: (i) smooth or nodular thickening of the peribronchovascular interstitium surrounding vessels and bronchi in the perihilar lung, (ii) smooth or nodular interlobular septal thickening, (iii) smooth or nodular subpleural interstitial thickening, (iv) thickening of the peribronchovascular axial interstitium in the centrilobular regions, and (v) preservation of normal lung architecture at the lobular level despite the presence of these findings [15,16,19–21] (Table 5-1).

Peribronchovascular interstitial thickening or peribronchial cuffing is commonly visible on HRCT in the perihilar lung, and can be diffuse, focal, or asymmetric (Figs. 5-1 through 5-5) [15,22,23]. The thickened peribronchovascular interstitium may be smooth, closely mimicking the appearance of bronchial wall thickening (see Fig. 3-4), or it can be nodular (see Figs. 3-51 and 3-52; Fig. 5-3) [15]; in both instances, the thickened interstitium is sharply marginated from the adjacent aerated lung. In patients who have peribronchovascular interstitial thickening from PLC, pulmonary artery branches adjacent to the bronchi also appear larger than normal, and nodular [15]; in other words, the size relationship of the thick-walled bronchi and adjacent vessels is maintained.

Stein et al. [20] performed an extensive analysis of the CT patterns of lymphangitic carcinomatosis, and found a localized or diffuse increase in reticular opacities and an increase in the number and thickness of interlobular septa in all patients who had PLC (Figs. 5-1 through 5-6). In patients who had PLC, interlobular septal thickening is often most pronounced in the peripheral lung regions. In the study by Stein et al., thickened septa appeared 1 to 2 cm in length, usually contacted the pleural surface, and were more numerous and thicker than similar septa seen in healthy control subjects. In lymphatic spread of carcinoma, the thickened septa usually appear smooth in contour. However, these may also have a beaded appearance resulting from tumor growth in the lymphatics, as contrasted with the irregular septal thickening seen in patients who have fibrosis (Figs. 5-1 through 5-3) [15,16]. In an HRCT study of postmortem lung specimens, 19 of 22 cases with interstitial pulmonary metastases showed the appearance of beaded or nodular septal thickening. The beaded septa corresponded directly to the presence of tumors growing in pulmonary capillaries, lymphatics, and the septal interstitium [16]. Smooth or nodular thickening of the subpleural interstitium is also commonly seen; this is easiest to recognize adjacent to the fissures.

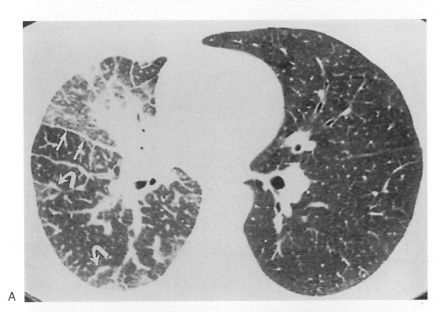

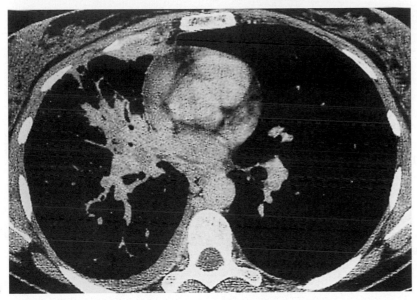

FIG. 5-1. Septal thickening in unilateral lymphangitic carcinomatosis. **A:** HRCT at a lung window setting in a 44-year-old woman who has adenocarcinoma demonstrates thickening of the interlobular septa (*curved arrows*) and major fissure (*straight arrows*), which is both smooth and nodular or beaded. Intralobular vessels appear abnormally prominent because of centrilobular interstitial thickening. There is also perihilar peribronchovascular interstitial thickening, as evidenced by apparent thickening of the bronchial wall and increased diameter of the hilar vessels. Note that even though there is septal thickening, there is no distortion of pulmonary architecture, as would be typical of pulmonary fibrosis. **B:** A mediastinal window setting demonstrates nodular thickening of the right peribronchovascular interstitium, right anterior pleural thickening, and a small right pleural effusion.

Stein et al. [20] observed septal thickening that outlined distinct pulmonary lobules (polygonal arcades) in approximately 50% of patients who had PLC (Figs. 5-3, 5-5, and 5-6). These lobules usually contained a visible central branching opacity, or dot, representing the centrilobular artery branch or branches, surrounded by the thickened centrilobular peribronchovascular interstitium. This appearance is one of the most characteristic HRCT features of PLC [20]. Prominence of the centrilobular artery is commonly seen in regions of lung in which septal thickening is present. In a distinct minority of patients who have PLC, centrilobular interstitial thickening predominates [7].

Five factors may account for thickening of the peribronchovascular interstitium, interlobular septa, and centrilobular axial interstitium seen on HRCT in patients who have PLC: (i) tumor-filling pulmonary vessels or lymphatics, (ii) the presence of tumor within the interstitium, (iii) distention of ves-

sels or lymphatic channels distal to central vascular or lymphatic tumor emboli, (iv) interstitial pulmonary edema secondary to tumor obstruction of the lymphatics, and (v) interstitial fibrosis secondary to the presence of interstitial tumor or secondary to long-standing interstitial edema [1,12,15,16]. In patients who have HRCT findings of PLC, pathologic studies [15,16] have shown that the visible thickening of the interlobular septa and peribronchovascular interstitium was caused mainly by interstitial tumor growth, rather than by vascular distension, edema, or fibrosis, although these abnormalities were also present [15,16].

In approximately 50% of patients, the abnormalities of PLC appear focal or unilateral, rather than diffuse. Focal disease may involve the axial interstitium mainly or exclusively, leading to thickening of the bronchovascular bundles, or mainly the peripheral interstitium, leading to thickening of the interlobular septa [23].

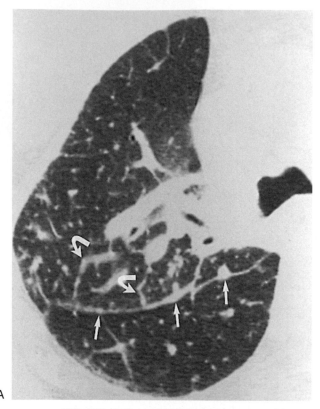

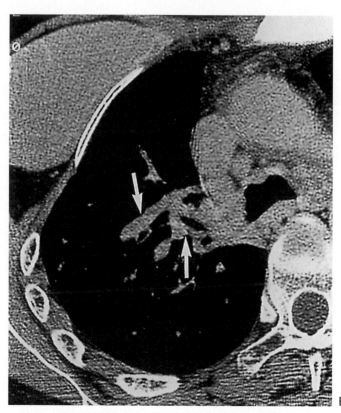

A   B

FIG. 5-2. Unilateral pulmonary lymphangitic carcinomatosis. HRCT at the level of the aortic arch in a 44-year-old woman who had a previous right mastectomy for adenocarcinoma, now presenting with unilateral right pulmonary lymphangitic carcinomatosis. **A:** Lung windows demonstrate nodular thickening of the interlobular septa (*curved arrows*) and interlobar fissure (*straight arrows*). **B:** Mediastinal windows show mediastinal lymphadenopathy and nodular thickening of the central peribronchovascular interstitium (*arrows*). Incidental note is made of right breast implant and right paratracheal lymphadenopathy.

It is characteristic of PLC that lung architecture appears normal despite the presence of abnormal reticular opacities; pulmonary lobules surrounded by thick septa are easily identified because the lobules appear normal in size and shape (Figs. 5-5 and 5-6). There is no distortion of lobular size or dimensions in PLC, as is typically seen in patients who have

interstitial fibrosis. The importance of this finding cannot be overemphasized; if there is lung distortion associated with findings that would otherwise be typical of PLC, another diagnosis should be considered. Although it is typical for abnormalities to progress, even in patients receiving chemotherapy, stable or slowly progressing abnormalities can be seen in some patients [24].

Hilar lymphadenopathy is visible on HRCT in only 50% of patients who have PLC, supporting the supposition that PLC is often the result of hematogenous spread of tumor to the interstitium, rather than central lymphatic obstruction with retrograde spread of tumor or edema [20]. In a study by Grenier et al. [25], lymphadenopathy was visible in 38% to 54% of patients who had lymphangitic carcinomatosis. Mediastinal lymph node enlargement can also be seen. Lymph node enlargement can be symmetric or asymmetric. Pleural effusion may also be present.

Utility of High-Resolution Computed Tomography

In patients who have PLC, characteristic HRCT findings can be seen in patients who have normal chest radiographs. In such cases, the HRCT findings tend to be focal and more

TABLE 5-1. *HRCT findings in lymphangitic spread of carcinoma*

Smooth or nodular peribronchovascular interstitial thickening (peribronchial cuffing)[a,b]

Smooth or nodular interlobular septal thickening[a,b]

Smooth or nodular thickening of fissures[a]

Normal lung architecture; no distortion[a,b]

Prominence of centrilobular structures

Diffuse, patchy, or unilateral distribution

Lymph node enlargement

Pleural effusion[b]

[a]Most common findings.
[b]Findings most helpful in differential diagnosis.

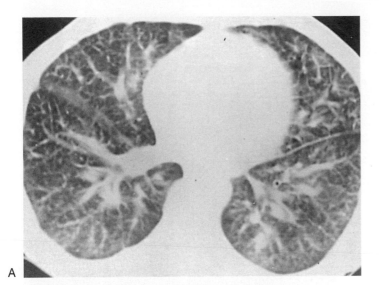

A

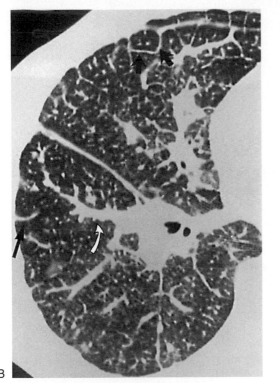

B

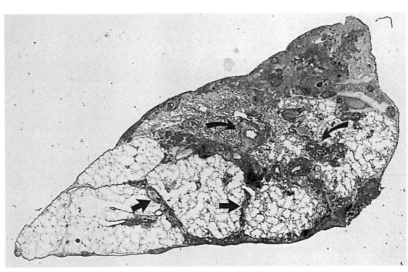

C

FIG. 5-3. Lymphangitic carcinomatosis and septal thickening in a 52-year-old man. **A:** Conventional 10-mm collimation CT scan shows prominence of the peribronchovascular interstitium and an ill-defined increase in the attenuation of both lungs. The appearance is nonspecific. **B:** HRCT at the same level targeted to the right lung demonstrates thickening of the peribronchovascular interstitium (bronchovascular bundles) which appears nodular (*curved arrow*), and shows septal thickening (*long arrow*) and thickening of septa surrounding lobules (i.e., polygonal arcades) (*short arrow*). **C:** Scanning micrograph of open-lung biopsy specimen shows thickening of the interlobular septa (*arrows*) and peribronchovascular interstitium (*curved arrows*), largely due to tumor deposits rather than fibrous tissue or edema. (From Munk PL, Müller NL, Miller RR, et al. Pulmonary lymphangitic carcinomatosis: CT and pathologic findings. *Radiology* 1988;166:705, with permission.)

pronounced in peripheral lung regions not well-visualized on chest radiographs [20]. Furthermore, conventional CT is not adequate for assessing the lung parenchyma in patients who have PLC; findings such as interlobular septal thickening, which are characteristic of PLC, are not often visible on scans obtained with 10-mm collimation [15,20].

Mathieson et al. [26] compared the diagnostic accuracy of HRCT to that of chest radiography in a study of 118 consecutive patients who had various chronic diffuse interstitial lung diseases. The CT and radiographic findings were independently assessed by three observers without knowledge of clinical or pathologic data. Of 18 patients who had lymphangitic carcinomatosis, a confident diagnosis was made on the chest radiograph in 20% of cases; this interpretation was correct in 64% of readings. By contrast, a confident diagnosis of lymphangitic carcinomatosis was suggested on CT in 54% of readings, the interpretation being correct in 93% of cases. Grenier et al. [25] assessed the relative value of clinical, chest radiographic, and CT findings in making a specific diagnosis of chronic diffuse interstitial lung diseases in 208 consecutive patients, of whom 13 had pathologically proven lymphangitic carcinomatosis. A confident diagnosis was made based on a combination of clinical and radiographic findings in 54% of patients who had lymphangitic carcinomatosis (the assessment being correct in 92%), and on a combination of clinical, radiographic, and CT findings in 92% (correct in all instances).

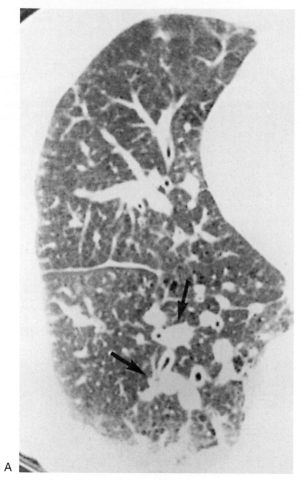
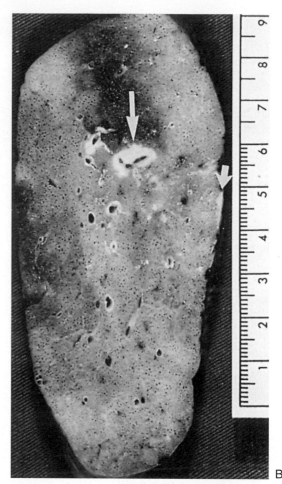

A

B

FIG. 5-4. Pulmonary lymphangitic carcinomatosis. **A:** HRCT in a patient who has lymphangitic carcinomatosis shows thickening of the peribronchovascular interstitium (*arrows*) and interlobular septa. **B:** Pathologic specimen in a different patient who has localized lymphangitic carcinomatosis. Note thickening of the peribronchovascular interstitium (*long arrow*) and subpleural interstitium (*short arrow*), due to lymphatic spread of tumor. (From Munk PL, Müller NL, Miller RR, et al. Pulmonary lymphangitic carcinomatosis: CT and pathologic findings. *Radiology* 1988;166:705, with permission.)

In a patient who has a known tumor and symptoms of dyspnea, HRCT findings typical of PLC are usually considered diagnostic, and a lung biopsy is usually not performed in clinical practice. In patients without a known neoplasm, HRCT can be helpful in directing lung biopsy to the most productive sites, as PLC is often focal [15]. Also, because transbronchial biopsy is usually positive in PLC, typical HRCT findings can also serve to suggest this as the most appropriate procedure.

Differential Diagnosis

Although peribronchovascular interstitial thickening and smooth septal thickening, often seen in patients with PLC, can also be seen in association with pulmonary edema, the differentiation of these entities can be made on clinical grounds. Also, nodular or beaded interstitial thickening is characteristic of PLC, but not pulmonary edema. In the study by Ren et al. [16], nodular septal thickening was not noted in

any pathologic specimens of patients who had pulmonary edema, fibrosis, or normal lungs.

However, it is clear that the presence of nodular septal thickening is a nonspecific finding that reflects a perilymphatic distribution of abnormalities, commonly seen in patients who have sarcoidosis [15,16] and less often visible in CWP or silicosis, lymphocytic interstitial pneumonia (LIP), and amyloidosis [6]. In sarcoidosis and CWP, although septal nodules are commonly seen, septal thickening is usually less extensive than that seen in patients who have lymphangitic spread of tumor; only an occasional patient who has sarcoidosis shows extensive nodular septal thickening. Moreover, in sarcoidosis and CWP, distortion of lung architecture and secondary pulmonary lobular anatomy may be visible, particularly if septal thickening is present; this distortion is not seen in patients who have PLC [27]. On the other hand, the presence of pleural effusion would be more in keeping with PLC than sarcoidosis or silicosis. The differentiation of PLC, sarcoidosis, silicosis, and CWP is discussed in greater detail in the discussion of sarcoidosis below.

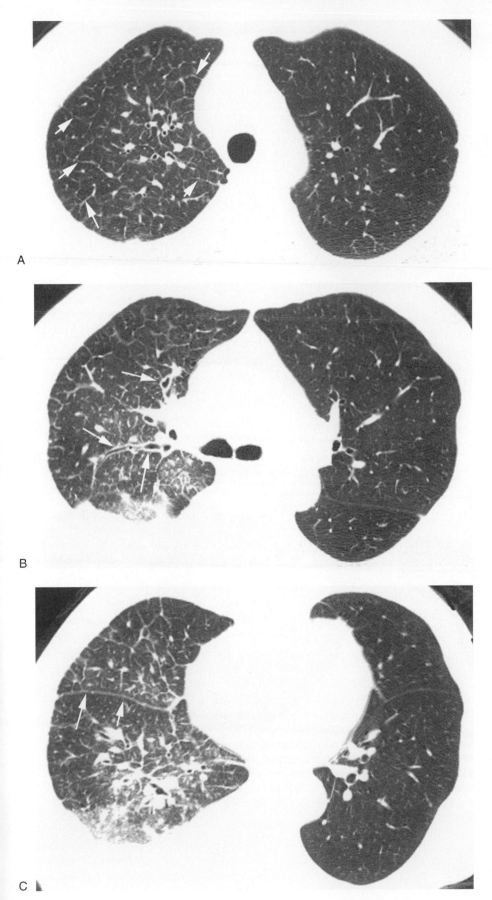

FIG. 5-5. A–C: HRCT in a 73-year-old man who has cough and shortness of breath. Smooth interlobular septal thickening is visible on the right (*arrows*, **A**), typical of pulmonary lymphangitic carcinomatosis. Thickening of the peribronchovascular interstitium (*arrows*, **B**) and right major fissure are also visible (*arrows*, **C**). Right pleural effusion is present. Bronchogenic carcinoma was diagnosed on bronchoscopy.

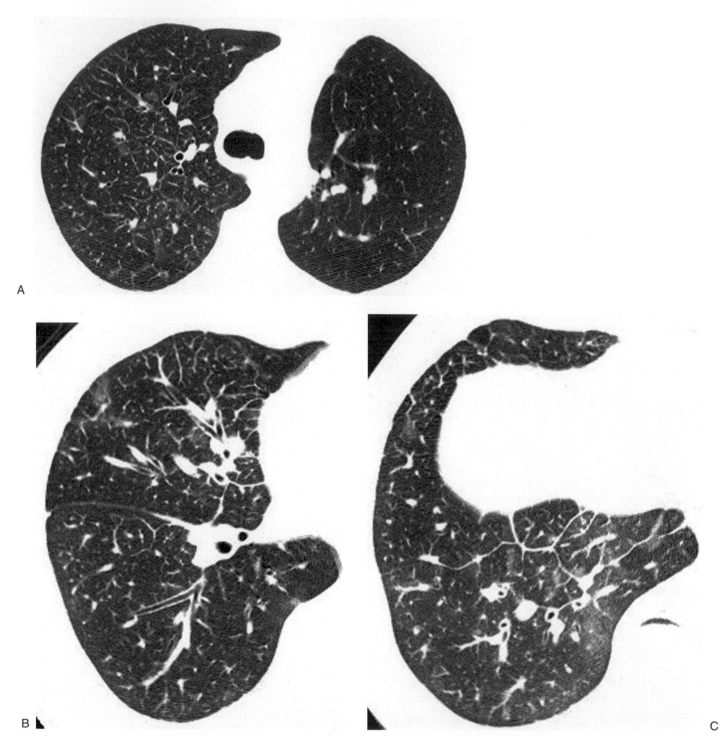

FIG. 5-6. A–C: HRCT at three levels in a patient who had prior partial left pneumonectomy for lung carcinoma. **A:** Scan through the right upper lobe shows smooth interlobular septal thickening and thickening of the peribronchovascular interstitium. There is no distortion of lung anatomy on the right, and lobules appear to be of normal size and shape. The left lung is reduced in volume because of surgery. **B,C:** Scans through the right lung at lower levels show a similar appearance. Transbronchial biopsy showed lymphatics invaded by tumor.

In pulmonary fibrosis, nodular septal thickening is uncommon, and the margins of the thickened interlobular septa are irregular. Distortion of the lung architecture and lung destruction (honeycombing) are common in patients who have fibrosis [21,28].

HEMATOGENOUS METASTASES

In many patients, hematogenous tumor metastases to the lung result in the presence of localized tumor nodules, rather than interstitial invasion, as occurs in PLC. Hematogenous metastases typically result in multiple large, well-defined nodules; in patients who have a history of carcinoma, this appearance on plain radiographs is usually sufficient for diagnosis. In some patients, however, widespread hematogenous metastases occur in the absence of a known primary tumor, resulting in the appearance of numerous small nodules. In such patients, HRCT may be obtained to define the abnormality, and may be valuable in suggesting the correct diagnosis.

High-Resolution Computed Tomography Findings

In patients who have hematogenous metastases, HRCT typically shows small discrete nodules with a basal predominance. When limited in number, nodules may be seen primarily in the lung periphery [11]; in patients who have innumerable metastases, a uniform or random distribution throughout the lung may be seen (Figs. 5-7 through 5-9) (Table 5-2) [17,29]. Typically, hematogenous metastases lack the specific relationship to lobular structures and interlobular septa that is seen in patients who have PLC. Nodules tend to appear evenly distributed with respect to lobular anatomy, or random in distribution [29,30]. Some nodules, however, may be seen as related to small branches of pulmonary vessels,

and this finding can be helpful in diagnosis. Although interlobular septal thickening and peribronchovascular interstitial thickening, common findings in PLC, are typically lacking in patients who have hematogenous metastases (Figs. 5-7 through 5-9), some overlap between the appearances of PLC and hematogenous metastases is not uncommon. This overlap in patterns is uncommon in other diseases and may be used to suggest the correct diagnosis (see Fig. 3-51).

To elucidate the HRCT characteristics of pulmonary metastatic nodules, Murata et al. [30] compared HRCT and pathology in five lungs obtained at autopsy from patients who had metastatic neoplasms. The relationship of metastatic nodules to lobular structures was studied using HRCT, specimen radiographs, and stereomicroscopy. Nodules were widely distributed throughout pulmonary lobules as seen on HRCT, and no predominance in specific lobular regions was noted. Eleven percent of small nodules (smaller than 3 mm in diameter) appeared centrilobular, 68% were intralobular, and 21% were seen in relation to interlobular septa. Similar results were reported by Hirakata and coworkers [29,31]. Occasionally, intravascular tumor emboli may result in nodular or beaded thickening of the peripheral pulmonary arteries (see Fig. 9-3) [32].

Detection of pulmonary nodules and assessment of their relationship to vascular structures is improved with the use of sliding thin-slab maximum-intensity projection technique (see Fig. 1-20) [33,34]. Using 1- to 3-mm sections and spiral CT, Napel et al. [33] devised a method for rapidly computing a series of either overlapping maximum- or minimum-intensity projection images through a thin slab of lung, retaining a normal superoinferior or axial orientation. This results in images of high contrast resolution allowing enhanced visualization of peripheral blood vessels in particular using maximum-intensity projection reconstructions. This approach has proved of some value for detecting micronodules in patients who have diffuse infiltrative lung disease [34].

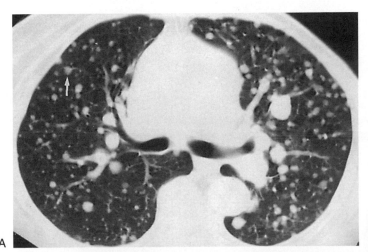
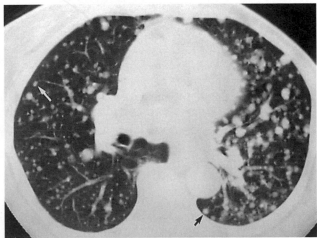

A   B

FIG. 5-7. A,B: Hematogenous metastases. The nodules are sharply defined. Although some nodules (*arrows*) appear to be related to small vascular branches, most nodules lack a specific relationship to lobular structures and appear to be random in distribution. Subpleural nodules are visible. Septal thickening is absent.

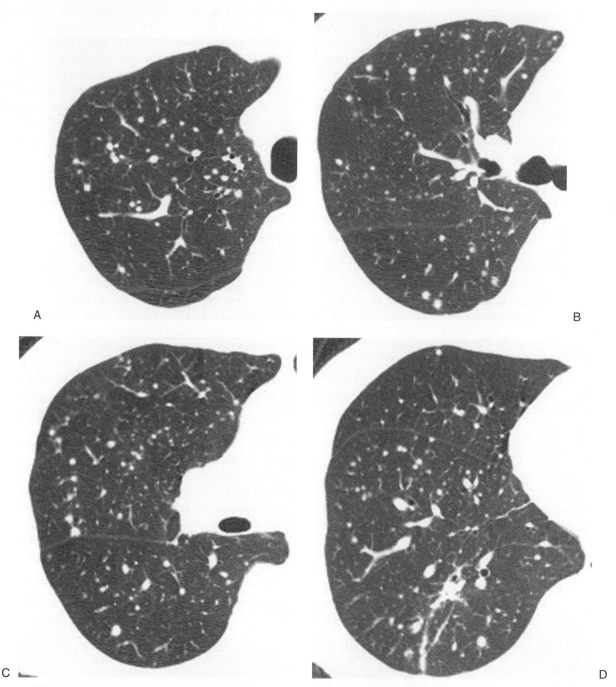

A

B

C

D

FIG. 5-8. A–D: Targeted views of the right lung in a patient who has hematogenous metastases. The nodules are small and sharply defined. There is involvement of the pleural surfaces, but overall the nodules appear to involve the lung diffusely. This pattern of distribution is termed *random*. Septal thickening is absent.

Utility of Computed Tomography and High-Resolution Computed Tomography

CT is clearly more sensitive than plain radiographs in detecting lung metastases [11]. In one study [35], plain radiographs, CT, and surgery were compared as to the number of nodules detected in 100 lungs from 84 patients who had previously treated extrathoracic malignancies and showed new lung nodules. Of 237 nodules resected, 173 (73%) were identified with CT. Chest radiography disclosed all resected nodules in 44% of cases, whereas CT disclosed all nodules in 78%. Two hundred and seven (87%) of the resected nodules were of metastatic origin, 21 (9%) were benign, and nine (4%) were bronchogenic carcinomas. Of those nodules seen with CT and not with radiography of the chest, 84% were of metastatic origin.

Several studies have shown that spiral CT is superior to conventional CT in the detection of pulmonary nodules. Costello et al. [36] documented in a study of 19 patients that spiral CT,

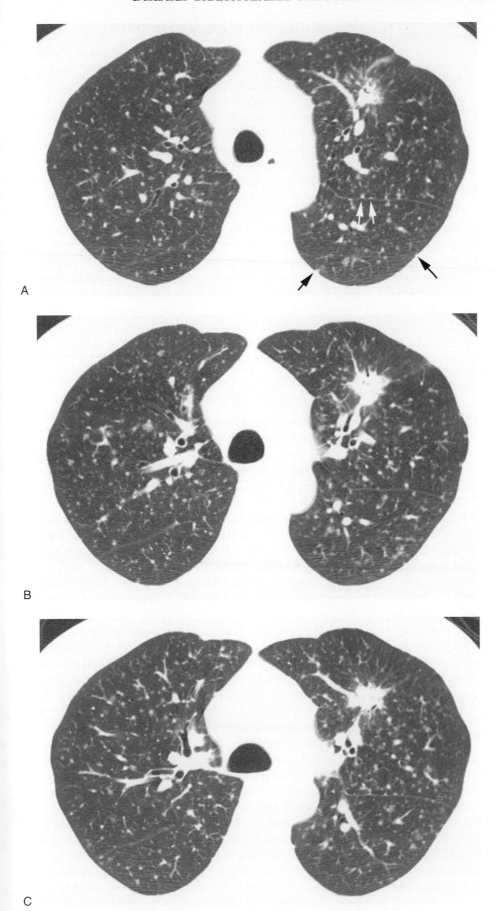

A

B

C

FIG. 5-9. A–C: Hematogenous metastases from a left upper lobe adenocarcinoma. The nodules are very small and sharply defined. Subpleural nodules are visible at the costal pleural surface (*black arrows*) and adjacent to the major fissure (*white arrows*). Lung involvement is diffuse.

TABLE 5-2. *HRCT findings in hematogenous metastases*

Smooth, well-defined nodules with a random and uniform distribution[a,b]

Some nodules visible in relation to vessels or pleural surfaces[a,b]

Features of lymphangitic spread of carcinoma may be present[a,b]

[a]Most common findings.
[b]Findings most helpful in differential diagnosis.

using 10-mm slice thickness with a pitch of one, detected 22% more nodules than conventional CT, using contiguous 8-mm sections. Remy-Jardin et al. [37] compared standard CT using sequential 10-mm sections to spiral CT using 10-mm sections with a pitch of one. In a series of 39 patients, the mean number of nodules detected per patient was significantly higher with spiral as compared to conventional CT (18 ± 4.5 vs. 12.6 ± 3.2), as were the number of nodules smaller than 5 mm (12.7 ± 3.7 vs. 8.4 ± 2.3) [37].

Munden et al. [38] assessed the clinical importance of nodules 1 cm or smaller detected on CT in 64 patients who had 65 nodules resected. Of the 64 patients, 37 (58%) had no known previous malignancy, and 27 (42%) had previous malignancy. Overall, 58% of these lesions were malignant. Among the patients without previous malignancy, 14 (38%) had lung carcinoma [10 (27%) primary bronchogenic carcinoma, four (11%) carcinoid]. In patients who had a previous malignancy, malignant lesions were diagnosed in 81% (22 of 27 patients). This included seven (26%) patients who had bronchogenic carcinoma as a second primary carcinoma. In patients who did not have previous malignancy, benign lesions were diagnosed in 59% (22 of 37 patients); in patients who had previous malignancy, benign lesions were diagnosed in 18% (5 of 27 patients).

Although HRCT may be used to characterize the distribution and morphology of lung nodules visible on chest radiographs in patients who have hematogenous pulmonary metastases, conventional or spiral CT technique, with contiguous or overlapping thick slices, is of more value in detecting pulmonary metastases in patients who have normal chest films [11].

Although spiral CT is superior to conventional CT in the detection of pulmonary nodules, it should be noted that small nodules can be missed, regardless of CT technique. Diederich and coworkers [39] assessed the sensitivity of spiral CT in 13 patients who underwent surgical exploration and resection of 90 nodules. Spiral CT was performed using 5-mm collimation and reconstruction intervals of 3- and 5-mm, and interpreted by two independent observers. For lesions detected by at least one observer, the sensitivity of helical CT was 69% for intrapulmonary nodules smaller than 6 mm in diameter, and 95% for intrapulmonary nodules larger than or equal to 6 mm in diameter. For lesions smaller than or equal to 10 mm in diameter, sensitivity was better using a reconstruction interval of 3 mm rather than 5 mm [39].

BRONCHIOLOALVEOLAR CARCINOMA

Bronchoalveolar carcinoma (BAC) can present as a solitary nodule or mass (43% of patients), as an area of focal or diffuse consolidation (30% of patients), or as a diffuse abnormality characterized by ill-defined nodules (27% of patients) [40]. In patients who have BAC, diffuse lung involvement may represent multifocal origin, endobronchial spread of tumor from a primary focus, hematogenous metastases, or a combination of these.

The most common presentation of BAC is as a solitary pulmonary nodule [40,41]. Solitary nodules have a typical spiculated appearance [42]. In 50% to 60% of patients, the nodules contain bubblelike lucencies or air bronchograms [41,42]. On HRCT, the nodule may be of soft-tissue attenuation, may be associated with both soft-tissue opacity and areas of ground-glass opacity, or present as a focal area of ground-glass opacity [41]. Ground-glass opacity results from the tendency of the tumor to spread locally using the lung structure as a stroma (lepidic growth) [41,43]. Focal BAC may progress to diffuse pulmonary involvement by bronchogenic spread [41].

High-Resolution Computed Tomography Findings of Diffuse Bronchioloalveolar Carcinoma

Patients who have diffuse lung involvement from BAC can show (i) patchy areas of consolidation, sometimes associated with air bronchograms or air-filled cystic spaces (Fig. 5-10) [44], (ii) patchy or multifocal ground-glass opacity with or without interlobular septal thickening (i.e., crazy-paving) (see Fig. 3-101) [45] (iii) extensive centrilobular airspace nodules (Figs. 5-10 and 5-11), or (iv) diffuse small nodules mimicking the appearance of hematogenous metastases (Fig. 5-10) (Table 5-3) [42,46]. In a study by Akira et al. [46] of 38 patients who had diffuse BAC, the predominant finding on HRCT was consolidation in 22 (58%), multiple nodules in 12 (32%), and ground-glass opacity in four (10%), although most patients showed a combination of these findings. Overall, HRCT findings in the series by Akira et al. [46] included consolidation (76%), ground-glass opacity (76%), nodules (74%), centrilobular nodules (68%), air bronchograms (47%), pleural effusion (13%), and lymph node enlargement (8%). A peripheral distribution was seen in 50% and a lower lobe predominance in 48%.

In patients who had multiple nodules as the predominant finding, nodule size ranged from 1 mm to 3 cm in diameter. The nodule margin was most often ill-defined, or associated with a halo sign, but well-defined nodules were also seen. The predominant nodule distribution most often appeared centrilobular, a finding likely reflecting endobronchial spread of tumor. Bronchocentric nodules were also common and may be due to lymphatic spread [46]. Nodules with a random distribution were less often visible; these may reflect hematogenous spread of the tumor. Cavitation of nodules was sometimes present.

Areas of consolidation or ground-glass opacity associated with BAC can represent the presence of intra-alveolar tumor growth, and mucin and fluid produced by the tumor; air bron-

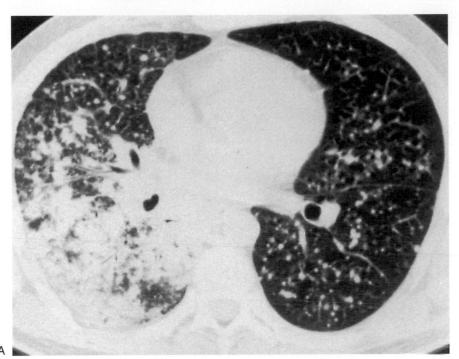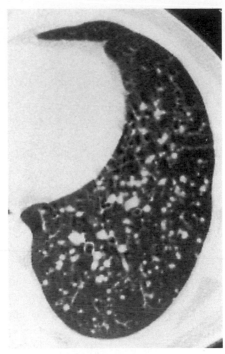

A   B

FIG. 5-10. Bronchioloalveolar carcinoma in a 34-year-old man. **A:** HRCT demonstrates areas of consolidation in the right lower lobe; ill-defined nodules, some of which appear to be centrilobular; and multiple, small, well-defined nodules. **B:** Targeted view of the left lung shows numerous small nodules, particularly in the left lower lobe. At least some of these nodules show a random distribution, similar to hematogenous metastases. Note the presence of subpleural nodules.

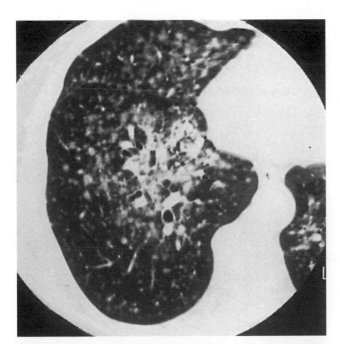

FIG. 5-11. Bronchioloalveolar carcinoma. Targeted HRCT image through the right lung. Ill-defined nodules are visible throughout the lung, and most appear centrilobular in location. Transbronchial biopsy was diagnostic.

chograms are commonly visible [42,47]. Centrilobular nodules are commonly associated, seen in 73% of patients in one study [46]. Also, because fluid and mucus produced by the tumor are of low attenuation, if CT is performed with contrast infusion, the *CT angiogram sign* can be seen. The CT angiogram sign is said to be present if contrast-enhanced pulmonary vessels appear denser than the surrounding opacified lung. In a study by Im et al. [48], the CT scans of 12 patients who had lobular or segmental BAC were reviewed; the CT angiogram sign was seen in nearly all of the patients. However, this sign is dependent on the volume and concentration of contrast injected and has been observed in bacterial pneumonia, lipoid

TABLE 5-3. *HRCT findings in diffuse bronchioloalveolar carcinoma*

Diffuse, patchy, or multifocal consolidation[a,b]
Ill-defined centrilobular nodules[a,b]
Combination of first two findings[a,b]
CT angiogram sign on enhanced scan[a]
Features of hematogenous metastases[a]

[a]Most common findings.
[b]Findings most helpful in differential diagnosis.

pneumonia, pulmonary lymphoma, pulmonary infarction, and pulmonary edema [49]. The CT angiogram sign is therefore of limited value in differential diagnosis.

Utility of High-Resolution Computed Tomography

In some patients who have consolidative or nodular lung disease, HRCT findings allow BAC and other diseases to be distinguished. In a study by Aquino et al. [50], the CT findings of consolidative BAC were compared to those of pneumonia to determine if CT findings allow distinction between these diseases. Findings seen more often on CT scans of patients who had consolidative BAC included coexisting nodules ($p = .001$) and a peripheral distribution of consolidation ($p = .001$) [50].

Akira et al. [46] also compared the findings of diffuse BAC with those seen in patients who had other diffuse lung diseases. In patients who had a nodular form of BAC, a centrilobular distribution was significantly more common than in patients who had miliary tuberculosis or pulmonary metastases. In patients who had consolidative BAC, a lower lung predominance was more common than in patients who had eosinophilic pneumonia and bronchogenic spread of tuberculosis (TB). Also, narrowing of involved bronchi, cavitation, heterogeneous consolidation, bulging of a fissure, and associated nodules were significantly more common in patients who had BAC than in those who had eosinophilic pneumonia.

CT can play a crucial role in the initial evaluation of patients who have BAC who appear to have limited and potentially resectable lesions, based on their plain radiographic appearance. CT can show the presence of diffuse disease when unrecognizable on plain films, indicating unresectability [51]. However, as pointed out by Zwirewich and others [52], CT is only 65% sensitive in detecting multiple adenocarcinomas.

KAPOSI'S SARCOMA

Approximately 15% to 20% of patients who have acquired immunodeficiency syndrome (AIDS) develop Kaposi's sarcoma (KS). KS is much more common among subjects who acquire AIDS through sexual contact; almost all cases occur in homosexual or bisexual men, and KS in intravenous drug users or patients exposed to HIV by different means is less frequent [53].

Pulmonary involvement occurs in 20% to 50% of AIDS patients who have KS [54] and is usually, but not always, preceded by recognized cutaneous or visceral involvement. Endobronchial lesions detected at bronchoscopy tend to predict the presence of pulmonary disease [55]. Chest radiographs typically show bilateral and diffuse abnormalities, characterized by the presence of interstitial opacities that are predominantly peribronchovascular, poorly defined nodules which can be several centimeters in diameter, and ill-defined areas of consolidation (Fig. 5-12) [53,55]. Pleural effusions that are usually bilateral are seen in 30% of cases. Hilar or mediastinal lymph node enlargement is apparent on the chest radiograph in approximately 10% of patients.

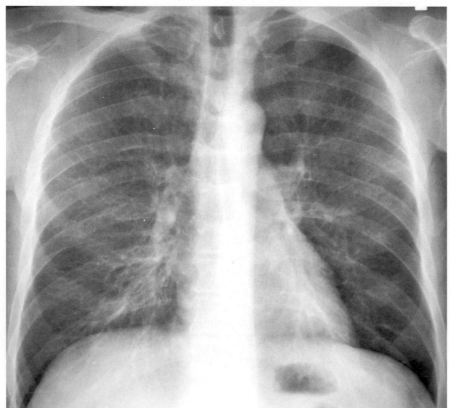

FIG. 5-12. Kaposi's sarcoma. **A:** Chest radiograph in a patient who has acquired immunodeficiency syndrome (AIDS) and Kaposi's sarcoma (KS) shows an increase in interstitial opacities, particularly in the right lung base. *Continued*

A

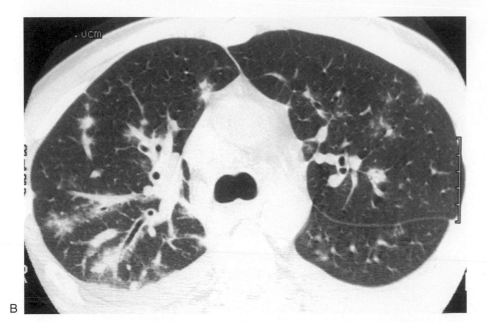

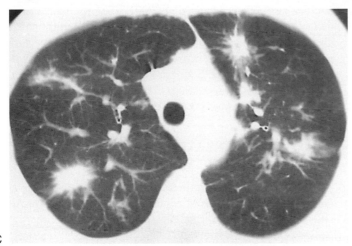

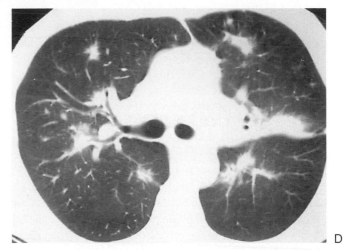

FIG. 5-12. *Continued* **B:** HRCT in this patient shows irregular peribronchovascular infiltration typical of this disease. Posteriorly, the opacities appear flame-shaped. The more abnormal right lung can be contrasted with the more normal appearance on the left. **C,D:** CT in a different patient who has AIDS and KS shows typical findings of ill-defined and irregular or flame-shaped nodules occurring predominantly in the perihilar and peribronchovascular regions. Several nodules surround bronchi or contain air bronchograms. There is also evidence of peribronchovascular interstitial thickening.

Computed Tomography and High-Resolution Computed Tomography Findings

Pathologically, pulmonary involvement in KS is patchy but has a distinct relationship to vessels and bronchi in the perihilar regions [54,56]. Early CT findings include thickening of the peribronchovascular interstitium, particularly at the lung bases, mimicking the appearance of infectious AIDS-related airways disease [54]. Typical CT features of KS in more advanced cases include irregular and ill-defined (flame-shaped) nodules that often predominate in the peribronchovascular regions, peribronchovascular interstitial thickening, interlobular septal thickening, pleural effusion, and lymphadenopathy (Figs. 5-12 and 5-13) (Table 5-4) [57]. The presence of these nodules is helpful in distinguishing the appearance of KS from that of AIDS-related airways disease [54].

In a study [53] of radiographs and CT in 24 patients who had intrathoracic KS, 22 of 24 patients (92%) had radiographic findings of bilateral perihilar opacities. CT scans obtained in 16 patients confirmed the presence of perihilar opacities in 14 patients (88%), with extension into the lung parenchyma along the peribronchovascular interstitium (Figs. 5-12 and 5-13). In a separate CT study of 13 patients who had KS [58], all had multiple flame-shaped or nodular lesions with ill-defined margins, which were usually symmetric (11 of 13 patients), and peribronchovascular and perihilar in distribution (9 of 13 patients). Ten also had pleural effusion, which was bilateral in nine. Five had mediastinal adenopathy, and two had hilar adenopathy. In a study by Hartman et al. [57] of 26 patients who had KS, the most common CT findings included nodules (85%), a peribronchovascular distribution of disease (81%), lymphadenopathy (50%), interlobular septal thickening (38%), consolidation (35%) or ground-glass opacity (23%), and pleural effusion (35%).

Utility of High-Resolution Computed Tomography

In most patients, the presence of typical nodules on CT and a perihilar distribution of abnormalities allow KS to be

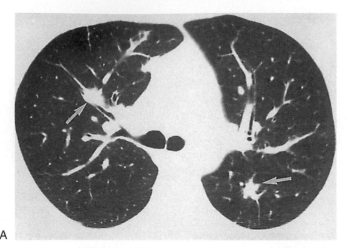
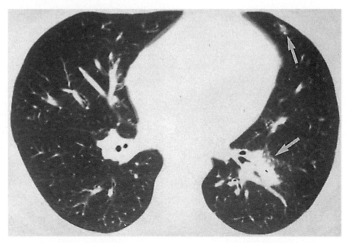

A

B

FIG. 5-13. A,B: Kaposi's sarcoma. HRCT in an acquired immunodeficiency syndrome patient with Kaposi's sarcoma (KS) shows ill-defined nodules (*arrows*) in the perihilar and peribronchovascular regions. This appearance and distribution is typical of KS.

distinguished from other thoracic complications of AIDS [54]. In the study by Hartman et al. [57], which included 102 patients who had thoracic complications of AIDS, the accuracy of CT in diagnosing KS was assessed in a blinded fashion. In patients who had KS, this diagnosis was listed first in 83% of cases and was listed among the top three choices in 92% [57]. Kang and coworkers [59] assessed the diagnostic accuracy of CT in 139 patients who had AIDS. The CT scans were interpreted by two independent observers. When the observers were confident in the diagnosis of KS, they were correct in 91% of cases (31 of 34 interpretations).

However, a number of other diseases in AIDS patients can be associated with the presence of pulmonary nodules and may therefore mimic the findings seen in KS. These include lymphoma, bronchogenic carcinoma, *Pneumocystis carinii* pneumonia (PCP), TB, nontuberculous mycobacterial infection, and bacterial, fungal, or viral infections [57,60]. Despite this, a correct distinction of KS from infection may often be made. In a study by Edinburgh et al. [61], CT scans in 60 HIV-infected patients who had multiple pulmonary nodules were evaluated for nodule size, distribution, and morphology. Thirty-six of 43 patients (84%) with opportunistic infection had a predominance of nodules smaller than 1 cm, whereas 14 of 17 patients (82%) with neoplasm had a predominance of

nodules larger than 1 cm (*p* <.00001). Twenty-eight of 43 patients (65%) with opportunistic infection had a centrilobular distribution of nodules, whereas only one of 17 patients (6%) with neoplasm had this distribution (*p* <.00001). Seven of eight patients (88%) with a peribronchovascular distribution of nodules had KS (*p* <.00001). This finding in association with nodule size of larger than 1 cm strongly predicted KS.

LYMPHOPROLIFERATIVE DISORDERS, LYMPHOMA, AND LEUKEMIA

Pulmonary lymphoproliferative disorders comprise a complex group of diseases, resulting in a spectrum of focal and diffuse lung abnormalities associated with either a benign or malignant course [62–65]. Many of these diseases are related to abnormal proliferation of submucosal lymphoid follicles distributed along distal bronchi and bronchioles, termed *mucosa-associated lymphoid tissue* (MALT) or, more specifically, *bronchus-associated lymphoid tissue* (BALT) [63,64]. BALT consists primarily of B lymphocytes, although T lymphocytes are also present.

Proliferations of BALT may be either hyperplastic or neoplastic, but a distinction between them may be difficult without analysis of cell populations, using immunohistochemical techniques. Polyclonal cellular proliferations demonstrated in this manner are usually hyperplastic and benign, whereas most monoclonal cellular proliferations are malignant [62]. However, in some cases, hyperplasia and neoplasia may both be present, and some conditions formerly thought of as benign have been shown to contain malignant elements or have malignant potential. Many examples of diffuse lymphoid hyperplasia or lymphoma occur in immunosuppressed patients or patients who have AIDS and appear to be associated with the Epstein-Barr virus (EBV) [66].

In patients who have lymphoid hyperplasia, the extent of lesions can vary, presenting as (i) a focal lesion or nodule (focal

---

TABLE 5-4. *HRCT findings in Kaposi's sarcoma*

Irregular and ill-defined peribronchovascular nodules[a,b]
Peribronchovascular interstitial thickening[a,b]
Interlobular septal thickening[a]
Pleural effusions[a]
Lymphadenopathy

[a]Most common findings.
[b]Findings most helpful in differential diagnosis.

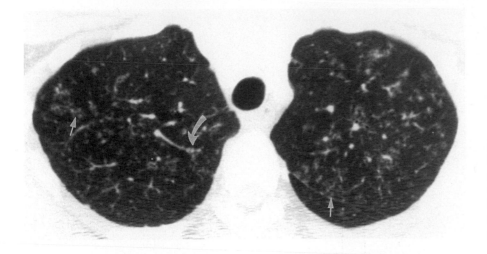

FIG. 5-14. Follicular bronchiolitis. HRCT in a patient who has rheumatoid arthritis shows small nodules in a centrilobular (*straight arrows*) and peribronchovascular (*curved arrow*) distribution. Also noted are subpleural nodules and nodules adjacent to the left interlobular fissure.

or nodular lymphoid hyperplasia), (ii) a multifocal proliferation largely limited to the airway walls (follicular bronchiolitis or follicular hyperplasia), or (iii) multifocal or diffuse lymphoid hyperplasia with interstitial involvement (lymphoid interstitial pneumonitis) [63,64]. Malignant pulmonary lymphoproliferative diseases and those having at least some malignant potential include: (i) angioimmunoblastic lymphadenopathy (AILD), (ii) primary pulmonary lymphoma, including MALToma and high-grade lymphoma, (iii) secondary pulmonary lymphoma, (iv) AIDS-related lymphoma (ARL), (v) posttransplantation lymphoproliferative disorder (PTLD), (vi) lymphomatoid granulomatosis, and (vii) leukemia.

Focal Lymphoid Hyperplasia

Focal lymphoid hyperplasia is an uncommon benign condition, characterized histologically by localized, polymorphous proliferation of benign mononuclear cells consisting of a mixture of polyclonal lymphocytes, plasma cells, and histiocytes [64]. The term *focal lymphoid hyperplasia* is used by some authors as synonymous with pseudolymphoma [62,64]. It is likely, however, that many lesions previously called *pseudolymphomas* are currently classified as MALTomas (see below) [63,67]; therefore, the term *pseudolymphoma* is not currently recommended.

The most frequent radiologic manifestation of focal lymphoid hyperplasia consists of a solitary nodule or a focal area of consolidation [62,68]. The nodules or nodular areas of consolidation usually measure 2 to 5 cm in diameter and contain air bronchograms [68]. There is no associated lymphadenopathy.

Follicular Bronchiolitis

Follicular bronchiolitis, defined as hyperplasia of BALT, is characterized histologically by the presence of diffuse proliferation of lymphoid follicles in the interstitial tissue adjacent to bronchi and bronchioles [63,69]. Follicular

bronchiolitis is commonly present in patients who have chronic bronchial inflammation (i.e., bronchiectasis), and is a common incidental finding on lung biopsy; this is termed *secondary follicular bronchiolitis*. Primary follicular bronchiolitis is much less common and is usually seen in patients who have a history of an underlying immunodeficiency (including AIDS), connective tissue disease (particularly Sjögren's syndrome or rheumatoid arthritis), or eosinophilia [63,69,70]. Primary follicular bronchiolitis is commonly associated with worsening dyspnea. Prognosis is related to age, with younger patients often having progressive disease [69]. Response to steroid treatment is variable [69].

In patients who have follicular bronchiolitis, chest radiographs characteristically show a diffuse reticular or reticulonodular pattern [69]. HRCT typically demonstrates small nodular opacities in a centrilobular and peribronchovascular distribution (see Fig. 4-21; Fig. 5-14) [70,71]. In the majority of cases, these measure 1 to 3 mm in diameter, although occasionally they can measure as much as 1 cm in diameter [70].

Howling and coworkers reviewed the HRCT findings in 12 patients who had biopsy-proved follicular bronchiolitis [70]. The predominant abnormalities consisted of small nodules and areas of ground-glass opacity. The nodules had a centrilobular distribution in all 12 patients, corresponding to the location of small bronchioles. In some patients, the centrilobular opacities had a branching appearance, reflecting the morphology of the small airways involved. Additional peribronchial nodules were present in five (42%) and subpleural nodules in three (25%) of the 12 patients. The nodules were diffuse but mainly involved the lower lung zones. Nine (75%) patients had patchy bilateral areas of ground-glass opacity. Additional findings seen in a small number of patients included mild interlobular septal thickening, bronchial wall thickening, and peribronchial consolidation [70]. Diffuse air-trapping on expiratory HRCT has also been reported in association with follicular bronchiolitis [72].

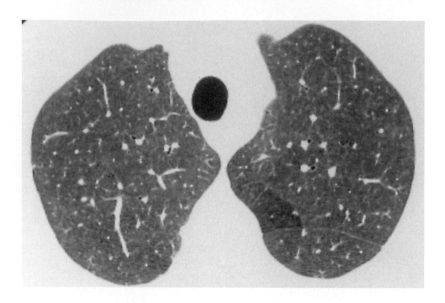

FIG. 5-15. Lymphocytic interstitial pneumonia in a 75-year-old man who has acquired immunodeficiency syndrome. HRCT demonstrates extensive bilateral areas of ground-glass opacity and small poorly defined nodules, some of which appear centrilobular.

Lymphocytic Interstitial Pneumonia

LIP is a benign lymphoproliferative disorder, characterized histologically by a diffuse interstitial infiltrate of mononuclear cells consisting predominantly of lymphocytes and plasma cells [63,73,74]. It is distinguished from follicular bronchiolitis in that the abnormality is not limited to the airways. LIP frequently occurs in association with other conditions, most commonly Sjögren's syndrome, AIDS, primary biliary cirrhosis, or multicentric Castleman disease [73,75,76]. Except for patients who have AIDS, in which affected patients are most often children, the majority of patients who have LIP are adults, with the mean age at presentation being approximately 50 years. The main clinical symptoms are cough and dyspnea.

The radiographic findings consist of a reticular or reticulonodular pattern involving mainly the lower lung zones [73,77,78]. Less common abnormalities include a nodular pattern, ground-glass opacities, and airspace consolidation.

High-Resolution Computed Tomography Findings

The predominant abnormalities on HRCT consist of diffuse bilateral areas of ground-glass opacity and poorly defined centrilobular nodules (Figs. 5-15 and 5-16); other common findings include subpleural nodules, thickening of the bronchovascular bundles (Figs. 5-17 and 5-18), cystic airspaces (see Fig. 4-36; Fig. 5-19), and patchy ground-glass opacity (Fig. 5-20) (Table 5-5) [76,79,80]. In some patients, the appearance of LIP may closely mimic that of lymphangitic spread of carcinoma (Fig. 5-18).

Johkoh and coworkers reviewed the HRCT findings in 22 patients who had LIP [76]. All patients had areas of ground-glass opacity and poorly defined centrilobular nodules. Small subpleural nodules were seen in 19 (86%) patients, thickening of the peribronchovascular interstitium in 19 (86%), mild interlobular septal thickening in 18 (82%), and cystic airspaces in 15 (68%) (Figs. 5-15 through 5-20) [76]. The cystic airspaces had thin walls, measured 1 to 30 mm in diameter, and involved

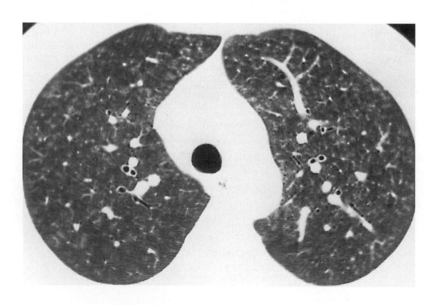

FIG. 5-16. Lymphocytic interstitial pneumonia in a 38-year-old woman who has acquired immunodeficiency syndrome. Ill-defined centrilobular nodules are visible diffusely.

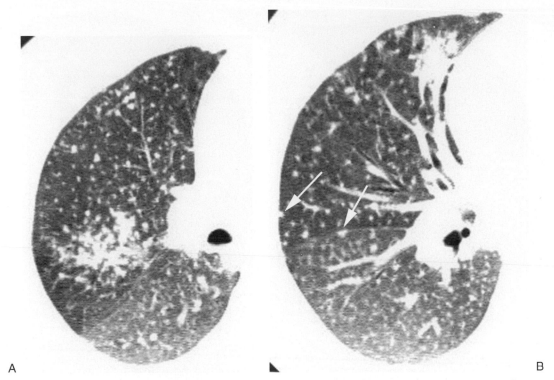

FIG. 5-17. Lymphocytic interstitial pneumonia in an 11-year-old boy who has acquired immunodeficiency syndrome. **A:** Extensive peribronchovascular nodules are visible. **B:** At a lower level, small nodules are visible in relation to the pleural surfaces and major fissure (*arrows*), and a large nodule is also present.

less than 10% of the lung parenchyma (see Fig. 4-36). Less common manifestations seen on HRCT include nodules 1 to 2 cm in diameter, airspace consolidation, bronchiectasis, and, occasionally, honeycombing [76,81]. Although lymph node enlargement is seldom evident on the chest radiograph, mediastinal lymphadenopathy was present on CT in 15 of the 22 (68%) patients reported on by Johkoh et al. [76].

Correlation of HRCT with pathologic findings has demonstrated that centrilobular nodules are due to peribronchiolar infiltration with lymphocytes and plasma cells, whereas the ground-glass opacities reflect a diffuse interstitial infiltration. The pathogenesis of the cystic airspaces is not clear, although it has been postulated that they may be due to partial airway obstruction by the peribronchiolar cellular infiltration [79]. Supporting this contention is a report of severe air-trapping in a patient with follicular hyperplasia of BALT [72].

In a study by Honda et al. [82], HRCT findings of LIP were compared to those in patients who had malignant lymphoma. Several significant differences in the appearances of these diseases were found. Cysts were more common in patients who had LIP (82%) than in patients who had malignant lymphoma (2%), whereas airspace consolidation and large nodules (11 to 30 mm in diameter) were more common in patients who had malignant lymphoma (66% and 41%, respectively) than in patients who had LIP (18% and 6%) ($p < .001$). Pleural effusions (25%) were seen only in patients who had malignant lymphoma.

Angioimmunoblastic Lymphadenopathy

Angioimmunoblastic lymphadenopathy (AILD) is an uncommon systemic disease that commonly results in intrathoracic lymph node enlargement [62,63,65]. In some cases, the lung and pleura are also involved. Histologically, abnormal lymph nodes show a proliferation of vessels and infiltration by a heterogeneous population of lymphocytes, plasma cells, and immunoblasts. T-cell proliferation is most common, and the Epstein-Barr virus genome has been detected in most cases. An association with drug treatment suggests that a hypersensitivity reaction may also be involved in the development of AILD. Progression to malignant lymphoma may occur, a condition termed *AILD-like T-cell lymphoma*.

AILD patients are usually over 50. Constitutional symptoms are typical with fever and weight loss; other findings include hepatomegaly, splenomegaly, rash, generalized lymph node enlargement, polyclonal hypergammopathy, and Coombs'-positive anemia [65]. The clinical course is variable with three distinct patterns being identified. Fifty percent of patients have rapid progression to death, 25% have prolonged survival with steroid and antineoplastic treatment, and 25% have prolonged survival without treatment.

The radiographic appearance of AILD is similar to that of lymphoma [62,63,83]. Approximately 55% of cases show extensive mediastinal and hilar lymph node enlargement. One-third of cases show lung involvement. Interstitial infiltration in the lower lobes associated with septal thickening or patchy con-

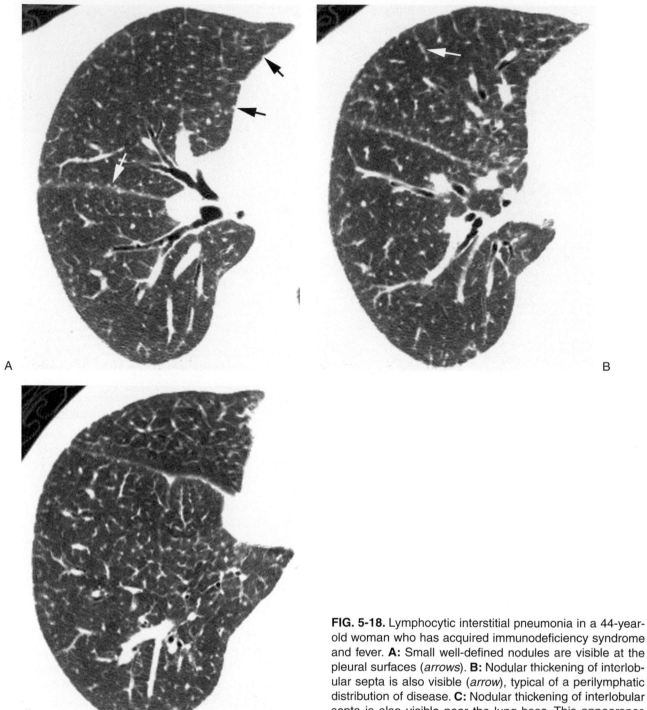

FIG. 5-18. Lymphocytic interstitial pneumonia in a 44-year-old woman who has acquired immunodeficiency syndrome and fever. **A:** Small well-defined nodules are visible at the pleural surfaces (*arrows*). **B:** Nodular thickening of interlobular septa is also visible (*arrow*), typical of a perilymphatic distribution of disease. **C:** Nodular thickening of interlobular septa is also visible near the lung base. This appearance mimics that of lymphangitic spread of carcinoma.

solidation are typical (Fig. 5-21) [83,84]. Pleural effusion may be present [62]. Enlarged lymph nodes may be enhanced if contrast infusion is used [85].

Primary Pulmonary Lymphoma

A pulmonary lymphoma can be considered primary if it shows no evidence of extrathoracic dissemination for at least 3 months after the initial diagnosis [65,86]. Primary pulmonary lymphoma is an uncommon neoplasm; in one study of 1,269 cases of lymphoma, less than 1% were deemed to have a pulmonary origin [87]. Primary pulmonary lymphoma is generally classified as a low-grade B-cell lymphoma (MALToma or BALToma) or high-grade lymphoma. Primary T-cell lymphomas may occasionally be seen but are relatively rare.

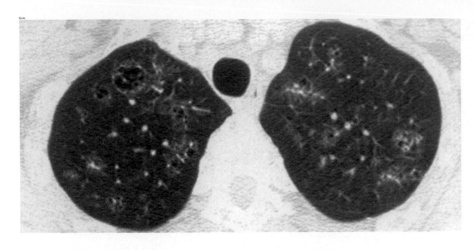

FIG. 5-19. Lymphocytic interstitial pneumonitis. HRCT demonstrates patchy ground-glass opacities and cystic spaces in both upper lobes.

Low-Grade B-Cell Lymphoma (MALToma or BALToma)

Low-grade (small lymphocytic) lymphomas account for more than 80% of primary pulmonary lymphomas. The majority is derived from MALT, hence the term *MALToma*, often used to describe the tumors [64]. In the lung, these tumors are believed to arise from cells present in BALT [88]. At least some of these tumors were previously classified as pseudolymphomas [63,67,68]. As the name suggests, patients who have primary pulmonary low-grade B-cell lymphoma generally have a good prognosis. For example, in one study of 43 cases, the overall 5-year survival rate was 84% [89].

The most common radiologic manifestation of primary low-grade B-cell lymphoma consists of a solitary nodule or a focal area of consolidation measuring from 2 to 8 cm in diameter (Fig. 5-22) [90–93]. Air bronchograms are visible in approximately 50% of cases [86]. Other patterns of lung involvement include a localized area of consolidation, which may range from a small subsegmental area to an entire lobe, or, less commonly, multiple nodules or multifocal areas of consolidation [94,95]. The parenchymal abnormalities typi-

cally show an indolent course, with slow growth over months or years [86,96].

On HRCT, multiple or solitary masses or areas of consolidation are most typical (Table 5-6). They may be seen as primarily peribronchial in location, and bronchi within the affected lung parenchyma may appear stretched and slightly narrowed [91,95,97]. Rarely, airway involvement is manifested by bronchial wall thickening and marked narrowing of the bronchial lumen [98]. Other findings seen on HRCT include centrilobular nodules, interlobular septal thickening, ground-glass opacities, or cystic or bubblelike lesions [92,97]. Pleural effusion is present in approximately 10% of cases, usually in association with evidence of parenchymal involvement [86,90]. Lymphadenopathy is evident radiographically in 5% to 30% of cases at presentation [90,97].

High-Grade Lymphoma

Most cases of primary high-grade pulmonary lymphoma are of B-cell type; occasional cases of anaplastic (Ki-1) lym-

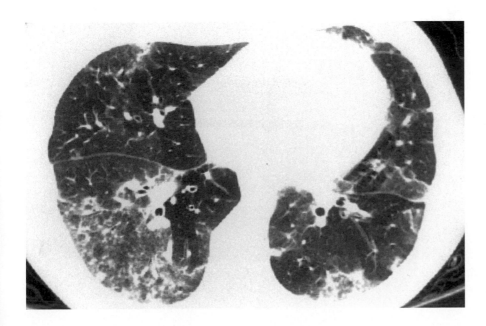

FIG. 5-20. 26-year-old woman who has lymphocytic interstitial pneumonia. HRCT demonstrates patchy bilateral ground-glass opacities and a few poorly defined centrilobular and subpleural nodules, best seen in the right lower lobe.

TABLE 5-5. *HRCT findings in lymphocytic interstitial pneumonia*

Ground-glass opacity[a]
Poorly defined centrilobular nodules[a]
Subpleural nodules[a]
Interlobular septal thickening or nodules[a]
Thickening of peribronchovascular interstitium[a]
Cystic airspaces[a,b]
Lymph node enlargement[a]

[a]Most common findings.
[b]Findings most helpful in differential diagnosis.

phoma or peripheral T-cell lymphoma have also been reported [99]. Some tumors occur in patients who have AIDS or organ transplants (posttransplant lymphoproliferative disorder); these are described below. The most common radiographic presentation consists of solitary or multiple nodules (Figs. 5-23 and 5-24) [91,96]. Lymph node enlargement may be present. Other manifestations include bilateral consolidation or a diffuse reticulonodular pattern.

Secondary Pulmonary Lymphoma

Pulmonary involvement in association with extrathoracic or diffuse lymphoma is more common than primary pulmonary lymphoma. In one review of 651 patients who had lymphoma, 54 (8%) had histologically documented pulmonary involvement [100]. Of these 54, the lung was the primary site of involvement in 21 (39%), whereas in 33 (61%), the lung was secondarily involved by tumor originating in a variety of distant sites [100].

Intrathoracic abnormalities are common in patients who have lymphoma, being seen at presentation in 67% to 87% of patients who have Hodgkin's disease (HD), and 43% to 45% of patients who have non-Hodgkin's lymphoma (NHL) [101–103]. In the majority of patients, intrathoracic disease is limited to lymph nodes. Pulmonary involvement is apparent radiographically at presentation in approximately 5% to 10% of patients who have NHL, and 10% to 15% of patients who have HD [101–105]. In patients who have HD, lung involvement at presentation is almost always associated with hilar or mediastinal lymph node enlargement [105]; this is not the case with NHL. However, radiographic and CT appearances of lung disease in HD and NHL are quite similar [96,100,106].

The most frequent CT and HRCT finding in secondary pulmonary lymphoma consists of solitary or multiple nodules, masses, or masslike consolidation, usually ranging from 0.5 to 8 cm in diameter, well-defined or ill-defined, and sometimes cavitary (Fig. 5-25) [100,102–104,106]. In one study, air bronchograms were visible in 47% of masses of NHL and 32% of masses of HD [106].

A diffuse reticular pattern with thickening of the interlobular septa may also be seen, closely mimicking the appearance of lymphangitic carcinomatosis (Fig. 5-26) [91,96]. This pattern may reflect interstitial tumor infiltration or lymphatic or venous obstruction by mediastinal or hilar tumor. Thickening of the peribronchovascular interstitium is seen in as many as 55% of cases [106], often associated with other findings. Patchy airspace consolidation with air bronchograms may also be seen [91,96,100] and is associated with a poor prognosis [100].

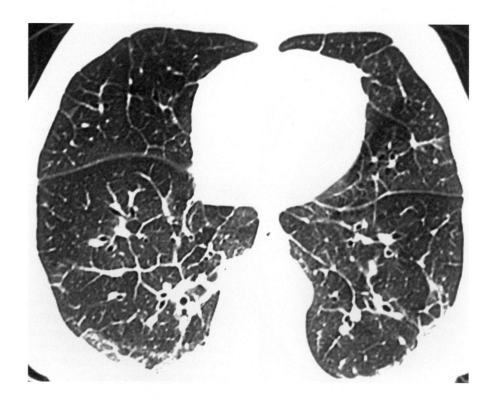

FIG. 5-21. Angioimmunoblastic lymphadenopathy-like lymphoma. HRCT shows extensive interlobular septal thickening. The appearance mimics that of lymphangitic spread of carcinoma.

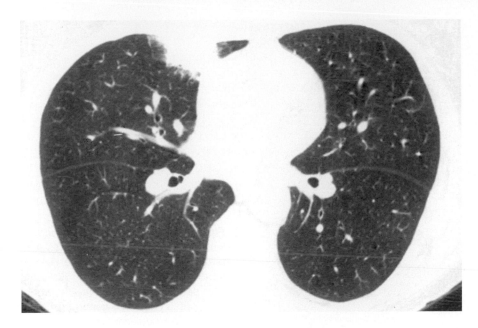

FIG. 5-22. MALToma. HRCT shows focal area of consolidation in the right middle lobe. Follow-up 6 months later showed no interval change. The diagnosis was proven at surgical resection. The patient was a 69-year-old woman.

Lewis and coworkers reviewed the conventional CT findings in 31 patients who had secondary pulmonary lymphoma [106]. The most common pulmonary parenchymal manifestations were nodules or masses larger than 1 cm in diameter or masslike areas of consolidation (68% of patients), and nodules less than 1 cm in diameter (61% of patients) [106]. The nodules often contained air bronchograms and had shaggy borders. Pleural effusion and lymph node enlargement were visible in 42% and 35% of cases, respectively.

Acquired Immunodeficiency Syndrome–Related Lymphoma

Lymphoma has an incidence of approximately 5% in patients who have AIDS [107]. The most common cell type is B-cell non-Hodgkin's lymphoma (NHL) [108]. Ioachim et al. [108] reviewed 111 cases of AIDS-related lymphoma (ARL), and 100 represented NHL, whereas 11 were Hodgkin's disease (HD). EBV has been implicated in some cases of both NHL and Hodgkin's lymphoma [108,109].

ARL is typically characterized by advanced clinical stage and high histologic grades. NHL in AIDS patients originates predominantly in extranodal locations and frequently involves multiple sites, including bone marrow, central nervous system, lung, liver, and bowel [108]. ARL is associated with advanced AIDS and low CD_4 counts [110]. ARL is characterized by high aggressiveness, frequent posttreatment relapse, and short periods of survival [108,109].

Thoracic involvement is common in patients who have ARL and is present in up to 70% of cases at autopsy [110]. In a study of 116 consecutive cases of ARL, 20 (17%) patients were considered to have thoracic involvement, and in 15 cases the thorax was the major site of disease [111]. In another study, 11 (31%) of 35 patients who had ARL had biopsy-proved thoracic involvement [112]. Primary pulmonary ARL is less frequent, and accounts for only 8% to 15% of cases [91].

Pulmonary nodules or masses are the most common radiographic and CT finding in ARL, typically ranging in size from 0.5 to 5 cm in diameter, although most nodules are larger than 1 cm (Fig. 5-27) [56,91,109,111–113]. The nodules are usually multiple and well-defined but may appear spiculated, and cavitation may be present. Localized consolidation or reticular opacities may also be seen. Pleural effusion is common, usually in combination with multiple nodules; this appearance is considered typical of ARL [112].

Mediastinal lymph node enlargement is more common in patients who have lung involvement occurring in association with disseminated ARL than it is in patients who have primary or localized pulmonary ARL. Node enlargement in association with thoracic ARL was seen in three of 11 patients studied by Sider et al. [112], and in 54% of patients studied by Eisner et al. [110], but it was not seen in two recent studies of primary ARL of the lung [109,113].

The clinical, radiographic, and autopsy features of 38 patients who had AIDS-related NHL associated with pulmonary involvement were reviewed by Eisner et al. [110]. Most patients had respiratory symptoms (87%) and signs (84%).

TABLE 5-6. *HRCT findings in low-grade B-cell lymphoma (MALToma or BALToma)*

Multiple or solitary nodules[a,b]
Multiple or localized areas of consolidation[a]
Air bronchograms[a]
Peribronchial distribution[a,b]
Slow growth[a,b]
Pleural effusion

BALT, bronchus-associated lymphoid tissue; MALT, mucosa-associated lymphoid tissue.
[a]Most common findings.
[b]Findings most helpful in differential diagnosis.

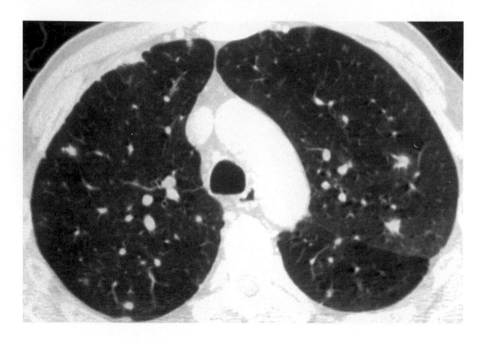

FIG. 5-23. High-grade non-Hodgkin's lymphoma. HRCT demonstrates bilateral nodules with irregular margins and focal areas of subpleural thickening. The patient was a 70-year-old woman who presented with generalized high-grade non-Hodgkin's lymphoma.

The majority of patients had advanced HIV infection, with a mean CD_4 count of 67 (± 65). Thoracic CT revealed pulmonary nodules (50%), lobular consolidation (27%), and lung mass (19%) as the most common parenchymal abnormalities. Pleural effusion was visible in 68% of cases.

Posttransplantation Lymphoproliferative Disorders

Several histologic patterns of lymphocyte proliferation, known collectively as *posttransplantation lymphoproliferative disorder (PTLD)*, can occur after bone marrow or solid organ transplantation [114,115]. The histologic patterns range from benign hyperplastic proliferation of lymphocytes to malignant lymphoma.

Most cases of PTLD have been associated with EBV infection, and it is likely that such infection is an essential step in the development of the majority of cases [114,116,117]. PTLD affects approximately 2% of transplant recipients [118]. The incidence is highest after lung transplantation, with PTLD being seen in approximately 6% to 9% of lung transplant recipients [66,119]. The majority of patients present in the first year after transplantation. PTLD can manifest as localized or disseminated disease, and has a predilection for extranodal involvement [66]. Lung involvement may occur as part of multiorgan disease or in isolation.

High-Resolution Computed Tomography Findings

The most common CT findings in PTLD include (i) single or multiple, small or large pulmonary nodules, which may be well-defined, ill-defined, or associated with the halo sign; (ii) patchy or focal consolidation or ground-glass opacity; (iii) a pre-

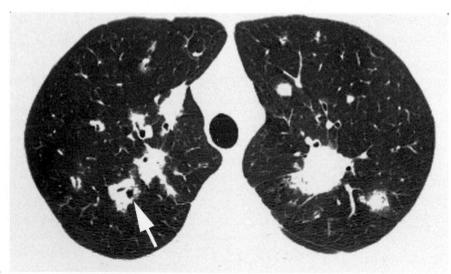

A

FIG. 5-24. A–C: High-grade T-cell lymphoma in a 33-year-old man. HRCT demonstrates well-defined nodules surrounding bronchi or containing air bronchograms (*arrows*). *Continued*

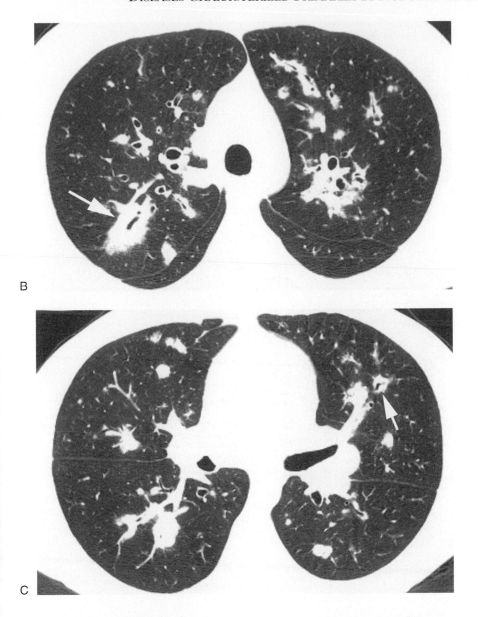

FIG. 5-24. *Continued*

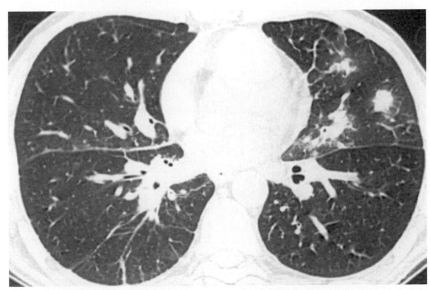

FIG. 5-25. Recurrent lymphoma. HRCT shows nodules in the lingula. Also noted is interlobular septal thickening in the lingula and right lower lobe. The patient was a 38-year-old woman who had recurrent non-Hodgkin's lymphoma.

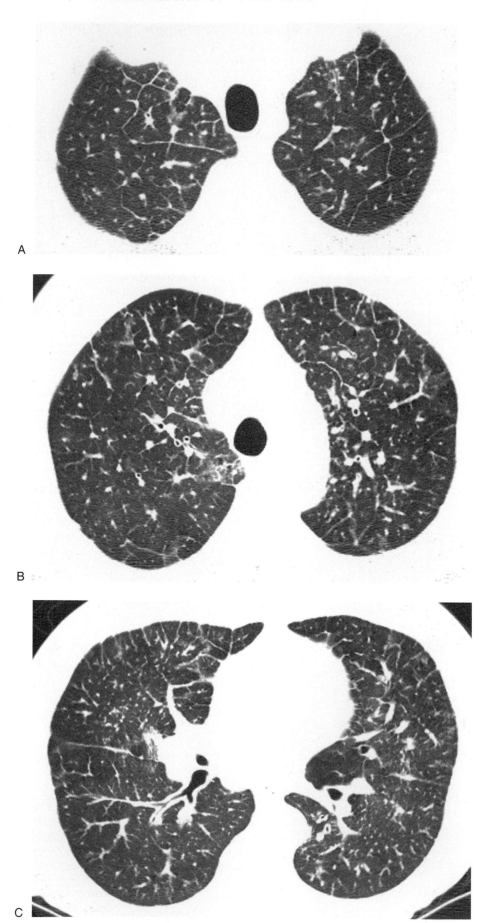

FIG. 5-26. A–C: Lymphoma with secondary lung involvement in a 79-year-old man. HRCT demonstrates extensive interlobular septal thickening, thickening of interlobar fissures, and peribronchovascular interstitial thickening identical in appearance to that of lymphangitic spread of carcinoma.

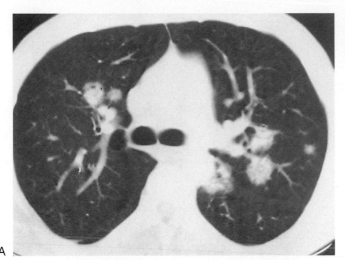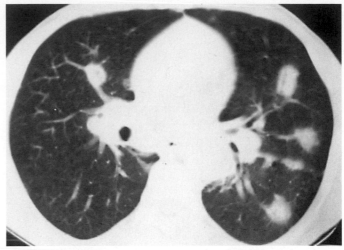

A
B

FIG. 5-27. A,B: Non-Hodgkin's lymphoma. CT in an acquired immunodeficiency syndrome patient who has non-Hodgkin's lymphoma shows ill-defined nodules, many of which are perihilar and peribronchovascular, or contain air bronchograms. This appearance mimics that of Kaposi's sarcoma.

dominantly peribronchial and subpleural or diffuse distribution of parenchymal abnormalities; and (iv) hilar or mediastinal lymphadenopathy (Fig. 5-28) (Table 5-7) [91,115,120,121]. In a review of the radiologic manifestations in 28 patients by Dodd and coworkers, nodules were identified on the chest radiograph or CT in 16 patients (57%) [120,121]. The nodules were well-circumscribed, measured between 0.3 and 5 cm in diameter, and were usually multiple and distributed randomly throughout the lungs. Patchy, predominantly peribronchial airspace consolidation associated with air bronchograms was seen in three patients, two of whom also had lung nodules. Mediastinal and hilar lymphadenopathy was seen in 17 of 28 (60%) patients, thymic

involvement in two, pericardial thickening or effusion in two, and pleural effusion in four.

Carignan et al. [121] reviewed the HRCT findings in four patients who had PTLD. All four patients had nodules on HRCT, two had hilar and mediastinal lymphadenopathy, and one had pleural effusion. In three of the four patients, a halo of ground-glass opacity was seen surrounding the lung nodules; this finding has been reported in other studies [115], and pathologic correlation showed the halo to be related to infiltration of the adjacent lung by a less dense infiltrate of lymphoid cells (Fig. 5-28) [122]. In another investigation of 17 patients who had PTLD, 15 (88%) had multiple nodules on CT, six (35%) had interlobular septal thickening, five

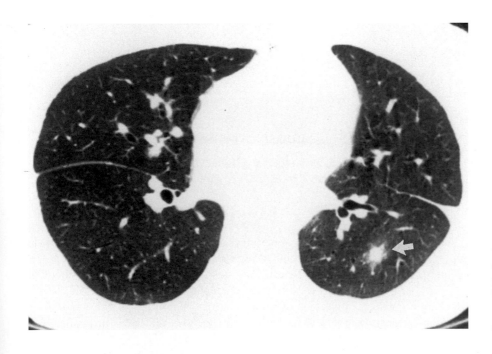

FIG. 5-28. Posttransplantation lymphocytic disorder after double lung transplant. HRCT demonstrates left lower lobe nodule with irregular margins and halo of ground-glass attenuation (*arrow*). Also noted is a small left pleural effusion.

TABLE 5-7. *HRCT findings in posttransplantation lymphoproliferative disorder*

Single or multiple nodules, well-defined or ill-defined[b]
Halo sign
Patchy or focal consolidation or ground-glass opacity[a]
Peribronchial, subpleural, or random distribution[a]
Lymph node enlargement

[a]Most common findings.
[b]Findings most helpful in differential diagnosis.

(29%) had areas of ground-glass opacity, four (23%) had areas of airspace consolidation, and five had hilar or mediastinal lymphadenopathy [66]. The nodules had a predominantly peribronchovascular or subpleural distribution.

Lymphomatoid Granulomatosis (Angioimmune Proliferative Lesion)

The term *lymphomatoid granulomatosis (angioimmune proliferative lesion)* is used to refer to a group of angiocentric, angiodestructive abnormalities characterized by a lymphoid infiltrate and a variable degree of cellular atypia [62,64,65]. Three grades are considered to exist based on the degree of cytologic abnormalities and necrosis, and their response to treatment [62]. Progression to histologically overt lymphoma may occur. B cells appear to constitute the primary neoplastic proliferation in patients who have lymphomatoid granulomatosis, although an exuberant T-cell reaction is present [64,123]. EBV has been detected in most cases investigated [62,123]. The lung is the primary site of disease, although other organs, including skin, brain, kidneys, and heart, may be involved.

Radiographic and CT findings consist primarily of bilateral, poorly defined nodular lesions, ranging from 0.5 to 8 cm in diameter, with a basal predominance [62,78,124]. Lesions may progress rapidly and cavitate, mimicking Wegener's granulomatosis. Pleural effusion may be present.

Leukemia

Pleuropulmonary infiltration is evident at autopsy in 20% to 40% of patients who have leukemia [125,126]. However, the radiographic abnormalities in these patients are seldom due to pleuropulmonary leukemic infiltration alone. In the majority of patients, parenchymal abnormalities seen on the radiograph are due to pneumonia, hemorrhage, drug-induced lung damage, or heart failure [127,128]. In an autopsy review of 60 patients who died from acute or chronic myelogenous or lymphocytic leukemia, radiographically demonstrable disease was related to hemorrhage in 74%, infection in 67%, edema or congestion in 57%, and leukemic infiltration in 26%; only 5% were radiographically normal [127].

The radiographic findings of pulmonary leukemic infiltration in the absence of other pulmonary complications

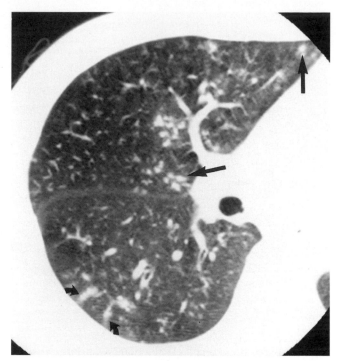

FIG. 5-29. Leukemia. HRCT targeted to the right lung demonstrates nodules (*straight arrows*) and nodular thickening of the interlobular septa (*curved arrows*). (Case courtesy of Dr. Takeshi Johkoh, Osaka University Medical School, Osaka, Japan.)

consist of bilateral reticulation that resembles interstitial edema or lymphangitic carcinomatosis. Heyneman and coworkers reviewed the HRCT findings of pulmonary leukemic infiltrates in ten patients who had histopathologically proven disease and no other concomitant pulmonary complications [129]. The predominant abnormalities consisted of interlobular septal thickening, seen in all patients, and thickening of the bronchovascular bundles, seen in nine patients. The septal thickening was smooth in six patients and nodular in four patients. Nodules measuring 5 to 10 mm in diameter were present in eight patients (Fig. 5-29). Less common findings included focal areas of ground-glass attenuation or consolidation [129].

SARCOIDOSIS

Sarcoidosis is a systemic disorder of unknown cause, characterized by the presence of noncaseating granulomas. These may resolve spontaneously or progress to fibrosis [130]. Sarcoidosis may involve almost any organ, but most morbidity and mortality is the result of pulmonary disease [131]. Pulmonary manifestations are present in 90% of patients, 20% to 25% of whom have permanent functional impairment [131].

Pathologically, the most characteristic feature of sarcoidosis is the presence of noncaseating granulomas in a lymphatic or perilymphatic distribution [17]. The granulomas are well formed, with histiocytes centrally, surrounded by a

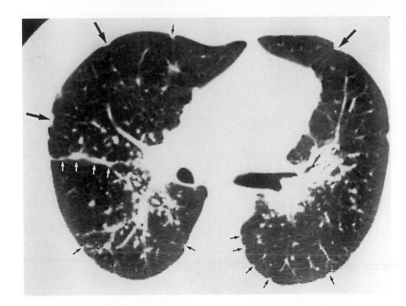

FIG. 5-30. Sarcoidosis with a perilymphatic distribution of nodules. Numerous small nodules are seen in relation to the perihilar, bronchovascular interstitium. Bronchial walls appear irregularly thickened. Subpleural nodules (*small arrows*) are seen bordering the costal pleural surfaces and right major fissure. This appearance is virtually diagnostic of sarcoidosis. Clusters of subpleural granulomas (*large arrows*) have been termed *pseudoplaques*.

collarette of lymphocytes and mononuclear cells [132,133]. Although some investigators believe that alveolitis is the initial pathologic lesion in sarcoidosis, and that alveolitis is essential to the development of sarcoid granulomas and lung fibrosis in these patients [133–136], this hypothesis is based primarily on indirect evidence from findings on bronchoalveolar lavage (BAL) and gallium scintigraphy [135,136]. The lung parenchyma between granulomas is usually normal in patients who have sarcoidosis, and although there may be a mononuclear infiltrate in the alveolar walls immediately adjacent to a granuloma, there is usually no discernible evidence of a diffuse alveolitis [137].

Approximately 60% to 70% of patients who have sarcoidosis have characteristic radiologic findings. These consist of symmetric, bilateral hilar and paratracheal lymphadenopathy, with or without concomitant parenchymal abnormalities [138–140]. In 25% to 30% of cases, however, the radiologic findings are nonspecific or atypical, and in 5% to 10% of patients, the chest radiograph is normal [130,131,138–142].

Sarcoid granulomas, which are the hallmark of this disease, are distributed primarily along the lymphatics in the peribronchovascular interstitial space (both in the perihilar regions and lobular core), and, to a lesser extent, in the interlobular septa and subpleural interstitial space. This characteristic perilymphatic distribution of sarcoid granulomas is difficult to recognize on plain radiographs, but is clearly seen on HRCT (see Figs. 3-44 through 3-47; Figs. 5-30 through 5-32) and in macroscopic illustrations of the pathology of this disease [18,130,133,143–146]. The perilymphatic distribution of granulomas is one of the features of sarcoidosis that is most helpful in making a pathologic diagnosis, and is also responsible for the high rate of success of diagnosis by bronchial and transbronchial biopsy [130]. Although sarcoid granulomas are microscopic, they often coalesce to form macroscopic nodules several millimeters in diameter.

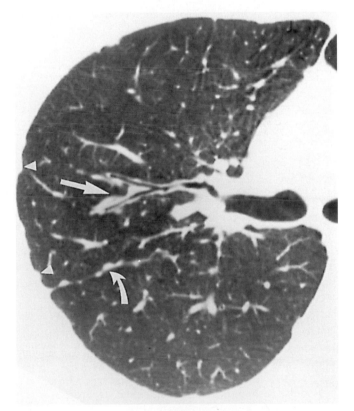

FIG. 5-31. Perilymphatic nodules in a 41-year-old man with sarcoidosis. HRCT at the level of the right upper lobe bronchus shows nodular thickening of the peribronchovascular interstitium (*straight arrow*) and right major fissure (*curved arrow*). Also visible are numerous subpleural nodules (*arrowheads*). (From Müller NL, Kullnig P, Miller RR. The CT findings of pulmonary sarcoidosis: analysis of 25 patients. *AJR Am J Roentgenol* 1989;152:1179, with permission.)

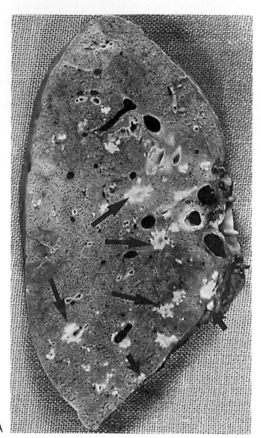
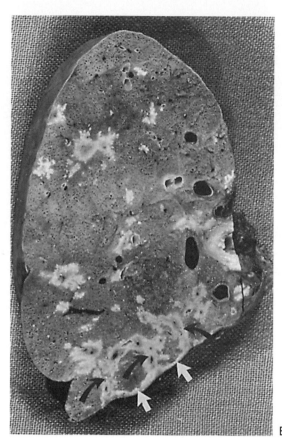

FIG. 5-32. Sarcoidosis with perilymphatic nodules. **A,B:** Gross pathologic specimen cut in the transverse plane, at two levels through the right upper lobe in a 55-year-old woman who has sarcoidosis. Noncaseating sarcoid granulomas are located within the peribronchovascular interstitium (*long arrows*), subpleural regions (*short arrows*), and to a lesser extent in relation to interlobular septa containing veins (*curved arrows*) in **B**. (From Müller NL, Kullnig P, Miller RR. The CT findings of pulmonary sarcoidosis: analysis of 25 patients. *AJR Am J Roentgenol* 1989;152:1179; and Müller NL, Miller RR. Computed tomography of chronic diffuse infiltrative lung disease: part 2. *Am Rev Respir Dis* 1990;142:1440, with permission.)

High-Resolution Computed Tomography Findings

The most characteristic HRCT abnormality in patients who have sarcoidosis consists of small nodules in a perilymphatic distribution, visible in relation to (i) the peribronchovascular regions, adjacent to the perihilar vessels and bronchi, (ii) the fissures, (iii) the costal subpleural regions, (iv) interlobular septa, and (v) the centrilobular regions (Figs. 5-30 through 5-34) [27,143,147–150] (Table 5-8). However, the degree to which these structures are involved varies considerably among individual patients (Figs. 5-35 through 5-41).

Nodules visible on HRCT can appear as small as a few millimeters in diameter; they tend to be sharply defined despite their small size. In most cases, these nodules represent coalescent groups of microscopic granulomas (Figs. 5-32 through 5-41) [148,151,152], although nodules visible on HRCT can also represent nodular areas of fibrosis [148]. The nodules may be numerous and distributed throughout both lungs. However, in up to 50% of patients, the nodularity may be scanty or focal, localized to small areas in one or both

lungs (Fig. 5-36). An upper lobe predominance is common (Fig. 5-36), but not invariable (Fig. 5-37).

Sarcoid granulomas frequently cause nodular thickening of the perihilar, peribronchovascular interstitium as seen on HRCT, and extensive peribronchovascular nodularity is characteristic and highly suggestive of this disease (Figs. 5-30, 5-32, 5-35, 5-39). Subpleural nodules are also typical of sarcoidosis [18,143]. Irregular or nodular interlobular septal thickening is apparent in the majority of patients (Figs. 5-34, 5-37, 5-38), but in most patients is not extensive [142,153]. On the other hand, in some patients, interlobular septal thickening may be a predominant feature of this disease (Figs. 5-37 and 5-38). Granulomas occurring in relation to the peribronchovascular interstitium in the lobular core can be seen as centrilobular nodules on HRCT, but other findings indicative of a perilymphatic distribution are usually visible (see Fig. 3-45) [7].

Confluence of granulomas may result in large opacities with ill-defined contours or areas of frank consolidation (Figs. 5-34, 5-39, 5-40) [27,150]. Large nodules measuring from 1 to 4 cm in diameter were seen in 15% to 25% of

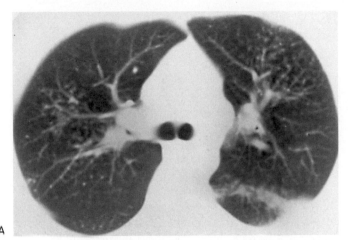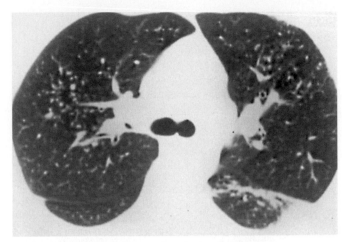

A B

FIG. 5-33. Sarcoidosis in a 28-year-old man. **A:** A 10-mm collimation scan at the level of the tracheal carina shows bilateral hilar lymphadenopathy and nodules in a predominantly peribronchovascular distribution. **B:** A 1.5-mm collimation scan (standard algorithm) at the same level. The peribronchovascular distribution of the nodules is more difficult to appreciate, but the individual nodules are more clearly seen. Note the patchy distribution of the abnormalities. An area of increased attenuation in the superior segment of the left lower lobe is presumably due to conglomeration of subpleural granulomas. (From Müller NL, Kullnig P, Miller RR. The CT findings of pulmonary sarcoidosis: analysis of 25 patients. *AJR Am J Roentgenol* 1989;152:1179, with permission.)

patients in several studies (see Fig. 3-48) [143,147,151,154]. Grenier et al. [155] reported the presence of confluent nodules larger than 1 cm in 53% of patients who had sarcoidosis. In our experience, these predominate in the upper lobes and the peribronchovascular regions. Air bronchograms may be seen within these nodules. Large nodules can also cavitate, but this is uncommon; Grenier et al. [155] reported this finding in only 3% of cases.

Patients who have sarcoidosis sometimes show patchy areas of ground-glass opacity on HRCT (Figs. 5-40 through 5-42), which may be superimposed on a background of interstitial nodules or fibrosis. Correlation of ground-glass opacity in patients who have sarcoidosis with pathologic specimens has been obtained in a small number of patients [143,151,156]. The results of these correlations suggest that areas of ground-glass opacity usually are due to the presence

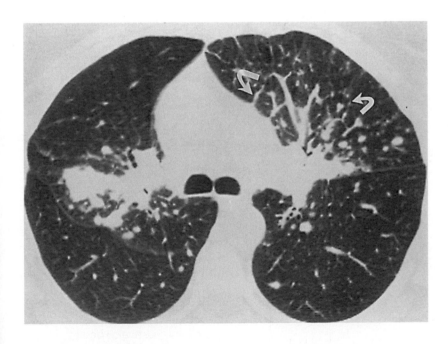

FIG. 5-34. Septal thickening in a 68-year-old woman with sarcoidosis. HRCT at the level of the tracheal carina shows bilateral hilar lymphadenopathy and nodules in a central peribronchovascular distribution. Nodular thickening of the interlobular septa is present, particularly on the left side (*arrows*).

TABLE 5-8. *HRCT findings in sarcoidosis*

Smooth or nodular peribronchovascular interstitial thickening (peribronchial cuffing)[a,b]

Small, well-defined nodules in relation to the pleural surfaces, interlobular septa, centrilobular structures[a,b]

Peribronchovascular distribution of nodules in the central lung and upper lobes[a,b]

Large nodules (>1 cm) or consolidation[a]

Ground-glass opacity

Findings of fibrosis: septal thickening, traction bronchiectasis,[a] honeycombing

Conglomerate masses associated with bronchiectasis[a,b]

Patchy distribution

Lymph node enlargement, usually symmetric[a]

---

[a]Most common findings.
[b]Findings most helpful in differential diagnosis.

of extensive interstitial sarcoid granulomas rather than alveolitis. Leung et al. [156] correlated CT findings with findings in pathologic specimens in 29 patients who had chronic infiltrative lung disease. Their study included two patients who had sarcoidosis in whom ground-glass opacity was present in an area in which open-lung biopsy was performed. At pathologic examination, extensive interstitial sarcoid granulomas were the only finding in one patient, and fine honeycombing and diffuse sarcoid granulomas were found in the other. In neither case was there evidence of alveolitis. The absence of alveolitis in two other patients who had sarcoidosis who underwent lobectomy because of concomitant bronchogenic carcinoma was also reported by Müller et al. [143]. Nishimura et al. [151] reviewed the CT and pathologic findings in eight patients who had sarcoidosis. The most frequent feature on CT was the presence of small nodules along bronchi, vessels, and subpleural regions and thickening of the bronchovascular bundles. Pathologically these findings were shown to be due to granulomas. Areas of ground-glass opacity were present in six cases (75%). Open-lung biopsy in an area of ground-glass opacity was obtained in one of these cases. Histopathologic analysis demonstrated only interstitial granulomas.

Histologically, airway involvement is common in sarcoidosis and can occur at any level from the epiglottis to the bronchioles [152]. Bronchial abnormalities have been reported in as many as 65% of sarcoidosis patients on HRCT, primarily consisting of regular or nodular bronchial wall thickening and bronchial luminal abnormalities [157]. However, in the absence of seeing distinct endobronchial lesions,

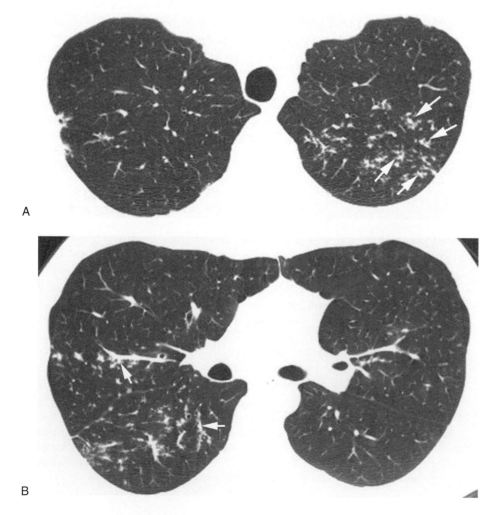

A

B

FIG. 5-35. Sarcoidosis with minimal involvement of the peribronchovascular interstitium. **A:** In the upper lobes, granulomas occurring in relation to the centrilobular peribronchovascular interstitium result in the appearance of clusters of nodules (*arrows*). **B:** At a lower level, peribronchovascular nodules are visible in relation to larger arteries (*arrows*). Nodules in relation to the major fissures are also seen.

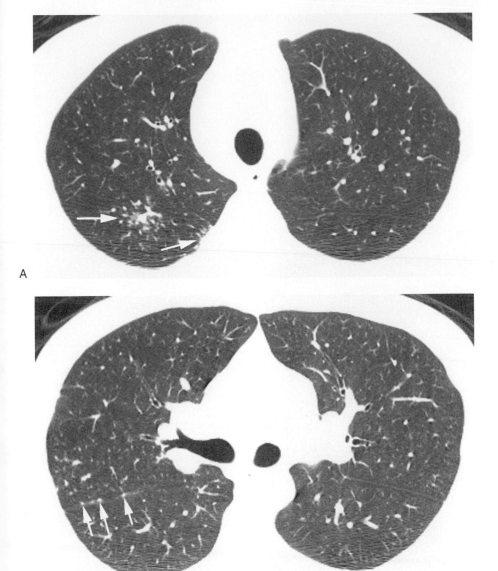

FIG. 5-36. Sarcoidosis with minimal parenchymal involvement. **A:** Several clusters of granulomas are visible in the peribronchovascular and subpleural regions (*arrows*). **B:** At a lower level, a few nodules are visible in relation to the major fissure (*arrows*). Hilar lymph node enlargement is visible.

it may be difficult to distinguish a true bronchial wall abnormality from thickening of the peribronchovascular interstitium. In a study by Lenique et al. [157], when HRCT showed a luminal abnormality, bronchoscopy showed mucosal thickening in 86% of patients and a positive transbronchial biopsy in 93%. However, in patients thought to show bronchial wall thickening on HRCT, only 59% had mucosal thickening on bronchoscopy. This differs little from the 43% incidence of mucosal thickening seen at bronchoscopy in patients who had normal-appearing airways on HRCT.

HRCT manifestations of bronchial or bronchiolar obstruction are uncommon but may be seen. Obstruction of lobular or segmental bronchi resulting in collapse may occur because of endobronchial granulomas or enlarged peribronchial lymph nodes. In a small number of patients, focal areas of decreased attenuation and vascularity (i.e., mosaic perfusion) may be seen on inspiratory HRCT in patients who have sarcoidosis. Air-trapping on expiratory HRCT due to endolu-

minal or submucosal sarcoid granulomas or fibrotic obstruction of small airways is more common (Fig. 5-42) [158] and was observed in 40 of 45 (89%) patients in one study [159].

In patients who have sarcoidosis and have been followed using HRCT, areas of nodularity, consolidation, and ground-glass opacity tend to decrease over time (Fig. 5-43). Although fibrosis need not occur with healing of granulomatous lesions, findings of fibrosis tend to become more prominent over time. As fibrosis develops, irregular reticular opacities, including irregular septal thickening, often become a predominant feature (see Fig. 3-16; Figs. 5-44 and 5-45). Reticular opacities, as with the nodules, are frequently seen along the perihilar bronchovascular bundles [143,147,160]. The most common early HRCT finding of fibrosis with lung distortion is posterior displacement of the main and upper lobe bronchi (see Fig. 3-82; Fig. 5-45); this finding indicates loss of volume in the posterior segments of the upper lobes [27,150].

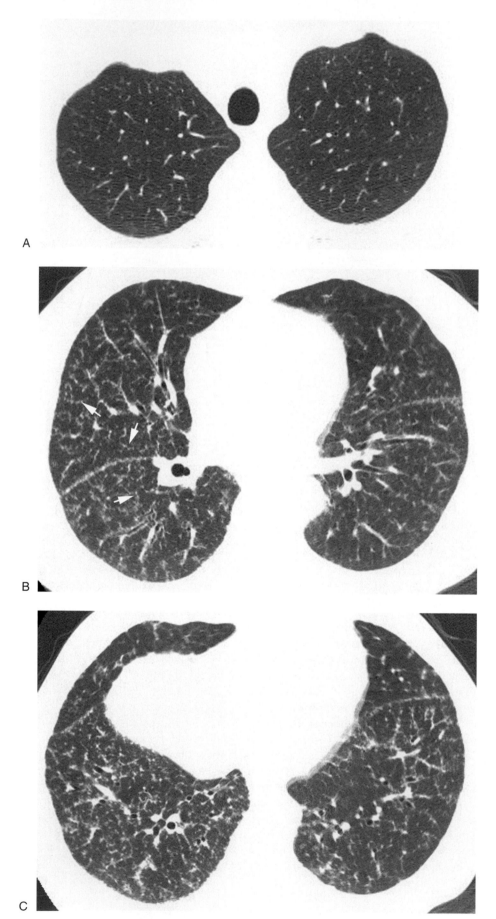

A

B

C

FIG. 5-37. Sarcoidosis with interlobular septal thickening and a basal distribution. **A:** The upper lobes appear normal. **B:** In the lower lobes, nodular thickening of the fissures is evident, and there is nodular thickening of interlobular septa (*arrows*). **C:** These findings are also visible at the lung base.

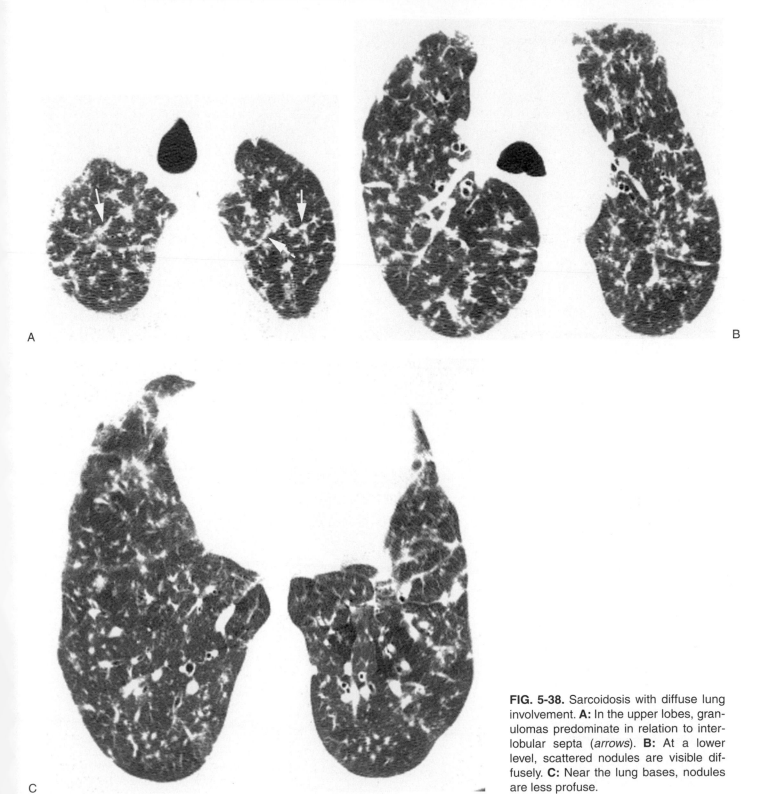

FIG. 5-38. Sarcoidosis with diffuse lung involvement. **A:** In the upper lobes, granulomas predominate in relation to interlobular septa (*arrows*). **B:** At a lower level, scattered nodules are visible diffusely. **C:** Near the lung bases, nodules are less profuse.

Progressive fibrosis also leads to abnormal central conglomeration of perihilar bronchi and vessels associated with masses of fibrous tissue, typically most marked in the upper lobes (see Fig. 3-82; Figs. 5-46 and 5-47) [142,161]. Fibrotic masses are frequently associated with bronchial dilation, a finding referred to as *traction bronchiectasis* [28,162], and this combination typical of sarcoidosis. The only other diseases that commonly result in conglomerate massive fibrosis are silicosis, TB, and talcosis.

Honeycombing or lung cysts can be present in patients who have sarcoidosis but are less common than in other

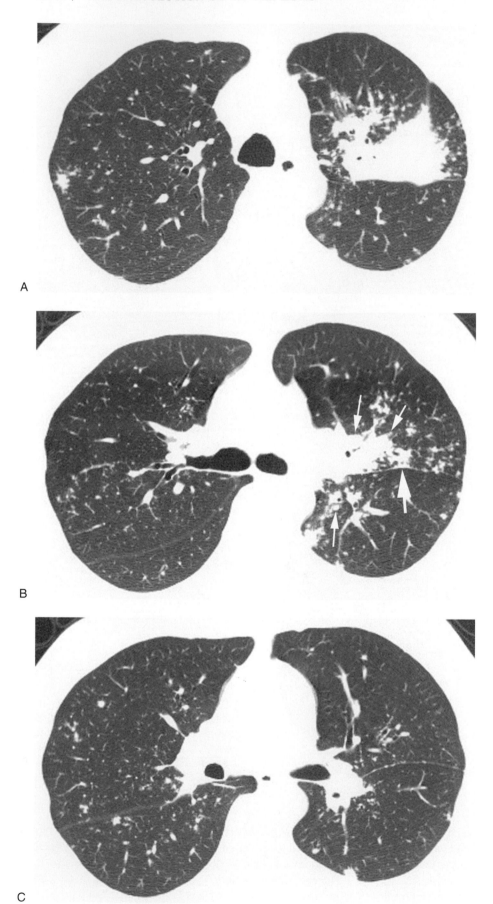

FIG. 5-39. Sarcoidosis with a conglomerate mass of granulomas. **A:** A large mass is visible in the left upper lobe, with smaller nodules seen at its periphery and in other lung regions. **B:** At a lower level, peribronchovascular involvement typical of sarcoidosis is more easily identified (*small arrows*) as is involvement of the major fissure (*large arrow*). **C:** At a level below the carina, fewer abnormalities are visible. As in this patient, sarcoidosis often has an upper lobe predominance.

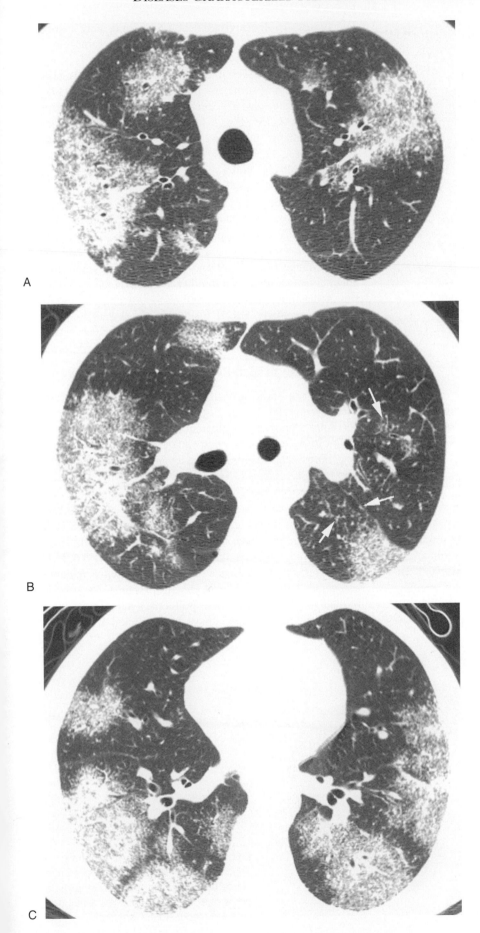

FIG. 5-40. A–C: Sarcoidosis with patchy lung involvement by small nodules and ground-glass opacity. Large foci of confluent granulomas may mimic consolidation. In less abnormal regions (*arrows*, **B**), small clusters of granulomas and fissural nodules can be identified.

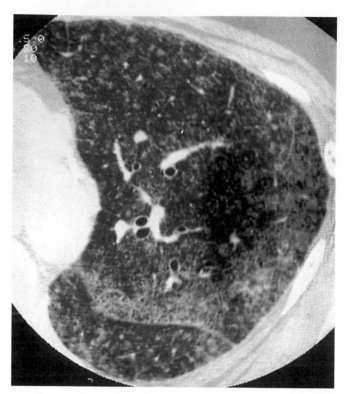

FIG. 5-41. Sarcoidosis with small nodules and ground-glass opacity. Very small nodules are present diffusely. Within the lung periphery, ground-glass opacity likely reflects the presence of confluence of multiple small nodules.

fibrotic lung diseases such as idiopathic pulmonary fibrosis. The cysts vary in diameter from 3 mm to 2 cm, with walls smaller than 1 mm in thickness, and are invariably subpleural in location (Figs. 5-46 and 5-48) [148]. Honeycombing is usually limited to patients who have severe fibrosis and central conglomeration of bronchi [148]. The honeycombing seen in patients who have sarcoidosis involves mainly the middle and upper lung zones, with relative sparing of the

lung bases [163]. Rarely, the honeycombing may involve mainly the lower lung zones and mimic the appearance seen in idiopathic pulmonary fibrosis [164].

CT has also been shown to be helpful in assessing the presence and extent of some complications of sarcoidosis [141]. Even though true cavitary sarcoidosis is rare, pseudocavities representing bullae (Fig. 5-47) or bronchiectasis are common in patients who have extensive fibrosis [165,166]. Superimposed bacterial infection and saprophytic fungal infection with mycetoma formation can be readily detected with CT (Fig. 5-47) [141,150,152].

HRCT demonstrates the characteristic symmetric hilar and paratracheal lymphadenopathy better than plain chest radiographs, despite the spacing of scans (Fig. 5-49). Lymph node calcification is not uncommon, and can be eggshell-like in appearance (Figs. 5-49 and 5-50). On CT, lymph node enlargement is often seen in other locations, including anterior mediastinum, axilla, internal mammary chain and retrocrural region [141]. HRCT may be useful in detecting hilar lymphadenopathy in lungs distorted by fibrosis.

Clinical Utility of High-Resolution Computed Tomography

HRCT can show parenchymal abnormalities in patients who have normal chest radiographs, and in patients in whom only hilar adenopathy is apparent [143]. HRCT also has been shown to be superior to chest radiographs in demonstrating early fibrosis and distortion of the lung parenchyma in patients who have sarcoidosis [154]. However, CT cannot be used to rule out parenchymal involvement; HRCT can be normal in patients who have pulmonary involvement by sarcoidosis proved by transbronchial biopsy or lobectomy [143,148,167].

In patients who have sarcoidosis, as in those who have other chronic infiltrative lung diseases, ground-glass opacity usually reflects the presence of active, potentially treatable, or reversible disease [151,154,156,168]. Serial CT scans performed in patients who have pulmonary sarcoidosis, both with and without treatment, have demonstrated that nodules,

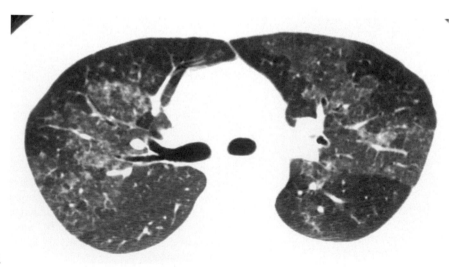

FIG. 5-42. Sarcoidosis with ground-glass opacity and air-trapping. **A:** The primary abnormality in this patient is ground-glass opacity, although a few small nodules are also visible. *Continued*

A

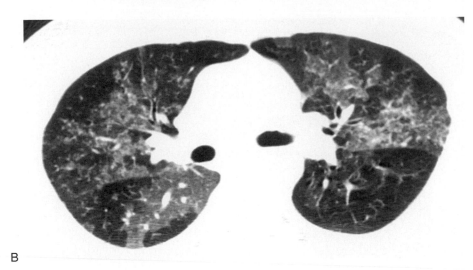

FIG. 5-42. *Continued* B: An expiratory image shows areas of air-trapping in the lung periphery.

ground-glass opacity, consolidation, and interlobular septal thickening usually represent potentially treatable or reversible disease [149,154,168]. The extent of nodules and consolidation in sarcoidosis has been shown to correlate with the intensity of lung gallium uptake [148,169] and with serum angiotensin-converting enzyme levels [169]. Although one study showed correlation between the extent of ground-glass attenuation and gallium uptake [148], this was not confirmed in subsequent studies [149,169]. Irregular lines and reticular opacities are usually irreversible but may occasionally improve or resolve [168]. Architectural distortion and honeycombing represent irreversible disease [149,154,168].

Most investigators believe that HRCT has a very limited role, if any, in assessing or predicting pulmonary function in patients who have sarcoidosis [170]. Although CT provides a superior pictorial assessment of disease pattern, extent, and

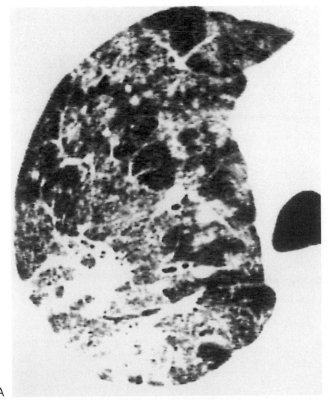

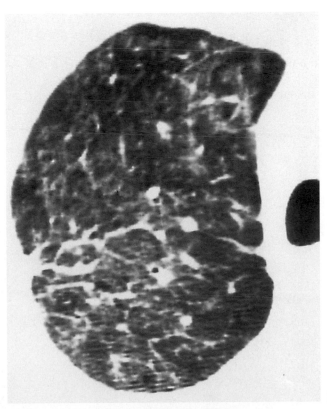

FIG. 5-43. Sarcoidosis before and after treatment. A: Before treatment, multiple nodules, areas of ground-glass opacity, and dense consolidation are present. B: After treatment, there has been a significant decrease in nodularity and consolidation. Ground-glass opacity, septal thickening, and parenchymal bands persist. At least some of these findings reflect residual fibrosis.

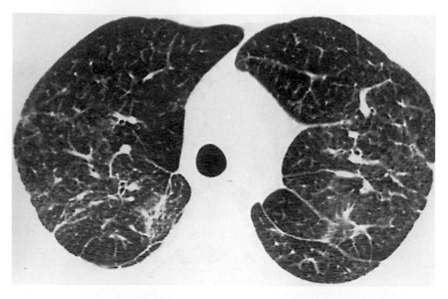

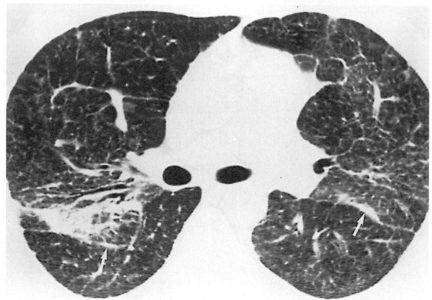

FIG. 5-44. Pulmonary sarcoidosis and findings of pulmonary fibrosis in a 32-year-old man. HRCT at the level of the tracheal carina shows extensive irregular or nodular septal thickening (*arrows*), irregular interfaces, and traction bronchiectasis. Posterior displacement of the upper lobe bronchi is an early sign of lung distortion. Extensive bilateral ground-glass opacities correlated with increased ^{67}Ga uptake reflecting the presence of active inflammation.

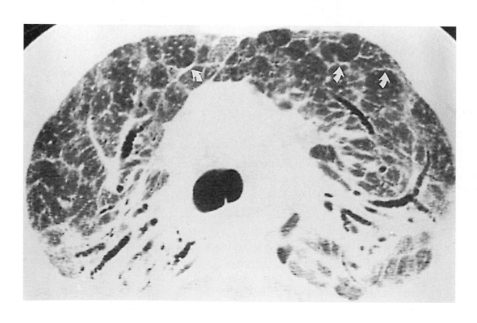

FIG. 5-45. Pulmonary sarcoidosis and findings of pulmonary fibrosis in a 32-year-old man. HRCT at the level of the tracheal carina shows extensive irregular or nodular septal thickening (*arrows*), irregular interfaces, and traction bronchiectasis. Posterior displacement of the upper lobe bronchi is an early sign of lung distortion. Extensive bilateral ground-glass opacities correlated with increased ^{67}Ga uptake.

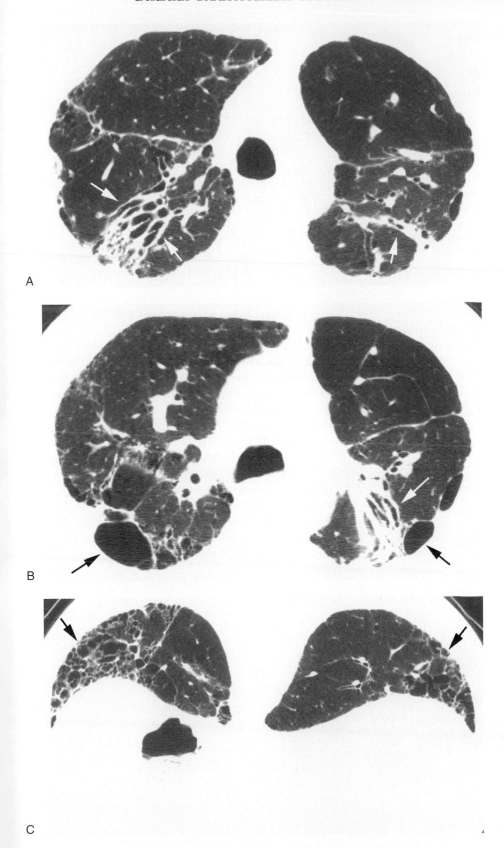

FIG. 5-46. Extensive pulmonary fibrosis due to sarcoidosis. **A:** In the upper lobes, fibrous masses associated with traction bronchiectasis and posterior displacement of bronchi are visible (*white arrows*). **B:** At a lower level, a fibrous mass (*white arrow*) is visible on the left. Subpleural bullae (*black arrows*) reflect adjacent fibrosis. **C:** Near the lung base, small areas of subpleural honeycombing (*arrows*) are visible.

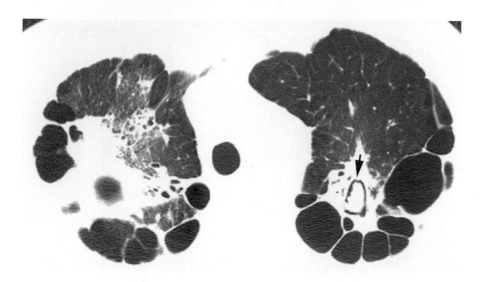

FIG. 5-47. End-stage sarcoidosis with upper lobe fibrous masses, adjacent emphysema, and a mycetoma (*arrow*).

distribution, it is controversial whether it correlates better than chest radiographs with clinical and functional impairment in patients who have sarcoidosis [170]. In a review of 27 patients who had sarcoidosis, Müller et al. [171] demonstrated that CT and radiographic assessment of disease extent had similar correlations with the severity of dyspnea ($r = 0.61$ and 0.58, respectively; $p <.001$), total lung capacity ($r = -0.54$ and -0.62, respectively; $p <.01$), and with gas transfer as assessed by the carbon monoxide diffusing capacity (DL_{CO}) ($r = -0.62$ and -0.52, respectively; $p <.01$). In a prospective HRCT study of 44 patients, Brauner et al. [27] found that the CT visual score had a lower correlation than did the radiographic score with total lung capacity (TLC) ($r = -0.30$ and -0.49, respectively), forced expiratory volume at one second (FEV_1) ($r = -0.41$ and -0.40, respectively), and DL_{CO} ($r = -0.41$ and -0.46, respectively). Bergin et al. [147], on the other hand, found that the CT scores

of disease correlated better with functional impairment (all r >0.49) than the radiographic scores (all r <0.15).

Remy-Jardin et al. [149] have also reported low, but statistically significant, correlations between the HRCT extent of various findings of sarcoidosis, with the exception of nodules and pulmonary function test (PFT) results. The best correlations were between the overall extent of abnormalities seen on HRCT, and forced vital capacity (FVC) ($r = -0.40$), FEV_1 ($r = -0.37$), TLC ($r = -0.48$), and DL_{CO} ($r = -0.49$; all $p <.0001$). Specific HRCT findings having the best correlations with PFTs were consolidation, ground-glass opacity, and lung distortion, although these correlations were generally low.

Recognizing that some patients who have sarcoidosis show PFT findings of airflow obstruction, and some show findings of air-trapping on expiratory HRCT, Hansell et al. [159] attempted to identify HRCT findings correlating with

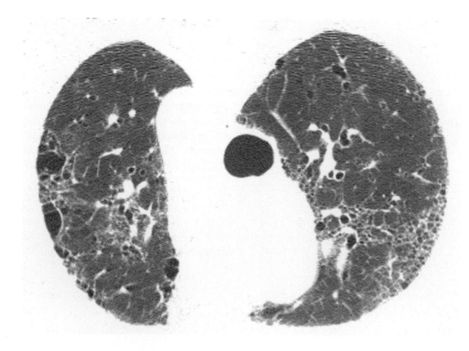

FIG. 5-48. Prone HRCT in a patient who has end-stage sarcoidosis manifested by upper lobe honeycombing.

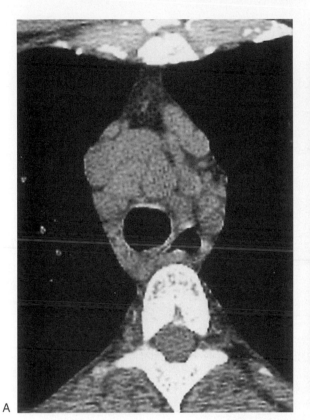

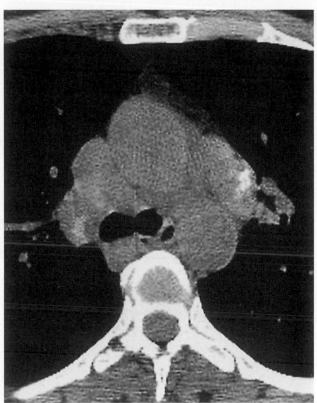

A   B

FIG. 5-49. A,B: Extensive mediastinal and hilar lymph node enlargement with calcification, seen on HRCT in a patient who has sarcoidosis.

functional airway obstruction. Against expectations, the extent of reticular abnormalities shown on HRCT, rather than the extent of air-trapping, correlated best with airflow obstruction, as shown by inverse relationships with the FEV_1 ($p < .001$), FEV_1/FVC ($p < .01$), and maximum expiratory flow rates ($p < .001$), and a positive relationship with the residual volume–total lung capacity ratio ($p < .001$).

Carrington et al. [146] have suggested that poor correlation between the radiographic severity of disease and the functional impairment in patients who have sarcoidosis may be due to the fact that the nodular lesions, although easily seen and quantitated, cause minimal dysfunction. This situation is similar to that seen in patients who have silicosis, in whom the severity of interstitial fibrosis rather than the number or size of nodules is responsible for impaired function [146]. In the study by Müller et al. [171], patients who had predominantly irregular reticular opacities had more severe dyspnea and lower lung volumes than patients who had predominantly nodular opacities ($p < .05$). Also, as indicated above, Remy-Jardin et al. [149] found that the extent of nodular opacities seen on HRCT in patients who had sarcoidosis lacked a significant correlation with PFTs.

Differential Diagnosis

Conditions that most closely mimic the HRCT appearance of sarcoidosis are pulmonary lymphangitic carcinomatosis (PLC), silicosis or coal worker's pneumoconiosis (CWP), and berylliosis. Each of these can result in a perilymphatic distribution of nodules, with nodules being seen in relation to the perihilar peribronchovascular interstitium, interlobular septa, the subpleural regions, and lobular core. However, the predominant distribution of each of these in relation to these compartments is somewhat different.

In sarcoidosis, nodules tend to predominate in the peribronchovascular and subpleural regions; in PLC, nodules are most frequently septal and peribronchovascular [20,26,148]; in silicosis and CWP, nodules usually appear centrilobular and subpleural in location on HRCT [6,18,172–174]. Furthermore, in patients who have silicosis and CWP, nodules tend to appear bilaterally symmetric and uniformly distributed or with a posterior predominance, findings that are much less frequent with sarcoidosis.

When septal thickening is present in patients who have sarcoidosis, it is usually less extensive than that seen in patients who have PLC. Distortion of lobular architecture, a finding indicative of fibrosis, may be seen in patients who have end-stage sarcoidosis and septal thickening; lung distortion is not seen with PLC [143,175]. Conglomerate masses and other evidence of fibrosis such as honeycombing can be seen with either sarcoidosis or with silicosis and CWP [142], but are not seen in PLC. In some patients who have sarcoidosis, however, the pattern of parenchymal involvement may be quite similar to that of lymphatic spread of tumor [26,143].

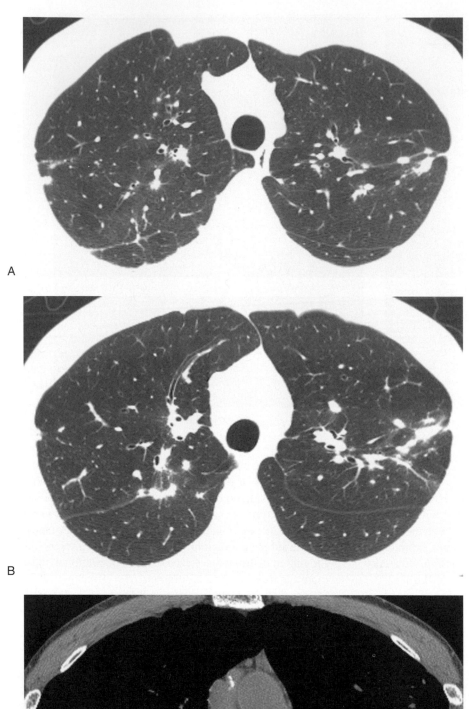

A

B

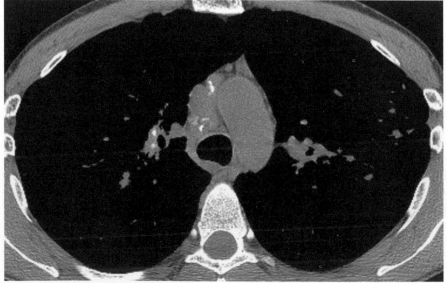

C

FIG. 5-50. Lung windows **(A,B)** and soft-tissue window **(C)** scans in a patient with sarcoidosis, lung nodules, and hilar and mediastinal lymph node enlargement and calcification. **A,B:** Small, well-defined nodules are visible with a distribution characteristic of sarcoidosis. Nodules are patchy in distribution. **C:** Mediastinal and hilar lymph node calcification is easily seen.

BERYLLIUM DISEASE (BERYLLIOSIS)

Berylliosis is a chronic granulomatous lung disease resulting from occupational exposure to beryllium; it is indistinguishable from sarcoidosis histologically [176,177]. Exposure to beryllium can occur in the ceramics industry, in nuclear weapons production, or in fluorescent lamp manufacture. Berylliosis is characterized by a beryllium-specific, cell-mediated immune response, which can be diagnosed in its early stages by the use of a blood test, called the *beryllium lymphocyte transformation test* [176].

HRCT findings in patients who have berylliosis are similar to those reported in patients who have sarcoidosis. The most common findings are parenchymal nodules (57% of patients) and interlobular septal thickening (50% of patients). As in patients who have sarcoidosis, nodules often predominate in the peribronchovascular regions, or along interlobular septa. Other HRCT findings include ground-glass opacity (32% of patients), honeycombing (7% of patients), conglomerate masses (7% of patients), bronchial wall thickening (46% of patients), and hilar or mediastinal lymphadenopathy (39% of patients) [176]. Occasionally, the parenchymal nodules may calcify [178]. In a study of 28 patients [176] who had berylliosis detected using the beryllium lymphocyte transformation test and confirmed by lung biopsy, chest radiographs were abnormal in 54% of patients, whereas HRCT showed at least one abnormality in 89% of patients. Although HRCT did not detect abnormalities in all patients, many subjects in this study had preclinical disease without symptoms of respiratory dysfunction.

SILICOSIS AND COAL WORKER'S PNEUMOCONIOSIS

Silicosis and coal worker's pneumoconiosis (CWP) are distinct diseases with differing histology, resulting from the inhalation of different inorganic dusts. However, the radiographic and HRCT appearances of silicosis and CWP are quite similar, and they cannot be easily or reliably distinguished in individual cases.

Silicosis is caused by inhalation of dust-containing silicon dioxide [179–184]. In North America, heavy-metal mining and hard-rock mining are the occupations most frequently associated with chronic silicosis.

The diagnosis of silicosis requires the combination of an appropriate history of silica exposure and characteristic findings on the chest radiograph. Pathologically, the pulmonary lesions seen in patients who have silicosis are centrilobular, peribronchiolar nodules, consisting of layers of laminated connective tissue. The nodules measure from 1 to 10 mm in diameter and are scattered diffusely throughout the lungs, although they are usually most numerous in the upper lobes and perihilar regions. Focal emphysema (also known as focal-dust emphysema) surrounding the nodule is common.

As indicated by its name, CWP results from inhalation of coal dust. Because a small amount of silica is present in coal mine dust, it was long assumed that CWP represented a form of silicosis, but this is not usually the case [185]. CWP can be seen in workers exposed to washed coal, which is nearly free of silica, and a very similar pneumoconiosis occurs with inhalation of pure carbon. As with silicosis, a history of significant exposure (10 years or more) is necessary to consider the diagnosis [180,185]. The characteristic lesion of CWP is the coal macule, a 1- to 5-mm diameter focal accumulation of coal dust, surrounded by a small amount of fibrous tissue [185]. Histologically, the coal macule consists of numerous pigment-laden macrophages in the interstitium adjacent to respiratory bronchioles. As the disease progresses, coal macules are surrounded by small areas of focal emphysema. As in patients who have silicosis, these abnormalities tend to surround respiratory bronchioles in the lobular core, and are therefore primarily centrilobular in location [180,185].

The characteristic radiologic abnormality seen in patients who have both silicosis and CWP consists of small, well-circumscribed nodules, usually measuring 2 to 5 mm in diameter, but ranging from 1 to 10 mm, mainly involving the upper and posterior lung zones [6,174,180,185]; although there is a tendency for the nodules of silicosis to be better defined than those of CWP, this is not necessarily true in individual cases. These small nodules indicate the presence of simple or uncomplicated silicosis or CWP.

The appearance of large opacities, also known as *conglomerate masses* or *progressive massive fibrosis*, indicates the presence of complicated silicosis or complicated CWP. A large opacity is considered to be larger than 1 cm in diameter [180,185]. These masses tend to develop in the middle portion or periphery of the upper lung zones and migrate toward the hila, leaving overinflated emphysematous spaces between the conglomerate mass and the pleura [186,187]. Although the appearance of the conglomerate masses seen in silicosis and CWP are quite similar, their histology is different. In patients who have silicosis, these masses represent a conglomeration of numbers of silicotic nodules associated with fibrous tissue; in CWP, they consist of an amorphous black mass surrounded by fibrous tissue. In both silicosis and CWP, these masses can undergo necrosis and cavitation.

Although simple silicosis and simple CWP cause few symptoms and little clinical impairment, the development of complicated silicosis or complicated CWP is associated with the appearance of respiratory symptoms and a deterioration of lung function [180,185]. However, patients who have silicosis usually have greater respiratory impairment for a given degree of radiographic abnormality than do patients who have CWP. Furthermore, the complicated form of silicosis has a poorer prognosis than does simple silicosis, but this is not necessarily the case with CWP [185,188]. In patients who have silicosis, the size of the conglomerate masses is often related to the severity of symptoms.

Hilar lymphadenopathy is present in many patients. The lymph nodes are often calcified. A characteristic peripheral eggshell calcification is seen in approximately 5% of cases of

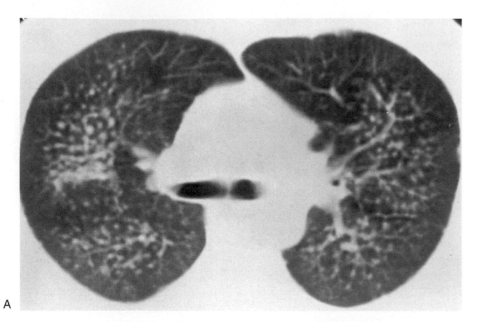

A

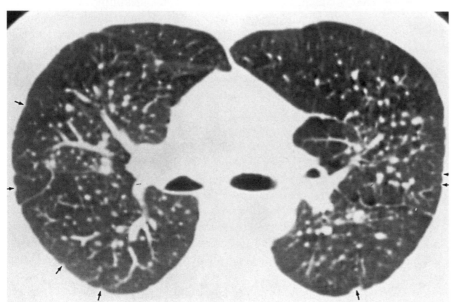

B

FIG. 5-51. Silicosis and nodules in a 50-year-old man. **A:** Conventional 10-mm collimation CT scan shows numerous lung nodules bilaterally, with relative sparing of the lung periphery. **B:** HRCT at the same level. The HRCT more clearly defines the presence of subpleural nodules (*small arrows*). The nodules are smoothly marginated and sharply defined. Nodule profusion is more easily evaluated on the conventional CT.

silicosis and is almost pathognomonic of this entity. When eggshell calcification is seen in a patient who has CWP, it reflects the presence of silica in the coal dust.

Computed Tomography and High-Resolution Computed Tomography Findings

On CT, as on the radiograph, the most characteristic feature of either simple silicosis or simple CWP is the presence of small nodules (see Fig. 3-49; Figs. 5-51 through 5-54) that are centrilobular or subpleural in location (Table 5-9) [5,6,18,174,189,190]. The nodules vary in size, but usually measure 2 to 5 mm in diameter as seen on HRCT, and can be calcified. Nodules occurring in relation to thickened interlobular septa, as are seen in patients who have PLC or sarcoidosis,

are few or lacking. The nodules seen in patients who have silicosis tend to be more sharply defined than those seen in CWP (Figs. 5-53 and 5-54).

Nodules are present diffusely and bilaterally, but in patients who have mild silicosis or CWP, they may be seen only in the upper lobes. The nodules tend to be most numerous in the right upper lobe (Fig. 5-52). A posterior predominance of nodules is also often visible on CT (see Fig. 3-49) [6,174] (Table 5-9). More severe silicosis is characterized on CT by an increase in the number and size of nodules. Nodules often appear to be uniformly distributed throughout the involved lung regions, rather than being clustered.

Akira et al. [172] reviewed the HRCT scans in 90 patients who had pneumoconiosis with small, rounded opacities on chest radiographs; 61 of these 90 had silicosis, and 12 had CWP. The 90 patients were divided into three groups on the

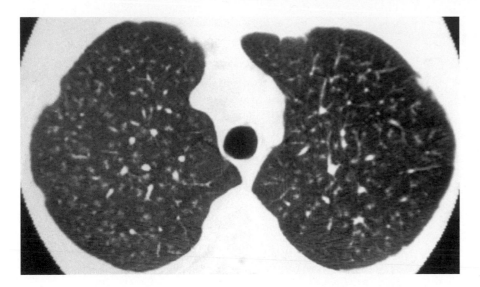

FIG. 5-52. Silicosis. HRCT in a patient who has mild silicosis shows bilateral upper lobe nodules, with predominant involvement of the right upper lobe. The nodules have a predominantly centrilobular distribution. Also note presence of subpleural nodules giving an appearance that superficially resembles that of pleural plaques, thus the designation pseudoplaques. (Courtesy of Dr. Juan Jimenez, Hospital General de Asturias, Oviedo, Spain.)

basis of the type of opacity that was visible. The first group consisted of 55 patients whose radiographs predominantly showed International Labor Organization (ILO) type p rounded opacities (nodules smaller than 1.5 mm in diameter), including 32 patients who had silicosis; six patients who had CWP; and 17 patients who had talcosis, welder's lung, and graphite pneumoconiosis. The second group consisted of 29 patients whose radiographs showed predominantly ILO type q rounded opacities (nodules 1.5 to 3 mm in diameter), including 23 patients who had silicosis and six patients who had CWP. The third group consisted of six patients who had silicosis whose radiographs showed predominantly ILO type r rounded opacities (nodules greater than 3 mm in diameter).

In those patients who had radiographic type p pneumoconiosis, HRCT showed ill-defined centrilobular, peribronchiolar opacities (Fig. 5-53), sometimes having the appearance of small branching structures or a few closely spaced dots [172]. In 21 of the 55 patients, Akira et al. [172] also demonstrated small intralobular areas of abnormally low attenuation. CT-pathologic correlation in two postmortem specimens showed that the small branching opacities and the areas of low attenuation corresponded, respectively, to areas of irregular fibrosis around and along the respiratory bronchioles and to focal areas of associated centrilobular emphysema.

Opacities of the q and r types were characterized by sharply demarcated, rounded nodules or irregular, contracted nodules [172]. Appearances with CT differed among the three types of opacities, but no differences were noted between the CT appearances of silicosis and the other pneumoconioses with the same size of nodules. Focal centrilobular emphysema was more commonly found with type p pneumoconiosis than with these two types.

In studies by Remy-Jardin et al. [6,18] of 86 patients who had CWP, parenchymal nodules 7 mm or less in diameter were seen on CT and HRCT in 81% of patients; in 3%, the nodules were calcified. In half of the patients, the nodules were low in attenuation; they usually had irregular borders. Subpleural nodules were frequently seen (Fig. 5-54), representing mac-

ules or focal areas of visceral pleural thickening [6,18]. Coalescence of subpleural nodules into pseudoplaques was visible in some; pseudoplaques can mimic the appearance of an asbestos-related pleural plaque.

Increased reticular opacities are not a prominent feature of silicosis or CWP. However, Remy-Jardin et al. [6,18] reported the occurrence of lower lobe honeycombing in 8% of 86 patients who had CWP. The significance of this finding is unclear.

Progressive massive fibrosis is always associated with a background of small nodules visible on HRCT [6]. In the patients who had CWP reported on by Remy-Jardin et al. [6], conglomerate masses were usually oval, and nearly all had irregular borders (Figs. 5-55 and 5-56). Distortion of lung architecture and vascular anatomy was also evident. The most prom-

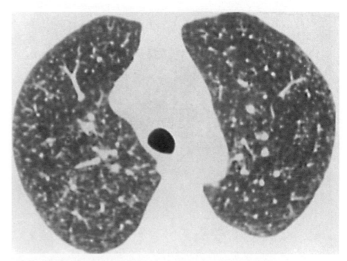

FIG. 5-53. Coal worker's pneumoconiosis (CWP) in a 56-year-old man. HRCT at the level of the aortic arch shows numerous small nodules. The nodules are less well-defined than those seen in silicosis. These involve both lungs diffusely at this level. A diffuse distribution is more typical of CWP or silicosis than it is of sarcoidosis.

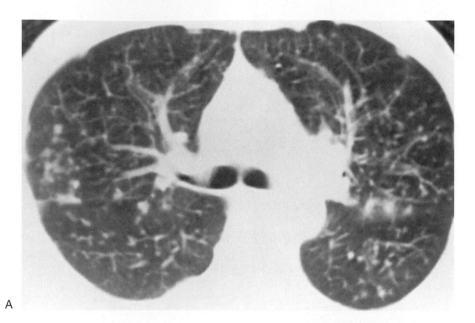

A

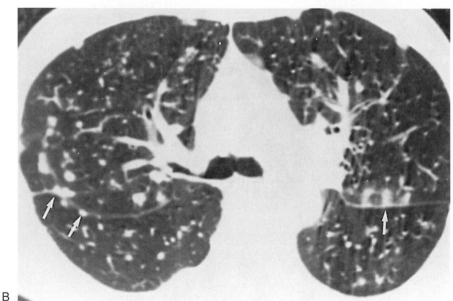

B

FIG. 5-54. Silicosis in a 60-year-old man. **A:** Conventional 10-mm collimation CT scan at the level of the right upper lobe bronchus shows nodules bilaterally. A few subpleural nodules are also visible. Groups of subpleural nodules (so-called pseudoplaques) mimic the appearance of the pleural plaques that occur in patients with asbestos exposure. **B:** HRCT at the same level better delineates the nodule margins, as well as nodular thickening of the subpleural interstitium adjacent to the major fissures (*arrows*).

TABLE 5-9. *HRCT findings in silicosis and coal worker's pneumoconiosis*

Small nodules, 2–5 mm in diameter, ill-defined or well-defined, centrilobular and subpleural[a]

Reticular opacities inconspicuous[a]

Diffuse distribution, with upper lobe and posterior predominance[a,b]

Conglomerate masses, irregular in shape, containing areas of necrosis[a,b]

Focal centrilobular emphysema[a]

Irregular or cicatricial emphysema in silicosis

Lymph node enlargement or calcification

[a]Most common findings.
[b]Findings most helpful in differential diagnosis.

---

inent CT feature of progressive massive fibrosis associated with silicosis is masslike consolidation associated with apical parenchymal scarring and adjacent bullae (irregular or cicatricial emphysema); emphysema seems to be more conspicuous in patients who have silicosis than in those who have CWP [6]. Calcification in association with conglomerate masses is common. In patients who had CWP, conglomerate masses larger than 4 cm always contained areas of necrosis, visible as low attenuation, with or without cavitation [6]. Thickening of extrapleural fat adjacent to peripheral conglomerate masses was also reported by Remy-Jardin et al. [6]. Although these masses are typically seen in the upper lobes, conglomerate masses in the lower lobes have also been reported [190].

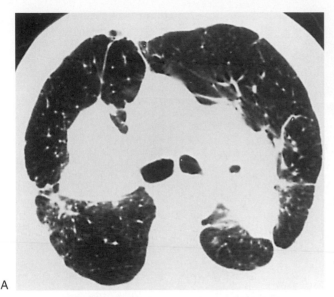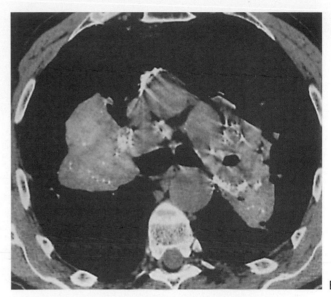

A   B

FIG. 5-55. Progressive massive fibrosis due to silicosis in a 70-year-old man. **A:** HRCT using lung window settings at the level of the main bronchi shows bilateral conglomerate masses and emphysema. **B:** Mediastinal window settings at the same level shows areas of calcification within the conglomerate masses, hila, and mediastinal nodes.

Hilar and/or mediastinal lymph node enlargement was visible in 15% to 38% of patients who had silicosis studied by Grenier et al. [25]. Eggshell calcification can sometimes be seen (Fig. 5-57).

Utility of Computed Tomography and High-Resolution Computed Tomography

HRCT has been shown to be superior to both conventional CT and chest radiography in the detection of small nodules in patients who have silicosis [5] and CWP [6,174]. Bégin et al. [5] compared HRCT to conventional CT and chest radiographs in the detection of early silicosis in 49 patients and two normal controls. The patients had been exposed to silica dust for an average of 29 years and had chest radiograph scores of 0 or 1 as determined by the ILO criteria. In this study, chest radiographs were interpreted as normal in 32 patients, indeterminate in six, and abnormal in 13. Thirteen of the 32 (41%) cases interpreted as normal on radiographs had evidence of silicosis on CT or HRCT. Furthermore, in 10% of the patients who had silicosis, abnormalities were visible only on HRCT [5]; in the remaining cases, abnormalities were more clearly defined using HRCT than on the conventional CT studies.

Remy-Jardin et al. [6] reviewed the chest radiographs and CT scans in miners exposed to coal dust. Nodules were detected on HRCT in 11 out of 48 patients (23%), with no evidence of pneumoconiosis on chest radiographs (ILO profusion score <1/0). Similarly, Gevenois et al. [191] demonstrated nodules on CT in 16 of 40 (40%) coal workers with no evidence of pneumoconiosis on chest radiography (ILO profusion score <1/0). A combination of 10-mm collimation conventional CT

and 1-mm collimation HRCT scans was superior to either technique alone in the detection of pulmonary nodules. Inter-reader agreement in the assessment of lung opacities, as assessed by kappa statistics, is also significantly better for the readings of CT scans than chest radiographs ($p < .001$) [5].

CT and HRCT can provide significant information regarding the stage of the disease in patients who have silicosis and CWP because they can detect coalescence of nodules and the development of conglomerate masses that may not be apparent on plain radiographs [173,174]. Also, in some patients who appear to have this finding on chest radiographs, HRCT shows that progressive massive fibrosis is not present [6].

It has been shown that in patients who have silicosis, pulmonary function abnormalities correlate more closely with the severity of emphysema than the profusion of small nodules. A major advantage of CT relative to chest radiographs is in the evaluation of emphysema extent. Chest radiographs may detect large bullae but are notably insensitive in detecting more diffuse emphysema. In the ILO classification, the presence of bullae is denoted by the symbol "bu," but there is no system for quantitating bullous changes. CT, on the other hand, allows quantitation of the severity and extent of emphysema seen in association with silicotic nodules.

For example, Bergin et al. [174] compared the qualitative and quantitative CT assessment of silicosis with chest radiographs and PFTs in 17 patients who had silicosis and in six controls. The CT scans were visually graded as to the extent of silicosis, mean attenuation values were measured, and the extent of any associated emphysema was determined. Significant correlation was found between the ILO category of nodule profusion recorded from the radiograph,

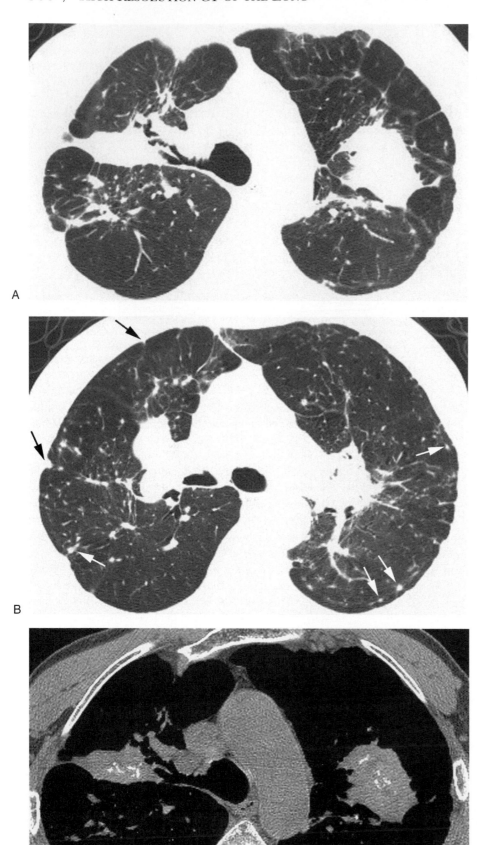

A

B

C

FIG. 5-56. Progressive massive fibrosis due to silicosis. **A:** HRCT using lung window settings show bilateral conglomerate masses. **B:** At a lower level, small centrilobular nodules (*white arrows*) and subpleural nodules (*black arrows*) are typical of silicosis. **C:** Tissue window settings at the level of **A** shows areas of calcification within the conglomerate masses.

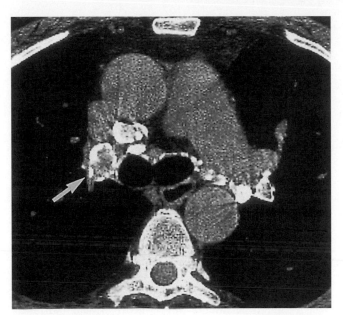

FIG. 5-57. Eggshell calcification (*arrow*) on HRCT in a patient who has silicosis.

and both the mean attenuation values ($r > 0.62$; $p < .001$) and the visual CT scores ($r > 0.84$; $p < .001$) for extent. Although there was poor correlation between the PFT results and the nodule profusion determined using the chest radiographs and CT, there was a significant correlation between the CT emphysema score and measurements of airflow obstruction and impairment of gas transfer. Emphysema associated with silicosis was easily detected on CT, but not on the radiographs.

Also, Kinsella et al. [187] reviewed PFT and chest CT scans in 30 subjects who had silicosis. The extent of emphysema was the strongest independent predictor of pulmonary function impairment; the extent of small nodules was also an independent predictor of pulmonary function impairment, albeit a weaker one. It was also shown in this study that in the absence of progressive massive fibrosis, smokers had more extensive emphysema and more severe functional impairment than did nonsmokers [187]. In the absence of progressive massive fibrosis, silicosis was not associated with significant emphysema.

To investigate the relationship of lung function, airflow limitation, and lung injury in silica-exposed workers, Begin et al. [192] analyzed the clinical, functional, and radiologic data of 94 long-term workers exposed in the granite industry or in foundries. In those workers who had coalescence of nodules and conglomerate masses seen on chest radiographs or CT scans, there was a significant loss of lung volume, impairment in gas exchange, and increased airflow obstruction compared to patients who did not show this finding. Furthermore, in 40% of the patients who had conglomeration, this finding was visible only on CT.

Differential Diagnosis

As indicated earlier, patients who have silicosis can show HRCT findings similar to those seen with sarcoidosis and PLC [174], although the diseases can usually be distinguished on the basis of history and a careful examination of the CT scans. The HRCT features that suggest sarcoidosis include a central clustering of nodules in relation to perihilar vessels and bronchi and the presence of focal or multifocal abnormalities intermixed with normal or almost normal areas of lung; in silicosis and CWP, nodules usually appear bilaterally symmetric and more uniformly distributed. Also, the development of reticular opacities is much less common with silicosis than with sarcoidosis. Beaded septa as seen in patients who have PLC and sarcoidosis are generally inconspicuous or lacking in patients who have silicosis.

OTHER NODULAR PNEUMOCONIOSES

Graphite Worker's Pneumoconiosis

Exposure to graphite dust may produce pathologic and radiographic abnormalities similar to those seen in coal workers [172,193]. HRCT findings include small centrilobular nodules, nodules along interlobular septa, and nodules in a subpleural location. In a study of 19 graphite workers [193], small centrilobular nodules were seen in all, appearing as ill-defined clusters of small nodules or branching opacities, corresponding to macular lesions along the course of bronchioles, or larger, better-defined nodules representing larger macular lesions. Interlobular septal thickening was present in 11 patients, and clusters of subpleural nodules were seen in eight of the 19 patients. Reticulation was a predominant finding in three patients.

Welder's Pneumoconiosis

Electric-arc welders and oxyacetylene welders may inhale fine particles of iron oxide during the course of their work. Little fibrosis results, but the particles accumulate in macrophages aggregated in relation to perivascular and peribronchial lymphatics. Plain radiographs show small nodules with a perihilar predominance; these may clear with time [193].

HRCT scan findings in 21 arc welders have been reported by Akira [193]. The predominant finding consisted of diffuse, ill-defined centrilobular micronodules in 15 patients (71%); some of these had a fine-branching appearance. Emphysema was seen in seven, likely related to smoking. Focal areas of consolidation may appear very high in attenuation due to the presence of iron.

TALCOSIS

Talcosis secondary to intravenous injection of talc is seen almost exclusively in drug users who inject medications intended for oral use [194,195]. The talc (magnesium sili-

TABLE 5-10. *HRCT findings in talcosis secondary to intravenous drug abuse*

Randomly distributed nodules 1 mm or less in diameter[a]

Diffuse granular appearance[a]

Ground-glass opacities

Perihilar conglomerate masses

Increased attenuation within conglomerate masses[b]

Panacinar emphysema[a,c]

[a]Most common findings.
[b]Findings most helpful in differential diagnosis.
[c]Seen almost exclusively in methylphenidate (Ritalin) users.

cate) acts as a filler and lubricant in tablets containing oral medications. When drug users crush the tablets, dissolve them in water, and inject the solution intravenously, numerous talc particles become trapped within pulmonary arterioles and capillaries. The particles result in small granulomas composed of multinucleated giant cells surrounded by a small amount of fibrous tissue [196]. Talc can be identified within the giant cells as irregular, birefringent crystals. Oral medications and drugs commonly injected intravenously include pentazocine (Talwin), meperidine, propoxyphene (Darvon), heroin, cocaine, amphetamines, and methylphenidate hydrochloride (Ritalin) [196,197].

The initial radiologic manifestations of talcosis consist of numerous discrete nodules measuring 1 mm or smaller in diameter [196]. Follow-up chest radiographs show gradual coalescence of the nodules toward the perihilar regions of the upper lobes. Eventually, talcosis results in conglomerate masses in the upper lobes that closely resemble the progressive massive fibrosis seen in silicosis [195,196].

Intravenous injection of methylphenidate hydrochloride (Ritalin) may result in talcosis and panacinar emphysema, which is clinically, radiologically, and pathologically similar to that seen in patients who have alpha-1-antitrypsin deficiency [196–198]. The mechanism for the development of panacinar emphysema in these patients is not clear.

High-Resolution Computed Tomography Findings

Padley et al. [199] described the HRCT findings in three patients who had pulmonary talcosis secondary to chronic intravenous drug abuse. One patient had diffuse ground-glass opacities, and two had small nodules and confluent perihilar masses resembling progressive massive fibrosis (Table 5-10) (Fig. 5-58). The confluent masses contained high-attenuation material consistent with talc. Nodules may be centrilobular in location [7].

Stern et al. [198] reviewed the chest radiographs and available CT scans in 21 patients who injected crushed methylphenidate (Ritalin) tablets. The radiographs showed predominantly basilar emphysema in all cases. In

11 patients who had serial radiographs, the basilar emphysema was seen to progress over a 2- to 7-year period. CT scans available in three patients showed panacinar emphysema that was diffuse, but involved predominantly the lower lung zones. Autopsy results available in four patients demonstrated severe panacinar emphysema, and numerous talc granulomas measuring 0.5 mm or less in diameter. The talc granulomas were not evident on the radiographs or CT scans.

Ward and coworkers [196] reviewed the conventional and HRCT findings in 12 patients who had talcosis. The study included seven patients who had abused methylphenidate (Ritalin) either alone or in combination with other drugs, and five patients who abused substances other than methylphenidate. The main abnormalities consisted of innumerable small nodules in five patients (42%), ground-glass opacities in two patients (17%), and emphysema in five patients (42%) (Table 5-10). The nodules measured smaller than 1 mm in diameter, and were distributed diffusely throughout both lungs, resulting in a fine granular appearance. In three of the five patients who had nodules, conglomerate masses were present in the perihilar regions of the upper lobes. In two of the patients, the conglomerate masses contained high-attenuation material consistent with talc. The authors found no significant difference in the prevalence of nodules and ground-glass attenuation between Ritalin and non–Ritalin abusers. However, lower lobe panacinar emphysema was seen more commonly in Ritalin abusers (6 of 7, 86% of patients) than in non–Ritalin abusers (1 of 5, 20% of patients).

DIFFUSE PARENCHYMAL AMYLOIDOSIS

The term *amyloidosis* refers to a group of conditions characterized by extracellular deposition of abnormal protein [200,201]. It can be classified into localized, primary systemic, and secondary systemic forms [200]. A retrospective review of the Mayo Clinic experience from 1980 to 1993 identified 55 patients who had biopsy-proven pulmonary amyloidosis [200]. Sixty-four percent of patients had primary systemic amyloidosis, 31% had localized amyloidosis, and 5% had secondary amyloidosis.

Radiologically, primary systemic amyloidosis usually results in a reticular or reticulonodular pattern due to diffuse interstitial parenchymal involvement [200]. This presentation is also known as diffuse parenchymal or alveolar septal amyloidosis. The abnormal areas can calcify or, rarely, show frank ossification [202]. Less commonly, primary systemic amyloidosis may present as a small nodular pattern mimicking sarcoidosis or miliary TB. The localized form of amyloidosis may manifest as single or, less commonly, multiple lung nodules or masses (nodular parenchymal amyloidosis), or as thickening of the airway wall (tracheobronchial amyloidosis) [201]. Deposition of other types of protein may result in similar disease. An example is light-chain disease [203].

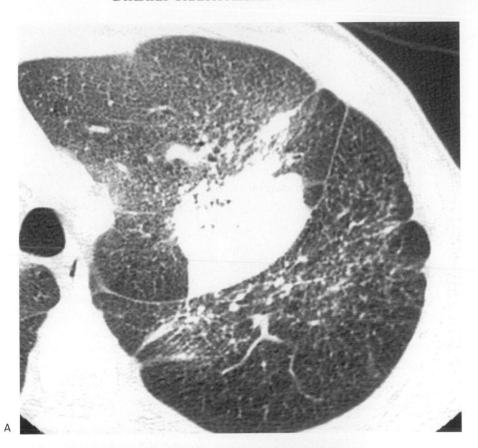

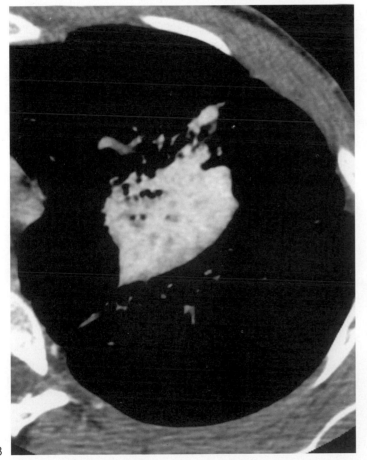

FIG. 5-58. Talcosis. **A:** HRCT targeted to the left lung demonstrates numerous small nodules giving a fine granular appearance. Conglomeration of nodules is present in the left upper lobe. Also noted are irregular linear opacities and architectural distortion. **B:** Soft-tissue windows show increased attenuation within the conglomerate mass due to accumulation of talc. The patient was a 27-year-old intravenous drug user.

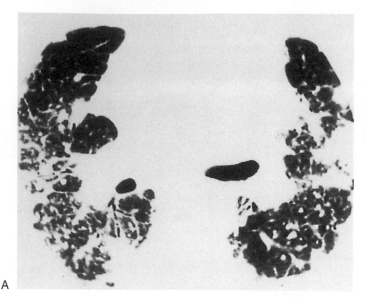
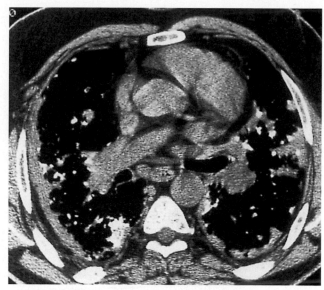

A B

FIG. 5-59. Diffuse alveolar septal amyloidosis. **A:** Lung window shows interlobular septal thickening, small, well-defined nodules, and subpleural masses. **B:** Soft-tissue window setting shows the subpleural masses to best advantage. Many small nodules are calcified. This study was performed 16 months after that shown in Fig. 3-53.

High-Resolution Computed Tomography Findings

Pickford and coworkers reviewed the CT findings in 18 patients who had proven amyloidosis [201]. The most common pulmonary parenchymal manifestation of primary systemic amyloidosis consisted of multiple pulmonary nodules ranging from 2 to 15 mm in diameter, interlobular septal thickening, and intralobular linear opacities (Figs. 5-59 and 5-60). Less common findings included areas of ground-glass attenuation, consolidation, traction bronchiectasis, honeycombing, and foci of calcification within nodules. The main manifestations of localized amyloidosis consisted of single or multiple discrete nodules or masses (nodular amyloidosis), 20% of which had foci of calcification, and thickening of the larynx, trachea, or bronchus (tracheobronchial amyloidosis). Other findings seen in some patients who had amyloidosis included lymphadenopathy and pleural effusion.

Desai et al. [81] described three patients who had a combination of benign pulmonary lymphocytic infiltrate and amyloidosis. The HRCT appearances of the three cases were strikingly similar, consisting of multiple pulmonary nodules and thin-walled cysts of varying sizes. Many of the nodules had bizarre shapes and abutted the cysts (Fig. 5-61), and calcification of nodules was visible.

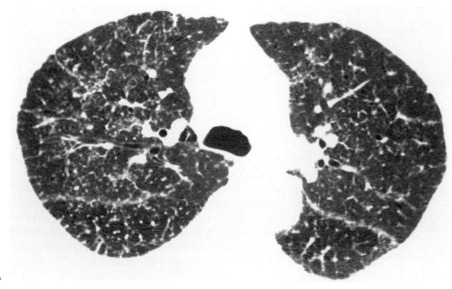

A

FIG. 5-60. **A,B:** Multiple myeloma with light chain protein deposition. HRCT shows multiple small nodules involving interlobular septa and the subpleural interstitium adjacent to fissures. Biopsy revealed protein deposition initially thought to represent amyloidosis but confirmed to represent light chains. *Continued*

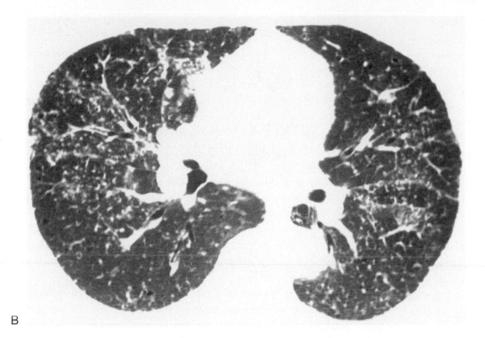

B

FIG. 5-60. *Continued*

Graham et al. [204] reported the initial and follow-up HRCT findings in one patient who had diffuse parenchymal amyloidosis. The diagnosis of amyloidosis was initially suggested because of HRCT findings of small interstitial nodules associated with dense calcification. HRCT findings in this patient included abnormal reticular opacities; interlobular septal thickening; small, well-defined nodules 2 to 4 mm in diameter; and confluent consolidative opacities that predominated in the subpleural regions of the middle and lower lung zones (see Fig. 3-53; Fig. 5-59). Some nodules were densely calcified, and some of the areas of consolidation contained punctate foci of calcification. These calcifications were not visible on chest radiographs. Follow-up HRCT studies (Fig. 5-59)

performed more than one year after the initial examination (see Fig. 3-53) showed progression of the diffuse parenchymal disease, including an increase in the reticular opacities, septal thickening, the size and number of nodules and consolidative opacities, and an increase in the size and number of the multiple calcifications.

Calcification of small interstitial nodules on HRCT has a limited differential diagnosis. Multifocal lung calcification, often associated with lung nodules, has also been reported in association with infectious granulomatous diseases such as TB [205], sarcoidosis [18], silicosis and CWP [6,18], talcosis [199], fat embolism associated with ARDS [206], metastatic calcification (see Fig. 3-106) [207], and alveolar microlithiasis (see Fig. 3-107) [208,209].

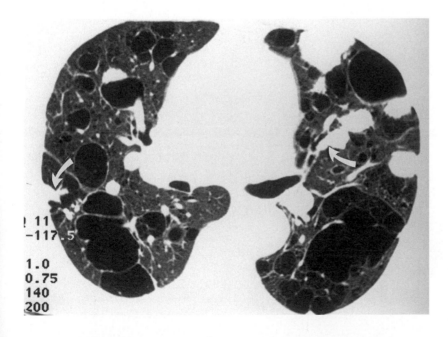

! 11
−117.5
1.0
0.75
140
200

FIG. 5-61. Thin-walled cysts and nodules in a 68-year-old woman with Sjögren's syndrome and amyloidosis. The nodules were partially calcified, and some had unusual shapes (*arrows*). Biopsy revealed a lymphocytic infiltrate and amyloid deposits. Some overlap with the appearance of lymphocytic interstitial pneumonia with cysts seems likely. (From Desai SR, Nicholson AG, Stewart S, et al. Benign pulmonary lymphocytic infiltration and amyloidosis: computed tomographic and pathologic features in three cases. *J Thorac Imag* 1997;12:215, with permission.)

WEGENER'S GRANULOMATOSIS

Wegener's granulomatosis is a rare, multisystem disease that may be associated with involvement of the upper and lower respiratory tracts, glomerulonephritis, and necrotizing vasculitis of a variety of organs and tissues. Criteria of value in diagnosis include (i) nasal or oral inflammation, (ii) an abnormal chest radiograph, (iii) an abnormal urinary sediment, and (iv) granulomatous inflammation on biopsy or hemoptysis [210]. In some patients, the disease may be limited to the respiratory tract.

Wegener's granulomatosis most commonly affects patients between the ages of 30 and 60 years. Most patients have sinusitis and cough, and hemoptysis is common. Renal disease associated with hematuria, proteinuria, and renal failure is present or develops in most. Lung disease associated with Wegener's granulomatosis is characterized by a neutrophilic capillaritis, granulomatous inflammation, and necrotizing vasculitis affecting larger vessels. The presence of serum antineutrophilic cytoplasmic antibody (C-ANCA) is characteristic, being seen in as many as 90% of cases.

Radiographic manifestations include multiple pulmonary nodules or masses, often cavitary; solitary nodule or mass; and focal or diffuse consolidation [211–213]. Abnormalities are identified on the initial chest radiograph in 45% of patients, and are seen at some time in the course of disease in 85%.

Computed Tomography and High-Resolution Computed Tomography Findings

CT findings in Wegener's granulomatosis have been reported in several studies [213–216]. The typical appearance is that of multiple nodules, usually limited in number, ranging in size from a few millimeters to 10 cm in diameter, without a zonal predominance, and having a random distribution (Fig. 5-62) [212–214]. Masses may also appear peribronchial or peribronchovascular in distribution [217]. In a study of ten patients [214], CT scans revealed multiple pulmonary nodules in seven patients, and a single nodule in one. The nodules ranged in diameter from 2 mm to 7 cm, and most had irregular margins. Ill-defined centrilobular nodules, likely reflecting the presence of vasculitis, have also been reported [216]. Cavitation of nodules is common, being present in all nodules larger than 2 cm in one study [214]; the cavity walls are often thick and irregular or shaggy, although thin-walled cavities may also be seen.

Consolidation or ground-glass opacity is also a common manifestation of Wegener's granulomatosis, usually related to pulmonary hemorrhage. Consolidation may occur as an isolated finding or in association with pulmonary nodules. The distribution of consolidation is variable, being lobular, patchy, or diffuse in different patients. Cavitation may be present. Additional CT findings include pleural thickening, pleural effusion, and hilar or mediastinal lymph node enlargement.

Pulmonary abnormalities may clear completely with treatment, or some scarring may result. In a study of ten patients who had Wegener's granulomatosis [215], the reversibility of pulmonary lesions after treatment was assessed using serial CT, during a period ranging from 6 to 54 months (mean, 20 months). Follow-up CT showed a decrease in the extent of disease in all cases. Ground-glass opacity cleared without residual scarring as did 69% of nodules, and 40% of areas of pulmonary consolidation. Masses cleared in all cases, but some scarring resulted; scarring was less common with clearing of nodules or consolidation. Some nodules and areas of consolidation persisted.

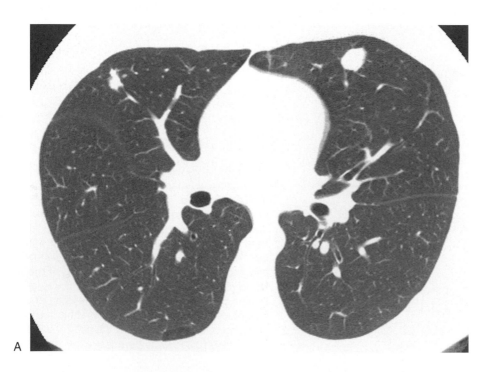

FIG. 5-62. A,B: Wegener's granulomatosis. HRCT shows multiple well-defined nodules. *Continued*

A

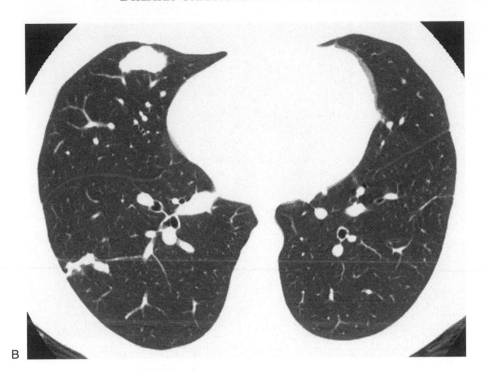

B

FIG. 5-62. *Continued*

Utility of High-Resolution Computed Tomography

CT may provide information not available on chest radiographs in patients who have Wegener's granulomatosis. In a study of ten cases [214], CT scans contributed additional information in seven. CT may demonstrate nodules and cavitation not apparent in radiographs or may exclude the possibility of nodules in treated patients.

HRCT may be a useful adjunct to the clinical assessment of pulmonary disease activity. The utility of HRCT for monitoring pulmonary disease activity was assessed in 73 patients who had Wegener's granulomatosis [218]. In this study, the status of pulmonary disease activity at the time of examination was scored according to clinical, bronchoscopic, BAL, and radiographic findings. Lung nodules and masses and areas of parenchymal opacification were significantly associated with active disease; these were seen in 60% of patients thought to have active disease and 20% of patients who had past lung disease. Parenchymal bands and septal thickening were observed in both groups with pulmonary involvement, but no significant difference was found between patients who had active or past disease in frequency of these findings; these findings were seen in 32% to 48% of patients who had active disease, and 13% to 22% of patients who had past disease.

TUBERCULOSIS

Although the prevalence of TB has declined since the advent of modern chemotherapy, pulmonary TB remains an important cause of disease worldwide and has experienced a resurgence in the United States [219]. In 1990, there were an estimated 7.5 million cases of TB and 2.5 million deaths reported to the World Health Organization [220]. In 1997, new cases of TB were estimated at 8 million, including 3.5 million cases (44%) of infectious pulmonary disease [221]. The global burden of TB remains enormous, mainly because of poor control in southeast Asia, sub-Saharan Africa, and eastern Europe [221]. Factors leading to an increased incidence of TB in the United States include the high incidence of TB among the AIDS population, an increase in immigrants from countries with a high incidence of TB, and the emergence of drug-resistant strains [219]. In industrialized countries, TB is seen most commonly in nonwhite, immigrant, or debilitated patients [222,223]. Of concern is the increasing prevalence of multidrug-resistant TB (MDR-TB) [224,225].

Primary and Postprimary Tuberculosis

Traditionally, TB infection has been considered in two stages: primary infection and reactivation or postprimary disease. In fact, however, in individual cases, a clear distinction between these two types of disease may be impossible to make in the absence of prior chest radiographs or, more important, a recent history of exposure or skin test conversion [226–230]. Nonetheless, given the widespread use of these terms, awareness of their definitions remains important.

Primary pulmonary TB is acquired by the inhalation of airborne organisms. The initial site of lung infection is variable, but often, the middle and lower lung zones are first involved [223,226,231–233]. A focal pneumonitis typically results, with subsequent caseous necrosis and lymphatic spread of organisms to hilar and mediastinal lymph nodes. In 90% to 95% of subjects, development of immunity results in healing of the lesions, with development of pulmonary and hilar granulomas. Hematogenous spread of infection also occurs in patients who have primary TB, but these organisms are inactivated as immunity develops.

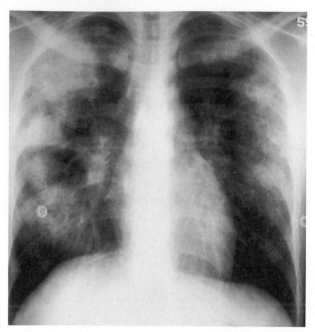
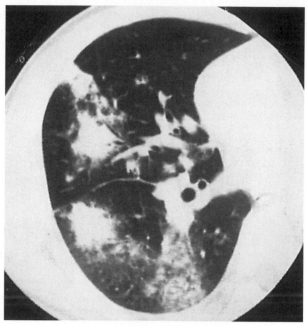

FIG. 5-63. Primary tuberculosis with patchy consolidation. **A:** Posteroanterior chest radiograph shows the presence of bilateral peripheral areas of consolidation. Initially, this pattern suggested the possibility of chronic eosinophilic pneumonia. **B:** Target reconstructed HRCT image through the right lower lobe shows patchy and nodular consolidation both centrally and peripherally. Transbronchial biopsy proved tuberculosis.

Radiographically, in a series reported by Woodring et al. [226], primary TB was associated with consolidation (50% of patients) that often involved the middle or lower lobes (Fig. 5-63), cavitation (29% of patients), segmental or lobar atelectasis (18% of patients), hilar and mediastinal lymphadenopathy (35% of patients), and miliary disease (6% of patients). These findings may occur alone or in combination, but in up to 15% of patients who have documented TB, chest radiographs may be normal [226,227]. Hilar lymph node enlargement is common, particularly in young children [223].

In most subjects, the primary infection is localized and clinically inapparent. However, in 5% to 10% of patients who have primary TB, the infection is poorly contained and dissemination occurs; this is termed *progressive primary TB*. Extensive cavitation of the tuberculous pneumonia can occur with endobronchial spread of the infection; rupture of necrotic lymph nodes into the bronchi can also result in endobronchial dissemination [223,231,232]. Hematogenous spread can also occur as a result of progressive primary TB.

With the development of delayed hypersensitivity, pulmonary granulomas heal with fibrosis. However, viable organisms often survive, and reactivation of lung disease (reactivation or postprimary TB) may occur at a later date [232]. Patients who have reactivation or postprimary TB characteristically show radiographic evidence of apical abnormalities, identifiable in up to 90% of cases [230]. The apical predominance of reactivation TB is usually attributed to the oxygen-rich environment existing in the lung apices, but may in fact result from diminished apical lymphatic drainage [234]. In patients who had postprimary TB

described by Woodring et al. [226], radiographic findings included patchy consolidation, streaky opacities, or both (100% of patients), primarily in the apical and posterior segments of the upper lobes (91% of patients), cavitation (45% of patients), bronchogenic spread of disease with ill-defined nodules (21% of patients), evidence of fibrosis (29% of patients), and pleural effusion (18% of patients) (Fig. 5-64).

Radiographic signs of active TB, regardless of its stage, include focal consolidation, generally apical or, less commonly, in the superior segments of the lower lobes, and cavitation [223,230] (Figs. 5-64 through 5-66). Endobronchial spread of infection also indicates activity, and may occur in the absence of radiographically demonstrable cavitation. Endobronchial spread is associated with poorly defined pulmonary nodules varying between 5 and 10 mm in size, so-called airspace or acinar nodules. Disease activity may also be inferred in those patients treated empirically in whom radiographic resolution can be documented. Although radiographic findings cannot generally be relied on to indicate inactive disease, a lack of change in the appearance of opacities on radiographs over a 6-month period has proved valuable in determining disease to be inactive [235].

Pleural effusions are common in patients who have primary TB, being seen in as many as 25% of patients; these effusions are thought to represent a hypersensitivity reaction to TB proteins, and organisms are uncommonly isolated from the fluid. The effusions may be large, unilateral, and unassociated with obvious parenchymal disease on chest radiographs [226]. Pleural effusion is also associated with postprimary TB, although it is less frequent than in primary

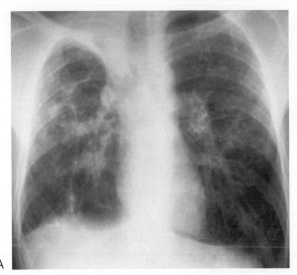 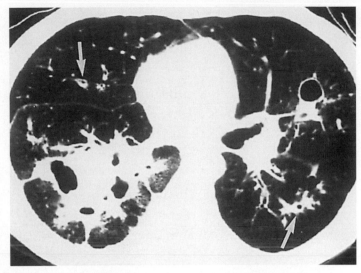

FIG. 5-64. Reactivation tuberculosis with cavitation. **A:** Posteroanterior radiograph shows evidence of significant volume loss in the right upper lobe associated with cavitation. Although there is a suggestion of cavitation in the middle and lower lobes bilaterally, precise delineation of the number and extent of cavities is difficult. **B:** HRCT through the midlung zones shows both thick- and thin-walled cavities bilaterally, associated with focal areas of airspace consolidation. The number and appearance of these are much more easily evaluated in cross section as is bronchiectasis (*arrows*).

TB; pleural effusion has been reported in 18% of patients who have postprimary TB [226]. Pleural effusion can be caused by rupture of a tuberculous cavity into the pleural space, causing empyema. Bronchopleural fistula can also result, leading to a pleural air-fluid level.

In many cases of advanced cavitary TB, extensive pleural abnormalities are present, with pleural thickening and calcification being most common. Pleural thickening has been reported in up to 41% of patients studied who had postprimary TB [226]. Usually, pleural abnormalities represent the sequela of underlying parenchymal disease and are apical in location; in occasional cases, pleural thickening is attributable to prior pneumothorax therapy.

Computed Tomography and High-Resolution Computed Tomography Findings

The CT and HRCT findings seen in association with TB are numerous and varied and reflect the protean manifestations of this disease [205,223,233,236–244] (Table 5-11). Findings include (i) airspace consolidation of varying degrees (Fig. 5-63); (ii) cavitation (Figs. 5-64 and 5-65); (iii) centrilobular nodules and branching linear opacities (tree-in-bud appearance) that reflect endobronchial spread of infection (Figs. 5-65 through 5-67); (iv) small, well-defined, randomly distributed nodules that indicate miliary or hematogenous spread of infection (see Fig. 3-55; Fig. 5-68); (v) pleural effusion; and (vi) lymph node enlargement with central necrosis (Fig. 5-69) [205,236,245]. A combination of these findings is most helpful in making a diagnosis of TB; most commonly, TB is associated with poorly defined centrilobular nodular

and branching linear opacities, and parenchymal consolidation, cavitation, or both (Figs. 5-63 through 5-65). Although most tuberculous cavities are thick-walled, thin walled cavities are frequently seen as well, especially in patients undergoing treatment.

Im et al. [205] reported the HRCT findings in 41 patients who had newly diagnosed active TB (29 patients) or recent reactivation of disease (12 patients). In the 29 patients who had newly diagnosed active TB, HRCT findings included cavitary nodules (69% of patients), lobular consolidation (52% of patients), interlobular septal thickening (34% of patients), bronchovascular distortion (17% of patients), bronchial impaction (17% of patients), and fibrotic bands (17% of patients). Mediastinal lymph node enlargement was seen in nine (31%) patients who had newly diagnosed disease. Patients having follow-up HRCT during treatment showed a gradual decrease in lobular consolidation. On the other hand, bronchovascular distortion, emphysema, fibrosis, and bronchiectasis increased on follow-up scans, indicating the presence of fibrosis [205]. In most cases, parenchymal abnormalities have a clearly segmental distribution. In a study of 71 patients who had TB, Ikezoe et al. [240] found that a pattern of segmental distribution of abnormalities was present in 97% of cases. In addition, satellite lesions were identified in 93% of cases, whereas single cavities were seen in 95%.

In the 12 patients who had reactivation of disease reported by Im et al. [205], CT findings of distortion of bronchovascular structures (58% of patients), bronchiectasis (58% of patients), emphysema (50% of patients), and fibrotic bands (50% of patients) were more frequent than in the patients who had

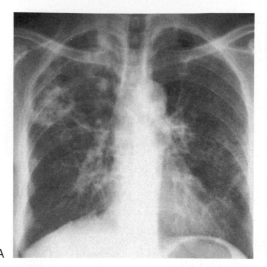

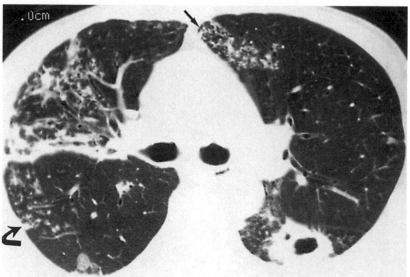

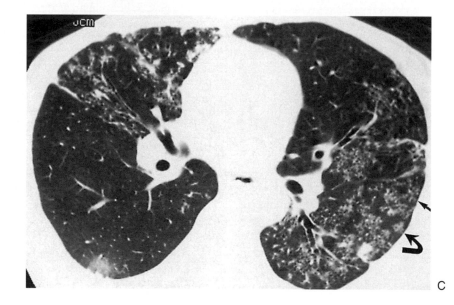

FIG. 5-65. Reactivation tuberculosis with cavitation and endobronchial spread of infection. **A:** Posteroanterior radiograph shows a thick-walled cavity in the right upper lobe associated with ill-defined nodular opacities in both lungs, suggestive of endobronchial spread of infection. HRCT images through the carina **(B)** and lower lobes **(C)** show focal clusters of poorly defined nodular opacities ranging between 2 and 10 mm in size, some of which are clearly centrilobular in distribution (*curved arrows* in **B** and **C**). Peripheral branching structures also can be identified (*straight arrows* in **B** and **C**), an appearance caused by impaction of infected material in distal airways (so-called tree-in-bud appearance). In this case, HRCT also disclosed an unexpected thick-walled cavity in the superior segment of the left lower lobe.

newly diagnosed disease, and indicative of prior infection with scarring. Lobular consolidation was less common in this group than in patients who had newly diagnosed active disease.

Of greatest importance in making an accurate HRCT diagnosis of active TB are findings of endobronchial spread of infection [205,246–248]. On HRCT, endobronchial spread of TB can result in poorly defined centrilobular nodules or rosettes of nodules, 2 to 10 mm in diameter, branching centrilobular opacities, appropriately described as tree-in-bud, or both (see Figs. 3-66 and 3-67; Figs. 5-65 through 5-67) [205,233,247,248].

Pathologically, the centrilobular nodules reflect the presence of intra- and peribronchiolar inflammatory exudate, whereas the branching tree-in-bud correlates with the presence of solid caseous material filling or surrounding terminal or respiratory bronchioles or alveolar ducts (see Fig. 3-66) [205]. With more extensive disease, coalescence of the centrilobular opacities occurs, resulting in focal areas of bron-

chopneumonia. In the study by Im et al. [205], the earliest HRCT findings of endobronchial dissemination were the presence of centrilobular nodules, 2 to 4 mm in diameter (see Figs. 3-67 and 3-68; Figs. 5-65 and 5-66), or centrilobular tree-in-bud (Figs. 5-65 and 5-66). These findings invariably resolved within 5 to 9 months of beginning treatment, and thus indicated reversible disease.

Im et al. [205] stress the high frequency of HRCT findings of endobronchial spread of infection in their patients who have newly diagnosed active TB or recent reactivation of disease. Of the 29 patients who had newly diagnosed active TB [205], 28 (97% of patients) had HRCT findings of endobronchial spread of infection, with centrilobular nodules or centrilobular branching structures (97% of patients) or a tree-in-bud appearance (72% of patients), bronchial wall thickening with or without bronchiectasis (79% of patients), or poorly defined nodules 5 to 8 mm in diameter (69% of patients). Findings of bronchogenic spread were also seen in 11 of 12

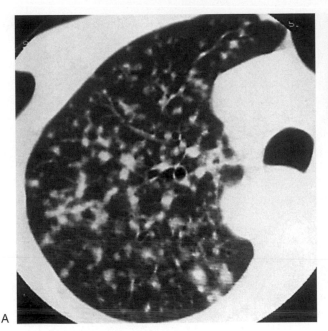

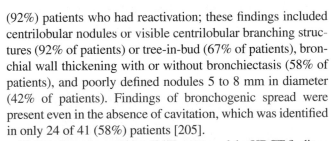

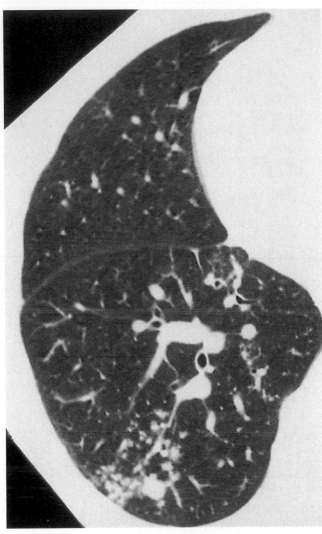

FIG. 5-66. Endobronchial spread of tuberculosis in reactivation tuberculosis. **A:** Targeted HRCT through the right upper lobe shows numerous, diffuse, poorly defined nodules typical of endobronchial spread of infection, some appearing perivascular and centrilobular in location. Chest radiographs (not shown) showed this process to be present diffusely throughout both lungs, without evidence of cavitation. Transbronchial biopsy proved tuberculosis. **B:** HRCT through the right lower lobe in a different patient shows clusters of small nodules with a focal distribution. These are also typical of endobronchial spread of infection.

(92%) patients who had reactivation; these findings included centrilobular nodules or visible centrilobular branching structures (92% of patients) or tree-in-bud (67% of patients), bronchial wall thickening with or without bronchiectasis (58% of patients), and poorly defined nodules 5 to 8 mm in diameter (42% of patients). Findings of bronchogenic spread were present even in the absence of cavitation, which was identified in only 24 of 41 (58%) patients [205].

Hatipoglu and coworkers [247] compared the HRCT findings in 32 patients who had newly diagnosed active pulmonary TB and 34 patients who had inactive disease. Findings seen only in patients who had active TB included centrilobular nodules, branching linear opacities, or both in 91% of patients, tree-in-bud appearance (71% of patients), nodules 5 to 8 mm in diameter (69% of patients), and consolidation (44% of patients). Cavitation was present in 50% of patients who had active TB and 12% of patients who had inactive disease. Similarly, in a study of 27 patients who had TB, centrilobular nodules (n = 17) and poorly marginated nodules (n = 21) were present only before treatment [248]. Centrilobular nodules and tree-in-bud are also commonly seen in children who have active TB [243].

Miliary TB results in a very fine nodular or reticulonodular pattern on HRCT [236,239,243,244,249,250] (see Fig. 3-55; Fig. 5-68). In a review of the HRCT findings in 25 patients who had proven miliary TB, HRCT demonstrated miliary nodules in 24 patients [249]. The majority of nodules mea-

TABLE 5-11. *HRCT findings in active tuberculosis*

Patchy unilateral or bilateral airspace consolidation, frequently peribronchial in distribution[a]

Cavitation, thin- or thick-walled[a]

Scattered airspace (acinar) nodules, centrilobular branching structures, tree-in-bud[a]

Superimposition of first three findings[a,b]

Miliary disease: small, well-defined nodules

Pleural effusion, bronchopleural fistula, empyema necessitatis

Low-density hilar/mediastinal lymph nodes[a,b]

[a]Most common findings.
[b]Findings most helpful in differential diagnosis.

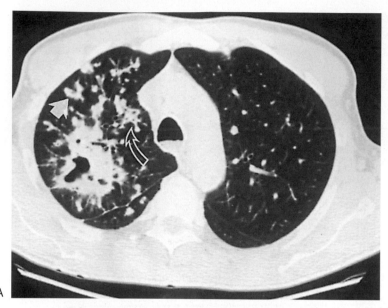

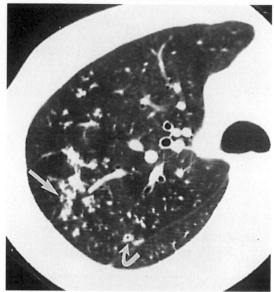

FIG. 5-67. Cavitary tuberculosis with endobronchial spread of infection. **A:** HRCT shows an irregular, thick-walled cavity in the posterior segment of the right upper lobe. Scattered nodules and clusters of nodules (*curved arrow*) are typical of endobronchial spread of infection. Branching opacities in the peripheral lung (*straight arrow*) are typical of dilated bronchioles filled with infected material, so-called tree-in-bud. **B:** Targeted reconstruction shows clustered nodules (*straight arrow*). A small nodular opacity with a central lucency (*curved arrow*) may represent a cavitary nodule, or bronchiolectasis with surrounding inflammation.

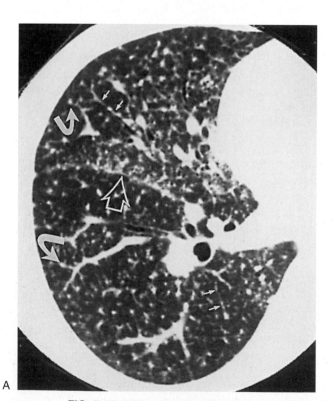

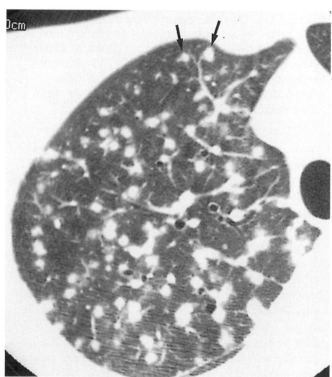

FIG. 5-68. Miliary tuberculosis (TB). **A:** HRCT with targeted reconstruction through the right lower lobe shows numerous well-defined 1- to 2-mm nodules that are diffuse in distribution. Some nodules appear septal (*arrows*) or subpleural (*open arrow*), whereas others appear to be associated with small feeding vessels, suggesting a hematogenous origin (*curved arrows*). Transbronchial biopsy proved tuberculosis. **B:** Miliary TB in another patient shows larger nodules, but the same distribution is noted as that seen in **A**. Nodules appear uniformly distributed and of similar size. Some nodules appear septal, subpleural, or associated with small vessels (*arrows*). *Continued*

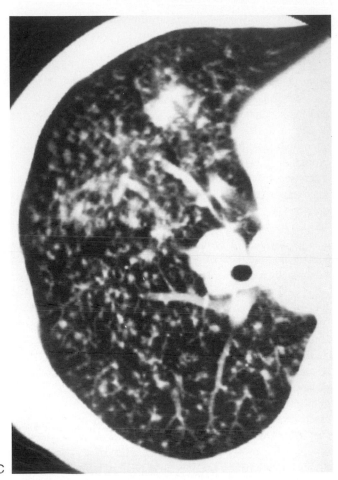

sured 1 to 3 mm in diameter, but some of the nodules reached 5 mm in diameter. The nodules had a random distribution within the lung, without cephalocaudad, central-to-peripheral, or intralobular predominance. In all patients, nodules were present in the subpleural and perivascular regions (see Fig. 3-55; Fig. 5-68). Other findings included ground-glass opacities present in 23 patients (92%), interlobular septal thickening and intralobular reticulation in 11 patients (44%), mediastinal lymphadenopathy in eight patients (32%), and pleural effusions in four patients (16%). Miliary nodules can be distinguished from nodules seen in association with endobronchial spread because of their smaller size, uniform diameter, even distribution throughout the lung, and because they are unassociated with evidence of bronchial wall thickening [205] (see Fig. 3-55).

Patients who have active TB and disseminated disease may occasionally present with acute respiratory failure. In a study by Choi et al. [242] of 1,010 patients who had active pulmonary TB, 17 patients (1.7%) presented with acute respiratory failure, and nine of the 17 (53%) patients died. The most common chest radiographic appearances were small nodular lesions (16 of 17; 94%), consolidation (13 of 17; 76%), and ground-glass opacity (12 of 17; 70%). On HRCT in 11 patients, miliary nodules were seen in six patients (55%), whereas bronchogenic spread of TB with disseminated centrilobular nodules and a tree-in-bud appearance was seen in five patients (45%). Diffuse areas of ground-glass attenuation were seen in all six patients who had miliary nodules, and four of five patients who had bronchogenic spread of TB.

Hilar and mediastinal lymph node enlargement is commonly seen on HRCT in patients who have active TB

FIG. 5-68. *Continued* **C:** Miliary TB in a patient with acquired immunodeficiency syndrome.

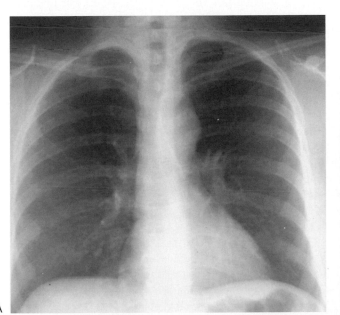

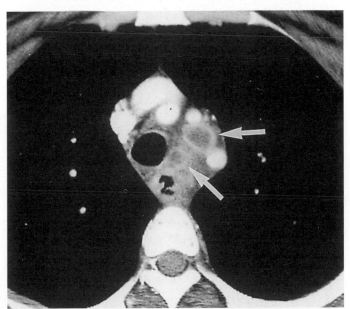

FIG. 5-69. Tuberculous lymphadenopathy. **A:** Posteroanterior radiograph shows subtle prominence of the mediastinum. **B:** Contrast-enhanced CT at the level of the great vessels shows several low-density, rim-enhancing lymph nodes (*arrows*) typical of mycobacterial infection. In this case, the diagnosis of *Mycobacterium* tuberculosis was established by transbronchial needle aspiration of subcarinal nodes (not shown).

[233,251] and is particularly common in children, seen in 83% of patients in one study [243]. In the study by Im et al. [205], mediastinal lymph node enlargement was seen on HRCT in nine of 29 patients who had newly diagnosed disease, and in 2 of 12 patients who had reactivation. Right paratracheal and tracheobronchial nodes preponderate [245,251]. In another study by Im et al. [245] of patients who had active TB, nodes larger than 2 cm in diameter invariably showed central areas of low attenuation on contrast-enhanced CT, with peripheral rim enhancement; this finding is considered strongly suggestive of active TB (Fig. 5-69). As further documented by Pastores et al. [252], rim-enhancing lymph nodes can be identified in nearly 85% of AIDS patients and 67% of HIV-positive patients who have culture or histologically verified TB. Moon et al. [253] further assessed the role of CT in the diagnosis of tuberculous mediastinal lymphadenitis in 37 patients who had active disease and 12 patients who had inactive disease. In the 37 patients who had active disease, mediastinal lymph nodes varied in size from 1.5 to 6.7 cm (mean, 2.8 ± 1.0 cm), and all had central low-attenuation and peripheral rim enhancement. Node calcifications were seen in seven patients (19%). In the 12 patients who had inactive disease, the nodes were usually smaller than nodes in patients who had active disease, and they appeared homogeneous without low-attenuation areas. Calcifications within the nodes were seen in 10 of the 12 (83%) patients who had inactive disease. Low-attenuation areas within the lymph nodes in patients who had active TB corresponded pathologically to areas of caseous necrosis. In all 25 patients followed after treatment, enlarged mediastinal nodes decreased in size and low-attenuation areas within the nodes disappeared. Other mediastinal abnormalities visible using CT include fibrosing mediastinitis and endotracheal or endobronchial disease [231].

Pleural abnormalities are also common on HRCT [233,243,254]. In patients who have active TB, pleural effusions can be small or large, and are often associated with parietal pleural thickening visible on CT; associated visceral pleural thickening may indicate emphysema, whereas air collections within the pleural fluid indicate the presence of bronchopleural fistula and empyema. Empyema necessitatis with chest wall involvement can also result. In patients who have long-standing pleural thickening, calcification may be present; residual loculated pleural fluid collections identified with CT in patients who have chronic pleural thickening frequently harbor viable bacilli [255]. Apical pleural thickening and extrapleural fat thickening are common in patients who have postprimary TB and apical lung abnormalities [238].

Utility of High-Resolution Computed Tomography

Chest radiographs play a major role in the diagnosis and management of patients who have TB infection, but have limitations [226–229,231,256]. Radiographic misdiagnosis of primary TB is frequent, occurring in over 30% of cases [226]. Also, findings of reactivation or postprimary TB are frequently overlooked on chest radiographs. In the study by Woodring et al. [226], reactivation TB was correctly diagnosed in only 59% of cases.

CT and HRCT can be valuable in several settings. CT is more sensitive than chest radiography in the detection and characterization of both subtle parenchymal [205,239,250,256] and mediastinal disease [245,252]. In patients clinically suspected of having TB with normal or equivocal radiographic abnormalities, the increased sensitivity of CT may allow prompt diagnosis before results of culture [252]. In a study of 41 consecutive children who had confirmed TB with both chest radiographs and CT [243], a diagnosis of TB was suggested only on CT scans in eight patients (20%), based on the appearance of low-attenuation nodes with rim enhancement, calcifications, nodules of bronchogenic spread, or miliary nodules. Furthermore, in 37% of patients, CT scans provided information that altered clinical management [243].

CT and HRCT are especially efficacious in detecting small foci of parenchymal cavitation, both in areas of confluent pneumonia and in areas of dense fibrocalcific disease associated with distortion of the underlying lung parenchyma (Figs. 5-64 and 5-65) [231,250,256]. In one study of 41 patients who had active TB [205], HRCT showed cavities in 58%, whereas chest radiographs showed cavities in only 22%. HRCT is also helpful in distinguishing parenchymal cavities from areas of cystic bronchiectasis occurring in association with lung fibrosis [162]. Although no specific correlation exists between the radiographic or CT appearance of tuberculous cavities and disease activity [257], CT is an especially effective method for determining the stability of cavities when present. Cavities in patients who have TB usually disappear after chemotherapy; however, healed cavities sometimes persist.

CT and particularly HRCT may also be of value in detecting the presence of diffuse lung involvement when corresponding chest radiographs are normal, or show minimal or limited disease [205,231,236,256]. It has been shown that CT and HRCT are more sensitive than plain radiographs in detecting endobronchial spread of TB, a finding that, in our experience and in that of others, invariably indicates the presence of activity (Fig. 5-65). In one series, endobronchial TB was identifiable by CT alone in 40% of cases [256]. Occasionally, endobronchial spread is so extensive and diffuse that the appearance mimics diffuse malignancy, especially that resulting from disseminated bronchoalveolar cell carcinoma. Although in most cases the clinical history and course are sufficiently different to avoid confusion, the correct diagnosis may require histologic verification.

CT can also reveal miliary disease when the chest radiograph is normal [239,244]. It should be emphasized, however, that a number of disease entities, in addition to TB, can result in miliary disease, especially in immunocompromised patients [258]. These include both fungal and viral infections. Less commonly, miliary nodules may be the primary finding in HIV-positive patients who have *Pneumocystis carinii* pneumonia (PCP).

HRCT is helpful in the differential diagnosis of TB from other lung diseases, in the distinction of active from inactive

TB, and in assessing antituberculous treatment efficiency [247,248,259]. Lee et al. [259] reviewed the HRCT scans in 188 patients being assessed for suspicion of pulmonary TB. Based on the pattern and distribution of findings on CT, 133 of 146 (91%) patients who had TB were correctly diagnosed as having TB whereas 32 of 42 (76%) patients who did not have TB were correctly excluded. HRCT allowed correct identification of 71 of 89 (80%) of patients who had active TB and 51 of 57 (89%) of patients who had inactive TB. Hatipoglu et al. [247] demonstrated that the most helpful findings to distinguish active from inactive TB are centrilobular nodules, branching linear opacities, or both, a tree-in-bud appearance, nodules 5 to 8 mm in diameter, and airspace consolidation. In their study, these findings were seen only in patients who had active TB. Pocy et al. [248] performed HRCT scans before, during, and after 6 months of antituberculous treatment in 27 patients who had postprimary TB. Before treatment, poorly defined 5 to 10 mm diameter airspace nodules were present in 80% of patients and centrilobular nodules in 65% of patients. In all cases, these nodules disappeared after 6 months of treatment. Cavities, present in 45% of patients, developed smooth borders and thinner walls after treatment. Interlobular septal thickening, intralobular lines and traction bronchiectasis were seen both before and after treatment.

CT more accurately defines the presence and extent of lymph node disease than does routine chest radiography (Fig. 5-69). In particular, the finding of low-attenuation necrotic lymph nodes with rim enhancement after contrast infusion strongly suggests a diagnosis of mycobacterial infection, both in immunocompetent patients and in patients who are HIV-positive [57,243,245,252,260]. This appearance is more easily seen on contrast-enhanced CT than on HRCT obtained without contrast enhancement. Although a similar appearance may be seen in patients who have fungal infections, especially cryptococcosis and histoplasmosis, this appearance is less frequent in patients who have lymphadenopathy secondary to metastatic neoplasm, KS, or lymphoma, and in our experience almost always indicates the presence of a treatable infection [53]. In some cases, CT can serve as a guide for determining the best sites for node biopsy and can help determine whether mediastinoscopy or parasternal mediastinotomy is most appropriate. Other mediastinal abnormalities have also been described, including fibrosing mediastinitis as well as endotracheal or bronchial lesions [231]. Generally, these too are easily identified with CT.

CT can be valuable in such cases in which pleural disease is not visible on plain films [250,255]. Residual loculated pleural fluid collections may be identified with CT; these frequently harbor viable bacilli [255]. CT can also be valuable in diagnosing bronchopleural fistula.

Complications associated with TB, including intracavitary mycetoma, and pleural disease such as empyema and bronchopleural fistulas, can also be diagnosed using CT. Mycetomas (fungus balls) are common in patients who have cavitary TB, and colonization of cavities by *Aspergillus* species is most frequent. Conventional CT and HRCT are far more efficacious

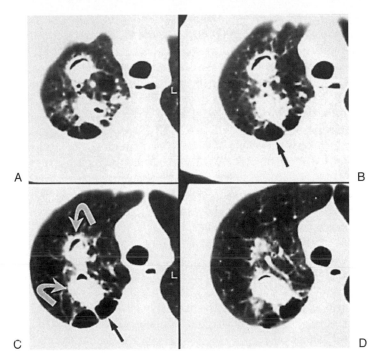

FIG. 5-70. Cavitary tuberculosis associated with an aspergilloma. **A–D:** Enlargements of sequential HRCT images obtained through the right upper lobe, from above-downwards in a patient whose chest radiograph (not shown) suggested the presence of a poorly defined nodule or mass. Two separate cavities can be identified; within both, discrete filling defects can be seen (*curved arrows*, **C**). Note that these do not represent air-fluid levels. Posteriorly, several bullae can be identified as well, easily distinguished from the adjacent cavities (*straight arrows*, **B,C**). Subsequent scans obtained in the prone position (not shown) confirmed that the filling defects were free-moving. These findings are characteristic of intracavitary fungus balls. Aspergillomas were subsequently documented bronchoscopically.

than chest radiographs in detecting intracavitary mycetoma (Fig. 5-70), and its HRCT appearance has been well-described [261]. A mature fungus ball is easily identified as a well-circumscribed intracavitary mass or opacity, associated with an air-crescent sign (Fig. 5-70). Typically, the position of the intracavitary opacity (and therefore the air crescent) changes when the patient is scanned in prone and supine positions. Thickening of the wall of a tuberculous cavity can be a finding of superimposed fungal infection before the development of a fungus ball. In select cases, these findings may lead to earlier and hence more efficacious therapy, including the localization of cavities before surgical resection.

Tuberculosis in the Human Immunodeficiency Virus–Positive Patient

The incidence of *Mycobacterium tuberculosis* (MTB) in the United States has dramatically increased as a result of the AIDS epidemic. Mycobacterial infections occur in approximately 10% of AIDS patients [56,262]. The incidence of TB in the AIDS population is 200 to 500 times that of the general population [263]; although it is one of the most curable diseases in these patients, it is also one of the most contagious. TB is an AIDS indicator disease in HIV-positive patients who have CD_4 cell counts below 200 cells per mm^3 [264].

The diagnosis of TB is frequently problematic, especially in patients who have AIDS [265]. The tuberculin skin test remains positive in approximately one-third of AIDS patients previously exposed to TB, whereas positive acid-fast sputum smears occur in less than 50% of HIV-positive patients who have active TB [266,267]. Additionally, the likelihood of a positive smear has been shown to be independent of both the presence of parenchymal cavitation on chest radiographs and the CD_4 cell count [267,268]. BAL is only positive in approximately 20% of cases. Delay in establishing the correct diagnosis in this patient population is hazardous. Kramer and coworkers [269], in a series of 52 AIDS patients, found that the diagnosis of TB was delayed in 48% of patients. Furthermore, 45% of those in whom the diagnosis was delayed died of TB, as compared with 19% of patients who had timely diagnoses. Other studies suggest that TB infection may accelerate the course of HIV infection, in terms of both increased concurrent opportunistic infections and decreased survival [270].

The pattern of TB in HIV-positive patients differs from that in non-AIDS patients [265,271–273]. Specifically, diffuse disease (Fig. 5-68C), atypical patterns, and lymphadenopathy (Fig. 5-69) are seen more commonly in the HIV-positive population. The radiographic manifestations of TB in HIV-positive patients reflect the extent of cellular immune compromise [265,267,271,274,275]. Early in the course of infection, especially in patients who have CD_4 cell counts greater than 200 per mm^3, TB is usually indistinguishable from that which occurs in non–HIV-positive patients. Cutaneous reactivity to tuberculin is generally preserved, and radiographic manifestations include upper lobe cavitary infiltrates [265,274,276]. In contrast, in more severely immunocompromised patients, sputum culture is more likely to be positive, and radiographs are usually suggestive of primary infection. Long et al. [274] found that a pattern typical of primary TB was identified on chest radiographs in 80% of AIDS patients, as compared to 30% of HIV-positive patients who did not have clinical AIDS and only 11% of HIV-negative patients who had TB. In a study of 97 HIV-infected patients who had TB, Jones et al. [271] found that mediastinal adenopathy was noted in 20 of 58 (34%) patients who had CD_4 counts less than 200 cells per mm^3, compared with only four of 29 (14%) patients who had CD_4 counts greater than 200 cells per mm^3.

Dissemination of infection is also more common in patients who have greater degrees of immunocompromise. As documented by Hill et al. [277] in a study of 51 AIDS patients who had disseminated disease, chest radiographs showed evidence of miliary disease in nearly half of the patients, and intrathoracic lymphadenopathy in one-third of patients.

Up to 85% of HIV-positive patients who have documented TB have abnormal radiographs. These findings have led the Centers for Disease Control and Prevention to recommend routine radiographic screening of all HIV-seropositive patients [278]. In addition, as delay in diagnosis may cause a significant increase in mortality in this population, it has been suggested that empiric therapy be initiated in all patients who had chest radiographic findings suggestive of TB [269].

Despite a close correlation between radiographic findings and the level of immunocompromise, a normal radiograph does not preclude active disease. Normal chest radiographs have been reported in as many as 15% of cases with documented sputum culture positive TB, even in patients who had CD_4 counts less than 200 per mm^3 [264,269]. In a retrospective study of 133 AIDS patients who had culture-positive TB, chest radiographs failed to suggest the correct diagnosis in 32% of cases [267]. In this study, the failure to diagnose TB resulted when radiographs appeared normal (13% of cases), showed minimal radiographic abnormalities such as linear opacities or calcified granulomas, or showed atypical patterns of disease, such as diffuse reticulonodular infiltrates mimicking infection with PCP [267].

Evaluation of this population is further complicated by the increasing frequency of multidrug-resistant organisms (MDR-TB). The result either of initial infection with a drug-resistant organism (primary resistance) or inadequate treatment (secondary resistance), infection with drug-resistant organisms frequently results in rapidly progressive disease in the absence of appropriate therapy. Although patients who have MDR-TB are more likely to have infiltrates and cavities, these findings are nonspecific. Nonetheless, it has been suggested that chest radiographs may play an indispensable role in the early diagnosis of drug-resistance by confirming a lack of response to routine antituberculous chemotherapy. As reported by Lessnau et al. [279] in a study of 72 patients, 33 of whom had sensitive MTB and 39 of whom had single-drug–resistant [3] or MDR-TB [57], initial radiographs were of little value in distinguishing these groups. However, after 2 weeks of therapy, 20 of 35 (57%) patients who had MDR-TB showed progression of disease, whereas this was not the case in patients who had sensitive MTB. Based on these data, the authors suggested that pending drug sensitivity results, evidence of worsening on chest radiographs after 2 weeks of routine antituberculous therapy could be interpreted as presumptive evidence of MDR-TB [279]. On the other hand, as documented by others, disease progression on treatment may not indicate MDR-TB but coexistent infection. Small et al., for example, in a study of 33 HIV-positive patients who had TB found that although all 25 patients who had pulmonary TB alone exhibited radiographic improvement after appropriate therapy, in eight patients, radiographic evidence of progression was found to correlate with a newly acquired nontuberculous pulmonary disease.

Computed Tomography and High-Resolution Computed Tomography Findings

As would be expected, differences have been reported in the HRCT appearances of TB occurring in HIV-positive patients as compared to patients that are HIV-negative; TB in HIV-positive patients tends to resemble primary TB, at least in association with AIDS. CT findings found to be less common in HIV-positive patients include cavitation, findings of endobronchial spread of infection, nodules 10 to 30 mm in diameter, consolidation, bronchial wall thickening, and findings typical of postprimary infection [272,273,280]. Findings more frequently seen in HIV-positive patients include mediastinal lymph node enlargement, atypical infiltrates, and miliary spread.

The results of several studies comparing the frequency of CT findings in HIV-positive and HIV-negative patients who have TB have been quite consistent [272,273,280]. Leung et al. [272] compared the CT findings of 42 HIV-positive and 42 HIV-seronegative patients who had pulmonary TB. Findings seen with significantly lower frequency in HIV-positive compared to HIV-negative patients were cavitation (19% vs. 55%), consolidation (43% vs. 69%), and endobronchial spread (57% vs. 90%). Conversely, a miliary pattern was seen in 17% of seropositive patients and in none of the seronegative cases.

Laissy et al. [280] compared the conventional and HRCT findings in 29 HIV-positive and 47 HIV-negative patients who had newly diagnosed pulmonary TB. As shown by Leung et al. [272], HIV-positive patients demonstrated significantly lower frequency of cavitation (24% vs. 49%). Furthermore, in HIV-positive patients, cavitation was significantly more common in patients who had more than 200 CD_4 T cells per mm^3 (50% vs. 13%). Other findings less frequent in HIV-positive patients included nodules 10 to 30 mm in diameter (14% vs. 47%), and bronchial wall thickening (14% vs. 45%). In HIV-positive patients, lymphadenopathy was significantly less common in patients who had more than 200 CD_4 T cells per mm^3 (33% vs. 70%).

Haramati and coworkers [273] compared the chest radiographic and CT findings in 67 HIV-positive and 31 HIV-negative patients. On chest radiographs, HIV-positive patients had significantly greater frequency of mediastinal lymphadenopathy (60% vs. 23%) and atypical infiltrates (55% vs. 10%). Conversely, HIV-negative patients had infiltrates typical for reactivation TB (77% vs. 30%) and cavitation (52% vs. 18%) significantly more commonly than HIV-positive patients. The chest CT scans showed a similar trend, but the only significant differences were the more frequent bilateral mediastinal lymphadenopathy in HIV-positive patients and more frequent cavitation in HIV-negative patients.

As in immunocompetent patients who have TB, CT and HRCT can be valuable in diagnosis when plain radiographs are nonspecific. Hartman et al. [57] assessed the accuracy of CT interpretation in 102 AIDS patients who had proven intrathoracic disease. On CT, mycobacterial infection was correctly suggested as the first choice diagnosis in 44% of patients, and among the top three choices in 77% of 26 patients who had TB or *Mycobacterium avium* complex (MAC) infection.

NONTUBERCULOUS MYCOBACTERIAL INFECTIONS

Nontuberculous mycobacteria (NTMB) are ubiquitous in the environment, being found in soil, lakes, streams, various food sources, and in domestic animals. Unlike TB, which is transmitted by person-to-person contact, NTMB infection is believed to be acquired through environmental exposure. Pulmonary infection results predominantly from inhalation of organisms along with dust or aerosolized water droplets. In patients who have AIDS, organisms can be acquired through the gastrointestinal tract, with resultant bacteremia and secondary lung involvement [234,281]. As with TB, the frequency of pulmonary infection resulting from NTMB is increasing at least partially because of the AIDS epidemic [234,282,283].

A number of species of NTMB have been identified, but pulmonary disease is usually the result of *Mycobacterium kansasii* or organisms classified as belonging to *Mycobacterium avium* complex (MAC) [232,234,281,284]. Because NTMB cultured from the sputum can be a contaminant rather than a pathogen or can reflect the presence of inconsequential airway colonization in patients who have morphologic abnormalities such as bronchiectasis, emphysema, or pneumoconiosis, criteria for the diagnosis of NTMB lung disease have been established by the American Thoracic Society [285], and were updated in 1997 [286]. These criteria apply only to symptomatic patients who have radiographic evidence of infiltrative, nodular, or cavitary lung disease, or HRCT showing multifocal bronchiectasis and/or multiple small nodules. In general terms, the American Thoracic Society criteria for NTMB infection require (i) three positive cultures, or two positive cultures and one positive smear for acid-fast bacilli (AFB) from three sputum samples or bronchial washings obtained in the preceding 12 months, (ii) a positive bronchial washing with a 2+ to 4+ AFB smear or 2+ to 4+ growth on solid media, or (iii) a transbronchial or open-lung biopsy yielding NTMB or showing histopathologic features of mycobacterial infection (granulomatous inflammation, AFB, or both) and one or more positive sputum or bronchial washing samples for an NTMB, even in low numbers [286]. Other suggested criteria for diagnosis include bronchoscopic washings demonstrating *M. kansasii*, as this organism is only rarely present as a contaminant or positive cultures obtained from bronchoscopic washings in association with positive blood or marrow cultures in AIDS patients [287]. It cannot be overemphasized that definite diagnosis is a prerequisite for good patient management, as treatment usually requires a prolonged course of multidrug therapy.

NTMB infection can be associated with a variety of clinical and radiographic presentations, but two common patterns are seen in immunocompetent individuals [234,281]. The first of these, so-called classic NTMB infection, closely resembles TB; the second form of infection, which has been termed the *nonclassic* form of NTMB, has distinct radiographic and clinical features [234].

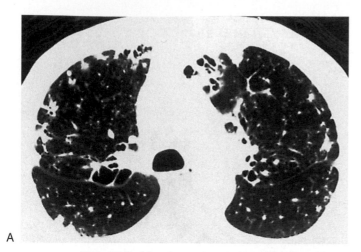
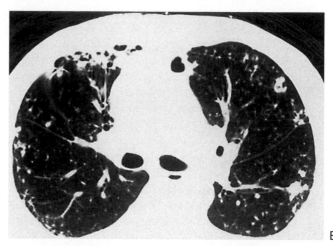

A
B

FIG. 5-71. *Mycobacterium avium* complex (MAC) infection. **A,B:** HRCT at two levels in a 63-year-old man shows findings of bronchiectasis and small nodules and clusters of nodules in the peripheral lung. This combination of findings is suggestive of MAC infection.

Classic NTMB infection is seen predominantly in men, most commonly in their 50s, 60s, and 70s, and many patients have an underlying lung disease, such as chronic obstructive pulmonary disease (COPD) or emphysema, or other risk factors such as smoking, alcohol abuse, diabetes, or nonpulmonary malignancies [234,288,289]. Symptoms are often insidious, and include cough, hemoptysis, and weight loss; fever is present in a minority of patients. Radiographs typically show apical opacities that are nodular or consolidative, and are associated with scarring and volume loss [234,281,287,288,290]. As seen on chest radiographs, cavitation occurs in the majority (90%) of cases and is frequently associated with pleural thickening (40%) or endobronchial spread of infection (60%) [288,290]. Pleural effusion and lymph node enlargement are less common. Disseminated infection with an appearance mimicking miliary TB is uncommon, being seen in a few percent of cases [281].

The second form of NTMB occurs in 20% to 30% of immunocompetent patients who have NTMB and is typically produced by infection with MAC [234]. Patients generally lack predisposing conditions. Women constitute approximately 80% of cases, and many are in their seventies [234,241,291–294]. As with classic NTMB, the onset of disease is insidious, with chronic cough and hemoptysis being the most common symptoms. Fever is uncommon [234]. Typical pathologic findings include bronchiectasis, extensive granuloma formation throughout the airways, bronchiolitis, centrilobular lesions, consolidation, and cavitation [295]. Typical radiographic findings include multiple, bilateral, poorly defined nodules, which involve the lung in a patchy fashion and lack the upper lobe predominance seen in patients who have classic disease. Patchy bronchiectasis is commonly visible radiographically, being most common in the middle lobe and lingula.

Also at risk are immunocompromised patients, especially those who have AIDS. Unlike the preceding two groups, radiographs may be normal in this group. To date, MAC has been identified in up to 20% of AIDS patients, with estimates as high as 50% of patients infected at autopsy [284].

Computed Tomography and High-Resolution Computed Tomography Findings

The HRCT appearance of pulmonary NTMB infection has been reported by several authors [234,241,291–294] and varies with the form of disease. As would be expected, the CT appearance of classical NTMB mimics that seen in patients who have TB. Findings include apical opacities, cavities that may be smooth or irregular in appearance, bronchiectasis in regions of severe lung damage, pleural thickening adjacent to abnormal lung regions, and nodules (0.5 to 2.0 cm in diameter) in areas of lung distant to the dominant focus of infection [234], probably representing endobronchial spread of infection.

The CT appearance of nonclassic NTMB infection caused by MAC has been reported by several authors [291–293]. Although patients who have NTMB infections can show a variety of CT findings, there is a propensity for such patients to have bronchiectasis in combination with small nodules, although not necessarily in the same lobe; these small nodules may have the appearance of tree-in-bud (Figs. 5-72 through 5-76) (Table 5-12) [241,291,292]. These findings correlate with typical pathologic findings of bronchiectasis, bronchiolitis, centrilobular involvement, and nodules [295]. In a study by Hartman et al. [291], CT scans were reviewed in 62 patients who had positive MAC cultures. Of the 62 patients, 60 had pulmonary opacities, which were nodular in 39 patients, and 40 patients had bronchiectasis. Most significant, all 35 patients who had small nodular infiltrates also had bronchiectasis (Figs. 5-72 and 5-73). None of these 35 patients was immunocompromised, and 29 (83%) of them were women, with a mean age of 66 years. Of the 27 patients

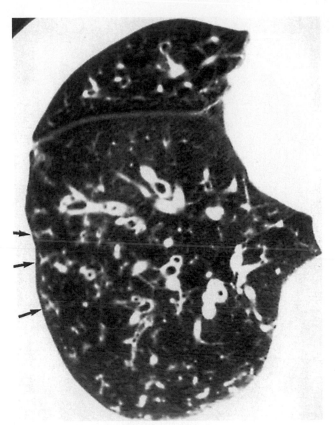

FIG. 5-72. *Mycobacterium avium* complex (MAC). Targeted HRCT through the right lower lobe of an elderly white female who has a chronic cough shows focal areas of bronchiectasis associated with scattered, poorly defined centrilobular nodular and tubular branching structures (*arrows*). Not infrequently, as in this case, these HRCT findings are the first to suggest possible infection by a nontuberculous mycobacterium. Subsequent sputum samples revealed heavy growth of MAC.

who did not have small nodular infiltrates and bronchiectasis, 25 had underlying malignancy or immunocompromise. Findings of bronchiectasis, tree-in-bud, and nodules are most common in the middle lobe and lingula (Figs. 5-73 through 5-75). The presence of reduced lung attenuation as a result of air-trapping and mosaic perfusion has also been stressed as an important finding in MAC, occurring with or without bronchiectasis or small nodules in 41% of lung zones assessed in one study [296].

Moore [292] reviewed the CT and HRCT findings in 40 patients who had cultures positive for NTMB. Common findings included bronchiectasis (80% of patients) (Figs. 5-71 through 5-74); consolidation or ground-glass opacity (73% of patients) (Fig. 5-75); nodules (70% of patients); and evidence of scarring, volume loss, or both (28% of patients). Less commonly observed were cavities, lymphadenopathy, and pleural disease. Both small (less than 1 cm in diameter), well-defined nodules and large, ill-defined nodules were seen; some small nodules were centrilobular and associated with a tree-in-bud appearance (Figs. 5-76 and 5-77). In some

patients, bronchiectasis was seen to develop in previously normal lung regions, suggesting that this finding results from the mycobacterial infection and does not represent a preexisting or predisposing condition; this has been confirmed by others [295,297]. It was concluded that some combination of bronchiectasis, consolidation, and nodules on CT scans should raise the possibility of atypical mycobacterial infection; 30 of the 40 patients showed two or three of these findings. Similar results were reported in a study of 70 patients who had MAC. CT findings included bronchiectasis (97% of patients), small nodules (89% of patients), parenchymal distortion (60% of patients), bronchial wall thickening (56% of patients), consolidation (50% of patients), and cavity formation (49% of patients) [298].

Swensen et al. [293] tested the hypothesis that bronchiectasis and multiple small lung nodules seen on chest CT are indicative of MAC infection or colonization by reviewing the CT scans of 100 patients who had a CT diagnosis of bronchiectasis; 24 of these 100 patients also had multiple pulmonary nodules visible on CT. Mycobacterial cultures were performed in 15 of the 24 patients who had lung nodules seen in combination with bronchiectasis, and 48 of the 76 patients who had bronchiectasis without lung nodules. Of the 15 patients who had bronchiectasis and lung nodules, eight (53%) had cultures positive for MAC, as did two of the 48 (4%) patients who had no CT evidence of lung nodules. Thus, the authors found that CT findings of small lung nodules in association with bronchiectasis had a sensitivity of 80%, a specificity of 87%, and an accuracy of 86% in predicting positive cultures for MAC. Similar findings were documented by Tanaka et al. [299] in a prospective study of 26 patients evaluated over a 4-year period who had findings on CT suggestive of MAC pulmonary disease, including clusters of small nodules in the lung periphery and bronchiectasis. Thirteen (50%) of these patients proved to have positive MAC cultures from bronchial washings [299], and epithelioid granulomas were demonstrated on biopsy in 8 of the 13.

Lynch et al. [294] also correlated CT findings with presence or absence of a positive sputum culture in patients who had known MAC. Although in other studies, the presence of positive sputum cultures has been clearly associated with bronchiectasis and nodules in patients who have MAC, Lynch et al. found a stronger association with the presence of cavities. Thirty-one of 34 subjects (91%) who had MAC with cavities on CT had a positive sputum culture within 3 weeks of the CT study, compared with 7 of 12 subjects (58%) without cavities ($p = .001$). Similarly, 36 of 42 subjects (85%) with airspace disease, but only two of eight subjects (25%) without airspace disease grew MAC from their sputum ($p < .001$). In this study, sputum positivity was not associated with the presence of bronchiectasis ($p = .156$) or nodules ($p = .377$) in patients who had MAC.

CT findings of MAC may progress, improve, or remain stable on follow-up studies [297]. In a study of 18 women and seven men with a median age of 66 years who had a diagnosis of MAC, the initial chest CT examination showed find-

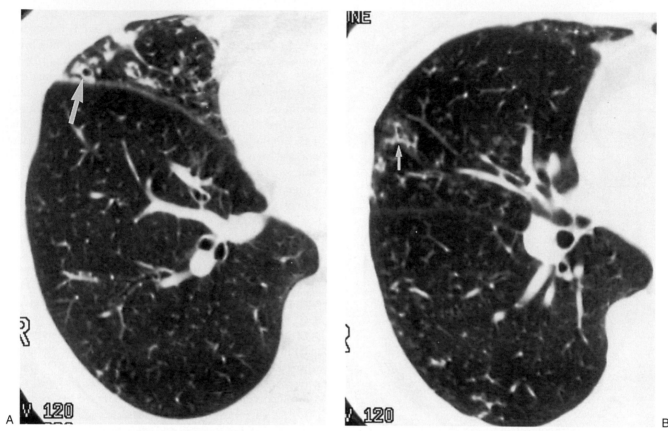

FIG. 5-73. *Mycobacterium avium* complex (MAC). **A,B:** HRCT in an elderly white female shows focal bronchiectasis (*large arrow*) associated with a tree-in-bud appearance (*small arrow*) and small centrilobular nodules. These abnormalities are largely limited to the right middle lobe.

ings typical of MAC, including bronchiectasis (visible in 53% of lung regions examined), centrilobular nodules (69%), nodules (32%), airspace disease (12%), and cavities in 4%. The middle lobe and lingula were most frequently involved. Bronchiectasis scores were significantly higher on CT studies obtained an average of 28 months after the initial examination; bronchiectasis progressed in 15 patients and improved in four patients. Centrilobular nodules progressed in nine patients and improved in seven during follow-up.

In another study, CT scans before and during follow-up were also reviewed [296]. Pretreatment CT scans showed small nodules in 47% of the lung zones studied in ten patients, reduced lung attenuation in 41%, and bronchiectasis in 27%. In patients who had not received treatment, or who received noncurative treatment, bronchiectasis developed or worsened in 46% of lung zones. In contrast, after curative treatment, small nodules disappeared completely in 48% of lung zones.

In a study [241] comparing the frequency of bronchiectasis in patients who had TB to that seen with MAC infection, although small nodules, consolidation, and cavity formation were seen with similar frequency in both diseases, bronchiectasis was found to be significantly more common in patients who had MAC (94% vs. 27% for patients who had TB). Similar results were reported by Lynch et al. [294] in a study of 15 subjects who had TB, and 55 subjects who had

MAC. Bronchiectasis involving four or more lobes (often associated with centrilobular nodules) and the combination of right middle lobe and lingular bronchiectasis were seen only in MAC. Kasahara et al. [298] found bronchiectasis and parenchymal distortion to be significantly more common in patients who had MAC, as compared to those with TB.

TABLE 5-12. *HRCT findings in nontuberculous mycobacterial infection*
Bronchiectasis[a]
Small or large nodules[a]
Combination of first two findings[a,b]
Patchy unilateral or bilateral airspace consolidation[a]
Cavitation, thin- or thick-walled
Scattered airspace (acinar) nodules, centrilobular branching structures, tree-in-bud[a]
Scarring and volume loss
Pleural effusion or thickening
Hilar/mediastinal lymph node enlargement
[a]Most common findings. [b]Findings most helpful in differential diagnosis.

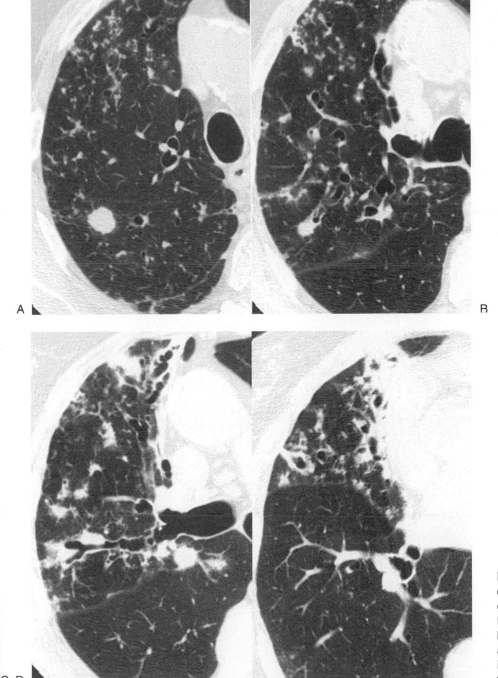

FIG. 5-74. A–D: *Mycobacterium avium* complex (MAC) infection in a 72-year-old woman who had a chronic cough. HRCT at four levels shows findings of bronchiectasis, large and small nodules, and tree-in-bud, characteristic of MAC infection. Abnormalities predominate in the upper and middle lobes.

Nontuberculous Mycobacterial Infection in the Human Immunodeficiency Virus–Positive Patient

Although less commonly identified as a cause of pulmonary disease than *M. tuberculosis*, the incidence of NTMB infections, and MAC in particular, is increasing, especially in HIV-positive homosexual men [300]. Because the main portal of infection in patients who have MAC is the gastrointestinal tract, infection is typically disseminated at the time of

diagnosis. Intrathoracic involvement typically occurs late in the course of infection, with significant chest radiographic changes occurring in only 5% of cases.

Unfortunately, radiographic findings are indistinguishable from those caused by *M. tuberculosis* and include intrathoracic lymphadenopathy, pulmonary infiltrates, nodules, and miliary disease. In most cases, these findings probably represent secondary infection in patients who have disseminated disease, although primary infection may also occur. In addition to MAC, patients who have AIDS also may become infected with other NMTB [301–304]. In particular, *M. kansasii* may result in treatable pulmonary disease that otherwise resembles reactivation TB. As shown by Levine and Chaisson [301], 14 of 19 patients who had proven *M. kansasii* infection had exclusive pulmonary disease. Nine of these patients showed marked improvement after initiation of antituberculous chemotherapy, whereas autopsies performed on another three treated patients showed no evidence of residual infection.

Computed Tomography and High-Resolution Computed Tomography Findings

Only a few reports of CT findings in AIDS patients who had NTMB infections have been published [57,304,305]. Findings are nonspecific and may closely resemble those of TB occurring in an AIDS patient (Fig. 5-78).

However, several differences in the appearance of TB and MAC in AIDS patients have been described. Laissy et al. compared the CT and HRCT scans of 29 AIDS patients who

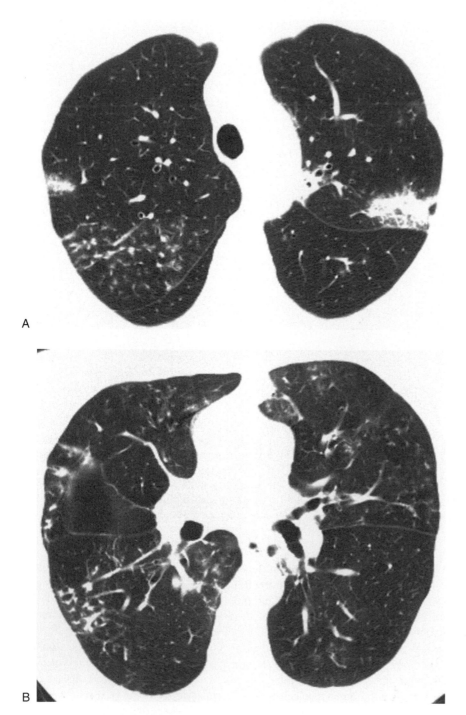

A

B

FIG. 5-75. A–C: *Mycobacterium avium* complex (MAC) infection in a 70-year-old woman who has cough and hemoptysis. Several areas of consolidation are seen. A patchy distribution of centrilobular nodules and tree-in-bud are typical of MAC. Large airway abnormalities are visible in the right middle lobe and lingula. *Continued*

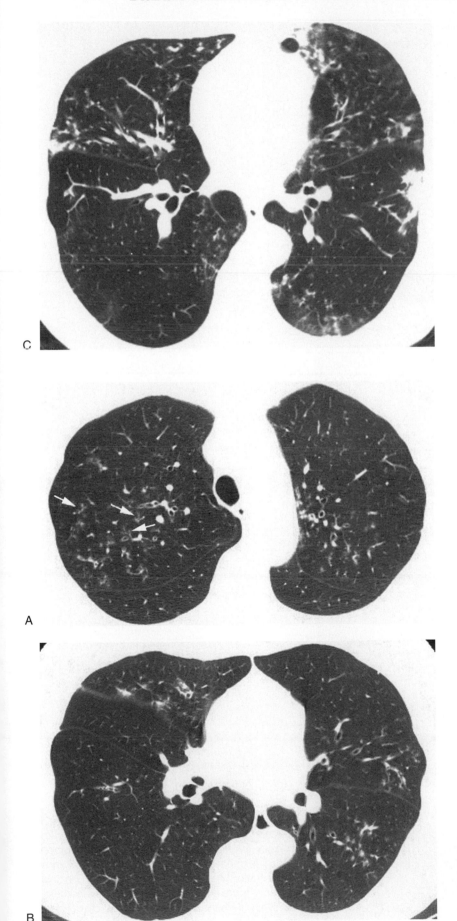

FIG. 5-75. *Continued*

FIG. 5-76. *Mycobacterium avium* complex (MAC) infection in a 70-year-old woman who has a chronic cough. **A:** In the upper lobes, small clusters of nodules and tree-in-bud (*arrows*) are visible. **B:** At a lower level, similar findings are visible. These findings are nonspecific but typical of MAC in a woman of this age.

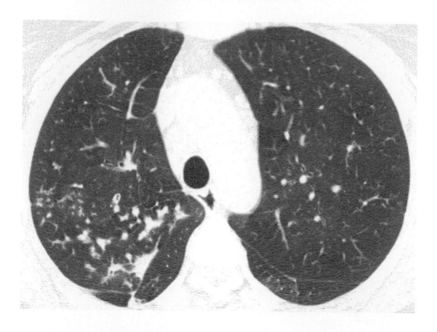

FIG. 5-77. *Mycobacterium avium* complex infection in a 62-year-old woman. Clusters of small and large nodules are visible in the right upper lobe.

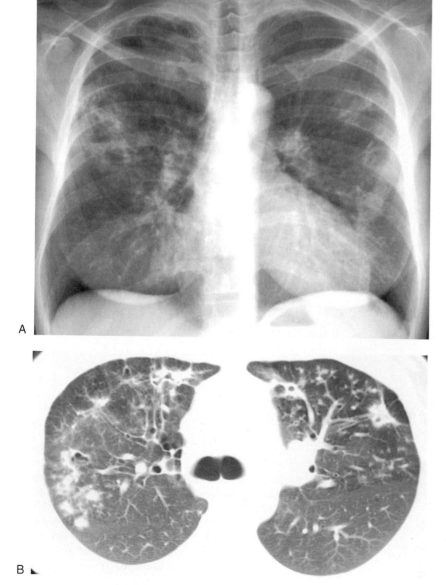

A

B

FIG. 5-78. *Mycobacterium avium* complex (MAC) infection in two patients with acquired immunodeficiency syndrome (AIDS). **A:** Chest radiograph shows ill-defined nodular opacities with evidence of cavitation in the right lung. **B:** HRCT in this patient shows findings typical of active tuberculosis, with ill-defined centrilobular opacities, tree-in-bud, and cavitary nodules. *Continued*

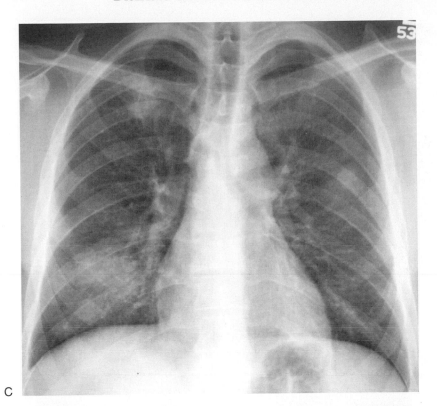

C

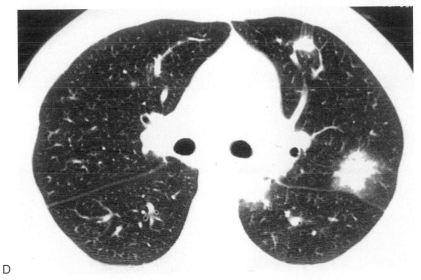

D

FIG. 5-78. *Continued* **C:** In another patient with MAC infection and AIDS, chest radiograph also shows ill-defined nodular opacities. **D:** HRCT shows poorly marginated lung nodules. The larger of these is associated with a halo sign.

had culture proven TB and 23 AIDS patients who had NTMB infection. Patients who had NTMB were more likely to have areas of ground-glass attenuation (48% vs. 17%) and a lower lobe predominance of centrilobular nodules than patients who had TB. Conversely, patients who had TB were more likely to have unilateral lung involvement (44% vs. 5%) and lymphadenopathy (76% vs. 43%) than patients who had NTMB. The lower prevalence of mediastinal lymphadenopathy in NTMB had also been previously shown in the study by Hartman et al. [57]. Furthermore, unlike in patients who have TB, low-density lymphadenopathy is relatively uncommon in NTMB infection, being identified in one series in only three of 11 patients who had documented lymphade-

nopathy and infection with MAC [57]. Although the majority of AIDS patients who have MAC have disseminated disease, occasional pulmonary involvement may occur without evidence of dissemination [306]. The radiologic abnormalities in these patients may consist only of focal, patchy, or diffuse airspace consolidation [306].

MILIARY BACILLE CALMETTE-GUÉRIN

Bacille Calmette-Guérin is usually a nonpathogenic mycobacterium. Instillation of bacille Calmette-Guérin into the urinary bladder is an effective treatment for superficial bladder carcinoma, heightening the body's immune response [307,308]. Systemic side effects including fever, chills, sepsis, and hepatitis occur in up to 5% of cases, but pulmonary complications are less common, being reported in less than 1% [309]. Hematogenous dissemination of the organism to the lung may occur [310].

On HRCT, this results in an appearance of small, well-defined, randomly distributed nodules indistinguishable from the appearance of miliary TB (Fig. 5-79) [307,308]. Resolution occurs after treatment with antituberculous medication [307].

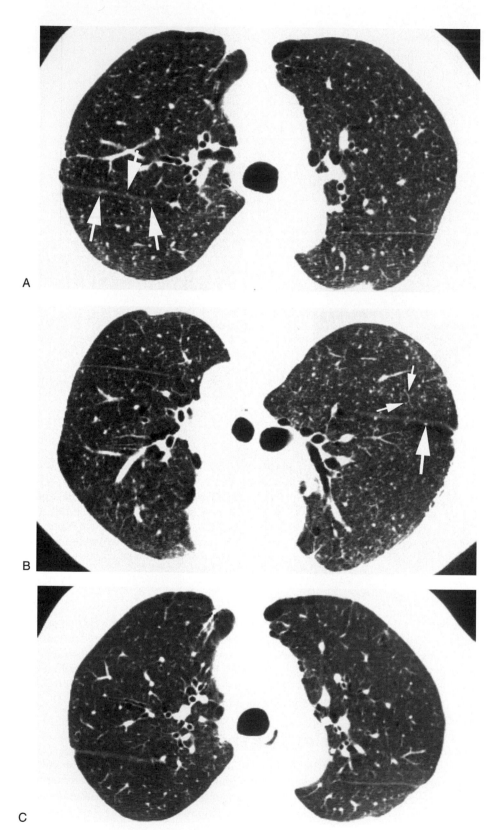

FIG. 5-79. Hematogenous dissemination of Bacille Calmette-Guérin after immunotherapy for bladder carcinoma. Supine **(A)** and prone **(B)** HRCT obtained because of cough and fever show numerous, small, sharply defined nodules having a random distribution. Nodules are visible adjacent to the major fissure (*large arrows*) and small vessels (*small arrows*). This appearance is identical to that of miliary TB. Bronchoscopy showed noncaseating granulomas. **C:** Eight weeks after **A** and **B**, after treatment with antituberculous medication, HRCT is near normal.

BRONCHOPNEUMONIA

Bronchopneumonia is usually associated with infection by *Staphylococcus aureus,* gram-negative bacteria (i.e., *Pseudomonas, Haemophilus*), and some fungi, particularly *Aspergillus* [311,312]. Similar abnormalities may be seen in patients who have atypical pneumonia, and viral and mycoplasma infections [313–315]. Involvement of small airways is the predominant pathologic feature (i.e., an infectious bronchiolitis or bronchitis), with the exudation of numerous polymorphonuclear leukocytes into the airway lumen. The inflammatory reaction also involves the airway wall, resulting in ulceration and destruction, and may involve the peribronchial or peribronchiolar alveoli secondarily. With progression, the inflammatory exudate may involve entire secondary lobules, resulting in confluent bronchopneumonia or lobular pneumonia. Radiographs typically show focal or multifocal, peribronchial or patchy areas of consolidation, often multilobular [316–318].

High-Resolution Computed Tomography Findings

In patients who have bronchopneumonia, HRCT shows findings similar to those of endobronchial spread of TB or MAC. Ill-defined centrilobular nodular opacities measuring from 4 to 10 mm in diameter are often seen on HRCT, representing consolidation involving or surrounding bronchioles (see Figs. 3-64, 3-65, 3-70, 3-71; Fig. 5-80) [314,315,319–321]. Lobular con-

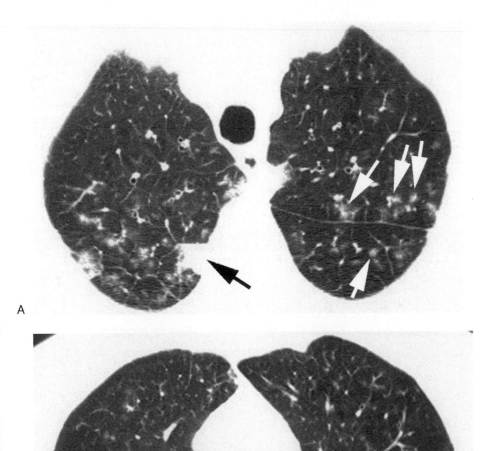

A

B

FIG. 5-80. Bronchopneumonia due to infection with *Haemophilus influenzae.* **A:** Ill-defined centrilobular opacities (*white arrows*) reflect peribronchiolar inflammation and consolidation. Lobular consolidation (*black arrow*) may also be seen (so-called lobular pneumonia is a synonym). **B:** Similar centrilobular nodules are seen at a lower level, but are less numerous. A patchy distribution is typical of bronchopneumonia. *Continued*

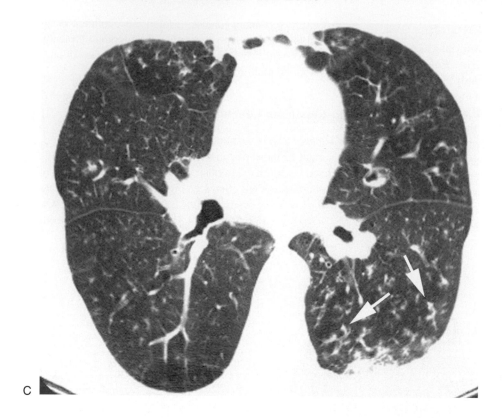

C

FIG. 5-80. *Continued* C: Near the lung base, several focal areas of consolidation are visible, along with areas of tree-in-bud due to infectious bronchiolitis.

solidation may also be present, and confluence of opacified lobules may result in larger areas of consolidation (see Fig. 3-65; Figs. 5-80 through 5-82). Tree-in-bud may be visible, reflecting the presence of the bronchiolar luminal exudate (see Fig. 3-71; Fig. 5-80). If the organisms involved are sufficiently virulent, as in patients who have *Staphylococcus*, tissue destruction may result, with radiographic findings of necrosis, abscess formation, and pneumatocele formation [316]. HRCT is better able to show typical findings of bronchopneumonia than are chest radiographs [321].

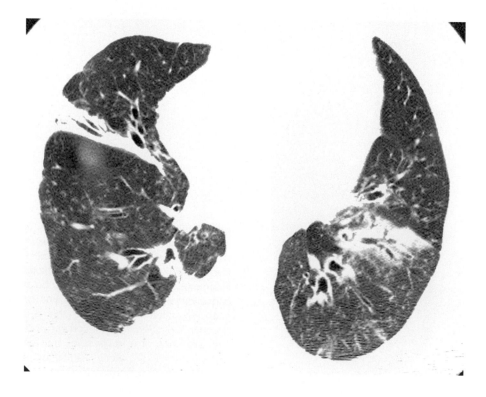

FIG. 5-81. Bronchopneumonia due to infection with *Pseudomonas*. Patchy areas of consolidation are present, related to airways. Bronchial wall thickening and small nodular opacities representing tree-in-bud reflect infectious bronchitis and bronchiolitis.

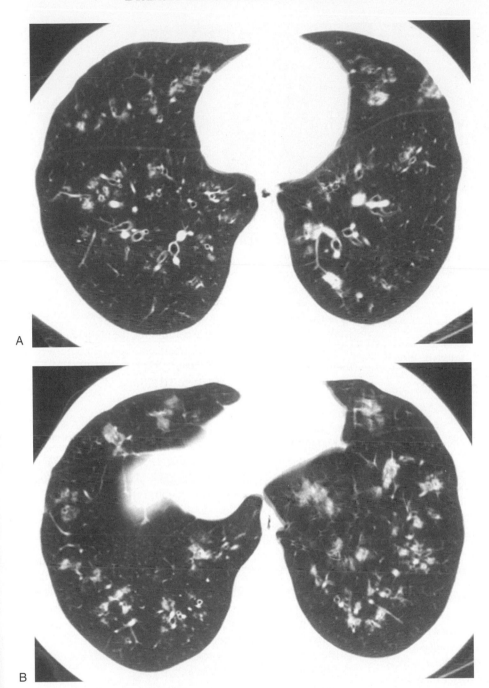

FIG. 5-82. A,B: Bacterial bronchopneumonia. HRCT at two levels shows a combination of patchy ill-defined centrilobular nodules and larger areas of consolidation, some of which appear lobular.

ASPERGILLUS-RELATED LUNG DISEASE

Aspergillus can cause a broad spectrum of pulmonary diseases, usually occurring in patients who have preexisting lung disease or some degree of immunological abnormality, either hypersensitivity or immunosuppression [322,323]. It may be associated with various forms of eosinophilic lung disease or hypersensitivity pneumonitis, discussed in Chapter 6. In asthmatic patients, it may lead to a hypersensitivity reaction associated with bronchiectasis and mucoid impaction (allergic bronchopulmonary aspergillosis) discussed in detail in Chapter 8, or granulo-

matous inflammation (bronchocentric granulomatosis) discussed in Chapter 6 [324,325]. It may colonize preexisting cavities to form a mycetoma [261]. In patients who have preexisting disease such as COPD, chronic necrotizing aspergillosis or semiinvasive aspergillosis may result [326,327]. In the immunocompromised host, *Aspergillus* may invade blood vessels, causing hemorrhagic infarction (angioinvasive aspergillosis) [328–330], or it may cause tracheobronchitis, bronchiolitis, or pneumonia (airway invasive aspergillosis) [312]. Often, there is some overlap between these various manifestations of *Aspergillus*-related lung disease in an individual patient.

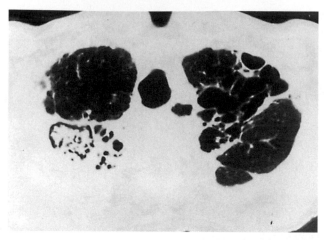
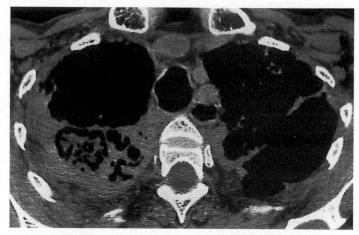

A

B

FIG. 5-83. Developing aspergilloma. Lung **(A)** and soft-tissue **(B)** window settings in a patient who has end-stage sarcoidosis and upper lobe cystic disease. A developing aspergilloma in the right upper lobe shows a typical, irregular, spongelike appearance.

Aspergilloma

An aspergilloma represents a mass of tangled fungal hyphae, fibrin, mucus, and cellular debris [322]. It typically is found in immunocompetent hosts. It is most often associated with preexisting cavities resulting from TB or sarcoidosis, although it may be seen in a variety of lung diseases [331]. In a study of 100 patients who had sarcoidosis and were followed for 10 years, ten developed an aspergilloma; furthermore, these ten cases occurred in only 19 patients who had cystic lung disease [332]. Although most are saprophytic, *Aspergillus* mycetoma may be associated with hypersensitivity reactions or limited tissue invasion, in some cases [333]. Hemoptysis, which may be massive, is a common complication.

Radiographic and HRCT findings of aspergilloma have been well described [322]. The presence of a well-defined homogenous nodular opacity within a thin- or thick-walled cavity associated with an air crescent sign is typical (Fig. 5-47) [261]. The mycetoma may be seen to move if decubitus or prone scans are obtained. However, in many cases, the appearance of an aspergilloma is atypical, being nonmobile, appearing as focal thickening or fronds in association with the cavity wall or as an irregular spongelike opacity containing airspaces and filling the preexisting cavity (Fig. 5-83) [261,322]. Presumably, this appearance reflects the presence of irregular fronds of fungal mycelia mixed with some residual intracavitary air.

Because the fungus incites an inflammatory response in the cavity wall and surrounding lung, a rich network of vessels and granulation tissue is often present in association with the cavity. Therefore, hemoptysis is a common symptom in patients who have aspergilloma, and it may be massive and life-threatening. Serum precipitins are usually positive for *Aspergillus*, whereas sputum culture reveals organisms in approximately half.

Pulmonary aspergilloma may also occur in immunosuppressed patients or patients who have HIV infection. In one study of 25 patients who had aspergilloma, the clinical presentation, progression of disease, treatment, and outcome were related to the patient's HIV status [331]. Of the 25 patients who had aspergilloma, ten were HIV-infected and 15 were HIV-negative. Predisposing diseases included TB (18 of 25 patients, 72%), sarcoidosis (4 of 25 patients, 16%), and *Pneumocystis carinii* pneumonia (PCP) (3 of 25 patients, 12%). All 25 patients had evidence of aspergilloma on chest CT. In addition, 17 of 25 patients had evidence of *Aspergillus* species in fungal culture, pathologic specimens, or immunoprecipitins. Although progressive disease was more common in the HIV-positive patients, hemoptysis was more frequent in patients that were HIV-negative. Hemoptysis was present in 15 of 25 (60%) patients [11 of 15 (73%) patients in the HIV-negative group, vs. 4 of 10 (40%) patients in the HIV-infected group]. Severe hemoptysis occurred in 5 of 15 (33%) patients in the HIV-negative group, versus 1 of 10 (10%) of the HIV-infected group. Disease progression occurred more frequently among the HIV-infected group [4 of 8 patients (50%) vs. 1 of 13 patients (8%) in HIV-negative individuals]. Four of eight (50%) patients in the HIV-infected group died, versus one of 13 (8%) patients in the HIV-negative group.

Chronic Necrotizing (Semiinvasive) Aspergillosis

Chronic necrotizing aspergillosis is typically associated with slowly progressive upper lobe abnormalities. Most patients have underlying chronic lung disease, including TB, COPD, fibrosis, or pneumoconiosis [322,326,327]. Patients may be mildly immunocompromised (e.g., chronic disease, advanced age, diabetes, poor nutrition, alcoholism, low-dose steroid treatment) but lack the severe immune deficiencies typical of patients who have invasive aspergillosis. Pathology reveals a combination of granulomatous inflammation, necrosis, and fibrosis similar to that seen in TB [333]. Symptoms are nonspecific, consisting of cough, sputum production, weight

TABLE 5-13. *HRCT findings in pulmonary aspergillosis*

Chronic necrotizing (semi-invasive) aspergillosis
  Upper lobe consolidation mimicking tuberculosis[a,b]
  One or more large nodules[a]
  Cavitation of consolidation or nodules[a,b]
  Intracavitary mycetoma
  Pleural thickening
Angioinvasive aspergillosis
  Ill-defined nodules or focal consolidation with a halo sign (early)[a,b]
  Cavitary nodules with an air-crescent sign (late)[a,b]
Airway-invasive aspergillosis
  Patchy peribronchial consolidation[a]
  Small ill-defined nodules centrilobular nodules or tree-in-bud[a,b]
  Areas of ground-glass opacity
  Lobar consolidation

[a]Most common findings.
[b]Findings most helpful in differential diagnosis.

loss, fever, and hemoptysis. The course is often indolent and progressive over a period of weeks to months; progressive disease may be fatal. Radiographs typically show upper lobe consolidation, with progressive cavitation over a period of weeks to months, indistinguishable from TB [322,326,327].

Franquet et al. [327] reviewed the radiographic and HRCT findings in nine patients who had semiinvasive aspergillosis associated with COPD. The radiologic and HRCT findings consisted of parenchymal consolidation (n = 6) and multiple nodules larger than 1 cm in diameter (n = 3) (Table 5-13). Parenchymal consolidation involved the upper lobes in five patients and was bilateral in four. Cavitation was present in two of the six patients who had consolidation, and in two of the three patients who had nodular opacities (Fig. 5-84). Adjacent pleural thickening was shown by HRCT in four patients. Histologically, the areas of consolidation represented active inflammation, and intraalveolar hemorrhage containing *Aspergillus* organisms. In the three patients who had multiple cavitary nodules, a variable degree of central necrosis was observed. The inflammatory infiltrate extended into the surrounding lung parenchyma, and adjacent areas of hemorrhage were also seen. *Aspergillus* colonies were identified within the lung tissue. Aspergillomas may develop in patients who have chronic necrotizing aspergillosis, having a typical or atypical appearance. With progressive disease, chest wall involvement may be present [322].

Invasive Aspergillosis

Invasive aspergillosis is characterized by involvement of normal lung tissue by *Aspergillus* organisms, usually resulting in significant tissue damage and necrosis [322,323]. It almost always occurs in immunosuppressed patients and is

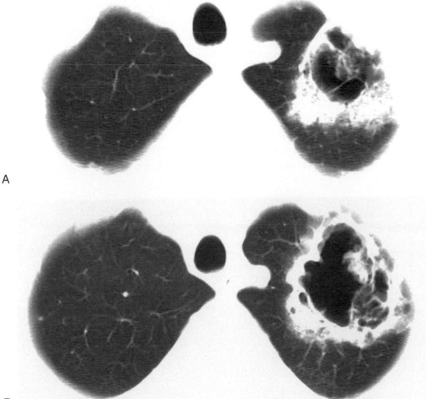

A

B

FIG. 5-84. A,B: Chronic necrotizing aspergillosis. A large cavitary mass is visible at the left lung apex, resembling cavitary tuberculosis. Irregular opacity within the cavity represents proliferating fungus.

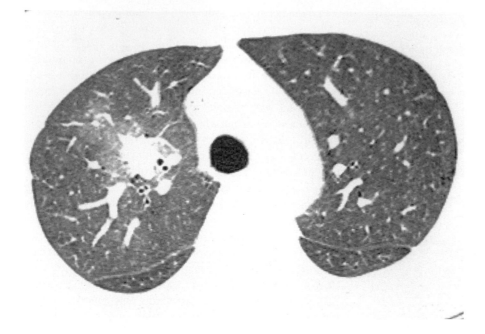

FIG. 5-85. Invasive pulmonary aspergillosis. HRCT at the level of the aortic arch shows right upper nodule surrounded by a halo of ground glass attenuation (halo sign). The patient was a 54-year-old man who had severe neutropenia after chemotherapy for chronic myelogenous leukemia. In this clinical setting, the findings are virtually diagnostic of angioinvasive aspergillosis.

particularly common in neutropenic patients who have acute leukemia, use corticosteroids or other immunosuppressive agents, or who have organ transplantation or malignancies [322,328,329,334]. Although it may be seen in patients who have AIDS, it is relatively uncommon, and usually associated with neutropenia or steroid therapy [335]. Invasive aspergillosis may occur in several forms.

Angioinvasive Aspergillosis

This is the most common form of invasive aspergillosis. Pathologic examination shows infiltration of lung tissue by fungus, with invasion of small arteries, vascular occlusion, and, often, infarction of involved lung [322,336]. Ill-defined nodules or focal areas of consolidation are typically seen on chest radiographs, but radiographic findings of invasive pulmonary aspergillosis are nonspecific until healing of the lesions has begun; during healing, nodules often cavitate, and air crescents characteristically develop. The presence of an air crescent (i.e., an air-crescent sign) in angioinvasive aspergillosis reflects the presence of lung necrosis, with the presence of a sequestrum or ball of devitalized and necrotic lung within the cavity. Although this appearance mimics that of a mycetoma within a preexisting cavity, the two conditions are unrelated.

Cavitation, when present, generally occurs approximately 2 weeks after appearance of the nodular opacities and is associated with a white blood cell count of more than 1,000. Thus, the presence of cavitation is generally considered to be a good prognostic sign. In one study, the most frequent symptoms associated with invasive pulmonary aspergillosis were cough (92% of patients), chest pain (76% of patients), and hemoptysis (54% of patients) [337]. Its prognosis is poor, unless promptly treated using antifungal agents or surgery [337,338].

In patients who have invasive pulmonary aspergillosis, CT can show characteristic findings that strongly suggest the diagnosis early in the course of disease [328,339]. Clinically, this diagnosis may be extremely difficult to make. This problem is further compounded by the potentially severe side effects associated with routine antifungal therapy.

High-Resolution Computed Tomography Findings

Invasive pulmonary aspergillosis commonly results in scattered foci of pulmonary parenchymal inflammation, infarction, and necrosis, which reflect hematogenous dissemination of the fungal organism associated with vascular obstruction. As documented by Kuhlman et al. [328] in patients who had acute leukemia who have early invasive aspergillosis, CT predictably shows a halo of opacity surrounding focal dense parenchymal nodules (Table 5-13). The halo surrounding the nodule is characteristically lower in attenuation than the nodule itself; in other words, the halo is of ground-glass opacity. This appearance has been termed the *halo sign* (Figs. 5-85 and 5-86). Many of these characteristic lesions are associated with vessels.

Hruban et al. [336] have obtained radiologic-pathologic correlation in patients who have documented invasive pulmonary aspergillosis and have clarified the etiology of the halo sign. In their patients, the halo and central nodule reflected a rim of coagulation necrosis or hemorrhage surrounding a central fungal nodule or infarct, respectively; an association of the halo sign with hemorrhagic nodules has been confirmed by others [340]. As shown on chest radiographs, an air-crescent sign may be seen after necrosis of lung (Fig. 5-87).

Some authors [328,336] have concluded that, in an appropriate population, the CT appearance of early invasive

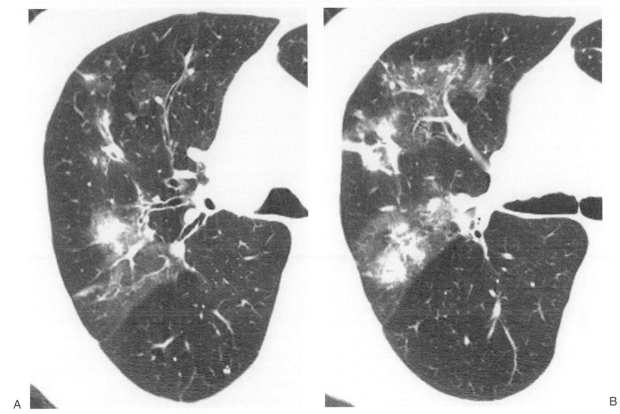

FIG. 5-86. A,B: Invasive pulmonary aspergillosis in a neutropenic patient with leukemia. Multiple pulmonary nodules are associated with the halo sign.

aspergillosis with a visible halo sign is sufficiently characteristic to justify a presumptive diagnosis and treatment. In one study, a halo sign was seen in 5 of 21 bone marrow transplantation patients who had a fungal infection [341]. However, others have emphasized that this finding can be associated with a variety of infectious and noninfectious processes. The halo sign has been reported in association with TB [342], candidiasis, *Legionella* pneumonia, cytomegalovirus, herpes simplex, Wegener's granulomatosis, BAC [43], metastatic angiosarcoma, and KS [340].

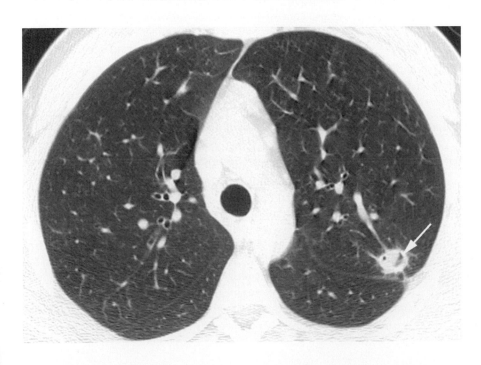

FIG. 5-87. Invasive pulmonary aspergillosis in a patient who has leukemia. A nodule in the left lung shows an air crescent (*arrow*) outlining a ball of necrotic lung.

Utility of High-Resolution Computed Tomography

The utility of CT in assessing immunosuppressed patients who have fever has been stressed by several investigators; in this setting, CT is more sensitive in detecting nodules suggestive of fungal infection and in characterizing their appearance. In a study [341] of febrile bone marrow transplant recipients, nodules were visible on CT in 20 of 21 patients who had fungal infections, and CT also showed cavitation (n = 7), the halo sign (n = 4), ill-defined margins (n = 5), air bronchograms (n = 2), or a cluster of fluffy nodules (n = 1). Chest radiographs showed nodules in 17 patients, and cavitation in five patients. In none of the nine episodes of fever resulting from bacteremia were there opacities on chest radiographs or CT studies. The authors concluded that CT studies demonstrating complicated nodules in febrile BMT patients strongly suggest a fungal infection, whereas negative CT studies suggest bacteremia or infection of nonpulmonary origin.

In another study, Won et al. [343] assessed the usefulness of HRCT in predicting the presence of invasive pulmonary aspergillosis in neutropenic patients. In five of ten (50%) patients who had suspected angioinvasive pulmonary aspergillosis, this diagnosis proved to be correct. In these five, the most common CT findings were segmental areas of consolidation associated with ground-glass opacity (four of five cases), and at least one nodule with a halo sign (two of five cases). Segmental areas of consolidation plus ground-glass attenuation were seen as isolated findings in three, and mixed findings with nodules that had a surrounding halo were seen in one case. Similar findings were seen in patients who had mucormycosis, organizing pneumonia, and pulmonary hemorrhage.

Early antifungal treatment, combined with surgical resection if necessary, may dramatically improve the prognosis of patients who have angioinvasive aspergillosis [337]. CT scans performed promptly in febrile neutropenic patients who have pulmonary x-ray infiltrates may reveal findings (i.e., the halo sign) that allow early diagnosis and treatment. In one study [337], the time to diagnosis was reduced dramatically from 7 days to 1.9 days with the use of CT.

The diagnosis of angioinvasive aspergillosis may be difficult to make at bronchoscopy, and transbronchial or open lung biopsies are frequently hazardous in immunosuppressed patients because of profound bone marrow suppression [322]. Brown et al. [311] compared the utility of HRCT and BAL in making this diagnosis. BAL was positive for fungi in only two of 11 patients who had HRCT findings consistent with angioinvasive aspergillosis. CT findings of angioinvasive aspergillosis included nodules measuring 1 to 3.5 cm in diameter in six patients, segmental consolidation in three patients, and both nodules and segmental consolidation in two patients. Furthermore, BAL may be positive for *Aspergillus* in immunosuppressed patients in the absence of invasive disease, and HRCT may be valuable in separating patients who have colonization from those who have significant disease [334].

In AIDS patients, CT can also be of value in the diagnosis of fungal infections [57]. Fungal infections, however, are rel-atively uncommon in this setting, being seen in less than 5% of patients [56]. Fungal infections in AIDS patients usually accompany disseminated disease. CT findings reported in AIDS patients include lymphadenopathy, nodules, masses, and consolidation [57].

Airway Invasive Aspergillosis (**Aspergillus Bronchopneumonia**)

Invasive aspergillosis associated with the airways, known as *airway invasive aspergillosis* or *Aspergillus bronchiolitis* and *bronchopneumonia*, is characterized by patchy peribronchial consolidation, centrilobular nodules, and in some cases, the finding of tree-in-bud (Figs. 5-88 and 5-89) [312,344]. Invasion of pulmonary arteries may be present but is much less conspicuous than with angioinvasive disease. Airway invasive aspergillosis accounts for approximately 15% of cases of invasive aspergillosis in immunocompromised patients.

In a study of nine patients who had pathologically proved airway invasive aspergillosis [312], CT findings included patchy bilateral consolidation predominantly peribronchial in location (n = 3), centrilobular nodules smaller than 5 mm in diameter (n = 2), lobular consolidation (n = 1), and ground-glass opacity (n = 1) (Table 5-13). At pathologic examination, the peribronchial infiltrates represented bronchopneumonia, and the nodules represented *Aspergillus* bronchiolitis, with a variable degree of peribronchiolar organizing pneumonia and hemorrhage [312].

In another study [311], CT findings of *Aspergillus* bronchopneumonia included peribronchial consolidation in five patients, small centrilobular micronodules in one patient, and both in four patients. In patients who have *Aspergillus* bronchopneumonia, BAL is more likely to be positive than in patients who have angioinvasive disease. In one study, BAL was positive for fungi in eight of ten patients who had CT scans consistent with *Aspergillus* bronchopneumonia, but was positive in only two of 11 patients who had HRCT findings consistent with angioinvasive aspergillosis [311].

Acute Tracheobronchitis

A less severe manifestation of airway invasion by *Aspergillus* is acute tracheobronchitis, in which organisms are limited to the large airways with little if any extension to involve the lung parenchyma and pulmonary arteries [322,323,345,346]. Tracheobronchitis accounts for approximately 5% of cases of invasive pulmonary aspergillosis and has a predilection for transplant patients and patients who have AIDS [345]. It is associated with multiple ulcerative, plaquelike, or nodular inflammatory lesions involving the trachea, mainstem, and segmental bronchi. Smaller airways may be involved, and this abnormality may progress to involve lung parenchyma. Symptoms include dyspnea, cough, and hemoptysis. Because abnormalities are limited to the airways, chest radiographs and CT are usually nonspecific or normal [346].

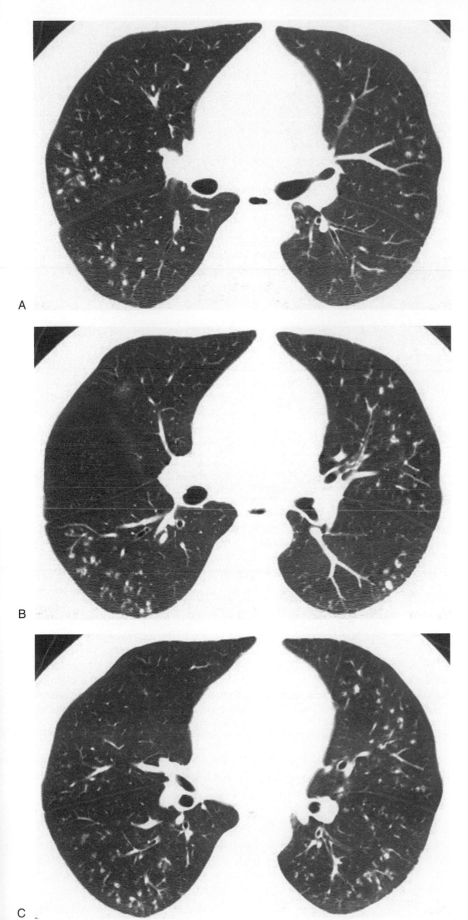

FIG. 5-88. A–C: Airway invasive pulmonary aspergillosis in an immunosuppressed patient with leukemia. HRCT shows multiple centrilobular nodules and clusters of nodules, with some opacities having the appearance of tree-in-bud. This appearance is nonspecific, but in an immunosuppressed patient, it suggests this diagnosis.

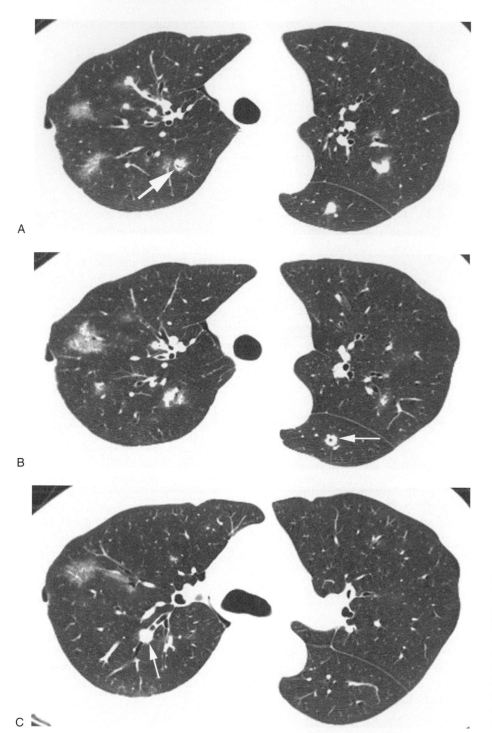

A

B

C

FIG. 5-89. A–C: Airway invasive pulmonary aspergillosis in an immunosuppressed patient who had a bone marrow transplant. HRCT shows multiple centrilobular nodules. Some of these (*arrows*, **A** and **B**) contain a lucency representing a centrilobular bronchiole or focal cavitation. The close relationship of these nodules to an airway is clearly seen (*arrow*, **C**). Patchy areas of ground-glass opacity are also visible.

Similar but distinct from acute tracheobronchitis is *obstructing bronchial aspergillosis* [54,347], a condition most frequent in patients who have AIDS. Obstructing bronchial aspergillosis is characterized by the acute onset of fever, dyspnea, and cough associated with the expectoration of bronchial casts consisting of mucus and *Aspergillus*. Airways are occluded by these casts, but the wall is not inflamed or invaded. CT scans show bilateral focal lower lobe consolidation or mucous plugging [54,348].

FUNGAL INFECTIONS OTHER THAN ASPERGILLOSIS

Fungal infection is a serious cause of morbidity and mortality in immunocompromised patients, occurring most often in patients who have chemotherapy-induced neutropenia, after solid organ or bone marrow transplantation, or in association with AIDS [341,348]. *Aspergillus* and *Cryptococcus* are among the most important opportunistic infections involving the lung. *Candida* may also affect the lung, but pulmonary involvement is usually secondary, and associated with sepsis and diffuse disease.

Most fungal diseases result in CT and HRCT patterns of disease indistinguishable from those described for mycobacterial infections and aspergillosis, including both focal and diffuse parenchymal infiltrates, cavitation, nodules, hilar and mediastinal adenopathy, miliary nodules (see Fig. 3-56), and pleural abnormalities [341,348].

Cryptococcal infection is usually limited to the lung in immunocompetent patients, and symptoms are relatively mild. However, as many as 70% of cryptococcal infections occur in immunocompromised subjects [348–350]. In these patients, lung involvement is typical, but dissemination often occurs. In immunocompromised patients who have *Cryptococcus* infection, radiographs typically show more extensive abnormalities than in immunocompetent hosts. In a study of 24 cases of proven pulmonary cryptococcosis [350], immunocompetent subjects tended to have radiographic findings of a peripheral nodule or nodules. Immunocompromised hosts, on the other hand, demonstrated a wider variety of radiographic abnormalities, including single nodules; multiple nodules that progressed to confluence, cavitation, or both; segmental consolidation; bilateral bronchopneumonia; or mixed patterns. In this study, adenopathy, cavitation, and pleural effusions were limited to the immunocompromised hosts. In a study of chest radiographs and CT in patients who had AIDS and cryptococcosis, abnormalities consisted of patchy ill-defined consolidation, well-defined consolidation with air bronchograms, or large nodules [351]. A predominance of abnormalities in the lung periphery has been reported [352]. Small centrilobular nodules similar to those seen with endobronchial spread of TB have been reported on HRCT with endobronchial spread of cryptococcal pneumonia [246,320].

Mucormycosis and *Zygomycosis* are general terms used to describe infections by fungi of the class *Zygomycetes*, including *Rhizopus* and *Mucor*, among others [353]. These infections usually occur in the setting of hematologic malignancy and neutropenia, or diabetes, and have a high mortality [348]. In one study of 32 cases, 20 patients were immunosuppressed and nine had diabetes mellitus [354]. As with invasive *Aspergillus*, invasion of pulmonary arteries may occur with thrombosis, infarction, and pulmonary hemorrhage. In patients who have neutropenia, pulmonary mucormycosis mimics the clinical, radiographic, and pathologic manifestations of invasive aspergillosis [348,354,355]. Patients typically present with fever, cough, bloody sputum, dyspnea, and chest pain.

CT findings in mucormycosis include lobular, multilobar, wedge-shaped, or masslike consolidation, and solitary or multiple nodules or masses [354,355]. Also seen in some patients are the halo sign, central areas of low attenuation, cavitation, and the presence of an intracavitary mass with an air-crescent sign [354,355]. Associated radiographic findings include hilar or mediastinal adenopathy, and unilateral or bilateral pleural effusion [354].

HRCT features of some other fungal infections have been described. For example, peribronchovascular interstitial thickening, centrilobular opacities, consolidation, cavities, traction bronchiectasis, and paracicatricial emphysema have been described in patients who have South American blastomycosis [356]. In general, the accurate diagnosis of a fungal infection requires confirmation by histologic examination of a biopsy specimen or culture.

SEPTIC EMBOLISM AND INFARCTION

Septic pulmonary emboli, with or without infarction, generally result in diffuse parenchymal abnormalities; only rarely do they present as solitary lesions within the lungs. The correct radiographic diagnosis usually is suggested by the finding of well-defined, bilateral peripheral nodules with various degrees of cavitation, especially in the setting of known intravenous drug abuse or some other known source of sepsis. In a significant percentage of cases, however, these findings may not be readily apparent on the radiograph [357]. Cavitary parenchymal nodules presumably result from septic occlusion of small, peripheral pulmonary arterial branches, resulting in the development of metastatic lung abscesses. The finding of triangular, wedge-shaped regions most likely results from infarction complicated by infection, presumably caused by larger emboli than those that result in simple nodular lung abscesses.

Computed Tomography and High-Resolution Computed Tomography Findings

The CT appearance of septic pulmonary emboli and infarcts has been well described (Table 5-14) [357–360]. In patients who have septic embolism, peripheral nodules in varying stages of cavitation are often present, presumably due to intermittent seeding of the lungs by infected material. Especially characteristic is the finding of identifiable feeding vessels in association with peripheral nodules (Fig. 5-90); this was visible in ten of 15 cases (67%) studied by Huang et al. [357]. Similar findings have been reported by Kuhlman et al. [359] in a series of 18 patients who had documented septic pulmonary emboli; these authors found nodules associ-

---

TABLE 5-14. *HRCT findings in septic embolism and infarction*

Bilateral peripheral nodules in varying stages of cavitation[a]

Peripheral wedge-shaped triangular opacities abutting pleural surfaces, with or without cavitation[a]

Relationship of opacities to vessels[a]

Superimposition of first three findings[a,b]

Associated pleural and/or pericardial effusions

Indwelling venous catheters

[a]Most common findings.
[b]Findings most helpful in differential diagnosis.

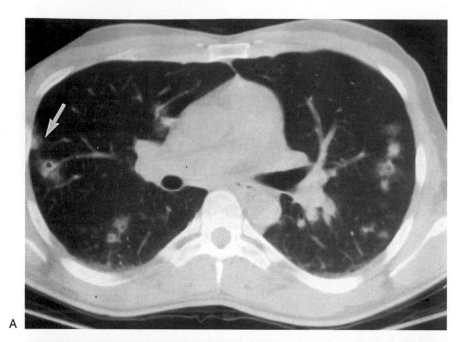

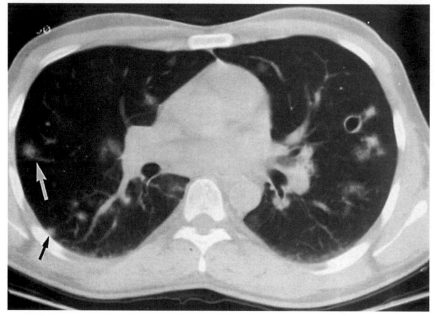

FIG. 5-90. Septic pulmonary emboli. **A,B:** CT sections through the midlungs of a known intravenous drug abuser show scattered, mostly peripheral, poorly defined foci of airspace consolidation, many of which contain varying degrees of cavitation. Note that a number of these appear to be associated with feeding vessels (*arrows*, **A,B**), suggesting a hematogenous origin. Subsequent blood cultures confirmed staphylococcal septicemia.

ated with vessels in 67% of cases. CT can be helpful in suggesting the diagnosis of septic embolism. Compared with plain radiographs, CT scans provided useful additional information in 8 of 15 cases (53%) in one study [357]. Furthermore, the diagnosis of septic embolism was first suggested on CT in 7 of 15 cases, and in 6 of 18 cases [357,359].

Septic emboli may also result in pulmonary infarction. An infarction is recognizable as a triangular, wedge-shaped opacity with its base oriented at the pleural surface. After the administration of a bolus of intravenous-contrast medium, the perimeter of an infarct characteristically enhances, possibly owing to collateral blood flow from adjacent bronchial arteries, whereas the center of the lesion remains lucent. Cystic changes within an area of infarction may signify either necrosis or infection. Unfortunately, this appearance is not entirely diagnostic, because pneumonias may occasionally have a similar appearance. As suggested by Balakrishnan et al. [360], in a CT-pathologic correlative study of 12 proven pulmonary infarcts in ten patients, specificity increases when a vessel can be identified at the apex of the infarct.

It should be noted that especially septic emboli, but rarely the appearance of pulmonary infarcts, may be mimicked either by a vasculitis, such as Wegener's granulomatosis, or even cavitary metastases. In these cases, however, confusion with septic emboli in particular is rare because of the differences in clinical presentation.

REFERENCES

1. Trapnell DH. The radiological appearance of lymphangitic carcinomatosis of the lung. *Thorax* 1964;19:251–260.

2. Heitzman ER. Pattern recognition in pulmonary radiology. In: *The lung: radiologic-pathologic correlations*, 2nd ed. St. Louis: CV Mosby, 1984:70–105.

3. Genereux GP. Pattern recognition in diffuse lung disease: a review of theory and practice. *Med Radiogr Photog* 1985;61:2–31.

4. Carstairs LS. The interpretation of shadows in a restricted area of a lung field on the chest radiograph. *Proc R Soc Med* 1961;54:1961.

5. Bégin R, Ostiguy G, Fillion R, et al. Computed tomography scan in the early detection of silicosis. *Am Rev Respir Dis* 1991;3:1.

6. Remy-Jardin M, Degreef JM, Beuscart R, et al. Coal worker's pneumoconiosis: CT assessment in exposed workers and correlation with radiographic findings. *Radiology* 1990;177:363–371.

7. Gruden JF, Webb WR, Warnock M. Centrilobular opacities in the lung on high-resolution CT: diagnostic considerations and pathologic correlation. *AJR Am J Roentgenol* 1994;162:569–574.

8. Gruden JF, Webb WR, Naidich DP, et al. Multinodular disease: anatomic localization at thin-section CT—multireader evaluation of a simple algorithm. *Radiology* 1999;210:711–720.

9. Reittner P, Müller NL, Heyneman L, et al. Mycoplasma pneumoniae pneumonia: radiographic and high-resolution CT features in 28 patients. *AJR Am J Roentgenol* 1999;174:37–41.

10. Fraser RS, Müller NL, Colman N, Paré PD, eds. *Diagnosis of diseases of the chest*. Philadelphia: WB Saunders, 1999:1381–1417.

11. Davis SD. CT evaluation for pulmonary metastases in patients with extrathoracic malignancy. *Radiology* 1991;180:1–12.

12. Heitzman ER. Lymphangitic metastasis to lung. In: *The lung: radiologic-pathologic correlations*, 2nd ed. St. Louis: Mosby, 1984:413–421.

13. Janower ML, Blennerhasset JB. Lymphangitic spread of metastatic tumor to lung. *Radiology* 1971;101:267–273.

14. Goldsmith SH, Bailey HD, Callahan EL, et al. Pulmonary metastases from breast carcinoma. *Arch Surg* 1967;94:483–488.

15. Munk PL, Müller NL, Miller RR, et al. Pulmonary lymphangitic carcinomatosis: CT and pathologic findings. *Radiology* 1988;166:705–709.

16. Ren H, Hruban RH, Kuhlman JE, et al. Computed tomography of inflation-fixed lungs: the beaded septum sign of pulmonary metastases. *J Comput Assist Tomogr* 1989;13:411–416.

17. Colby TV, Swensen SJ. Anatomic distribution and histopathologic patterns in diffuse lung disease: correlation with HRCT. *J Thorac Imag* 1996;11:1–26.

18. Remy-Jardin M, Beuscart R, Sault MC, et al. Subpleural micronodules in diffuse infiltrative lung diseases: evaluation with thin-section CT scans. *Radiology* 1990;177:133–139.

19. Zerhouni EA, Naidich DP, Stitik FP, et al. Computed tomography of the pulmonary parenchyma: part 2. interstitial disease. *J Thorac Imag* 1985;1:54–64.

20. Stein MG, Mayo J, Müller N, et al. Pulmonary lymphangitic spread of carcinoma: appearance on CT scans. *Radiology* 1987;162:371–375.

21. Meziane MA, Hruban RH, Zerhouni EA, et al. High resolution CT of the lung parenchyma with pathologic correlation. *Radiographics* 1988;8:27–54.

22. Webb WR. High-resolution CT of the lung parenchyma. *Radiol Clin North Am* 1989;27:1085–1097.

23. Johkoh T, Ikezoe J, Tomiyama N, et al. CT findings in lymphangitic carcinomatosis of the lung: correlation with histologic findings and pulmonary function tests. *AJR Am J Roentgenol* 1992;158:1217–1222.

24. Ikezoe J, Godwin JD, Hunt KJ, et al. Pulmonary lymphangitic carcinomatosis: chronicity of radiographic findings in long-term survivors. *AJR Am J Roentgenol* 1995;165:49–52.

25. Grenier P, Chevret S, Beigelman C, et al. Chronic diffuse infiltrative lung disease: determination of the diagnostic value of clinical data, chest radiography, and CT with Bayesian analysis. *Radiology* 1994;194:383–390.

26. Mathieson JR, Mayo JR, Staples CA, et al. Chronic diffuse infiltrative lung disease: comparison of diagnostic accuracy of CT and chest radiography. *Radiology* 1989;171:111–116.

27. Brauner MW, Grenier P, Mompoint D, et al. Pulmonary sarcoidosis: evaluation with high-resolution CT. *Radiology* 1989;172:467–471.

28. Webb WR, Stein MG, Finkbeiner WE, et al. Normal and diseased isolated lungs: high-resolution CT. *Radiology* 1988;166:81–87.

29. Hirakata K, Nakata H, Nakagawa T. CT of pulmonary metastases with pathological correlation. *Semin Ultrasound CT MR* 1995;16:379–394.

30. Murata K, Takahashi M, Mori M, et al. Pulmonary metastatic nodules: CT-pathologic correlation. *Radiology* 1992;182:331–335.

31. Hirakata K, Nakata H, Haratake J. Appearance of pulmonary metastases on high-resolution CT scans: comparison with histopathologic findings from autopsy specimens. *AJR Am J Roentgenol* 1993;161:37–43.

32. Shepard JA, Moore EH, Templeton PA, et al. Pulmonary intravascular tumor emboli: dilated and beaded peripheral pulmonary arteries at CT. *Radiology* 1993;187:797–801.

33. Napel S, Rubin GD, Jeffrey Jr RB. STS-MIP: a new reconstruction technique for CT of the chest. *J Comput Assist Tomogr* 1993;17:832–838.

34. Remy-Jardin M, Remy J, Artaud D, et al. Diffuse infiltrative lung disease: clinical value of sliding-thin-slab maximum intensity projection CT scans in the detection of mild micronodular patterns. *Radiology* 1996;200:333–339.

35. Peuchot M, Libshitz HI. Pulmonary metastatic disease: radiologic-surgical correlation. *Radiology* 1987;164:719–722.

36. Costello P, Anderson W, Blume D. Pulmonary nodule: evaluation with spiral volumetric CT. *Radiology* 1991;179:875–876.

37. Remy-Jardin M, Remy J, Giraud F, et al. Pulmonary nodules: detection with thick-section spiral CT versus conventional CT. *Radiology* 1993;187:513–520.

38. Munden RF, Pugatch RD, Liptay MJ, et al. Small pulmonary lesions detected at CT: clinical importance. *Radiology* 1997;202:105–110.

39. Diederich S, Semik M, Lentschig MG, et al. Helical CT of pulmonary nodules in patients with extrathoracic malignancy: CT-surgical correlation. *AJR Am J Roentgenol* 1999;172:353–360.

40. Hill CA. Bronchioloalveolar carcinoma: a review. *Radiology* 1984;150:15–20.

41. Lee KS, Kim Y, Han J, et al. Bronchioloalveolar carcinoma: clinical, histopathologic, and radiologic findings. *Radiographics* 1997;17:1345–1357.

42. Adler B, Padley S, Miller RR, et al. High-resolution CT of bronchioloalveolar carcinoma. *AJR Am J Roentgenol* 1992;159:275–277.

43. Kuriyama K, Seto M, Kasugai T, et al. Ground-glass opacity on thin-section CT: value in differentiating subtypes of adenocarcinoma of the lung. *AJR Am J Roentgenol* 1999;173:465–469.

44. Naidich DP, Zerhouni EA, Hutchins GM, et al. Computed tomography of the pulmonary parenchyma: part 1. Distal air-space disease. *J Thorac Imag* 1985;1:39–53.

45. Tan RT, Kuzo RS. High-resolution CT findings of mucinous bronchioloalveolar carcinoma: a case of pseudopulmonary alveolar proteinosis. *AJR Am J Roentgenol* 1997;168:99–100.

46. Akira M, Atagi S, Kawahara M, et al. High-resolution CT findings of diffuse bronchioloalveolar carcinoma in 38 patients. *AJR Am J Roentgenol* 1999;173:1623–1629.

47. Hommeyer SH, Godwin JD, Takasugi JE. Computed tomography of air-space disease. *Radiol Clin North Am* 1991;29:1065–1084.

48. Im JG, Han MC, Yu EJ, et al. Lobar bronchioloalveolar carcinoma: "angiogram sign" on CT scans. *Radiology* 1990;176:749–753.

49. Gaeta M, Caruso R, Barone M, et al. Ground-glass attenuation in nodular bronchioloalveolar carcinoma: CT patterns and prognostic value. *J Comput Assist Tomogr* 1998;22:215–219.

50. Aquino SL, Chiles C, Halford P. Distinction of consolidative bronchioloalveolar carcinoma from pneumonia: do CT criteria work? *AJR Am J Roentgenol* 1998;171:359–363.

51. Metzger RA, Multhern CB, Arger PH, et al. CT differentiation of solitary from diffuse bronchioloalveolar carcinoma. *J Comput Assist Tomogr* 1981;5:830–833.

52. Zwirewich CV, Miller RR, Müller NL. Multicentric adenocarcinoma of the lung: CT-pathologic correlation. *Radiology* 1990;176:185–190.

53. Naidich DP, Tarras M, Garay SM, et al. R. Kaposi sarcoma: CT-radiographic correlation. *Chest* 1989;96:723–728.

54. McGuinness G, Gruden JF, Bhalla M, et al. AIDS-related airway disease. *AJR Am J Roentgenol* 1997;168:67–77.

55. Gruden JF, Huang L, Webb WR, et al. AIDS-related Kaposi sarcoma of the lung: radiographic findings and staging system with bronchoscopic correlation. *Radiology* 1995;195:545–552.

56. Naidich DP, McGuinness G. Pulmonary manifestations of AIDS: CT and radiographic correlations. *Radiol Clin North Am* 1991;29:999–1017.

57. Hartman TE, Primack SL, Müller NL, et al. Diagnosis of thoracic complications in AIDS: accuracy of CT. *AJR Am J Roentgenol* 1994;162:547–553.

58. Wolff SD, Kuhlman JE, Fishman EK. Thoracic Kaposi sarcoma in AIDS: CT findings. *J Comput Assist Tomogr* 1993;17:60–62.

59. Kang EY, Staples CA, McGuinness G, et al. Detection and differential diagnosis of pulmonary infections and tumors in patients with AIDS: value of chest radiography versus CT. *AJR Am J Roentgenol* 1996;166:15–19.

60. Gruden JF, Klein JS, Webb WR. Percutaneous transthoracic needle biopsy in AIDS: analysis in 32 patients. *Radiology* 1993; 189:567–571.

61. Edinburgh KJ, Jasmer RM, Huang L, et al. Multiple pulmonary nodules in AIDS: usefulness of CT in distinguishing among potential causes. *Radiology* 2000;214:427–432.

62. Bragg DG, Chor PJ, Murray KA, et al. Lymphoproliferative disorders of the lung: histopathology, clinical manifestations, and imaging features. *AJR Am J Roentgenol* 1994;163:273–281.

63. Gibson M, Hansell DM. Lymphocytic disorders of the chest: pathology and imaging. *Clin Radiol* 1998;53:469–480.

64. Koss MN. Pulmonary lymphoid disorders. *Semin Diagn Pathol* 1995;12:158–171.

65. Thompson GP, Utz JP, Rosenow EC, et al. Pulmonary lymphoproliferative disorders. *Mayo Clin Proc* 1993;68:804–817.

66. Collins J, Müller NL, Leung AN, et al. Epstein-Barr-virus-associated lymphoproliferative disease of the lung: CT and histologic findings. *Radiology* 1998;208:749–759.

67. Bolton-Maggs PH, Colman A, Dixon GR, et al. Mucosa associated lymphoma of the lung. *Thorax* 1993;48:670–672.

68. Holland EA, Ghahremani GG, Fry WA, et al. Evolution of pulmonary pseudolymphomas: clinical and radiologic manifestations. *J Thorac Imag* 1991;6:74–80.

69. Yousem SA, Colby TV, Carrington CB. Follicular bronchitis/bronchiolitis. *Hum Pathol* 1985;16:700–706.

70. Howling SJ, Hansell DM, Wells AU, et al. Follicular bronchiolitis: thin-section CT and histologic findings. *Radiology* 1999;212:637–642.

71. Kinoshita M, Higashi T, Tanaka C, et al. Follicular bronchiolitis associated with rheumatoid arthritis. *Intern Med* 1992;31:674–677.

72. Oh YW, Effmann EL, Redding GJ, et al. Follicular hyperplasia of bronchus-associated lymphoid tissue causing severe air-trapping. *AJR Am J Roentgenol* 1999;172:745–747.

73. Koss MN, Hochholzer L, Langloss JM, et al. Lymphoid interstitial pneumonia: clinicopathological and immunopathological findings in 18 cases. *Pathology* 1987;19:178–185.

74. Fishback N, Koss M. Update on lymphoid interstitial pneumonitis. *Curr Opin Pulm Med* 1996;2:429–433.

75. Travis WD, Fox CH, Devaney KO, et al. Lymphoid pneumonitis in 50 adult patients infected with the human immunodeficiency virus: lymphocytic interstitial pneumonitis versus nonspecific interstitial pneumonitis. *Hum Pathol* 1992;23:529–541.

76. Johkoh T, Müller NL, Pickford HA, et al. Lymphocytic interstitial pneumonia: thin-section CT findings in 22 patients. *Radiology* 1999;212:567–572.

77. Julsrud PR, Brown LR, Li CY, et al. Pulmonary processes of mature-appearing lymphocytes: pseudolymphoma, well-differentiated lymphocytic lymphoma, and lymphocytic interstitial pneumonitis. *Radiology* 1978;127:289–296.

78. Glickstein M, Kornstein MJ, Pietra GG, et al. Nonlymphomatous lymphoid disorders of the lung. *AJR Am J Roentgenol* 1986;147:227–237.

79. Ichikawa Y, Kinoshita M, Koga T, et al. Lung cyst formation in lymphocytic interstitial pneumonia: CT features. *J Comput Assist Tomogr* 1994;18:745–748.

80. McGuinness G, Scholes JV, Jagirdar JS, et al. Unusual lymphoproliferative disorders in nine adults with HIV or AIDS: CT and pathologic findings. *Radiology* 1995;197:59–65.

81. Desai SR, Nicholson AG, Stewart S, et al. Benign pulmonary lymphocytic infiltration and amyloidosis: computed tomographic and pathologic features in three cases. *J Thorac Imag* 1997;12:215–220.

82. Honda O, Johkoh T, Ichikado K, et al. Differential diagnosis of lymphocytic interstitial pneumonia and malignant lymphoma on high-resolution CT. *AJR Am J Roentgenol* 1999;173:71–74.

83. Limpert J, MacMahon H, Variakojis D. Angioimmunoblastic lymphadenopathy: clinical and radiological features. *Radiology* 1984; 152:27–30.

84. Zylak CJ, Banerjee R, Galbraith PA, et al. Lung involvement in angioimmunoblastic lymphadenopathy (ail). *Radiology* 1976; 121:513–519.

85. Locksmith JP, Brannon MH. Diffuse CT contrast enhancement of cervical lymph nodes in angioimmunoblastic lymphadenopathy. *J Comput Assist Tomogr* 1991;15:703–704.

86. Cordier JF, Chailleux E, Lauque D, et al. Primary pulmonary lymphomas: a clinical study of 70 cases in nonimmunocompromised patients. *Chest* 1993;103:201–208.

87. Rosenberg SA, Diamond HD, Jaslowitz B, et al. Lymphosarcoma: a review of 1269 cases. *Medicine* 1961;40:31–84.

88. Harris NL. Low-grade B-cell lymphoma of mucosa-associated lymphoid tissue and monocytoid B-cell lymphoma: related entities that are distinct from other low-grade B-cell lymphomas [editorial;comment]. *Arch Pathol Lab Med* 1993;117:771–775.

89. Li G, Hansmann ML, Zwingers T, et al. Primary lymphomas of the lung: morphological, immunohistochemical and clinical features. *Histopathology* 1990;16:519–531.

90. Koss MN, Hochholzer L, Nichols PW, et al. Primary non-Hodgkin's lymphoma and pseudolymphoma of lung: a study of 161 patients. *Hum Pathol* 1983;14:1024–1038.

91. Lee KS, Kim Y, Primack SL. Imaging of pulmonary lymphomas. *AJR Am J Roentgenol* 1997;168:339–345.

92. McCulloch GL, Sinnatamby R, Stewart S, et al. High-resolution computed tomographic appearance of MALToma of the lung. *Eur Radiol* 1998;8:1669–1673.

93. Knisely BL, Mastey LA, Mergo PJ, et al. Pulmonary mucosa-associated lymphoid tissue lymphoma: CT and pathologic findings. *AJR Am J Roentgenol* 1999;172:1321–1326.

94. Bosanko CM, Korobkin M, Fantone JC, et al. Lobar primary pulmonary lymphoma: CT findings. *J Comput Assist Tomogr* 1991;15:679–682.

95. O'Donnell PG, Jackson SA, Tung KT, et al. Radiological appearances of lymphomas arising from mucosa-associated lymphoid tissue (MALT) in the lung. *Clin Radiol* 1998;53:258–263.

96. Au V, Leung AN. Radiologic manifestations of lymphoma in the thorax. *AJR Am J Roentgenol* 1997;168:93–98.

97. Lee DK, Im JG, Lee KS, et al. B-cell lymphoma of bronchus-associated lymphoid tissue (BALT): CT features in 10 patients. *J Comput Assist Tomogr* 2000;24:30–34.

98. Gollub MJ, Castellino RA. Diffuse endobronchial non-Hodgkin's lymphoma: CT demonstration. *AJR Am J Roentgenol* 1995; 164:1093–1094.

99. Close PM, Macrae MB, Hammond JM, et al. Anaplastic large-cell Ki-1 lymphoma: pulmonary presentation mimicking miliary tuberculosis. *Am J Clin Pathol* 1993;99:631–636.

100. Mentzer SJ, Reilly JJ, Skarin AT, et al. Patterns of lung involvement by malignant lymphoma. *Surgery* 1993;113:507–514.

101. Castellino RA, Blank N, Hoppe RT, et al. Hodgkin's disease: contributions of chest CT in the initial staging evaluation. *Radiology* 1986;160:603–605.

102. Filly R, Blank N, Castellino R. Radiographic distribution of intrathoracic disease in previously untreated patients with Hodgkin's disease and non-Hodgkin's lymphoma. *Radiology* 1976;120:277.

103. Castellino RA, Hilton S, O'Brien JP, et al. Non-Hodgkin lymphoma: contribution of chest CT in the initial staging evaluation. *Radiology* 1996;199:129–132.

104. Castellino RA. The non-Hodgkin lymphomas: practical concepts for the diagnostic radiologist. *Radiology* 1991;178:315–321.

105. Castellino RA. Hodgkin's disease: practical concepts for the diagnostic radiologist. *Radiology* 1986;157:305–310.

106. Lewis ER, Caskey CI, Fishman EK. Lymphoma of the lung: CT findings in 31 patients. *AJR Am J Roentgenol* 1991;156:711–714.

107. Polish LB, Cohn DL, Ryder JW, et al. Pulmonary non-Hodgkin's lymphoma in AIDS. *Chest* 1989;96:1321–1326.

108. Ioachim HL, Dorsett B, Cronin W, et al. Acquired immunodeficiency syndrome-associated lymphomas: clinical, pathologic, immunologic, and viral characteristics of 111 cases. *Hum Pathol* 1991;22:659–673.

109. Ray P, Antoine M, Mary-Krause M, et al. AIDS-related primary pulmonary lymphoma. *Am J Respir Crit Care Med* 1998;158:1221–1229.

110. Eisner MD, Kaplan LD, Herndier B, et al. The pulmonary manifestations of AIDS-related non-Hodgkin's lymphoma. *Chest* 1996; 110:729–736.

111. Blunt DM, Padley SP. Radiographic manifestations of AIDS related lymphoma in the thorax. *Clin Radiol* 1995;50:607–612.

112. Sider L, Weiss AJ, Smith MD, et al. Varied appearance of AIDS-related lymphoma in the chest. *Radiology* 1989;171:629–632.

113. Bazot M, Cadranel J, Benayoun S, et al. Primary pulmonary AIDS-related lymphoma: radiographic and CT findings. *Chest* 1999;116:1282–1286.

114. Craig FE, Gulley ML, Banks PM. Posttransplantation lymphoproliferative disorders. *Am J Clin Pathol* 1993;99:265–276.

115. Rappaport DC, Chamberlain DW, Shepherd FA, et al. Lymphoproliferative disorders after lung transplantation: imaging features. *Radiology* 1998;206:519–524.

116. Schenkein DP, Schwartz RS. Neoplasms and transplantation—trading swords for plowshares [editorial;comment]. *N Engl J Med* 1997;336:949–950.

117. Donnelly LF, Frush DP, Marshall KW, et al. Lymphoproliferative disorders: CT findings in immunocompromised children. *AJR Am J Roentgenol* 1998;171:725–731.

118. Nalesnik MA, Makowka L, Starzl TE. The diagnosis and treatment of posttransplant lymphoproliferative disorders. *Curr Probl Surg* 1988;25:367–472.

119. Aris RM, Maia DM, Neuringer IP, et al. Post-transplantation lymphoproliferative disorder in the Epstein-Barr virus-naive lung transplant recipient. *Am J Respir Crit Care Med* 1996;154:1712–1717.

120. Dodd GD, Ledesma-Medina J, Baron RL, Fuhrman CR. Posttransplant lymphoproliferative disorder: intrathoracic manifestations. *Radiology* 1992;184:65–69.

121. Carignan S, Staples CA, Müller NL. Intrathoracic lymphoproliferative disorders in the immunocompromised patient: CT findings. *Radiology* 1995;197:53–58.

122. Brown MJ, Miller RR, Müller NL. Acute lung disease in the immunocompromised host: CT and pathologic examination findings. *Radiology* 1994;190:247–254.

123. Myers JL, Kurtin PJ, Katzenstein AL, et al. Lymphomatoid granulomatosis. Evidence of immunophenotypic diversity and relationship to Epstein-Barr virus infection. *Am J Surg Pathol* 1995;19:1300–1312.

124. Prenovault JM, Weisbrod GL, Herman SJ. Lymphomatoid granulomatosis: a review of 12 cases. *Can Assoc Radiol J* 1988;39:263–266.

125. Doran HM, Sheppard MN, Collins PW, et al. Pathology of the lung in leukaemia and lymphoma: a study of 87 autopsies. *Histopathology* 1991;18:211–219.

126. Rollins SD, Colby TV. Lung biopsy in chronic lymphocytic leukemia. *Arch Pathol Lab Med* 1988;112:607–611.

127. Maile CW, Moore AV, Ulreich S, et al. Chest radiographic-pathologic correlation in adult leukemia patients. *Invest Radiol* 1983;18:495–499.

128. Tenholder MF, Hooper RG. Pulmonary infiltrates in leukemia. *Chest* 1980;78:468–473.

129. Heyneman LE, Johkoh T, Ward S, et al. Pulmonary leukemic infiltrates: high-resolution CT findings in 10 patients. *AJR Am J Roentgenol* 2000;174:517–521.

130. Colby TV, Carrington CB. Infiltrative lung disease. In: Thurlbeck WM, ed. *Pathology of the lung*. New York: Thieme Medical Publishers, 1988:425–518.

131. Crystal RG, Bitterman PB, Rennard SI, et al. Interstitial lung diseases of unknown cause: disorders characterized by chronic inflammation of the lower respiratory tract. *N Engl J Med* 1984;310:154–166.

132. Colby T, Carrington C. Interstitial lung disease. In: Thurlbeck WM, Churg AM, eds. *Pathology of the lung*. New York: Thieme Medical Publishers, 1994:589–737.

133. Thomas PD, Hunninghake GW. Current concepts of the pathogenesis of sarcoidosis. *Am Rev Respir Dis* 1987;135:747–760.

134. Rosen Y, Athanassiades TJ, Moon S, et al. Nongranulomatous interstitial pneumonitis in sarcoidosis. *Chest* 1978;74:122–125.

135. Crystal RG, Gadek JE, Ferrans VJ, et al. Interstitial lung disease: current concepts of pathogenesis, staging and therapy. *Am J Med* 1981;70:542–568.

136. Keogh BA, Hunninghake GW, Line BR, et al. The alveolitis of pulmonary sarcoidosis: evaluation of natural history and alveolitis-dependent changes in lung function. *Am Rev Respir Dis* 1983;128:256–265.

137. Müller NL, Miller RR. Ground-glass attenuation, nodules, alveolitis, and sarcoid granulomas (editorial). *Radiology* 1993;189:31–32.

138. Hillerdal G, Neu E, Osterman K, et al. Sarcoidosis: epidemiology and prognosis, a 15-year European study. *Am Rev Respir Dis* 1984;130:29–32.

139. McLoud TC, Epler GR, Gaensler EA, et al. A radiographic classification for sarcoidosis: physiologic correlation. *Invest Radiol* 1982;17:129–138.

140. Scadding JG, Mitchell DN. Sarcoidosis. London: Chapman and Hall Medical, 1985:101–180.

141. Hamper UM, Fishman EK, Khouri NF, et al. Typical and atypical CT manifestations of pulmonary sarcoidosis. *J Comput Assist Tomogr* 1986;10:928–936.

142. Dawson WB, Müller NL. High-resolution computed tomography in pulmonary sarcoidosis. *Semin Ultra CT MR* 1990;11:423–429.

143. Müller NL, Kullnig P, Miller RR. The CT findings of pulmonary sarcoidosis: analysis of 25 patients. *AJR Am J Roentgenol* 1989;152:1179–1182.

144. Müller NL, Miller RR. Computed tomography of chronic diffuse infiltrative lung disease: part 1. *Am Rev Respir Dis* 1990;142:1206–1215.

145. Heitzman ER. Sarcoidosis. In: *The lung: radiologic-pathologic correlations*. St. Louis: CV Mosby, 1984:294–310.

146. Carrington CB, Gaensler EA, Mikus JP, et al. Structure and function in sarcoidosis. *Ann N Y Acad Sci* 1976;278:265–283.

147. Bergin CJ, Bell DY, Coblentz CL, et al. Sarcoidosis: correlation of pulmonary parenchymal pattern at CT with results of pulmonary function tests. *Radiology* 1989;171:619–624.

148. Lynch DA, Webb WR, Gamsu G, et al. Computed tomography in pulmonary sarcoidosis. *J Comput Assist Tomogr* 1989;13:405–410.

149. Remy-Jardin M, Giraud F, Remy J, et al. Pulmonary sarcoidosis: role of CT in the evaluation of disease activity and functional impairment and in prognosis assessment. *Radiology* 1994;191:675–680.

150. Traill ZC, Maskell GF, Gleeson FV. High-resolution CT findings of pulmonary sarcoidosis. *AJR Am J Roentgenol* 1997;168:1557–1560.

151. Nishimura K, Itoh H, Kitaichi M, et al. Pulmonary sarcoidosis: correlation of CT and histopathologic findings. *Radiology* 1993;189:105–109.

152. Miller BH, Rosado-de-Christenson ML, McAdams HP, et al. From the archives of the AFIP. Thoracic sarcoidosis: radiologic-pathologic correlation. *Radiographics* 1995;15:421–437.

153. Müller NL, Miller RR. Computed tomography of chronic diffuse infiltrative lung disease: part 2. *Am Rev Respir Dis* 1990;142:1440–1448.

154. Brauner MW, Lenoir S, Grenier P, et al. Pulmonary sarcoidosis: CT assessment of lesion reversibility. *Radiology* 1992;182:349–354.

155. Grenier P, Valeyre D, Cluzel P, et al. Chronic diffuse interstitial lung disease: diagnostic value of chest radiography and high-resolution CT. *Radiology* 1991;179:123–132.

156. Leung AN, Miller RR, Müller NL. Parenchymal opacification in chronic infiltrative lung diseases: CT-pathologic correlation. *Radiology* 1993;188:209–214.

157. Lenique F, Brauner MW, Grenier P, et al. CT assessment of bronchi in sarcoidosis: endoscopic and pathologic correlations. *Radiology* 1995;194:419–423.

158. Gleeson FV, Traill ZC, Hansell DM. Evidence of expiratory CT scans of small-airway obstruction in sarcoidosis. *AJR Am J Roentgenol* 1996;166:1052–1054.

159. Hansell DM, Milne DG, Wilsher ML, et al. Pulmonary sarcoidosis: morphologic associations of airflow obstruction at thin-section CT. *Radiology* 1998;209:697–704.

160. Bergin CJ, Müller NL. CT of interstitial lung disease: a diagnostic approach. *AJR Am J Roentgenol* 1987;148:9–15.

161. Lynch DA, Brasch RC, Hardy KA, et al. Pediatric pulmonary disease: assessment with high-resolution ultrafast CT. *Radiology* 1990;176:243–248.

162. Westcott JL, Cole SR. Traction bronchiectasis in end-stage pulmonary fibrosis. *Radiology* 1986;161:665–669.

163. Primack SL, Hartman TE, Hansell DM, et al. End-stage lung disease: CT findings in 61 patients. *Radiology* 1993;189:681–686.

164. Padley SP, Padhani AR, Nicholson A, et al. Pulmonary sarcoidosis mimicking cryptogenic fibrosing alveolitis on CT. *Clinical Radiology* 1996;51:807–810.

165. Miller BH, Rosado-de-Christenson ML, McAdams HP, et al. Thoracic sarcoidosis: radiologic-pathologic correlation [published erratum appears in *Radiographics* 1997 Nov–Dec;17(6):1610]. *Radiographics* 1995;15:421–437.

166. Ichikawa Y, Fujimoto K, Shiraishi T, et al. Primary cavitary sarcoidosis: high-resolution CT findings [letter]. *AJR Am J Roentgenol* 1994;163:745.

167. Nakata H, Kimoto T, Nakayama T, et al. Diffuse peripheral lung disease: evaluation by high-resolution computed tomography. *Radiology* 1985;157:181–185.
168. Murdoch J, Müller NL. Pulmonary sarcoidosis: changes on follow-up CT examinations. *AJR Am J Roentgenol* 1992;159:473–477.
169. Leung AN, Brauner MW, Caillat-Vigneron N, et al. Sarcoidosis activity: correlation of HRCT findings with those of 67Ga scanning, bronchoalveolar lavage, and serum angiotensin-converting enzyme assay. *J Comput Assist Tomogr* 1998;22:229–234.
170. Austin JHM. Pulmonary sarcoidosis: what are we learning from CT? *Radiology* 1989;171:603–604.
171. Müller NL, Mawson JB, Mathieson JR, et al. Sarcoidosis: correlation of extent of disease at CT with clinical, functional, and radiographic findings. *Radiology* 1989;171:613–618.
172. Akira M, Higashihara T, Yokoyama K, et al. Radiographic type p pneumoconiosis: high-resolution CT. *Radiology* 1989;171:117–123.
173. Bégin R, Bergeron D, Samson L, et al. CT assessment of silicosis in exposed workers. *AJR Am J Roentgenol* 1987;148:509–514.
174. Bergin CJ, Müller NL, Vedal S, et al. CT in silicosis: correlation with plain films and pulmonary function tests. *AJR Am J Roentgenol* 1986;146:477–483.
175. Bergin C, Roggli V, Coblentz C, et al. The secondary pulmonary lobule: normal and abnormal CT appearances. *AJR Am J Roentgenol* 1988;151:21–25.
176. Newman LS, Buschman DL, Newell JD, et al. Beryllium disease: assessment with CT. *Radiology* 1994;190:835–840.
177. Harris KM, McConnochie K, Adams H. The computed tomographic appearances in chronic berylliosis. *Clin Radiol* 1993;47:26–31.
178. Gevenois PA, Vande Weyer R, De Vuyst P. Beryllium disease: assessment with CT [letter;comment]. *Radiology* 1994;193:283–284.
179. Seaton A. Silicosis. In: Morgan WKC, Seaton A, eds. *Occupational lung diseases*, 2nd ed. Philadelphia: WB Saunders, 1984:250–294.
180. Sargent EN, Morgan WKC. Silicosis. In: Preger L, ed. *Induced disease. Drug, irradiation, occupation.* New York: Grune & Stratton, 1980:297–315.
181. Balaan MR, Weber SL, Banks DE. Clinical aspects of coal workers' pneumoconiosis and silicosis. *Occup Med* 1993;8:19–34.
182. Davis GS. The pathogenesis of silicosis: state of the art. *Chest* 1986;89:166S–169S.
183. Mossman BT, Churg A. Mechanisms in the pathogenesis of asbestosis and silicosis. *Am J Respir Crit Care Med* 1998;157:1666–1680.
184. Wagner GR. Asbestosis and silicosis. *Lancet* 1997;349:1311–1315.
185. Sargent EN, Morgan WKC. Coal workers' pneumoconiosis. In: Preger L, ed. *Induced disease. Drug, irradiation, occupation.* New York: Grune & Stratton, 1980:275–295.
186. Pendergrass EP. Caldwell Lecture 1957: silicosis and a few of the other pneumoconioses: observations of certain aspects of the problem, with emphasis on the role of the radiologist. *AJR Am J Roentgenol* 1958;80:1–41.
187. Kinsella N, Müller NL, Vedal S, et al. Emphysema in silicosis: a comparison of smokers with nonsmokers using pulmonary function testing and computed tomography. *Am Rev Respir Dis* 1990;141:1497–1500.
188. Parkes WR. Diseases due to free silica. In: *Occupational lung disorders*, 2nd ed. London: Butterworth, 1982:134–158.
189. Bégin R, Ostiguy G, Groleau S, et al. Computed tomographic scanning of the thorax in workers at risk of or with silicosis. *Semin Ultrasound CT MR* 1990;11:380–392.
190. Shida H, Chiyotani K, Honma K, et al. Radiologic and pathologic characteristics of mixed dust pneumoconiosis. *Radiographics* 1996;16:483–498.
191. Gevenois PA, Pichot E, Dargent F, et al. Low-grade coal worker's pneumoconiosis: comparison of CT and chest radiography. *Acta Radiol* 1994;35:351–356.
192. Bégin R, Ostiguy G, Cantin A, et al. Lung function in silica-exposed workers: a relationship to disease severity assessed by CT scan. *Chest* 1988;94:539–545.
193. Akira M. Uncommon pneumoconioses: CT and pathologic findings. *Radiology* 1995;197:403–409.
194. Pare JA, Fraser RG, Hogg JC, et al. Pulmonary "mainline" granulomatosis: talcosis of intravenous methadone abuse. *Medicine (Baltimore)* 1979;58:229–239.
195. Pare JP, Cote G, Fraser RS. Long-term follow-up of drug abusers with intravenous talcosis. *Am Rev Respir Dis* 1989;139:233–241.
196. Ward S, Heyneman LE, Reittner P, et al. Talcosis secondary to IV abuse of oral medications: CT findings. *AJR Am J Roentgenol* 2000;174:789–793.
197. Schmidt RA, Glenny RW, Godwin JD, et al. Panlobular emphysema in young intravenous Ritalin abusers. *Am Rev Respir Dis* 1991;143:649–656.
198. Stern EJ, Frank MS, Schmutz JF, et al. Panlobular pulmonary emphysema caused by i.v. injection of methylphenidate (Ritalin): findings on chest radiographs and CT scans. *AJR Am J Roentgenol* 1994;162:555–560.
199. Padley SPG, Adler BD, Staples CA, et al. Pulmonary talcosis: CT findings in three cases. *Radiology* 1993;186:125–127.
200. Utz JP, Swensen SJ, Gertz MA. Pulmonary amyloidosis: the Mayo Clinic experience from 1980 to 1993. *Ann Intern Med* 1996; 124:407–413.
201. Pickford HA, Swensen SJ, Utz JP. Thoracic cross-sectional imaging of amyloidosis. *AJR Am J Roentgenol* 1997;168:351–355.
202. Ayuso MC, Gilabert R, Bombi JA, et al. CT appearance of localized pulmonary amyloidosis. *J Comput Assist Tomogr* 1987;11:197–199.
203. Buxbaum J. Mechanisms of disease: monoclonal immunoglobulin deposition. Amyloidosis, light chain deposition disease, and light and heavy chain deposition disease. *Hematol Oncol Clin North Am* 1992;6:323–346.
204. Graham CM, Stern EJ, Finkbeiner WE, et al. High-resolution CT appearance of diffuse alveolar septal amyloidosis. *AJR Am J Roentgenol* 1992;158:265–267.
205. Im JG, Itoh H, Shim YS, et al. Pulmonary tuberculosis: CT findings—early active disease and sequential change with antituberculous therapy. *Radiology* 1993;186:653–660.
206. Hamrick-Turner J, Abbitt PL, Harrison RB, et al. Diffuse lung calcification following fat emboli and adult respiratory distress syndromes: CT findings. *J Thorac Imag* 1994;9:47–50.
207. Hartman TE, Müller NL, Primack SL, et al. Metastatic pulmonary calcification in patients with hypercalcemia: findings on chest radiographs and CT scans. *AJR Am J Roentgenol* 1994;162:799–802.
208. Cluzel P, Grenier P, Bernadac P, et al. Pulmonary alveolar microlithiasis: CT findings. *J Comput Assist Tomogr* 1991;15:938–942.
209. Korn MA, Schurawitzki H, Klepetko W, et al. Pulmonary alveolar microlithiasis: findings on high-resolution CT. *AJR Am J Roentgenol* 1992;158:981–982.
210. Leavitt RY, Fauci AS, Bloch DA, et al. The American College of Rheumatology 1990 criteria for the classification of Wegener's granulomatosis. *Arthritis Rheum* 1990;33:1101–1107.
211. Cordier JF, Valeyre D, Guillevin L, et al. Pulmonary Wegener's granulomatosis: a clinical and imaging study of 77 cases. *Chest* 1990;97:906–912.
212. Aberle DR, Gamsu G, Lynch D. Thoracic manifestations of Wegener granulomatosis: diagnosis and course. *Radiology* 1990;174:703–709.
213. Hoffman GS, Kerr GS, Leavitt RY, et al. Wegener granulomatosis: an analysis of 158 patients. *Ann Intern Med* 1992;116:488–498.
214. Weir IH, Müller NL, Chiles C, et al. Wegener's granulomatosis: findings from computed tomography of the chest in 10 patients. *Can Assoc Radiol J* 1992;43:31–34.
215. Attali P, Begum R, Ban Romdhane H, et al. Pulmonary Wegener's granulomatosis: changes at follow-up CT. *European Radiology* 1998;8:1009–1113.
216. Connolly B, Manson D, Eberhard A, et al. CT appearance of pulmonary vasculitis in children. *AJR Am J Roentgenol* 1996; 167:901–904.
217. Foo SS, Weisbrod GL, Herman SJ, et al. Wegener granulomatosis presenting on CT with atypical bronchovasocentric distribution. *J Comput Assist Tomogr* 1990;14:1004–1006.
218. Reuter M, Schnabel A, Wesner F, et al. Pulmonary Wegener's granulomatosis: correlation between high-resolution CT findings and clinical scoring of disease activity. *Chest* 1998;114:500–506.
219. Miller WT. Tuberculosis in the 1990s. *Radiol Clin North Am* 1994;32:649–661.
220. Raviglione MC, Snider Jr DE, Kochi A. Global epidemiology of tuberculosis. Morbidity and mortality of a worldwide epidemic. *JAMA* 1995;273:220–226.
221. Dye C, Scheele S, Dolin P, et al. Consensus statement. Global burden of tuberculosis: estimated incidence, prevalence, and mortality by country. WHO Global Surveillance and Monitoring Project. *JAMA* 1999;282:677–686.

222. Centers for Disease Control and Prevention. Tuberculosis morbidity: United States. *MMWR Morb Mortal Wkly Rep* 1996;46:695–700.

223. Leung AN. Pulmonary tuberculosis: the essentials. *Radiology* 1999;210:307–322.

224. Bradford WZ, Daley CL. Multiple drug-resistant tuberculosis. *Infect Dis Clin North Am* 1998;12:157–172.

225. Cohn DL, Bustreo F, Raviglione MC. Drug-resistant tuberculosis: review of the worldwide situation and the WHO/IUATLD Global Surveillance Project. International Union Against Tuberculosis and Lung Disease. *Clin Infect Dis* 1997;24[Suppl 1]:S121–S130.

226. Woodring JH, Vandiviere HM, Fried AM, et al. Update: the radiographic features of pulmonary tuberculosis. *AJR Am J Roentgenol* 1986;146:497–506.

227. Krysl J, Korzeniewska-Koesela M, Müller NL, et al. Radiologic features of pulmonary tuberculosis: an assessment of 188 cases. *Can Assoc Radiol J* 1994;45:101–107.

228. Buckner CB, Walker CW. Radiologic manifestations of adult tuberculosis. *J Thorac Imag* 1990;5:28–37.

229. Leung AN, Müller NL, Pineda PR, et al. Primary tuberculosis in childhood: radiographic manifestations. *Radiology* 1992;182:87–91.

230. McAdams HP, Erasmus J, Winter JA. Radiologic manifestations of pulmonary tuberculosis. *Radiol Clin North Am* 1995;33:655–678.

231. Kuhlman JE, Deutsch JH, Fishman EK, et al. CT features of thoracic mycobacterial disease. *Radiographics* 1990;10:413–431.

232. Haque AK. The pathology and pathophysiology of mycobacterial infections. *J Thorac Imag* 1990;5:8–16.

233. Lee KS, Im JG. CT in adults with tuberculosis of the chest: characteristic findings and role in management. *AJR Am J Roentgenol* 1995;164:1361–1367.

234. Miller Jr WT. Spectrum of pulmonary nontuberculous mycobacterial infection. *Radiology* 1994;191:343–350.

235. American Thoracic Society. Diagnostic standards and classification of tuberculosis. *Am Rev Respir Dis* 1990;142:725–735.

236. Lee KS, Song KS, Lim TH, et al. Adult-onset pulmonary tuberculosis: findings on chest radiographs and CT scans. *AJR Am J Roentgenol* 1993;160:753–758.

237. Lee KS, Kim YH, Kim WS, et al. Endobronchial tuberculosis: CT features. *J Comput Assist Tomogr* 1991;15:424–428.

238. Im J-G, Webb WR, Han MC, et al. Apical opacity associated with pulmonary tuberculosis: high-resolution CT findings. *Radiology* 1991;178:727–731.

239. McGuinness G, Naidich DP, Jagirdar J, et al. High resolution CT findings in miliary lung disease. *J Comput Assist Tomogr* 1992;16:384–390.

240. Ikezoe J, Takeuchi N, Johkoh T, et al. CT appearance of pulmonary tuberculosis in diabetic and immunocompromised patients: comparison with patients who had no underlying disease. *AJR Am J Roentgenol* 1992;159:1175–1179.

241. Primack SL, Logan PM, Hartman TE, et al. Pulmonary tuberculosis and Mycobacterium avium-intracellulare: a comparison of CT findings. *Radiology* 1995;194:413–417.

242. Choi D, Lee KS, Suh GY, et al. Pulmonary tuberculosis presenting as acute respiratory failure: radiologic findings. *J Comput Assist Tomogr* 1999;23:107–113.

243. Kim WS, Moon WK, Kim IO, et al. Pulmonary tuberculosis in children: evaluation with CT. *AJR Am J Roentgenol* 1997;168:1005–1009.

244. Oh YW, Kim YH, Lee NJ, et al. High-resolution CT appearance of miliary tuberculosis. *J Comput Assist Tomogr* 1994;18:862–866.

245. Im J-G, Song KS, Kang HS, et al. Mediastinal tuberculous lymphadenitis: CT manifestations. *Radiology* 1987;164:115–119.

246. Murata K, Itoh H, Todo G, et al. Centrilobular lesions of the lung: demonstration by high-resolution CT and pathologic correlation. *Radiology* 1986;161:641–645.

247. Hatipoglu ON, Osma E, Manisali M, et al. High resolution computed tomographic findings in pulmonary tuberculosis. *Thorax* 1996;51:397–402.

248. Poey C, Verhaegen F, Giron J, et al. High resolution chest CT in tuberculosis: evolutive patterns and signs of activity. *J Comput Assist Tomogr* 1997;21:601–607.

249. Hong SH, Im JG, Lee JS, et al. High resolution CT findings of miliary tuberculosis. *J Comput Assist Tomogr* 1998;22:220–224.

250. Sharma SK, Mukhopadhyay S, Arora R, et al. Computed tomography in miliary tuberculosis: comparison with plain films, bronchoalveolar lavage, pulmonary functions and gas exchange. *Australas Radiol* 1996;40:113–118.

251. Codecasa LR, Besozzi G, De Cristofaro L, et al. Epidemiological and clinical patterns of intrathoracic lymph node tuberculosis in 60 human immunodeficiency virus-negative adult patients. *Monaldi Arch Chest Dis* 1998;53:277–280.

252. Pastores SM, Naidich DP, Aranda CP, et al. Intrathoracic adenopathy associated with pulmonary tuberculosis in patients with human immunodeficiency virus infection. *Chest* 1993;103:1433–1437.

253. Moon WK, Im JG, Yeon KM, et al. Mediastinal tuberculous lymphadenitis: CT findings of active and inactive disease. *AJR Am J Roentgenol* 1998;170:715–718.

254. Moon WK, Kim WS, Kim IO, et al. Complicated pleural tuberculosis in children: CT evaluation. *Pediatr Radiol* 1999;29:153–157.

255. Hulnick DH, Naidich DP, McCauley DI. Pleural tuberculosis evaluated by computed tomography. *Radiology* 1983;149:759–765.

256. Naidich DP, McCauley DI, Leitman BS, et al. Computed tomography of pulmonary tuberculosis. In: Siegelman SS, ed. *Computed tomography of the chest*. New York: Churchill Livingstone, 1984:175–217.

257. Centers for Disease Control. Tuberculosis, final data: United States, 1986. *MMWR Morb Mortal Wkly Rep* 1988;36:817–820.

258. Wasser LS, Brown E, Talavera W. Miliary PCP in AIDS. *Chest* 1989;96:693–695.

259. Lee KS, Hwang JW, Chung MP, et al. Utility of CT in the evaluation of pulmonary tuberculosis in patients without AIDS. *Chest* 1996;110:977–984.

260. Naidich DP, Garay SM, Goodman PC, et al. Pulmonary manifestations of AIDS. In: *Radiology of acquired immune deficiency syndrome*. New York: Raven, 1988:47–77.

261. Roberts CM, Citron KM, Strickland B. Intrathoracic aspergilloma: role of CT in diagnosis and treatment. *Radiology* 1987;165:123–128.

262. Goodman PC. Tuberculosis and AIDS. *Radiol Clin North Am* 1995;33:707–717.

263. Markowitz N, Hansen NI, Hopewell PC, et al. Incidence of tuberculosis in the United States among HIV-infected persons. The Pulmonary Complications of HIV Infection Study Group. *Ann Intern Med* 1997;126:123–132.

264. Centers for Disease Control. 1993 revised classification system for HIV infection and expanded surveillance case definition for AIDS among adolescents and adults. *MMWR Morb Mortal Wkly Rep* 1992;41:1–11.

265. Barnes PF, Bloch AB, Davidson PT, et al. Tuberculosis in patients with human immunodeficiency virus infection. *N Engl J Med* 1991;324:1644–1650.

266. Fitzgerald JM, Grzybowski S, Allen EA. The impact of human immunodeficiency virus infection on tuberculosis and its control. *Chest* 1991;100:191–200.

267. Greenberg SD, Frager D, Suster B, et al. Active pulmonary tuberculosis in patients with AIDS: spectrum of radiographic findings (including a normal appearance). *Radiology* 1994;193:115–119.

268. Smith RL, Yew K, Berkowitz KA, et al. Factors affecting the yield of acid-fast sputum smears in patients with HIV and tuberculosis. *Chest* 1994;106:684–686.

269. Kramer F, Modilevsky T, Waliany AR, et al. Delayed diagnosis of tuberculosis in patients with human immunodeficiency virus infection. *Am J Med* 1990;89:451–456.

270. Whalen C, Horsburgh CR, Hom D, et al. Accelerated course of human immunodeficiency virus infection after tuberculosis. *Am J Respir Crit Care Med* 1995;151:129–135.

271. Jones BE, Young SMM, Antoniskis D, et al. Relationship of the manifestations of tuberculosis to CD4 cell counts in patients with human immunodeficiency virus infection. *Am Rev Respir Dis* 1993;148:1292–1297.

272. Leung AN, Brauner MW, Gamsu G, et al. Pulmonary tuberculosis: comparison of CT findings in HIV-seropositive and HIV-seronegative patients. *Radiology* 1996;198:687–691.

273. Haramati LB, Jenny-Avital ER, Alterman DD. Effect of HIV status on chest radiographic and CT findings in patients with tuberculosis. *Clin Radiol* 1997;52:31–35.

274. Long R, Maycher B, Scalcini M, et al. The chest roentgenogram in pulmonary tuberculosis patients seropositive for human immunodeficiency virus type 1. *Chest* 1991;99:123–127.

275. Goodman PC. Pulmonary tuberculosis in patients with acquired immunodeficiency syndrome. *J Thorac Imag* 1990;1990:38–45.

276. Pitchenik AE, Rubinson HA. The radiographic appearance of tuberculosis in patients with the acquired immune deficiency syndrome (AIDS) and pre-AIDS. *Am Rev Respir Dis* 1985;131:393–396.

277. Hill AR, Somasundaram P, Brustein S, et al. Disseminated tuberculosis in the acquired immunodeficiency syndrome. *Am Rev Respir Dis* 1991;144:1164–1170.

278. Centers for Disease Control. Screening for tuberculosis and tuberculous infection in high risk populations and the use of preventive therapy for tuberculous infection in the United States: recommendations of the Advisory Committee for Elimination of Tuberculosis. *MMWR Morb Mortal Wkly Rep* 1990;39:1–12.

279. Lessnau KD, Gorla M, Talavera W. Radiographic findings in HIV-positive patients with sensitive and resistant tuberculosis. *Chest* 1994;106:687–689.

280. Laissy JP, Cadi M, Boudiaf ZE, et al. Pulmonary tuberculosis: computed tomography and high-resolution computed tomography patterns in patients who are either HIV-negative or HIV-seropositive. *J Thorac Imag* 1998;13:58–64.

281. Woodring JH, Vandiviere HM. Pulmonary disease caused by nontuberculous mycobacteria. *J Thorac Imag* 1990;5:64–76.

282. O'Brien RJ. The epidemiology of nontuberculous mycobacterial disease. *Clin Chest Med* 1989;10:407–418.

283. Buckner CB, Leithiser RE, Walaker CW, et al. The changing epidemiology of tuberculosis and other mycobacterial infections in the United States: implications for the radiologist. *AJR Am J Roentgenol* 1991;156:255–264.

284. Patz EF Jr, Swensen SJ, Erasmus J. Pulmonary manifestations of nontuberculous Mycobacterium. *Radiol Clin North Am* 1995;33:719–729.

285. American Thoracic Society. Diagnosis and treatment of disease caused by nontuberculous mycobacteria. *Am Rev Respir Dis* 1990;142:940–953.

286. Diagnosis and treatment of disease caused by nontuberculous mycobacteria. This official statement of the American Thoracic Society was approved by the Board of Directors, March 1997. Medical Section of the American Lung Association. *Am J Respir Crit Care Med* 1997;156:S1–S25.

287. Albelda SM, Kern JA, Marinelli DL, et al. Expanding spectrum of pulmonary disease caused by nontuberculous mycobacteria. *Radiology* 1985;157:289–296.

288. Christensen EE, Dietz GW, Ahn CH, et al. Pulmonary manifestations of Mycobacterium intracellularis. *AJR Am J Roentgenol* 1979;133:59–66.

289. Rubin SA. Tuberculosis and atypical mycobacterial infections in the 1990s. *Radiographics* 1997;17:1051–1059.

290. Christensen EE, Dietz GW, Ahn CH, et al. Radiographic manifestations of pulmonary Mycobacterium kansasii infections. *AJR Am J Roentgenol* 1978;131:985–993.

291. Hartman TE, Swensen SJ, Williams DE. Mycobacterium avium-intracellulare complex: evaluation with CT. *Radiology* 1993;187:23–26.

292. Moore EH. Atypical mycobacterial infection in the lung: CT appearance. *Radiology* 1993;187:777–782.

293. Swensen SJ, Hartman TE, Williams DE. Computed tomography in diagnosis of Mycobacterium avium-intracellulare complex in patients with bronchiectasis. *Chest* 1994;105:49–52.

294. Lynch DA, Simone PM, Fox MA, et al. CT features of pulmonary Mycobacterium avium complex infection. *J Comput Assist Tomogr* 1995;19:353–360.

295. Fujita J, Ohtsuki Y, Suemitsu I, et al. Pathological and radiological changes in resected lung specimens in Mycobacterium avium intracellulare complex disease. *Eur Respir J* 1999;13:535–540.

296. Maycher B, O'Connor R, Long R. Computed tomographic abnormalities in Mycobacterium avium complex lung disease include the mosaic pattern of reduced lung attenuation. *Can Assoc Radiol J* 2000;51:93–102.

297. Obayashi Y, Fujita J, Suemitsu I, et al. Successive follow-up of chest computed tomography in patients with Mycobacterium avium-intracellulare complex. *Respir Med* 1999;93:11–15.

298. Kasahara T, Nakajima Y, Niimi H, et al. [HRCT findings of pulmonary Mycobacterium avium complex: a comparison with tuberculosis]. *Nihon Kokyuki Gakkai Zasshi* 1998;36:122–127.

299. Tanaka E, Amitani R, Niimi A, et al. Yield of computed tomography and bronchoscopy for the diagnosis of Mycobacterium avium complex pulmonary disease. *Am J Respir Crit Care Med* 1997;155:2041–2046.

300. Katz MH, Hessol NA, Buchbinder SP, et al. Temporal trends of opportunistic infections and malignancies in homosexual men with AIDS. *J Infect Dis* 1994;170:198–202.

301. Levine B, Chaisson RE. Mycobacterium kansasii: a cause of treatable pulmonary disease associated with advanced human immunodeficiency virus (HIV) infection. *Ann Int Med* 1991;114:861–868.

302. Bamberger DM, Driks MR, Gupta MR, et al. Mycobacterium kansasii among patients infected with human immunodeficiency virus in Kansas City. *Clin Infect Dis* 1994;18:395–400.

303. Barber TW, Craven DE, Farber HW. Mycobacterium gordonae: a possible opportunistic respiratory tract pathogen in patients with advanced human immunodeficiency virus, Type 1 infection. *Chest* 1991;100:716–720.

304. Rigsby MO, Curtis AM. Pulmonary disease from nontuberculous mycobacteria in patients with human immunodeficiency virus. *Chest* 1994;106:913–919.

305. Laissy JP, Cadi M, Cinqualbre A, et al. Mycobacterium tuberculosis versus nontuberculous mycobacterial infection of the lung in AIDS patients: CT and HRCT patterns. *J Comput Assist Tomogr* 1997;21:312–317.

306. Hocqueloux L, Lesprit P, Herrmann JL, et al. Pulmonary Mycobacterium avium complex disease without dissemination in HIV-infected patients. *Chest* 1998;113:542–548.

307. Jasmer RM, McCowin MJ, Webb WR. Miliary lung disease after intravesical bacillus Calmette-Guerin immunotherapy. *Radiology* 1996;201:43–44.

308. Rabe J, Neff KW, Lehmann KJ, et al. Miliary tuberculosis after intravesical bacille Calmette-Guerin immunotherapy for carcinoma of the bladder. *AJR Am J Roentgenol* 1999;172:748–750.

309. Lamm DL, van der Meijden PM, Morales A, et al. Incidence and treatment of complications of bacillus Calmette-Guerin intravesical therapy in superficial bladder cancer. *J Urol* 1992;147:596–600.

310. McParland C, Cotton DJ, Gowda KS, et al. Miliary Mycobacterium bovis induced by intravesical bacille Calmette-Guerin immunotherapy. *Am Rev Respir Dis* 1992;146:1330–1333.

311. Brown MJ, Worthy SA, Flint JD, et al. Invasive aspergillosis in the immunocompromised host: utility of computed tomography and bronchoalveolar lavage. *Clin Radiol* 1998;53:255–257.

312. Logan PM, Primack SL, Miller RR, et al. Invasive aspergillosis of the airways: radiographic, CT, and pathologic findings. *Radiology* 1994;193:383–388.

313. Tanaka H, Shibusa T, Sugaya F, et al. [A case of influenza B viral bronchopneumonia followed by CT]. *Nippon Kyobu Shikkan Gakkai Zasshi* 1992;30:947–951.

314. Lee KS, Kim TS, Han J, et al. Diffuse micronodular lung disease: HRCT and pathologic findings. *J Comput Assist Tomogr* 1999;23:99–106.

315. Tanaka N, Matsumoto T, Kuramitsu T, et al. High resolution CT findings in community-acquired pneumonia. *J Comput Assist Tomogr* 1996;20:600–608.

316. Macfarlane J, Rose D. Radiographic features of staphylococcal pneumonia in adults and children. *Thorax* 1996;51:539–540.

317. Itoh H, Tokunaga S, Asamoto H, et al. Radiologic-pathologic correlations of small lung nodules with special reference to peribronchiolar nodules. *AJR Am J Roentgenol* 1978;130:223–231.

318. Heitzman ER, Markarian B, Berger I, et al. The secondary pulmonary lobule: a practical concept for interpretation of radiographs. II. application of the anatomic concept to an understanding of roentgen pattern of in disease states. *Radiology* 1969;93:514–520.

319. Itoh H, Murata K, Konishi J, et al. Diffuse lung disease: pathologic basis for the high-resolution computed tomography findings. *J Thorac Imag* 1993;8:176–188.

320. Murata K, Khan A, Herman PG. Pulmonary parenchymal disease: evaluation with high-resolution CT. *Radiology* 1989;170:629–635.

321. Syrjälä H, Broas M, Suramo I, et al. High-resolution computed tomography for the diagnosis of community-acquired pneumonia. *Clin Infect Dis* 1998;27:358–363.

322. Gefter WB. The spectrum of pulmonary aspergillosis. *J Thorac Imag* 1992;7:56–74.

323. Logan PM, Müller NL. High-resolution computed tomography and pathologic findings in pulmonary aspergillosis: a pictorial essay. *Can Assoc Radiol J* 1996;47:444–452.

324. Angus RM, Davies ML, Cowan MD, et al. Computed tomographic scanning of the lung in patients with allergic bronchopulmonary

aspergillosis and in asthmatic patients with a positive skin test to Aspergillus fumigatus. *Thorax* 1994;49:586–589.

325. Panchal N, Bhagat R, Pant C, et al. Allergic bronchopulmonary aspergillosis: the spectrum of computed tomography appearances. *Respir Med* 1997;91:213–219.

326. Gefter WB, Weingrad TR, Epstein DM, et al. "Semi-invasive" pulmonary aspergillosis: a new look at the spectrum of Aspergillus infections of the lung. *Radiology* 1981;140:313–321.

327. Franquet T, Müller NL, Gimenez A, et al. Semiinvasive pulmonary aspergillosis in chronic obstructive pulmonary disease: radiologic and pathologic findings in nine patients. *AJR Am J Roentgenol* 2000;174:51–56.

328. Kuhlman JE, Fishman EK, Burch PA, et al. Invasive pulmonary aspergillosis in acute leukemia: the contribution of CT to early diagnosis and aggressive management. *Chest* 1987;92:95–99.

329. Kuhlman JE, Fishman EK, Siegelman SS. Invasive pulmonary aspergillosis in acute leukemia: characteristic findings on CT, the CT halo sign, and the role of CT in early diagnosis. *Radiology* 1985;157:611–614.

330. Staples CA, Kang EY, Wright JL, et al. Invasive pulmonary aspergillosis in AIDS: radiographic, CT, and pathologic findings. *Radiology* 1995;196:409–414.

331. Addrizzo-Harris DJ, Harkin TJ, McGuinness G, et al. Pulmonary aspergilloma and AIDS. A comparison of HIV-infected and HIV-negative individuals. *Chest* 1997;111:612–618.

332. Wollschlager C, Khan F. Aspergillomas complicating sarcoidosis: a prospective study in 100 patients. *Chest* 1984;86:585–588.

333. Yousem SA. The histological spectrum of chronic necrotizing forms of pulmonary aspergillosis. *Hum Pathol* 1997;28:650–656.

334. Diederich S, Scadeng M, Dennis C, et al. Aspergillus infection of the respiratory tract after lung transplantation: chest radiographic and CT findings. *Eur Radiol* 1998;8:306–312.

335. Klapholz A, Salomon N, Perlman DC, et al. Aspergillosis in the acquired immunodeficiency syndrome. *Chest* 1991;100:1614–1618.

336. Hruban RH, Meziane MA, Zerhouni EA, et al. Radiologic-pathologic correlation of the CT halo sign in invasive pulmonary aspergillosis. *J Comput Assist Tomogr* 1987;11:534–536.

337. Caillot D, Casasnovas O, Bernard A, et al. Improved management of invasive pulmonary aspergillosis in neutropenic patients using early thoracic computed tomographic scan and surgery. *J Clin Oncol* 1997;15:139–147.

338. Robinson LA, Reed EC, Galbraith TA, et al. Pulmonary resection for invasive Aspergillus infections in immunocompromised patients. *J Thorac Cardiovasc Surg* 1995;109:1182–1196; discussion, 1196–1197.

339. Kuhlman JE, Fishman EK, Burch PA, et al. CT of invasive pulmonary aspergillosis. *AJR Am J Roentgenol* 1988;150:1015–1020.

340. Primack SL, Hartman TE, Lee KS, et al. Pulmonary nodules and the CT halo sign. *Radiology* 1994;190:513–515.

341. Mori M, Galvin JR, Barloon TJ, et al. Fungal pulmonary infections after bone marrow transplantation: evaluation with radiography and CT. *Radiology* 1991;178:721–726.

342. Gaeta M, Volta S, Stroscio S, et al. CT "halo sign" in pulmonary tuberculoma. *J Comput Assist Tomogr* 1992;16:827–828.

343. Won HJ, Lee KS, Cheon JE, et al. Invasive pulmonary aspergillosis: prediction at thin-section CT in patients with neutropenia—a prospective study. *Radiology* 1998;208:777–782.

344. Seely JM, Effmann EL, Müller NL. High-resolution CT of pediatric lung disease: imaging findings. *AJR Am J Roentgenol* 1997;168:1269–1275.

345. Kemper CA, Hostetler JS, Follansbee SE, et al. Ulcerative and plaque-like tracheobronchitis due to infection with Aspergillus in patients with AIDS. *Clin Infect Dis* 1993;17:344–352.

346. Machida U, Kami M, Kanda Y, et al. Aspergillus tracheobronchitis after allogeneic bone marrow transplantation. *Bone Marrow Transplant* 1999;24:1145–1149.

347. Hummel M, Schuler S, Hempel S, et al. Obstructive bronchial aspergillosis after heart transplantation. *Mycoses* 1993;36:425–428.

348. Connolly Jr JE, McAdams HP, Erasmus JJ, et al. Opportunistic fungal pneumonia. *J Thorac Imag* 1999;14:51–62.

349. Boyars MC, Zwischenberger JB, Cox Jr CS. Clinical manifestations of pulmonary fungal infections. *J Thorac Imag* 1992;7:12–22.

350. Khoury MB, Godwin JD, Ravin CE, et al. Thoracic cryptococcosis: immunologic competence and radiologic appearance. *AJR Am J Roentgenol* 1984;141:893–896.

351. Sider L, Westcott MA. Pulmonary manifestations of cryptococcosis in patients with AIDS: CT features. *J Thorac Imag* 1994;9:78–84.

352. Kurasawa T, Ikeda N, Sato A, et al. [A clinical study of pulmonary cryptococcosis. The Study Group of Respiratory Mycosis in Kyoto]. *Kansenshogaku Zasshi* 1998;72:352–357.

353. Rubin SA, Chaljub G, Winer-Muram HT, et al. Pulmonary zygomycosis: a radiographic and clinical spectrum. *J Thorac Imag* 1992;7:85–90.

354. McAdams HP, Rosado de Christenson M, Strollo DC, et al. Pulmonary mucormycosis: radiologic findings in 32 cases. *AJR Am J Roentgenol* 1997;168:1541–1548.

355. Jamadar DA, Kazerooni EA, Daly BD, et al. Pulmonary zygomycosis; CT appearance. *J Comput Assist Tomogr* 1995;19:733–738.

356. Funari M, Kavakama J, Shikanai-Yasuda MA, et al. Chronic pulmonary paracoccidioidomycosis (South American blastomycosis): high-resolution CT findings in 41 patients. *AJR Am J Roentgenol* 1999;173:59–64.

357. Huang RM, Naidich DP, Lubat E, et al. Septic pulmonary emboli: CT-radiographic correlation. *AJR Am J Roentgenol* 1989;153:41–45.

358. Müller-Leisse C, Klosterhalfen B, Hauptmann S, et al. Computed tomography and histologic results in the early stages of endotoxin-injured pig lungs as a model for adult respiratory distress syndrome. *Invest Radiol* 1993;28:39–45.

359. Kuhlman JE, Fishman EK, Teigen C. Pulmonary septic emboli: diagnosis with CT. *Radiology* 1990;174:211–213.

360. Balakrishnan J, Meziane MA, Siegelman SS, et al. Pulmonary infarction: CT appearance with pathologic correlation. *J Comput Assist Tomogr* 1989;13:941–945.

CHAPTER 6

Diseases Characterized Primarily by Parenchymal Opacification

The diseases reviewed in this chapter produce ground-glass opacity or airspace consolidation as primary high-resolution computed tomography (HRCT) abnormalities. *Ground-glass opacity* is defined as a hazy increase in lung attenuation that does not obscure underlying vessels; if vessels within the area of abnormality are obscured, the term *consolidation* is used [1,2].

Ground-glass opacity results from morphologic abnormalities below the resolution of HRCT and can reflect minimal thickening of the pulmonary interstitium or alveolar walls, the presence of cells or fluid within the alveolar airspaces, or an increase in the capillary blood volume [3–7]. Ground-glass opacity is the main abnormality seen in patients who have hypersensitivity pneumonitis [extrinsic allergic alveolitis (EAA)], desquamative interstitial pneumonia (DIP), respiratory bronchiolitis–interstitial lung disease (RB-ILD), acute interstitial pneumonia (AIP), nonspecific interstitial pneumonia (NSIP), alveolar proteinosis, and diffuse pneumonias, such as *Pneumocystis carinii* pneumonia (PCP).

Parenchymal consolidation is seen most commonly in patients who have bronchiolitis obliterans organizing pneumonia (BOOP) or chronic eosinophilic pneumonia, or in bacterial pneumonias [8]. Parenchymal opacification ranging from ground-glass opacity to consolidation may also be seen in patients who have pulmonary edema [3,9–11]; adult respiratory distress syndrome (ARDS) [12–14]; viral, tuberculous, and fungal pneumonias [14,15]; radiation pneumonitis [16–18]; infarction [14]; or bronchioloalveolar carcinoma [14,19]. The clinical findings and plain radiographic appearances of many of these diseases are sufficient for diagnosis.

However, in selected cases, HRCT may contribute to patient management by detecting abnormalities when corresponding chest radiographs are normal, clarifying confusing or equivocal radiographic findings, or delineating the extent of disease. As is discussed, HRCT can play an especially important role in detecting infections in immunocompromised patients.

HYPERSENSITIVITY PNEUMONITIS (EXTRINSIC ALLERGIC ALVEOLITIS)

Hypersensitivity pneumonitis (HP), also known as Extrinsic allergic alveolitis (*EAA*), is an allergic lung disease caused by the inhalation of antigens contained in a variety of organic dusts [20,21]. Farmer's lung, which is the best-known HP syndrome, results from the inhalation of fungal organisms (thermophilic actinomycetes) that grow in moist hay. Many other HP syndromes also result from fungi, but as with farmer's lung, they are usually named after the setting in which exposure occurs or the organic substance involved; several examples are bird breeder's lung, mushroom worker's lung, malt worker's lung, maple-bark disease, and hot-tub lung. Acute exposure of susceptible individuals to an offending antigen produces fever, chills, dry cough, and dyspnea; long-term exposure can produce progressive shortness of breath with few or minimal systemic symptoms [22]. Recurrent acute episodes are common with recurrent exposure.

The radiographic and pathologic abnormalities that are seen in patients who have HP are quite similar, regardless of the organic antigen responsible (Fig. 6-1); these abnormalities can be classified into acute, subacute, and chronic stages. In the *acute stage*, heavy exposure to the inciting antigen can cause diffuse ill-defined airspace consolidation visible on radiographs; this reflects alveolar filling by a neutrophilic inflammatory infiltrate or pulmonary edema due to diffuse alveolar damage (DAD) [23,24]. It should be recognized, however, that not all patients who have clinical symptoms of HP show acute radiographic abnormalities of airspace disease. Ill-defined airspace nodules can also be seen with acute exposure.

After resolution of the acute abnormalities, which may take several days, or between episodes of acute exposure, a fine nodular pattern is often visible on radiographs. This pattern is characteristic of the *subacute stage* of HP, but, as with acute disease, it is not always seen [25]. The nodular appearance correlates with the presence of alveolitis, interstitial infiltrates, small granulomas, and cellular bronchiolitis; histologic abnormalities are usually most severe in a peribronchiolar distribution [23,26]. Unlike the granulomas seen in patients who have sarcoidosis, the granulomas in HP are irregular in shape and poorly defined [22].

The *chronic stage* of HP is characterized by the presence of fibrosis, which may develop months or years after the initial exposure [25]. The fibrosis can be patchy in distribution and can mimic radiographically and pathologically the appearance of IPF with honeycombing [27].

It is commonly believed that the chronic stage of HP is characterized by fibrosis that mainly involves the upper lung zones [25,28]. This conclusion, however, is based on the radiographic findings in a small number of cases, most of them from a single study [28], and in most cases, radiographic findings of fibrosis predominate in the middle lung or lower lung zones [29,30].

The radiographic appearance of recurrent, transient ground-glass opacities or ill-defined consolidation superimposed on a pattern of small nodules is considered typical and highly suggestive of HP. However, it should be emphasized that the plain radiologic findings seen in this disease are nonspecific, and there have been conflicting reports as to the radiologic pattern and distribution of disease [25,30,31]. Also, repeated exposure to the offending antigen can lead to a confusing superimposition of different radiographic patterns and stages of the disease process. Acute and subacute changes and chronic fibrosis can all be present at the same time.

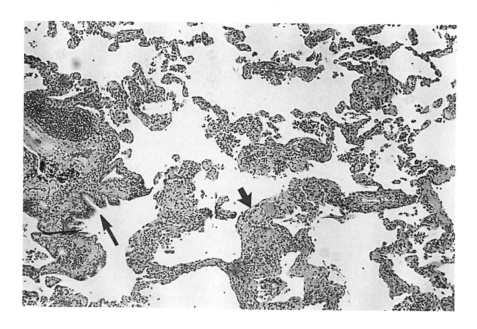

FIG. 6-1. Microscopic view of an open-lung biopsy specimen from a patient who had subacute hypersensitivity pneumonitis. A diffuse interstitial mononuclear cell infiltrate is present. This interstitial infiltrate accounts for the ground-glass opacity seen on HRCT. Also noted are localized areas of bronchiolitis (*large arrow*) and small ill-defined granulomas (*small arrow*).

TABLE 6-1. *HRCT findings in hypersensitivity pneumonitis*

Subacute

Patchy or diffuse ground-glass opacity[a]

Small centrilobular nodular opacities[a,b]

Superimposition of first two findings[a,b]

Lobular areas of decreased attenuation (mosaic perfusion)[a,b]

Lobular areas of air-trapping on expiratory scans[a,b]

Findings of fibrosis

Chronic

Findings of fibrosis (intralobular interstitial thickening, irregular interfaces, irregular interlobular septal thickening, honeycombing, traction bronchiectasis, or bronchiolectasis)[a]

Superimposed ground-glass opacity or centrilobular nodules[a]

Patchy distribution of abnormalities[a,b]

No zonal predominance of fibrosis, relative sparing of the costophrenic angles[a,b]

[a]Most common findings.
[b]Findings most helpful in differential diagnosis.

High-Resolution Computed Tomography Findings

Acute Stage

The HRCT findings of HP depend on the stage of disease (Table 6-1). Silver et al. [26] described the HRCT findings in two patients who had acute HP. Both of these had bilateral airspace consolidation and small (1 to 3 mm in diameter), ill-defined, rounded opacities on both radiographs and on HRCT. In these two patients, the HRCT and radiographic findings were considered to be identical, and HRCT added no further information.

Subacute Stage

Much more commonly, HRCT is performed in the subacute stage of HP, weeks to months after first exposure to the antigen. Typical findings include patchy ground-glass opacity, small ill-defined centrilobular nodules, or both (Figs. 6-2 through 6-5) (Table 6-1). In the study by Silver et al. [26], three of the patients had clinically subacute HP at the time of their CT study. Their symptoms had been present for 3 to 7 months before CT. These three patients had poorly defined nodules, 1 to 5 mm in diameter, visible on their chest radiographs and CT scans. CT also showed bilateral areas of ground-glass opacity that were not apparent on the radiograph. The ground-glass opacity was seen in the same distribution as the small, rounded opacities. Correlation with pathologic specimens demonstrated that the findings on HRCT reflected the presence of mononuclear cell bronchiolitis, mononuclear cell interstitial infiltrates, and scattered, poorly defined, nonnecrotizing granulomas (Fig. 6-3) [26].

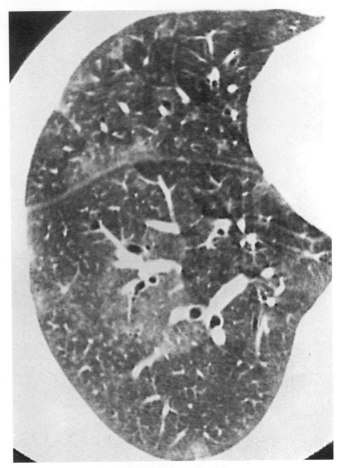

FIG. 6-2. Subacute hypersensitivity pneumonitis. HRCT through the right lung base shows patchy ground-glass opacity.

Hansell and Moskovic [32] reviewed the HRCT findings in 15 patients who had subacute HP. The most common abnormality on HRCT was the presence of diffuse bilateral ground-glass opacity, present in 11 (73%) of the patients. The diffuse ground-glass opacity was recognized on HRCT by the presence of abnormally prominent bronchial walls, and a marked contrast between the attenuation of the lung parenchyma and the air in the major airways. Although the ground-glass opacity was diffuse, it was most marked in the middle and lower lung zones. The second most common finding, present in six patients (40%), was the presence of poorly defined nodules measuring approximately 4 mm in diameter and being most numerous in the middle and lower lung zones.

Remy-Jardin et al. [33] reviewed the HRCT findings in 21 patients who had subacute bird-breeder's HP. The most common finding, seen in 16 (76%) of the patients, was the presence of nodules. These measured less than 5 mm in diameter, were bilateral, and involved all three lung zones to a comparable degree. The nodules were poorly defined and had a characteristic centrilobular distribution (Figs. 6-3 and 6-4). The second most common finding, seen in eleven (52%) of the patients, was the presence of areas of ground-glass opacity. The ground-glass opacity was seen in conjunction with

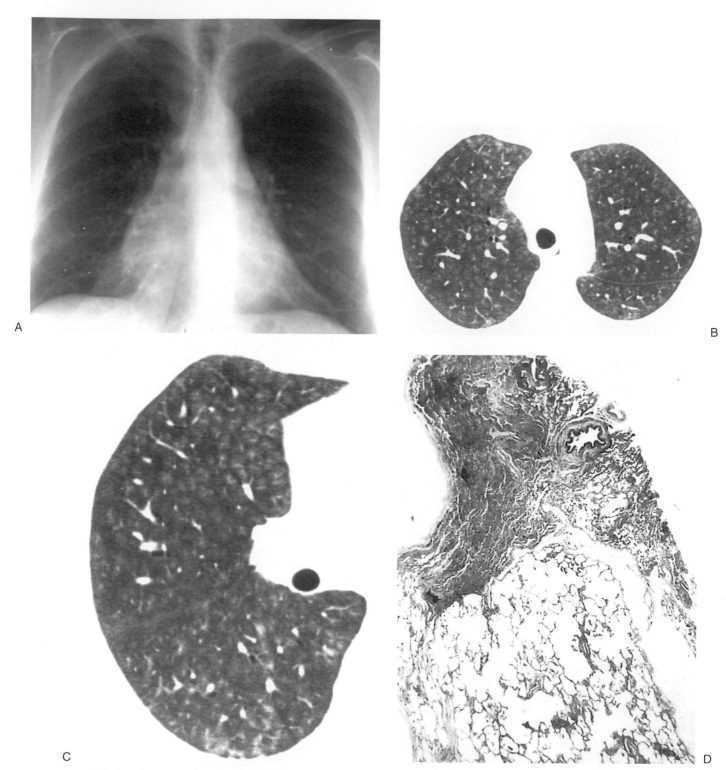

FIG. 6-3. Subacute hypersensitivity pneumonitis in a bird fancier. **A:** Chest radiograph is normal despite progressive shortness of breath. **B:** HRCT through the upper lobes shows diffuse ill-defined nodules of ground-glass opacity. **C:** HRCT in the right midlung shows that the nodules spare the pleural surfaces. Some of the nodules surround or are associated with small vascular branches. These findings indicate the centrilobular location of the nodules. This appearance is frequently seen in patients who have subacute hypersensitivity pneumonitis. **D:** open-lung biopsy specimen shows a focal area of infiltration, corresponding to a centrilobular nodule. A small bronchiole is visible in the region of abnormality.

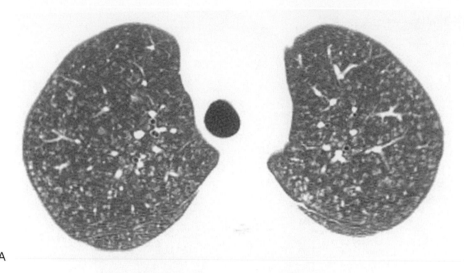

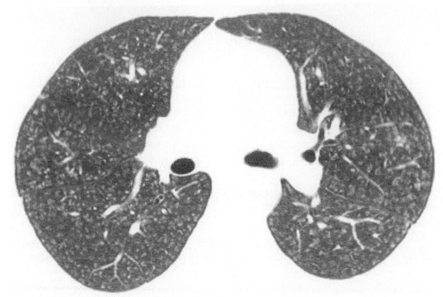

FIG. 6-4. A,B: Subacute hypersensitivity pneumonitis in a young woman exposed to fungus while having her bathroom remodeled. HRCT shows innumerable centrilobular nodules. Note that nodules spare the fissures and pleural surfaces.

nodules or, less commonly, as an isolated finding. The ground-glass opacity involved all three lung zones but was slightly more marked in the lower lung zones. It was patchy in distribution in eight patients and diffuse in three patients.

Another common manifestation of subacute HP is the presence of focal areas of decreased attenuation on inspiratory HRCT (Figs. 6-5 through 6-8), air-trapping on expiratory HRCT (Figs. 6-9 and 6-10), or both [34,35]. These areas usually have sharply defined margins and a configuration consistent with involvement of single or multiple adjacent pulmonary lobules (Figs. 6-7 through 6-10). In a review of the HRCT findings in 22 patients who had HP, Hansell et al. found that 19 patients (86%) had focal areas of decreased attenuation, 18 patients (82%) had ground-glass opacities, and 12 patients (55%) had centrilobular nodules [34]. In the study by Small et al., 15 of 20 (75%) patients had focal areas of decreased attenuation on inspiratory HRCT, and 11 of 12 (92%) of the patients who had expiratory scans had focal areas of air-trapping [35]. The areas of decreased attenuation and air-trapping are presumably

caused by small airway obstruction due to the bronchiolitis seen in patients with HP [34,35]. A combination of increased lung attenuation (ground-glass opacity) and decreased lung attenuation (mosaic perfusion) on inspiratory scans (i.e., the head-cheese sign) is common in HP [36]. In some patients who have HP, evidence of expiratory air-trapping may be seen in the absence of inspiratory scan abnormalities (Fig. 6-10) [37].

Chronic Stage

Chronic HP is characterized by the presence of fibrosis, although findings of active disease are often superimposed (Table 6-1). Silver et al. [26] described the HRCT findings in six patients who had subacute symptoms superimposed on chronic HP. In these patients, symptoms had been present for 1 to 6 years. The chest radiographs and CT scans in these six patients showed irregular reticular opacities representing fibrosis (Figs. 6-11 and 6-12). The CT scans also showed patchy bilateral areas of ground-glass opacity (Figs. 6-11

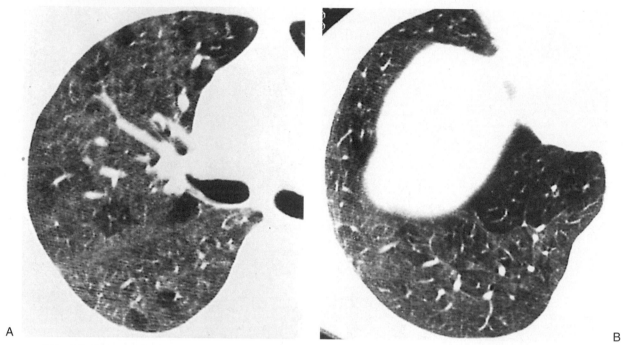

A

B

FIG. 6-5. Subacute hypersensitivity pneumonitis. HRCT in a 68-year-old woman at the levels of the right upper lobar bronchus **(A)** and at the right base **(B)**. Patchy ground-glass opacities are seen at both levels. At the level in **A**, some individual lobules appear lucent, a finding that likely reflects air-trapping and mosaic perfusion.

and 6-12), and scattered, small nodules (Fig. 6-13). As in patients who have subacute disease, areas of reduced lung attenuation due to mosaic perfusion may be seen on inspiratory scans, and air-trapping may be seen on expiratory scans.

Adler et al. [38] reviewed the HRCT scans in 16 patients who had chronic HP. All patients showed findings of fibrosis with irregular opacities and distortion of the lung parenchyma. The distribution of the fibrosis in the transverse plane was variable, being patchy in distribution in some cases and predominantly subpleural or peribronchovascular in others (Fig. 6-14). Honeycombing, when present, was usually subpleural in distribution (Fig. 6-15) [38]. In a study by Grenier et al.

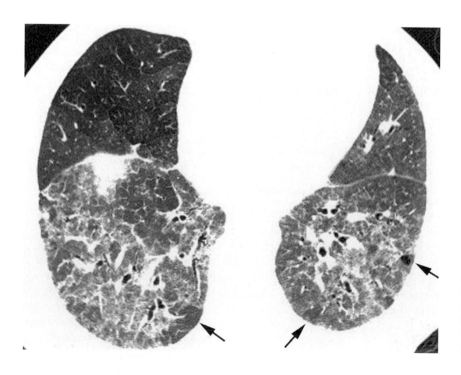

FIG. 6-6. Subacute hypersensitivity pneumonitis in a bird fancier. Patchy ground-glass opacity is visible in the lower lobes. Some lobules (*arrows*) appear relatively lucent, a finding that reflects air-trapping and mosaic perfusion.

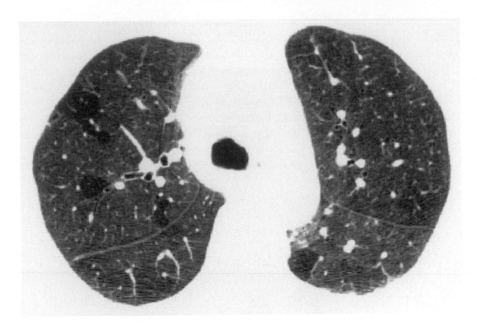

FIG. 6-7. Subacute hypersensitivity pneumonitis in a bird fancier. HRCT demonstrates bilateral ground-glass opacities. Note localized areas of decreased attenuation and vascularity with a size and configuration corresponding to a secondary pulmonary lobule. These localized areas of decreased attenuation are presumably due to bronchiolitis associated with hypersensitivity pneumonitis.

[31], honeycombing was seen in 23% of patients who had HP. Other findings in the patients studied by Adler et al. [38], indicative of active disease, included poorly defined, small nodular opacities seen in ten cases (62%), and areas of ground-glass opacity seen in 15 (94%) of the cases. The nodules and areas of ground-glass opacity involved mainly the middle and lower lung zones. In another study [32] of six patients who had chronic HP, HRCT revealed ill-defined nodular centrilobular and peribronchiolar opacities in all six cases and areas of ground-glass density in four; in patients who have HP, these findings are usually indicative of active disease.

Findings of fibrosis in patients who have chronic HP most often show a middle lung or lower lung zone predominance, or are evenly distributed throughout the upper, middle, and lower lung zones [38,39]. Relative sparing of the lung bases, seen in a majority of cases of chronic HP, allows distinction of this entity from IPF, in which the fibrosis usually predominates in the lung bases. It should be noted, however, that two of the 16 cases reported by Adler et al. [38] showed a lower lung zone predominance of abnormalities. Furthermore, Grenier et al. [40] report a lower lobe predominance of disease in 31% of patients who have HP. In the study by Lynch

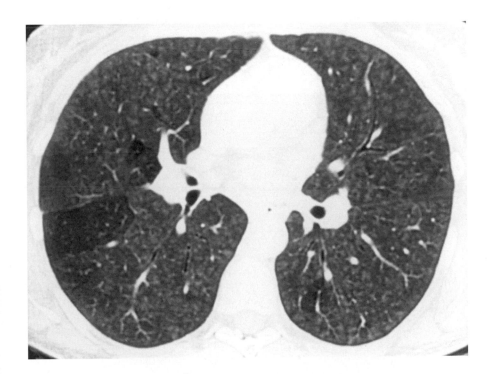

FIG. 6-8. Subacute hypersensitivity pneumonitis in a farmer. HRCT demonstrates bilateral poorly defined small nodular opacities in a characteristic centrilobular distribution. Also note localized areas of decreased attenuation and vascularity with a size and configuration corresponding to one or more adjacent secondary pulmonary lobules.

et al., the fibrosis in chronic HP had an upper lung zone predominance in three of 19 (16%) patients, a middle zone predominance in three patients (16%), lower lung zone predominance in eight patients (42%), and no zonal predominance in five patients (26%) [39]; five patients (26%) had both a peripheral and lower lung zone predominance of the fibrosis [39]. Therefore, in some patients with chronic HP, HRCT findings are identical to those of IPF. In clinical practice, the differential diagnosis of HP and IPF is facilitated by the clinical history and laboratory findings.

Utility of High-Resolution Computed Tomography

Several studies have demonstrated that HRCT is more sensitive than chest radiographs in the assessment of patients who have HP (Fig. 6-3), although the sensitivity of HRCT is not 100%. In a study by Remy-Jardin et al. [33], seven of 21 patients who had subacute HP (33%) had normal chest radiographs, and all patients had abnormal HRCT scans. Lynch et al. [41] assessed the sensitivity of HRCT and chest radiographs in the detection of HP diagnosed in a population of

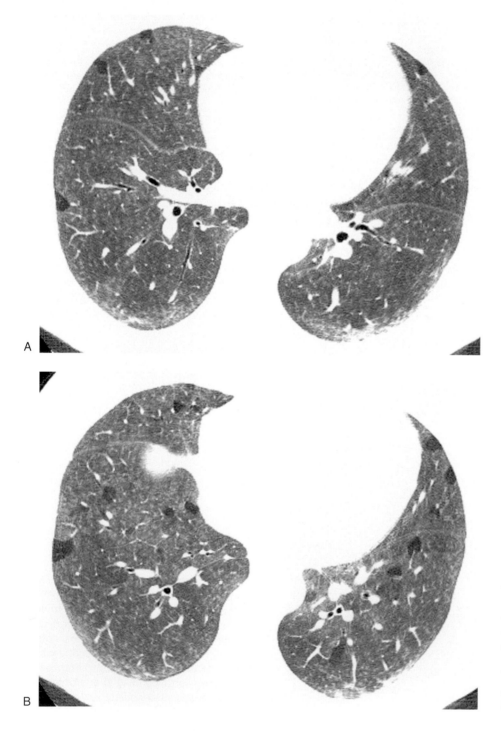

FIG. 6-9. Subacute hypersensitivity pneumonitis in a bird fancier. Inspiratory HRCT at three levels **(A–C)** show ill-defined centrilobular nodules, patchy ground-glass opacity, and lobular areas of lucency. A postexpiratory scan **(D)** shows air-trapping in relation to the lucent lobules and in other lung regions. This finding reflects the bronchiolitis associated with hypersensitivity pneumonitis. *Continued*

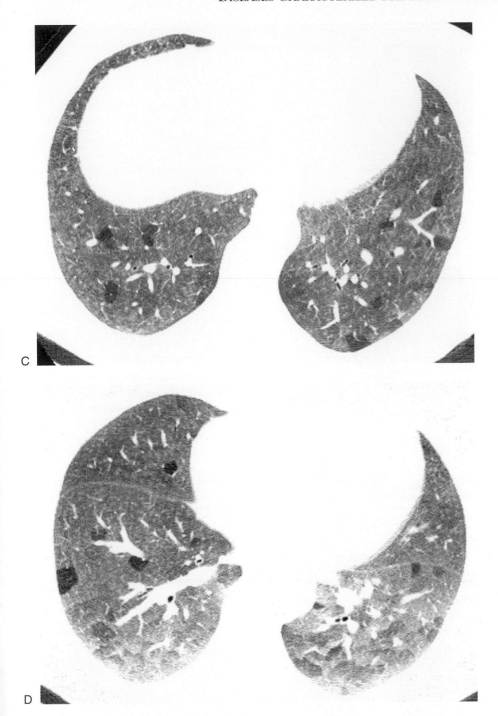

FIG. 6-9. *Continued*

swimming pool employees. The diagnosis of HP was based on two or more work-related signs or symptoms, abnormal results on transbronchial biopsies, or abnormal lymphocytosis on bronchoalveolar lavage (BAL) fluid. Only one of 11 subjects (9%) had abnormal findings on the chest radiographs, whereas five (45%) had abnormal HRCT findings. The abnormality on HRCT in each case consisted of small, poorly defined centrilobular nodules. This population-based study allowed assessment of patients with relatively mild disease. Pulmonary function tests (PFTs) were either normal or only minimally abnormal in all cases. It should be pointed out

that in this study, HRCT scans were performed at 4-cm slice intervals, so that mild localized abnormalities might have been missed on HRCT [41]. It cannot be overemphasized that optimal assessment of infiltrative lung disease requires HRCT scans at 1-cm intervals in the supine position, or at 2-cm intervals in both supine and prone positions. In another study [42], six patients who had chronic HP were examined using PFTs, BAL, lung biopsy, chest radiographs, and HRCT. The chest radiographs showed a variety of findings, including a mixed alveolar/interstitial pattern, peribronchiolar thickening, a diffuse granular pattern, or linear fibrosis. In general,

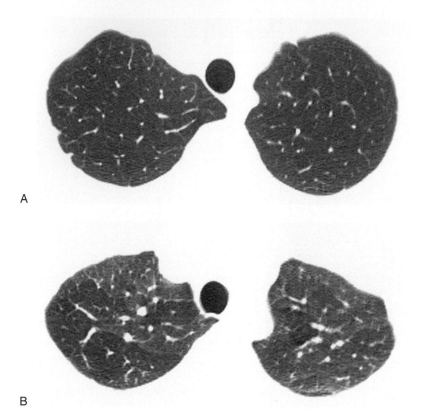

A

B

FIG. 6-10. Subacute hypersensitivity pneumonitis
A: The inspiratory HRCT scan is normal. **B:** An
expiratory scan shows patchy air-trapping.

HRCT showed more abnormalities than were apparent on the plain chest radiographs and demonstrated findings of active disease not suggested on the chest radiographs.

In addition to its increased sensitivity, the pattern and distribution of lung abnormalities are better assessed on HRCT than on conventional CT or chest radiographs [26,32]. The CT appearance of ill-defined centrilobular nodules smaller than 5 mm in diameter amid patchy areas of ground-glass opacity is characteristic of the subacute stage of HP [26,32,41]. Swensen et al. [43] assessed the diagnostic accu-

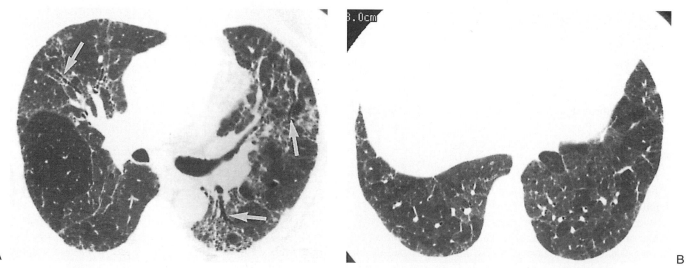

A

B

FIG. 6-11. A 54-year-old man who had recurrent episodes of hypersensitivity pneumonitis over 10 years. **A:** HRCT at the level of the bronchus intermedius demonstrates evidence of fibrosis with irregular reticular opacities, traction bronchiectasis (*arrows*), and architectural distortion. Localized honeycombing is present in the subpleural lung regions of the left lower lobe. Also noted are bilateral areas of ground-glass opacity in a patchy distribution. These may represent subacute hypersensitivity pneumonitis superimposed on chronic fibrosis. **B:** HRCT scan through the lung bases shows areas of ground-glass opacity in a patchy distribution but no definite evidence of fibrosis.

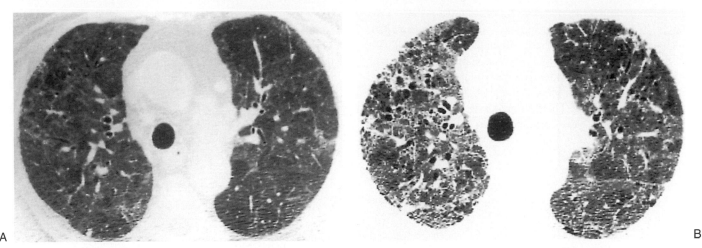

A   B

FIG. 6-12. Progression of hypersensitivity pneumonitis. **A.** HRCT at the level of the upper lobes shows patchy ground-glass opacity, but findings of reticulation and fibrosis are minimal. **B:** On an HRCT obtained 1 year later, there is extensive evidence of fibrosis with irregular reticular opacities, traction bronchiectasis, and some areas of honeycombing. Patchy ground-glass opacity remains visible, particularly in the left lung.

racy of HRCT in 85 patients undergoing surgical biopsy for diagnosis of diffuse lung disease, including nine patients who had HP. Based on the pattern and distribution of parenchymal abnormalities, the correct diagnosis of HP was made as a first-choice diagnosis in seven of the nine (78%) patients who had HP, and the correct diagnosis was included in the top three diagnostic choices in all nine patients.

In HP, small nodules and areas of ground-glass opacity represent potentially treatable or reversible disease. Remy-Jardin et al. [33] performed sequential CT scans several months apart in 14 patients who had subacute bird-breeder's lung and in 13 patients who had chronic bird-breeder's lung. After cessation of exposure to the avian antigen, the HRCT scans in patients who had subacute HP showed marked improvement in the areas of ground-glass opacity or small nodules, or returned to normal. Patients who continued to be exposed to the avian antigen showed no interval change in the HRCT scans. Similarly, in patients who had chronic HP, there was improvement in the small nodules and in the areas of ground-glass opacity in patients who were no longer exposed to the avian antigen. Findings of fibrosis such as irregular linear areas of attenuation, architectural distortion, and honeycombing are irreversible.

In a patient presenting with a several-month history of dry cough, progressive shortness of breath, and an HRCT scan showing bilateral areas of ground-glass opacity, the differential diagnosis includes HP, nonspecific interstitial pneumonia (NSIP), desquamative interstitial pneumonia (DIP), and alveolar proteinosis [32,44–46]. A careful clinical history and serologic testing can often confirm the diagnosis of HP, thus precluding the need for open-lung biopsy. DIP and NSIP often have a subpleural predominance of areas of ground-glass opacity and are rarely associated with centrilobular nodules, as is HP [39,47]. Alveolar proteinosis, also rare, is characterized by the presence of smoothly thickened interlobular septa within

the areas of hazy increased opacity that give a crazy-paving appearance [44,45]. It can be readily diagnosed by BAL.

PFTs in patients who have HP can show both restrictive and obstructive patterns. In the acute phase, reduction in lung volume, diffusing capacity, and static lung compliance are the

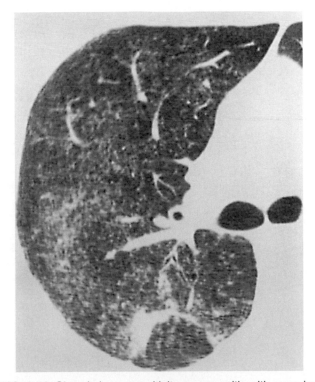

FIG. 6-13. Chronic hypersensitivity pneumonitis with superimposed subacute disease. HRCT at the level of the tracheal carina in a 31-year-old man shows ill-defined small nodular opacities and ground-glass opacities. Mild fibrosis is present posteriorly due to intermittent chronic exposure to the antigen.

most common findings [31,48]. An obstructive pattern is frequent in the subacute and chronic phases, as indicated by increased residual volume and total lung capacity and slowing of forced expiratory flow, and can be seen in combination with a restrictive pattern [31,48]. To some extent, functional abnormalities correlate with HRCT findings. In one series of 22 patients who had HP, HRCT scans with limited number of expiratory images were correlated with PFTs [34]. Areas of

decreased attenuation, mosaic perfusion, and air-trapping were seen in 19 patients and were the most frequent findings. The extent of decreased attenuation correlated well with severity of functional index of air-trapping as indicated by increased residual volume ($r = .58$; $p < .01$). The authors concluded that areas of decreased attenuation and mosaic perfusion are important CT findings and are probably related to pathologic findings of bronchiolitis [34].

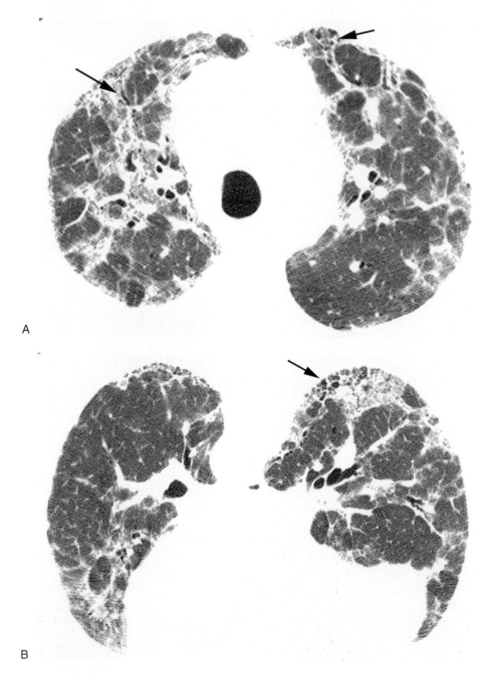

A

B

FIG. 6-14. Chronic hypersensitivity pneumonitis with fibrosis and superimposed subacute disease in a bird fancier. **A:** HRCT at the level of the upper lobes shows interlobular septal thickening, intralobular interstitial thickening, and some traction bronchiolectasis (*arrows*). Ground-glass opacity is superimposed. **B:** Prone scan at the lung bases shows patchy ground-glass opacity and findings of fibrosis, including mild honeycombing (*arrow*).

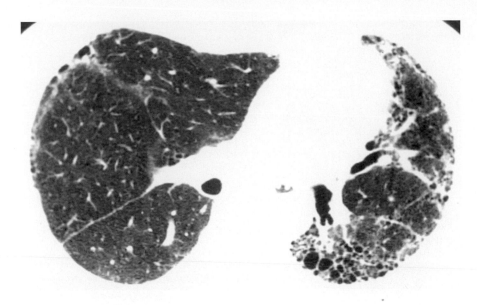

FIG. 6-15. Chronic hypersensitivity pneumonitis with fibrosis resulting from exposure to *Penicillium* mold used in the curing of sausages. Peripheral honeycombing is visible, with a left sided predominance. This appearance is indistinguishable from that of Idiopathic pulmonary fibrosis.

EOSINOPHILIC LUNG DISEASE

The term *eosinophilic lung disease* describes a group of entities characterized by abundant accumulation of eosinophils in the pulmonary interstitium and airspaces [49,50]. Peripheral blood eosinophilia is commonly present. Diagnostic criteria include (i) radiographic or CT findings of lung disease in association with peripheral eosinophilia, (ii) biopsy confirmed lung tissue eosinophilia, or (iii) increased eosinophils at BAL [49]. The disorders can be classified into those of unknown cause and those with a known etiology [51].

Idiopathic Eosinophilic Lung Disease

Common idiopathic eosinophilic lung diseases include (i) simple pulmonary eosinophilia, (ii) acute eosinophilic pneumonia, (iii) chronic eosinophilic pneumonia, (iv) hypereosinophilic syndrome (HES), and (v) Churg-Strauss syndrome. These conditions reflect a spectrum of diseases having mild to severe symptoms and focal to diffuse radiographic abnormalities. Idiopathic connective tissue diseases may also be associated with blood or tissue eosinophilia. These include Wegener's granulomatosis (see Chapter 5), rheumatoid disease (see Chapter 4), and polyarteritis [52,53].

Simple Pulmonary Eosinophilia

Simple pulmonary eosinophilia, also known as *Loeffler's syndrome*, is characterized by blood eosinophilia and focal areas of consolidation, usually transient, visible on chest radiographs. Although similar findings can be seen in association with a number of etiologic agents, particularly parasites and drug reactions, ideally the term should be limited to cases in which the etiology is unknown. Approximately one-third of cases are idiopathic.

Patients typically have cough and mild shortness of breath [50]. Pathologically, eosinophils and histiocytes accumulate in alveolar walls and alveoli [49]. The radiographic manifestations are characteristic, and consist of transient and migratory areas of consolidation that typically clear spontaneously within one month [50]. These are nonsegmental, may be single or multiple, and usually have ill-defined margins [49,50]. On radiographs and HRCT, the areas of consolidation often have a predominantly peripheral distribution [49]. On HRCT, areas of ground-glass opacity may be seen, and focal areas of consolidation or large nodules may be associated with a halo sign [51].

Chronic Eosinophilic Pneumonia

Chronic eosinophilic pneumonia is an idiopathic condition characterized by extensive filling of alveoli by a mixed inflammatory infiltrate consisting primarily of eosinophils. A similar interstitial infiltrate is often present [54]. Chronic eosinophilic pneumonia is usually associated with an increased number of eosinophils in the peripheral blood. Clinically, patients present with fever, cough, weight loss, malaise, and shortness of breath. Symptoms are often severe and last 3 months or longer [54–57]. Life-threatening respiratory compromise may occur, but this is unusual [58].

Radiographically, chronic eosinophilic pneumonia is characterized by the presence of homogeneous peripheral airspace consolidation, "the photographic negative of pulmonary edema" [54]. This pattern can remain unchanged for weeks or months unless steroid therapy is given; chronic eosinophilic pneumonia responds promptly to the administration of steroids.

The combination of blood eosinophilia, peripheral consolidation visible on the radiograph, and rapid response to steroid therapy are often sufficiently characteristic to obviate the need for lung biopsy [50,54,57]. The diagnosis, however,

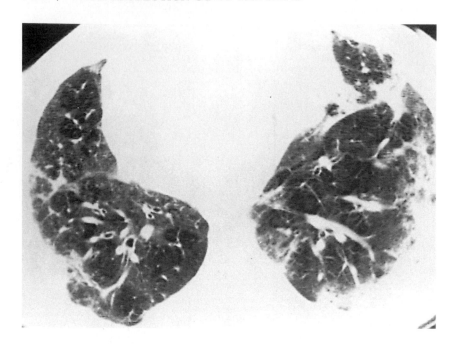

FIG. 6-16. Chronic eosinophilic pneumonia. HRCT through the lung bases in a 43-year-old woman shows subpleural airspace consolidation.

may be difficult in patients who have minimal blood eosinophilia or in whom the peripheral distribution of infiltrates is not apparent. This classic radiologic picture, however, is seen only in approximately 50% of cases [50,57].

High-Resolution Computed Tomography Findings

Chronic eosinophilic pneumonia is characterized by (i) consolidation, often peripheral and patchy in distribution (see Figs. 3-103 and 3-104; Figs. 6-16 through 6-18), (ii) patchy or peripheral ground-glass opacity, sometimes associated with crazy-paving, (iii) linear or bandlike opacities, usually seen during resolution, and (iv) an upper lobe predominance of abnormalities (Table 6-2). Mayo et al. [59] reviewed the

chest radiographs and CT scans in six patients who had chronic eosinophilic pneumonia. All patients had patchy airspace consolidation, and in five of the six cases, the consolidation was most marked in the middle and upper lung zones. In only one of the six patients was the classic pattern of airspace consolidation confined to the outer third of the lungs readily apparent on the plain radiographs; however, in all six, a characteristic peripheral airspace consolidation was clearly demonstrated on CT. This study suggests that CT may be helpful in making the diagnosis of chronic eosinophilic pneumonia when the clinical findings are suggestive, but the radiographic pattern is nonspecific.

Ebara et al. [60] reviewed the radiographic and CT findings in 17 patients who had chronic eosinophilic pneumonia.

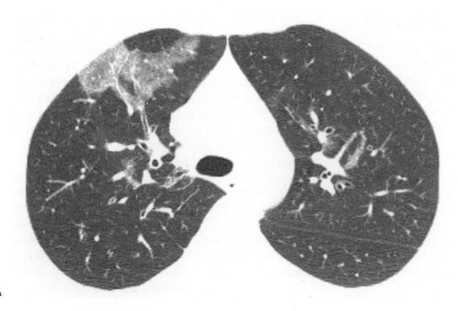

A

FIG. 6-17. A–C: Chronic eosinophilic pneumonia. Patchy areas of ground-glass opacity and consolidation have a distinct peripheral distribution. *Continued*

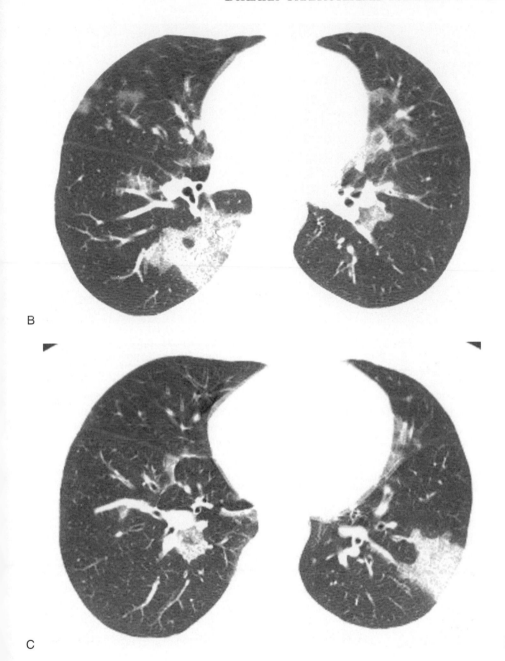

B

C

FIG. 6-17. *Continued*

A peripheral predominance of areas of consolidation or ground-glass opacities was evident on the radiograph in eleven patients (65%) and on CT in 16 patients (94%). The abnormalities on CT included ground-glass opacities in 82% of patients, confluent consolidation in 47%, patchy consolidation or airspace nodules in 29%, and streaky or bandlike opacities in 6% (Fig. 6-18) [60]. All seven patients in whom the CT scans were performed within 4 weeks of the onset of clinical symptoms had dense confluent subpleural consolidation with or without ground-glass opacities. Five of the seven patients in whom the initial CT was performed 1 to 2 months from the onset of symptoms had inhomogeneous patchy consolidation or focal ground-glass opacities. One of the three patients in whom the CT scans were performed more than 2 months after the onset of symptoms had dense subpleural consolidation, one had patchy consolidation and areas of atelectasis, and one had subpleural bandlike opacities [60]. These bandlike opacities are often seen in patients who have clearing of disease and likely reflect atelectasis. The pattern of crazy-paving may also be seen in patients who have chronic eosinophilic pneumonia.

An appearance identical to that of chronic eosinophilic pneumonia can be seen in patients who have simple pulmonary eosinophilia or Loeffler's syndrome. Simple pulmonary eosinophilia, however, is usually self-limited and associated with pulmonary infiltrates that are transient or fleeting [8,50]. With simple pulmonary eosinophilia, areas of consolidation can appear and disappear within days; chronic eosinophilic pneumonia has a more protracted course, and areas of consolidation remain unchanged over weeks or months.

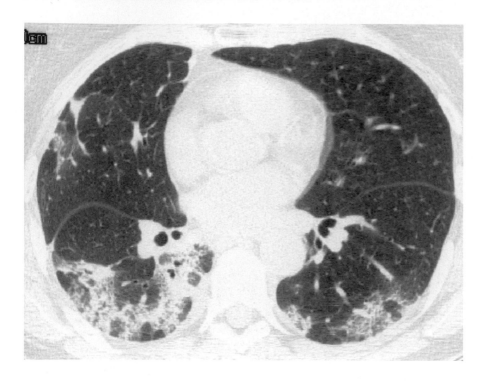

FIG. 6-18. Chronic eosinophilic pneumonia. HRCT in a 73-year-old woman demonstrates patchy bilateral subpleural ground-glass opacities, consolidation, and linear opacities.

The presence of peripheral airspace consolidation can be considered suggestive of chronic eosinophilic pneumonia only in the appropriate clinical setting; that is, in patients who have eosinophilia. An identical appearance of peripheral airspace consolidation can be seen in BOOP (see Fig. 3-102; Figs. 6-22, 6-23, and 6-25) [61]. However, whereas virtually all cases of chronic eosinophilic pneumonia have a predominantly upper lobe distribution, the consolidation in BOOP often involves the lower lung zones to a greater degree [61]. On the other hand, some patients who have lung disease have pathologic features of both chronic eosinophilic pneumonia and BOOP [59,61]. Therefore, it is not surprising that they can have identical radiologic and CT findings [59,61–63]. A peripheral distribution of disease, mimicking chronic eosinophilic pneumonia, can sometimes be seen in patients who have sarcoidosis [64], NSIP, and DIP (Figs. 6-37 through 6-39).

Acute Eosinophilic Pneumonia

Acute eosinophilic pneumonia is an acute febrile illness associated with rapidly increasing shortness of breath and

TABLE 6-2. *HRCT findings in chronic eosinophilic pneumonia*

Patchy unilateral or bilateral airspace consolidation[a]
Peripheral, middle, and upper lung predominance[a,b]
Ground-glass opacity ± superimposed septal thickening (i.e., crazy-paving)
Linear or bandlike subpleural opacities

[a]Most common findings.
[b]Findings most helpful in differential diagnosis.

hypoxemic respiratory failure [49,65]. The diagnosis is based on clinical findings of acute respiratory failure and presence of markedly elevated numbers of eosinophils in BAL fluid [65].

The radiographic manifestations are similar to those of pulmonary edema [49,66]. The earliest radiographic manifestation consists of reticular opacities, frequently with Kerley B lines. This progresses over a few hours or days to bilateral interstitial infiltrates, and airspace consolidation involving mainly the lower lung zones [49]. Small bilateral pleural effusions are present in the majority of patients [67].

The HRCT findings of acute eosinophilic pneumonia have been described in a small number of patients. The primary HRCT manifestations include bilateral areas of ground-glass opacity, smooth interlobular septal thickening, small pleural effusions, and, occasionally, areas of consolidation [51,67,68]. The combination of ground-glass opacity and septal thickening may result in the appearance of crazy-paving.

Hypereosinophilic Syndrome

HES is a condition characterized by blood eosinophilia present persistently for at least 6 months, associated with multiorgan tissue infiltration by mature eosinophils [49,50,69]. An underlying cause may or may not be evident.

The main causes of morbidity and mortality are cardiac and central nervous system involvement [69]. Pulmonary and pleural involvement occurs in approximately 40% of cases [65]. Pulmonary symptoms include cough, wheezing, and shortness of breath. The radiographic manifestations are nonspecific and consist of transient hazy opacities or areas of consolidation [69]. Cardiac involvement eventually leads to cardiomegaly, pulmonary edema, and pleural effusion [70]. The prognosis is poor.

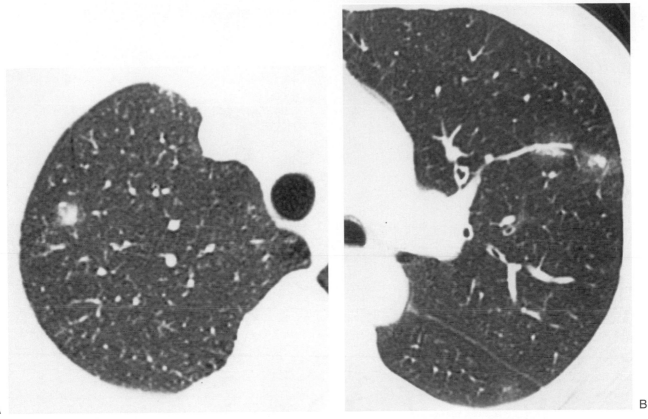

FIG. 6-19. Hypereosinophilic syndrome. Views of the right **(A)** and left **(B)** upper lobes from an HRCT demonstrate small nodules surrounded by a halo of ground glass attenuation. (Courtesy of Dr. Eun-Young Kang, Korea University Guro Hospital, Seoul.)

Kang and coworkers described the HRCT findings in five patients who had idiopathic HES and pulmonary involvement [71]. The predominant abnormality in all five patients was the presence of bilateral pulmonary nodules measuring 1 cm or smaller in diameter (Fig. 6-19). The majority of nodules had a halo of ground-glass opacity and involved mainly the peripheral lung regions. Two patients had small pleural effusions.

Churg-Strauss Syndrome

Churg-Strauss syndrome is a multisystem disorder characterized by the presence of necrotizing vasculitis, extravascular granuloma formation, and eosinophilic infiltration of various organs, particularly the lungs, skin, heart, nerves, gastrointestinal tract, and kidneys [49–51]. Patients often have a history of allergic diseases including asthma, nasal polyps, or sinusitis. Criteria helpful in the diagnosis of Churg-Strauss syndrome in a patient who has vasculitis include (i) asthma, (ii) eosinophilia of greater than 10% of the white blood cell count, (iii) neuropathy, (iv) migratory or transient pulmonary opacities, (v) sinus abnormalities, and (vi) extravascular eosinophils on biopsy [72]. Cough and hemoptysis are common, but symptoms may reflect the involvement of various organs, including skin rash, diarrhea, neuropathy, and congestive heart failure.

Radiographic abnormalities are common. Pulmonary opacities have been identified in as many as 70% of cases, having the appearance of simple pulmonary eosinophilia, chronic eosinophilic pneumonia, pulmonary hemorrhage, or pulmonary edema [50].

HRCT findings are variable and nonspecific, reflecting the different pulmonary manifestations of this disease. Findings include (i) consolidation or ground-glass opacity (59%), which may have peripheral distribution or be patchy and geographic (Fig. 6-20), (ii) pulmonary nodules (12%) ranging from 0.5 to 3.5 cm in diameter, which may contain air bronchograms or cavitate, (iii) centrilobular nodules (12%), (iv) bronchial wall thickening or bronchiectasis (35%), and (v) interlobular septal thickening due to edema (6%) (Table 6-3) [52,53,73,74].

Eosinophilic Lung Disease of Specific Etiology

Known causes of eosinophilic lung disease include drugs, parasites, and fungi [51].

Drug-Related Diseases

Drugs are an important cause of eosinophilic lung disease [49,50]. A large number of drugs have been reported to be associated with eosinophilic lung disease; implicated drugs include

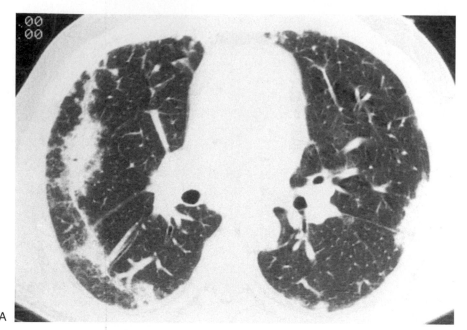

A

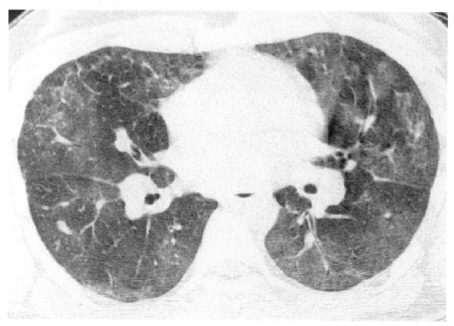

B

FIG. 6-20. Churg-Strauss syndrome in two patients. **A:** In a 52-year-old man, Churg-Strauss syndrome is associated with peripheral areas of consolidation. This appearance is nonspecific, but common in this condition. **B:** In a 21-year-old man, patchy ground-glass opacity with a light peripheral predominance is the predominant finding.

antibiotics, nonsteroidal antiinflammatory agents, drugs used for inflammatory bowel disease, and inhaled illicit drugs such as cocaine and heroin [49,50]. Reactions range from those sim-

ilar to simple pulmonary eosinophilia to those imitating acute eosinophilic pneumonia. CT findings can include consolidation, ground-glass opacity, or pulmonary edema. Drug reactions are discussed in detail in Chapter 4.

Parasitic Infestations

Parasites most commonly result in findings similar to simple pulmonary eosinophilia [51]. The majority of cases are due to roundworms such as *Ascaris lumbricoides*, *Toxocara*, *Ancylostoma*, and *Strongyloides stercoralis* [49–51]. Tropical pulmonary eosinophilia is caused by the worms *Wuchereria bancrofti* and *Brugia malayi*, with most cases being reported in India, Africa, South America, and Southeast Asia

TABLE 6-3. *HRCT findings in Churg-Strauss syndrome*

Consolidation or ground-glass opacity[a]
Peripheral or patchy distribution[a]
Small or large nodules, sometimes cavitary
Bronchial wall thickening or bronchiectasis
Interlobular septal thickening

[a]Most common findings.

[75]. In the Far East, the lung fluke *Paragonimus westermani* is typically responsible. Symptoms are nonspecific but include fever, weight loss, dyspnea, cough, and hemoptysis. CT findings reported in *Paragonimiasis* include patchy lung consolidation, cystic lesions filled with air or fluid, pneumothorax, and pleural effusion [76].

Fungal Disease

The primary fungal disease associated with pulmonary eosinophilia is allergic bronchopulmonary aspergillosis (ABPA), characterized by asthma, peripheral eosinophilia, central bronchiectasis, mucous plugging, and an allergic reaction to *Aspergillus fumigatus* (see Figs. 8-37 and 8-38). It is described in detail in Chapter 8. However, other patterns of disease may result from exposure to fungus, including IIP, eosinophilic pneumonia, and bronchocentric granulomatosis.

Bronchocentric Granulomatosis

The characteristic histologic abnormality seen in patients who have bronchocentric granulomatosis is the presence of necrotizing granulomatous inflammation centered around bronchioles and small bronchi [50,51,77–79]. It may be associated with complete destruction of the airway mucosa and filling of the airway lumen with necrotic material [80]. In asthmatic subjects, bronchocentric granulomatosis is most commonly associated with *Aspergillus*, and fungal hyphae are often present within these lesions. Bronchocentric granulomatosis may also be seen in immunosuppressed patients and in patients who have mycobacterial infection and noninfectious inflammatory diseases such as rheumatoid arthritis [51,79].

Bronchocentric granulomatosis is generally considered to be a hypersensitivity reaction. Patients are usually young, one-third have a history of asthma, and peripheral eosinophilia is seen in one-half of cases [77]; tissue eosinophilia is also present in asthmatic patients. This process may be asso-

ciated with ABPA in asthmatic patients, but abnormalities in bronchocentric granulomatosis tend to be more focal than those seen with ABPA. Symptoms are often mild, with fever, cough, chest pain, and hemoptysis. Chest radiographs may show a focal nodule or area of consolidation, most often in an upper lobe [50,51].

CT findings in a small number of patients who had bronchocentric granulomatosis have been reported [51,79]. In a study of five patients [79], common appearances were a spiculated mass lesion (three patients) and lobular consolidation with associated mild volume loss (two patients). One of the two patients with consolidation also had extensive mucoid impaction [79]. The abnormalities predominantly involved an upper lobe in four patients and a lower lobe in one. In the four cases in which the lesion was resected, the macroscopic pathological appearance was that of consolidation (n = 2) or a mass lesion (n = 2). *Aspergillus* hyphae were identified in two cases, and *Nocardia* was cultured in one. Patchy lung attenuation due to airway obstruction and mosaic perfusion may also be seen [81]. Masses and consolidation represent necrotic tissue associated with consolidation or eosinophilic pneumonia.

BRONCHIOLITIS OBLITERANS ORGANIZING PNEUMONIA

BOOP is a disease characterized pathologically by the presence of granulation tissue polyps within the lumina of bronchioles and alveolar ducts and patchy areas of organizing pneumonia, consisting largely of mononuclear cells and foamy macrophages, in the surrounding lung (Fig. 6-21) [82,83]. Most cases are idiopathic, but a BOOP-like reaction may also be seen in patients who have pulmonary infection, drug reactions, collagen-vascular diseases, Wegener's granulomatosis, and after toxic fume inhalation [84–88].

Since its original description, a number of names have been used to describe this entity [83]. "BOOP" is generally

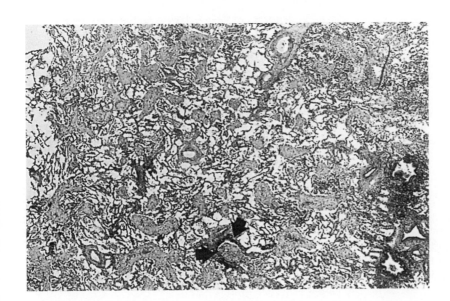

FIG. 6-21. Bronchiolitis obliterans organizing pneumonia (BOOP)/cryptogenic organizing pneumonia. A microscopic view of an open-lung biopsy specimen from a patient who has BOOP and findings of ground-glass opacity on HRCT. The specimen shows the presence of granulation tissue polyps in bronchioles and alveolar ducts (*arrows*) and areas of consolidation.

used in the United States. However, because the clinical, functional, radiologic, and HRCT findings in BOOP are primarily the result of an organizing pneumonia, it has been suggested that the term *cryptogenic organizing pneumonia* (COP) more accurately reflects the true nature of this disease [89–92]). COP and, simply, organizing pneumonia have been suggested as alternative designations for this disease by the American Thoracic Society/European Respiratory Society Multidisciplinary Consensus Classification Committee [93]. The terms *bronchiolitis obliterans with intraluminal polyps* and *proliferative bronchiolitis* have also been used to describe the principal bronchiolar abnormality present in patients who have BOOP [94]. However, because of its wide acceptance in the clinical, radiologic, and pathologic literature, and the number of possible alternative designations available, for simplicity we use the term *BOOP* in this book.

Patients who have BOOP typically present with a several-month history of nonproductive cough [63,92,95,96]. They often have a low-grade fever, malaise, and shortness of breath. PFTs characteristically show a restrictive pattern. Clinically and functionally, the findings may be similar to IPF, although the duration of symptoms in patients who have BOOP is shorter, systemic symptoms are more common, and finger clubbing is rarely seen [63,92,95,96]. The patients

usually respond well to corticosteroid therapy and have a good prognosis [95].

The characteristic radiologic features of BOOP consist of patchy, nonsegmental, unilateral, or bilateral areas of airspace consolidation [63,92,95,96]. Irregular reticular opacities may be present, but they are rarely a major feature. Small nodular opacities may be seen as the only finding or, more commonly, are seen in association with areas of airspace consolidation.

Although the radiologic findings of BOOP are nonspecific, in the majority of cases, the presence of areas of consolidation and the paucity or absence of reticular opacities allows an easy distinction of BOOP from UIP [63,96]. In some patients, the consolidation may be peripheral, a pattern similar to that seen in chronic eosinophilic pneumonia [62,63].

High-Resolution Computed Tomography Findings

The CT and HRCT findings in patients who have BOOP have been described by a number of authors [61,63,97–99], and these descriptions are remarkably similar. Typical HRCT features of this entity include: (i) patchy consolidation (seen in 80% of cases) or ground-glass opacity (in 60% of cases), often with a subpleural and/or peribronchial distribution (Figs. 6-22 through 6-27); (ii) small, ill-defined nodules (30%

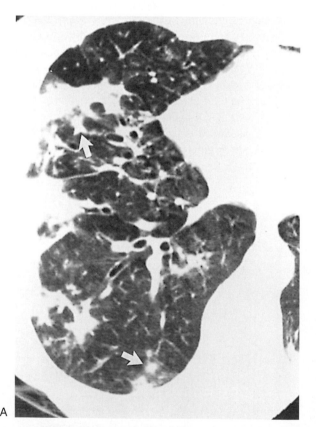

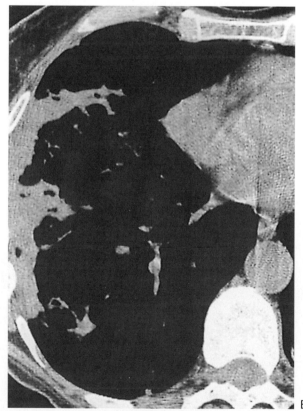

FIG. 6-22. Bronchiolitis obliterans organizing pneumonia/cryptogenic organizing pneumonia. **A:** HRCT through the right lower lung zone in a 64-year-old woman shows airspace consolidation mainly in the subpleural regions. Some small nodules of consolidation are seen to be centrilobular (*arrows*). **B:** Mediastinal window settings better delineate the dense subpleural consolidation.

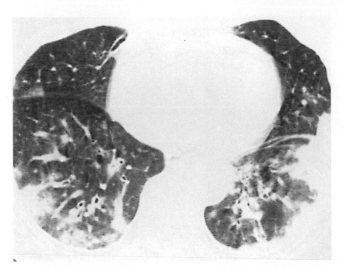

FIG. 6-23. Bronchiolitis obliterans organizing pneumonia/cryptogenic organizing pneumonia. HRCT through the lower-lung zones in a 68-year-old woman shows subpleural and peribronchial distribution of the airspace consolidation. Some areas of consolidation are nodular.

to 50% of cases) that may be peribronchial or peribronchiolar (see Fig. 3-76; Figs. 6-28 and 6-29); (iii) large nodules or masses (Fig. 6-30) [100]; and (iv) bronchial wall thickening or dilatation in abnormal lung regions (Fig. 6-27) (Table 6-4). Crazy-paving, with a superimposition of ground-glass opacity and interlobular septal thickening, may also be seen in patients who have BOOP. BOOP often involves the lower lung zones to a greater degree than the upper lung zones [61].

Müller et al. [61] reviewed the radiographic and CT features of 14 patients who had biopsy-proven BOOP. Ten of the 14 patients had patchy unilateral or bilateral airspace consolidation. A predominantly subpleural distribution of the airspace consolidation was apparent on CT in six patients (Figs. 6-22 and 6-23), whereas this appearance was seen on radio-

graphs in two patients. In some patients, the airspace consolidation was more marked in a peribronchial distribution (Fig. 6-27). Areas of ground-glass opacity were also seen (Figs. 6-25 and 6-26). Nishimura and Itoh [101] correlated findings on 5-mm collimated CT scans with open-lung biopsy in eight patients who had BOOP. Biopsies from areas of dense consolidation showed filling of the terminal airspaces with branching granulation tissue buds.

Consolidation was also the most common HRCT abnormality seen in a study of 43 patients with biopsy-proven BOOP [99]. This study included 32 immunocompetent patients and 11 immunocompromised patients. Consolidation was visible in 79% of the cases reviewed (Table 6-4); it was present alone in nine cases and as part of a mixed pattern in 25 cases. In 32 cases, the consolidation was bilateral, with a nonsegmental, patchy distribution. The consolidation was predominantly subpleural in ten cases, predominantly peribronchovascular in ten cases (Fig. 6-27), and in seven cases had areas of both subpleural and peribronchovascular consolidation. Thus, 27 (63%) of 43 cases had either a predominantly subpleural distribution of consolidation, predominantly peribronchovascular distribution of consolidation, or both. The consolidation had no zonal or anterior-posterior predominance. Consolidation was more common in immunocompetent patients, being seen in 29 of 32 (91%) compared to 5 of 11 immunocompromised patients (45%) ($p < .01$).

Areas of ground-glass opacity were present in 26 of 43 (60%) cases in a study by Lee et al. [99]. In all but two cases, the areas of ground-glass opacity were seen as part of a mixed pattern. The areas of ground-glass opacity were bilateral and random in distribution. Areas of ground-glass opacity were present in eight of 11 (73%) immunocompromised patients, as compared to 18 of 32 (56%) immunocompetent patients ($p < .25$). In the CT-pathologic study performed by Nishimura and Itoh [101], ground-glass opacity correlated with alveolar septal inflammation, but little granulation tissue, in the terminal airspaces.

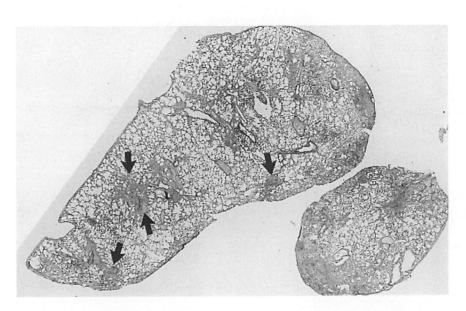

FIG. 6-24. Open-lung biopsy specimen from a patient who has bronchiolitis obliterans organizing pneumonia/cryptogenic organizing pneumonia viewed at low power. In this patient, ill-defined nodular opacities were seen on HRCT. The pathologic specimen shows that the nodular opacities seen on HRCT are due to small localized areas of organizing pneumonia (*arrows*) surrounding areas of bronchiolitis obliterans.

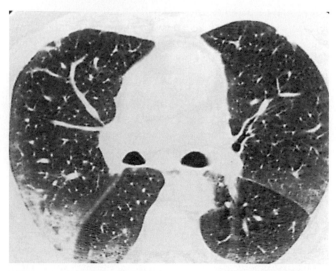

FIG. 6-25. Bronchiolitis obliterans organizing pneumonia/cryptogenic organizing pneumonia in a 55-year-old man. HRCT shows patchy, bilateral ground-glass opacities and airspace consolidation mainly in the subpleural regions.

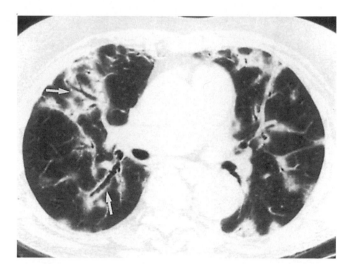

FIG. 6-27. An 81-year-old woman who has bronchiolitis obliterans organizing pneumonia/cryptogenic organizing pneumonia. HRCT demonstrates bilateral areas of consolidation. The consolidation is predominantly peribronchial in distribution. Note bronchial dilatation in the areas of consolidation (*arrows*).

Nodular opacities measuring 1 to 10 mm in diameter are common and were seen in 50% of patients studied by Müller et al. [61]; these nodules were typically ill-defined (Figs. 6-28 and 6-29). In two patients, these were more numerous along the bronchovascular bundles. On pathologic examination, the parenchymal nodules were found to represent localized zones of organizing pneumonia, which were centered around abnormal bronchioles (Fig. 6-24) [61]. Individual abnormal regions were separated from other involved areas by relatively normal parenchyma. Nodules were also present in 13 (30%) of 43 cases studied by Lee et al. [99]. They were the only finding in four cases and were part of a mixed pattern in nine cases. They were bilateral in ten cases and unilateral in three. The nodules were smaller than 5 mm in diameter in five cases and larger than 5 mm in diameter in

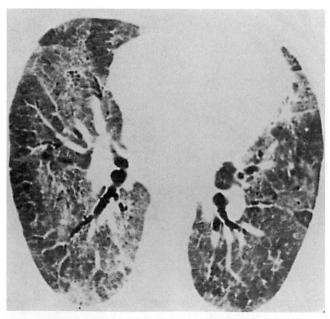

FIG. 6-26. Bronchiolitis obliterans organizing pneumonia/cryptogenic organizing pneumonia in a 65-year-old woman. Extensive bilateral ground-glass opacities show relative sparing of the subpleural region.

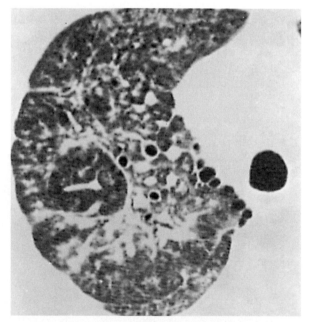

FIG. 6-28. Bronchiolitis obliterans organizing pneumonia (BOOP)/cryptogenic organizing pneumonia. HRCT through the right upper lobe in a patient with BOOP shows ground-glass opacities, bronchial wall thickening, and small nodules. Many of the nodules are centrilobular.

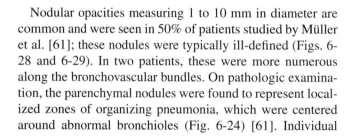

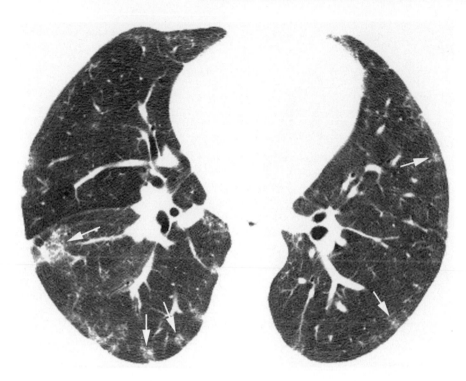

FIG. 6-29. Nodular areas of bronchiolitis obliterans organizing pneumonia/cryptogenic organizing pneumonia. Ill-defined nodular areas of ground-glass opacity and consolidation appear predominantly centrilobular in location.

eight cases. Most of the nodules had well-defined, smooth margins. Nodules were more frequently observed in immunocompromised patients (6 of 11, 55%) than in immunocompetent patients (seven of 32, 22%) (p <.025). Nodules in BOOP sometimes appear to be predominantly centrilobular [102]. Occasionally, the nodules in BOOP may be large.

Large nodules or masses may be the predominant HRCT finding in some patients who have BOOP [100]. Akira et al. [100] reviewed the HRCT scans and clinical records of 59 consecutive patients who had histologically proven BOOP; 12 patients had multiple large nodules or masses, 8 mm to 5 cm in diameter, as the primary manifestation of disease (Fig. 6-30). The number of large nodules ranged from two to eight per patient. Of 60 lesions in the 12 patients, 53 (88%) had an irregular margin, 27 (45%) had an air bronchogram, 23 (38%) had a pleural tail, and 21 (35%) had a spiculated margin. Ancillary findings included focal thickening of the interlobular septa in 5 of the 12 (42%) patients, pleural thickening in four (33%) patients, and parenchymal bands in three (25%) patients.

Bronchial wall thickening and dilatation may be seen on HRCT in patients who have extensive consolidation and is usually restricted to these areas (Fig. 6-27) [61]. In a study of 43 patients who had BOOP [99], bronchial dilatation was present in association with areas of consolidation in 24 cases and with areas of ground-glass opacity and nodules in two cases each. The significance of this finding is unclear; it is not known whether these bronchial abnormalities are reversible or whether they represent cylindrical bronchiectasis.

Other findings in patients who have BOOP include small pleural effusions, present in 30% to 35% of cases [61,99]. They may be unilateral or bilateral [99]. Irregular linear opacities were seen in 2 of 14 (14%) patients studied by Müller et al. [61] and 3 of 43 (7%) cases studied by Lee et al. [99]. They were associated with consolidation and located in the subpleural regions of the lower lung zones. Mild honeycombing in the subpleural regions of the lower lung zones was present in 2 of 43 cases studied by Lee et al. [99].

TABLE 6-4. *HRCT findings in bronchiolitis obliterans organizing pneumonia*

Patchy bilateral airspace consolidation (80%)[a]
Ground-glass opacity (60%) or crazy-paving[a]
Subpleural and/or peribronchovascular distribution[a]
Combination of first three findings[a,b]
Bronchial wall thickening, dilatation in abnormal areas[a]
Small nodular opacities, often centrilobular
Large nodules
Pleural effusion
Honeycombing (uncommon)

[a]Most common findings.
[b]Findings most helpful in differential diagnosis.

Utility of High-Resolution Computed Tomography

The CT and the plain film findings of BOOP are nonspecific and may be seen in a variety of infections and neoplastic diseases [100]. However, BOOP can usually be readily distinguished from other chronic interstitial and airspace lung

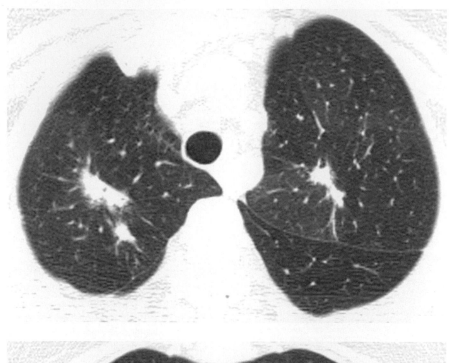

A

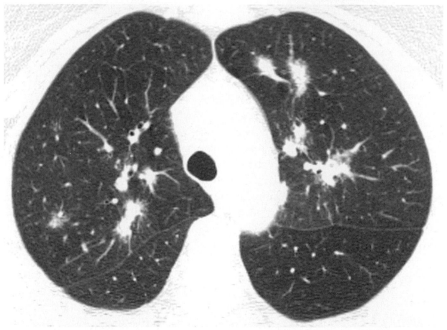

B

FIG. 6-30. A,B: Nodular areas of bronchiolitis obliterans organizing pneumonia/cryptogenic organizing pneumonia. Irregular nodular areas of consolidation are predominantly peribronchial in location.

diseases on HRCT. Johkoh et al. [103] reviewed the HRCT findings in 129 patients who had various idiopathic interstitial pneumonias, including 24 with BOOP. On average, based on the pattern and distribution of abnormalities on HRCT, two independent observers made a correct first-choice diagnosis in 79% of 24 cases of BOOP, 71% of 35 cases of UIP, 63% of 23 cases of DIP, 65% of 20 cases of AIP, and 9% of 27 cases of NSIP [103]. CT also provides a better assessment of disease pattern and distribution than do chest radiographs and is therefore superior to plain film in determining optimal biopsy site. HRCT is recommended routinely as a guide to optimal biopsy site in all patients undergoing open-lung biopsy.

NONSPECIFIC INTERSTITIAL PNEUMONIA

NSIP is an interstitial lung disease characterized by inflammation and fibrosis involving predominantly the alveolar walls but lacking any specific features that would allow a diagnosis of UIP, DIP, BOOP, or AIP [104,105]. It is therefore largely a diagnosis of exclusion [6]. NSIP may be idiopathic or represent a reaction pattern seen in patients with collagen-vascular diseases or HP [104,105]. In contradistinction to the heterogeneous histology seen in patients who have UIP, histologic lesions in patients who have NSIP are temporally homogeneous, appearing to represent the same stage in the evolution of the disease (see Table 4-1).

TABLE 6-5. *HRCT findings of nonspecific interstitial pneumonia*

Patchy ground-glass opacity[a]

Airspace consolidation[a]

Irregular reticular opacities[a]

Honeycombing (uncommon)

Peripheral and lower lung zone predominance[a,b]

[a]Most common findings.
[b]Findings most helpful in differential diagnosis.

Clinically, patients present with symptoms similar to IPF: dyspnea and cough with an average duration of 8 months [105]. It has been described in patients ranging from 9 to 78 years of age, the average age being approximately 50 years [105,106].

The radiographic findings consist mainly of ground-glass opacities or consolidation involving predominantly the lower lung zones [106]. Other manifestations include a reticular pattern or a combination of interstitial and airspace patterns [105,106]. In approximately 10% of cases, the chest radiograph is normal [104].

High-Resolution Computed Tomography Findings

In patients who have NSIP, HRCT usually shows patchy areas of ground-glass opacity, often with a peripheral predominance, patchy consolidation, and irregular reticular opacities [107] (Table 6-5). Although honeycombing may be present, it tends to be inconspicuous, particularly in comparison to UIP.

Park et al. [106] described the HRCT findings in seven patients who had NSIP. The predominant abnormality seen in all cases was bilateral ground-glass opacity, which sometimes showed a peripheral predominance (see Fig. 3-94; Fig. 6-31). Seventy-one percent of patients had associated areas of consolidation involving the lower lung zones, and 29% had irregular linear opacities (Figs. 6-32 and 6-33). After treatment, the abnormalities seen on HRCT completely resolved in 43% of patients, improved in 43%, and progressed in 14% [106]. Similar findings were reported by Cottin et al. [108] in eleven patients. In the latter study, nine of 11 patients had ground-glass opacities, six patients had patchy areas of consolidation, and five patients had thickening of the interlobular septa. Ten patients improved or stabilized after treatment with corticosteroids or immuno-

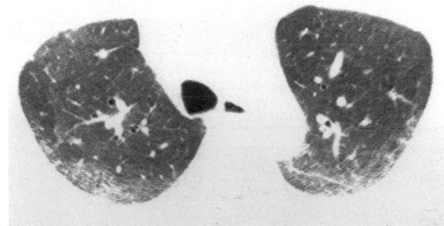

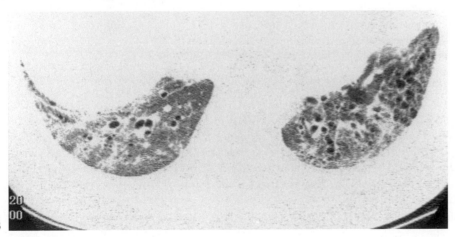

FIG. 6-31. A 58-year-old woman who had nonspecific interstitial pneumonia. A: HRCT at the level of the aortic arch demonstrates patchy bilateral ground-glass opacities. B: HRCT through the lung bases shows ground-glass opacities, mild reticulation, and marked traction bronchiectasis.

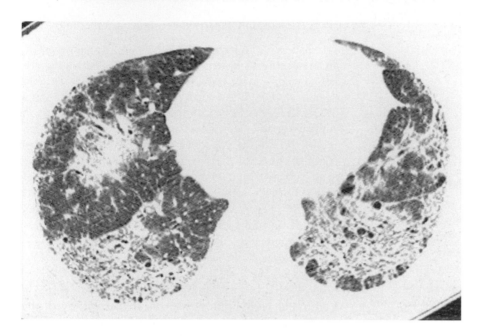

FIG. 6-32. A 39-year-old woman who had nonspecific interstitial pneumonia. HRCT demonstrates intralobular linear opacities and irregular interlobular septal thickening resulting in a fine bilateral reticular pattern. Also noted are patchy ground-glass opacities, traction bronchiectasis, and small focal areas of honeycombing. The appearance resembles that of idiopathic pulmonary fibrosis.

suppressive agents. All patients were alive a mean of 4 years after diagnosis [108].

Kim et al. [109] compared HRCT with the pathologic findings in 23 patients who had NSIP. The predominant HRCT abnormality seen in all patients was bilateral ground-glass opacity, with (35%) or without (65%) consolidation. Other common findings included irregular linear opacities (87%), thickening of bronchovascular bundles (65%), and bronchial dilatation (52%). All parenchymal abnormalities showed a subpleural predominance. Ground-glass opacities corresponded histologically to interstitial thickening by inflammation and fibrosis, whereas areas of consolidation corresponded to areas of BOOP, or, occasionally, microscopic honeycombing with mucin stasis [109].

It should be noted that there is considerable overlap between the HRCT findings seen in NSIP and those present in other interstitial pneumonias (see Table 4-1). Abnormalities seen on HRCT in patients who have NSIP can mimic those of DIP (predominantly ground-glass opacities), BOOP, or AIP (predominantly airspace consolidation), and, occasionally, those of UIP (predominantly lower lobe reticulation with or without honeycombing) [103]. For example, Johkoh et al. [103] reviewed the HRCT findings in 129 patients who had various idiopathic interstitial pneumonias, including 27 patients who had NSIP. The main abnormalities in patients who had NSIP included ground-glass opacities seen in 100% of patients, intralobular linear opacities in 93% of patients, airspace consolidation in 41% of patients, and honeycombing seen in 26% of patients [103]. Two independent observers made a correct first-choice diagnosis, on average, in 71% of cases of UIP, 79% of cases of BOOP, and 63% of cases of DIP, but in only 9% of cases of NSIP. In none of the cases of NSIP was the diagnosis made with a high degree of confidence on HRCT.

Utility of High-Resolution Computed Tomography

Although an accurate diagnosis of interstitial pneumonia cannot always be made using HRCT, the HRCT appearance is often used to determine further evaluation. In a patient who has suspected idiopathic interstitial pneumonia, the HRCT finding of patchy or subpleural ground-glass opacity, with or without reticulation, should suggest a likely diagnosis of NSIP rather than UIP. Generally, lung biopsy is recommended in this setting. On the other hand, if honeycombing is a predominant feature of disease, UIP is much more likely than NSIP, and lung biopsy is often avoided.

HRCT may also be valuable in the follow-up of disease. In patients who have NSIP, areas of ground-glass opacity decrease on follow-up HRCT, and the extent of decrease correlates significantly with that of functional improvement. Kim et al. [110] assessed serial changes on HRCT and PFTs in 13 patients who had NSIP (mean follow-up period, 11 months). On initial HRCT, all patients had areas of ground-glass opacity and irregular linear opacities. The areas of ground-glass opacity decreased significantly on follow-up CT, whereas areas of irregular linear opacity decreased slightly. Initial forced vital capacity (FVC) (69%) also improved significantly on follow-up examination (84%) ($p = .003$). The decrease in the extent of ground-glass opacity on CT correlated significantly with changes in FVC ($r = -.70, p = .007$) and diffusing capacity for carbon monoxide ($r = -.60, p = .031$).

In a study by Nishiyama et al. [107] of 15 patients who had proven NSIP, initial HRCT findings included a mixed pattern of ground-glass opacity and consolidation (n = 11), peribronchovascular interstitial thickening (n = 6), parenchymal bands (n = 8), intralobular interstitial thickening (n = 12), and traction bronchiectasis (n = 14). On follow-up HRCT in 14 cases, the abnormalities had disappeared completely in three cases, improved in nine cases, persisted in one case, and worsened in one case.

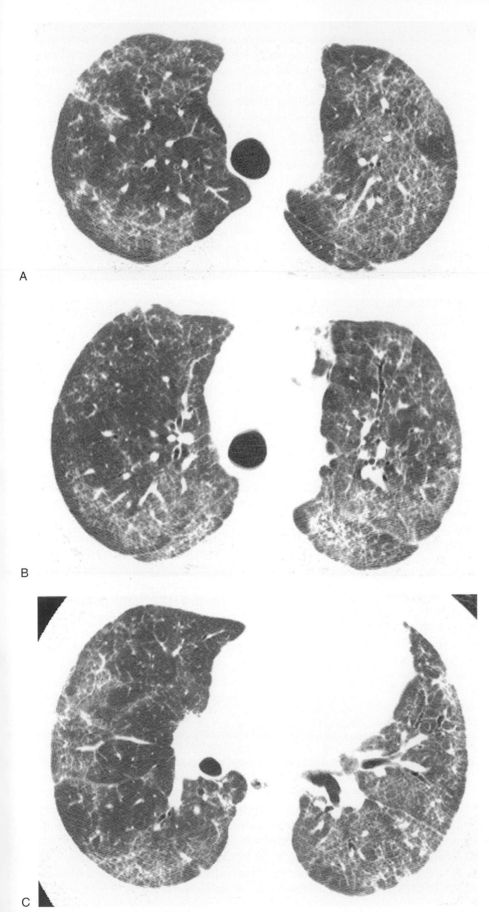

FIG. 6-33. A–C: Nonspecific interstitial pneumonia in a 60-year-old man who had dyspnea. HRCT findings consist of ground-glass opacity associated with some irregular reticulation. Although the subpleural regions are involved, lung involvement is diffuse and patchy.

RESPIRATORY BRONCHIOLITIS AND RESPIRATORY BRONCHIOLITIS–INTERSTITIAL LUNG DISEASE

Respiratory bronchiolitis (RB), also known as *smokers' bronchiolitis*, is a common incidental histologic finding in cigarette smokers [111,112]. RB is usually unassociated with specific symptoms [112,113]. However, smokers who have findings of RB who are symptomatic have also been described. These patients typically present with clinical findings mimicking those of interstitial lung disease and are generally referred to as having respiratory bronchiolitis and respiratory bronchiolitis–interstitial lung disease (RB-ILD) [114–116].

RB is characterized histologically by the presence of numerous macrophages filling respiratory bronchioles and adjacent alveolar ducts and alveoli [111,112]. The macrophages contain periodic acid-Schiff–positive brown pigment; this pigment represents particulate matter unique to cigarette smoke, contained within cytoplasmic phagolysosomes. In patients who have symptomatic RB-ILD, peribronchiolar and alveolar wall inflammation is more pronounced than in patients who are asymptomatic [115]. RB-ILD typically involves the lung parenchyma in a patchy fashion, with some areas spared, whereas adjacent lobules may be severely involved.

Patients who have RB-ILD are typically young—usually in their 30s and 40s—and complain of chronic cough and progressive shortness of breath, often of 1 or 2 years' duration. PFT results are variable but usually show a restrictive abnormality. A reduced diffusing capacity, averaging 62% of predicted in the series reported by Yousem et al. [116], is the most consistent abnormality in patients who have RB-ILD. Chest radiographs can be normal or can show nonspecific bilateral, irregular, opacities, usually with a lower zonal predominance [116].

The prognosis of patients who have RB-ILD is good; progression to pulmonary fibrosis, respiratory failure, or death has not been reported during follow-up periods of several years [116]. Smoking cessation leads to amelioration of symptoms. Patients who continue to smoke may improve clinically, but those with persistent complaints may benefit from oral steroid therapy. Despite symptomatic regression, histologic changes may not resolve completely. Some authors have suggested that RB may be the precursor to chronic airway abnormalities or centrilobular emphysema in susceptible individuals.

High-Resolution Computed Tomography Findings

Respiratory Bronchiolitis

In the majority of patients who have RB, the histologic abnormalities are too mild to be detected on HRCT [113,117,118]. When present, HRCT findings consist of poorly defined centrilobular nodules and multifocal ground-glass opacities [117–119]. These findings can be diffuse but tend to involve mainly the upper lung zones [113,117,118].

Remy-Jardin et al. [117] reviewed the HRCT scans in 39 heavy smokers (mean smoking index of 41 pack-years) who had the diagnosis of RB proved at lung resection for solitary nodules. Eleven (28%) had ground-glass opacities and four (10%) had poorly defined centrilobular nodules [117]. Correlation with the histologic findings showed that the areas of ground-glass opacity could be attributed to intraalveolar macrophages, alveolar wall thickening by inflammation or fibrosis, or organizing alveolitis [117].

In a study by Heyneman et al. [118], the main abnormalities seen in 16 patients who had RB were centrilobular nodules present in 12 (75%) patients, and ground-glass opacities seen in six patients (38%) (Fig. 6-34). The nodules were usually poorly defined and measured 3 to 5 mm in diameter. The nodules were either diffuse throughout the lungs or located predominantly or exclusively in the middle and upper lung zones. The ground-glass opacities were usually patchy in distribution and present in all lung zones. Centrilobular emphysema was evident on HRCT in nine (56%) of the patients who had RB [118].

Respiratory Bronchiolitis–Interstitial Lung Disease

Not all patients with RB-ILD show abnormalities on HRCT. The most common HRCT findings consist of (i) centrilobular nodules, (ii) ground-glass opacities, (iii) thickening of bronchial walls, and (iv) an upper lobe predominance (Figs. 6-35 and 6-36) (Table 6-6) [118,120,121]. Upper lobe emphysema is commonly present due to smoking. A small percentage of patients have a reticular pattern due to fibrosis [112,118,121]. The fibrosis in RB-ILD is mild and tends to involve mainly the lower lung zones.

Holt et al. [121] described the HRCT findings in five patients with RB-ILD. The findings were variable and ranged from no detectable abnormality to atelectasis, ground-glass opacities, emphysema, and reticular interstitial opacities [121]. Heyneman et al. [118] reviewed the HRCT findings in eight patients who had RB-ILD. Seven of the eight (87%) patients had ground-glass opacities, and seven had centrilobular nodules. Only two (25%) of the patients showed evidence of fibrosis, as determined by the presence of intralobular linear opacities and honeycombing in the lower lobes. Emphysema was evident on HRCT in 50% of cases [118].

Park et al. [120] correlated HRCT findings with pathologic findings in 17 patients who had RB-ILD. All patients were current or former cigarette smokers. The predominant HRCT findings consisted of bronchial wall thickening in 16 patients (94%), centrilobular nodules in 13 patients (76%), ground-glass opacities in 14 patients (82%), and upper lobe predominant emphysema in ten patients (59%). The extent of centrilobular nodules correlated with the severity of inflammation and extent of macrophages in respiratory bronchioles, whereas the ground-glass opacities correlated with macrophage accumulation in alveolar ducts and alveoli [120].

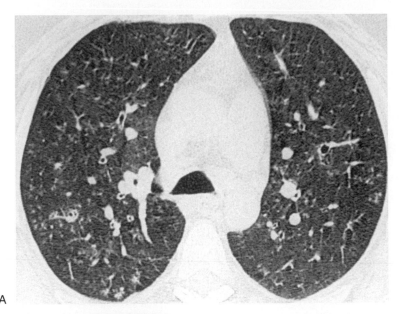

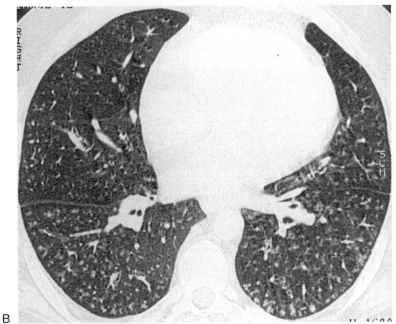

FIG. 6-34. Respiratory bronchiolitis. **A:** HRCT at the level of the aortic arch demonstrates patchy bilateral ground-glass opacities. Also noted are a few centrilobular nodules and bronchial wall thickening. **B:** HRCT at the level of the inferior pulmonary veins demonstrates centrilobular nodules and branching linear opacities, giving a tree-in-bud appearance. (Courtesy of Dr. Martine Remy-Jardin, Hôpital Calmette, Universitaire de Lille, France.)

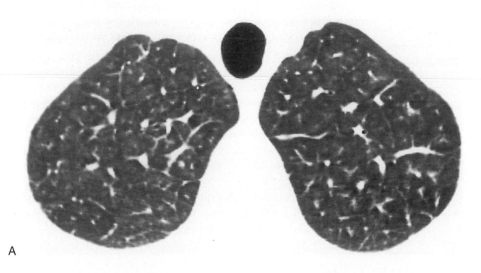

FIG. 6-35. Respiratory bronchiolitis–interstitial lung disease. **A:** HRCT through the upper lobes shows patchy areas of ground-glass opacity, many of which appear to be centrilobular, and surround small vascular branches. (From Gruden JF, Webb WR. CT findings in a proved case of respiratory bronchiolitis. *AJR Am J Roentgenol* 1993;161:44–46, with permission.) *Continued*

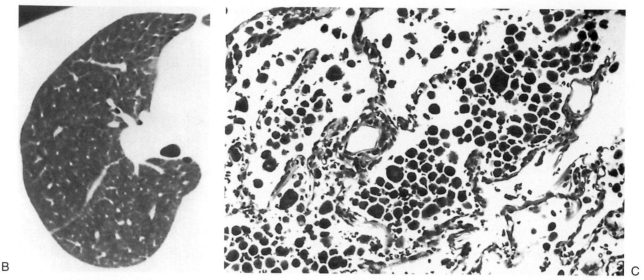

B

C

FIG. 6-35. *Continued* B: HRCT at a lower level also shows small, ill-defined areas of ground-glass opacity. C: Open-lung biopsy specimen shows numerous dark-pigmented macrophages filling alveoli, typical of respiratory bronchiolitis.

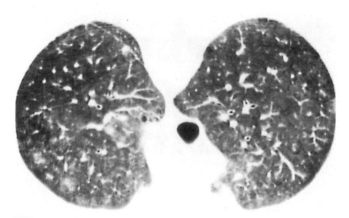

FIG. 6-36. Respiratory bronchiolitis–interstitial lung disease in a 29-year-old female smoker who had 6 months of progressive dyspnea and cough. Prone HRCT shows patchy areas of ground-glass opacity, some of which appear nodular.

TABLE 6-6. *HRCT findings of respiratory bronchiolitis–interstitial lung disease*

No visible abnormality
Centrilobular nodular opacities[a]
Patchy ground-glass opacity[a]
Bronchial wall thickening[a]
Upper lobe predominance[a,b]
Findings of fibrosis usually absent
Associated centrilobular emphysema

[a]Most common findings.
[b]Findings most helpful in differential diagnosis.

DESQUAMATIVE INTERSTITIAL PNEUMONIA

DIP is an uncommon condition, characterized histologically by the presence of numerous macrophages filling the alveolar airspaces, mild inflammation of the alveolar walls, and minimal fibrosis [23]. Because the histologic lesion consists primarily of an accumulation of alveolar macrophages, *alveolar macrophage pneumonia* has been suggested as an alternative designation for DIP by the American Thoracic Society/European Respiratory Society Multidisciplinary Consensus Classification Committee [93]. DIP can be seen in association with a variety of conditions, including drug reactions, Langerhans cell histiocytosis, leukemia, asbestosis, and hard-metal pneumoconiosis [23]. Approximately 90% of patients who have DIP are cigarette smokers [118,122]. In some patients who have DIP, the macrophage accumulation may have a peribronchiolar predominance similar to that seen in RB-ILD, the only distinction being the presence of more diffuse involvement of the airspaces in DIP [104,116]. However, there is a continuum of the extent of airspace macrophage accumulation between RB-ILD and DIP, sometimes making it difficult to distinguish between these two entities. Therefore, it is likely that RB-ILD and DIP are highly related conditions, representing different degrees of small airway and parenchymal reaction to cigarette smoke [104,118]. Although it was previously thought that DIP represented the active phase of UIP, these entities are now considered to be unrelated.

DIP occurs most commonly in patients between 30 and 50 years of age [47,122]. The clinical symptoms usually consist of slowly progressive exertional dyspnea and dry cough [122]. The most common finding on chest radiographs in

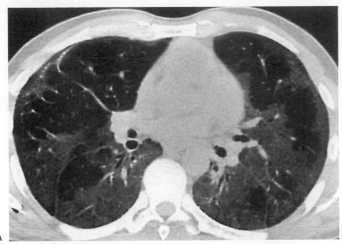

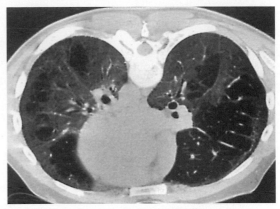

FIG. 6-37. HRCT scans from a 39-year-old man who has biopsy-proved desquamative interstitial pneumonia. **A:** HRCT at the level of the superior segmental bronchi shows areas of ground-glass opacity in a predominantly subpleural distribution. **B:** HRCT obtained at the same level as in **A** with the patient in the prone position shows that the ground-glass opacity is not secondary to dependent atelectasis. (From Hartman TE, Primack SL, Swensen SJ, et al. Desquamative interstitial pneumonia: thin-section CT findings in 22 patients. *Radiology* 1993;187:787–790, with permission.)

patients who have DIP is the presence of ground-glass opacities in the lower-lung zones [122,123]. However, in 3% to 22% of patients who have biopsy-proven DIP, the chest radiograph has been reported as being normal [122,124].

High-Resolution Computed Tomography Findings

On HRCT, the predominant abnormality in patients who have DIP is the presence of areas of ground-glass opacity [46,47] (Figs. 6-37 through 6-39) (Table 6-7). This is not surprising, considering that the predominant histologic findings in patients who have DIP are filling of the alveolar airspaces with macrophages, relative preservation of the underlying pulmonary anatomy, and minimal fibrosis. A subpleural and

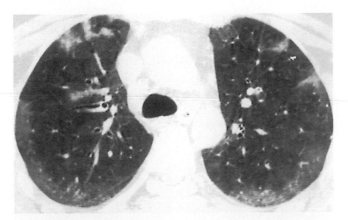

FIG. 6-38. A 45-year-old patient who has desquamative interstitial pneumonia. HRCT at the level of the tracheal carina demonstrates bilateral areas of ground-glass opacity. The ground-glass opacity is most marked in the subpleural lung regions.

basal predominance is often present, and although reticular opacities may be associated with the ground-glass opacity, honeycombing is uncommon. Because of its association with smoking, centrilobular emphysema may also be present.

Hartman et al. [47] reviewed the HRCT scans in 22 patients who had biopsy-proven DIP. The predominant abnormality in this group was the presence of areas of ground-glass opacity. The areas of ground-glass opacity were seen mainly in the lower-lung zones in 16 patients (73%), the middle lung zones in three patients (14%), and the upper lung zones in three patients (14%). The areas of ground-glass opacity had a predominantly peripheral distribution in 13 patients (59%), a patchy distribution in five patients (23%), and a diffuse distribution in four patients (18%) (Figs. 6-37 through 6-39).

Irregular linear opacities were seen in 13 of 22 (59%) patients. These were more marked in the lower lung zones in 11 patients, middle lung zones in one patient, and upper lung zones in one patient. In 11 of the 13 patients with irregular linear opacities, there was associated architectural distortion, indicating the presence of fibrosis. Honeycombing was identified in seven patients. The honeycombing was present only in the lower lung zones, was peripheral, and involved less than 10% of the lung bases.

Heyneman et al. [118] reviewed the HRCT findings in 16 patients who had RB, eight patients who had RB-ILD, and 6 patients who had DIP. The predominant abnormalities in patients who had RB consisted of centrilobular nodules seen in 75% of patients, and ground-glass opacities seen in 38% of patients. The main findings in patients who had RB-ILD were ground-glass opacities seen in 50% of patients, centrilobular nodules in 38%, and mild fibrosis present in 25% of patients. All patients who had DIP had extensive ground-

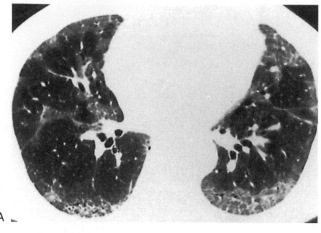

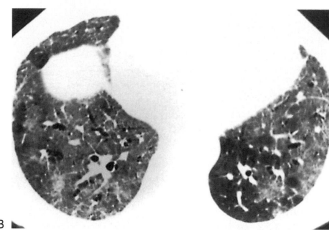

FIG. 6-39. A 71-year-old man who has desquamative interstitial pneumonia. **A:** HRCT at the level of the inferior pulmonary veins demonstrates bilateral areas of ground-glass opacity involving mainly the subpleural lung regions. **B:** HRCT through the lung bases demonstrates more extensive bilateral involvement. There is a mild increase in reticulation.

glass opacities, and 63% showed evidence of mild fibrosis. All patients who had RB and RB-ILD and 85% of patients who had DIP had a smoking history. The authors concluded that the considerable overlap between the HRCT findings of RB, RB-ILD, and DIP is consistent with the concept that these entities are part of the spectrum of the same disease

TABLE 6-7. *HRCT findings in desquamative interstitial pneumonia*

Bilateral, patchy ground-glass opacity[a]
Subpleural and basal predominance[a]
Superimposition of first two findings[b]
Reticular opacities
Honeycombing (uncommon)
Associated centrilobular emphysema

[a]Most common findings.
[b]Findings most helpful in differential diagnosis.

process, representing different degrees of severity of reaction to cigarette smoke [118].

ACUTE INTERSTITIAL PNEUMONIA

AIP is a fulminant disease of unknown etiology that usually occurs in a previously healthy person and produces histologic findings of diffuse alveolar damage (DAD) [125]. There is often a prodromal illness associated with symptoms of a viral upper respiratory infection, followed by rapidly increasing dyspnea and respiratory failure. Patients who have AIP usually require mechanical ventilation within 1 to 2 weeks from the onset of symptoms. The majority of patients die within 6 months of presentation [125–127]. The pathologic abnormalities consist of thickening of the alveolar walls due to edema, inflammatory cells, and active fibroblast proliferation, but little mature collagen deposition. There is extensive alveolar damage with hyaline membrane formation. Because the acute presentation and the histologic features are identical with those of ARDS, AIP has also been referred to as idiopathic ARDS [127].

Primack et al. [126] reviewed the radiographic and HRCT findings in nine patients who had AIP. Bilateral airspace opacification was present on the chest radiographs of all nine patients. The airspace opacification was diffuse in five patients (56%), involved mainly the upper lung zones in two patients (22%), and involved mainly the lower lung zones in two patients (22%). Honeycombing was identified on the radiographs in two patients.

High-Resolution Computed Tomography Findings

In the early stages of AIP, HRCT findings consist primarily of patchy bilateral ground-glass opacity and consolidation, which tend to be diffuse and lack a specific distribution (Figs. 6-40 through 6-43) (Table 6-8) [126,128]. In a study by Primack et al. [126], bilateral, symmetric areas of

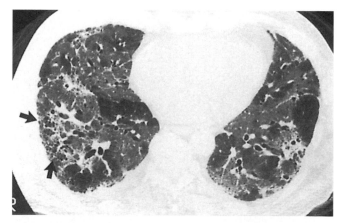

FIG. 6-40. A 74-year-old man who has acute interstitial pneumonia. HRCT through the lung bases demonstrates extensive bilateral areas of ground-glass opacity. Also noted are a reticular pattern and fine honeycombing involving mainly the subpleural lung regions of the right lower lobe (*arrows*).

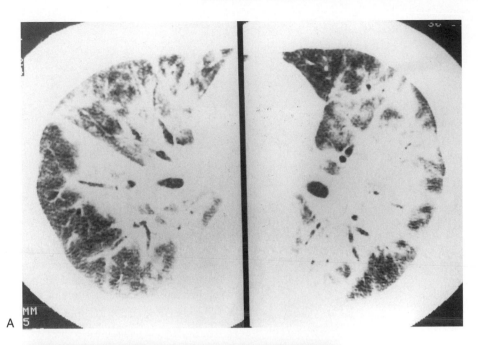

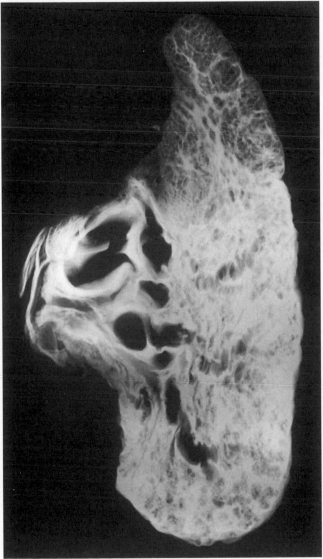

FIG. 6-41. Acute interstitial pneumonia in a 47-year-old man. **A:** HRCT scan shows areas of consolidation having a peribronchovascular distribution. **B:** Low-kilovoltage radiograph of inflated and fixed postmortem lung reveals extensive consolidation. *Continued*

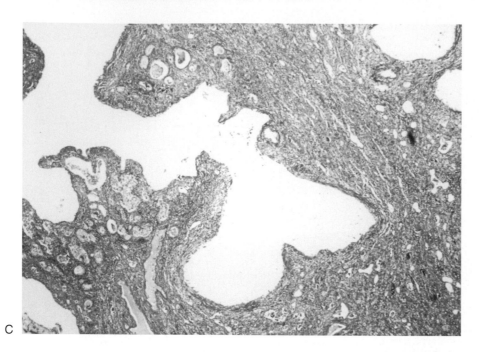

C

FIG. 6-41. *Continued* C: Histologic specimen shows dilated alveolar ducts lined by hyaline membranes and prominent associated interstitial fibrosis (elastica-van Gieson stain, ×25). (From Akira M. Computed tomography and pathologic findings in fulminant forms of idiopathic interstitial pneumonia. *J Thorac Imag* 1999;14:76–84, with permission.)

ground-glass opacity were present on HRCT in all nine cases (Fig. 6-40). The areas of ground-glass opacity involved all lung zones to a similar extent in seven patients (78%), and had an upper lung zone predominance in the other two patients. In six patients (67%), the areas of ground-glass opacity had a patchy distribution with focal areas of sparing, giving a geographic appearance, and three patients had diffuse involvement. In none of the cases did the areas of ground-glass opacity involve mainly the central or subpleural lung regions.

Bilateral areas of airspace consolidation were identified on HRCT in six of nine cases (Figs. 6-41 through 6-43) [126]. The consolidation had a predominantly basilar distribution in three patients (Figs. 6-42 and 6-43), a diffuse distribution in two patients, and an upper lung zone predominance in one patient. A predominantly subpleural distribution of consolidation was present in two cases, the distribution in the other four cases being random.

Architectural distortion and traction bronchiectasis may be seen as the disease evolves and fibrosis develops. In a study by Akira et al. [128], these findings were observed only on CT scans obtained more than 7 days after the onset of symptoms. Subpleural honeycombing was seen at HRCT in three of nine patients reviewed by Primack et al. [126], including two cases in which this finding was apparent on the radiographs. The areas of honeycombing involved less than 10% of the lung parenchyma.

Eight of the nine patients studied by Primack et al. [126] died within 3 months of presentation. The surviving patient underwent a follow-up HRCT study that showed only mild residual peripheral reticulation 2 months after the initial HRCT study. Repeat open-lung biopsy at the time of the follow-up HRCT study in this case showed inactive fibrosis.

Johkoh et al. reviewed the HRCT findings in 36 patients who had AIP [129]. The main abnormalities consisted of extensive areas of ground-glass attenuation present in all patients and areas of consolidation seen in 33 (92%) patients (Table 6-8). Other common findings included architectural distortion, traction bronchiectasis, thickening of the bronchovascular bundles, and thickening of the interlobular septa. The abnormalities involved mainly the lower lung zones in 13 patients (39%) and the upper lung zones in five patients (14%); in the remaining patients there was equal

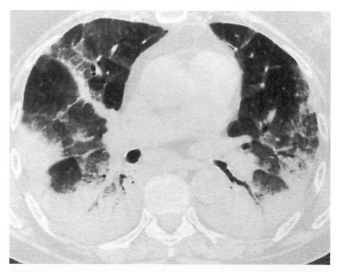

FIG. 6-42. An 83-year-old woman who has acute interstitial pneumonia. HRCT at the level of the bronchus intermedius demonstrates extensive bilateral consolidation involving the dependent regions of the lower lobes. Patchy areas of ground-glass opacity are present anteriorly.

involvement of all three lung zones. A predominant dependent distribution was present in nine patients (25%) and a peripheral distribution in three patients (8%) [129].

Ichikado et al. correlated the HRCT findings with lung pathology in 14 patients who had AIP [130]. Areas of ground-glass attenuation and consolidation without traction bronchiectasis were present in the exudative or early proliferative phase of AIP. Traction bronchiectasis was seen in the late proliferative and fibrotic phases of AIP [130]. Honeycombing, present in a small percentage of patients with AIP, correlates with the presence of dense interstitial fibrosis and restructuring of distal airspaces [126,130].

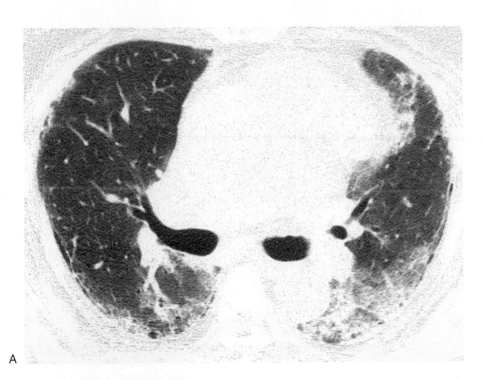

A

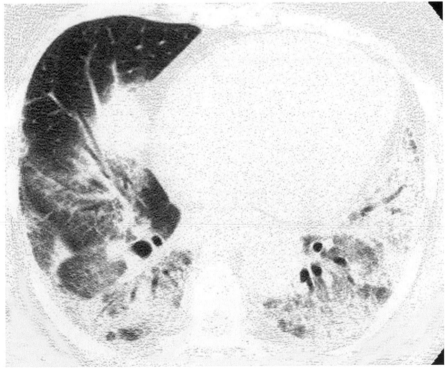

B

FIG. 6-43. A–C: Acute interstitial pneumonia in a 70-year-old woman who subsequently died. HRCT findings are nonspecific, with patchy consolidation and ground-glass opacity predominating in the subpleural lung regions and at the lung bases. *Continued*

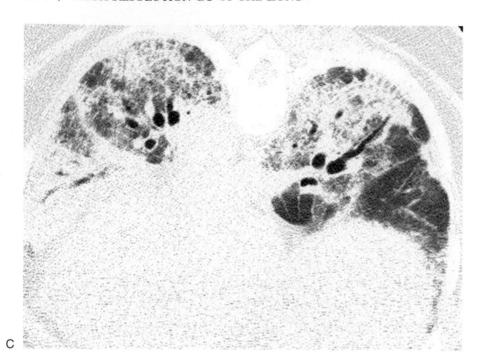

C

FIG. 6-43. *Continued*

TABLE 6-8. *HRCT findings of acute interstitial pneumonia*

Extensive bilateral ground-glass opacities[a]
Airspace consolidation[a]
Architectural distortion[a]
Combination of first three findings[a]
Consolidation predominantly basilar and dependent

[a]Most common findings.

ALVEOLAR PROTEINOSIS

Pulmonary alveolar proteinosis (PAP) is a disease characterized by filling of the alveolar spaces with a periodic acid-Schiff–positive proteinaceous material, rich in lipid [131,132]. The pathogenesis of this disease is poorly understood, and the majority of cases are considered to be idiopathic. Some cases result from exposure to dusts (particularly silica) or from immunologic disturbances due to immunodeficiency, hematologic and lymphatic malignancies, or chemotherapy [132–138].

In patients who have PAP, men outnumber women by a ratio of 4:1. Patients range in age from a few months to more than 70 years, with two-thirds of patients being between 30 and 50 years old [139]. Symptoms are usually mild and of insidious onset. They include nonproductive cough, fever, and mild dyspnea on exertion.

The prognosis of patients who have PAP has improved considerably since the advent of treatment using BAL [131,136,140]. After lavage, many patients remain in remission, but others relapse; patients who relapse require retreatment every 6 to 24 months, and a few become refractory to treatment [141].

Usual radiographic manifestations of PAP are those of airspace consolidation or ground-glass opacity; air bronchograms are rare. The typical radiograph shows a bilateral, patchy, diffuse, or perihilar ill-defined nodular or confluent airspace pattern, which is usually most severe in the lung bases [132,142–144]. Although reticular opacities may be seen, they are usually mild [145]. The radiographic appearance often resembles that of pulmonary edema, except for the absence of cardiomegaly and pleural effusion.

High-Resolution Computed Tomography Findings

HRCT findings in patients who have PAP include (i) bilateral areas of ground-glass opacity, (ii) smooth interlobular septal thickening in lung regions showing ground-glass opacity (i.e., crazy-paving), (iii) consolidation, and (iv) a patchy or geographic distribution [44,45,145]. In a study by Godwin et al. [44], abnormalities ranged from ill-defined nodular opacities (airspace nodules) to large areas of ground-glass opacity or confluent airspace consolidation (Table 6-9).

In many patients, areas of ground-glass opacity or consolidation are sharply demarcated from the surrounding normal

---

TABLE 6-9. *HRCT findings in alveolar proteinosis*

Bilateral ground-glass opacity[a]
Smooth septal thickening in abnormal areas[a]
Superimposition of first two findings (i.e., crazy-paving)[a,b]
Consolidation
Patchy or geographic distribution

[a]Most common findings.
[b]Findings most helpful in differential diagnosis.

parenchyma, giving the abnormal areas a geographic appearance. In some of these cases, the sharp margination of areas of lung opacity reflect lobular or lobar boundaries; in other cases, there is no apparent anatomic reason to account for this sharp edge. The distribution of disease is variable [44,45,145], sometimes being mainly central and sometimes peripheral. CT, and particularly HRCT, commonly shows smooth thickening of the interlobular septa that is not apparent on chest radiographs.

A geographic distribution of consolidation or ground-glass opacity and smooth thickening of the interlobular septa (see Figs. 3-11 and 3-96; Figs. 6-44 and 6-45) was visible on CT in all six cases reported by Murch and Carr [45]. The thickened interlobular septa were present only within areas of consolidation, and were shown on open-lung biopsy to reflect septal edema. Interstitial abnormalities characterized by the presence of alveolar wall infiltration by lymphocytes and macrophages,

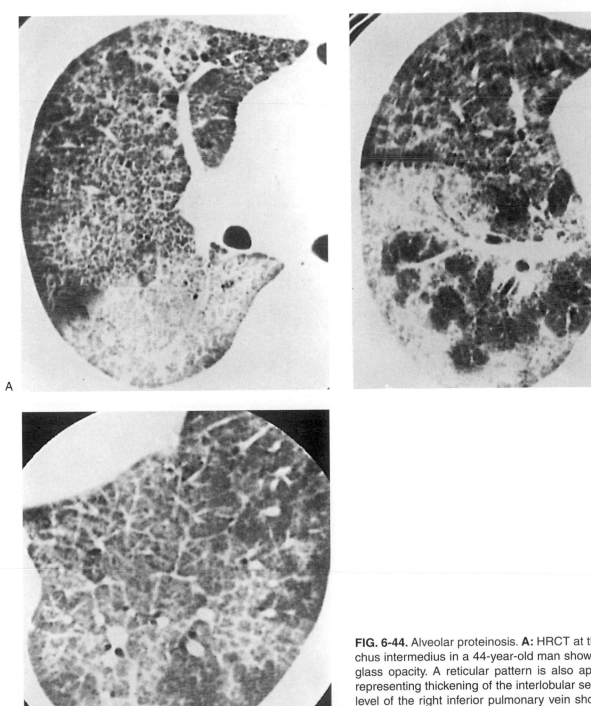

FIG. 6-44. Alveolar proteinosis. **A:** HRCT at the level of the bronchus intermedius in a 44-year-old man shows extensive ground-glass opacity. A reticular pattern is also apparent, presumably representing thickening of the interlobular septa. **B:** HRCT at the level of the right inferior pulmonary vein shows similar findings. **C:** HRCT through the left lower lobe shows ground-glass opacities and thickened interlobular septa. This is the typical crazy-paving appearance of alveolar proteinosis.

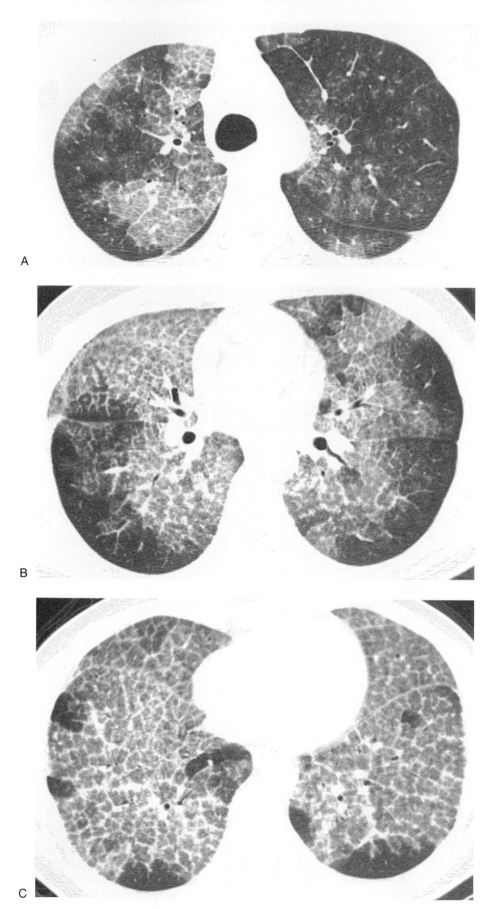

FIG. 6-45 A–C: Alveolar proteinosis. Patchy areas of ground-glass opacity and associated reticular opacities (i.e., crazy-paving). There is a basal predominance of abnormalities. This patient was treated with bronchoalveolar lavage with significant improvement.

and interstitial edema, have also been reported in other studies. These findings probably reflect interstitial inflammation [143,146]. Septal thickening can also represent interstitial accumulation of the proteinaceous material. It should be emphasized that in patients with alveolar proteinosis, septal thickening is usually visible only in regions of ground-glass opacity.

Lee et al. [145] reviewed the radiographic and HRCT findings present on 25 occasions in seven patients who had PAP. On chest radiographs, ground-glass opacities were the predominant abnormality. On HRCT, ground-glass opacities or consolidation was seen in 96% of the images analyzed, and reticular opacities in 94%. In the majority of cases, reticular opacities were visible only in areas also showing ground-glass opacification. The ground-glass opacities were diffuse in 76% of cases and focal or patchy in 24%. A distinct central or peripheral predominance was not present in any of the cases [145]. CT may show parenchymal abnormalities even in patients who have normal radiographs [147].

The demarcation of normal and abnormal lung regions and the demonstration of thickened interlobular septa are much better seen on HRCT than on conventional CT. The combination of a geographic distribution of areas of ground-glass opacity with smoothly thickened interlobular septa within the areas of airspace disease, resulting in a crazy-paving appearance, is strongly suggestive of alveolar proteinosis in patients with subacute or chronic symptoms (see Figs. 3-11 and 3-96; Fig. 6-45) [45,132], although this appearance can be seen in a number of other diseases associated with the presence of ground-glass opacity, including PCP, bacterial pneumonia, lipoid pneumonia, and ARDS (see Table 3-10) [148,149].

Utility of High-Resolution Computed Tomography

In patients having bronchoalveolar lavage for treatment of PAP, HRCT may be used to localize the most abnormal lung regions for selective lavage and is also helpful in following the course of disease on a regional basis. It has also been shown that the extent of radiographic and HRCT abnormalities, most notably ground-glass opacity, correlates with the presence of a restrictive ventilatory defect, reduced diffusing capacity, and hypoxemia both before and after BAL [145].

CT can demonstrate focal pneumonia in patients who have PAP that is not apparent on plain radiographs [44]. Superimposed infection, often by *Nocardia asteroides*, is a common complication of alveolar proteinosis; on plain radiographs it can be difficult or impossible to distinguish infection from the airspace consolidation due to alveolar proteinosis. By detecting focal areas of dense consolidation or abscess formation, CT may confirm a clinical suspicion of superimposed infection [44]. In early studies, infection with *Nocardia* was reported in as many as 8% of patients who had alveolar proteinosis [136]. It is now less common, presumably owing to the use of BAL in treatment of affected patients [132,140,142]. More recently, some investigators have noted an association of pulmonary alveolar proteinosis with *Mycobacterium avium-intracellulare* and *P. carinii* infections [132].

LIPOID PNEUMONIA

Exogenous lipoid pneumonia results from the chronic aspiration or inhalation of animal, vegetable, or petroleum-based oils or fats. The degree of lung inflammation or fibrosis associated with the aspirated oil is related to the amount of free fatty acid that is present. Animal fats generally result in more inflammation and fibrosis than vegetable or mineral oils because they are hydrolyzed by lung lipases, releasing fatty acids. A large quantity of oily material must usually be aspirated before symptoms develop. Lower lobe opacities or ill-defined masses are typical on chest radiographs [8,150].

High-Resolution Computed Tomography Findings

If a large amount of lipid has been aspirated, CT can show low-attenuation consolidation [–35 to –75 Hounsfield units (HU)] or ground-glass opacity (Figs. 6-46 through 6-48) (Table 6-10) [150,151]; this appearance is most common in patients with chronic mineral oil aspiration. An appearance of ground-glass opacity in association with interlobular septal thickening and intralobular lines (crazy-paving) has also been reported (Fig. 6-48) [148]. Pathologic correlation in patients who had crazy-paving showed the ground-glass

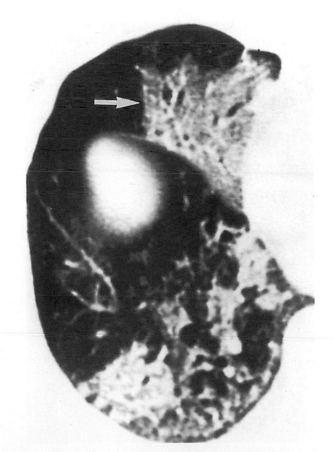

FIG. 6-46. Lipoid pneumonia from chronic mineral oil aspiration. HRCT at the right lung base shows patchy areas of consolidation and ground-glass opacity (*arrow*). Centrilobular opacities are visible posteriorly.

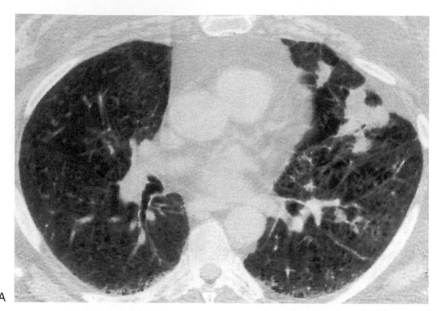

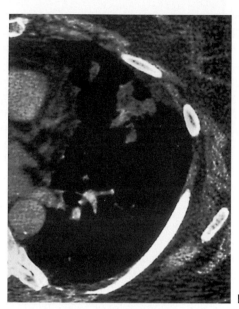

A

B

FIG. 6-47. Extrinsic lipoid pneumonia in a 66-year-old woman who presented with a chronic cough. The chest radiograph demonstrated ill-defined bilateral infiltrates and a nodular opacity in the lingula. **A:** HRCT shows patchy areas of consolidation in the lingula and left lower lobe. **B:** Soft-tissue window setting scan shows the presence of fat in the areas of consolidation. Attenuation values range from −70 to −90 HU. A history of mineral oil ingestion was obtained after the CT.

opacity to be due to aspirated oil, intraalveolar macrophages, and hyperplasia of alveolar lining cells. Interlobular septal thickening and intralobular lines reflected infiltration by lipid-laden macrophages, inflammation, and fibrosis in one patient [148]. Centrilobular opacities may also be seen.

However, because inflammation or fibrosis may accompany the presence of the lipid material, the CT attenuation of the consolidation need not be low. In some patients, necrosis and cavitation may be present [152]. Huggosson et al. [152] reported a series of nine infants who had a history of animal or

vegetable fat intake, and a lung biopsy or BAL diagnosis of lipoid pneumonia. Eight had aspiration of animal fats. Pathologic findings were an intense lymphocytic infiltration, with scattered lipid-containing granulomas. Plain films and CT showed areas of consolidation in the medial-posterior parts of the lungs. CT attenuation measurements did not reveal fat.

Lee et al. [153] reviewed the chest radiographs and HRCT scans in six patients who had proven lipoid pneumonia. Lipoid pneumonia was related to the ingestion of mineral oil in three patients, and shark liver oil (as a restorative) in three

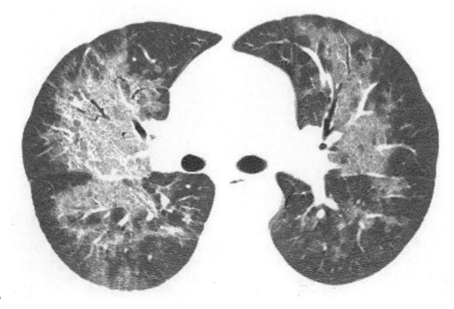

A

FIG. 6-48. A–C: Lipoid pneumonia resulting from chronic mineral oil aspiration. Patchy areas of ground-glass opacity are visible bilaterally, with a predominant central distribution. There is associated intralobular interstitial thickening, resulting in an appearance of crazy-paving. *Continued*

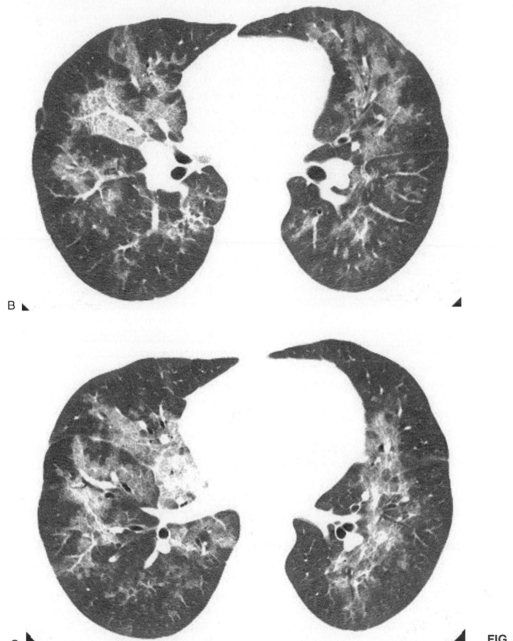

FIG. 6-48. *Continued*

patients. Clinical symptoms included cough, mild fever, and chest discomfort. Chest radiographs demonstrated bilateral airspace consolidation in three patients, irregular masslike opacities in two patients, and a reticular pattern in one patient.

CT and HRCT demonstrated diffuse parenchymal consolidation in three cases, localized areas of irregular consolidation in two cases, and subpleural pulmonary fibrosis and honeycombing in one case [153]. The areas of consolidation primarily involved the lower lung zones, whereas the irregular areas of consolidation were in the lingula. In the three patients who had consolidation, CT and HRCT demonstrated attenuation lower than that of chest wall musculature, but slightly higher than that of subcutaneous fat. These three

cases were all related to the intake of large amounts of shark liver oil. The two cases of lipoid pneumonia appearing as irregular masslike opacities on chest radiographs were shown on HRCT to represent localized areas of consolidation containing fat (Fig. 6-47). In these two patients, the masslike lesions were surrounded by findings suggestive of fibrosis, including reticular opacities and architectural distortion. In one patient who had findings of subpleural fibrosis and honeycombing, no areas of low attenuation were visible on CT. It should be pointed out, however, that the diagnosis of lipoid pneumonia in this patient was based on history and transbronchial biopsy, and may not have been related to the findings of fibrosis seen on CT.

TABLE 6-10. *HRCT findings in lipoid pneumonia*

Patchy unilateral or bilateral airspace consolidation[a]
Consolidation low in attenuation[a,b]
Ground-glass opacity or crazy-paving[a]
Lower lung predominance[a,b]

[a]Most common findings.
[b]Findings most helpful in differential diagnosis.

DIFFUSE PNEUMONIA

The CT and HRCT findings of various causes of pneumonia have been described [8,144,154–157]. Generally, focal pneumonias, with the exception of multinodular diseases, are not assessed using CT, and plain radiographs in combination with clinical findings are sufficient for diagnosis. The appearances of mycobacterial infections, fungal infections, and bronchopneumonia appearing as lung nodules are described in Chapter 5.

Diffuse parenchymal opacification resulting from pneumonia can be seen with a variety of organisms. Diffuse pneumonia is most common in immunocompromised patients, including those who have malignancy, acquired immunodeficiency syndrome (AIDS), or are transplant recipients, but occasionally occurs in subjects who have normal immunity. Although the clinical and chest radiographic findings associated with different types of diffuse pneumonias have been extensively described, in many cases, a timely diagnosis proves elusive based on radiographs alone. On the other hand, many infectious processes have distinctive CT appearances, often allowing a presumptive diagnosis to be made, especially in the immunocompromised population [158,159]. Also, in patients who have an established diagnosis, CT may play an important role in assessing individual response to therapy. Lastly, identification of the varied manifestations of pulmonary infection is necessary to avoid confusion with noninfectious infiltrative diseases.

The use of CT to diagnose diffuse pulmonary infection has received relatively little attention [8,159]. However, the CT appearances of some pneumonias, notably PCP, cytomegalovirus (CMV) pneumonia, and *Mycoplasma* pneumonia have been well described, and it is important to be familiar with the typical HRCT appearances of these diseases.

Pneumocystis carinii Pneumonia

PCP is the most common opportunistic infection in human immunodeficiency virus (HIV)–infected patients [160,161]. Although the overall incidence of PCP has markedly decreased since the institution of prophylactic therapy, approximately 60% of HIV-infected patients continue to have an episode of PCP during the course of their illness [160–162]. It should be noted, however, that in recent years PCP has been supplanted by bacterial infections as the most common lung infection in patients with AIDS [161,163–

165]. In contradistinction to the decreasing incidence in AIDS, the incidence of PCP in immunocompromised patients who do not have AIDS has been increasing, with mortality in this population approaching 50% [165,167].

Pathologically, PCP results in the presence of foamy, intraalveolar exudates. Atypical patterns of presentation, however, are not unusual [167,168]. As documented by Travis et al. [168] in a study of atypical pathologic findings in 123 lung biopsy specimens, PCP also may result in cavitation, vascular invasion, vasculitis, and even noncaseating, calcified granulomas. A definitive diagnosis of PCP requires the demonstration of organisms in sputum or BAL fluid [169]. Sputum induction has variously been reported to detect PCP in 50% to 90% of cases, and is indicated in all patients considered at high risk for PCP.

Radiographically, PCP has been reported to cause diffuse bilateral interstitial or alveolar infiltrates, or both, in up to 85% of cases [169–172]; however, it should be emphasized that, in as many as 15% of proven cases, radiographs remain normal (Fig. 6-49). The most characteristic appearance on chest radiographs is the finding of fine to medium reticular or nodular opacities, or ill-defined hazy consolidation; these appearances can be diagnostic in many cases [173]. Atypical features include asymmetric or nodular infiltrates, or both, apical disease, lobular pneumonia, cavitary nodules and cysts, miliary nodules, adenopathy, effusions, and pneumothoraces [174–179].

Of particular interest is the frequency of cystic abnormalities and associated pneumothoraces in AIDS patients who have PCP [174,175,180]. It has been estimated that 10% or more of patients who have PCP demonstrate either air-filled cysts or pneumatoceles, typically involving the upper lobes [174]. Chow et al. [181], in a report of 100 patients who had proven PCP, found radiographic evidence of cysts in 34 (34%) patients. Of these, 32 had multiple cysts varying between 1 and 5 cm in diameter. Although present throughout the lungs in more than 50% of patients, cysts predominated in the upper lung zones. A clear association between cysts and pneumothorax was also shown, and 35% of the 34 patients who had cysts developed pneumothorax. With therapy, cysts typically shrink or resolve entirely within 5 months [174,181]. In most series, there is a greater tendency for patients receiving aerosolized pentamidine for prophylaxis to develop upper lobe infiltrates and cysts, but this is not always the case [181].

High-Resolution Computed Tomography Findings

HRCT findings in patients who have PCP have been reported by a number of authors and are varied. Common findings include (i) patchy or diffuse ground-glass opacity, (ii) consolidation, (iii) thick-walled, irregular, or septated cysts or cavities, (iv) centrilobular opacities, (v) interlobular septal thickening, (vi) small or large nodules, and (vii) a central, perihilar, or upper lobe distribution in many cases (Table 6-11) [158,159,179,182–184]. For example, Bergin et al. [184], in a study of 14 patients who had PCP, showed that the predominant

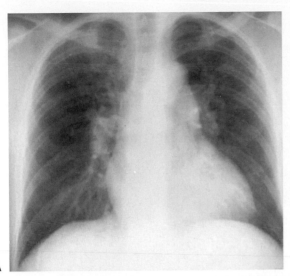
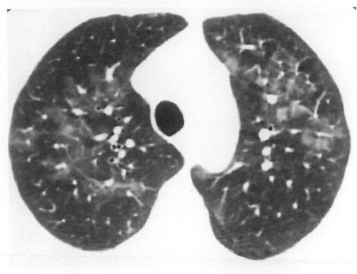

A

B

FIG. 6-49. *Pneumocystis carinii* pneumonia (PCP)—acute phase. **A:** Posteroanterior chest radiograph shows no evidence of parenchymal consolidation. Hilar fullness bilaterally is secondary to enlarged pulmonary arteries in this patient with known pulmonary artery hypertension (PH). An association between acquired immunodeficiency syndrome and PH has been noted. **B:** HRCT section through the upper lobes in the same patient as in **A**, obtained at the same time, shows typical foci of ground-glass opacification bilaterally, compatible with the early intraalveolar, exudative phase of infection. Note that despite the increased lung opacity, normal parenchymal architectural detail can still be identified. Transbronchial biopsy-proven PCP.

CT finding was areas of ground-glass opacity or consolidation, or both (Figs. 6-49 through 6-52). In many cases, in addition to diffuse, bilateral disease, a distinct mosaic pattern could be identified, with areas of normal lung intervening between scattered, focal areas of parenchymal involvement (Figs. 6-51 and 6-52). In seven cases, thickened septal lines were seen in association with areas of ground-glass opacity, presumably reflecting a combination of fluid and cellular debris within alveoli, as well as thickening of the alveolar interstitium either by edema or cellular infiltration (see Fig. 3-98; Fig. 6-53) [184].

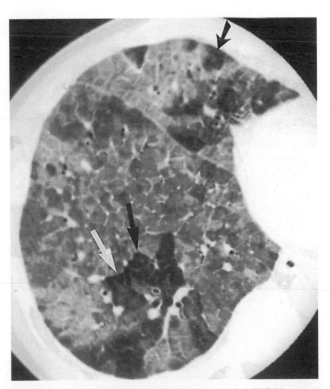

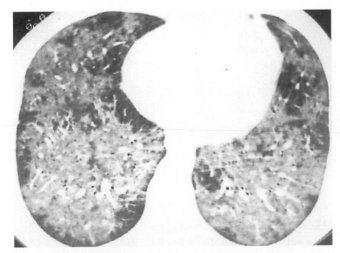

FIG. 6-50. *Pneumocystis carinii* pneumonia (PCP)—acute phase. HRCT section through the lower lobes in a patient who has documented PCP shows evidence of both diffuse ground-glass opacification and consolidation.

FIG. 6-51. *Pneumocystis carinii* pneumonia (PCP)—acute phase. Retrospectively targeted HRCT section through the right lung in a patient who had documented acute PCP shows a mosaic pattern of ground-glass opacification. Note that there is clear sparing of isolated secondary lobules (*arrows*).

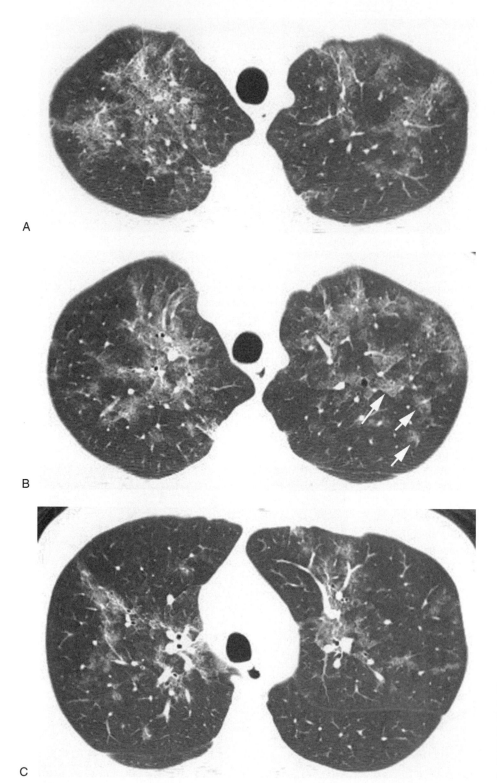

A

B

C

FIG. 6-52. A–C: Acute *Pneumocystis carinii* pneumonia in a patient with acquired immunodeficiency syndrome. Patchy areas of ground-glass opacity have an upper lobe predominance. Some areas of opacity (*arrows*, **B**) have a lobular or centrilobular distribution.

A similar spectrum of CT findings has also been described by Kuhlman et al. and Hartman et al. [158,183]. In a retrospective study of 39 patients [184], Kuhlman et al. found three patterns of CT involvement, including a ground-glass pattern, a patchwork pattern, and an interstitial or reticular pattern in 26%, 56%, and 18% of cases, respectively. Associated CT findings included nodular densities in 18% of cases, adenopathy or effusions, or both, in another 18% of cases, and cystic abnormalities in 38% of cases [183]. Hartman et al. [158] studied 24 patients who had PCP; CT findings included ground-glass opacity in 92% of patients, consolidation in 38% of patients, cystic changes in 33% of patients, nodules in 25%

TABLE 6-11. *HRCT findings in* Pneumocystis carinii *pneumonia*

Patchy or diffuse bilateral ground-glass opacity[a]

Central, perihilar, or upper lobe predominance[a]

Thick-walled, irregular, septated cavities; thin-walled cysts[a]

Superimposition of first three findings[a,b]

Pneumothorax related to cysts

Consolidation

Reticulation and septal thickening (resolving disease)

Bronchiectasis or bronchiolectasis

Small nodules, centrilobular or diffuse

Large nodules or masses (rare)

[a]Most common findings.
[b]Finding most helpful in differential diagnosis.

of patients, lymphadenopathy in 25% of patients, and pleural effusion in 17% of patients. Interlobular septal thickening and reticular abnormalities were present in 17% of patients.

A central or perihilar predominance of ground-glass opacity may be present and is considered typical of PCP (see Fig. 3-93). In recent years, however, a predominance of abnormalities in the upper lobes has also been recognized as a common occurrence (Fig. 6-52) [179]. In a study by Gruden et al. [185] of patients who had PCP not showing typical features on chest radiographs, all had an upper lobe predominance of parenchymal opacities.

HRCT findings in patients who have PCP reflect the stage of disease [165,184]. Initially, scattered foci of ground-glass opacity or airspace consolidation can be identified, corresponding to the presence of intraalveolar exudates as well as some degree of thickening of the alveolar septa; this can be termed the *acute phase of PCP* (Figs. 6-49 through 6-52). In our experience, CT is considerably more sensitive than routine chest radiographs for the detection of early parenchymal disease. Occasionally, areas of dense consolidation or coalescence may be identified, especially in patients who have more extensive parenchymal inflammation (Fig. 6-49). With time, interstitial abnormalities predominate in patients who have PCP. In treated patients who have resolving or subacute infection, reticular opacities representing thickened interlobular septa and intralobular lines can be seen in association with ground-glass opacity (i.e., crazy-paving) (see Fig. 3-98; Figs. 6-53 and 6-54). Reticulation reflects organization of intraalveolar exudates with resultant thickening of the pulmonary interstitium; it typically occurs in areas in which ground-glass opacity was visible during the acute phase of disease.

After therapy, residual changes generally can be appreciated on CT scans (Fig. 6-55). Rarely, infection with *P. carinii* results in diffuse parenchymal fibrosis (Fig. 6-56) [186]. In our experience, this appearance is generally distinguishable from acute infection, due to the absence of CT evidence of ground-glass opacity or consolidation. Less frequently, PCP results in mild, peripheral bronchiectasis and/or bronchiolectasis, presumably the result of PCP bronchiolitis [187].

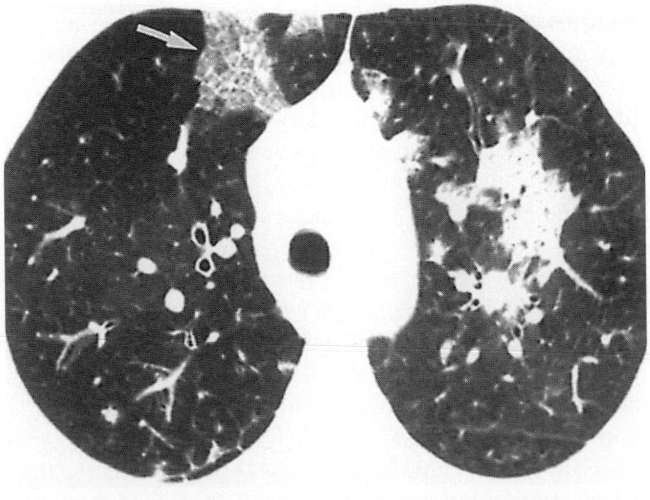

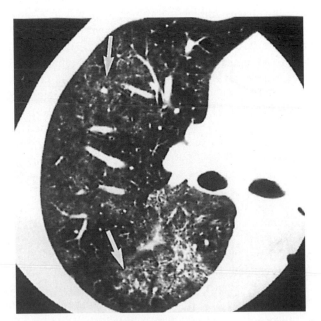

FIG. 6-53. Subacute *Pneumocystis carinii* pneumonia (PCP) with septal thickening. HRCT section through the distal trachea shows focal areas of ground-glass opacification in both upper lobes in a patient who has documented PCP. Note that within these areas, intralobular septal thickening is apparent (*arrow*), presumably resulting from the organization of acute intraalveolar exudates.

FIG. 6-54. *Pneumocystis carinii* pneumonia (PCP)—subacute phase. Target-reconstructed HRCT image through the right middle lung in a patient receiving therapy for documented *P. carinii* pneumonia. Discrete foci of increased density can be seen, many of which have a slightly reticular configuration (*arrows*). These findings are compatible with organization of previous intraalveolar exudates, resulting in infiltration of the pulmonary interstitium.

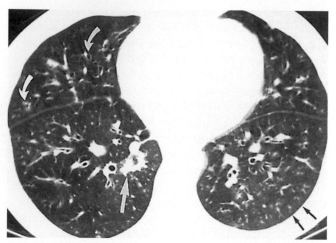

FIG. 6-55. *Pneumocystis carinii* pneumonia (PCP). HRCT section through the lower lobes in a patient who had previously treated PCP. Note that in addition to residual areas of consolidation (*white arrow*), a few centrilobular opacities can be identified (*black arrows*) as well as mild bronchiectasis (*curved arrows*), presumably the result of bronchiolitis. These changes were not identifiable on the accompanying chest radiograph (not shown).

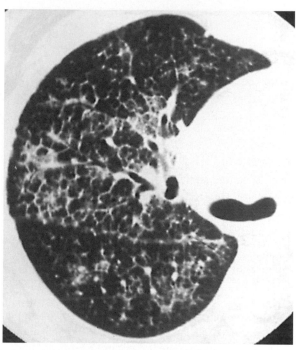

FIG. 6-56. Targeted-HRCT image through the right lung shows diffuse, coarse reticulation in the central portions of the lung in a patient with previously diagnosed and treated *Pneumocystis carinii* pneumonia (PCP). In this case, infection with PCP has resulted in a pattern of diffuse fibrosis largely confined to the central portions of the lung.

Cystic changes are frequently identified with CT in patients who have PCP, with an incidence of approximately 35% in several studies [158,179,182,188,189]. Cysts associated with PCP are variable in appearance, being of different sizes and shapes and having a thick or thin wall. Complex cysts, cysts occurring in clusters, and cysts with an irregular shape are common. Although cysts may affect any lung region, an upper lobe predominance is common [181]. Thick-walled cavitary nodules may also be seen in patients who have PCP, reflecting granulomatous inflammation [190] or bronchiectasis [191].

Kuhlman et al. [189] have also noted the appearance of premature bullous disease in AIDS patients. Using criteria previously established for the CT diagnosis of emphysema, these authors found bullous changes in 23 of 55 (42%) patients, despite an average age of only 37 years. In 70% of these cases, these changes were preceded by one or more documented episodes of infection [189]. Gurney and Bates also have reported identifying upper lobe cystic disease both in AIDS patients as well as in intravenous drug abusers [188]. Frequently indistinguishable radiographically, bullous lung disease secondary to intravenous drug abuse resulted in peripheral cystic abnormalities with sparing of the central portions of the lungs, whereas well-defined cysts randomly distributed throughout the lungs were more characteristic in patients who had documented PCP [188].

Feuerstein et al. have described cystic lung disease in five patients who had PCP, in whom radiographic-CT/pathologic correlation was obtained [192]. In two patients, *P. carinii* organisms and chronic inflammation were demonstrated in the walls of necrotic, thin-walled cavities. However, large apical and subpleural cysts lined by fibrous tissue could also be identified without evidence either of inflammation or infection. Importantly, cystic abnormalities were only identified by CT in two of five patients, even in retrospect [192]. These findings suggest a spectrum of cystic changes in AIDS patients, with larger subpleural cysts potentially arising from rupture of intraparenchymal necrotizing cavities [193]. In our experience, cystic changes in the lung appear to follow a predictable evolution. Initially, cysts appear as small foci in areas of parenchymal consolidation, often associated with clearly dilated, thick-walled bronchi (see Fig. 3-131; Figs. 6-57 and 6-58). With time, these coalesce to form bizarre-shaped, thick-walled cysts that often appear septated. There is a tendency for subpleural cysts to communicate with the pleura, accounting for the high incidence of pneumothoraces developing in these patients (see Fig. 3-132; Fig. 6-59). After therapy, these lesions eventually regress, resulting either in complete disappearance, or residual nodules or masses, or both (Fig. 6-60). In addition to suggesting the proper diagnosis, CT can be of value in select cases by differentiating these lesions from those caused by other cavitary diseases potentially occurring in this population, especially septic emboli and fungal infections [194,195].

Spontaneous pneumothorax may accompany the presence of cystic disease and may be the first radiographic manifestation of PCP, and this finding in an AIDS patient is virtually diagnostic of this disease (see Fig. 3-132; Fig. 6-59). It is

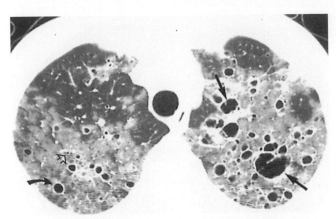

FIG. 6-57. *Pneumocystis carinii* pneumonia—cystic disease. HRCT section through the upper lobes shows extensive cystic changes throughout the lungs. These cysts are variable in size and are most often thick-walled (*curved arrow*). Many are septated, probably the result of coalescence (*straight arrows*). Note that cystic changes occur only in areas of ground-glass opacification, and that within these same areas there are also clearly dilated bronchi (*open arrow*). These findings suggest that many of the cysts probably represent pneumatoceles.

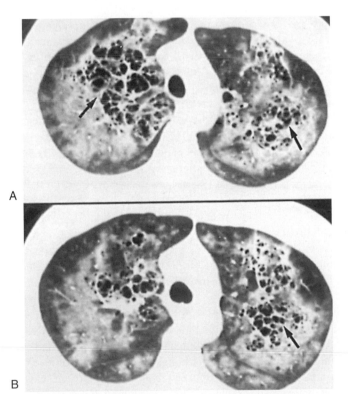

FIG. 6-58. *Pneumocystis carinii* pneumonia (PCP)—cystic disease. **A,B:** HRCT images in a patient who had documented PCP show the presence of innumerable cysts, superimposed on a background of diffuse airspace consolidation bilaterally. Note that many of the cysts are thick-walled, and many have become confluent (*arrows*). In our experience, the finding of bizarre, multiseptated, thick-walled cysts scattered throughout the parenchyma arising in foci of airspace disease should strongly suggest the diagnosis of cystic PCP.

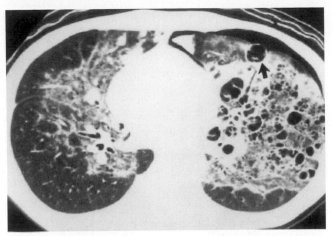

FIG. 6-59. *Pneumocystis carinii* pneumonia—cystic disease. HRCT section through the middle lungs shows extensive cystic disease primarily within areas of ground-glass opacification. Note that one of these in the lung periphery is communicating with the pleural space, resulting in a bronchopleural fistula (*arrow*). Not surprisingly, these often prove difficult to treat.

likely that pneumothorax is related to the presence of subpleural cysts. In a study by Chow et al. [181], 34% of patients who had PCP and lung cysts visible on chest radiographs developed a pneumothorax, as compared to 7% of patients who did not have visible cysts.

Hilar or mediastinal lymph node enlargement, or both, may be seen in approximately 20% of patients who have PCP, although the enlargement is usually mild [158,183,196]. Pathologic examination of nodes [196] has shown numerous PCP organisms to be present. Calcification may also occur, although this is more typical of disseminated PCP.

Less typical manifestations of PCP may also be encountered [179]. PCP may present with a variety of nodular patterns; in one study, these were visible on HRCT in 28% of cases [197]. The presence of a large nodule or mass (i.e., a pneumocystoma) may occasionally be seen in HIV-positive patients, mimicking the appearance of bronchogenic carcinoma and leading to needle aspiration biopsy for diagnosis [198]. Large quantities of organisms may be found within these masses. Solitary nodules or masses in patients who have PCP often reflect the presence of a granulomatous reaction to the presence of the organism and are usually seen early in the course of HIV infection [161,190]. These masses may cavitate [190]. Calcification is rare [161].

Small nodules, a few millimeters to a centimeter in diameter, may rarely be seen in patients who have PCP. As with larger nodules in this disease, this appearance may reflect the presence of a granulomatous response to the infection early in the course of HIV disease. Its appearance may mimic sarcoidosis. PCP may also result in poorly defined centrilobular nodules and tree-in-bud. These are presumably the result of distal airway involvement and may account for the occasional presence of either bronchiectasis or bronchiolectasis [187,199]. It should be kept in mind, however, that the

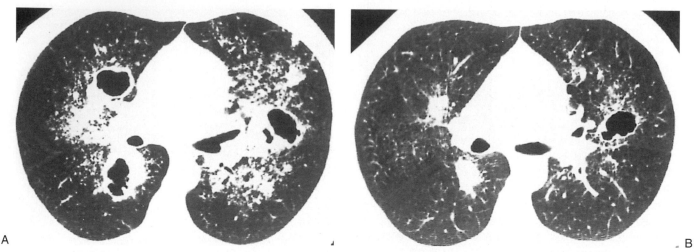

A

B

FIG. 6-60. *Pneumocystis carinii* pneumonia (PCP)—cystic disease. **A:** HRCT section through the middle lungs shows bilateral thick-walled cysts in association with ill-defined nodular opacities in a patient who has documented PCP. This case is somewhat atypical in that cysts usually form within areas of ground-glass opacification or consolidation. **B:** Follow-up scan at the same level as **A**, obtained several weeks following initiation of successful therapy, shows that the two cysts on the right have collapsed and are identifiable only as focal areas of dense consolidation. On the left side, the residual cyst is smaller and thinner-walled. Previously identified nodular infiltrate has largely resolved.

appearance of small nodules is uncommonly the result of PCP in patients who have AIDS. It is much more likely the result of bacterial or mycobacterial infection [200].

Some patients who have PCP present with a relatively chronic and indolent course, with stable or slowly progressive clinical and radiographic abnormalities over a period of months to years [160,179]. This has been termed *chronic PCP*, and is associated with interstitial fibrosis, honeycombing, and a giant cell and granulomatous reaction [201].

Utility of Computed Tomography

The accuracy of CT in the diagnosis of PCP and other pulmonary complications of AIDS was assessed by Hartman et al. [158]. The CT and HRCT scans of 102 patients who had AIDS and proven thoracic complications were reviewed, along with those of 20 HIV-positive patients who did not have active intrathoracic disease. The CT scans were independently assessed by two observers without knowledge of clinical or pathologic data. Nineteen of the 20 cases without active disease were correctly identified by one observer, and 18 by the other. All 102 cases with active disease were correctly identified as abnormal by one observer, and 101 cases by the second observer. Furthermore, without benefit of clinical or pathologic information, a confident diagnosis was achieved using CT in 48% of the cases, and this diagnosis was correct in 92% of these.

The most common pulmonary complication in the patients who had AIDS studied by Hartman et al. was PCP, present in 35 cases. Based on the CT findings, the two observers made a confident diagnosis of PCP in 25 cases, and this diagnosis was correct 94% of the time. The diagnosis of PCP in these

cases was based on the presence of areas of ground-glass opacity. False-positive diagnoses in 6% of the cases were due to motion or poor inspiratory effort resulting in apparent areas of ground-glass opacity. Although the appearance of ground-glass opacity can be seen in immunosuppressed patients as a result of other pneumonias, they are much less common.

Kang et al. [202] compared the sensitivity and specificity of chest radiography and CT in the detection of pulmonary infections and tumors in 139 patients who had AIDS. Of the 106 patients who had intrathoracic complications, 90% were correctly identified on the radiograph and 96% on CT. Of 33 patients who did not have intrathoracic disease, 73% were correctly identified at radiography and 86% at CT. A confident first-choice diagnosis by two independent observers was most often correct in Kaposi's sarcoma (31 of 34 interpretations, 91%), PCP (33 of 38 interpretations, 87%), and lymphoma (four of four interpretations, 100%).

Furthermore, HRCT may be quite valuable in detecting PCP when clinical and plain film assessment is inconclusive. Gruden et al. [185] studied the utility of HRCT in 51 AIDS patients who had a high clinical probability of PCP, and in whom chest radiographic findings were normal, equivocal, or nonspecific. In this study, patchy or nodular ground-glass attenuation visible on HRCT was considered to indicate possible PCP. The sensitivity of HRCT in detecting PCP was 100%, with a specificity of 89%, and an accuracy of 90% ($p <.005$); no case of PCP was missed on HRCT. The authors conclude that HRCT may allow exclusion of PCP in patients who have normal, equivocal, or nonspecific findings on chest radiographs, and that bronchoscopy can be avoided in many patients on the basis of the HRCT findings. In a similar study [203], HRCT findings were compared with BAL results in

13 HIV-positive patients who had a strong clinical suspicion of PCP and a normal chest radiograph. The patients all had a CD_4 count of less than 200 cells per mm^3, a nonproductive cough or nonpurulent sputum, fever, and dyspnea or decreased exercise tolerance. Four patients had patchy ground-glass opacities visible on HRCT, and one also showed interstitial thickening. All four proved to have PCP on BAL. None of the nine patients who were negative for PCP on BAL had ground-glass opacity on HRCT. It has also been reported that HRCT is more accurate than gallium scintigraphy in patients who have equivocal disease [204].

Although the presence of areas of ground-glass opacity in patients with AIDS is most suggestive of PCP, in immunocompromised patients who do not have AIDS, ground-glass opacity is a less specific finding. Brown et al. [205] compared the findings on HRCT with pathologic specimens in 33 immunocompromised patients who had acute pulmonary complications. Fourteen patients who did not have AIDS had ground-glass opacity as their main abnormality. In these 14 patients, PCP accounted for the areas of ground-glass opacity in three cases, cytotoxic drug reaction in four, COP in four, lymphoma in two, and CMV pneumonia in one.

Cytomegalovirus Pneumonia

CMV pneumonia frequently occurs in immunosuppressed patients, especially after organ transplantation [165,206–211]. After allogeneic bone marrow transplantation, for example, CMV pneumonitis characteristically causes fever, pulmonary infiltrates, and hypoxia resulting in ARDS [206,212]; it typically occurs more than 2 months after transplantation. Patients who have severe graft-versus-host disease are usually at highest risk. Crawford et al., in a study of 111 open lung biopsies performed on 109 marrow transplant recipients who had diffuse pulmonary infiltrates, identified infection in 63% of cases; 90% of these proved to be caused by CMV infection [207]. Bacterial or yeast infections were identified in only 4% of cases, whereas PCP was identified in only 6%. With the use of CMV-negative blood products in patients lacking cytomegalovirus antibodies, as well as the intravenous administration of CMV immune globulin and prophylactic administration of antiviral agents, including acyclovir or ganciclovir, the incidence of serious CMV infection has been reduced. A similar approach is also now used in patients after heart-lung or lung transplantation [210].

CMV infection also has been frequently identified in renal transplantation patients. Moore et al. [211], in a study of patients treated with cyclosporin-prednisone immunosuppression after renal transplantation, found that CMV was present in eight of 17 cases of pneumonia, including five of six patients with diffuse pulmonary infiltrates and all six patients with multiple-organism infections. It has been speculated that CMV infection itself may compromise T-cell function causing further immunocompromise in this population.

CMV is well-recognized as the most common viral organism to be identified in patients who have AIDS [165]; however, there is considerable controversy concerning the clinical significance of this finding [213]. CMV is frequently detected by cytology, histopathology, or by culture in AIDS patients, without causing recognizable disease, and is present in up to 80% of patients at autopsy [214–216]. Proven cases of clinically significant CMV pneumonitis are relatively uncommon and have been rarely reported antemortem. However, with the increasing length of patient survival, largely the result of prophylaxis for PCP, CMV pneumonitis is more often being recognized in late-stage disease, especially in patients with CD_4 counts smaller than 50 per mm^3 [217].

High-Resolution Computed Tomography Findings

The CT findings in patients who have CMV pneumonitis are quite variable and include (i) patchy or diffuse consolidation, (ii) ground-glass opacities, (iii) small centrilobular nodular opacities, (iv) bronchial wall thickening, (v) pleural effusion, and (vi) a combination of consolidation and reticular opacities (Table 6-12) [165,218–221]. Aafedt et al. [219] described the CT findings in eight immunocompromised non-AIDS patients, seven of whom had received solid organ or bone marrow transplant. The most common CT findings consisted of a combination of airspace consolidation and interstitial patterns seen in seven patients, and airspace consolidation alone in one patient.

Kang et al. [219] reviewed the CT findings in ten solid organ or bone marrow transplant patients who had CT and pathologically proven isolated pulmonary CMV infection. Nine of the ten patients had parenchymal abnormalities evident on CT, and one patient had a normal CT. The findings in the nine patients included small nodules present in six patients, consolidation in four patients, ground-glass opacities in four patients, and reticulation in one patient. Centrilobular areas of ground-glass opacity tend to be an early finding of CMV [221].

McGuinness et al. [220] reviewed the CT and pathologic findings in 21 AIDS patients who had CMV pneumonitis. The parenchymal abnormalities were heterogeneous and included ground-glass opacities, airspace consolidation, nodules or masslike infiltrates, and reticulation. Ground-glass opacities were present in nine patients (21%) but were the predominant abnormality in only four patients (Figs. 6-61 and 6-62). Con-

TABLE 6-12. *HRCT findings in cytomegalovirus pneumonia*

Patchy bilateral foci of ground-glass opacification, consolidation, or both[a]

Scattered, poorly defined nodules, masses, or both[a]

Superimposition of first two findings[a,b]

Reticulation and septal thickening (resolving disease)

Small nodules, diffuse

[a]Most common findings.
[b]Findings most helpful in differential diagnosis.

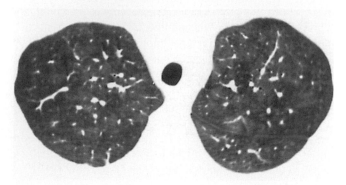

FIG. 6-61. Cytomegalovirus (CMV) pneumonitis—acute phase. HRCT section through the upper lobes shows subtle diffuse ground-glass opacification in an acquired immunodeficiency syndrome patient with histologically documented CMV pneumonitis. Note that this appearance is indistinguishable from that caused by acute *Pneumocystis carinii* pneumonia.

solidation was present in seven patients (33%) but was the predominant abnormality in only one patient. Pathologically, these changes corresponded primarily to the presence of DAD. Similar to HRCT findings in patients who have resolving PCP, reticular changes were identified in six cases, corresponding histologically to the presence of alveolar wall thickening, intralobular interstitial thickening, and interlobular septal thickening (Fig. 6-63). Most striking, in this same population, nodules (including one patient with diffuse miliary nodules), masses, or both were identified in 62% of cases, including five cases in which ground-glass opacification could be seen.

Abnormalities tend to be bilateral and symmetric in patients who have CMV. In the study by Kang et al. [219], nodular opacities had a bilateral and symmetric distribution and involved all lung zones, whereas consolidation primarily involved the lower lung zones. In a study by Abe et al. [221], areas of ground-glass opacity were bilateral in all cases and

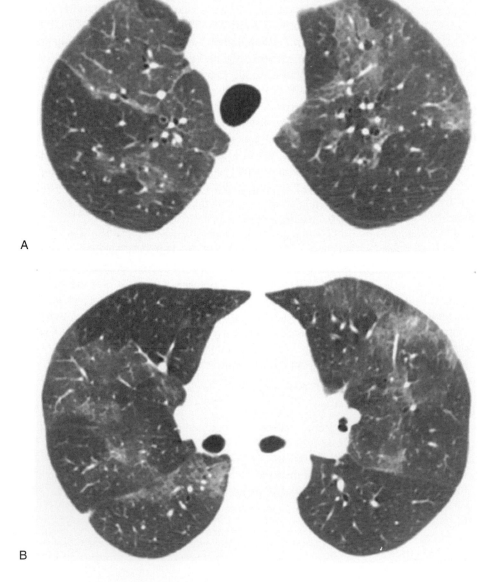

A

B

FIG. 6-62. A,B: Acute phase cytomegalovirus pneumonia in an immunosuppressed patient. Patchy ground-glass opacity is visible bilaterally.

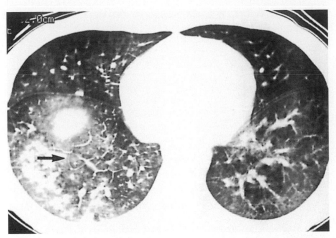

FIG. 6-63. Cytomegalovirus (CMV) pneumonitis—subacute phase. HRCT section through the lung bases shows diffuse ground-glass opacification most marked in the right lower lobe in a patient who has proven CMV pneumonitis. Thickened interlobular septa are clearly identifiable in the right lower lobe (*arrow*), consistent with dilated lymphatics resulting from organization of intraalveolar exudates.

were diffuse in 67%; the subpleural lung regions were spared in 83%. Areas of consolidation were bilateral in 67%, nonsegmental in 67%, and involved the lower lobes in all cases.

Viral Pneumonias Other Than Cytomegalovirus

In addition to CMV, other viral infections may occur in immunosuppressed patients [165,222,223]. These may be associated with similar radiographic findings. HRCT findings have been reported in a limited number of cases.

Herpes simplex virus pneumonia is rare and usually occurs after clinically apparent mucocutaneous disease in patients that are immunosuppressed as a result of organ transplantation, bone marrow transplantation, or advanced AIDS [165]. Poorly defined nodular opacities and areas of ground-glass opacity have been reported on HRCT [165].

Varicella-zoster infection usually results in chicken pox, occurring in children and being self-limited. Varicella-zoster pneumonia is most common in adults and immunocompromised patients [224,225]. Symptoms range from mild to severe, and a significant number of adults with pneumonia die as a result of their disease. HRCT findings of varicella-zoster pneumonia have been reported in a few cases [226,227] and include small well-defined or ill-defined nodules, centrilobular nodules, nodules with surrounding ground-glass opacity, patchy ground-glass opacity, and coalescence of nodules; the disappearance of these findings on imaging studies corresponded to healing of skin lesions in patients after antiviral chemotherapy [226].

Respiratory syncytial virus (RSV) infection is a common cause of lower respiratory tract infection in children. In older children and adults, RSV can cause either upper or lower airway infection. RSV can occur in a more virulent form in recipients of bone marrow, solid organ, or lung transplants [223,228]. The most common presenting complaints are those of a lower respiratory infection with dyspnea, fever, cough, and purulent sputum. The severity of disease and clinical course are variable, but PFTs often show evidence of airway obstruction [228]. Chest radiographs may show heterogeneous unilateral or bilateral opacities [222,228]. In one study [229], HRCT findings before, during, and after acute infection with RSV infection were reviewed in nine lung transplant recipients. CT findings included ground-glass opacity (n = 7), airspace consolidation (n = 5), and tree-in-bud (n = 4) (Fig. 6-64). Bronchial wall thickening and dilatation were also seen. Five of seven patients with follow-up examinations showed new air-trapping (n = 3), persistent bronchial dilatation (n = 3), or thickening (n = 2). Two patients developed bronchiolitis obliterans, and three developed bronchiolitis obliterans syndrome with evidence of airway obstruction. The authors suggested that RSV infection may be associated with the development of bronchiolitis obliterans in these patients [229].

Mycoplasma pneumoniae Pneumonia

Mycoplasma pneumonia is a common cause of community-acquired pneumonia, accounting for up to 30% of all pneumonias in the general population [230–232]. Clinical symptoms include fever, cough, sputum production, fatigue, malaise, and myalgia [233,234]. Histologically, *M. pneumoniae* infection is characterized by the presence of an acute cellular bronchiolitis, which may progress to bronchopneumonia [112].

The radiographic manifestations are nonspecific, consisting of patchy areas of airspace consolidation, reticular interstitial infiltrates, nodular opacities, and bronchial wall thickening [233–236].

High-Resolution Computed Tomography Findings

Reittner et al. [235] reviewed the radiographic and HRCT findings in 28 patients who had serologically proven *M. pneumoniae* pneumonia. The most common finding on the radiograph was the presence of airspace opacification, either ground-glass opacity or consolidation (n = 24) which was patchy and segmental (n = 9) or nonsegmental (n = 15) in distribution (Fig. 6-65). On HRCT, areas of ground-glass opacity were seen in 24 patients (85%), and airspace consolidation was seen in 22 patients (79%) (Table 6-13). In 13 patients (59%), the areas of consolidation had a lobular distribution evident on HRCT (Fig. 6-66). Nodules were seen more commonly on HRCT (25 of 28 patients, 89%) than on radiographs (14 patients, 50%) (*p* <.01). In 24 patients (86%), the nodules had a predominantly centrilobular distribution on HRCT. Thickening of the bronchovascular bundles was identified on HRCT in 23 of 28 patients (82%), compared to five patients (18%) on the radiograph (*p* <.01) (Fig. 6-67).

The high prevalence of centrilobular nodules in patients who had *M. pneumoniae* pneumonia in the study by Reittner

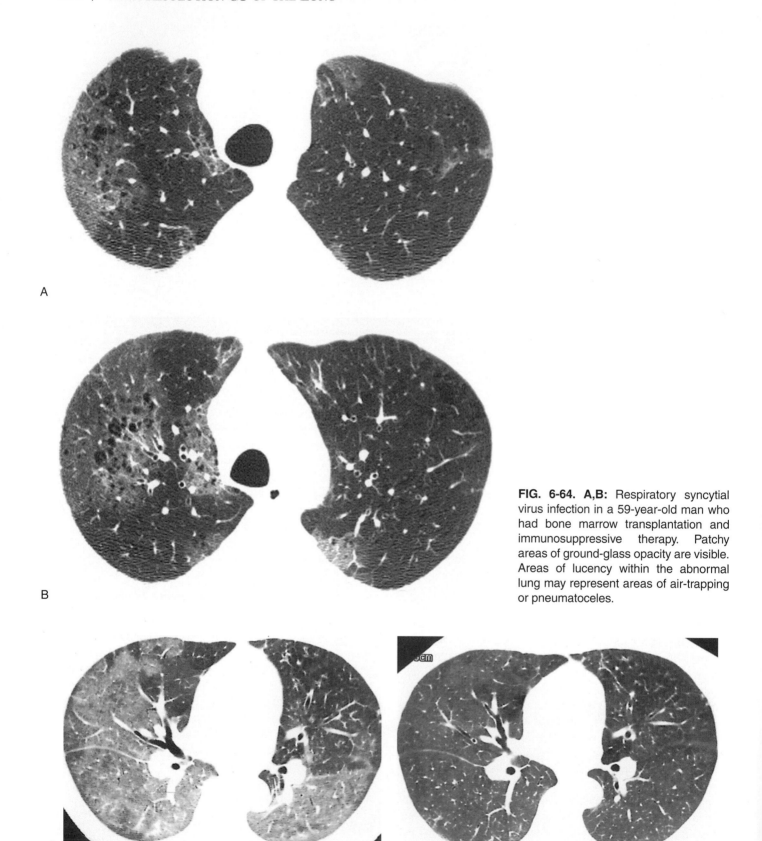

A

B

FIG. 6-64. A,B: Respiratory syncytial virus infection in a 59-year-old man who had bone marrow transplantation and immunosuppressive therapy. Patchy areas of ground-glass opacity are visible. Areas of lucency within the abnormal lung may represent areas of air-trapping or pneumatoceles.

A   B

FIG. 6-65. *Mycoplasma* pneumonia with patchy ground-glass opacity. **A:** HRCT section at the level of the middle lobe bronchus demonstrates ground-glass opacification of the right lung and superior segment of the left lower lobe in a patient who had proven *Mycoplasma* pneumonia. **B:** Follow-up HRCT at the same level as in **A** shows only minimal residual ground-glass opacification.

TABLE 6-13. *HRCT findings in* Mycoplasma *pneumonia*

Patchy or nodular ground-glass opacity, consolidation, or both[a]

Lobular distribution of opacities[a]

Ill-defined centrilobular nodules[a]

Thickening of the peribronchovascular interstitium[a]

Patchy or lobular areas of mosaic perfusion

Patchy or lobular air-trapping on expiratory scans[a,b]

[a]Most common findings.
[b]Findings most helpful in differential diagnosis.

et al. [235], as well as the patchy distribution of the nodules, confirms findings reported by Gruden et al. [102] in other infectious causes of bronchiolitis and bronchopneumonia. Bronchiolitis and bronchiolitis obliterans may occur in a variety of infections, including mycoplasma and viral pneumonias [112,236,237].

Because of the presence of bronchiolitis in patients who have *Mycoplasma* pneumonia, airway obstruction with mosaic perfusion and expiratory air-trapping may be seen on HRCT in addition to findings of ground-glass opacity, consolidation, and centrilobular nodules (Table 6-13) (see Fig. 3-146) [238]. Furthermore, a considerable proportion of children who have a history of prior *Mycoplasma* pneumonia have abnormal findings on HRCT, suggestive of small airway obstruction [239]. In a study of 38 children requiring hospitalization for *Mycoplasma* pneumonia, HRCT performed after an interval of 1 to 2 years commonly showed findings of small airway obstruction. Abnormal HRCT find-

ings were present in 37% (14/38) of these patients. These abnormalities included mosaic perfusion (n = 12), bronchiectasis (n = 8), bronchial wall thickening (n = 4), decreased vascularity (n = 1), and air-trapping on expiratory scans (9 of 29 tested). The area affected by these abnormalities, usually involving two or more lobes, corresponded in all cases to the location of infiltrate seen on chest radiographs at the time of the acute pneumonia. There is evidence to suggest that these abnormalities are more likely to occur in younger subjects and those with a higher antibody titer at the time of pneumonia [239].

In the majority of patients who have community-acquired pneumonia, chest radiography provides adequate imaging information, and HRCT is not warranted. However, an increasing number of patients undergo CT, especially HRCT, when there is a high clinical suspicion for pneumonia with normal or questionable radiographic findings. Syrjälä and coworkers prospectively compared HRCT with chest radiography in 47 patients who had clinical symptoms and signs suggestive of community-acquired pneumonia [240]. Evidence of pneumonia was identified on HRCT in 26 patients, compared with 18 on radiography (*p* <.01). Furthermore, in a study by Tanaka et al. [231], the HRCT appearances of community-acquired bacterial and atypical pneumonias (largely *Mycoplasma*) were compared and found to be quite different. In 14 cases of atypical pneumonia [*Mycoplasma* pneumonia (n = 12), *Chlamydia* pneumonia (n = 1), and influenza viral pneumonia (n = 1)], HRCT showed centrilobular opacities (64%), acinar shadows (71%), airspace consolidation (57%), and ground-glass opacity with a lobular distribution (86%). Bacterial pneumonias, on the other hand, frequently showed airspace consolidation with a segmental distribution (72%).

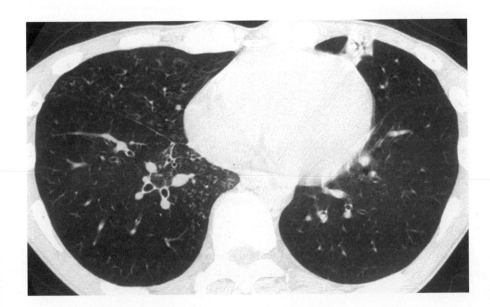

FIG. 6-66. *Mycoplasma* pneumonia. HRCT demonstrates lobular area of consolidation in the lingula and centrilobular nodules in the right middle and lower lobes.

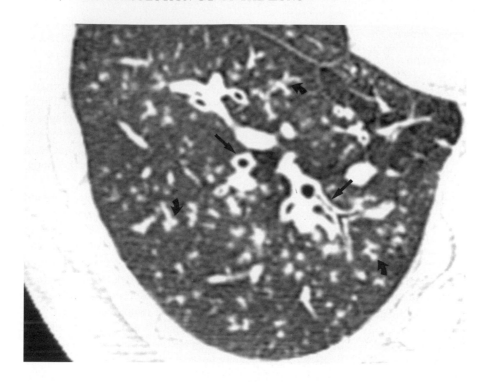

FIG. 6-67. *Mycoplasma* pneumonia. HRCT targeted to the right lung demonstrates extensive bronchial wall thickening (*straight arrows*), centrilobular nodules, and branching linear and nodular opacities (tree-in-bud appearance) (*curved arrows*). (Courtesy of Dr. Jay Soung Park, Department of Radiology, Soonchunhyang University, Seoul, Korea.)

DIFFUSE PULMONARY HEMORRHAGE

Diffuse pulmonary hemorrhage can result from a variety of diseases, and making a specific diagnosis may be difficult [241,242]. Chest radiographic findings are often nondiagnostic, and hemoptysis may be lacking even in patients who have sufficient hemorrhage to result in anemia [243]. If possible, diffuse pulmonary hemorrhage should be distinguished from focal pulmonary hemorrhage occurring as a result of bronchiectasis, chronic bronchitis, active infection (e.g., tuberculosis), chronic infection, neoplasm, or pulmonary embolism [242,244].

The differential diagnosis of diffuse pulmonary hemorrhage includes antiglomerular basement membrane disease (Goodpasture's syndrome), collagen-vascular disease such as Wegener's granulomatosis and lupus erythematosus, idiopathic pulmonary hemosiderosis (IPH), drug reactions, anticoagulation, and thrombocytopenia [244,245]. In general, HRCT shows consolidation or ground-glass opacity in the presence of acute hemorrhage; ill-defined centrilobular nodules may predominate in some patients (Table 6-14) (Fig. 6-68). Within days of an acute episode of hemorrhage, the presence of inter-lobular septal thickening may be seen in association with ground-glass opacity (i.e., crazy-paving) as hemosiderin-laden macrophages accumulate in the interstitium (Fig. 6-68).

Goodpasture's Syndrome

Antiglomerular basement membrane disease (Goodpasture's syndrome) most typically occurs in young men [241]. It is usually associated with symptoms of cough, mild hemoptysis, dyspnea, weakness, and anemia. Findings of renal disease are usually, but not always present, including hematuria, proteinuria, and renal failure. Although plain radiographs may be normal, they usually show diffuse airspace consolidation or ground-glass opacity, usually bilateral and symmetric and often with a perihilar predominance. After an acute episode of hemorrhage, there is a tendency for the airspace opacities to resolve, being superseded by an interstitial abnormality or septal thickening. HRCT usually shows consolidation or ground-glass opacity and may be abnormal in the face of subtle plain film findings (see Fig. 3-87) [242,244].

Idiopathic Pulmonary Hemosiderosis

IPH is a disease of unknown origin, characterized by recurrent episodes or diffuse pulmonary hemorrhage without associated glomerulonephritis or serologic abnormality [244,245]. IPH most commonly occurs in young children or young adults. IPH is sometimes associated with celiac disease or immunoglobulin A gammopathy. Symptoms include cough, hemoptysis, dyspnea, and anemia. Plain radiographic and CT findings are similar to those of Goodpasture's syndrome. Cheah et al. [243] reported the HRCT findings in four

---

TABLE 6-14. *HRCT findings in pulmonary hemorrhage*

Patchy or diffuse ground-glass opacity, consolidation, or both[a]

Ill-defined centrilobular nodules

Interlobular septal thickening developing over days[a]

Superimposition of first two findings with third finding (crazy-paving)[a,b]

[a]Most common findings.
[b]Findings most helpful in differential diagnosis.

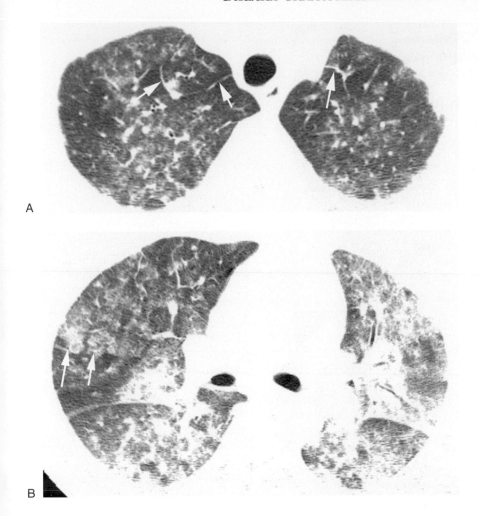

A

B

FIG. 6-68. Pulmonary hemorrhage associated with thrombotic thrombocytopenic purpura. Interlobular septal thickening is visible (*arrows*, **A**). Patchy areas of ground-glass opacity and consolidation are typical of pulmonary hemorrhage. In some regions, opacities appear to be lobular or centrilobular (*arrows*, **B**).

patients who had IPH. Predominant findings in the acute phase of disease included diffuse nodules and diffuse ground-glass opacity (Fig. 6-69); ill-defined centrilobular nodules were also reported by Seely et al. [245] in this disease. Pathologic findings include alveolar hemorrhage, hemosiderin-laden macrophages, and a variable degree of interstitial fibrosis.

Collagen-Vascular Disease

Diffuse pulmonary hemorrhage may occur with many collagen diseases, most commonly lupus erythematosus and Wegener's granulomatosis [244,245]. Hemoptysis is common and may be massive. HRCT findings are similar to other causes of diffuse pulmonary hemorrhage (Fig. 6-70).

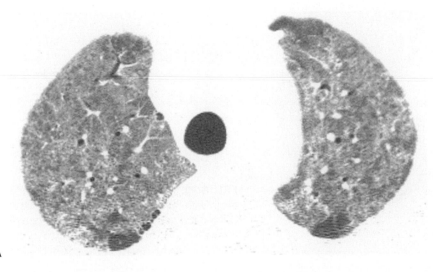

A

FIG. 6-69. A–C: Pulmonary hemorrhage associated with idiopathic pulmonary hemosiderosis. Diffuse ground-glass opacity associated with fine reticulation is typical of pulmonary hemorrhage. *Continued*

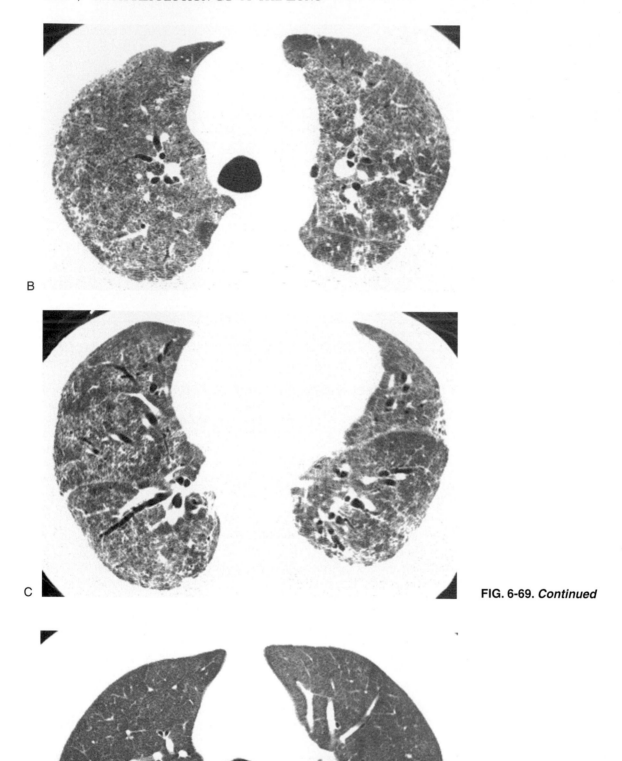

B

C

FIG. 6-69. *Continued*

FIG. 6-70. Pulmonary hemorrhage associated with systemic lupus erythematosus. Diffuse but geographic ground-glass opacity is visible.

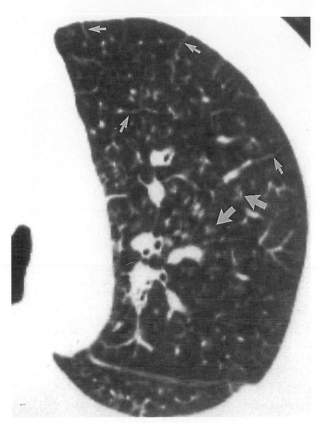

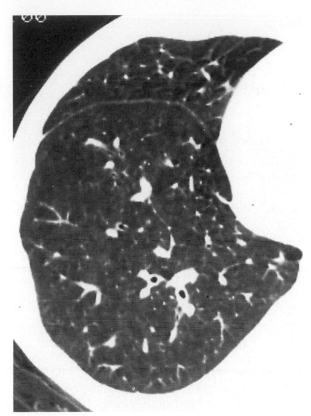

FIG. 6-71. Pulmonary edema associated with cardiomyopathy. Both interlobular septal thickening (*small arrows*) and ill-defined centrilobular opacities (*large arrows*) are visible. Also note thickening of the peribronchovascular interstitium, with peribronchial cuffing.

FIG. 6-72. Pulmonary edema in a patient who had renal failure and chronic dyspnea. Hazy, ground-glass opacities are present, some of which are centrilobular in location. Despite the lack of thickened septa, pleural fluid, or prominent pulmonary vessels, open-lung biopsy (not illustrated) showed only pulmonary edema. (From Gruden JF, Webb WR, Warnock M. Centrilobular opacities in the lung on high-resolution CT: diagnostic considerations and pathologic correlation. *AJR Am J Roentgenol* 1994;162:569–574, with permission.)

PULMONARY EDEMA AND ADULT RESPIRATORY DISTRESS SYNDROME

Patients who have pulmonary edema, either hydrostatic (cardiogenic) or increased permeability (noncardiogenic), and ARDS are not generally imaged using HRCT, as their diagnosis is usually based on a combination of clinical and chest radiographic findings. However, a knowledge of their HRCT appearances may sometimes be of value in diagnosis.

Pulmonary edema is often classified as being either hydrostatic, or due to increased permeability. It should be recognized, however, that a simple distinction between hydrostatic and permeability edema is not entirely appropriate; permeability edema may occur with or without DAD or may be associated with hydrostatic edema [246,247]. A classification of pulmonary edema as (i) hydrostatic edema, (ii) permeability edema associated with DAD, (iii) permeability edema without associated DAD, or (iv) mixed edema [246,247] agrees better with pathology, physiology, and radiology. Although these types of edema cannot always be distinguished on the basis of plain film or CT findings [8,159], their appearances tend to differ [246,247].

Hydrostatic Pulmonary Edema

Hydrostatic pulmonary edema results from alterations in the normal relationship between intra- and extravascular hydrostatic and oncotic pressures. In most cases, an increased intravascular pressure reflecting pulmonary venous hypertension is the predominant cause, resulting in loss of fluid into the interstitium. Low intravascular oncotic pressure resulting from hypoalbuminemia can also result in increased interstitial transudation of fluid.

On HRCT, hydrostatic edema generally results in a combination of septal thickening and ground-glass opacity (see Fig. 3-10; Figs. 6-71 through 6-74), but septal thickening (see Fig. 3-10) or ground-glass opacity (Figs. 6-72 through 6-74) can predominate in individual cases (Table 6-15) [10,246,248,249]. In some patients, ill-defined perivascular and centrilobular opacities can also be seen (see Fig. 3-41; Figs. 6-71 and 6-72) [102]. There is a tendency for hydrostatic edema to have a perihilar and gravitational distribution [250], but this is not always present. Thickening of the peri-

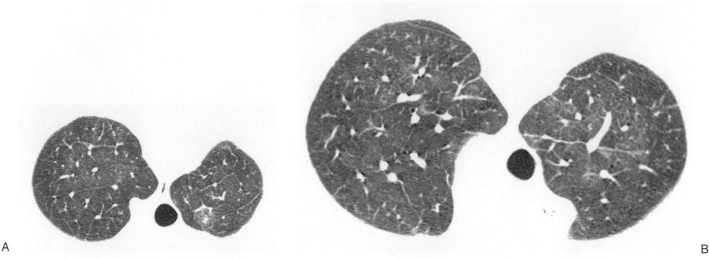

A

B

FIG. 6-73. A,B: Cardiogenic pulmonary edema. Hazy, ground-glass opacities are associated with interlobular septal thickening.

hilar peribronchovascular interstitium (peribronchial cuffing) and fissural thickening are also common (Fig. 6-71). In studies of hydrostatic edema in dog lungs, HRCT has shown a predominantly central, peribronchovascular, and posterior distribution of edema, associated with an increased thickness of bronchial walls [251,252]. It has been suggested that a perihilar or bat-wing distribution of edema is most typical in patients who have a rapid accumulation of fluid [247].

Storto et al. [253] reviewed the HRCT findings in seven patients who had hydrostatic pulmonary edema. Abnormalities visible on HRCT included ground-glass opacities in six patients, interlobular septal thickening in five patients, peribronchovascular interstitial thickening in five patients, increased vascular caliber in four patients, and pleural effusion or thickening of the interlobar fissures in

four patients. The ground-glass opacities were diffuse or patchy in distribution and often had a subtle gravitational predominance. The interlobular septal thickening was smooth and uniform, except for a focal nodular appearance due to prominent septal veins [253].

Permeability Edema with Diffuse Alveolar Damage and Adult Respiratory Distress Syndrome

ARDS is characterized by diffuse lung injury, with progressive dyspnea and hypoxemia over a period of hours to days. Injury to capillary endothelium with permeability edema and injury to the respiratory epithelium are present histologically. Specific criteria for the diagnosis of ARDS include an acute onset, hypoxemia with $PaO_2/FIO_2 \leq 200$ mm Hg, characteris-

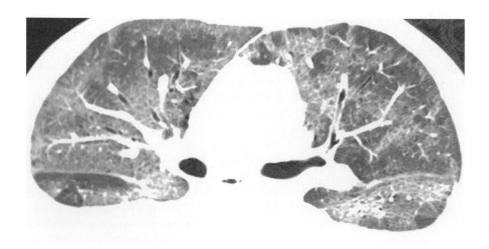

FIG. 6-74. Cardiogenic pulmonary edema. Hazy ground-glass opacity, interlobular septal thickening, intralobular interstitial thickening, thickening of fissures, and large pleural effusions are present.

TABLE 6-15. *HRCT findings in pulmonary edema*

Hydrostatic edema
Smooth interlobular septal thickening[a]
Patchy ground-glass opacity[a]
Smooth peribronchovascular interstitial thickening[a]
Smooth subpleural or fissural thickening[a]
Superimposition of first four findings[a,b]
Ill-defined centrilobular nodules
Dependent, perihilar, or lower lung predominance
Increased permeability edema without diffuse alveolar damage (DAD)
Findings of hydrostatic edema
Increased permeability edema with DAD (adult respiratory distress syndrome)
Diffuse or patchy ground-glass opacity or consolidation[a,b]
Centrilobular opacities[a]
Interlobular septal thickening
Dependent predominance[a]
Peripheral distribution
Anterior lung fibrosis with healing[a,b]

[a]Most common findings.
[b]Findings most helpful in differential diagnosis.

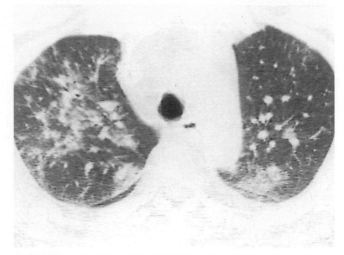

FIG. 6-75. Adult respiratory distress syndrome due to cytotoxic drug reaction in a 44-year-old man. HRCT demonstrates patchy bilateral areas of consolidation and ground-glass opacity in the upper lobes. Diffuse consolidation was present in the lower lobes. The diagnosis was proved by open-lung biopsy.

tic bilateral radiographic abnormalities, and a normal pulmonary artery wedge pressure or clinical absence of elevated left atrial pressure [254]. ARDS can result from one of a number of toxic agents or insults, including infection, inhalation of toxic fumes or gases, aspiration of gastric acid (Mendelson syndrome), sepsis, shock, extrathoracic trauma, fat embolism, pneumonia, and any cause of DAD. Typically, radiographs show multiple, diffuse, poorly circumscribed alveolar opacities that increase in size and eventually become confluent.

Permeability edema is a manifestation of capillary endothelial injury with resultant loss of fluid and protein into the lung interstitium. It is often associated with DAD and ARDS. However, it is important to recognize that, in patients who have ARDS, the abnormalities seen on HRCT not only reflect the presence of pulmonary edema, but also reflect abnormalities associated with DAD, including epithelial damage, epithelial hyperplasia, inflammation, and fibrosis [246,255].

On HRCT, pulmonary edema occurring secondary to lung injury or ARDS is generally associated with ground-glass opacity or consolidation, and a predominance in dependent lung regions is common (Table 6-15) (Fig. 6-75). Opacities can be diffuse or patchy, affecting the lung in a geographic fashion, and sometimes involve the centrilobular regions [9,256,257]. Interlobular septal thickening is less common than in hydrostatic edema, but can be seen [256]. Depending on the etiology of the edema, opacities can predominate in

the peripheral and subpleural regions [246,257], or can spare the lung periphery [9,256]. For example, Tagliabue et al. [258] reviewed the CT findings in 74 patients who had ARDS. The main abnormalities consisted of airspace consolidation or a combination of consolidation and ground-glass opacities. In 86% of patients, the opacities mainly involved the dependent lung regions. Other common findings included air bronchograms seen in 89% of patients, and small unilateral (22% of patients) or bilateral (28% of patients) pleural effusions.

Goodman et al. [259] compared the CT appearances of patients who had ARDS due to pulmonary disease (most due to pneumonia) to those who had ARDS resulting from extrapulmonary causes (most often sepsis), and significant differences were found. In patients who had ARDS due to pulmonary disease, consolidation and ground-glass opacity were equally prevalent and lung disease was often asymmetric. On the other hand, in patients who had an extrathoracic cause of ARDS, ground-glass opacity was predominant, and symmetric lung involvement was the rule.

The CT findings in patients who had pulmonary fat embolism syndrome, a cause of ARDS, include diffuse ground-glass opacity, focal areas of consolidation or ground-glass opacity, or nodules [257]. Focal abnormalities predominated in the upper lobes. Gravity-dependent opacities predominated in the lower lobes. Follow-up CT scans showed rapid improvement in half of patients. The extent of abnormalities on CT correlated with oxygenation [257].

Over time, consolidation clears in patients who have ARDS, but ground-glass opacity and cystic areas of lung destruction persist [246]. Owens et al. [260] assessed serial HRCT scans in eight patients who had ARDS. Ini-

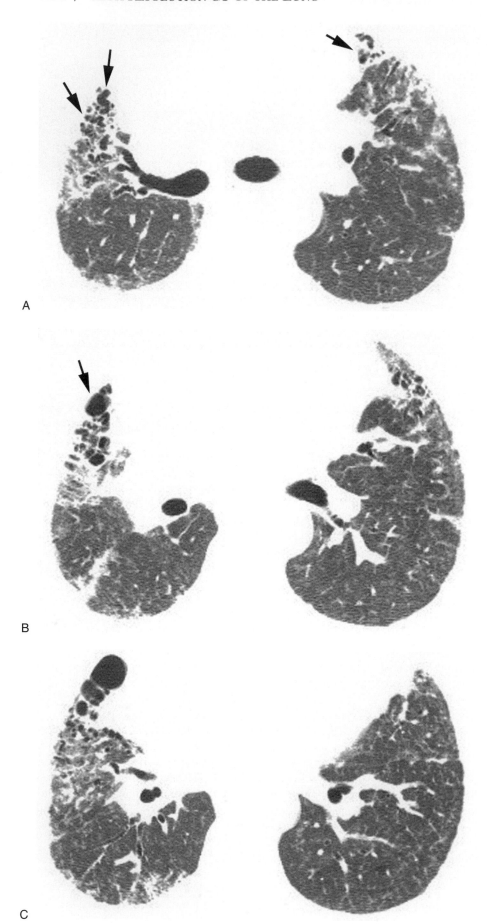

A

B

C

FIG. 6-76. A–C. Pulmonary fibrosis following adult respiratory distress syndrome. Traction bronchiectasis (*arrows*, **A**), subpleural cystic areas of lung destruction (*arrow*, **B**), and irregular reticular opacities are visible within the anterior lungs. The posterior lungs appear relatively normal.

tial HRCT scans showed ground-glass opacities and parenchymal distortion in all eight patients, multifocal areas of consolidation in six patients, reticular opacities in six patients, and linear opacities in five patients. Follow-up scans during convalescence showed clearing of the consolidation in all patients, but persistence of ground-glass opacification in four of the eight patients. The reticular pattern persisted unchanged in five of eight patients, became more extensive in two, and developed in one. Parenchymal distortion was present initially in all eight patients and persisted in six patients. One patient developed HRCT findings suggestive of emphysema. Overall, 77% of the lung was abnormal during the acute phase of ARDS, and 35% on follow-up. There was significant correlation between the extent of abnormalities on HRCT and the lung injury score [260].

In patients who have pulmonary fibrosis resulting from ARDS [261], abnormalities on follow-up HRCT have a striking anterior distribution (Fig. 6-76). This unusual distribution likely reflects the fact that patients who have ARDS typically develop posterior lung atelectasis and consolidation; it is thought that consolidation protects the posterior lung regions from the effects of mechanical ventilation, including high ventilatory pressures and high oxygen tension [261].

Permeability Edema without Diffuse Alveolar Damage

Permeability pulmonary edema may occur without accompanying DAD in patients who have drug reactions, interleukin-2 treatment [262], transfusion reaction, *Hantavirus* pulmonary syndrome [263], or as a result of a mild insult usually resulting in ARDS, such as air embolism or toxic shock syndrome [246]. It has been suggested that the absence of a pulmonary epithelial injury in such patients reduces the extent of alveolar edema [246].

In patients who have pulmonary edema occurring in the absence of DAD, pulmonary edema typically resembles hydrostatic edema, with interlobular septal thickening being a predominant feature, and consolidation is less conspicuous or absent (Table 6-15). Edema may clear rapidly because of the absence of epithelial injury.

Mixed Edema

Mixed permeability and hydrostatic edema may be seen in the presence of diseases resulting in increased intravascular pressure and capillary endothelial injury. A mixed etiology is thought to occur in patients who have high-altitude pulmonary edema [264], neurogenic pulmonary edema, reperfusion edema, reexpansion edema, edema associated with tocolytic therapy, posttransplantation edema, postpneumonectomy or postvolume reduction edema, and in patients with edema related to air embolism [246,247]. As would be expected, the CT appearances of patients having these types of edema are variable [264].

REFERENCES

1. Webb WR, Müller NL, Naidich DP. Standardized terms for high-resolution computed tomography of the lung: a proposed glossary. *J Thorac Imag* 1993;8:167–185.
2. Austin JH, Müller NL, Friedman PJ, et al. Glossary of terms for CT of the lungs: recommendations of the Nomenclature Committee of the Fleischner Society. *Radiology* 1996;200:327–331.
3. Remy-Jardin M, Remy J, Giraud F, et al. Computed tomography assessment of ground-glass opacity: semiology and significance. *J Thorac Imag* 1993;8:249–264.
4. Remy-Jardin M, Giraud F, Remy J, et al. Importance of ground-glass attenuation in chronic diffuse infiltrative lung disease: pathologic-CT correlation. *Radiology* 1993;189:693–698.
5. Leung AN, Miller RR, Müller NL. Parenchymal opacification in chronic infiltrative lung diseases: CT-pathologic correlation. *Radiology* 1993;188:209–214.
6. Müller NL, Colby TV. Idiopathic interstitial pneumonias: high-resolution CT and histologic findings. *Radiographics* 1997;17:1016–1022.
7. Gay SE, Kazerooni EA, Toews GB, et al. Idiopathic pulmonary fibrosis: predicting response to therapy and survival. *Am J Respir Crit Care Med* 1998;157:1063–1072.
8. Hommeyer SH, Godwin JD, Takasugi JE. Computed tomography of air-space disease. *Radiol Clin North Am* 1991;29:1065–1084.
9. Murata K, Herman PG, Khan A, et al. Intralobular distribution of oleic acid-induced pulmonary edema in the pig: evaluation by high-resolution CT. *Invest Radiol* 1989;24:647–653.
10. Todo G, Herman PG. High-resolution computed tomography of the pig lung. *Invest Radiol* 1986;21:689–696.
11. Primack SL, Hartman TE, Lee KS, et al. Pulmonary nodules and the CT halo sign. *Radiology* 1994;190:513–515.
12. Greene R. Adult respiratory distress syndrome: acute alveolar damage. *Radiology* 1987;163:57–66.
13. Webb WR. High-resolution CT of the lung parenchyma. *Radiol Clin North Am* 1989;27:1085–1097.
14. Naidich DP, Zerhouni EA, Hutchins GM, et al. Computed tomography of the pulmonary parenchyma: part 1. Distal air-space disease. *J Thorac Imag* 1985;1:39–53.
15. Meziane MA, Hruban RH, Zerhouni EA, et al. High resolution CT of the lung parenchyma with pathologic correlation. *Radiographics* 1988;8:27–54.
16. Ikezoe J, Takashima S, Morimoto S, et al. CT appearance of acute radiation-induced injury in the lung. *AJR Am J Roentgenol* 1988;150:765–770.
17. Ikezoe J, Morimoto S, Takashima S, et al. Acute radiation induced pulmonary injury: computed tomographic evaluation. *Semin Ultrasound CT MR* 1990;11:409–416.
18. Logan PM. Thoracic manifestations of external beam radiotherapy. *AJR Am J Roentgenol* 1998;171:569–577.
19. Adler B, Padley S, Miller RR, et al. High-resolution CT of bronchioloalveolar carcinoma. *AJR Am J Roentgenol* 1992;159:275–277.
20. Ando M, Suga M. Hypersensitivity pneumonitis. *Curr Opin Pulm Med* 1997;3:391–395.
21. Chryssanthopoulos C, Fink JN. Hypersensitivity pneumonitis. *J Asthma* 1983;20:285–296.
22. Fraser RS, Müller NL, Colman N, et al. Inhalation of organic dusts. In: Fraser RS, Müller NL. Colman N, et al., eds. *Diagnosis of diseases of the chest*, 3rd ed. Philadelphia: WB Saunders, 1999:2361–2385.
23. Colby T, Carrington C. Interstitial Lung Disease. In: Thurlbeck WM, ed. *Pathology of the lung*. New York: Thieme Medical Publishers, 1995:589–737.
24. Tasaka S, Kanazawa M, Kawai C, et al. Fatal diffuse alveolar damage from bird fanciers' lung. *Respiration* 1997;64:307–309.
25. Cook PG, Wells IP, McGavin CR. The distribution of pulmonary shadowing in farmer's lung. *Clin Radiol* 1988;39:21–27.
26. Silver SF, Müller NL, Miller RR, et al. Hypersensitivity pneumonitis: evaluation with CT. *Radiology* 1989;173:441–445.
27. Seal RME, Hapke EJ, Thomas GO, et al. The pathology of the acute and chronic stages of farmer's lung. *Thorax* 1968;23:469.
28. Hargreave F, Hinson KF, Reid L, et al. The radiological appearances of allergic alveolitis due to bird sensitivity (bird fancier's lung). *Clin Radiol* 1972;23:1–6.
29. Mindell HJ. Roentgen findings in farmer's lung. *Radiology* 1970;97:341–346.

30. Yoshizawa Y, Ohtani Y, Hayakawa H, et al. Chronic hypersensitivity pneumonitis in Japan: a nationwide epidemiologic survey. *J Allergy Clin Immunol* 1999;103:315–320.
31. Hapke EJ, Seal RME, Thomas GO, et al. Farmer's lung: a clinical, radiographic, functional and serologic correlation of acute and chronic stages. *Thorax* 1968;23:451–468.
32. Hansell DM, Moskovic E. High-resolution computed tomography in extrinsic allergic alveolitis. *Clin Radiol* 1991;43:8–12.
33. Remy-Jardin M, Remy J, Wallaert B, et al. Subacute and chronic bird breeder hypersensitivity pneumonitis: sequential evaluation with CT and correlation with lung function tests and bronchoalveolar lavage. *Radiology* 1993;198:111–118.
34. Hansell DM, Wells AU, Padley SP, et al. Hypersensitivity pneumonitis: correlation of individual CT patterns with functional abnormalities. *Radiology* 1996;199:123–128.
35. Small JH, Flower CD, Traill ZC, et al. Air-trapping in extrinsic allergic alveolitis on computed tomography. *Clin Radiol* 1996;51:684–688.
36. Chung MH, Edinburgh KJ, Webb EM, et al. Mixed infiltrative and obstructive disease on high-resolution CT: differential diagnosis and functional correlates in a consecutive series. *J Thorac Imaging*
37. Arakawa H, Webb WR. Air-trapping on expiratory high-resolution CT scans in the absence of inspiratory scan abnormalities: correlation with pulmonary function tests and differential diagnosis. *AJR Am J Roentgenol* 1998;170:1349–1353.
38. Adler BD, Padley SP, Müller NL, et al. Chronic hypersensitivity pneumonitis: high-resolution CT and radiographic features in 16 patients. *Radiology* 1992;185:91–95.
39. Lynch DA, Newell JD, Logan PM, et al. Can CT distinguish hypersensitivity pneumonitis from idiopathic pulmonary fibrosis? *AJR Am J Roentgenol* 1995;165:807–811.
40. Grenier P, Valeyre D, Cluzel P, et al. Chronic diffuse interstitial lung disease: diagnostic value of chest radiography and high-resolution CT. *Radiology* 1991;179:123–132.
41. Lynch DA, Rose CS, Way D, et al. Hypersensitivity pneumonitis: sensitivity of high-resolution CT in a population-based study. *AJR Am J Roentgenol* 1992;159:469–472.
42. Buschman DL, Gamsu G, Waldron JA, et al. Chronic hypersensitivity pneumonitis: use of CT in diagnosis. *AJR Am J Roentgenol* 1992;159:957–960.
43. Swensen SJ, Aughenbaugh GL, Myers JL. Diffuse lung disease: diagnostic accuracy of CT in patients undergoing surgical biopsy of the lung. *Radiology* 1997;205:229–234.
44. Godwin JD, Müller NL, Takasugi JE. Pulmonary alveolar proteinosis: CT findings. *Radiology* 1988;169:609–613.
45. Murch CR, Carr DH. Computed tomography appearances of pulmonary alveolar proteinosis. *Clin Radiol* 1989;40:240–243.
46. Müller NL, Staples CA, Miller RR, et al. Disease activity in idiopathic pulmonary fibrosis: CT and pathologic correlation. *Radiology* 1987;165:731–734.
47. Hartman TE, Primack SL, Swensen SJ, et al. Desquamative interstitial pneumonia: thin-section CT findings in 22 patients. *Radiology* 1993;187:787–790.
48. Warren CP, Tse KS, Cherniack RM. Mechanical properties of the lung in extrinsic allergic alveolitis. *Thorax* 1978;33:315–321.
49. Allen JN, Davis WB. Eosinophilic lung diseases. *Am J Respir Crit Care Med* 1994;150:1423–1438.
50. Bain GA, Flower CD. Pulmonary eosinophilia. *Eur J Radiol* 1996;23:3–8.
51. Kim Y, Lee KS, Choi DC, et al. The spectrum of eosinophilic lung disease: radiologic findings. *J Comput Assist Tomogr* 1997;21:920–930.
52. Connolly B, Manson D, Eberhard A, et al. CT appearance of pulmonary vasculitis in children. *AJR Am J Roentgenol* 1996;167:901–904.
53. Primack SL, Müller NL. Radiologic manifestations of the systemic autoimmune diseases. *Clin Chest Med* 1998;19:573–586.
54. Gaensler EA, Carrington CB. Peripheral opacities in chronic eosinophilic pneumonia: the photographic negative of pulmonary edema. *AJR Am J Roentgenol* 1977;128:1–13.
55. Pearson DJ, Rosenow EC. Chronic eosinophilic pneumonia (Carrington's): a follow-up study. *Mayo Clin Proc* 1978;53:73–78.
56. Dines DE. Chronic eosinophilic pneumonia: a roentgenographic diagnosis [editorial]. *Mayo Clin Proc* 1978;53:129–130.
57. Jederlinic PJ, Sicilian L, Gaensler EA. Chronic eosinophilic pneumonia: a report of 19 cases and a review of the literature. *Medicine* 1988;67:154–162.
58. Libby DM, Murphy TF, Edwards A, et al. Chronic eosinophilic pneumonia: an unusual cause of acute respiratory failure. *Am Rev Respir Dis* 1980;122:497–500.
59. Mayo JR, Müller NL, Road J, et al. Chronic eosinophilic pneumonia: CT findings in six cases. *AJR Am J Roentgenol* 1989;153:727–730.
60. Ebara H, Ikezoe J, Johkoh T, et al. Chronic eosinophilic pneumonia: evolution of chest radiograms and CT features. *J Comput Assist Tomogr* 1994;18:737–744.
61. Müller NL, Staples CA, Miller RR. Bronchiolitis obliterans organizing pneumonia: CT features in 14 patients. *AJR Am J Roentgenol* 1990;154:983–987.
62. Bartter T, Irwin RS, Nash G, et al. Idiopathic bronchiolitis obliterans organizing pneumonia with peripheral infiltrates on chest roentgenogram. *Arch Intern Med* 1989;149:273–279.
63. Müller NL, Guerry-Force ML, Staples CA, et al. Differential diagnosis of bronchiolitis obliterans with organizing pneumonia and usual interstitial pneumonia: clinical, functional, and radiologic findings. *Radiology* 1987;162:151–156.
64. Glazer HS, Levitt RG, Shackelford GD. Peripheral pulmonary infiltrates in sarcoidosis. *Chest* 1984;86:741–744.
65. Allen JN, Pacht ER, Gadek JE, et al. Acute eosinophilic pneumonia as a reversible cause of noninfectious respiratory failure. *N Engl J Med* 1989;321:569–574.
66. Hayakawa H, Sato A, Toyoshima M, et al. A clinical study of idiopathic eosinophilic pneumonia. *Chest* 1994;105:1462–1466.
67. Cheon JE, Lee KS, Jung GS, et al. Acute eosinophilic pneumonia: radiographic and CT findings in six patients. *AJR Am J Roentgenol* 1996;167:1195–1199.
68. King MA, Pope-Harman AL, Allen JN, et al. Acute eosinophilic pneumonia: radiologic and clinical features. *Radiology* 1997;203:715–719.
69. Winn RE, Kollef MH, Meyer JI. Pulmonary involvement in the hypereosinophilic syndrome. *Chest* 1994;105:656–660.
70. Epstein DM, Taormina V, Gefter WB, et al. The hypereosinophilic syndrome. *Radiology* 1981;140:59–62.
71. Kang EY, Shim JJ, Kim JS, et al. Pulmonary involvement of idiopathic hypereosinophilic syndrome: CT findings in five patients. *J Comput Assist Tomogr* 1997;21:612–615.
72. Masi AT, Hunder GG, Lie JT, et al. The American College of Rheumatology 1990 criteria for the classification of Churg-Strauss syndrome (allergic granulomatosis and angiitis). *Arthritis Rheum* 1990;33:1094–1100.
73. Buschman DL, Waldron Jr JA, King Jr TE. Churg-Strauss pulmonary vasculitis: high-resolution computed tomography scanning and pathologic findings. *Am Rev Respir Dis* 1990;142:458–461.
74. Worthy SA, Müller NL, Hansell DM, et al. Churg-Strauss syndrome: the spectrum of pulmonary CT findings in 17 patients. *AJR Am J Roentgenol* 1998;170:297–300.
75. Ottesen EA, Nutman TB. Tropical pulmonary eosinophilia. *Annu Rev Med* 1992;43:417–424.
76. Im JG, Whang HY, Kim WS, et al. Pleuropulmonary paragonimiasis: radiologic findings in 71 patients. *AJR Am J Roentgenol* 1992;159:39–43.
77. Gefter WB. The spectrum of pulmonary aspergillosis. *J Thorac Imag* 1992;7:56–74.
78. Logan PM, Müller NL. High-resolution computed tomography and pathologic findings in pulmonary aspergillosis: a pictorial essay. *Can Assoc Radiol J* 1996;47:444–452.
79. Ward S, Heyneman LE, Flint JD, et al. Bronchocentric granulomatosis: computed tomographic findings in five patients. *Clin Radiol* 2000;55:296–300.
80. Yousem SA. The histological spectrum of chronic necrotizing forms of pulmonary aspergillosis. *Hum Pathol* 1997;28:650–656.
81. Lynch DA, Hay T, Newell Jr JD, et al. Pediatric diffuse lung disease: diagnosis and classification using high-resolution CT. *AJR Am J Roentgenol* 1999;173:713–718.
82. Epler GR, Colby TV, McLoud TC, et al. Bronchiolitis obliterans organizing pneumonia. *N Engl J Med* 1985;312:152–158.
83. Myers JL, Colby TV. Pathologic manifestations of bronchiolitis, constrictive bronchiolitis, cryptogenic organizing pneumonia and diffuse panbronchiolitis. *Clin Chest Med* 1993;14:611–623.

84. Epler GR, Snider GL, Gaensler EA, et al. Bronchiolitis and bronchitis in connective tissue disease. *JAMA* 1979;242:528–532.
85. Colby TV, Myers JL. The clinical and histologic spectrum of bronchiolitis obliterans including bronchiolitis obliterans organizing pneumonia (BOOP). *Semin Respir Dis* 1992;13:119–133.
86. Epler GR. Bronchiolitis obliterans organizing pneumonia: definition and clinical features. *Chest* 1992;102(S):2–6.
87. Camus P, Lombard J-N, Perrichon M, et al. Bronchiolitis obliterans-organizing pneumonia in patients taking acebutolol or amiodarone. *Thorax* 1989;44:711–715.
88. Camp M, Mehta JB, Whitson M. Bronchiolitis obliterans and *Nocardia asteroides* infection of the lung. *Chest* 1987;92:1107–1108.
89. Geddes DM. BOOP and COP. *Thorax* 1991;46:545–547.
90. du Bois RM, Geddes DM. Obliterative bronchiolitis, cryptogenic organizing pneumonitis and bronchiolitis obliterans organizing pneumonia: three names for two different conditions. *Eur Respir J* 1991;4:774–775.
91. Hansell DM. What are bronchiolitis obliterans organizing pneumonia (BOOP) and cryptogenic organizing pneumonia (COP)? *Clin Radiol* 1992;45:369–370.
92. Davison AG, Heard BE, McAllister WC, et al. Cryptogenic organizing pneumonitis. *Quart J Med* 1983;52:382–393.
93. ATS/ERS International Multidisciplinary Consensus Classification of Idiopathic Interstitial Pneumonias: General Principles and Guidelines. American Thoracic Society, Toronto, May 2000.
94. King TE. Overview of bronchiolitis. *Clin Chest Med* 1993;14:607–610.
95. Epler GR, Colby TV, McLoud TC, et al. Idiopathic bronchiolitis obliterans with organizing pneumonia. *N Engl J Med* 1985;312:152–159.
96. Chandler PW, Shin MS, Friedman SE, et al. Radiographic manifestations of bronchiolitis obliterans with organizing pneumonia vs. usual interstitial pneumonia. *AJR Am J Roentgenol* 1986;147:899–906.
97. Miki Y, Hatabu H, Takahashi M, et al. Computed tomography of bronchiolitis obliterans. *J Comput Assist Tomogr* 1988;12:512–514.
98. Bouchardy LM, Kuhlman JE, Ball WC, et al. CT findings in bronchiolitis obliterans organizing pneumonia (BOOP) with radiographic, clinical, and histologic correlation. *J Comput Assist Tomogr* 1993;17:352–357.
99. Lee KS, Kullnig P, Hartman TE, et al. Cryptogenic organizing pneumonia: CT findings in 43 patients. *AJR Am J Roentgenol* 1994;162:543–546.
100. Akira M, Yamamoto S, Sakatani M. Bronchiolitis obliterans organizing pneumonia manifesting as multiple large nodules or masses. *AJR Am J Roentgenol* 1998;170:291–295.
101. Nishimura K, Itoh H. High-resolution computed tomographic features of bronchiolitis obliterans organizing pneumonia. *Chest* 1992;102:26S–31S.
102. Gruden JF, Webb WR, Warnock M. Centrilobular opacities in the lung on high-resolution CT: diagnostic considerations and pathologic correlation. *AJR Am J Roentgenol* 1994;162:569–574.
103. Johkoh T, Müller NL, Cartier Y, et al. Idiopathic interstitial pneumonias: diagnostic accuracy of thin-section CT in 129 patients. *Radiology* 1999;211:555–560.
104. Katzenstein AL, Myers JL. Idiopathic pulmonary fibrosis: clinical relevance of pathologic classification. *Am J Respir Crit Care Med* 1998;157:1301–1315.
105. Katzenstein AL, Fiorelli RF. Nonspecific interstitial pneumonia/fibrosis: histologic features and clinical significance. *Am J Surg Pathol* 1994;18:136–147.
106. Park JS, Lee KS, Kim JS, et al. Nonspecific interstitial pneumonia with fibrosis: radiographic and CT findings in seven patients. *Radiology* 1995;195:645–648.
107. Nishiyama O, Kondoh Y, Taniguchi H, et al. Serial high resolution CT findings in nonspecific interstitial pneumonia/fibrosis. *J Comput Assist Tomogr* 2000;24:41–46.
108. Cottin V, Donsbeck AV, Revel D, et al. Nonspecific interstitial pneumonia: individualization of a clinicopathologic entity in a series of 12 patients. *Am J Respir Crit Care Med* 1998;158:1286–1293.
109. Kim TS, Lee KS, Chung MP, et al. Nonspecific interstitial pneumonia with fibrosis: high-resolution CT and pathologic findings. *AJR Am J Roentgenol* 1998;171:1645–1650.
110. Kim EY, Lee KS, Chung MP, et al. Nonspecific interstitial pneumonia with fibrosis: serial high-resolution CT findings with functional correlation. *AJR Am J Roentgenol* 1999;173:949–953.
111. Colby TV. Bronchiolitis. Pathologic considerations. *Am J Clin Pathol* 1998;109:101–109.
112. Müller NL, Miller RR. Diseases of the bronchioles: CT and histopathologic findings. *Radiology* 1995;196:3–12.
113. Remy-Jardin M, Remy J, Gosselin B, et al. Lung parenchymal changes secondary to cigarette smoking: pathologic-CT correlations. *Radiology* 1993;186:643–651.
114. King TE. Respiratory bronchiolitis-associated interstitial lung disease. *Clin Chest Med* 1993;14:693–698.
115. Myers JL, Veal CF, Shin MS, et al. Respiratory bronchiolitis causing interstitial lung disease: a clinicopathologic study of six cases. *Am Rev Respir Dis* 1987;135:880–884.
116. Yousem SA, Colby TV, Gaensler EA. Respiratory bronchiolitis-associated interstitial lung disease and its relationship to desquamative interstitial pneumonia. *Mayo Clin Proc* 1989;64:1373–1380.
117. Remy-Jardin M, Remy J, Boulenguez C, et al. Morphologic effects of cigarette smoking on airways and pulmonary parenchyma in healthy adult volunteers: CT evaluation and correlation with pulmonary function tests. *Radiology* 1993;186:107–115.
118. Heyneman LE, Ward S, Lynch DA, et al. Respiratory bronchiolitis, respiratory bronchiolitis-associated interstitial pneumonia: different entities or part of the spectrum of the same disease process? *AJR Am J Roentgenol* 1999;173:1617-1622.
119. Gruden JF, Webb WR. CT findings in a proved case of respiratory bronchiolitis. *AJR Am J Roentgenol* 1993;161:44–46.
120. Park J, Tuder R, Brown KK, et al. Respiratory bronchiolitis-associated interstitial lung disease: CT-pathologic correlation. *Radiology* 1998;209:179.
121. Holt RM, Schmidt RA, Godwin JD, et al. High resolution CT in respiratory bronchiolitis-associated interstitial lung disease. *J Comput Assist Tomogr* 1993;17:46–50.
122. Carrington CB, Gaensler EA, Coute RE, et al. Natural history and treated course of usual and desquamative interstitial pneumonia. *N Engl J Med* 1978;298:801–809.
123. Gaensler EA, Goff AM, Prowse CM. Desquamative interstitial pneumonia. *N Engl J Med* 1966;274:113–128.
124. Feigin DS, Friedman PJ. Chest radiography in DIP: a review of 37 patients. *AJR Am J Roentgenol* 1980;134:91–99.
125. Katzenstein ALA, Myers JL, Mazur MT. Acute interstitial pneumonia: a clinicopathologic, ultrastructural, and cell kinetic study. *Am J Surg Pathol* 1986;10:256–267.
126. Primack SL, Hartman TE, Ikezoe J, et al. Acute interstitial pneumonia: radiographic and CT findings in nine patients. *Radiology* 1993;188:817–820.
127. Olson J, Colby TV, Elliott CG. Hamman-Rich syndrome revisited. *Mayo Clin Proc* 1990;65:1538–1548.
128. Akira M. Computed tomography and pathologic findings in fulminant forms of idiopathic interstitial pneumonia. *J Thorac Imag* 1999;14:76–84.
129. Johkoh T, Müller NL, Taniguchi H, et al. Acute interstitial pneumonia: thin-section CT findings in 36 patients. *Radiology* 1999;211:859–863.
130. Ichikado K, Johkoh T, Ikezoe J, et al. Acute interstitial pneumonia: high-resolution CT findings correlated with pathology. *AJR Am J Roentgenol* 1997;168:333–338.
131. Rosen SH, Castleman B, Liebow AA. Pulmonary alveolar proteinosis. *N Engl J Med* 1958;258:1123–1144.
132. Wang BM, Stern EJ, Schmidt RA, et al. Diagnosing pulmonary alveolar proteinosis: a review and an update. *Chest* 1997;111:460–466.
133. Sargent EN, Morgan WKC. Silicosis. In: Preger L, ed. *Induced disease. Drug, irradiation, occupation*. New York: Grune & Stratton, 1980:297–315.
134. Bedrossian CW, Luna MA, Conklin RH, et al. Alveolar proteinosis as a consequence of immunosuppression: a hypothesis based on clinical and pathologic observations. *Hum Pathol* 1980;11[Suppl]:527–535.
135. Carnovale R, Zornoza J, Goldman AM, et al. Pulmonary alveolar proteinosis: its association with hematologic malignancy and lymphoma. *Radiology* 1977;122:303–306.
136. Davidson JM, MacLeod WM. Pulmonary alveolar proteinosis. *Br J Dis Chest* 1969;63:13–28.
137. Teja K, Cooper PH, Squires JE, et al. Pulmonary alveolar proteinosis in four siblings. *N Engl J Med* 1981;305:1390–1392.

138. Miller RR, Churg AM, Hutcheon M, et al. Pulmonary alveolar proteinosis and aluminum dust exposure. *Am Rev Respir Dis* 1984;130:312–315.

139. Thurlbeck WM, Miller RR, Müller NL, et al. Chronic infiltrative lung disease. In: *Diffuse diseases of the lung: a team approach.* Philadelphia: Decker, 1991:102–115.

140. Kariman K, Kylstra JA, Spock A. Pulmonary alveolar proteinosis: prospective clinical experience in 23 patients for 15 years. *Lung* 1984;162:223–231.

141. Rogers RM, Levin DC, Gray BA, et al. Physiologic effects of bronchopulmonary lavage in alveolar proteinosis. *Am Rev Respir Dis* 1978;118:255–264.

142. Prakash UBS, Barham SS, Carpenter HA, et al. Pulmonary alveolar phospholipoproteinosis: experience with 34 cases and a review. *Mayo Clin Proc* 1987;62:499–518.

143. Ramirez RJ. Pulmonary alveolar proteinosis. *AJR Am J Roentgenol* 1964;92:571–577.

144. Genereux GP. CT of acute and chronic distal air space (alveolar) disease. *Semin Roentgenol* 1984;19:211–221.

145. Lee KN, Levin DL, Webb WR, et al. Pulmonary alveolar proteinosis: high-resolution CT, chest radiographic, and functional correlations. *Chest* 1997;111:989–995.

146. Miller PA, Ravin CE, Walker Smith GJ, et al. Pulmonary alveolar proteinosis with interstitial involvement. *AJR Am J Roentgenol* 1981;137:1069–1071.

147. Zimmer WE, Chew FS. Pulmonary alveolar proteinosis [clinical conference]. *AJR Am J Roentgenol* 1993;161:26.

148. Franquet T, Giménez A, Bordes R, et al. The crazy-paving pattern in exogenous lipoid pneumonia: CT-pathologic correlation. *AJR Am J Roentgenol* 1998;170:315–317.

149. Johkoh T, Itoh H, Müller NL, et al. Crazy-paving appearance at thin-section CT: spectrum of disease and pathologic findings. *Radiology* 1999;211:155–160.

150. Joshi RR, Cholankeril JV. Computed tomography in lipoid pneumonia. *J Comput Assist Tomogr* 1985;9:211–213.

151. Seo JB, Im JG, Kim WS, et al. Shark liver oil-induced lipoid pneumonia in pigs: correlation of thin-section CT and histopathologic findings. *Radiology* 1999;212:88–96.

152. Hugosson CO, Riff EJ, Moore CC, et al. Lipoid pneumonia in infants: a radiological-pathological study. *Pediatr Radiol* 1991;21:193–197.

153. Lee KS, Müller NL, Hale V, et al. Lipoid pneumonia: CT findings. *J Comput Assist Tomogr* 1995;19:48–51.

154. Murata K, Itoh H, Todo G, et al. Centrilobular lesions of the lung: demonstration by high-resolution CT and pathologic correlation. *Radiology* 1986;161:641–645.

155. Im JG, Itoh H, Shim YS, et al. Pulmonary tuberculosis: CT findings—early active disease and sequential change with antituberculous therapy. *Radiology* 1993;186:653–660.

156. Murata K, Khan A, Herman PG. Pulmonary parenchymal disease: evaluation with high-resolution CT. *Radiology* 1989;170:629–635.

157. Genereux GP. The Fleischner lecture: computed tomography of diffuse pulmonary disease. *J Thorac Imag* 1989;4:50–87.

158. Hartman TE, Primack SL, Müller NL, et al. Diagnosis of thoracic complications in AIDS: accuracy of CT. *AJR Am J Roentgenol* 1994;162:547–553.

159. Primack SL, Müller NL. High-resolution computed tomography in acute diffuse lung disease in the immunocompromised patient. *Radiol Clin North Am* 1994;32:731–744.

160. Kuhlman JE. Pneumocystic infections: the radiologist's perspective. *Radiology* 1996;198:623–635.

161. McGuinness G. Changing trends in the pulmonary manifestations of AIDS. *Radiol Clin North Am* 1997;35:1029–1082.

162. Hoover DR, Saah AJ, Bacellar H, et al. Clinical manifestations of AIDS in the era of *Pneumocystis* prophylaxis. Multicenter AIDS Cohort Study. *N Engl J Med* 1993;329:1922–1926.

163. Hirschtick RE, Glassroth J, Jordan MC, et al. Bacterial pneumonia in persons infected with the human immunodeficiency virus. Pulmonary Complications of HIV Infection Study Group. *N Engl J Med* 1995; 333:845–851.

164. Markowitz GS, Concepcion L, Factor SM, et al. Autopsy patterns of disease among subgroups of an inner-city Bronx AIDS population. *J Acquir Immune Defic Syndr Hum Retrovirol* 1996;13:48–54.

165. McGuinness G, Gruden JF. Viral and *Pneumocystis carinii* infections of the lung in the immunocompromised host. *J Thorac Imag* 1999;14:25–36.

166. Stover DE. Pneumocystis carinii: an update. *Pulmon Perspect* 1994;11:3–5.

167. Foley NM, Griffiths MH, Miller RF. Histologically atypical *Pneumocystis carinii* pneumonia. *Thorax* 1993;48:996–1001.

168. Travis WD, Pittaluga S, Lipschik GY, et al. Atypical pathologic manifestations of *Pneumocystis carinii* pneumonia in the acquired immune deficiency syndrome. *Am J Surg Path* 1990;14:615–625.

169. Murray JF, Mills J. Pulmonary infectious complications of human immunodeficiency virus infection. *Am Rev Respir Dis* 1990; 141:1356–1372.

170. Suster B, Ackerman M, Orenstein M, et al. Pulmonary manifestations of AIDS: review of 106 episodes. *Radiology* 1987;161:87–93.

171. DeLorenzo LJ, Huang CT, Maguire GP, et al. Roentgenographic patterns of *Pneumocystis carinii* pneumonia in 104 patients with AIDS. *Chest* 1987;91:323–327.

172. Naidich DP, Garay SM, Leitman BS, et al. Radiographic manifestations of pulmonary disease in the acquired immuno-deficiency syndrome (AIDS). *Semin Roentgenol* 1987;22:14–30.

173. Goodman PC. *Pneumocystis carinii* pneumonia. *J Thorac Imag* 1991;6:16–21.

174. Goodman PC, Daley C, Minagi H. Spontaneous pneumothorax in AIDS patients with *Pneumocystis carinii* pneumonia. *AJR Am J Roentgenol* 1986;147:29–31.

175. Sandhu JS, Goodman PC. Pulmonary cysts associated with *Pneumocystis carinii* pneumonia in patients with AIDS. *Radiology* 1989;173:33–35.

176. Barrio JL, Suarez M, Rodriguez JL, et al. *Pneumocystis carinii* pneumonia presenting as cavitating and noncavitating solitary pulmonary nodules in patients with the acquired immunodeficiency syndrome. *Am Rev Resp Dis* 1986;134:1094–1096.

177. Radin DR, Baker EL, Klatt EC, et al. Visceral and nodal calcification in patients with AIDS-related Pneumocystis carinii infection. *AJR Am J Roentgenol* 1990;154:27–31.

178. Wasser LS, Brown E, Talavera W. Miliary PCP in AIDS. *Chest* 1989;96:693–695.

179. Boiselle PM, Crans Jr CA, Kaplan MA. The changing face of *Pneumocystis carinii* pneumonia in AIDS patients. *AJR Am J Roentgenol* 1999;172:1301–1309.

180. Chaffey MH, Klein JS, Gamsu G, et al. Radiographic distribution of Pneumocystis carinii pneumonia in patients with AIDS treated with prophylactic inhaled pentamidine. *Radiology* 1990;175:715–719.

181. Chow C, Templeton PA, White CS. Lung cysts associated with Pneumocystis carinii pneumonia: radiographic characteristics, natural history, and complications. *AJR Am J Roentgenol* 1993;161:527–531.

182. Naidich DP, Garay SM, Goodman PC, et al. Pulmonary manifestations of AIDS. In: *Radiology of acquired immune deficiency syndrome.* New York: Raven, 1988:47–77.

183. Kuhlman JE, Kavuru M, Fishman EK, et al. Pneumocystis carinii pneumonia: spectrum of parenchymal CT findings. *Radiology* 1990;175:711–714.

184. Bergin CJ, Wirth RL, Berry GJ, et al. Pneumocystis carinii pneumonia: CT and HRCT observations. *J Comput Assist Tomogr* 1990;14:756–759.

185. Gruden JF, Huang L, Turner J, et al. High-resolution CT in the evaluation of clinically suspected Pneumocystis carinii pneumonia in AIDS patients with normal, equivocal, or nonspecific radiographic findings. *AJR Am J Roentgenol* 1997;169:967–975.

186. Schinella RA, Clancey J, Fazzini E, et al. Pneumocystis carinii as a cause of pulmonary fibrosis (abst). *Am Rev Res Dis* 1986;133A:180.

187. McGuinness G, Naidich DP, Garay SM, et al. AIDS associated bronchiectasis: CT features. *J Comput Assist Tomogr* 1993; 17:260–266.

188. Gurney JW, Bates FT. Pulmonary cystic disease: comparison of *Pneumocystis carinii* pneumatoceles and bullous emphysema due to intravenous drug abuse. *Radiology* 1989;173:27–31.

189. Kuhlman JE, Knowles MC, Fishman EK, et al. Premature bullous pulmonary damage in AIDS: CT diagnosis. *Radiology* 1989; 173:23–26.

190. Klein JS, Warnock M, Webb WR, et al. Cavitating and noncavitating granulomas in AIDS patients with Pneumocystis pneumonitis. *AJR Am J Roentgenol* 1989;152:753–754.

191. Sheikh S, Madiraju K, Steiner P, et al. Bronchiectasis in pediatric AIDS. *Chest* 1997;112:1202–1207.

192. Feuerstein I, Archer A, Pluda JM, et al. Thin-walled cavities, cysts, and pneumothorax in *Pneumocystis carinii* pneumonia: further observations with histopathologic correlation. *Radiology* 1990;174:697–702.

193. Panicek DM. Cystic pulmonary lesions in patients with AIDS [editorial]. *Radiology* 1989;173:12–14.

194. Huang RM, Naidich DP, Lubat E, et al. Septic pulmonary emboli: CT-radiographic correlation. *AJR Am J Roentgenol* 1989;153:41–45.

195. Kuhlman JE, Fishman EK, Teigen C. Pulmonary septic emboli: diagnosis with CT. *Radiology* 1990;174:211–213.

196. Mayor B, Schnyder P, Giron J, et al. Mediastinal and hilar lymphadenopathy due to *Pneumocystis carinii* infection in AIDS patients: CT features. *J Comput Assist Tomogr* 1994;18:408–411.

197. Bianco R, Arborio G, Mariani P, et al. [*Pneumocystis carinii* lung infections in AIDS patients: a study with high-resolution computed tomography (HRCT)]. *Radiol Med (Torino)* 1996;91:370–376.

198. Gruden JF, Klein JS, Webb WR. Percutaneous transthoracic needle biopsy in AIDS: analysis in 32 patients. *Radiology* 1993;189:567–571.

199. McGuinness G, Gruden JF, Bhalla M, et al. AIDS-related airway disease. *AJR Am J Roentgenol* 1997;168:67–77.

200. Edinburgh KJ, Jasmer RM, Huang L, et al. Multiple pulmonary nodules in AIDS: usefulness of CT in distinguishing among potential causes. *Radiology* 2000;214:427–432.

201. Wassermann K, Pothoff G, Kirn E, et al. Chronic *Pneumocystis carinii* pneumonia in AIDS. *Chest* 1993;104:667–672.

202. Kang EY, Staples CA, McGuinness G, et al. Detection and differential diagnosis of pulmonary infections and tumors in patients with AIDS: value of chest radiography versus CT. *AJR Am J Roentgenol* 1996;166:15–19.

203. Richards PJ, Riddell L, Reznek RH, et al. High resolution computed tomography in HIV patients with suspected Pneumocystis carinii pneumonia and a normal chest radiograph. *Clin Radiol* 1996;51:689–693.

204. Kirshenbaum KJ, Burke R, Fanapour F, et al. Pulmonary high-resolution computed tomography versus gallium scintigraphy: diagnostic utility in the diagnosis of patients with AIDS who have chest symptoms and normal or equivocal chest radiographs. *J Thorac Imag* 1998;13:52–57.

205. Brown MJ, Miller RR, Müller NL. Acute lung disease in the immunocompromised host: CT and pathologic examination findings. *Radiology* 1994;190:247–254.

206. Armitage JO. Bone marrow transplantation. *N Engl J Med* 1994;330:827–838.

207. Crawford SE, Hackman RC, Clark JG. Open-lung biopsy diagnosis of diffuse pulmonary infiltrates after marrow transplantation. *Chest* 1988;94:949–953.

208. Maurer JR, Tullis E, Grossman RF, et al. Infectious complications following isolated lung transplantation. *Chest* 1992;101:1056–1059.

209. Herman S, Rappaport D, Weisbrod G, et al. Single-lung transplantation: imaging features. *Radiology* 1989;170:89–93.

210. O'Donovan P. Imaging of complications of lung transplantation. *RadioGraphics* 1993;13:787–796.

211. Moore EH, Webb WR, Amend WJC. Pulmonary infections in renal transplantation patients treated with cyclosporin. *Radiology* 1988;167:97–103.

212. Winer-Muram HT, Gurney JW, Bozeman PM, et al. Pulmonary complications after bone marrow transplantation. *Radiol Clin North Am* 1996;34:97–117.

213. Millar AB, Patou GM, Miller RF, et al. Cytomegalovirus in the lungs of patients with AIDS: respiratory pathogen or passenger? *Am Rev Resp Dis* 1990;141:1474–1477.

214. Wallace MJ, Hannah J. Cytomegalovirus pneumonitis in patients with AIDS: findings in an autopsy series. *Chest* 1987;92:198–203.

215. Klatt EC, Shibata D. Cytomegalovirus infection in the acquired immunodeficiency syndrome: clinical and autopsy findings. *Arch Pathol Lab Med* 1988;112:540–544.

216. Miles PR, Baughman RP, Linnemann CC. Cytomegalovirus in the bronchoalveolar lavage fluid in patients with AIDS. *Chest* 1990;97:1072–1076.

217. Hoover DR, Saah AJ, Bacellar H, et al. Clinical manifestations of AIDS in the era of Pneumocystis prophylaxis. *N Engl J Med* 1993;329:1922–1926.

218. Aafedt BC, Halvorsen R, Tylen U, et al. Cytomegalovirus pneumonia: computed tomography findings. *Can Assoc Radiol J* 1990;41:276–280.

219. Kang EY, Patz EF, Jr., Müller NL. Cytomegalovirus pneumonia in transplant patients: CT findings. *J Comput Assist Tomogr* 1996;20:295–299.

220. McGuinness G, Scholes JV, Garay SM, et al. Cytomegalovirus pneumonitis: spectrum of parenchymal CT findings with pathologic correlation in 21 AIDS patients. *Radiology* 1994;192:451–459.

221. Abe K, Suzuki K, Kamata N, et al. [High-resolution CT findings in cytomegalovirus pneumonitis after bone marrow transplantation]. *Nippon Igaku Hoshasen Gakkai Zasshi* 1998;58:7–11.

222. Matar LD, McAdams HP, Palmer SM, et al. Respiratory viral infections in lung transplant recipients: radiologic findings with clinical correlation. *Radiology* 1999;213:735–742.

223. Palmer SM, Jr., Henshaw NG, Howell DN, et al. Community respiratory viral infection in adult lung transplant recipients. *Chest* 1998;113:944–950.

224. Feldman S. Varicella-zoster virus pneumonitis. *Chest* 1994;106:22S–27S.

225. Gogos CA, Bassaris HP, Vagenakis AG. Varicella pneumonia in adults. A review of pulmonary manifestations, risk factors and treatment. *Respiration* 1992;59:339–343.

226. Kim JS, Ryu CW, Lee SI, et al. High-resolution CT findings of varicella-zoster pneumonia. *AJR Am J Roentgenol* 1999;172:113–116.

227. Fraisse P, Faller M, Rey D, et al. Recurrent varicella pneumonia complicating an endogenous reactivation of chickenpox in an HIV-infected adult patient. *Eur Respir J* 1998;11:776–778.

228. Krinzman S, Basgoz N, Kradin R, et al. Respiratory syncytial virus-associated infections in adult recipients of solid organ transplants. *J Heart Lung Transplant* 1998;17:202–210.

229. Ko JP, Shepard JA, Sproule MW, et al. CT manifestations of respiratory syncytial virus infection in lung transplant recipients. *J Comput Assist Tomogr* 2000;24:235–241.

230. Mansel JK, Rosenow ECD, Smith TF, et al. *Mycoplasma pneumoniae* pneumonia. *Chest* 1989;95:639–646.

231. Tanaka N, Matsumoto T, Kuramitsu T, et al. High resolution CT findings in community-acquired pneumonia. *J Comput Assist Tomogr* 1996;20:600–608.

232. Chan ED, Kalayanamit T, Lynch DA, et al. *Mycoplasma pneumoniae*-associated bronchiolitis causing severe restrictive lung disease in adults: report of three cases and literature review. *Chest* 1999;115:1188–1194.

233. Putman CE, Curtis AM, Simeone JF, et al. *Mycoplasma pneumonia*. Clinical and roentgenographic patterns. *Am J Roentgenol Radium Ther Nucl Med* 1975;124:417–422.

234. Gückel C, Benz-Bohm G, Widemann B. Mycoplasmal pneumonias in childhood. Roentgen features, differential diagnosis and review of literature. *Pediatr Radiol* 1989;19:499–503.

235. Reittner P, Müller NL, Heyneman L, et al. *Mycoplasma pneumoniae* pneumonia: radiographic and high-resolution CT features in 28 patients. *AJR Am J Roentgenol* 1999;174:37–41.

236. Coultas DB, Samet JM, Butler C. Bronchiolitis obliterans due to Mycoplasma pneumoniae. *West J Med* 1986;144:471–474.

237. Wohl ME, Chernick V. State of the art: bronchiolitis. *Am Rev Respir Dis* 1978;118:759–781.

238. Arakawa H, Webb WR, McCowin M, et al. Inhomogeneous lung attenuation at thin-section CT: diagnostic value of expiratory scans. *Radiology* 1998;206:89–94.

239. Kim CK, Chung CY, Kim JS, et al. Late abnormal findings on high-resolution computed tomography after *Mycoplasma* pneumonia. *Pediatrics* 2000;105:372–378.

240. Syrjälä H, Broas M, Suramo I, et al. High-resolution computed tomography for the diagnosis of community-acquired pneumonia. *Clin Infect Dis* 1998;27:358–363.

241. Boyce NW, Holdsworth SR. Pulmonary manifestations of the clinical syndrome of acute glomerulonephritis and lung hemorrhage. *Am J Kidney Dis* 1986;8:31–36.

242. Cheah FK, Sheppard MN, Hansell DM. Computed tomography of diffuse pulmonary haemorrhage with pathological correlation. *Clin Radiol* 1993;48:89–93.

243. Witte R, Gurney J, Robbins R, et al. Diffuse pulmonary alveolar hemorrhage after bone narrow transplantation: radiographic findings in 39 patients. *AJR Am J Roentgenol* 1991;157:461–464.

244. Primack SL, Miller RR, Müller NL. Diffuse pulmonary hemorrhage: clinical, pathologic, and imaging features. *AJR Am J Roentgenol* 1995;164:295–300.

245. Seely JM, Effmann EL, Müller NL. High-resolution CT of pediatric lung disease: imaging findings. *AJR Am J Roentgenol* 1997; 168:1269–1275.

246. Ketai LH, Godwin JD. A new view of pulmonary edema and acute respiratory distress syndrome. *J Thorac Imag* 1998;13:147–171.

247. Gluecker T, Capasso P, Schnyder P, et al. Clinical and radiologic features of pulmonary edema. *Radiographics* 1999;19:1507–1531; discussion 1532–1533.

248. Webb WR, Stein MG, Finkbeiner WE, et al. Normal and diseased isolated lungs: high-resolution CT. *Radiology* 1988;166:81–87.

249. Bessis L, Callard P, Gotheil C, et al. High-resolution CT of parenchymal lung disease: precise correlation with histologic findings. *Radiographics* 1992;12:45–58.

250. Hedlund LW, Vock P, Effmann EL, et al. Hydrostatic pulmonary edema: an analysis of lung density changes by computed tomography. *Invest Radiol* 1984;19:254–262.

251. Forster BB, Müller NL, Mayo JR, et al. High-resolution computed tomography of experimental hydrostatic pulmonary edema. *Chest* 1992;101:1434–1437.

252. Scillia P, Delcroix M, Lejeune P, et al. Hydrostatic pulmonary edema: evaluation with thin-section CT in dogs. *Radiology* 1999;211:161–168.

253. Storto ML, Kee ST, Golden JA, et al. Hydrostatic pulmonary edema: high-resolution CT findings. *AJR Am J Roentgenol* 1995;165:817–820.

254. Bernard GR, Artigas A, Brigham KL, et al. The American-European Consensus Conference on ARDS. Definitions, mechanisms, relevant outcomes, and clinical trial coordination. *Am J Respir Crit Care Med* 1994;149:818–824.

255. Goodman LR. Congestive heart failure and adult respiratory distress syndrome. New insights using computed tomography. *Radiol Clin North Am* 1996;34:33–46.

256. Müller-Leisse C, Klosterhalfen B, Hauptmann S, et al. Computed tomography and histologic results in the early stages of endotoxin-injured pig lungs as a model for adult respiratory distress syndrome. *Invest Radiol* 1993;28:39–45.

257. Arakawa H, Kurihara Y, Nakajima Y. Pulmonary fat embolism syndrome: CT findings in six patients. *J Comput Assist Tomogr* 2000;24:24–29.

258. Tagliabue M, Casella TC, Zincone GE, et al. CT and chest radiography in the evaluation of adult respiratory distress syndrome. *Acta Radiol* 1994;35:230–234.

259. Goodman LR, Fumagalli R, Tagliabue P, et al. Adult respiratory distress syndrome due to pulmonary and extrapulmonary causes: CT, clinical, and functional correlations. *Radiology* 1999;213:545–552.

260. Owens CM, Evans TW, Keogh BF, et al. Computed tomography in established adult respiratory distress syndrome. Correlation with lung injury score. *Chest* 1994;106:1815–1821.

261. Desai SR, Wells AU, Rubens MB, et al. Acute respiratory distress syndrome: CT abnormalities at long-term follow-up. *Radiology* 1999;210:29–35.

262. Saxon RR, Klein JS, Bar MH, et al. Pathogenesis of pulmonary edema during interleukin-2 therapy: correlation of chest radiographic and clinical findings in 54 patients. *AJR Am J Roentgenol* 1991;156:281–285.

263. Ketai LH, Kelsey CA, Jordan K, et al. Distinguishing hantavirus pulmonary syndrome from acute respiratory distress syndrome by chest radiography: are there different radiographic manifestations of increased alveolar permeability? *J Thorac Imag* 1998;13:172–177.

264. Bartsch P. High altitude pulmonary edema. *Respiration* 1997;64:435–443.

CHAPTER 7

Diseases Characterized Primarily by Cysts and Emphysema

This disparate group of diseases has in common the presence of focal, multifocal, or diffuse parenchymal lucencies and lung destruction, which may be associated with the presence of lung cysts or emphysema. These diseases include pulmonary Langerhans cell histiocytosis (LCH), lymphangioleiomyomatosis (LAM), and different types of emphysema. Other causes of focal parenchymal lucencies or cysts, including airways diseases (both large and small), pulmonary fibrosis with honeycombing, and infectious diseases with resulting pneumatoceles or cavities, are discussed in Chapters 3, 4, 6, and 8.

PULMONARY LANGERHANS CELL HISTIOCYTOSIS (PULMONARY HISTIOCYTOSIS X)

Collectively, the term *Langerhans cell histiocytosis* (LCH) refers to a group of diseases of unknown etiology often recognized in childhood, in which Langerhans cell accumulations involve one or more body systems, including bone, lung, pituitary gland, mucous membranes and skin, lymph nodes, and liver [1,2]; this disease is also referred to as *histiocytosis X* or *eosinophilic granuloma*. Lung involvement in LCH is common and may be an isolated abnormality. In a review of 314 patients who had histologically proven LCH, pulmonary LCH was identified in 129 patients (40.8%), with isolated pulmonary involve-

ment occurring in 87 patients (28%) [1]. In patients who had multisystem disease in addition to pulmonary involvement, sites most often affected included bone and the pituitary gland [1].

Pathology

In its early stage, pulmonary LCH is characterized by the presence of granulomas containing large numbers of Langerhans cells and eosinophils, resulting in destruction of lung tissue [3]. LCH lesions are strikingly peribronchiolar in distribution, leading some to consider LCH a form of cellular bronchiolitis [2]. In its later stages, the cellular granulomas are replaced by fibrosis and the formation of lung cysts [4,5].

In normal subjects, Langerhans cells are exclusively found scattered among bronchial and bronchiolar epithelial cells. Functionally, they serve as antigen presenting cells or sentinels, processing and transporting antigens to regional lymph tissue with subsequent T-cell activation. Although studies have shown that LCH represents a clonal proliferation of cells [6], it is not thought that this disease is neoplastic. It is more likely that LCH in adults represents an uncontrolled or abnormal immune response initiated *in situ* by Langerhans cells in response to an unidentified antigenic stimulus [7]. Evidence that the lesions in LCH result from cellular recruitment rather than neoplastic cell proliferation include a lack of cellular atypia, absence of focal tissue invasion, and near-complete absence of Langerhans cells in late lesions.

In addition to peribronchiolar lesions, it has become apparent that in patients who have late-stage disease, LCH is also associated with a form of pulmonary vasculitis that leads to severe pulmonary hypertension in up to 80% of cases [3]. In one study of 21 patients who had end-stage pulmonary LCH associated with severe pulmonary hypertension, histopathologic evaluation revealed a proliferative vasculopathy involving muscular arteries and veins, with evidence of medial hypertrophy and intimal and subintimal fibrosis with resulting arterial obliteration in 60% of the cases [8]. Strikingly, these findings occurred in regions unaffected by Langerhans cells. Furthermore, follow-up histologic evaluation showed progression of vascular lesions in the absence of progression of granulomatous disease. In comparison to patients who have pulmonary hypertension due to end-stage idiopathic pulmonary fibrosis (IPF) or emphysema, pulmonary hypertension in patients who have LCH is significantly more severe despite significantly better expiratory function, suggesting that pulmonary hypertension in these patients represents a specific entity and not simply the result of chronic hypoxia. In addition to arterial disease, patients who have severe LCH are also predisposed to develop pulmonary venoocclusive disease [8,9].

Clinical Findings

LCH is an uncommon lung disease. Gaensler et al. [10] found LCH in only 3.4% of 502 patients who had open-lung biopsy for chronic, diffuse infiltrative lung disease.

More than 90% of patients who have pulmonary LCH are smokers, and this disease is considered to be related to smoking in most patients [3,11–16]. In a review of 87 patients who had isolated pulmonary involvement by LCH, only three were nonsmokers [1]. The majority of patients who have pulmonary LCH are young or middle-aged adults (average age, 32 years). Although previous reports have stressed a male preponderance, studies confirm that men and women are equally affected, likely the result of increasing tobacco use by women. Common presenting symptoms include cough and dyspnea [4,5]. Up to 20% of patients present with pneumothorax [11].

Compared to patients who have multisystem disease, the prognosis in patients who have isolated pulmonary involvement is good; the disease regresses spontaneously in 25% of patients and stabilizes clinically and radiographically in 50% of patients. In the remaining 25% of cases, the disease follows a progressive downhill course, resulting in diffuse cystic lung destruction. In a small minority of cases, death results from respiratory insufficiency, pulmonary hypertension, or both [1,2]. For example, in a review of 87 patients who had isolated pulmonary disease, 74 patients (85%) ultimately became disease-free, and three patients had progressive disease resulting in severe pulmonary fibrosis and pulmonary hypertension [1]. In two patients, coexisting lung carcinomas were also identified.

Although spontaneous regression of disease is common, disease recurrence has been documented to occur up to 7.5 years after the initial presentation [17]. Furthermore, there is no clear correlation between smoking history and recrudescence of disease, with nodules recurring in some patients after smoking cessation.

Radiographic Findings

The radiographic findings of LCH include reticular, nodular, and reticulonodular patterns, and honeycombing, often in combination [11–14,18]. Abnormalities are usually bilateral, predominantly involving the middle and upper lung zones, with relative sparing of the costophrenic angles [11,12]. Lung volumes are characteristically normal or increased.

High-Resolution Computed Tomography Findings

High-resolution computed tomography (HRCT) findings of pulmonary LCH have been reported by a number of authors [19–22]. HRCT findings closely mirror the gross pathologic appearances of this disease. In almost all patients, HRCT demonstrates cystic airspaces, which are usually less than 10 mm in diameter (see Figs 3-113 through 3-115; Figs. 7-1 and 7-2);

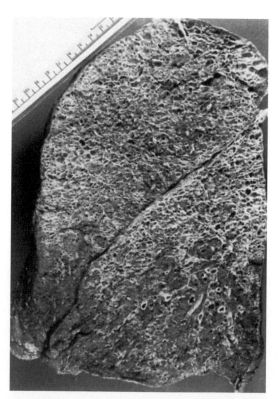

FIG. 7-1. Autopsy specimen from a patient who had pulmonary Langerhans cell histiocytosis. Fine cystic spaces predominate in the upper and middle lung zones. The lung bases are relatively spared. (From Müller NL, Miller RR. Computed tomography of chronic diffuse infiltrative lung disease: part 2. *Am Rev Respir Dis* 1990;142:1440–1448, with permission.)

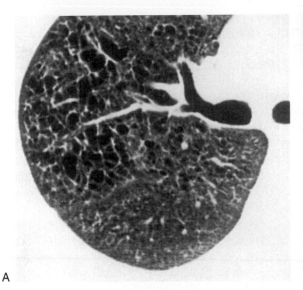

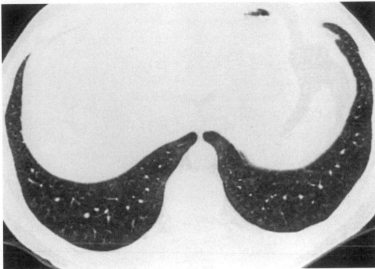

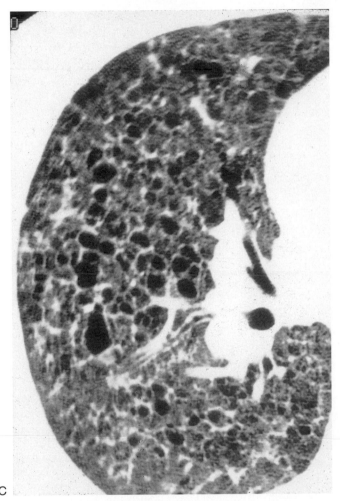

FIG. 7-2. Cystic pulmonary Langerhans cell histiocytosis (LCH). **A:** HRCT at the level of the right upper lobe bronchus in a 37-year-old man shows cystic airspaces with thin but well-defined walls. Some cysts are confluent or appear irregular in shape. Note the much milder disease in the superior segment of the right lower lobe. **B:** HRCT through the lung bases in the same patient shows that these are relatively spared. An upper-lobe predominance of abnormalities is characteristic of pulmonary LCH. **C:** Target-reconstructed image through the right lung in another patient who has documented LCH also showing extensive cystic lung disease. Note again the presence of bizarre-shaped cysts associated with architectural lung distortion.

these cysts are characteristic of LCH [19,20,23,24] and were seen in 17 of 18 patients studied by Brauner et al. [20] and all 12 patients studied by Giron et al. [24] (Table 7-1).

On HRCT, the lung cysts have walls that range from being thin and barely perceptible (see Fig. 3-113; Fig. 7-2) to being several millimeters in thickness (see Fig. 3-115;

Fig. 7-3). In a study by Grenier et al. [22], 88% of 51 patients who had LCH showed thin-walled (less than 2 mm) cysts on HRCT, whereas 53% of patients showed thick-walled (greater than 2 mm) cysts. The presence of distinct walls allows differentiation of these cysts from areas of emphysema, which can also be seen in some

TABLE 7-1. *HRCT findings in Langerhans cell histiocytosis*

Thin-walled lung cysts, some confluent or with bizarre shapes, usually smaller than 1 cm[a,b]

Thick-walled cysts[b]

Nodules, usually smaller than 1 to 5 mm, centrilobular and peribronchiolar, may be cavitary, may be seen in association with cysts[a,b]

Progression from 3 to 2 to 1[b]

Upper-lobe predominance in size and number of nodules or cysts, costophrenic angles spared[a,b]

Fine reticular opacities

Ground-glass opacity

Mosaic perfusion or air-trapping

[a]Findings most helpful in differential diagnosis.
[b]Most common findings.

patients. Although many cysts appear round, they can also have bizarre shapes, being bilobed, cloverleaf shaped, or branching in appearance (see Figs. 3-113 through 3-115; Fig. 7-2) [19]. These unusual shapes are postulated to occur because of fusion of several cysts, or perhaps because the cysts sometimes represent ectatic and thick-walled bronchi [19]; in the series reported by Brauner et al. [20], confluent or joined cysts with persisting septations were seen in more than two-thirds of patients. An upper lobe predominance in the size and number of cysts is common (see Fig. 3-113; Figs. 7-1 and 7-2). Large cysts or bullae (larger than 10 mm in diameter) are also seen in more than half of cases; some cysts are larger than 20 mm [20].

In some patients, cysts are the only abnormality visible on HRCT, but in the majority of cases, small nodules (usually smaller than 5 mm in diameter) are also present (see Fig. 3-59; Fig. 7-4) [19,20]; nodules were seen in 14 of 18

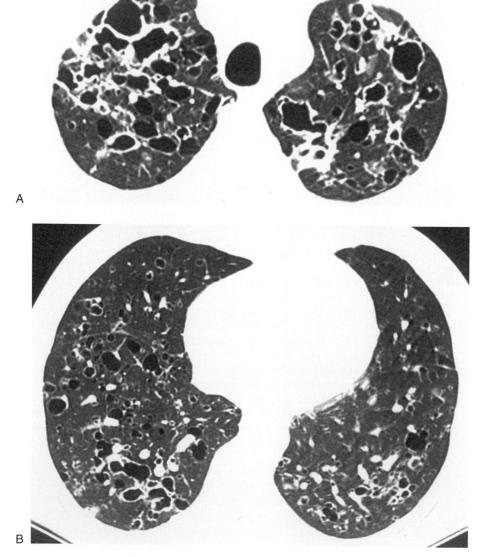

A

B

FIG. 7-3. HRCT in a 44-year-old man who has Langerhans cell histiocytosis and a history of cigarette smoking and shortness of breath. **A:** HRCT through the upper lobes shows numerous thick- and thin-walled lung cysts. Some cysts are very irregular in shape. The intervening lung parenchyma appears normal, and there is no evidence of diffuse fibrosis. **B:** Near the lung bases, cysts are smaller and less numerous. The presence of irregularly shaped cysts with an apical predominance is typical of Langerhans cell histiocytosis.

patients in Brauner's series, and in 14 of 17 patients in Moore's series [19,20]. Larger nodules, sometimes exceeding 1 cm, may also be seen, but they are less common. In the study by Grenier et al. [22], 47% of 51 patients who had LCH showed nodules smaller than 3 mm in diameter, whereas 45% of patients showed nodules ranging between 3 mm and 1 cm in diameter, and 24% of patients showed nodules exceeding 1 cm in size. Nodules can vary considerably in number in individual cases, probably depending on the activity of the disease; nodules can be few in number or myriad [19,20]. The margins of nodules are often irregular, particularly when there is surrounding cystic or reticular disease. On HRCT, many nodules can be seen to be peribronchial or peribronchiolar and therefore

centrilobular in location; in this disease, there is a tendency for granulomas to form around the bronchioles [20]. HRCT may be valuable in directing lung biopsy to areas showing lung nodules [20].

The nodules are usually homogeneous in appearance, but some nodules, particularly those larger than 1 cm in diameter, may show lucent centers, presumably corresponding to small cavities (Fig. 7-5) [25]. These cavities, however, may sometimes represent a dilated bronchiolar lumen surrounded by peribronchiolar granulomas and thickened interstitium [20]. In the study by Grenier et al. [22], 25% of 51 patients who had LCH showed cavitary nodules. In some patients, progression of cavitary nodules to cystic lesions has been observed [21,24]; this progression is characteristic and is described further below.

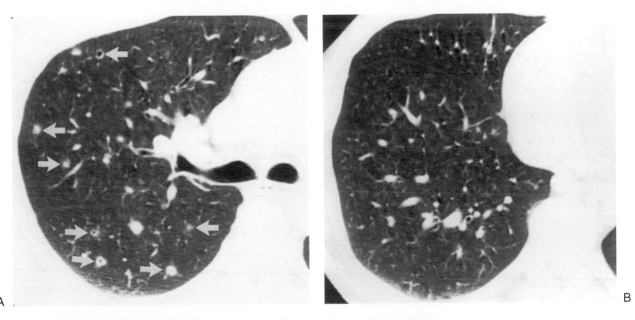

A

B

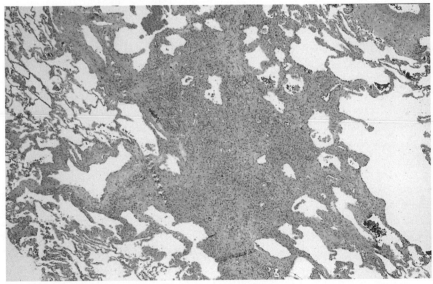

C

FIG. 7-4. Nodular Langerhans cell histiocytosis in a 30-year-old man. **A:** HRCT at the level of the right upper lobe bronchus shows several nodules (*arrows*). Some are solid, others are cavitated; some have smooth margins, others have irregular or poorly defined margins. **B:** HRCT through the right lower lung zone shows relative sparing of the lung bases. **C:** Histologic section from an open-lung biopsy shows a characteristic appearance of a poorly marginated granuloma surrounding a terminal bronchiole.

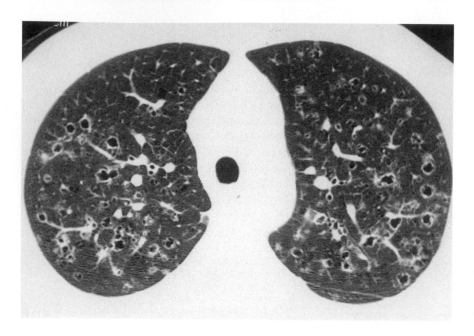

FIG. 7-5. Nodular Langerhans cell histiocytosis. Section below the carina showing diffuse, centrilobular thick-walled cavitary nodules in a more advanced state than that shown in Figure 7-3A.

In many patients who have cysts or nodules, the intervening lung parenchyma appears normal on HRCT, without evidence of fibrosis or septal thickening [19,20]. However, in a small percentage of cases, irregular interfaces (the interface sign) are present, or a fine reticular network of opacities is visible (Fig. 7-6) [20,24]. These fine reticular opacities may correlate with intralobular fibrosis or early cyst formation, or with the progression and confluence of cysts [24]. Ground-glass opacity is also sometimes seen but is not a prominent feature of this disease.

HRCT shows no consistent central or peripheral predominance of lesions [20,22], but in nearly all cases, the lung bases and the costophrenic sulci are relatively spared [19,26]. In Brauner's series [20] of 18 patients, two had abnormalities localized to the upper lobes and nine had disease that was predominant in the upper or middle lung zones; two patients had diffuse disease, but no patient had disease with a lower lung predominance. An upper lobar predominance was reported in 57% of Grenier's 51 patients [22], whereas a middle lung or basal predominance was never observed.

The evolution of lesions identified by CT has been reported. As documented by Brauner et al., in a study of 212 patients who had LCH, although nodular lesions were twice as frequent as cysts on initial CT studies, follow-up CT examinations showed cystic lesions twice as often as nodular disease [21]. Nodular opacities and thick-walled cysts typically underwent regression with time; at the same time, thin-walled cysts, linear densities, and emphysema either remained unchanged or progressed. These data support the previously noted conjecture that lesions in LCH undergo a predictable pathologic and radiologic evolution, beginning with centrilobular nodules (Fig. 7-4) and followed by cavitation (Fig. 7-5) and the formation of thick-walled cysts (Fig. 7-3), and, finally, the development of thin-walled cysts (Fig. 7-2). Whereas nodular lesions may regress spontaneously or be replaced by cysts, once formed, cystic lesions persist, eventually becoming indistinguishable from diffuse emphysema.

Evidence of mosaic perfusion on inspiratory scans and air-trapping on expiratory scans may also be seen in patients who have LCH and show nodular opacities or lung cysts (Fig. 7-7) [27]. This may reflect the presence of bronchiolar obstruction or air-trapping in cystic lung regions.

Utility of High-Resolution Computed Tomography

HRCT is superior to chest radiographs in demonstrating the morphology and distribution of lung abnormalities in patients who have LCH [19,20] and in making a specific diagnosis of this disease [22]. In fact, in many patients who have LCH and plain radiographic findings of reticular abnormalities, HRCT shows that the plain film findings reflect the presence of numerous superimposed lung cysts. As compared with chest radiographs, HRCT is significantly more sensitive in detecting small and large cysts and nodules smaller than 5 mm in diameter [20,22].

LCH is not associated with any consistent pattern of pulmonary function test (PFT) abnormalities, although airways obstruction is common [28] and probably related to peribronchiolar and bronchiolar luminal fibrosis [3]. In a study by Moore et al. [19], the extent of disease on HRCT correlated better ($r = -0.71$) with impairment in gas exchange, as assessed by the percent predicted carbon monoxide diffusing capacity, than did plain radiographic findings ($r = -0.57$). In another study [28], significant correlation ($r = 0.8$) between HRCT and diffusing capacity was also found. However, no correlation has been shown between CT findings and PFT findings of obstruction [19,28]. Air-trapping in association with lung cysts has

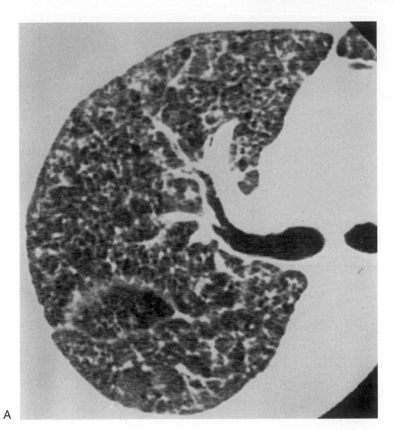

A

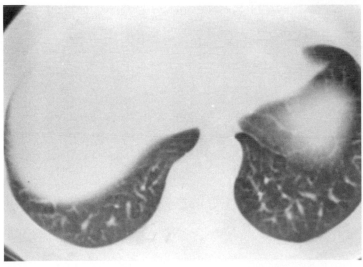

B

FIG. 7-6. End-stage pulmonary Langerhans cell histiocytosis in a 50-year-old woman. **A:** HRCT at the level of the right upper lobe bronchus shows extensive fibrosis with small honeycomb cysts. The disease involves the lung diffusely at this level. **B:** Conventional 10-mm collimation CT scan through the lung base is virtually normal.

been reported on expiratory HRCT in a patient who had LCH, despite the absence of evidence of airways obstruction on PFT [27].

Differential Diagnosis

In patients who show nodules as the only HRCT abnormality, the differential diagnosis is extensive; differentiation from sarcoidosis, silicosis, metastatic disease, and tuberculosis may be impossible, although the typical distribution of the nodules can be valuable [29]. Nodules in LCH tend to be centrilobular (Figs. 7-4 and 7-5), whereas septal, subpleural, and peribron-

chovascular nodules are typically seen in sarcoidosis, silicosis, and lymphangitic carcinomatosis [29]. Sparing of the costophrenic angles should raise the possibility of pulmonary LCH, but it can be seen in these diseases as well. The cystic changes that are seen, on the other hand, can be easily distinguished from the honeycombing that is seen in end-stage IPF. Pulmonary LCH characteristically involves the upper two-thirds of the lungs diffusely, with relative sparing of the costophrenic angles (Figs. 7-2 and 7-3) [19,20]; IPF and other causes of honeycombing primarily involve the subpleural lung regions and the lung bases [30]. Also, in patients who have IPF, the honeycomb cysts are surrounded by abnormal parenchyma, which

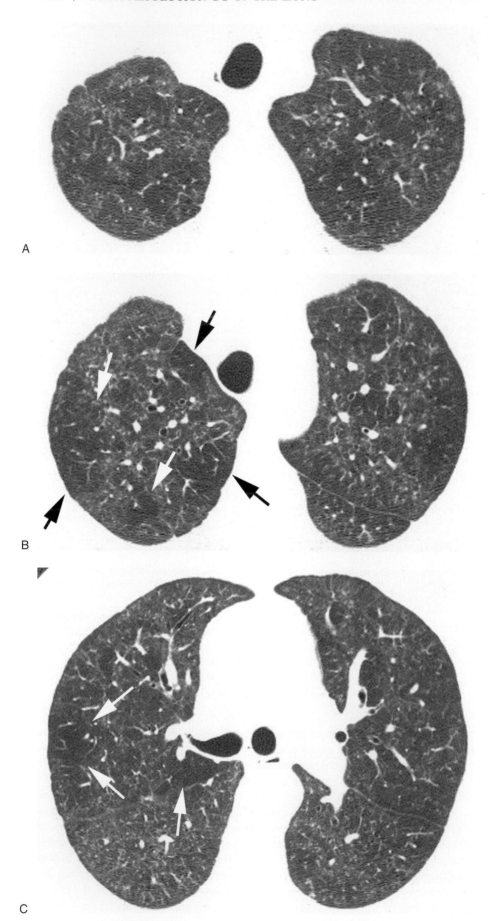

FIG. 7-7. Langerhans cell histiocytosis with small nodular opacities and mosaic perfusion due to air-trapping. HRCT at three levels **(A–C)** shows small nodular opacities associated with areas of relative lucency (*arrows*), representing mosaic perfusion due to air-trapping.

shows findings of extensive fibrosis, whereas most of the cysts in LCH are surrounded by normal lung. Lung volumes are normal or increased in cystic LCH, whereas they are generally reduced in patients who have IPF and show honeycombing.

In a woman, cystic lesions identical to those seen in pulmonary LCH can be seen in LAM or tuberous sclerosis (Figs. 7-11 through 7-13) [31–36]. LAM very rarely occurs in men. In patients who have LAM, the lower one-third of the lungs is usually involved, and nodules are rarely seen.

The cysts in pulmonary LCH, when adjacent to blood vessels, can mimic the signet ring sign of bronchiectasis (Fig. 7-5). However, distinction from bronchiectasis is straightforward because the cysts in LCH lack the characteristic continuity of dilated bronchi seen on contiguous slices in patients who have bronchiectasis [19].

Centrilobular emphysema typically has an upper lobe predominance similar to that seen in LCH. However, in many patients who have centrilobular emphysema, focal areas of lung destruction lack visible walls, distinguishing them from the lung cysts typical of this disease (Figs. 7-16, 7-17, and 7-19). On the other hand, in some patients who have centrilobular emphysema, areas of emphysema show very thin walls on HRCT, mimicking the appearance of LCH (Fig. 7-18). The presence of thick walls and large cystic spaces would favor a diagnosis of LCH.

Cystic airspaces are also common in a variety of fibrotic interstitial lung diseases, particularly end-stage IPF [30,37,38]. However, the upper lobe distribution of cysts in LCH is quite different from the basal distribution typical of IPF, and IPF typically shows a subpleural predominance that is lacking with LCH. The presence of findings of extensive fibrosis in patients who have IPF also allows their differentiation.

Multiple thin-walled lung cysts are also seen in patients who have lymphocytic interstitial pneumonia (see Figs. 4-36 and 5-19) [39–41]. Other findings in patients who have lymphocytic interstitial pneumonia include small subpleural nodules, centrilobular nodules, interlobular septal thickening, and ground-glass attenuation [41].

In patients with pneumonia particularly due to *Pneumocystis carinii*, lung cysts or pneumatoceles may be seen (see Figs. 6-57 through 6-60). These cannot be easily distinguished from cysts seen in patients who have LCH, other than by history or because of ancillary findings of pneumonia seen on HRCT [42–44].

Despite these similar appearances in various cystic lung diseases, the accuracy of HRCT in distinguishing three diseases that cause lung cysts (LCH, pulmonary LAM, and emphysema) was assessed in a study. Two radiologists were confident of the diagnosis of LCH in 84% of HRCT scans, of LAM in 79%, and of emphysema in 95% [45]. When confident, the observers were correct in 100% of the cases. Also, agreement between the observers was good for confident diagnoses (LCH, $\kappa = 0.77$; LAM, $\kappa = 0.88$; emphysema, $\kappa = 1$) [45]. Differentiation of LCH from other diseases is also possible in children [46], although disease progression may be more rapid than in adults [47].

LYMPHANGIOLEIOMYOMATOSIS

LAM is a rare multisystem disease characterized by progressive proliferation of immature-appearing smooth muscle cells (LAM cells) in the lung parenchyma (Fig. 7-8) and along axial lymphatic vessels in the chest and abdomen [48–50]. The hallmark of this disease is cystic destruction of the lung parenchyma (Fig. 7-9). Spindle cell proliferation can also involve the hilar, mediastinal, and extrathoracic lymph nodes, sometimes resulting in dilatation of intrapulmonary lymphatics and the thoracic duct. Involvement of the lymphatics can lead to chylous pleural effusions or ascites. Proliferation of cells in the walls of pulmonary veins may cause venous obstruction and lead to pulmonary venous hypertension with resultant hemoptysis.

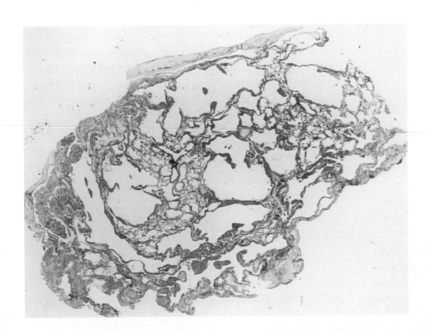

FIG. 7-8. Low-power microscopic view of an open-lung biopsy specimen from a patient who has lymphangioleiomyomatosis. Characteristic cystic spaces with atypical spindle cells lining their walls are seen throughout the specimen.

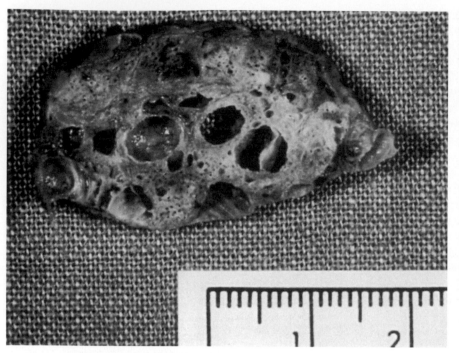
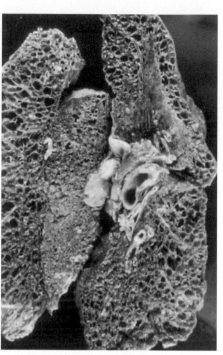

FIG. 7-9. Lymphangioleiomyomatosis. **A:** Open-lung biopsy specimen shows large cysts. (From Templeton PA, McLoud TC, Müller NL, et al. Pulmonary lymphangioleiomyomatosis: CT and pathologic findings. *J Comput Assist Tomogr* 1989;13:54–57, with permission.) **B:** Whole-lung specimen from a patient who had extensive cystic changes. (Case courtesy of Peter Kullnig, M.D., University of Graz, Graz, Austria.)

Pathology

The lesions of pulmonary LAM can be divided into early (active) and late phases [51,52]. In its early phases, LAM results in a proliferation of cells primarily in terminal bronchioles and alveolar walls (Fig. 7-8). Along the periphery of smooth muscle infiltrates, findings similar to those seen in other causes of emphysema are identified, due to the destructive effects of metalloproteinases expressed by the LAM cells. The result is proximal acinar and irregular emphysema, although similar changes may be seen resulting from more distal smooth muscle proliferation with normal-appearing proximal bronchioles [53].

Evidence of fibrogenesis, including the presence of abundant fibronectin, may also be identified. These changes result in dilated emphysema-like spaces, within which may be identified hyperplastic type II pneumocytes and hemosiderin-laden macrophages, presumably the result of hemorrhage [51,53]. Later in the course of disease, cellular infiltrates regress, leaving markedly dilated alveolar spaces associated with smooth muscle hyperplasia and diffuse collagen deposition.

Although proliferation of spindle cells causes circumferential narrowing and obstruction of bronchioles, leading to air-trapping and the development of thin-walled emphysematous cysts, airways obstruction with resulting emphysema also has been shown to result from loss of alveolar support. Using detailed morphometric analysis of postmortem lungs obtained from two patients who had LAM, Sobonya et al.

[54] have shown that of these two mechanisms, it is likely that the loss of parenchymal interdependence resulting from diffuse cystic disease and consequent loss of alveolar support may be the more important of the two.

The smooth muscle cells found in LAM have been shown to be phenotypically heterogeneous, smooth muscle, actin-positive cells derived from myoid precursors. Immunohistochemical studies show that approximately 80% of proliferating cells in LAM patients stain positively for estrogen receptors, whereas nearly all stain positively for progesterone receptors, in distinction to normal smooth muscle cells [53]. LAM cells also differ from normal smooth muscle cells because they react with HMB-45, a monoclonal antibody that identifies a 100-kDa glycoprotein (gp 100) that is located in premelanosome antigens in the cytoplasm of melanoma cell lines [50,51,53,55]. HMB-45 staining is also found in patients who have angiomyolipomas of the kidney, multifocal micronodular pneumocyte hyperplasia [56,57], and clear cell tumors of the lung [55]. Although the significance of immunohistochemical staining with HMB-45 remains uncertain, this finding has proved useful in improving the accuracy of transbronchial biopsy for diagnosing LAM.

Clinical Findings

LAM occurs almost exclusively in women of childbearing age, usually between 17 and 50 years old. However, rarely, it may be seen in postmenopausal women [58]. It has also been reported to occur in at least one male patient. Identical clinical, radiologic, and pathologic pulmonary changes may be seen in approximately 1% of patients who have tuberous sclerosis. Although tuberous sclerosis affects both genders equally, the pulmonary changes have been described almost exclusively in women.

The majority of patients presents with dyspnea and pneumothorax, cough, or both. The mean time interval from the onset of symptoms to diagnosis is typically between 3 and 5 years [50,59]. Sixty percent develop chylous pleural effusions, up to 80% develop pneumothoraces, and 30% to 40% develop blood-streaked sputum or frank hemoptysis at some time in the course of the disease [48,49,60]. Nearly all patients present with abnormal pulmonary function [50,59,61]. In a study of 35 patients who had LAM, the most common abnormality was decreased carbon monoxide–diffusing capacity (DLCO) occurring in 83% of patients, followed by hypoxemia in 57% of patients, airflow obstruction in 51% of patients, and combined obstruction, restriction, or both in 26% of patients [50]. Of these, the most important are measures of airflow obstruction, as these have been shown to most closely correlate with prognosis [61].

Although improvement has been reported clinically after treatment with progesterone, tamoxifen, or other antiestrogen agents, ablation of ovarian function after administration of luteinizing-release hormone analogues, radiotherapy, or oophorectomy, responses to such treatments are variable [51,58,59,62]. Most patients die within 5 to 10 years of the onset of symptoms. As a consequence, LAM is now listed as an indication for lung transplantation, with over 60 cases performed internationally as of 1997 [51]. Similar to patients who have sarcoidosis and giant cell interstitial pneumonia, disease recurrence in transplanted lungs has also now been reported [63].

Radiographic Findings

The plain radiographic manifestations of LAM include reticular, reticulonodular, miliary, and honeycomb patterns [60,64]. More than 50% of patients have radiographic evidence of pneumothorax at the time of first presentation [51]. Lung volumes can be increased in patients who have this disease. The radiologic findings may precede, accompany, or postdate other manifestations of the disease, such as pneumothorax and chylous pleural effusion. Not infrequently, radiographs fail to reveal the presence of diffuse lung cysts subsequently verified surgically [60]. As documented by Chu et al., chest radiographs were interpreted as normal in nine of 35 (26%) patients who had proven LAM [50].

High-Resolution Computed Tomography Findings

On HRCT, patients who have LAM characteristically show numerous thin-walled lung cysts, surrounded by relatively normal lung parenchyma (see Figs. 3-116 through 3-118; Figs. 7-10 through 7-13) [31–36,50,65–68] (Table 7-2). These cysts usually range from 2 mm to 5 cm in diameter, but

they can be larger. Their size tends to increase with progression of the disease [36]. In patients who have mild disease, the cysts usually measure smaller than 5 mm in diameter. In patients who have more extensive disease, in which 80% or more of the lung parenchyma is involved, the cysts tend to be larger, most being larger than 1 cm in diameter. The walls of the lung cysts are usually thin and faintly perceptible, but they may range up to 4 mm in thickness [32,36]. Irregularly shaped lung cysts, as are seen in patients who have LCH (Fig. 7-3), are uncommon. Lung cysts seen on HRCT correlate with the presence of the lung cysts that are common pathologically in this disease; these cysts are partially surrounded by the abnormal spindle cells typical of LAM.

In the majority of patients, the cysts are distributed diffusely throughout the lungs, and no lung zone is spared (Fig. 7-13); diffuse lung involvement is seen even in patients who have mild disease. In reported series [32,36], there is no evidence of lower lung zone, central, or peripheral predominance on CT scans. Thus, the HRCT findings do not support the previous impression that the lesions initially have a predominantly basal distribution [49].

In most patients, the lung parenchyma between the cysts appears normal on HRCT (Figs. 7-10 through 7-13). In some cases, however, a slight increase in linear interstitial markings [33,68], interlobular septal thickening [32,68], or patchy areas of ground-glass opacity [36] are also seen. The latter probably represent areas of pulmonary hemorrhage. Small nodules are occasionally seen but are not a prominent feature of this disease, as they are with LCH. Although these variations have led some to conclude that there is no pathognomonic CT appearance of LAM [68], in our experience, in the vast majority of cases, a specific CT diagnosis is warranted in the presence of characteristic diffuse lung cysts, especially when identified in women of childbearing age. Pneumothorax may be seen to be associated with cysts in patients who have this disease (Fig. 7-14).

Other features of LAM that can be seen on HRCT include hilar, mediastinal, and retrocrural adenopathy. Adenopathy was visible in four of the seven patients who had complete chest CT scans reported by Sherrier et al. [34]. Not surprisingly, pleural effusions, pneumothoraces, or both are frequently identified and can be helpful in distinguishing LAM from Langerhans histiocytosis. In one large series, they were identified in five [14%] and two [6%] patients, respectively [50]. Air-trapping on expiratory scans may also be seen [27].

Less well appreciated is the fact that abnormalities may also be frequently identified in the abdomen. Most important is the finding of renal angiomyolipomas. These have been noted to occur in up to 57% of patients who have LAM, and they are frequently bilateral. Chu et al. detected a total of 31 solid renal masses in 18 of 35 (51%) patients, including six patients (17%) who had multiple angiomyolipomas and four (11%) who had bilateral involvement. Typically, these are large at the time of diagnosis, usually larger than 4 cm in diameter, and have a well-known tendency to cause retroperitoneal bleeding. In addition to renal tumors, retroperito-

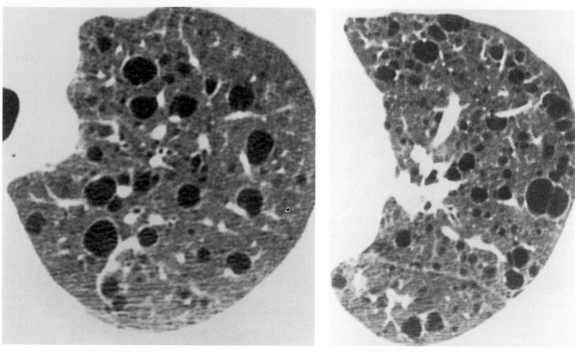

A
B

FIG. 7-10. Lymphangioleiomyomatosis in a 30-year-old woman. **A,B:** HRCT targeted to the left lung shows multiple cystic airspaces of varying sizes. These have walls ranging from being barely perceptible to 2 mm in thickness. The lung parenchyma between the cystic airspaces is normal. The cysts are primarily round in shape, but some are confluent. As contrasted with Langerhans cell histiocytosis, the upper and lower lobes are involved to a similar degree. (From Templeton PA, McLoud TC, Müller NL, et al. Pulmonary lymphangioleiomyomatosis: CT and pathologic findings. *J Comput Assist Tomogr* 1989;13:54–57, with permission.)

neal adenopathy is also frequent, occurring in up to three-quarters of patients in one report [50]. Ascites may also be identified, usually in conjunction with chylothoraces.

Utility of High-Resolution Computed Tomography

HRCT is superior to chest radiography in determining the extent and distribution of air cysts in this disease, and it can demonstrate extensive abnormalities in patients who have normal radiographic findings [32,34,36]. The cystic changes of LAM are also much easier to assess and are better defined on HRCT than on conventional CT (Fig. 7-12). Cysts visible on HRCT were rarely seen on chest radiographs, unless they were larger than 1 cm.

Disease extent as assessed on CT correlates better than do radiographic findings with clinical and functional impairment in patients who have LAM [51]. Typically, PFTs reveal decreased diffusing capacity and, less commonly, airflow obstruction with reduced forced expiratory volume in one second (FEV_1) and FEV_1/forced vital capacity (FVC) ratio, accompanied by a reduction in elastic recoil. Significant correlations have been documented between a reduced FEV_1/FVC ratio, increased total lung capacity (TLC), and prognosis [61]. On CT, the best correlations have been observed between the extent of disease and impairment in gas transfer as assessed by the carbon monoxide diffusing capacity [32,36,67]. Although significant correlations have also been

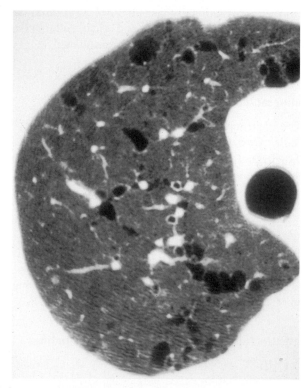

FIG. 7-11. HRCT targeted to the right lung in a patient who has documented tuberous sclerosis and lymphangioleiomyomatosis. Note the similarity between this case and that illustrated in Figure 7-10.

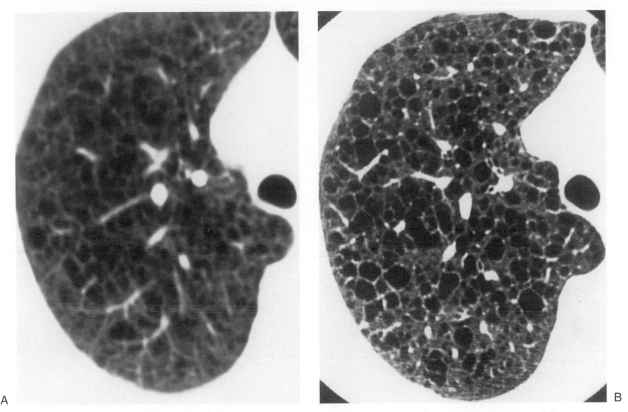

FIG. 7-12. Lymphangioleiomyomatosis in a 58-year-old woman. **A:** Conventional 10-mm collimation CT scan through the right upper lobe shows lucent areas. This appearance is similar to that of emphysema. **B:** HRCT demonstrates that the cystic airspaces have well-defined walls, allowing easy distinction from emphysema.

demonstrated between extent of cystic disease and severity of airways obstruction [32,67], this has proved more controversial. In the study by Aberle et al. [67], for example, good correlation was reported between CT scores and measures of airways obstruction, in particular the FEV_1/ FVC ratio ($r = -0.92$; $p < .002$). Similarly, Lenoir et al., in a study of 11 patients who had LAM (n = 9) and tuberous sclerosis (n = 2), found good correlation between CT findings and FEV_1/FVC ratios and DLCO [32]. In distinction, although good correlations between CT scores and DLCO have also been reported by Müller et al. in their study of 14 patients who had LAM, similar good correlation was not seen with lung volumes or airflow parameters [36].

Crausman et al. have assessed the use of quantitative CT (QCT) measurements as a means to predict prognosis in LAM patients [69,70]. Using two end-expiratory HRCT images (at the carina and just above the diaphragm), these authors used a density mask program using a threshold of –900 Hounsfield units (HU) to obtain a QCT index in ten patients who had documented LAM. Defined as the amount of cystic lung expressed as a percent of total lung area for the two slices combined, good correlation was found between the QCT index and the FEV_1 ($r = -0.9$; $p = .0005$), residual volume ($r = 0.7$; $p = .02$), DLCO ($r = -0.76$; $p = .01$), and exercise performance measured as maximum workload ($r = -0.84$; $p = .002$), among other measurements [69]. These

data are significant given previously noted correlations between measurements of airflow obstruction and prognosis [61]. As is discussed in greater detail later in this chapter, there are important limitations to the use of expiratory HRCT images for assessing both the extent and severity of emphysema that likely also apply to the use of expiratory CT for evaluating patients who have LAM [71].

The presence of many small, thin-walled, cystic airspaces scattered through both lungs in a young woman is highly suggestive of LAM. However, definitive diagnosis traditionally has required open-lung biopsy. This is because lung tissue from LAM patients, especially when obtained by transbronchial biopsy, may be mistaken for any disease that involves smooth muscle hyperplasia, including IPF. As previously discussed, it has been shown that immunohistochemical staining with HMB-45 is positive in patients who have LAM, improving the usefulness of transbronchial biopsy for this diagnosis [72,73]. CT is advantageous in demonstrating parenchymal abnormalities in symptomatic patients who have normal or questionably abnormal findings on chest radiographs, thus indicating the need for biopsy. It should be noted, however, that normal findings at CT examination do not rule out parenchymal disease in patients who have LAM [26].

Patients who have lung transplantation for LAM have increased morbidity and mortality due to complications

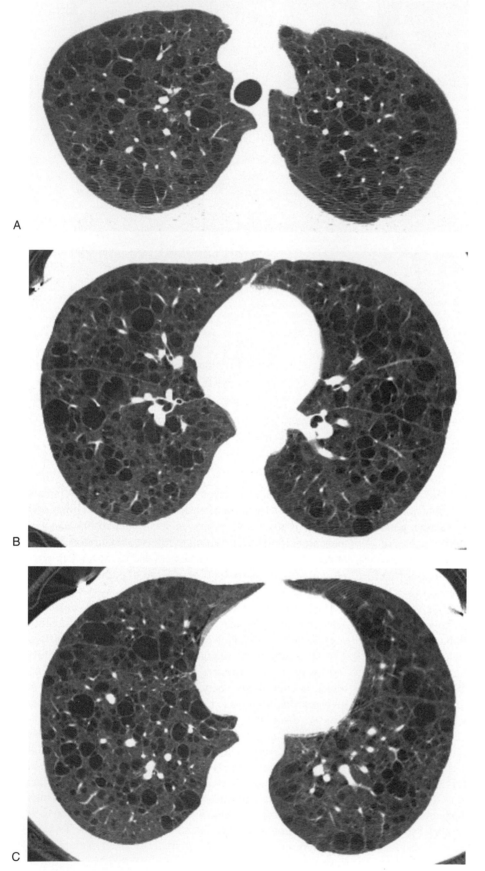

A

B

C

FIG. 7-13. A–C: Lymphangioleiomyomatosis in a 35-year-old woman with tuberous sclerosis. HRCT shows numerous discrete, round, thin-walled lung cysts. Cysts are thinner-walled and more regular in size and shape than those seen in patients who have Langerhans cell histiocytosis. Intervening lung parenchyma appears normal. Cysts are diffusely distributed, and cysts at the lung bases **(C)** are similar in size and number to those seen at the lung apices **(A)**. These abnormalities were associated with adenoma sebaceum, shortness of breath, airway obstruction on pulmonary function tests, and low diffusing capacity.

TABLE 7-2. *HRCT findings in lymphangioleiomyomatosis*

Thin-walled lung cysts, usually round in shape[a,b]
Diffuse distribution, costophrenic angles involved[a,b]
Mild septal thickening or ground-glass opacity
Adenopathy
Small nodules
Pleural effusion[b]

[a]Most common findings.
[b]Findings most helpful in differential diagnosis.

related to their underlying disease [74]; these LAM-related complications can be diagnosed or suggested with CT. In a review of 13 patients who had unilateral (n = 8) or bilateral (n = 5) lung transplantation for LAM, complications found during and after transplantation included excessive pleural adhesions (n = 4), native lung pneumothorax (n = 3) (Fig. 7-14), chylous effusion (n = 1), chylous ascites (n = 3), complications from renal angiomyolipomas (n = 4), and recurrent LAM (n = 1). One patient died as a result of complications of LAM [74].

Differential Diagnosis

Lung cysts very similar to those seen in LAM have also been described in patients who have pulmonary LCH [19,20]. However, three findings usually allow the differentiation of these two diseases. In many patients who have pulmonary LCH, a nodular component is also present (Fig. 7-5); this is uncommon with LAM. Irregularly shaped cysts, as are commonly seen in patients who have LCH (Figs. 7-2 and 7-3), are much less frequent with LAM. LCH characteristically involves the upper two-thirds of the lungs and spares the costophrenic angles (Fig. 7-3), whereas LAM involves the lungs diffusely [19,20]. In some patients, however, the HRCT findings of these two conditions can be identical.

A number of other cystic lung diseases and emphysema, delineated in the discussion of LCH above, may mimic the appearance of LAM. However, careful attention to the appearances of the cystic lesions, their distribution, and their clinical history can allow their distinction in many cases. The accuracy of HRCT in distinguishing LCH, LAM, and emphysema is excellent. In a study, two observers were confident of the diagnosis of LAM in 79% of cases and were correct in all of these [45].

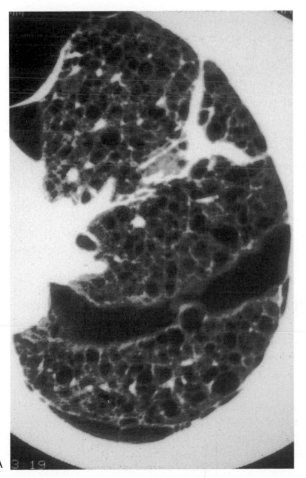

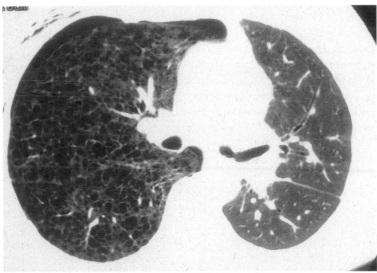

FIG. 7-14. Lymphangioleiomyomatosis before and after lung transplantation. **A:** Targeted reconstruction through the left lung shows diffuse lung cysts associated with a pneumothorax. Pneumothoraces occur commonly in this disease. **B:** Section in the same patient obtained following unilateral lung transplantation. Note subtle narrowing of the left upper lobe bronchus at the site of anastomosis. An occult right-sided pneumothorax is also identifiable anteriorly.

EMPHYSEMA

As defined by the American Thoracic Society, emphysema is "a condition of the lung characterized by permanent, abnormal enlargement of airspaces distal to the terminal bronchiole, accompanied by the destruction of their walls" [75–77]. This definition also includes the caveat "without obvious fibrosis" [78]; however, some observations have established that some degree of associated fibrosis is not uncommon [75,76].

It is generally accepted that emphysema results from an imbalance in the dynamic relationship between elastolytic and antielastolytic factors in the lung, usually related to smoking or enzymatic deficiency [79–81]. Abnormal or unopposed elastase activity in the lung is thought to lead to the tissue destruction representing the primary pathologic abnormality present in patients who have this disease.

Inhaled tobacco smoke attracts macrophages to distal airways and alveoli. Macrophages, in turn, along with airway epithelial cells, release chemotactic substances that serve to attract neutrophils and induce them to release elastases and other proteolytic enzymes [82,83]. Macrophages also release proteases in response to tobacco smoke. These elastases have the ability to cleave a variety of proteins, including collagen and elastin. Lung elastin is normally protected from excessive elastase-induced damage by alpha-1-protease inhibitor (alpha-1-antiprotease or antitrypsin) and other circulating antiproteinases. However, tobacco smoke tends to interfere with the function of alpha-1-antiprotease. In combination, these interactions result in structural damage in the distal airways and alveoli in smokers, leading to emphysema. Inherited deficiency in alpha-1-antiprotease may similarly result in lung destruction and emphysema.

Classification of Emphysema

Emphysema is usually classified into three main subtypes, based on the anatomic distribution of the areas of lung destruction, but the names applied to these subtypes by different investigators often differ [77,84]. These subtypes are: (i) proximal acinar, centriacinar, or centrilobular emphysema; (ii) panacinar or panlobular emphysema; and (iii) distal acinar or paraseptal emphysema. Although from an anatomic or pathologic point of view, it is most appropriate to refer to these types of emphysema relative to the presence and type of acinar abnormalities (i.e., proximal acinar, panacinar, and distal acinar), from the standpoint of understanding the use of HRCT, it is more appropriate to refer to them relative to the way in which we perceive them at the lobular level (i.e., centrilobular, panlobular, and paraseptal). As indicated in Chapter 2, acini cannot be resolved on HRCT. In the remainder of this chapter, the terms *centrilobular*, *panlobular*, and *paraseptal* are used to describe these three types of emphysema.

Centrilobular emphysema (proximal acinar emphysema, centriacinar emphysema) predominantly affects the respiratory bronchioles in the central portions of acini, and therefore involves the central portion of the lobule. Panlobular emphysema (panacinar emphysema) involves all the components of the acinus more or less uniformly, and therefore involves the entire lobule. Paraseptal (distal acinar emphysema) predominantly involves the alveolar ducts and sacs, with areas of destruction often marginated by interlobular septa.

Centrilobular emphysema usually results from cigarette smoking. It mainly involves the upper lung zones. In contrast, panlobular emphysema is classically associated with alpha-1-protease inhibitor (alpha-1-antitrypsin) deficiency, although it may also be seen without protease deficiency in smokers, in the elderly, distal to bronchial and bronchiolar obliteration, and associated with drug use [78]. Paraseptal emphysema can be an isolated phenomenon in young adults, often associated with spontaneous pneumothorax, or can be seen in older patients with centrilobular emphysema [78,85]. In their early stages, these three forms of emphysema can be easily distinguished morphologically. However, as they become more severe, their distinction becomes more difficult.

Bullae can develop in association with any type of emphysema, but they are most common with paraseptal or centrilobular emphysema. A *bulla*, by definition, is a sharply demarcated area of emphysema measuring 1 cm or larger in diameter and possessing a wall smaller than 1 mm in thickness [86]. In some patients who have emphysema, bullae can become quite large, resulting in significant compromise of respiratory function; this syndrome is sometimes referred to as *bullous emphysema*. Bullae have been classified by Reid according to their location and the type of emphysema with which they are associated [87]. According to this classification, type 1 bullae are subpleural in location and occur in patients who have paraseptal emphysema; type 2 bullae are also subpleural but are associated with generalized emphysema (centrilobular or panlobular); type 3 bullae are associated with generalized emphysema, but occur within the lung parenchyma rather than in a subpleural location.

Irregular airspace enlargement is an additional type of emphysema occurring in patients who have pulmonary fibrosis; this form of emphysema is also referred to as *paracicatricial* or *irregular* emphysema [78,84].

Emphysema, Chronic Obstructive Pulmonary Disease, and Clinical Findings

In patients who have emphysema, PFTs usually show findings of chronic airflow obstruction and reduced diffusing capacity. Airflow obstruction in patients who have emphysema is due to airways collapse on expiration, largely resulting from destruction of lung parenchyma and loss of airways tethering and support. Abnormal diffusing capacity is due to destruction of the lung parenchyma and the pulmonary vascular bed.

It is important to keep in mind that many patients who have emphysema also have chronic bronchitis, because both are smoking-related diseases. Chronic bronchitis is a poorly characterized entity that, for lack of a better definition, is considered to be present if a patient has chronic sputum production that is not caused by a specific disease such as bronchiectasis or tuberculosis [88]. Morphologic correlates with chronic bronchitis have been difficult to define, although common pathologic findings include bronchial wall thickening, mucous gland enlargement, smooth muscle hyperplasia, inflammation, and small airways abnormalities.

The term *chronic obstructive pulmonary disease* or *COPD* is often used to describe patients who have chronic and largely irreversible airways obstruction, most commonly associated with some combination of emphysema and chronic bronchitis [88]. The term indicates some uncertainty as to the exact pathogenesis of the functional abnormalities present [88]. Furthermore, COPD may be used to refer to diseases usually associated with airways obstruction, such as emphysema and chronic bronchitis, even if no obstruction is demonstrated on PFTs.

Respiratory symptoms in patients who have COPD usually include chronic cough, sputum production, and dyspnea. Although in patients who have COPD, cough and sputum production are largely manifestations of chronic bronchitis, the relative contributions of airways disease and emphysema to respiratory disability are often difficult to determine. However, in patients who have early alpha-1-protease inhibitor (alpha-1-antitrypsin) deficiency, airways disease is typically absent, and functional abnormalities primarily reflect the presence of emphysema. These include reduced FEV_1/FVC, FEV_1, and DLco [89]. In patients who have more long-standing emphysema associated with alpha-1-protease inhibitor deficiency, chronic cough and sputum production are common, likely due to increased susceptibility to infection [90] and the development of bronchiectasis [81].

Radiographic Findings

Radiographic abnormalities in patients who have emphysema generally reflect increased lung volume, lung destruction (reduced vascularity or bullae), or both [91–96]. When both findings are used as criteria for diagnosis, a sensitivity as high as 80% has been reported for chest films [91], although the likelihood of a positive diagnosis depends on the severity of disease [77]. When only findings of lung destruction are used for diagnosis, plain films are only 40% sensitive [96]. Although the accuracy of chest radiographs in diagnosing emphysema is somewhat controversial, it can be reasonably concluded from the studies performed that moderate to severe emphysema can be diagnosed radiographically, whereas mild emphysema is difficult to detect.

The presence of increased lung volume, or overinflation, can be very important in making the diagnosis of emphysema on plain radiographs, but overinflation is an indirect sign of this disease; findings of increased lung volume are nonspecific and can be lacking in some patients who have emphysema while being present in patients who have other forms of obstructive pulmonary disease. A number of plain radiographic findings of overinflation have been validated in patients who have COPD, although their sensitivity and specificity vary. These include (i) a lung height of 29.9 cm or more, measured from the dome of the right diaphragm to the tubercle of the first rib; (ii) flattening of the right hemidiaphragm on the lateral projection, with a height of less than 2.7 cm measured from anterior to posterior costophrenic angles; (iii) flattening of the right hemidiaphragm on a posteroanterior radiograph, with the highest level of the dome of the right hemidiaphragm less than 1.5 cm above a perpendicular line drawn between the costophrenic angle laterally and the vertebrophrenic angle medially; (iv) an increased retrosternal airspace, measuring more than 4.4 cm at a level 3 cm below the manubrial-sternal junction; and (v) the right hemidiaphragm at or below the level of the anterior end of the seventh rib [91,93–95,97–99].

The presence of bullae on chest radiographs is the only specific sign of emphysema, but this finding is infrequent and may not reflect the presence of generalized disease. A reduction in size of pulmonary vessels or vessel tapering can also reflect lung destruction, but this finding lacks sensitivity and can be unreliable.

High-Resolution Computed Tomography Findings

On HRCT, emphysema is characterized by the presence of areas of abnormally low attenuation, which can be easily contrasted with surrounding normal lung parenchyma if sufficiently low window means (–600 HU to –800 HU) are used [100–102]. In most instances, focal areas of emphysema can be easily distinguished from lung cysts or honeycombing; focal areas of emphysema often lack distinct walls (see Chapter 3) [45,100,101].

Although various CT findings of increased lung volume may also be seen in patients who have COPD and emphysema [103], their identification is usually secondary to the more direct observation of lung destruction characteristic of the various types of emphysema. In a study of 74 patients (44 who had normal lung function and 30 who had COPD), significant correlations were observed between FEV_1/FVC and the tracheal index (transverse/anteroposterior diameter; $r = 0.578$; $p < .0001$), anteroposterior/transverse thoracic diameters at the tracheal carina ($r = -0.523$; $p < .0001$) and 5 cm below ($r = -0.533$; $p < .0001$), and lung bulging in the intercostal spaces ($r = -0.462$; $p < .0001$) [103].

Centrilobular Emphysema

Centrilobular emphysema of mild to moderate degree is characterized on HRCT by the presence of multiple small, round areas of abnormally low-attenuation, several millimeters in diameter, distributed throughout the lung, but usually having an upper lobe predominance. Areas of lucency often appear to be grouped near the centers of secondary pulmonary lobules, surrounding the centrilobular artery branches (see Figs. 3-119 and 3-120; Figs. 7-15 through 7-17) (Table 7-3)

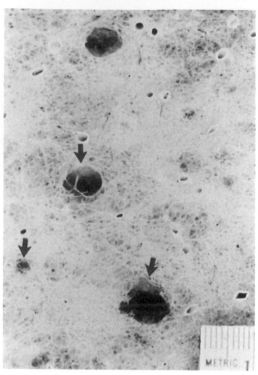

FIG. 7-15. Centrilobular or centriacinar emphysema. A low-power microscopic view of a lung specimen from a patient who has mild centrilobular emphysema. Areas of lung destruction measuring 3 to 10 mm in diameter are visible (*arrows*).

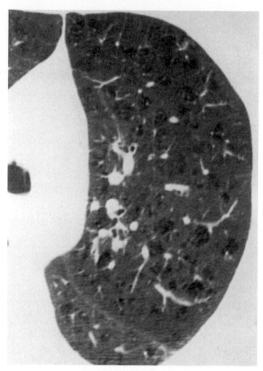

FIG. 7-16. Centrilobular emphysema in a 70-year-old smoker. HRCT at the level of the aortic arch shows localized areas of abnormally low attenuation measuring 2 to 10 mm in diameter, which can be seen to be centrilobular (they surround arteries in the lobular core). The areas of destruction lack recognizable walls.

[100–102,104,105]. These lucencies correspond to the well-circumscribed centrilobular or centriacinar areas of lung destruction seen pathologically in patients who have centrilobular emphysema [100,101,104–107]. Although the centrilobular location of lucencies cannot always be recognized on CT

or HRCT [101,104,105], the presence of multiple small areas of emphysema scattered throughout the lung is diagnostic of centrilobular emphysema (see Figs. 3-121 through 3-123; Figs. 7-16 through 7-18). In most cases, the areas of low-attenuation lack visible walls [45] (Figs. 7-16 and 7-17), although

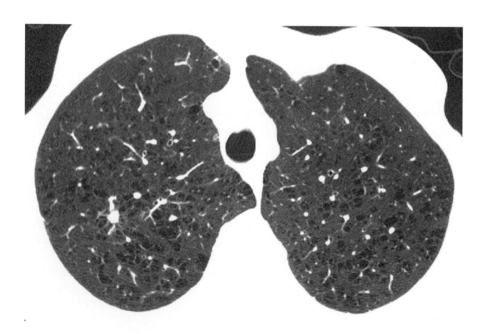

FIG. 7-17. Centrilobular emphysema with small focal lucencies. Lucencies lack visible walls, as is common in patients who have centrilobular emphysema. Some lucencies can be seen to surround small vessel branches. This appearance indicates that the emphysema has a centrilobular location. A small nodule in the right upper lobe represents an adenocarcinoma. See also Figure 7-36.

TABLE 7-3. *HRCT findings in centrilobular emphysema*

Multiple, small, spotty or centrilobular lucencies[a,b]
Upper-lobe predominance[a,b]
Lucencies may have thin walls
May be associated with paraseptal emphysema or bullae

[a]Most common findings.
[b]Findings most helpful in differential diagnosis.

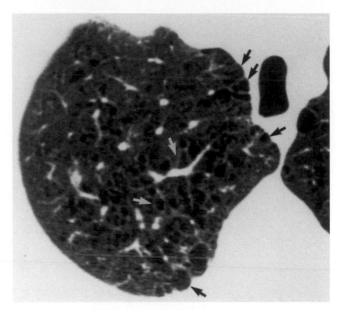

FIG. 7-18. Centrilobular emphysema. Some of the focal areas of lung destruction appear to be outlined by very thin walls (*white arrows*), probably due to fibrosis. Subpleural lucencies (*black arrows*) represent paraseptal emphysema, which can coexist with centrilobular emphysema.

very thin and relatively inconspicuous walls are occasionally seen on HRCT (Fig. 7-18), probably related to surrounding fibrosis; it has been shown that centrilobular emphysema is commonly associated with some fibrosis [75,76]. In patients who have centrilobular emphysema, bullae within the lung may have visible walls, and paraseptal emphysema and subpleural bullae are often seen (Figs. 7-19 and 7-20).

With more severe centrilobular emphysema, areas of destruction can become confluent. When this occurs, the centrilobular distribution of abnormalities is no longer recognizable on HRCT, or pathologically; the term *confluent centrilobular emphysema* is sometimes used to describe this occurrence (see Figs. 3-125 and 3-126; Figs. 7-21 and 7-22). This appearance can closely mimic the appearance of panlobular emphysema, and a distinction between these is of little clinical significance.

Panlobular Emphysema

Panlobular emphysema is characterized by uniform destruction of the pulmonary lobule, leading to widespread areas of abnormally low-attenuation (see Fig. 3-124; Figs. 7-23 through 7-27) (Table 7-4) [85,105,106,108]. Thurlbeck describes this entity as a "diffuse 'simplification' of the lung structure with progressive loss of tissue until little remains but the supporting framework of vessels, septa and bronchi" [84]. Involved lung appears abnormally lucent [108], a finding easy to appreciate in patients who have had unilateral lung transplantation (Figs. 7-24 and 7-26). Pulmonary vessels in the affected lung appear fewer and smaller than normal and may be quite inconspicuous. In contrast to centrilobular emphysema, panlobular emphysema almost always appears generalized or most severe in the lower lobes (Fig. 7-26).

Although it may lead to extensive destruction of the lung parenchyma, focal lucencies having the appearance of centrilobular emphysema are relatively uncommon, but they may be seen in less abnormal lung regions (Fig. 7-27). Associated paraseptal emphysema and bullae are relatively uncommon, despite the severity of lung destruction. In one study [108], frank bulla were seen in seven of 17 patients and were not considered a major feature of the disease.

In severe panlobular emphysema, the characteristic appearance of extensive lung destruction and the associated paucity of vascular markings are easily distinguished from normal lung parenchyma (Fig. 7-26). On the other hand, mild and even moderately severe panlobular emphysema can be very subtle and difficult to detect [107]. Furthermore, dif-

fuse panlobular emphysema unassociated with focal areas of lung destruction or bullae may be difficult to distinguish from diffuse small airways obstruction and air trapping resulting from bronchiolitis obliterans.

Alpha-1-antitrypsin deficiency may be associated with bronchiectasis or bronchial wall thickening (Fig. 7-26B) [109]. Presumably, as described previously, patients who have alpha-1-antitrypsin deficiency are more susceptible to airways damage during episodes of infection than are normal patients because of the same protease-antiprotease imbalance that leads to emphysema. In a study by King et al. [81], 6 of 14 (43%) patients who had alpha-1-antitrypsin deficiency had CT evidence of bronchiectasis, a finding associated with symptoms of infection. Two patients had diffuse cystic bronchiectasis. Similarly, in a study by Guest et al. [108], bronchial wall thickening, dilatation, or both were present in seven of 17 (41%) patients who had alpha-1-antitrypsin deficiency, with gross cystic bronchiectasis visible in one patient. Histologic findings in a patient who had alpha-1-antitrypsin deficiency and bronchiectasis visible on CT showed destruction of elastic lamina in ectatic bronchi and bronchioles [81].

The progression of panlobular emphysema associated with alpha-1-antitrypsin deficiency may be assessed using HRCT with densitometric measurements of lung attenuation [110,111] and has been found to be more sensitive than PFTs [111]. In one study [111], 23 patients were scanned twice at a 1-year interval. HRCT was obtained at 90% of the vital capacity (VC), at the level of the carina, 5 cm above the carina, and 5 cm below the carina. During the follow-up period, mean lung densities decreased by 14.2 ± 12.0 HU above the carina, by 18.1 ± 14.4 HU at the carina, and by 23.6 ± 15.0 HU below the carina. In another study [110], 22 patients who had moderate

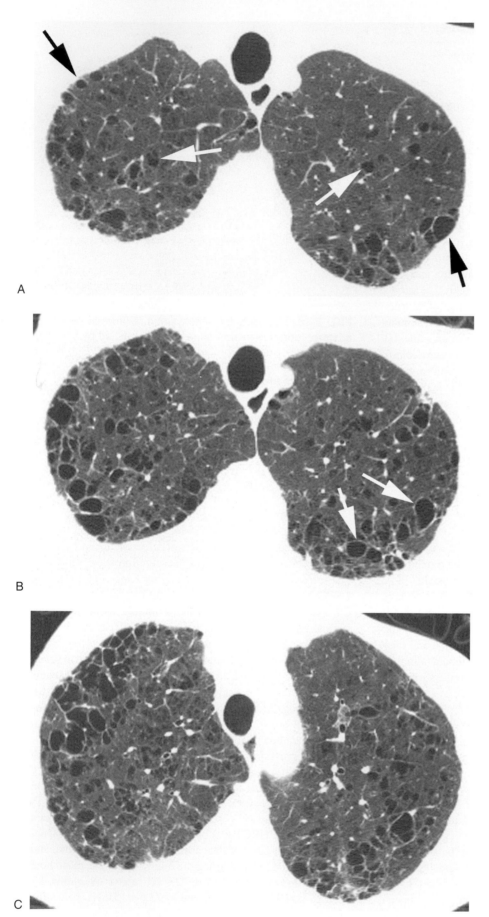

FIG. 7-19. Centrilobular and paraseptal emphysema. **A:** Areas of centrilobular emphysema (*white arrows*) are seen as focal lucencies in the central lung, without visible walls. Paraseptal emphysema in the subpleural regions (*black arrows*) is also visible, and thin walls are typically visible on HRCT. **B:** At a lower level, small bullae (*white arrows*) are associated with centrilobular emphysema. These have thin walls. **C:** At a level below **B**, centrilobular emphysema, intraparenchymal bullae, and paraseptal emphysema are all visible.

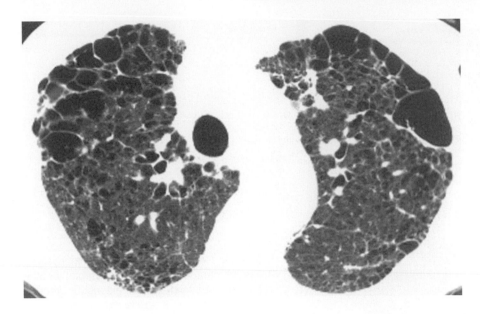

FIG. 7-20. Centrilobular emphysema with extensive paraseptal emphysema. Subpleural bullae and bullae within the lung parenchyma are both associated with centrilobular emphysema in this patient.

emphysema associated with alpha-1-antitrypsin deficiency were followed for 2 to 4 years with an annual lung CT. A highly significant decline in CT-measured lung density was found in low-density areas, corresponding to a mean annual loss of lung tissue of 2.1 g per L lung volume.

Paraseptal Emphysema

Paraseptal emphysema is characterized by involvement of the distal part of the secondary lobule and is therefore most striking in a subpleural location (see Figs. 3-127 through 3-129; Figs. 7-18 through 7-20 and 7-28 through 7-30). Areas of subpleural paraseptal emphysema often have visible walls, but these walls are very thin; they often correspond to inter-lobular septa. As with centrilobular emphysema, some fibrosis may be present. Even mild paraseptal emphysema is easily detected by HRCT (Table 7-5) [107].

When larger than 1 cm in diameter, areas of paraseptal emphysema are most appropriately termed *bullae* (Figs. 7-20 and 7-29 through 7-31). Subpleural bullae are frequently considered to be a manifestation of paraseptal emphysema, although they may be seen in all types of emphysema and as an isolated phenomenon; regardless of the cause of the subpleural bullae, they usually have thin walls that are visible on HRCT.

Lesur et al. [112] have shown that CT may be useful in the early detection of apical subpleural bullae in patients who have idiopathic spontaneous pneumothorax. This form of pneumothorax occurs most often in tall young adults [113] and is thought to be due to rupture of a subpleural bulla [112]. Out of 20 patients (mean age, 27 ± 7 years), CT demonstrated emphysema in 17 patients with a predominance in the lung apices, and in a subpleural location in 16 patients.

Bense et al. [114] have also demonstrated that emphysema is seen on CT in the majority of nonsmoking patients who have spontaneous pneumothorax. They compared the CT findings in 27 nonsmoking patients who had spontaneous pneumothorax to the CT findings in ten healthy subjects who had never smoked. Emphysema was present on CT in 22 of 27 nonsmoking patients who had spontaneous pneumothorax and in none of the 10 control subjects. The emphysema was present mainly in the periphery of the upper lung zones, a distribution consistent with paraseptal emphysema. In none of the cases was emphysema detected on a chest radiograph.

Similarly, in a prospective study of 35 patients who had primary spontaneous pneumothorax [115], the value of CT in detecting bullae was compared to that of chest radiographs. CT showed bullae or areas of subpleural emphysema in 31 of 35 (89%) patients, whereas chest radiographs showed these in only 11 patients (31%). Six patients had a recurrent pneumothorax during follow-up; no correlation between recurrence and the number, size, and distribution of bullae as assessed by CT was found.

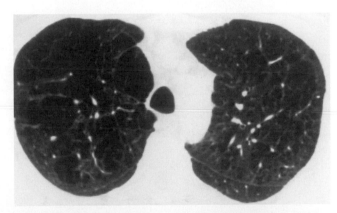

FIG. 7-21. Confluent centrilobular emphysema. Focal areas of centrilobular emphysema are visible on HRCT in the left upper lobe, whereas in the right upper lobe, areas of emphysema are large and confluent.

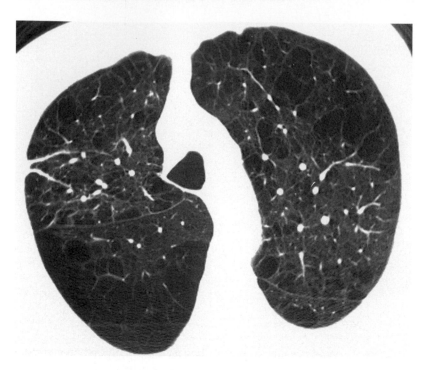

FIG. 7-22. Confluent centrilobular emphysema. Areas of centrilobular and paraseptal emphysema are associated with extensive areas of lung destruction. This appearance mimics that of panlobular emphysema, shown in Figure 7-27, but it is more patchy and was associated with a distinct upper lobe predominance.

Bullous Emphysema

The term *bullous emphysema* does not represent a specific pathologic entity but refers to the presence of emphysema associated with large bullae; it is generally seen in patients who have centrilobular emphysema, paraseptal emphysema, or both (Figs. 7-30 through 7-32) [87]. A syndrome of bullous emphysema, or giant bullous emphysema, has been described on the basis of clinical and radiologic features and is also known as *vanishing lung syndrome, type 1 bullous disease,* or *primary bullous disease of the lung* [116]. Giant bullous emphysema is often seen in young men and is characterized by the presence of large, progressive, upper lobe bullae, which occupy a significant volume of a hemithorax and are often asymmetric (Figs. 7-31 and 7-32). Arbitrarily, giant bullous emphysema is said to be present if bullae occupy at least one-third of a hemithorax [116].

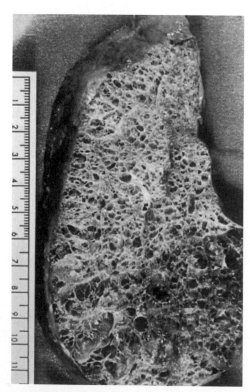

FIG. 7-23. Panlobular emphysema. A pathologic specimen shows diffuse involvement of the parenchyma with simplification of lung architecture.

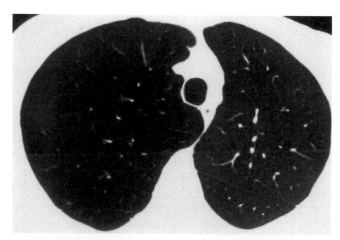

FIG. 7-24. Panlobular emphysema in a patient who had a left lung transplant. The emphysematous right lung is relatively large and lucent and shows fewer and smaller vessels than are visible on the left. This appearance is typical of panlobular emphysema.

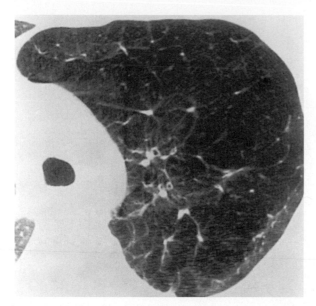

FIG. 7-25. Panlobular emphysema due to alpha-1-antiprotease deficiency in a 50-year-old woman. HRCT at the level of the aortic arch shows marked simplification of the architecture of the pulmonary parenchyma and areas of abnormally low attenuation. The areas of emphysema involve the entire secondary lobule and are easily distinguished from the localized 2- to 10-mm diameter areas of abnormally low attenuation seen in centrilobular emphysema.

Most patients who have giant bullous emphysema are cigarette smokers [117], but this entity may also occur in nonsmokers.

In nine patients who had giant bullous emphysema reported by Stern et al. [116], the most striking HRCT finding was the presence of multiple large bullae, varying in size from 1 to 20 cm in diameter, but usually between 2 and 8 cm in diameter (Figs. 7-31 and 7-32). Bullae were visible in a subpleural location and within the lung parenchyma, but subpleural bullae predominated. Bullae were often asymmetric, with one lung being involved to a greater degree. HRCT better depicted the presence of associated paraseptal and centrilobular emphysema than did chest radiographs. In this study [116], paraseptal emphysema was visible on HRCT in all subjects and was the predominant associated finding; centrilobular emphysema of varying degrees was present in eight of nine subjects.

Typically, bullae increase progressively in size. However, rarely, bullae may spontaneously decrease in size or disappear, usually as a result of secondary infection or obstruction of the proximal airways [118]. Spontaneous pneumothorax is common and may be recognized only on CT [112,115].

Irregular Airspace Enlargement

Irregular airspace enlargement, previously known as *irregular* or *cicatricial emphysema*, is commonly found adjacent to localized parenchymal scars, diffuse pulmonary fibrosis, and in the pneumoconioses, particularly progressive massive fibrosis (see Fig. 5-47) [119]. It is most easily recognized on CT when the associated fibrosis is identified. However, this type of emphysema may also be seen associated with microscopic fibrosis, in which case radiologic distinction between irregular and centrilobular emphysema may be impossible [120]

Quantitative Evaluation of Emphysema Using Computed Tomography

Technical Considerations

Our ability to diagnose and quantitate the extent and severity of emphysema using CT is influenced by a number of technical factors, including collimation, window settings,

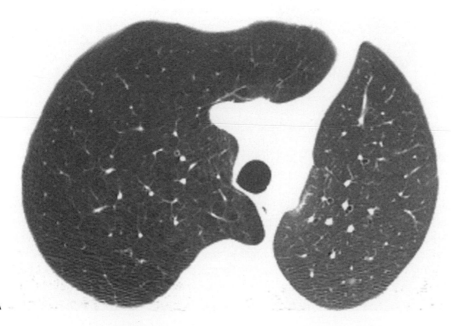

FIG. 7-26. Panlobular emphysema associated with alpha-1-antitrypsin deficiency in a patient who had left lung transplantation. **A:** The emphysematous lung is lucent compared to the normal transplant and contains fewer and smaller vessels. Focal lucencies, as are seen in patients who have centrilobular or paraseptal emphysema, are absent in this patient, as are paraseptal emphysema and bullae. *Continued*

A

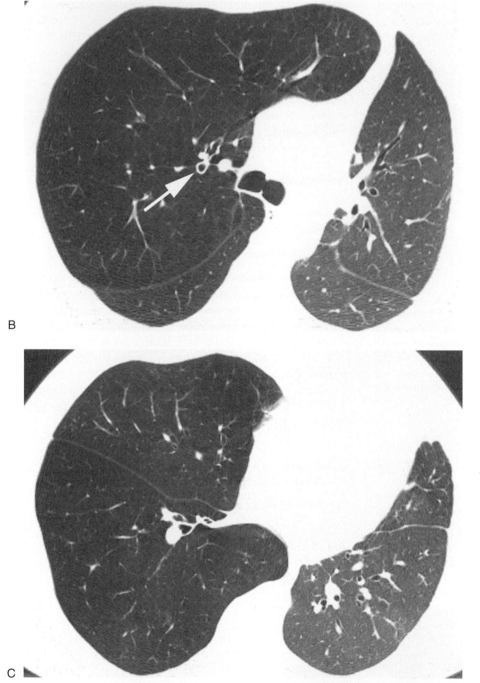

B

C

FIG. 7-26. *Continued* **B:** Findings of panlobular emphysema are also evident in the middle lung. Note bronchial wall thickening (*arrow*) as compared to the opposite side. The presence of bronchiectasis and bronchial wall thickening may be seen in patients who have alpha-1-antitrypsin deficiency. **C:** At the lung bases, findings of extensive emphysema are also visible. In panlobular emphysema, diffuse lung involvement is typical.

threshold values for diagnosing emphysema, radiation dose, reconstruction algorithm, phase of respiration, use of intravenous contrast media, number of sections assessed, and differences among individual scanners [71,121–128]. Awareness of these factors is a necessary prerequisite to accurate qualitative and quantitative evaluation of CT images.

Although emphysema may be detected using CT scans obtained using 10-mm collimation or spiral technique with collimation of 7 to 8 mm, thick collimation reduces the ability of CT to detect a mild degree of abnormality. Except when obtaining volumetric CT data, such techniques are not recommended for the diagnosis of emphysema.

It has been suggested that routine lung window settings, using a window level of approximately –700 HU and a window width of 1,000 HU, are acceptable for diagnosing emphysema [129]. Use of a window width of 1,500 HU is also satisfactory but reduces contrast between normal and emphysematous lung, making visual assessment more difficult. A narrow window width (e.g., 500 HU) with a low window mean (e.g., 800 HU) may be used to accentuate contrast between normal and emphysematous lung, although such a window setting would not be appropriate for routine HRCT [77,100,106].

At present, there is no generally agreed-on minimum number of sections necessary for accurate assessment of emphy-

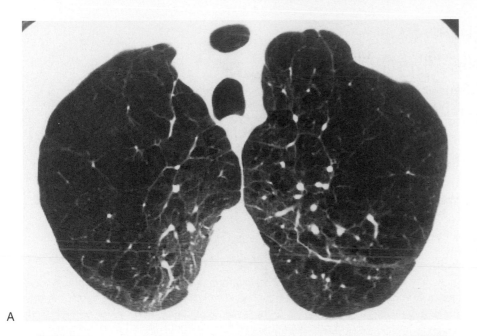

A

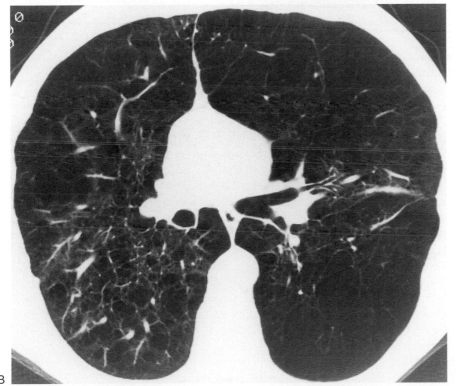

B

FIG. 7-27. A,B: Panlobular emphysema associated with alpha-1-antitrypsin deficiency. Although extensive lung destruction is present, some lung regions are less severely involved. In these regions, focal lucencies are visible, mimicking the appearance of centrilobular emphysema.

sema. Genevois et al., in an attempt to determine the least number of 1-mm sections necessary for accurate quantification, assessed progressively fewer sections obtained at 1-cm intervals and came to the conclusion that no standard number of HRCT images could be recommended due to wide variations from patient to patient [124]. Also, methods by which the lungs are segmented for the purposes of regional analysis also impact the accuracy of CT quantification. A variety of methods has been suggested, including manual, semiautomatic, and automated methods [130].

Milliampere (mA) settings used for HRCT are also important. Mishima et al. [126], in a study comparing a variety of mA scan settings ranging between 50 and 250, found that in patients who had mild emphysema, in whom the percent ratio of low-attenuation areas pathologically proved to be less than 30%, the mean low-attenuation area obtained by CT using less than 150 mA was significantly larger than that obtained using 250 mA; these authors concluded that a minimum current of greater than 200 mA is requisite for accurate quantification. These data may be pertinent in those cases in

TABLE 7-4. *HRCT findings in panlobular emphysema*

Lucent lung containing small pulmonary vessels[a,b]
Diffuse or lower lobe predominance[a,b]
Focal lucencies and bullae less common than with centrilobular emphysema[b]
Bronchiectasis or bronchial wall thickening

[a]Most common findings.
[b]Findings most helpful in differential diagnosis.

which an attempt is made to combine emphysema quantification with low-dose screening techniques.

Although possible variation among different scanners in lung densitometry also needs to be considered, as noted by Kemerink et al. in a comparison of a variety of different scanners, CT numbers for air proved independent of section thickness or reconstruction algorithm, suggesting that densitometric evaluation of moderate and severe emphysema is relatively immune to serious variations among scanners [122].

Morphologic Considerations

Despite widespread acceptance of the definition of emphysema as proposed by the American Thoracic Society, it should be noted that there is little consensus concerning how abnormal enlargement or destruction [78] should be quantified for the purpose of comparison with HRCT [77,131].

The extent and severity of emphysema may be assessed using either macroscopic or microscopic criteria [77,124,125,132,133]. Most CT studies have relied on the macroscopic morphometric panel grading system established by Thurlbeck et al. [77] for correlation [100,107,121,134–136]. Use of the panel grading system is based on a visual comparison of the extent of emphysema in a specific case to a series of 16 paper-mounted sagittal whole lung sections (Gough-Wentworth sections), arranged to provide visual standards of increasing disease severity. This approach has been criticized for its reliance on comparisons between different (axial and sagittal) planes, the visual detection of emphysema, and its subjective nature [125,133]. Despite these objections, the panel grading system remains an important validated standard for assessing QCT studies [131].

Gevenois and coworkers, in a series of reports, have recommended the use of computer-assisted evaluation of cross sectional Gough-Wentworth lung sections as a means for obtaining more accurate CT/pathologic correlations and as an alternative to a standard panel grading system [124,132,133,137,138]. Using this approach, macroscopic whole lung sections are divided into 7 × 7 cm fields, which are then digitized, enabling subsequent computer evaluation of the number of pixels in areas of emphysema identified by alterations in assigned gray scale. In turn, this allows direct comparison of the surface area of emphysema measured macroscopically, with macroscopic surface area measurements obtained by QCT analysis. Although the advantage of

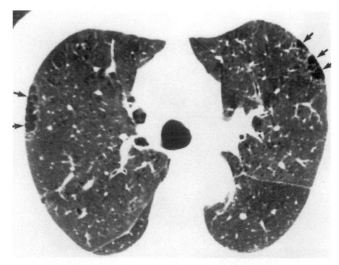

FIG. 7-28. Paraseptal emphysema. HRCT shows small, focal, subpleural lucencies (*arrows*) typical of paraseptal emphysema. These are commonly marginated by visible walls, usually representing interlobular septa. In some patients, areas of emphysema enlarge to form subpleural bullae.

this approach may seem intuitive, it has been noted that assigning gray-scale levels to emphysematous regions on lung sections remains subjective.

Alternative approaches have emphasized microscopic evaluation of emphysema. One such microscopic method involves a determination of the destructive index—a measurement of, among other findings, the number of breaks in alveolar walls identified microscopically [136,139]. This measurement has been shown to be increased in smokers in the absence of enlarged airspaces. Other measurements suggested as definitive are measurements of the mean linear intercept, mean interwall distance, and airspace wall per unit volume (AWUV) [77,125,131]. These latter point-counting techniques require placing a test line across a microscopic field and then counting the number of times the line crosses alveolar walls as a means to calculate alveolar surface area. As emphasized by Müller and Thurlbeck, however, these techniques are tedious to perform and are of less value in the presence of macroscopic emphysema [131].

It is apparent that there is little agreement as to which anatomic measurement or measurements of emphysema constitute a gold standard for determining disease extent and severity. Much of this controversy applies to defining minimal degrees of emphysema; the more extensive the disease, the less important are small differences between techniques. Most practical indications for the use of QCT involve assessing patients who have extensive disease [136].

Visual Quantification of Emphysema

The simplest method for estimating the severity of emphysema involves assigning a grade based on visual examination of CT scans [106,107,136,140–142]. Typically, this approach

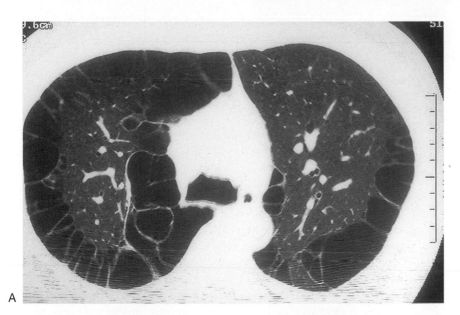

A

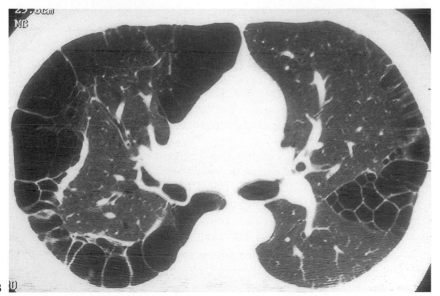

B

FIG. 7-29. A,B: HRCT sections through the carina and middle lung, respectively, show characteristic pattern of paraseptal emphysema with subpleural cystic changes resulting in a stacked coin appearance. Note that on the left side in **B**, subpleural cysts extend medially along the fissure. It is easy to see why chest radiographs in such patients have been described as having a "dirty lung" appearance. Cysts larger than 1 cm are best termed *bullae*.

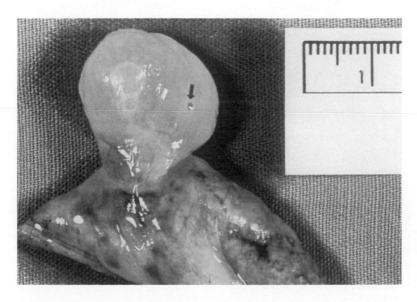

FIG. 7-30. Paraseptal emphysema with a large subpleural bulla. This patient presented with pneumothorax. The small hole in the bulla wall (*arrow*) was presumably the site of air leak.

TABLE 7-5. *HRCT findings in paraseptal emphysema*

Multiple, subpleural lucencies in a single layer, usually less than 1 cm[a,b]

Upper lobe predominance[a,b]

Thin walls are commonly visible[a,b]

May be associated with centrilobular emphysema or bullae

Pneumothorax may occur

[a]Most common findings.
[b]Findings most helpful in differential diagnosis.

calls for assessing individual HRCT sections, using a 4- or 5-point scale, as either normal or showing less than 25% lung involvement by emphysema, between 25% and 50% lung involvement, between 50% and 75% lung involvement, or greater than 75% involvement, with the total score expressed as percentage of total lung at that level [134]. Alternatively, a grid may be used to overlay the scan as a means of quantifying the extent of emphysema [107,143].

In general, visual inspection has yielded good correlations between CT and pathologic measures of the extent and severity, especially of centrilobular emphysema, in all but the mildest cases [137,143]. Bergin et al., for example, using areas of low-attenuation and vascular disruption as evidence of emphysema on contiguous 10-mm sections, reported good correlation between CT scores for the total lung assessed by three independent observers and pathologic scores of between .63 and .88 (all $p < .01$) [134].

Using HRCT in a study of postmortem lung specimens, Hruban et al. [100] were able to accurately identify centrilobular emphysema, even of a mild degree. The correlation between the *in vitro* CT emphysema score and the pathologic grade was excellent ($r = 0.91$). The ability of HRCT to accurately demonstrate the location and extent of emphysema in lung specimens was also shown by Webb et al. [101].

Although it may be possible to obtain a near one to one correlation between CT and pathologic specimens *in vitro*, it is not possible to obtain such a good correlation *in vivo*; minimal emphysema can sometimes be missed by HRCT. Miller et al. [107] found a CT-pathologic correlation of $r = 0.81$ when using 10-mm collimation scans and a correlation of $r = 0.85$ when using 1.5-mm collimation scans. In this series, 33 of 38 patients had emphysema; out of these 33, four patients who had mild centrilobular emphysema were interpreted as normal on CT. Although Kuwano et al. [136] found no significant difference between the HRCT and the pathology scores in 42 patients who had mild to moderate emphysema, with correlation between the CT scores and the pathology scores in this study ranging between 0.68 for 1-mm sections and 0.76 for 5-mm sections, respectively, the absence of patients who have minimal emphysema is a major limitation [77]. Furthermore, significant inter- and intraobserver variability was also reported.

Similar findings have been reported in patients who have panlobular emphysema. Spouge et al. [144] assessed the accuracy of CT in diagnosing and quantifying emphysema in ten patients who had pathologically proven panlobular emphysema and five normal controls. They compared the visual assessment and severity of emphysema on CT with pathologic assessment. The correlation between the assessment of extent of panlobular emphysema on CT and the pathologic grade was $r = 0.90$, $p < .01$ for conventional CT, and $r = 0.96$, $p < .01$ for HRCT. Also, there was significantly less interobserver variation in the grading of emphysema on HRCT than with conventional CT. The observers missed three cases of mild panlobular emphysema on conventional

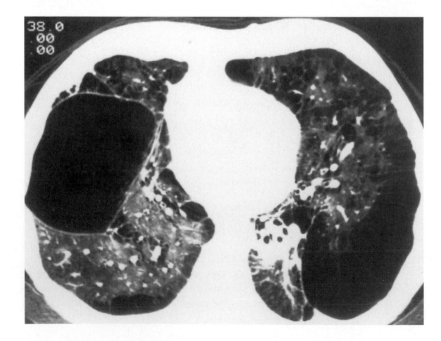

FIG. 7-31. Bullous emphysema. In this patient, HRCT shows large, bilateral subpleural bullae, associated with areas of paraseptal emphysema (best seen on the right) and centrilobular emphysema (best seen on the left).

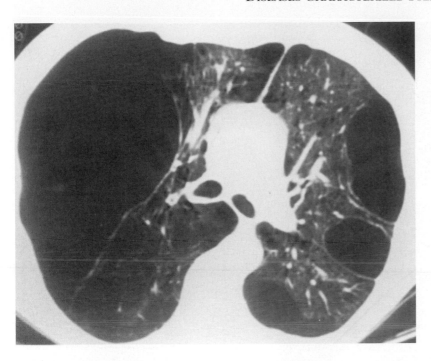

FIG. 7-32. Severe emphysema related to cigarette smoking in a 67-year-old man. Bullae are present bilaterally. Although there is extensive emphysema, the patient improved symptomatically after right bullectomy.

CT and two on HRCT. They concluded that HRCT allows improved correlation with the pathologic score, and decreased interobserver variation than conventional CT in patients with panlobular emphysema.

The accuracy of visual assessment of emphysema severity has been challenged [124]. Using a computer-assisted method for obtaining objective quantification of horizontal, paper-mounted lung sections as a gold standard, Bankier et al. compared HRCT densitometric evaluation of mean lung attenuation with subjective visual assessments by three readers in 62 consecutive patients evaluated before lung resection [138]. These authors found that subjective grading of emphysema was significantly less accurate than objective CT densitometric results ($r = 0.44$ to 0.51; $p < .05$ vs. $r = 0.56$ to 0.62; $p < .001$, respectively) when correlated to pathologic scores. Importantly, analysis of visual scoring data suggested systematic overestimation of emphysema by all three readers [138].

Computer-Assisted Quantification of Emphysema

Given the inherent limitations of subjective visual scoring, it is not surprising that early in the use of CT for emphysema assessment, attention was focused on the potential for direct analysis of digital data obtained from the CT scan [135,143,145–147]. In general, three different approaches have been used. These include: (i) use of a threshold value below which emphysema is considered to be present [density mask or pixel index (PI)] [135,147], (ii) assessment of the range of lung densities represented in a lung slice (histogram analysis) [146,148], and (iii) determining overall lung density, often in combination with volumetric imaging [111,130,149,150].

Hayhurst et al. first demonstrated the usefulness of a threshold attenuation value for the diagnosis of emphysema on CT scans by showing that patients who had pathologically proved emphysema contained more pixels between -900 HU and $-1,000$ HU than patients who did not have emphysema ($p < .001$) [145]. In a classic article, Müller et al. [135] made use of a standard software program called *density mask* that highlights voxels within any preselected range (Figs. 7-33 and 7-37). Using this technique with 10-mm-thick sections and highlighting all voxels less than -910 HU, these authors found good correlation ($r = 0.89$) between the extent and severity of emphysema, as measured preoperatively on a single section and a modified panel-grading system in 21 patients who had pathologic evidence of emphysema after lung resection. Three cases with emphysema scores less than ten were missed, however, and a diagnosis of emphysema was made in one normal patient. In comparison, the correlation between the mean of visual scores of two independent observers and the pathologic score was .90 ($p < .001$), leading these investigators and others to conclude that visual scoring was nearly as precise and clinically more practical than quantitative assessment [121,135].

The relationship between appropriate threshold values for diagnosing emphysema and slice thickness must be kept in mind. In the study described in the previous paragraph, using 10-mm collimation, Müller et al. compared the percentage of lung area with an attenuation level lower than three thresholds, -900, -910, and -920 HU, with pathologic grades of emphysema. They found that the highest correlation between CT and pathology made use of a threshold of -910 HU [135]. Similar good results using -910 HU have been reported by others. Gevenois et al. have shown that using 1-mm sections without intravenous contrast administration, the optimal threshold for HRCT images when compared to morphometric data is -950 HU, regardless of whether macroscopic or microscopic measures of emphysema were used for valida-

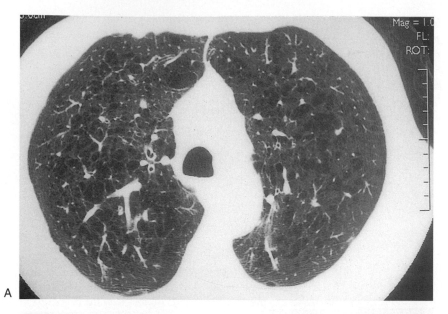

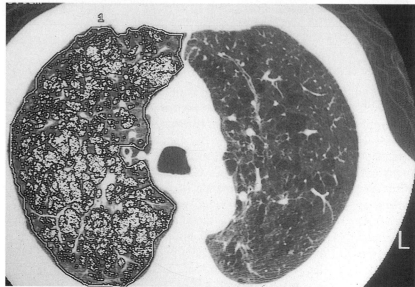

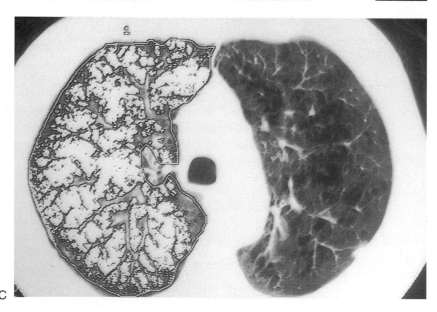

FIG. 7-33. Quantitative CT. **A:** A 1-mm section through the upper lobes shows evidence of confluent centrilobular emphysema. The right lung has been manually segmented. **B:** Density mask visually highlights all pixels measuring less than −950 HU. Mean lung density for the right lung measures −970 HU (SD, 13.5). **C:** A 7-mm section obtained in the same patient at approximately the same level as in **A** and **B**. The density mask highlights all pixels in the right lung less than −910 HU. Mean lung density measures −941 HU (SD, 21.3). Note that results differ dramatically depending on the choice of section thickness and threshold. In general, high-resolution images assessed with lower thresholds (i.e., −950 HU) have proved more accurate in assessing the extent and severity of emphysema on individual sections. This may prove important as multidetector-row scanners become more widely available, allowing whole lung volumes to be scanned with high-resolution techniques. *Continued*

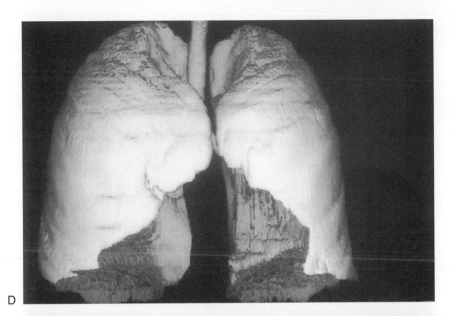

D

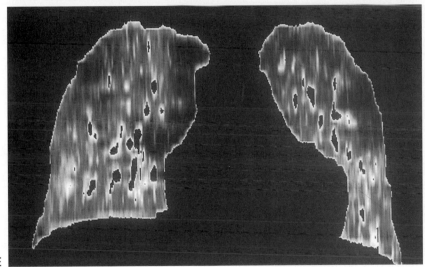

E

FIG. 7-33. *Continued* D: Three-dimensional rendering in this patient, obtained during a single breath hold using contiguous 7-mm sections (pitch = 2). **E:** Volumetrically rendered coronal section in the same patient shows marked heterogeneity of lung density with extensive emphysema largely restricted to the upper lobes. This patient subsequently underwent successful lung volume reduction surgery.

tion (Fig. 7-33) [71,124,125]. It should be kept in mind, however, that despite the fact that a threshold of –950 HU is generally accepted as appropriate for the diagnosis of emphysema, variation in lung density may be present in normal subjects. In a study by Gevenois et al. [151] of 42 healthy subjects ranging from 23 to 71 years in age, the authors found that lung density is influenced by TLC and, to a lesser degree, by age. In the healthy subjects, there was no significant difference between genders and no significant correlation between age and the mean lung density (MLD), but a significant correlation was found between age and the relative area of the lung with attenuation values lower than –950 HU. In addition, a significant correlation was found between the TLC expressed as absolute values and both the RA950 and the MLD. Similarly, as reported by Adams et al. [127] in an evaluation of factors affecting lung density in patients who did not have morphologic evidence of emphysema, the mean CT

lung density varied from –770 HU to –875 HU, and the cross-sectional area of pixels ranging between –900 and –1,000 HU varied from 9.6% to 58%.

Alternatively, computerized analysis of HRCT data may be used to produce a histogram of the frequency distribution of pixel density values in a given lung region (Fig. 7-34). All areas that have densities lower than the lowest fifth of the histogram or fall within a preselected range of densities may be defined as emphysematous [152]. Using this approach, it has been reported that the lowest fifth percentile of the histogram in patients who have emphysema correlates well with the surface area of walls of distal airspace wall per unit volume (AWUV) [146]. Using a similar approach in 28 patients who had emphysema, Gould et al. found significant correlations between the lowest fifth percentile of Hounsfield number values and both the mean value of the surface area of the walls of distal AWUV ($r = –0.77$) and the extent of emphysema ($r = 0.5$) [146].

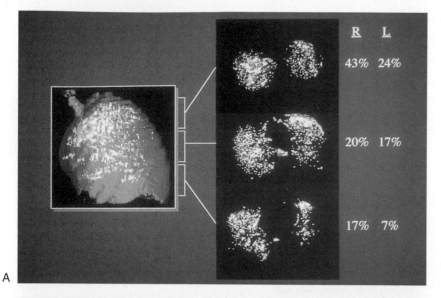

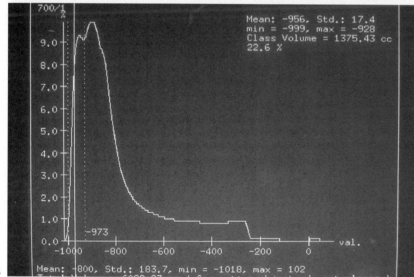

FIG. 7-34. Quantitative CT—three-dimensional evaluation. **A:** Whole-lung histogram with select axial images through the upper, middle, and lower lung fields shown to the left, respectively, obtained from a spiral CT study using 7-mm collimation and a pitch of 1.5. In this case, three separate lung volumes were independently analyzed. All pixels less than –910 HU are highlighted. The numbers to the right indicate the percentage of each of the three lung volumes with pixel densities below –910 HU. In this case, there is marked heterogeneity with more extensive disease in the upper lobes clearly identified. This patient subsequently had lung volume reduction surgery. **B:** Corresponding histogram of the entire right lung. The mean lung density measures –956 HU (SD, 17.4). Using –910 HU as a threshold, 22.6 percent of this lung is emphysematous. Note that whole-lung density measurements are less informative than quantitative evaluation of separate lung volumes for selecting optimal candidates for lung reduction surgery (compare with **A**). (Courtesy of Warren Gefter, M.D., Hospital of the University of Pennsylvania.)

An additional approach has been used, in which the MLD of either a given section or entire lung volumes may be computed as a means of defining the presence and extent of emphysema [110,111]. Good correlation has been reported between these methods and a variety of pathologic grading systems as well as measures of pulmonary function, especially DLCO. It should be emphasized that the development of sophisticated computer programs, coupled with spiral CT scanners, now allows practical quantitative three-dimensional (3D) CT assessment of either select regions or entire lung volumes in a single breath-hold period [130,149,150] (Figs. 7-33 and 7-34). Using 5- and 7-mm collimation with a pitch of 1.5, Park et al. [153] found good correlation between 3D assessment of both mean lung attenuation values and frequency distribution histograms of whole lungs compared with routine two-dimensional analysis ($r = 0.98$ to 0.99) and visual scoring ($r = 0.74$ to 0.82), respectively. Correlation was also noted to be reasonable between 3D densitometric

quantification and a range of physiologic parameters, including the DLCO ($r = -0.57$ to -0.64), the TLC ($r = 0.62$ to 0.71), and the ratio of FEV$_1$ to FVC ($r = -0.75$ to -0.82). It should be noted that the introduction of multidetector-row CT scanners now makes it feasible to reconstruct contiguous thin 1- to 2-mm sections through the entire lung volume. However, whether this will result in more accurate quantification of disease remains to be determined.

Although routine axial images typically suffice for evaluating emphysema, minimum intensity projection (MinIP) images may also be of value, especially in cases with subtle disease (Figs. 7-35 and 7-36) [154,155]. Comparing MinIP images with high-resolution 1-mm sections, Remy-Jardin found that in 13 patients who had subtle emphysema, MinIP was more sensitive than HRCT (81% vs. 62%, respectively) [155]. Furthermore, in four of 16 cases interpreted as normal on routine 1-mm images, subtle foci of emphysema could be identified on the corresponding minimum-intensity projec-

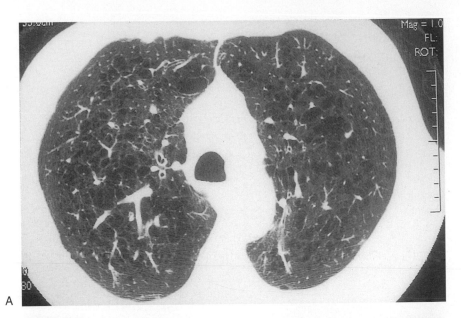

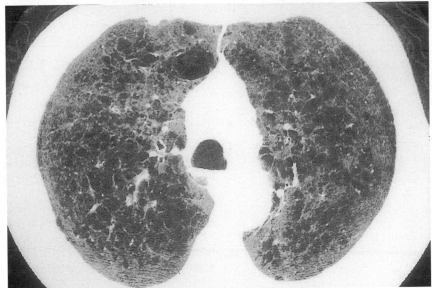

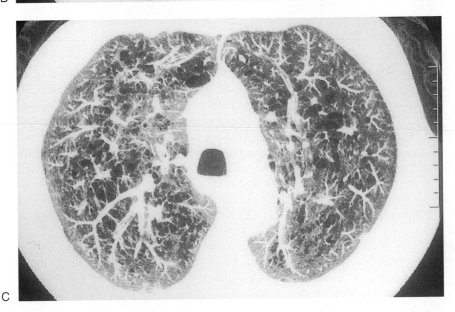

FIG. 7-35. Maximum- (MIP) and minimum- (MinIP) intensity projection imaging in emphysema in the same patient as shown in Figure 7-33. **A:** 1-mm section through the upper lobes shows diffuse centrilobular emphysema. **B,C:** MinIP and MIP images, respectively, derived from five contiguous 1-mm sections centered around the image shown in **A**. By suppressing vascular structures, MinIP images allow more precise definition of areas of low attenuation. In distinction, on MIP images **(C)**, visualization of the pulmonary vasculature is enhanced, allowing more precise anatomic localization of disease. In this case, note the presence of vessels crossing zones of low density characteristic of emphysema as distinct from other causes of focal low lung density **(C)**.

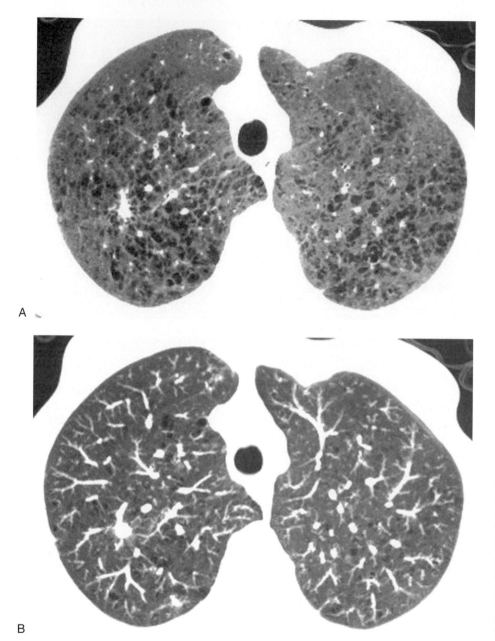

A

B

FIG. 7-36. Minimum- (MinIP) (**A**) and maximum- (MIP) (**B**) intensity projection images in a patient who has centrilobular emphysema. This is the same patient as shown in Figure 7-17. **A:** MinIP image formed from six adjacent 1-mm-thick HRCT scans shows focal lucencies typical of centrilobular emphysema. A small adenocarcinoma is visible in the right upper lobe. **B:** The emphysema is much less conspicuous on the MIP image, although the carcinoma and its relation to vascular structures are better seen.

tion images. In this study, minimum projection images obtained from 8-mm slabs (i.e., eight contiguous 1-mm sections) proved optimal for suppressing vascular structures. It should be noted that similar findings have been reported using MinIP images to identify subtle areas of decreased attenuation in patients who have small airways disease [156]. Comparing high-resolution images obtained in both inspiration and expiration with MinIP images through the lower lobes in 47 consecutive patients who had chronic sputum production, Fotheringham et al. showed that although expiratory images identified a greater extent of disease, interobserver variability was lowest for MinIP images. Although at present there is no indication for the routine use of MinIP images for diagnosing either emphysema or small airways disease, the likelihood of using these images may be

enhanced as multidetector-row scanners capable of routinely generating contiguous 1-mm sections gain widespread use.

To this point, densitometric evaluation primarily has focused on the use of mean lung attenuation, regional percent of emphysematous lung (so-called emphysema index), and histogram analysis of the distribution of CT numbers to detect and quantify the extent of emphysema. In fact, due to partial volume averaging, even using HRCT techniques, these simple density-based methods are relatively insensitive. As suggested by Uppaluri et al., these methods could be improved by additionally assessing the underlying pattern of disease [152]. Using an experimental automated so-called texture-based adaptive multiple feature methodology, these authors were able to merge adjacent pixels to form regions in which the difference between the gray levels of adjacent pixels was small.

This enabled a number of otherwise unfamiliar features to be analyzed, including first-order features such as variance, skewness, kurtosis, and gray level entropy, and second-order features such as gray level nonuniformity, entropy, inertia, and contrast, among others. Although this type of analysis is clearly in its infancy, it may be anticipated that with the aid of more and more sophisticated computed programs, at least some of these features may ultimately prove of clinical value.

Expiratory Imaging in Emphysema

The effect of differing phases of respiration on CT densitometry in patients who have emphysema has been evaluated by a number of investigators. In some studies, this is based on measurement of the pixel indent (PI). The *PI* is defined as the percentage of pixels in both lungs on a single scan that shows an attenuation lower than a predetermined threshold value (usually –900 HU) (see Fig. 3-155) [147,157]. Although the inspiratory PI has wide normal range, the expiratory PI is relatively constant. The normal PI at full inspiration ranges from 0.6 to as much as 58 when the threshold is –900 HU [127], although the mean value for PI ranges from 10 to 25, depending on the level scanned and on the CT scan collimation [157]. At full expiration with a threshold value of –900 HU, the normal range of PI is rather small, with a mean of less than 1.04 (SD, 1.30) [157]. Thus, in normals, the area of lung having an attenuation of less than –900 HU at full expiration in normals can generally be regarded as less than a few percent.

The expiratory PI can be used to quantitatively assess the area of low-attenuation lung in patients who have emphysema (see Fig. 3-155). In one study [147], 64 patients underwent both inspiratory and expiratory CT correlated with pulmonary physiology. There were 28 patients who had an inspiratory PI (measured as less than –900 HU) of more than 40, and 14 of these patients had an expiratory PI of more than 15. This group showed markedly abnormal PFT values suggestive of emphysema, whereas other patients showed normal lung function. Also, an expiratory PI over 15 accurately reflected and quantitated the degree of emphysema estimated by various PFTs.

Some researchers have attempted to standardize expiratory lung density measurements by use of spirometrically gated CT [123,147,158–160]. Lamers et al. [159] showed that images obtained 5 cm above and below the carina at both 90% and 10% of VC allowed accurate differentiation between patients who had emphysema on the one hand, and patients who had chronic bronchitis and controls on the other. Similarly, Beinert et al. [160] compared mean lung densities measured at three levels (at the carina and 5 cm above and below) at 20%, 50%, and 80% of VC in 11 patients who had emphysema and in 24 healthy controls. Although significant differences could be identified between emphysematous patients and controls at all levels, based on a twofold variation in the anteroposterior density gradient at 20% VC and for reasons of intra- and intersubjective comparability, these authors concluded that emphysema is best evaluated at an intermediate lung volume.

Although spirometric gating has not achieved widespread clinical use, the role of expiratory CT scans as a means for evaluating diffuse and focal air-trapping is widespread [149,161,162]. Although the use of expiratory scans to evaluate emphysema has been suggested [147], this has been discredited by Gevenois et al. [71]. In this latter study, 59 patients who had subsequently confirmed emphysema were scanned preoperatively with 1-mm-thick sections during both inspiration and expiration and subsequently evaluated with a variety of threshold values. Relative areas of low attenuation were then correlated to both macroscopic and microscopic indices of emphysema extent and severity to determine optimal expiratory CT thresholds. These proved to be –820 HU and –910 HU using microscopic and macroscopic standards of emphysema, respectively. Significantly, inspiratory scans using a previously validated threshold of –950 HU [124,125] proved superior to expiratory scans for quantifying emphysema, regardless of the method of pathologic correlation. Furthermore, although the relative area of decreased lung attenuation measured on inspiration scans most closely correlated with DLCO ($r = -0.49$; $p < .01$) (also measured in inspiration), the relative area of decreased lung attenuation on expiration most closely correlated with FEV_1/FVC ($r = -0.63$; $p < .001$) and residual volume ($r = 0.46$, $p < .001$). Based on these data, it can be concluded that the extent and severity of emphysema are best measured on scans obtained in inspiration, whereas expiratory scans are more accurate means of assessing airways obstruction with resulting air-trapping [71].

Utility of Computed Tomography

Standard chest radiography and PFTs are insensitive for the diagnosis of early emphysema [84,96]. CT is undoubtedly more sensitive than chest radiographs in diagnosing emphysema and in determining its type and extent. HRCT is also advantageous relative to conventional CT [77,100, 106,107,134,140,145,163,164]. However, before the development of surgical treatments for emphysema, HRCT was rarely indicated as a method for diagnosing emphysema. In fact, the combination of (i) a smoking history, (ii) a low DLCO, (iii) airways obstruction on PFTs, and (iv) an abnormal chest radiograph showing large lung volumes is usually sufficient to make the diagnosis.

On the other hand, some patients who have early emphysema can present with clinical findings more typical of interstitial lung disease or pulmonary vascular disease—namely, shortness of breath and low DLCO—without evidence of airways obstruction on PFTs [136,165]. In such patients, HRCT can be valuable in detecting the presence of emphysema and excluding an interstitial abnormality as a cause of respiratory dysfunction (Fig. 7-37). If significant emphysema is found on HRCT, no further evaluation is necessary; specifically, lung biopsy is not needed. For example, in a study of 470 HRCT examinations by Klein et al. [165], there were 47 cases in which emphysema was the dominant or sole

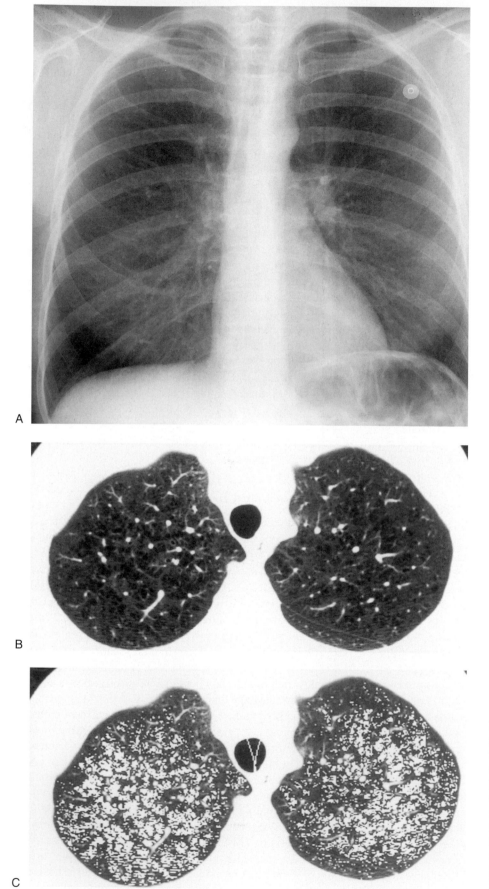

FIG. 7-37. HRCT diagnosis of emphysema in a patient who has a normal chest radiograph, reduced diffusing capacity (50% of predicted), normal expiratory flow, and clinical suspicion of either interstitial lung disease or pulmonary vascular disease. **A:** Chest radiograph appears normal. **B:** HRCT through the upper lobes shows patchy lucency typical of centrilobular emphysema, explaining the patient's disability. **C:** Density mask image highlights the extent of emphysema.

parenchymal abnormality. Of these 47 cases, 16 cases lacked chest radiographic findings of emphysema, and 10 of these 16 cases had decreased single breath diffusing capacity (DLCO <80% predicted) without evidence of airways obstruction (FEV_1/FVC and FEV_1 >80% predicted). In these patients, the severity of emphysema scored on the HRCT correlated closely ($r = 0.8$) with decreasing DLCO.

Furthermore, HRCT has a high specificity for diagnosing emphysema; emphysema is rarely overcalled in normal individuals or in patients who have severe hyperinflation due to other causes [166]. Also, emphysema is accurately distinguished from other causes of cystic lung disease [45]. In one study of patients who had cystic lung diseases, including emphysema [45], HRCT allowed two radiologists to be confident of the diagnosis of emphysema in 95% of cases. When confident, the observers were correct in 100% of the cases, and agreement between the observers was perfect for a confident diagnosis of emphysema ($\kappa = 1$).

It should also be noted that HRCT may be of value in differentiating between patients who have emphysema and those who have other obstructive airways diseases, such as asthma [151,157,166,167]. Although areas of low density may be identified in the lungs of asthmatic patients, these largely are a reflection of air-trapping and not anatomic emphysema. Newman et al. evaluated 18 asthmatics and 22 normal controls using a threshold of –900 HU, in both full inspiration and expiration using 1.5- and 10-mm sections, and found significantly more extensive low-attenuation areas in asthmatics as compared to controls, especially on high-resolution images obtained just above the diaphragm; however, the absence of low-attenuation lung on inspiratory scans excluded emphysema [157]. Gevenois et al. measured the extent of low-attenuation areas in ten mild asymptomatic asthmatics, seven severe asthmatics with documented airflow obstruction and hyperinflation, and 42 normal controls, using a density mask of –950 HU; no significant differences in the proportion of low-density regions was found between any of these groups [151].

Generally speaking, although PFT findings of airways obstruction are common in patients who have emphysema, the degree of airways obstruction correlates poorly with the anatomic extent of emphysema, with r values ranging from 0.40 to 0.70. Furthermore, emphysema can involve 30% of the lung parenchyma without airflow obstruction's being present [91–93,168]. At least partially, the lack of a close correlation between emphysema extent and airways obstruction reflects the fact that emphysema is often associated with chronic bronchitis, which may also contribute to lung function abnormalities in patients who have COPD and is more likely responsible for airways obstruction [131]. In one study of patients who had COPD and fixed expiratory airflow limitation, there was poor correlation between the extent of emphysema and FEV_1 ($r = -0.20$) or FEV_1/FVC ($r = -0.36$) [169], leading the authors to suggest that airflow obstruction in these patients is likely due to associated airways disease.

Similarly, in a study by Gevenois et al. [71] using inspiratory and expiratory HRCT, inspiratory scans were found to be most accurate in showing the extent of pathologic emphysema, whereas expiratory scans correlated best with PFT measures of airways obstruction, a fact which may be related to the presence of associated airways disease. The correlations between the extent of low-attenuation lung (< –950 HU) measured on inspiratory scans and FEV_1 and FEV_1/FVC were –0.50 and –0.63, respectively (both p <.001), whereas on expiratory scans correlation between the extent of low-attenuation lung (< –910 HU) increased to 0.68 and 0.72 (both p <.001), respectively. Abnormalities of diffusing capacity are also common in emphysema. In the study by Gevenois et al. [71], correlations between various measures of Dlco and low-attenuation lung measured on either inspiratory or expiratory scans ranged from –0.41 to –0.50 (p <.01 to p <.001).

Preoperative Assessment of Emphysema

HRCT can be valuable in the preoperative assessment of patients before surgical treatment of emphysema using bullectomy, lung transplantation, or volume reduction surgery [170,171]. HRCT has become routine in the evaluation of such patients before and after operation.

Bullectomy

Bullectomy refers to the surgical removal or decompression of large bullae, which have the effect of compressing relatively normal adjacent lung [172,173]. Most series show little postsurgical improvement when the bullae occupy less than one-third of a hemithorax [174]. However, bullectomy in appropriate patients may result in a decrease in lung volume, improved spirometry, and improved gas exchange [174].

CT has been reported to be of value in the preoperative assessment of patients who have bullous emphysema [175–177]. The majority of patients referred for bullectomy have well-demarcated bullae and varying degrees of emphysema [117]. CT allows for an assessment not only of the extent of bullous disease but also the degree of compression and the severity of emphysema in the remaining lung parenchyma (Figs. 7-31 and 7-32) [117,174,176–178]. In one study [175], CT showed well-defined bullae that were potentially resectable in 23 of 43 patients; 20 patients had bullae in association with generalized emphysema that were not amenable to surgical excision. Surgery is generally impossible if bullae are associated with extensive emphysema. Bullectomy is most effective when localized giant bullae are associated with localized paraseptal emphysema [117].

Lung Transplantation

Lung transplantation has become an important treatment for patients with severe emphysema. In 1998, 1,170 heart-lung (n = 103), single lung (n = 582), or double lung (n = 485) transplantations were registered with the International Heart-Lung Transplantation Registry (http://www.ishlt.org).

Approximately 6.7% of heart-lung transplants, 55.8% of single lung transplants, and 30.1% of double lung transplants were for emphysema.

Various criteria have been developed to enable selection of the most appropriate candidates for lung transplantation [170,171]. CT scans are routinely obtained to search for malignancy [179]. Furthermore, in patients who have a single lung transplantation, the side chosen for lung transplantation depends on the severity of the underlying disease in each lung, which may vary, and the presence of pleural disease, which may result from prior infection, thoracotomy, or other diseases [180]. Ideally, the more abnormal lung is removed, although the presence of markedly abnormal pleura would direct the surgeon to the opposite lung. In one study [179], the chest radiographs and CT scans of 190 transplant candidates were reviewed. CT prompted a change in the determination of which lung was more severely diseased in 27 of 169 (16%) patients. Of the 45 patients who subsequently underwent transplantation, CT prompted a change in the determination of which side to transplant from that made on the basis of plain radiography for four patients (9%). Solitary nodules detected in three patients proved to be bronchogenic carcinomas; two of these lesions were identified only on CT scans.

Lung Volume Reduction Surgery

First introduced by Brantigan in 1957, and reintroduced by Cooper, lung volume reduction surgery (LVRS) promises to transform our approach to the management of patients who have severe emphysema [181,182]. Currently, it is estimated that 2 million people have emphysema in the United States, accounting for more than 90,000 deaths annually, along with other forms of COPD [183]. Overall, it is the fourth-leading cause of death, with a mortality rate of approximately 50% [184].

Only cigarette smoking cessation has been shown to slow the progression of disease, whereas only oxygen therapy has been documented to decrease mortality in hypoxic patients [183]. Before LVRS, the only surgical options for the treatment of emphysema were bullectomy or lung transplantation. Although the precise mechanisms by which LVRS palliates the breathlessness of severe pulmonary emphysema are uncertain, it is likely that removal of nonfunctional lung tissue (downsizing) leads to decreased thoracic distension, allowing the chest wall and diaphragm to assume a more normal configuration. This results in a combination of increased elastic recoil, decreased air-trapping, improved expiratory airflow, and decreased ventilation-perfusion mismatching [148].

Although selection criteria for LVRS have been proposed, these are largely subjective and include patients who have an appropriate clinical presentation, radiographic evidence of bilateral emphysema, and poor pulmonary function despite optimal medical therapy (Table 7-6) [183]. Although PFTs are routinely obtained, usual criteria, including an FEV_1 of less than 30% predicted, residual volume greater than or

---

TABLE 7-6. *Lung volume reduction surgery: patient inclusion and exclusion criteria*

Inclusion criteria:

Radiographic evidence of bilateral emphysema

Studies demonstrating severe air-flow obstruction (FEV_1 = 10–40% of predicted; residual volume >180% of predicted; total lung capacity >110% of predicted)

Attainment of preoperative performance goals; smoking cessation

Exclusion criteria:

Age >80 yr

Previous thoracic surgery (sternotomy; lung resection)

Ischemic heart disease (arrhythmias; history of congestive failure or myocardial infarction within past 6 mo); uncontrolled hypertension

History of recurrent infections: bronchiectasis

Diffuse interstitial lung disease

Abnormal pulmonary function: $Paco_2$ >50 mm Hg; carbon monoxide diffusing capacity <20% of predicted; ventilator dependence; need for supplemental oxygen

Giant bullae

Pulmonary hypertension (peak systolic pressure >45 mm Hg)

Solitary pulmonary nodule (relative contraindication)

Chest wall deformities/pleural adhesions

Evidence of systemic disease/neoplasia felt to compromise survival during 5-year follow-up period

CT evidence for diffuse emphysema judged unsuitable for lung volume reduction surgery

---

Modified from Rationale and design of the National Emphysema Treatment Trial (NETT): a prospective randomized trial of lung reduction surgery. *J Thorac Cardiovasc Surg* 1999;118:518–528; Cleverley JR, Hansell DM. Imaging of patients with severe emphysema considered for lung reduction surgery. *Br J Radiol* 1999;72:227–235; and Kazerooni EA, Whyte RI, Flint A, et al. Imaging of emphysema and lung volume reduction surgery. *Radiographics* 1997;17:1023–1036.

---

equal to 180% of predicted, or TLC greater than or equal to 11% of predicted, have proved to be insensitive and unreliable predictors of response to surgery.

As a consequence, considerable attention has focused on the potential use of CT to improve selection criteria [148, 170,185–193]. Evaluating the relative merits of various studies is difficult due to the wide range of CT techniques and interpretive criteria used by different investigators (Table 7-7). In general, two broad approaches to the use of CT have been used. The first is based on visual inspection [187–189,191]. Typically, this combines estimates of disease severity as mild (<25% of the lung), moderate (25% to 50% of the lung), marked (50% to 75% of the lung), or severe (75% to 100% of the lung) with estimates of heterogeneity [188,194]. Alternatively, emphysema may be evaluated using QCT analysis, using a variety of measurements including MLD and the percent of lung involvement (so-called emphysema index), among others [148,185,186,190,192].

TABLE 7-7. *CT methods for lung volume reduction surgery assessment*

Study	Collimation	Phase of respiration	Technique: image analysis parameters
Bae (n = 10)[a]	Contiguous 10-mm scans; incremental	Inspiratory/expiratory scans	Quantitative CT: histogram evaluation (−900 HU); emphysema index
Holbert (n = 28)[b]	5 mm scans at 8 mm intervals; 10 mm scans at 10 mm intervals; incremental	Inspiratory scans	Quantitative CT: density mask (−910 HU); histogram display (mean CT number); three-dimensional modeling
Becker (n = 28)[c]	Contiguous 10-mm scans; spiral	Inspiratory scans	Quantitative CT: individual lung total capacity, residual volume, emphysema index, ratio of airspace to tissue volume
Gierada (n = 70)[d]	Contiguous 8- and 10-mm scans; spiral	Inspiratory scans	Quantitative CT: indices of global emphysema (−900 HU; −960 HU), regional emphysema severity, heterogeneity, and volume of lung tissue (−850 to −701 HU)
Gierada (n = 46)[e]	Contiguous 8- and 10-mm scans; incremental	Inspiratory scans	See above
Hunsacker (n = 20)[f]	Six select 1-mm HRCT scans	Inspiratory scans	Visual scoring: severity and extent (4-point scale); total emphysema score
Hamacher (n = 37)[g]	1-mm scans every 15 mm, contiguous 8-mm scans; spiral	Inspiratory scans	Visual scoring: degree of heterogeneity; upper versus lower lobe distribution
Slone (n = 50)[h]	Contiguous 8- and 10-mm scans; spiral	Inspiratory scans	Visual scoring: emphysema severity, degree of heterogeneity (5-point scale); degree of hyperinflation/lung compression

[a]Bae KT, Slone RM, Gierada DS, et al. Patients with emphysema: quantitative CT analysis before and after lung volume reduction surgery. Work in progress. *Radiology* 1997;203:705–714.
[b]Holbert JM, Brown ML, Sciurba FC, et al. Changes in lung volume and volume of emphysema after unilateral lung reduction surgery: analysis with CT lung densitometry. *Radiology* 1996;201:793–797.
[c]Becker MD, Borkmon YM, Austin JH, et al. Lung volumes before and after lung volume reduction surgery: quantitative CT analysis. *Am J Respir Crit Care Med* 1998;157:1593–1599.
[d]Gierada DS, Tusen RD, Villanueva IA, et al. Patient selection for lung volume reduction surgery: an objective model based on prior clinical decisions and quantitative CT analysis. *Chest* 2000;117:991–998.
[e]Gierada DS, Slone RM, Bae KT, et al. Pulmonary emphysema: comparison of preoperative quantitative CT and physiologic index values with clinical outcome after lung volume reduction surgery. *Radiology* 1997;205:235–242.
[f]Hunsaker A, Ingenito E, Topal U, et al. Preoperative screening for lung volume reduction surgery: usefulness of combining thin-section CT with physiologic assessment. *AJR Am J Roentgenol* 1998;170:309–314.
[g]Hamacher J, Bloch KE, Stammberger U, et al. Two years' outcome of lung volume reduction surgery in different morphologic emphysema types. *Ann Thorac Surg* 1999;68:1792–1798.
[h]Slone RM, Pilgram TK, Gierada DS, et al. Lung volume reduction surgery: comparison of preoperative radiologic features and clinical outcome [see comments]. *Radiology* 1997;204:685–693.

Hamacher et al., using a simplified morphologic classification, divided patients into three groups based on the pattern of distribution of disease as either homogeneous, moderately heterogeneous, or markedly heterogeneous [191]. By definition, *heterogeneous disease* implies marked regional variation in the severity of disease; patients who have centrilobular emphysema characteristically have more extensive involvement in the upper lobes, compared with patients who have alpha-1-antitrypsin deficiency and more extensive disease in the lung bases. Using this approach, these authors showed that functional improvement after LVRS was most pronounced in patients who had markedly heterogeneous disease, with an increase from preoperative FEV_1 of 31% predicted to 52% postoperatively [191]. In distinction, patients who had either moderately heterogeneous or homogeneous distribution showed significantly less improvement in their postoperative FEV_1 (from 29% to 44% and 26% to 38%, respectively). Interestingly, at 24 months, whereas improvement continued to be greatest in the group with markedly heterogeneous disease, significant improvement could still be identified in all three groups, suggesting that the ability of visual grading to accurately preoperatively predict individuals unlikely to improve is limited.

In this regard, Hunsaker et al. evaluated 20 preoperative patients using a four-point scale to visually assess the extent and severity of emphysema using six noncontiguous 1-mm sections (total score, 0 to 144) [189]. Using a postoperative change in FEV_1 of greater than or less than 150 mL to differentiate between responders and nonresponders, respectively, these authors showed that no patient who had mild emphysema (CT score <50) responded. However, in eight of the remaining 16 patients who had moderate to severe disease (CT scores >50) and in whom inspiratory resistance was measured, seven in whom inspiratory resistance measurement exceeded 8.5 cm H_2O per L per second failed to respond to surgery, suggesting to these investigators that optimal preoperative screening requires both radiologic and physiologic assessment [189]. It should be noted that the necessity to use esophageal balloon catheters to obtain these measurements has limited widespread acceptance of this approach.

Despite good results reported for visual grading, ideally, optimal preoperative evaluation should use more objective measurements of disease extent and severity. Currently, although not widely available, the use of QCT has been advocated as a more precise method for assessing morphologic alterations in the lung [148,185,186,190,192]. Bae et al., in an attempt to better define mechanisms of palliation after LVRS, assessed the accuracy of QCT by evaluating both inspiratory and expiratory images in ten patients before and after surgery using semiautomated segmentation methods [148]. Evaluating the frequency distribution of lung density histograms and measuring lung volumes, these authors found good correlation between CT emphysema indices and routine measurements of pulmonary function. In particular, postoperative changes in lung morphology were shown to correlate with improvement in exercise tolerance and pulmonary function.

Holbert et al., using density mask software to calculate the volume of the lungs and the volume of emphysema, also emphasized the ability of QCT to evaluate lung morphology [185]. In this study of 28 patients evaluated before and after LVRS, these authors showed that although the lung volume reduced surgically decreased by 22%, the remaining lung volume increased by only 4%, confirming that unilateral lung reduction does not cause statistically significant worsening of the remaining emphysematous lung. Similar results have been reported by Becker et al. [190].

In the most extensive study to date, Gierada et al. compared CT findings in 70 patients selected for bilateral LVRS with 32 patients denied LVRS based on subjective interpretation of the extent and severity of emphysema on chest radiographs, CT scans, and perfusion scintigraphy [192]. Using the percent of severe emphysema (defined as lung density less than

or equal to –960 HU), the ratio of upper lung to lower lung emphysema (threshold = –900 HU), and the residual volume to model selection decisions, these authors reported an overall correct prediction rate of 87%, including 91% of selected patients and 78% of excluded patients. Furthermore, patients who had higher selection probabilities based on QCT indices showed better postoperative improvements in physiologic measurements and exercise tolerance [192]. Based on these data, these authors concluded that QCT may play an important role in presurgical selection by improving the consistency by which selection criteria are applied.

In addition to improving selection of patients for LVRS, it should be emphasized that CT also plays an invaluable role in excluding potential candidates by identifying otherwise unsuspected pathology. Such patients include those who have bronchiectasis; unexpected coexisting interstitial lung disease, in particular IPF (Fig. 7-38); diseases that may radiographically mimic emphysema, such as bronchiolitis obliterans or end-stage LCH; dilated pulmonary arteries due to pulmonary hypertension; and subtle chest wall abnormalities (Table 7-6) [193]. It should be emphasized that the presence of emphysema may lead to a mistaken diagnosis of underlying interstitial disease, especially when complicated by acute airspace consolidation (Fig. 7-39). Awareness that acute pathologic processes may appear unusual in the presence of underlying emphysema usually obviates the problem clinically.

Most important is the identification of occult lung neoplasms (Figs. 7-17 and 7-36). It has now been shown that up to 7% of patients will have otherwise unsuspected neoplasms [179,195]. In one study of 148 patients selected for LVRS, 11% proved to have suspicious nodules; of these, nine lesions in eight patients proved to be malignant [196]. Most important, eight of these nine lesions proved to be Stage I cancers. Conversely, it should also be noted that in a significant percentage of cases evaluated for LVRS, lung cancers not identified on preoperative CT studies are often

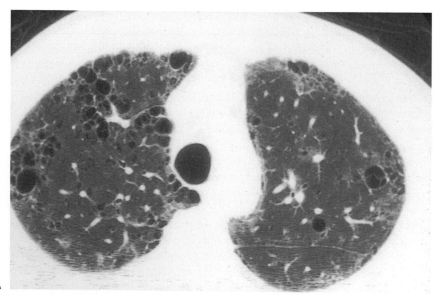

A

FIG. 7-38. A: HRCT section through the upper lobes in a patient being evaluated for lung volume reduction surgery (LVRS) shows extensive emphysema. *Continued*

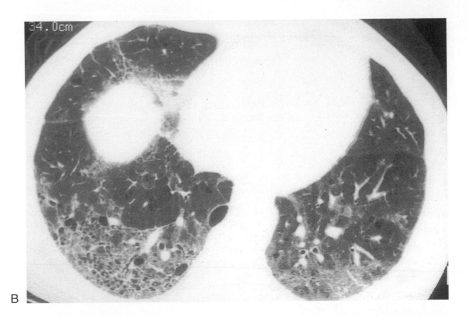

FIG. 7-38. *Continued* **B:** HRCT section through the lung bases in the same patient shows findings characteristic of diffuse lung fibrosis. CT is especially valuable in assessing potential candidates for LVRS by disclosing otherwise unexpected diffuse infiltrative lung diseases.

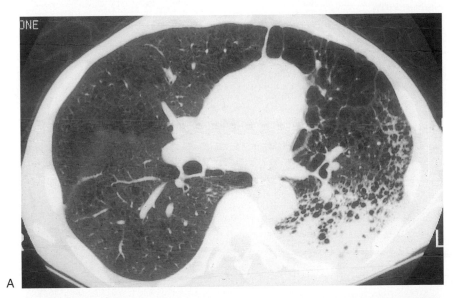

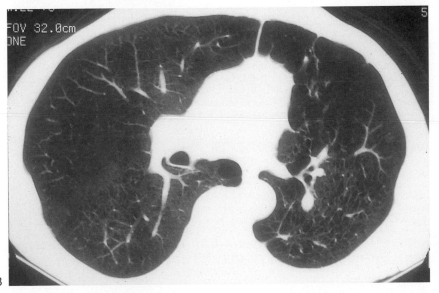

FIG. 7-39. A: HRCT section through the mid-lungs shows apparent honeycombing in the left lung. Extensive centrilobular emphysema is present on the right side. **B:** Section at the same level several weeks later, after a course of antibiotics, shows that apparent honey-combing in **A** actually represents acute air-space consolidation superimposed on severe underlying emphysema, in this case due to bacterial pneumonia.

identified at surgery. As documented by Hazelrigg et al. in a study of 281 patients having LVRS, 17 of 78 (22%) nodules proved malignant: of these, 14 were not identified prospectively by CT [197].

Despite these data, the role of CT as a means for preoperative evaluation of potential candidates for LVRS has yet to be determined. It should be noted that in several studies, chest radiographs have proven as accurate as CT in predicting response to LVRS [187,198]. Maki et al. assessed preoperative radiographs in 57 patients and showed that marked heterogeneity and unequivocal lung compression were 100% predictive of a favorable outcome (measured as a 30% improvement in either FEV_1, or the 6-minute walk test), whereas a lack of heterogeneity and lack of lung parenchymal compression were 94% and 92% predictive of an unfavorable outcome, respectively [198]. Based on these data, these authors concluded that chest radiographs alone may be sufficient to preoperatively evaluate potential LVRS candidates. Radiographic evidence of hyperinflation failed to prove a significant predictor of outcome [198]. Similarly, poor predictive values have also been noted for measurements of diaphragmatic excursion comparing inspiratory with expiratory radiographs [199]. It should be noted that, although similar evaluations have been performed using fast gradient-echo, breath-hold magnetic resonance imaging through the thorax in both full inspiration and expiration, this technique has not proved generally useful [200].

REFERENCES

1. Howarth DM, Gilchrist GS, Mullan BP, et al. Langerhans cell histiocytosis: diagnosis, natural history, management, and outcome. *Cancer* 1999;85:2278–2290.
2. Soler P, Tazi A, Hance AJ. Pulmonary Langerhans cell granulomatosis. *Curr Opin Pulm Med* 1995;1:406–416.
3. Travis WD, Borok Z, Roum JH, et al. Pulmonary Langerhans cell granulomatosis (histiocytosis X): a clinicopathologic study of 48 cases. *Am J Surg Pathol* 1993;17:971–986.
4. Marcy TW, Reynolds HY. Pulmonary histiocytosis X. *Lung* 1985;163:129–150.
5. Colby TV, Lombard C. Histiocytosis X in the lung. *Hum Pathol* 1983;14:847–856.
6. Willman CL, Busque L, Griffith BB, et al. Langerhans' cell histiocytosis (histiocytosis X)—a clonal proliferative disease. *N Engl J Med* 1994;331:154–160.
7. Brabencova E, Tazi A, Lorenzato M, et al. Langerhans cells in Langerhans cell granulomatosis are not actively proliferating cells. *Am J Pathol* 1998;152:1143–1149.
8. Fartoukh M, Humbert M, Capron F, et al. Severe pulmonary hypertension in histiocytosis X. *Am J Respir Crit Care Med* 2000;161:216–223.
9. Hamada K, Teramoto S, Narita N, et al. Pulmonary veno-occlusive disease in pulmonary Langerhans' cell granulomatosis. *Eur Respir J* 2000;15:421–423.
10. Gaensler EA, Carrington CB. Open biopsy for chronic diffuse infiltrative lung disease: clinical, roentgenographic, and physiologic correlations in 502 patients. *Ann Thorac Surg* 1980;30:411–426.
11. Lewis JG. Eosinophilic granuloma and its variants with special reference to lung involvement: a report of 12 patients. *QJM* 1964;33:337–359.
12. Lacronique J, Roth C, Battesti JP, et al. Chest radiological features of pulmonary histiocytosis X: a report based on 50 adult cases. *Thorax* 1982;37:104–109.
13. Friedman PJ, Liebow AA, Sokoloff J. Eosinophilic granuloma of lung: clinical aspects of primary pulmonary histiocytosis in the adult. *Medicine* 1981;60:385–396.
14. Basset F, Corrin B, Spencer H, et al. Pulmonary histiocytosis X. *Am Rev Respir Dis* 1978;118:811–820.
15. Hance AJ, Basset F, Saumon G, et al. Smoking and interstitial lung disease: the effect of cigarette smoking on the incidence of pulmonary histiocytosis X and sarcoidosis. *Ann N Y Acad Sci* 1986;465:643–656.
16. Winterbauer RH, Dreis DF, Jolly PC. Clinical correlation. In: Dail DH, Hammar SP, eds. *Pulmonary pathology*. New York: Springer-Verlag, 1988:1148–1151.
17. Tazi A, Montcelly L, Bergeron A, et al. Relapsing nodular lesions in the course of adult pulmonary Langerhans cell histiocytosis. *Am J Respir Crit Care Med* 1998;157:2007–2010.
18. Prophet D. Primary pulmonary histiocytosis X. *Clin Chest Med* 1982;3:643–653.
19. Moore AD, Godwin JD, Müller NL, et al. Pulmonary histiocytosis X: comparison of radiographic and CT findings. *Radiology* 1989; 172:249–254.
20. Brauner MW, Grenier P, Mouelhi MM, et al. Pulmonary histiocytosis X: evaluation with high resolution CT. *Radiology* 1989;172:255–258.
21. Brauner MW, Grenier P, Tijani K, et al. Pulmonary Langerhans cell histiocytosis: evolution of lesions on CT scans. *Radiology* 1997; 204:497–502.
22. Grenier P, Valeyre D, Cluzel P, et al. Chronic diffuse interstitial lung disease: diagnostic value of chest radiography and high-resolution CT. *Radiology* 1991;179:123–132.
23. Kulwiec EL, Lynch DA, Aguayo SM, et al. Imaging of pulmonary histiocytosis X. *Radiographics* 1992;12:515–526.
24. Giron J, Tawil A, Trussard V, et al. [Contribution of high resolution x-ray computed tomography to the diagnosis of pulmonary histiocytosis X: apropos of 12 cases]. *Ann Radiol (Paris)* 1990;33:31–38.
25. Taylor DB, Joske D, Anderson J, et al. Cavitating pulmonary nodules in histiocytosis-X high resolution CT demonstration. *Australas Radiol* 1990;34:253–255.
26. Müller NL, Miller RR. Computed tomography of chronic diffuse infiltrative lung disease: part 2. *Am Rev Respir Dis* 1990;142:1440–1448.
27. Stern EJ, Webb WR, Golden JA, et al. Cystic lung disease associated with eosinophilic granuloma and tuberous sclerosis: air-trapping at dynamic ultrafast high-resolution CT. *Radiology* 1992;182:325–329.
28. Kelkel E, Pison C, Brambilla E, et al. [Value of high-resolution tomodensitometry in pulmonary histiocytosis X: radiological, clinical and functional correlations]. *Rev Mal Respir* 1992;9:307–311.
29. Gruden JF, Webb WR, Naidich DP, et al. Multinodular disease: anatomic localization at thin-section CT—multireader evaluation of a simple algorithm. *Radiology* 1999;210:711–720.
30. Müller NL, Miller RR, Webb WR, et al. Fibrosing alveolitis: CT-pathologic correlation. *Radiology* 1986;160:585–588.
31. Guhl L. [Pulmonary involvement in lymphangioleiomyomatosis: studies using high-resolution computed tomography]. *Rofo* 1988;149:576–579.
32. Lenoir S, Grenier P, Brauner MW, et al. Pulmonary lymphangioleiomyomatosis and tuberous sclerosis: comparison of radiographic and thin-section CT findings. *Radiology* 1990;175:329–334.
33. Rappaport DC, Weisbrod GL, Herman SJ, et al. Pulmonary lymphangioleiomyomatosis: high-resolution CT findings in four cases. *AJR Am J Roentgenol* 1989;152:961–964.
34. Sherrier RH, Chiles C, Roggli V. Pulmonary lymphangioleiomyomatosis: CT findings. *AJR Am J Roentgenol* 1989;153:937–940.
35. Templeton PA, McLoud TC, Müller NL, et al. Pulmonary lymphangioleiomyomatosis: CT and pathologic findings. *J Comput Assist Tomogr* 1989;13:54–57.
36. Müller NL, Chiles C, Kullnig P. Pulmonary lymphangioleiomyomatosis: correlation of CT with radiographic and functional findings. *Radiology* 1990;175:335–339.
37. Aquino SL, Webb WR, Zaloudek CJ, et al. Lung cysts associated with honeycombing: change in size on expiratory CT scans. *AJR Am J Roentgenol* 1994;162:583–584.
38. Worthy SA, Brown MJ, Müller NL. Technical report: cystic air spaces in the lung: change in size on expiratory high-resolution CT in 23 patients. *Clin Radiol* 1998;53:515–519.
39. Ichikawa Y, Kinoshita M, Koga T, et al. Lung cyst formation in lymphocytic interstitial pneumonia: CT features. *J Comput Assist Tomogr* 1994;18:745–748.

40. Desai SR, Nicholson AG, Stewart S, et al. Benign pulmonary lymphocytic infiltration and amyloidosis: computed tomographic and pathologic features in three cases. *J Thorac Imag* 1997;12:215–220.

41. Johkoh T, Müller NL, Pickford HA, et al. Lymphocytic interstitial pneumonia: thin-section CT findings in 22 patients. *Radiology* 1999;212:567–572.

42. Feuerstein I, Archer A, Pluda JM, et al. Thin-walled cavities, cysts, and pneumothorax in *Pneumocystis carinii* pneumonia: further observations with histopathologic correlation. *Radiology* 1990;174:697–702.

43. Panicek DM. Cystic pulmonary lesions in patients with AIDS (editorial). *Radiology* 1989;173:12–14.

44. Gurney JW, Bates FT. Pulmonary cystic disease: comparison of *Pneumocystis carinii* pneumatoceles and bullous emphysema due to intravenous drug abuse. *Radiology* 1989;173:27–31.

45. Bonelli FS, Hartman TE, Swensen SJ, et al. Accuracy of high-resolution CT in diagnosing lung diseases. *AJR Am J Roentgenol* 1998;170:1507–1512.

46. Lynch DA, Hay T, Newell Jr JD, et al. Pediatric diffuse lung disease: diagnosis and classification using high-resolution CT. *AJR Am J Roentgenol* 1999;173:713–718.

47. Seely JM, Effmann EL, Müller NL. High-resolution CT of pediatric lung disease: imaging findings. *AJR Am J Roentgenol* 1997;168:1269–1275.

48. Colby TV, Carrington CB. Infiltrative lung disease. In: Thurlbeck WM, ed. *Pathology of the lung.* Stuttgart: Thieme Medical Publishers, 1988:425–518.

49. Corrin B, Liebow AA, Friedman PJ. Pulmonary lymphangioleiomyomatosis: a review. *Am J Pathol* 1975;79:348–382.

50. Chu SC, Horiba K, Usuki J, et al. Comprehensive evaluation of 35 patients with lymphangioleiomyomatosis. *Chest* 1999;115:1041–1052.

51. Kalassian KG, Doyle R, Kao P, et al. Lymphangioleiomyomatosis: new insights. *Am J Respir Crit Care Med* 1997;155:1183–1186.

52. Beck GJ, Sullivan EJ, Stoller JK, et al. Lymphangioleiomyomatosis: new insights [letter;comment]. *Am J Respir Crit Care Med* 1997;156:670.

53. Sullivan EJ. Lymphangioleiomyomatosis: a review. *Chest* 1998;114:1689–1703.

54. Sobonya RE, Quan SF, Fleishman JS. Pulmonary lymphangioleiomyomatosis: quantitative analysis of lesions producing airflow limitation. *Hum Pathol* 1985;16:1122–1128.

55. Flieder DB, Travis WD. Clear cell "sugar" tumor of the lung: association with lymphangioleiomyomatosis and multifocal micronodular pneumocyte hyperplasia in a patient with tuberous sclerosis. *Am J Surg Pathol* 1997;21:1242–1247.

56. Lantuejoul S, Ferretti G, Negoescu A, et al. Multifocal alveolar hyperplasia associated with lymphangioleiomyomatosis in tuberous sclerosis. *Histopathology* 1997;30:570–575.

57. Guinee D, Singh R, Azumi N, et al. Multifocal micronodular pneumocyte hyperplasia: a distinctive pulmonary manifestation of tuberous sclerosis. *Mod Pathol* 1995;8:902–906.

58. Braman SS, Mark EJ. A 32-year-old woman with recurrent pneumothorax. Massachusetts General Hospital Case Records, case 24-1988. *N Engl J Med* 1988;318:1601–1610.

59. Taylor JR, Ryu J, Colby TV, et al. Lymphangioleiomyomatosis. Clinical course in 32 patients. *N Engl J Med* 1990;323:1254–1260.

60. Carrington CB, Cugell DW, Gaensler EA, et al. Lymphangioleiomyomatosis: physiologic-pathologic-radiologic correlations. *Am Rev Respir Dis* 1977;116:977–995.

61. Kitaichi M, Nishimura K, Itoh H, et al. Pulmonary lymphangioleiomyomatosis: a report of 46 patients including a clinicopathologic study of prognostic factors. *Am J Respir Crit Care Med* 1995;151:527–533.

62. Adamson D, Heinrichs WL, Raybin DM, et al. Successful treatment of pulmonary lymphangioleiomyomatosis with oophorectomy and progesterone. *Am Rev Respir Dis* 1985;132:916–921.

63. Nine JS, Yousem SA, Paradis IL, et al. Lymphangioleiomyomatosis: recurrence after lung transplantation. *J Heart Lung Transplant* 1994;13:714–719.

64. Silverstein EF, Ellis K, Wolff M, et al. Pulmonary lymphangioleiomyomatosis. *AJR Am J Roentgenol* 1974;120:832–850.

65. Kullnig P, Melzer G, Smolle-Jüttner FM. High-resolution-computertomographie des thorax bei lymphangioleiomyomatose and tuberöser sklerose. *Rofo* 1989;151:32–35.

66. Merchant RN, Pearson MG, Rankin RN, et al. Computerized tomography in the diagnosis of lymphangioleiomyomatosis. *Am Rev Respir Dis* 1985;131:295–297.

67. Aberle DR, Hansell DM, Brown K, et al. Lymphangioleiomyomatosis: CT, chest radiographic, and functional correlations. *Radiology* 1990;176:381–387.

68. Kirchner J, Stein A, Viel K, et al. Pulmonary lymphangioleiomyomatosis: high-resolution CT findings. *Eur Radiol* 1999;9:49–54.

69. Crausman RS, Lynch DA, Mortenson RL, et al. Quantitative CT predicts the severity of physiologic dysfunction in patients with lymphangioleiomyomatosis. *Chest* 1996;109:131–137.

70. Crausman RS, Jennings CA, Mortenson RL, et al. Lymphangioleiomyomatosis: the pathophysiology of diminished exercise capacity. *Am J Respir Crit Care Med* 1996;153:1368–1376.

71. Gevenois PA, De Vuyst P, Sy M, et al. Pulmonary emphysema: quantitative CT during expiration. *Radiology* 1996;199:825–829.

72. Bonetti F, Chiodera PL, Pea M, et al. Transbronchial biopsy in lymphangioleiomyomatosis of the lung. HMB45 for diagnosis. *Am J Surg Pathol* 1993;17:1092–1102.

73. Guinee Jr DG, Feuerstein I, Koss MN, et al. Pulmonary lymphangioleiomyomatosis: diagnosis based on results of transbronchial biopsy and immunohistochemical studies and correlation with high-resolution computed tomography findings. *Arch Pathol Lab Med* 1994;118:846–849.

74. Collins J, Müller NL, Kazerooni EA, et al. Lung transplantation for lymphangioleiomyomatosis: role of imaging in the assessment of complications related to the underlying disease. *Radiology* 1999;210:325–332.

75. Cardoso WV, Thurlbeck WM. Pathogenesis and terminology of emphysema. *Am J Respir Crit Care Med* 1994;149:1383.

76. Snider GL. Pathogenesis and terminology of emphysema. *Am J Respir Crit Care Med* 1994;149:1382–1383.

77. Thurlbeck WM, Müller NL. Emphysema: definition, imaging, and quantification. *AJR Am J Roentgenol* 1994;163:1017–1025.

78. Snider GL, Kleinerman J, Thurlbeck WM, et al. The definition of emphysema: report of a National Heart, Lung, and Blood Institute, Division of Lung Diseases workshop. *Am Rev Respir Dis* 1985;132:182–185.

79. Janoff A. Elastases and emphysema. Current assessment of the protease-antiprotease hypothesis. *Am Rev Respir Dis* 1985;132:417–433.

80. Snider GL. The pathogenesis of emphysema—twenty years of progress. *Am Rev Respir Dis* 1981;124:321–324.

81. King MA, Stone JA, Diaz PT, et al. Alpha 1 antitrypsin deficiency: evaluation of bronchiectasis with CT. *Radiology* 1996;199:137–141.

82. Hunninghake GW, Crystal RG. Cigarette smoking and lung destruction: accumulation of neutrophils in the lungs of cigarette smokers. *Am Rev Respir Dis* 1983;128:833–838.

83. Blue ML, Janoff A. Possible mechanisms of emphysema in cigarette smokers: release of elastase from human polymorphonuclear leukocytes by cigarette smoke condensate in vitro. *Am Rev Respir Dis* 1978;117:317–325.

84. Thurlbeck WM. *Chronic airflow obstruction in lung disease.* Philadelphia: W. B. Saunders, 1976:12–30.

85. Stern EJ, Frank MS, Schmutz JF, et al. Panlobular pulmonary emphysema caused by i.v. injection of methylphenidate (Ritalin): findings on chest radiographs and CT scans. *AJR Am J Roentgenol* 1994;162:555–560.

86. Tuddenham WJ. Glossary of terms for thoracic radiology: recommendations of the Nomenclature Committee of the Fleischner Society. *AJR Am J Roentgenol* 1984;143:509–517.

87. Thurlbeck WM. Morphology of emphysema and emphysema-like conditions. In: *Chronic airflow obstruction in lung disease.* Philadelphia: W. B. Saunders, 1976:96–234.

88. American Thoracic Society. Standards for the diagnosis and care of patients with chronic obstructive pulmonary disease (COPD) and asthma. *Am Rev Respir Dis* 1987;136:225–243.

89. Bohadana AB, Peslin R, Uffholtz H, et al. Pulmonary function and clinical pattern in homozygous (PiZ) alpha1-antitrypsin deficiency. *Respiration* 1979;37:167–176.

90. Simonsson BG. Chronic cough and expectoration in patients with asthma and in patients with alpha1-antitrypsin deficiency. *Eur J Respir Dis Suppl* 1982;118:123–128.

91. Pratt PC. Role of conventional chest radiography in diagnosis and exclusion of emphysema. *Am J Med* 1987;82:998–1006.

92. Pratt PC. Conventional chest films can reveal emphysema, but not COPD (editorial). *Chest* 1987;92:8.

93. Burki NK. Conventional chest films can identify airflow obstruction (editorial). *Chest* 1988;93:675–676.

94. Burki NK. Roentgenologic diagnosis of emphysema: accurate or not? *Chest* 1989;95:1178–1179.

95. Sutinen S, Christoforidis AJ, Klugh GA, et al. Roentgenologic criteria for the recognition of nonsymptomatic pulmonary emphysema: correlation between roentgenologic findings and pulmonary pathology. *Am Rev Respir Dis* 1965;91:69–76.

96. Thurlbeck WM, Simon G. Radiographic appearance of the chest in emphysema. *AJR Am J Roentgenol* 1978;130:429–440.

97. Reich SB, Weinshelbaum A, Yee J. Correlation of radiographic measurements and pulmonary function tests in chronic obstructive pulmonary disease. *AJR Am J Roentgenol* 1985;144:695–699.

98. Simon G, Pride NB, Jones NL, et al. Relation between abnormalities in the chest radiograph and changes in pulmonary function in chronic bronchitis and emphysema. *Thorax* 1973;28:15–23.

99. Burki NL, Krumpelman JL. Correlation of pulmonary function with the chest roentgenogram in chronic airway obstruction. *Am Rev Respir Dis* 1980;121:217–223.

100. Hruban RH, Meziane MA, Zerhouni EA, et al. High resolution computed tomography of inflation fixed lungs: pathologic-radiologic correlation of centrilobular emphysema. *Am Rev Respir Dis* 1987;136:935–940.

101. Webb WR, Stein MG, Finkbeiner WE, et al. Normal and diseased isolated lungs: high-resolution CT. *Radiology* 1988;166:81–87.

102. Foster Jr WL, Gimenez EI, Roubidoux MA, et al. The emphysemas: radiologic-pathologic correlations. *Radiographics* 1993;13:311–328.

103. Arakawa H, Kurihara Y, Nakajima Y, et al. Computed tomography measurements of overinflation in chronic obstructive pulmonary disease: evaluation of various radiographic signs. *J Thorac Imag* 1998;13:188–192.

104. Murata K, Itoh H, Todo G, et al. Centrilobular lesions of the lung: demonstration by high-resolution CT and pathologic correlation. *Radiology* 1986;161:641–645.

105. Murata K, Khan A, Herman PG. Pulmonary parenchymal disease: evaluation with high-resolution CT. *Radiology* 1989;170:629–635.

106. Bergin CJ, Müller NL, Miller RR. CT in the qualitative assessment of emphysema. *J Thorac Imag* 1986;1:94–103.

107. Miller RR, Müller NL, Vedal S, et al. Limitations of computed tomography in the assessment of emphysema. *Am Rev Respir Dis* 1989;139:980–983.

108. Guest PJ, Hansell DM. High resolution computed tomography (HRCT) in emphysema associated with alpha-1-antitrypsin deficiency. *Clin Radiol* 1992;45:260–266.

109. Shin MS, Ho KJ. Bronchiectasis in patients with alpha 1-antitrypsin deficiency. A rare occurrence? *Chest* 1993;104:1384–1386.

110. Dirksen A, Friis M, Olesen KP, et al. Progress of emphysema in severe alpha 1-antitrypsin deficiency as assessed by annual CT. *Acta Radiol* 1997;38:826–832.

111. Zagers H, Vrooman HA, Aarts NJ, et al. Assessment of the progression of emphysema by quantitative analysis of spirometrically gated computed tomography images. *Invest Radiol* 1996;31:761–767.

112. Lesur O, Delorme N, Fromaget JM, et al. Computed tomography in the etiologic assessment of idiopathic spontaneous pneumothorax. *Chest* 1990;98:341–347.

113. Peters RM, Peters BA, Benirschke SK, et al. Chest dimensions in young adults with spontaneous pneumothorax. *Ann Thorac Surg* 1978;25:193–196.

114. Bense L, Lewander R, Eklund G, et al. Nonsmoking, non-alpha-1-antitrypsin deficiency induced emphysema in nonsmokers with healing spontaneous pneumothorax, identified by computed tomography of the lungs. *Chest* 1993;103:433–438.

115. Mitlehner W, Friedrich M, Dissmann W. Value of computer tomography in the detection of bullae and blebs in patients with primary spontaneous pneumothorax. *Respiration* 1992;59:221–227.

116. Stern EJ, Webb WR, Weinacker A, et al. Idiopathic giant bullous emphysema (vanishing lung syndrome): imaging findings in nine patients. *AJR Am J Roentgenol* 1994;162:279–282.

117. Gaensler EA, Jederlinic PJ, FitzGerald MX. Patient work-up for bullectomy. *J Thorac Imag* 1986;13:75–93.

118. Orton DF, Gurney JW. Spontaneous reduction in size of bullae (autobullectomy). *J Thorac Imag* 1999;14:118–121.

119. Kinsella N, Müller NL, Vedal S, et al. Emphysema in silicosis: a comparison of smokers with nonsmokers using pulmonary function testing and computed tomography. *Am Rev Respir Dis* 1990;141:1497–1500.

120. Akira M, Higashihara T, Yokoyama K, et al. Radiographic type p pneumoconiosis: high-resolution CT. *Radiology* 1989;171:117–123.

121. Stern EJ, Frank MS. CT of the lung in patients with pulmonary emphysema: diagnosis, quantification, and correlation with pathologic and physiologic findings. *AJR Am J Roentgenol* 1994;162:791–798.

122. Kemerink GJ, Lamers RJ, Thelissen GR, et al. Scanner conformity in CT densitometry of the lungs. *Radiology* 1995;197:749–752.

123. Kohz P, Stabler A, Beinert T, et al. Reproducibility of quantitative, spirometrically controlled CT. *Radiology* 1995;197:539–542.

124. Gevenois PA, de Maertelaer V, De Vuyst P, et al. Comparison of computed density and macroscopic morphometry in pulmonary emphysema. *Am J Respir Crit Care Med* 1995;152:653–657.

125. Gevenois PA, De Vuyst P, de Maertelaer V, et al. Comparison of computed density and microscopic morphometry in pulmonary emphysema. *Am J Respir Crit Care Med* 1996;154:187–192.

126. Mishima M, Itoh H, Sakai H, et al. Optimized scanning conditions of high resolution CT in the follow-up of pulmonary emphysema. *J Comput Assist Tomogr* 1999;23:380–384.

127. Adams H, Bernard MS, McConnochie K. An appraisal of CT pulmonary density mapping in normal subjects. *Clin Radiol* 1991;43:238–242.

128. Stoel BC, Vrooman HA, Stolk J, et al. Sources of error in lung densitometry with CT. *Invest Radiol* 1999;34:303–309.

129. Webb WR. Radiology of obstructive pulmonary disease. *AJR Am J Roentgenol* 1997;169:637–647.

130. Brown MS, McNitt-Gray MF, Goldin JG, et al. Automated measurement of single and total lung volume from CT. *J Comput Assist Tomogr* 1999;23:632–640.

131. Müller NL, Thurlbeck WM. Thin-section CT, emphysema, air-trapping, and airway obstruction [editorial]. *Radiology* 1996;199:621–622.

132. Gevenois PA, Koob MC, Jacobovitz D, et al. Whole lung sections for computed tomographic-pathologic correlations. Modified Gough-Wentworth technique. *Invest Radiol* 1993;28:242–246.

133. Gevenois PA, Zanen J, de Maertelaer V, et al. Macroscopic assessment of pulmonary emphysema by image analysis. *J Clin Pathol* 1995;48:318–322.

134. Bergin CJ, Müller NL, Nichols DM, et al. The diagnosis of emphysema: a computed tomographic-pathologic correlation. *Am Rev Respir Dis* 1986;133:541–546.

135. Müller NL, Staples CA, Miller RR, et al. "Density mask": an objective method to quantitate emphysema using computed tomography. *Chest* 1988;94:782–787.

136. Kuwano K, Matsuba K, Ikeda T, et al. The diagnosis of mild emphysema: correlation of computed tomography and pathology scores. *Am Rev Respir Dis* 1990;141:169–178.

137. Gevenois PA, Yernault JC. Can computed tomography quantify pulmonary emphysema? *Eur Respir J* 1995;8:843–848.

138. Bankier AA, De Maertelaer V, Keyzer C, et al. Pulmonary emphysema: subjective visual grading versus objective quantification with macroscopic morphometry and thin-section CT densitometry. *Radiology* 1999;211:851–858.

139. Saetta M, Shiner RJ, Angus GE, et al. Destructive index: a measurement of lung parenchymal destruction in smokers. *Am Rev Respir Dis* 1985;131:764–769.

140. Foster WL, Pratt PC, Roggli VL, et al. Centrilobular emphysema: CT-pathologic correlation. *Radiology* 1986;159:27–32.

141. Kinsella M, Müller NL, Abboud RT, et al. Quantitation of emphysema by computed tomography using a "density mask" program and correlation with pulmonary function tests. *Chest* 1990;97:315–321.

142. Dillon TJ, Walsh RL, Scicchitano R, et al. Plasma elastin-derived peptide levels in normal adults, children, and emphysematous subjects: physiologic and computed tomographic scan correlates. *Am Rev Respir Dis* 1992;146:1143–1148.

143. Sakai F, Gamsu G, Im J-G, et al. Pulmonary function abnormalities in patients with CT-defined emphysema. *J Comput Assist Tomogr* 1987;11:963–968.

144. Spouge D, Mayo JR, Cardoso W, et al. Panacinar emphysema: CT and pathologic correlation. *J Comput Assist Tomogr* 1993;17:710–713.

145. Hayhurst MD, MacNee W, Flenley DC, et al. Diagnosis of pulmonary emphysema by computerised tomography. *Lancet* 1984;2:320–322.

146. Gould GA, Macnee W, McLean A, et al. CT measurements of lung density in life can quantitate distal airspace enlargement-an essential defining feature of human emphysema. *Am Rev Resp Dis* 1988;137:380–392.

147. Knudson RJ, Standen JR, Kaltenborn WT, et al. Expiratory computed tomography for assessment of suspected pulmonary emphysema. *Chest* 1991;99:1357–1366.

148. Bae KT, Slone RM, Gierada DS, et al. Patients with emphysema: quantitative CT analysis before and after lung volume reduction surgery. Work in progress. *Radiology* 1997;203:705–714.

149. Kauczor HU, Heussel CP, Fischer B, et al. Assessment of lung volumes using helical CT at inspiration and expiration: comparison with pulmonary function tests. *AJR Am J Roentgenol* 1998;171:1091–1095.

150. Mergo PJ, Williams WF, Gonzalez-Rothi R, et al. Three-dimensional volumetric assessment of abnormally low-attenuation of the lung from routine helical CT: inspiratory and expiratory quantification. *AJR Am J Roentgenol* 1998;170:1355–1360.

151. Gevenois PA, Scillia P, de Maertelaer V, et al. The effects of age, sex, lung size, and hyperinflation on CT lung densitometry. *AJR Am J Roentgenol* 1996;167:1169 1173.

152. Uppaluri R, Mitsa T, Sonka M, et al. Quantification of pulmonary emphysema from lung computed tomography images. *Am J Respir Crit Care Med* 1997;156:248–254.

153. Park KJ, Bergin CJ, Clausen JL. Quantitation of emphysema with three-dimensional CT densitometry: comparison with two-dimensional analysis, visual emphysema scores, and pulmonary function test results. *Radiology* 1999;211:541–547.

154. Bhalla M, Naidich DP, McGuinness G, et al. Diffuse lung disease: assessment with helical CT—preliminary observations of the role of maximum and minimum intensity projection images. *Radiology* 1996;200:341–347.

155. Remy-Jardin M, Remy J, Gosselin B, et al. Sliding thin slab, minimum intensity projection technique in the diagnosis of emphysema: histopathologic-CT correlation. *Radiology* 1996;200:665–671.

156. Fotheringham T, Chabat F, Hansell DM, et al. A comparison of methods for enhancing the detection of areas of decreased attenuation on CT caused by airways disease. *J Comput Assist Tomogr* 1999;23:385–389.

157. Newman KB, Lynch DA, Newman LS, et al. Quantitative computed tomography detects air-trapping due to asthma. *Chest* 1994;106:105–109.

158. Kalender WA, Rienmuller R, Seissler W, et al. Measurement of pulmonary parenchymal attenuation: use of spirometric gating with quantitative CT. *Radiology* 1990;175:265–268.

159. Lamers RJ, Thelissen GR, Kessels AG, et al. Chronic obstructive pulmonary diseases. evaluation with spirometrically controlled CT lung densitometry. *Radiology* 1994;193:109–113.

160. Beinert T, Behr J, Mehnert F, et al. Spirometrically controlled quantitative CT for assessing diffuse parenchymal lung disease. *J Comput Assist Tomogr* 1995;19:924–931.

161. Stern EJ, Webb WR. Dynamic imaging of lung morphology with ultrafast high-resolution computed tomography. *J Thorac Imag* 1993;8:273–282.

162. Arakawa H, Webb WR. Expiratory high-resolution CT scan. *Radiol Clin North Am* 1998;36:189–209.

163. Sanders C, Nath PH, Bailey WC. Detection of emphysema with computed tomography: correlation with pulmonary function tests and chest radiography. *Invest Radiol* 1988;23:262–266.

164. Goddard PR, Nicholson EM, Laszlo E, et al. Computed tomography in pulmonary emphysema. *Clin Radiol* 1982;33:379–387.

165. Klein JS, Gamsu G, Webb WR, et al. High-resolution CT diagnosis of emphysema in symptomatic patients with normal chest radiographs and isolated low diffusing capacity. *Radiology* 1992;182:817–821.

166. Kinsella M, Müller NL, Staples C, et al. Hyperinflation in asthma and emphysema: assessment by pulmonary function testing and computed tomography. *Chest* 1988;94:286–289.

167. Goldin JG, McNitt-Gray MF, Sorenson SM, et al. Airway hyperreactivity: assessment with helical thin-section CT. *Radiology* 1998;208:321–329.

168. Müller NL. Clinical value of high-resolution CT in chronic diffuse lung disease. *AJR Am J Roentgenol* 1991;157:1163–1170.

169. Gelb AF, Schein M, Kuei J, et al. Limited contribution of emphysema in advanced chronic obstructive pulmonary disease. *Am Rev Respir Dis* 1993;147:1157–1161.

170. Slone RM, Gierada DS, Yusen RD. Preoperative and postoperative imaging in the surgical management of pulmonary emphysema. *Rad Clin North Am* 1998;36:57–89.

171. Erasmus JJ, McAdams HP, Tapson VF, et al. Radiologic issues in lung transplantation for end-stage pulmonary disease. *AJR Am J Roentgenol* 1997;169:69–78.

172. Connolly JE, Wilson A. The current status of surgery for bullous emphysema. *J Thorac Cardiovasc Surg* 1989;97:351–361.

173. Hazelrigg SR. Thoracoscopic management of pulmonary blebs and bullae. *Semin Thorac Cardiovasc Surg* 1993;5:327–331.

174. Snider GL. Reduction pneumoplasty for giant bullous emphysema: implications for surgical treatment of nonbullous emphysema. *Chest* 1996;109:540–548.

175. Morgan MD, Denison DM, Strickland B. Value of computed tomography for selecting patients with bullous lung disease for surgery. *Thorax* 1986;41:855–862.

176. Carr DH, Pride NB. Computed tomography in pre-operative assessment of bullous emphysema. *Clin Radiol* 1984;35:43–45.

177. Fiore DW, Biondetti PR, Sartori F, et al. The role of computer tomography in the evaluation of bullous lung disease. *J Comput Assist Tomogr* 1982;6:105–108.

178. Morgan MDL, Strickland B. Computed tomography in the assessment of bullous lung disease. *Br J Dis Chest* 1984;78:10–25.

179. Kazerooni EA, Chow LC, Whyte RI, et al. Preoperative examination of lung transplant candidates: value of chest CT compared with chest radiography. *AJR Am J Roentgenol* 1995;165:1343–1348.

180. Waters PF. Lung transplantation: recipient selection. *Semin Thorac Cardiovasc Surg* 1992;4:73–78.

181. Cooper JD, Trulock EP, Triantafillou AN, et al. Bilateral pneumectomy (volume reduction) for chronic obstructive pulmonary disease. *J Thorac Cardiovasc Surg* 1995;109:106–116; discussion 116–119.

182. Cooper JD, Patterson GA, Sundaresan RS, et al. Results of 150 consecutive bilateral lung volume reduction procedures in patients with severe emphysema. *J Thorac Cardiovasc Surg* 1996;112:1319–1329; discussion 1329–1330.

183. Rationale and design of the National Emphysema Treatment Trial (NETT): A prospective randomized trial of lung volume reduction surgery. *J Thorac Cardiovasc Surg* 1999;118:518–528.

184. Petty TL, Weinmann GG. Building a national strategy for the prevention and management of and research in chronic obstructive pulmonary disease. National Heart, Lung, and Blood Institute Workshop Summary. Bethesda, Maryland: August 29-31, 1995. *JAMA* 1997;277:246–253.

185. Holbert JM, Brown ML, Sciurba FC, et al. Changes in lung volume and volume of emphysema after unilateral lung reduction surgery: analysis with CT lung densitometry. *Radiology* 1996;201:793–797.

186. Gierada DS, Slone RM, Bae KT, et al. Pulmonary emphysema: comparison of preoperative quantitative CT and physiologic index values with clinical outcome after lung-volume reduction surgery. *Radiology* 1997;205:235–242.

187. Slone RM, Pilgram TK, Gierada DS, et al. Lung volume reduction surgery: comparison of preoperative radiologic features and clinical outcome. *Radiology* 1997;204:685–693.

188. Weder W, Thurnheer R, Stammberger U, et al. Radiologic emphysema morphology is associated with outcome after surgical lung volume reduction. *Ann Thorac Surg* 1997;64:313–319; discussion 319–320.

189. Hunsaker A, Ingenito E, Topal U, et al. Preoperative screening for lung volume reduction surgery: usefulness of combining thin-section CT with physiologic assessment. *AJR Am J Roentgenol* 1998;170:309–314.

190. Becker MD, Berkmen YM, Austin JH, et al. Lung volumes before and after lung volume reduction surgery: quantitative CT analysis. *Am J Respir Crit Care Med* 1998;157:1593–1599.

191. Hamacher J, Bloch KE, Stammberger U, et al. Two years' outcome of lung volume reduction surgery in different morphologic emphysema types. *Ann Thorac Surg* 1999;68:1792–1798.

192. Gierada DS, Yusen RD, Villanueva IA, et al. Patient selection for lung volume reduction surgery: An objective model based on prior clinical decisions and quantitative CT analysis. *Chest* 2000;117:991–998.

193. Cleverley JR, Hansell DM. Imaging of patients with severe emphysema considered for lung volume reduction surgery. *Br J Radiol* 1999;72:227–235.

194. Slone RM, Gierada DS. Radiology of pulmonary emphysema and lung volume reduction surgery. *Semin Thorac Cardiovasc Surg* 1996;8:61–82.

195. Pigula FA, Keenan RJ, Ferson PF, et al. Unsuspected lung cancer found in work-up for lung reduction operation. *Ann Thorac Surg* 1996;61:174–176.
196. Rozenshtein A, White CS, Austin JH, et al. Incidental lung carcinoma detected at CT in patients selected for lung volume reduction surgery to treat severe pulmonary emphysema. *Radiology* 1998;207:487–490.
197. Hazelrigg SR, Boley TM, Weber D, et al. Incidence of lung nodules found in patients undergoing lung volume reduction. *Ann Thorac Surg* 1997;64:303–306.
198. Maki DD, Miller WT Jr, Aronchick JM, et al. Advanced emphysema: preoperative chest radiographic findings as predictors of outcome following lung volume reduction surgery. *Radiology* 1999;212:49–55.
199. Takasugi JE, Wood DE, Godwin JD, et al. Lung volume reduction surgery for diffuse emphysema: radiologic assessment of changes in thoracic dimensions. *J Thorac Imag* 1998;13:36–41.
200. Gierada DS, Hakimian S, Slone RM, et al. MR analysis of lung volume and thoracic dimensions in patients with emphysema before and after lung volume reduction surgery. *AJR Am J Roentgenol* 1998;170:707–714.

CHAPTER 8

Airways Diseases

High-resolution computed tomography (HRCT) has revolutionized our understanding of diseases affecting the airways. HRCT not only allows direct, noninvasive visualization of structural changes involving both large, and medium-sized bronchi [1–8], but also allows a previously unattainable insight into airway physiology [9–17]. Furthermore, it is now possible to directly visualize a number of findings indicative of small airways disease using HRCT [18–22]. In this chapter, we review the HRCT diagnosis of large airway abnormalities specifically related to bronchiectasis and small airway abnormalities and bronchiolitis.

BRONCHIECTASIS

Bronchiectasis is defined as localized, irreversible dilatation of the bronchial tree. Bronchiectasis has been associated with a wide variety of causes (Table 8-1), the most frequent of which is acute, chronic, or recurrent infection [23–25]. In a review of 123 patients who had documented bronchiectasis, an antecedent potentially causative event, usually pneumonia, could be identified in 70% of cases [26]. In up to 40% of cases of bronchiectasis, however, an etiology cannot be established.

TABLE 8-1. *Bronchiectasis—associated conditions and possible mechanisms*

Condition	Mechanisms
Infection (bacteria, mycobacteria, fungus, virus)	Impaired mucociliary clearance, disruption of respiratory epithelium, microbial toxins, host-mediated inflammation
Immunodeficiency states [including acquired immunodeficiency syndrome (AIDS)]	Genetic or acquired predisposition to recurrent infection, associated with lymphocytic interstitial pneumonia in AIDS
Bronchial obstruction (tumor, foreign body, congenital abnormalities)	Impaired mucociliary clearance, recurrent infection
Alpha-1-antitrypsin deficiency	Proteinase-antiproteinase imbalance
Cystic fibrosis	Abnormal airway epithelial chloride transport, impaired mucus clearance, recurrent infection
Dyskinetic cilia syndrome (Kartagener's syndrome)	Genetic defect, absent or dyskinetic ciliary beating, impaired mucus clearance, recurrent infection
Young's syndrome (obstructive azoospermia)	Abnormal mucociliary clearance
Yellow nail–lymphedema syndrome	Unknown, lymphatic hypoplasia and sometimes immune deficiency, predisposition to recurrent infection?
Williams-Campbell syndrome	Congenital deficiency of bronchial cartilage, obstruction, impaired mucus clearance, recurrent infection
Tracheobronchomegaly (Mounier-Kuhn syndrome)	Congenital deficiency of membranous and cartilaginous parts of tracheal and bronchial walls, impaired mucus clearance, recurrent infection
Marfan syndrome	Unknown, genetic tissue defect, structural bronchial defect?
Asthma	Airway inflammation, mucous plugging
Allergic bronchopulmonary aspergillosis	Type I and Type III immune responses to fungus in airway lumen, mucous plugging
Bronchiolitis obliterans (e.g., postinfectious, lung transplant)	Bronchial wall inflammation, epithelial damage, recurrent infection in some cases
Aspiration, toxic fume inhalation	Inflammation
Systemic diseases (e.g., collagen-vascular diseases, inflammatory bowel disease, amyloidosis, endometriosis, sarcoidosis)	Various, including inflammation, infection, fibrosis
Chronic fibrosis	Traction bronchiectasis

Modified from Davis AL, Salzman SH. Bronchiectasis. In: Cherniack NS, ed. *Chronic obstructive pulmonary disease.* Philadelphia: WB Saunders, 1991:316–338.

Bronchiectasis can result from chronic or severe bacterial infection, especially with necrotizing infections such as *Staphylococcus*, *Klebsiella*, or *Bordetella pertussis* [25]. Granulomatous infections, including those caused by *Mycobacterium tuberculosis* [27], atypical mycobacteria, especially *Mycobacterium avium* complex (MAC) [28–30], and fungal organisms such as histoplasmosis are also associated with bronchiectasis. Furthermore, bronchiectasis is often present in patients who have bronchiolitis obliterans (BO) or the Swyer-James syndrome resulting from viral infection.

Bronchiectasis is commonly identified in patients infected with human immunodeficiency virus (HIV) [31]. A number of mechanisms have been proposed to account for accelerated bronchial wall destruction occurring in patients who have acquired immunodeficiency syndrome (AIDS), including recurrent infections, BO, and lymphocytic interstitial pneumonitis (LIP) [32,33]. King et al. [34] have shown that bronchial dilatation is common in HIV-positive patients, being seen in 36% of cases, and is associated with elevated levels of neutrophils in bronchoalveolar lavage fluid. Neutro-

phil elastase is associated with airway destruction in patients who have alpha-1-antitrypsin deficiency, and similarly may be an early mediator of bronchial wall destruction, even in asymptomatic HIV-positive patients.

Bronchiectasis may occur in association with a variety of genetic abnormalities, especially those with abnormal mucociliary clearance, immune deficiency, or structural abnormalities of the bronchus or bronchial wall (Table 8-1) [35]. In addition to cystic fibrosis (CF), causes of bronchiectasis having a genetic basis include alpha-1-antitrypsin deficiency; the dyskinetic cilia syndrome; Young's syndrome; Williams-Campbell syndrome (congenital deficiency of the bronchial cartilage); Mounier-Kuhn syndrome (congenital tracheobronchomegaly); immunodeficiency syndromes, including Bruton's hypogammaglobulinemia, immunoglobulin (Ig) A, and combined IgA-IgG subclass deficiencies; and the yellow nail syndrome (yellow nails, lymphedema, and pleural effusions). Chronic or recurrent infection is common in these conditions.

Noninfectious diseases that result in airway inflammation and mucous plugging can also result in bronchiectasis. These

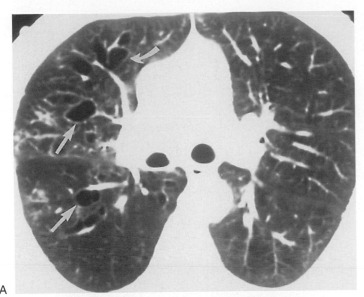
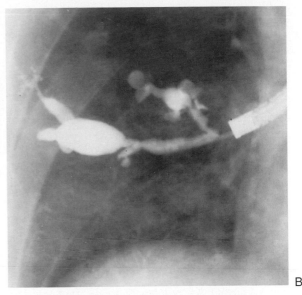

A   B

FIG. 8-1. Cystic bronchiectasis with bronchographic correlation. **A:** HRCT through the right upper lobe shows numerous thin-walled cysts (*straight arrows*). Note that despite their thin walls, many of these cysts lie adjacent to vessels and a few are obviously branching (*curved arrow*). Rarely, bronchiectasis can result in thin-walled cysts that nonetheless maintain a characteristic anatomic configuration. **B:** Coned-down radiograph after limited bronchography, performed through a centrally positioned bronchoscope, confirms presence of extensive cystic bronchiectasis. (From McGuinness G, Naidich DP, Leitman BS, et al. Bronchiectasis: CT evaluation. *AJR Am J Roentgenol* 1993;160:253–259, with permission.)

include allergic bronchopulmonary aspergillosis and, to a lesser extent, asthma [36–38]. Bronchiectasis may also occur in patients who have BO, regardless of its cause but including chronic rejection after heart-lung or lung transplantation [39–45] or bone marrow transplantation, most often as a result of rejection or chronic graft-versus-host disease (GVHD) [46].

Although the incidence of bronchiectasis is generally cited as decreasing in the United States, the true incidence of bronchiectasis has probably been underestimated [47]. In part, this may reflect decreased awareness in recent years of the protean manifestations of bronchiectasis, especially in an older population [23,26]. It should also be noted that documentation has traditionally relied on bronchography, which is rarely performed in current medical practice.

In general, a clinical diagnosis of bronchiectasis is possible only in the most severely affected patients, and differentiation from chronic bronchitis may be problematic even in this setting [48]. Most patients present with purulent sputum production and recurrent pulmonary infections [23,24,26]. Hemoptysis also is frequent, occurring in up to 50% of cases, and may be the only clinical finding [24,49,50]. Bronchitis, bronchiolitis, or emphysema frequently accompanies bronchiectasis and may cause obstructive abnormalities on pulmonary function tests.

Radiographic and Bronchographic Findings

The radiographic manifestations of bronchiectasis have been well described [51]. These include a loss of definition of vascular markings in affected lung segments, presumably secondary to peribronchial fibrosis and volume loss; evi-

dence of bronchial wall thickening; and, in more severely affected cases, the presence of discrete cysts occasionally containing air-fluid levels. It should be emphasized that most of these findings are nonspecific; a definitive radiographic diagnosis of bronchiectasis is generally considered difficult to make, except in the most advanced cases [48].

Woodring has suggested that a greater degree of accuracy may be achieved in the radiographic diagnosis of bronchiectasis by the use of additional radiographic criteria [52]. Most important of these is the assessment of bronchial dilatation, either by comparing the diameters of end-on bronchi in normal and abnormal areas of the lung or by direct measurement of bronchoarterial ratios in the same locations. Using these criteria, Woodring was able to accurately diagnose bronchiectasis in 38 patients who had either bronchographic or HRCT evidence of bronchiectasis. Specifically, bronchial dilatation was found to be present in 100% of cases, volume loss in 97%, bronchial wall thickening in 92%, a signet ring sign (abnormal bronchoarterial ratio) in 79%, compensatory hyperinflation in 45%, and discrete cysts in 42%. Also, radiographs identified 235 of 255 (92%) bronchiectatic lung segments [52]. Although there is no doubt that an accurate diagnosis of bronchiectasis may be made by using specific criteria, especially when films are closely correlated with clinical history, plain radiographs will likely remain of greatest value in those patients who have severe disease.

Bronchographic findings indicative of bronchiectasis include proximal or distal bronchial dilatation, or both; pruning or lack of normal tapering of peripheral airways; and luminal filling defects (Fig. 8-1). Although traditionally considered the gold standard, the reliability of bronchography in

TABLE 8-2. *HRCT findings in bronchiectasis*

Direct signs

Bronchial dilatation[a,b]

  Internal diameter > adjacent pulmonary artery[a,b]

Contour abnormalities[a,b]

  Signet ring sign (vertically oriented bronchi)

  Tram tracks (horizontally oriented bronchi)

  String of pearls (horizontally oriented bronchi)

  Cluster of cysts (especially in atelectatic lung)

Lack of tapering greater than 2 cm distal to bifurcation[b]

Visibility of peripheral airways[a,b]

  Within 1 cm of the costal pleura[a,b]

  Touching the mediastinal pleura[a,b]

Indirect signs

Bronchial wall thickening[a,b]

  Greater than 0.5 × diameter of an adjacent pulmonary artery (vertically oriented bronchi)[b]

Fluid- or mucus-filled bronchi[a,b]

Tubular or Y-shaped structures[a,b]

Branching or rounded opacities in cross section[a,b]

Air-fluid levels[b]

Mosaic perfusion[a]

Centrilobular nodules or tree-in-bud[a]

Atelectasis/consolidation[a]

Air-trapping on expiratory scans[a]

---

[a] Most common findings.
[b] Findings most helpful in differential diagnosis.

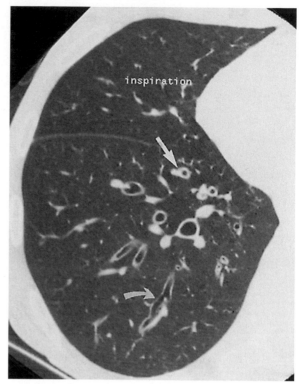

FIG. 8-2. Cylindrical bronchiectasis with bronchial dilatation and wall thickening. Target-reconstructed HRCT through the right lower lobe in a patient who has mild cylindrical bronchiectasis, obtained at full inspiration. Dilated bronchi have a signet ring appearance when sectioned vertically (*straight arrow*) and a tram track appearance when sectioned horizontally (*curved arrow*). Bronchial walls in the lower lobe are considerably thicker than in the middle lobe.

the diagnosis of bronchiectasis has been questioned. Currie et al. [48], in a study of 27 patients who had chronic sputum production evaluated bronchographically, showed that there was significant interobserver variability when studies were interpreted by two well-trained bronchographers. Agreement was reached in only 19 of 27 patients (70%) and 94 of 448 bronchopulmonary segments (21%). Bronchiectasis was identified in two additional patients (7%) by only one radiologist. These findings suggest that bronchography may be more limited in its utility than previously thought and should not be considered an absolute standard for diagnosis.

Computed Tomography and High-Resolution Computed Tomography Findings of Bronchiectasis

Bronchiectasis results in characteristic abnormalities, both direct and indirect, identifiable on HRCT (Table 8-2) [35,53]. Direct findings of bronchiectasis include bronchial dilatation [often described as cylindrical (Fig. 8-2), varicose (Fig. 8-3), or cystic (Figs. 8-3, 8-4, 8-6, and 8-7) depending on its appearance], lack of normal bronchial tapering, and visibility of airways in the peripheral lung zones (Fig. 8-6). Indirect signs include bronchial wall thickening and irregularity (Figs. 8-2, 8-3, and 8-9), as well as the presence of mucoid impaction of the

bronchial lumen (Figs. 8-10 and 8-11), bronchiolectasis, and tree-in-bud (TIB) (Figs. 8-16 and 8-17). Ancillary signs have also been described and include mosaic perfusion visible on inspiratory scans (Fig. 8-18), focal air-trapping identifiable on expiration scans (Fig. 8-18), tracheomegaly (Fig. 8-41), bronchial artery enlargement, and emphysema. A combination of these findings enables an accurate diagnosis in a large percentage of cases (Table 8-2).

Bronchial Dilatation

Because bronchiectasis is defined by the presence of bronchial dilatation, recognition of increased bronchial diameter is key to the CT diagnosis of this abnormality. Various sophisticated methods for measuring airway dimensions have been proposed. These include the use of digital image analysis programs, requiring operator-dependent definition of a "seed point" at the lumen-wall interface to obtain isocontour lines of the bronchial lumen [14], and automated thresholding to detect airway lumen area [54]. Whereas these approaches may allow precise quantitative assessment of airways and may prove particularly valuable in physiologic

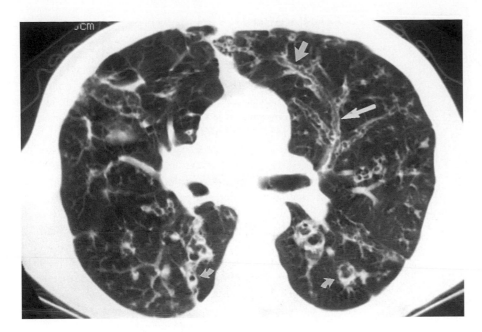

FIG. 8-3. Section through the middle lung fields in a patient who has varicose bronchiectasis in the left upper lobe (*straight arrows*). Note that there is also evidence of cystic bronchiectasis with a few air-fluid levels in the lower lobes (*curved arrows*).

studies, subjective visual criteria for establishing the presence of bronchial dilatation are most often used in the interpretation of scans [4,38,55–58].

For the purposes of the interpretation of HRCT, bronchial dilatation may be diagnosed using a comparison of bronchial size to that of adjacent pulmonary artery branches (i.e., the bronchoarterial ratio), by detecting a lack of bronchial tapering, and by identifying airways in the peripheral lung.

Bronchoarterial Ratio

In most cases, bronchiectasis is considered to be present when the internal diameter of a bronchus is greater than the diameter of the adjacent pulmonary artery branch—that is, the bronchoarterial ratio is greater than 1 (Figs. 8-2 through 8-4) [53]. The accuracy of this finding in diagnosing bronchiectasis has been validated in a number of studies comparing CT to

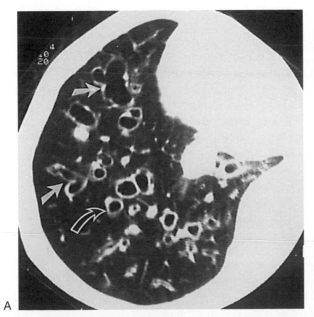

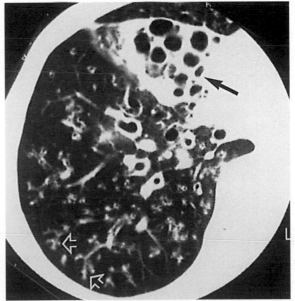

A   B

FIG. 8-4. Cystic bronchiectasis. **A,B:** Sequential target-reconstructed HRCT sections through the middle and right lower lobe. Markedly dilated airways are apparent diffusely, some obviously branching (*straight arrows*, **A**). Numerous signet rings are identifiable as well (*curved open arrow*, **A**). Note the cluster of cysts appearing within the collapsed middle lobe (*arrow*, **B**). A number of fluid-filled airways can be identified peripherally that are clearly centrilobular in distribution (*open arrows*, **B**); these represent dilated terminal bronchioles. (From Naidich DP. High-resolution computed tomography of cystic lung disease. *Semin Roentgenol* 1991;26:151–174, with permission.)

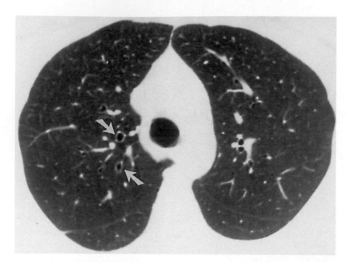

FIG. 8-5. Bronchial dilatation associated with asthma. HRCT section through the upper lobes in an asthmatic shows evidence of proximal bronchial dilatation, especially on the right (*arrows*), with bronchi being larger than adjacent vessels. This finding should be interpreted with caution in an asthmatic, as it may be reversible.

bronchography in patients who have bronchiectasis [59–62]. In patients who have bronchiectasis, the bronchial diameter is often much larger than the pulmonary artery diameter (i.e., greater than 1.5 times the artery diameter), a finding that not only reflects the presence of bronchial dilatation but also demonstrates some reduction in pulmonary artery size as a consequence of decreased lung perfusion in affected lung regions [56]. The association of a dilated bronchus with a much smaller adjacent pulmonary artery branch has been termed the *signet ring sign* (see Figs. 3-135 and 3-137; Figs. 8-2 through 8-4). This sign is valuable in recognizing bronchiectasis and in distinguishing it from other cystic lung lesions.

Although an increased bronchoarterial ratio is typical of bronchiectasis, it should be kept in mind that a bronchoarterial ratio of more than 1 need not always indicate the presence of bronchiectasis [4,38,56]. There are a number of instances in which airways may appear dilated in the absence of wall destruction, although this dilatation is usually minimal; this has been reported in asthmatic patients [36,38,63], in patients living at high altitudes [38,56], and in a small percentage of normals [64] (Fig. 8-5). For example, in an HRCT evaluation of 14 normal subjects [65], although the bronchoarterial ratio averaged 0.65 ± 0.16, 7% of interpretations showed some evidence of bronchial dilatation. Kim et al. [56] found that nine of 17 (53%) normal subjects living at an altitude of 1,600 meters had evidence of at least one bronchus equal to or larger in size than the adjacent pulmonary artery. These authors also found that two of 16 (12.5%) individuals living at sea level showed evidence of at least one abnormally dilated airway. Similarly, Lynch et al. [38] compared the internal diameters of lobular, segmental, subsegmental, and smaller bronchi to those of adjacent pulmonary artery branches in 27 normal subjects living in Denver. The authors

found that 37 of 142 (26%) bronchi evaluated and 59% of individuals had increased bronchoarterial ratios. Evaluation of the distribution of these abnormal airways has failed to identify any significant difference in the likelihood of abnormal bronchoarterial ratios in airways either by lobe or anteroposterior location within the lungs [56]. A similar lack of variation by segments, lobes, or lungs has been reported by Kim et al. [58].

It must be emphasized that bronchiectasis should not be diagnosed on the basis of an increased bronchoarterial ratio alone unless it is significant; in a study by Lynch et al. [38] of normal subjects and patients who had asthma, although bronchoarterial ratios of greater than 1 were frequently seen, in none of these was the bronchoarterial ratio greater than 1.5 [66]. Also, bronchial wall thickening is almost always seen in association with bronchial dilatation in patients who have bronchiectasis, as are irregularities in bronchial diameter and lack of bronchial tapering. In the normal subjects studied by Lynch et al. [38] who demonstrated an increased bronchoarterial ratio, bronchial wall thickening was relatively uncommon, and it is unlikely that any of the subjects in this study would have been diagnosed on clinical HRCT studies as having true bronchiectasis.

The definition of an *abnormal bronchoarterial ratio* varies widely among reported series [4,53,55,57,58,65,67], a fact that limits their comparison. In addition to variations in size criteria for considering a bronchus to be dilated (ranging from one to two times the diameter of the adjacent pulmonary artery) and the use of internal or external bronchial diameters for comparison to pulmonary artery diameter, important differences may also be attributable to the use of either visual inspection or objective measurements of bronchial and arterial dimensions. As emphasized by Kim et al. [56], visual inspection alone may lead to an overestimation of bronchoarterial ratios due to a subtle optical illusion, in which the diameter of hollow circles appears larger than solid circles despite their being identical in size. Considerable variation in bronchoarterial ratio may also be seen in normals. In a study by Kim et al. [58], the *arterobronchus ratio*, defined as the outer diameter of the pulmonary artery divided by the outer diameter of its accompanying bronchus measured at the subsegmental level, averaged 0.98 ± 0.14 but ranged from 0.53 to 1.39.

Despite variability in normal bronchial size and the methods by which bronchial diameter has been assessed, several studies have shown that measurements of bronchial diameter may be reliably made from HRCT [68,69]. Desai et al. [68] evaluated both inter- and intraobserver variation in CT measurements of bronchial wall circumference in 61 subsegmental bronchi and found the reproducibility of these measurements to be sufficiently clinically useful in demonstrating the progression of bronchiectasis. As emphasized by Diederich et al. [57], visual inspection remains the mainstay for assessing bronchial dilatation, as obtaining objective measurements (with or without the use of calipers) is time consuming and often clinically impractical. In this regard, use of visual inspection has been shown to

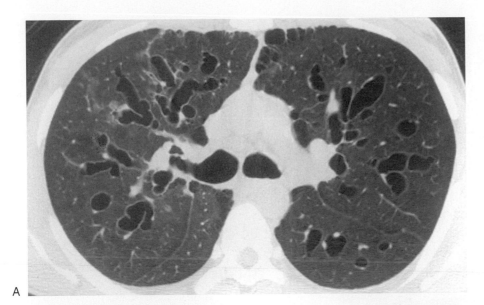

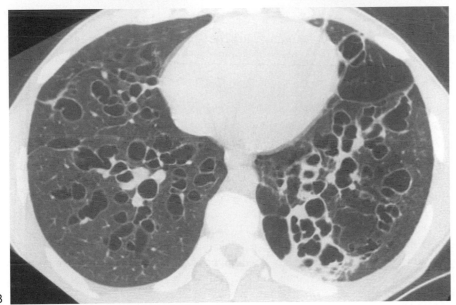

FIG. 8-6. Cystic bronchiectasis. **A,B:** Sections through the carina and lower lobes, respectively, show evidence of extensive cystic bronchiectasis. Bronchi are considerably larger than adjacent pulmonary artery branches (i.e., the bronchoarterial ratio is increased). In **A**, bronchi oriented in the plane of scan show a distinct lack of tapering. Note that despite marked dilatation, there is little evidence of bronchial wall thickening. In the left lower lobe, the cysts appear grouped together, giving the appearance of a cluster of grapes. In this region, the airway walls appear thickened, likely due to the presence of minimal consolidation in the posterior basilar segment. Note also the finding of a few bullae, most marked in the lingula but identifiable along the medial border of the left lower lobe as well.

have acceptable interobserver variability. Using visual inspection only, Diederich et al. [57] found close agreement among three readers both in the detection ($\kappa = 0.78$) and assessment of the severity ($\kappa = 0.68$) of bronchiectasis.

A potential limitation of the use of bronchoarterial ratios is the necessity of identifying both airways and accompanying arteries. This may not always be possible in patients who have coexisting parenchymal consolidation [4]. Kang et al. was unable to determine the bronchoarterial ratios in three cases in a study of 47 resected lobes with documented bronchiectasis due to the presence of parenchymal consolidation [4].

Lack of Bronchial Tapering

Lack of bronchial tapering has come to be recognized as an important finding in the diagnosis of bronchiectasis, and subtle cylindrical bronchiectasis in particular (Table 8-2)

(Fig. 8-6). It has been suggested that for this finding to be present, the diameter of an airway should remain unchanged for at least 2 cm distal to a branching point [56]. First emphasized by Lynch et al. [38] as a necessary finding for diagnosis, lack of bronchial tapering has been reported by some to be the most sensitive means for diagnosing bronchiectasis. Kang et al. [4], for example, in an assessment of 47 lobes with pathologically proved bronchiectasis, found lack of tapering of bronchial lumina in 37 cases (79%) as compared with increased bronchoarterial ratios seen in only 28 cases (60%). In another study [64], lack of tapering of bronchi was seen in 10% of HRCT interpretations in healthy subjects, compared with 95% of reviews in patients who had bronchiectasis. It should be emphasized that the accurate detection of this finding is difficult in the absence of contiguous HRCT sections, especially for vertically or obliquely oriented airways. The value of this sign is doubtful when HRCT scans are obtained

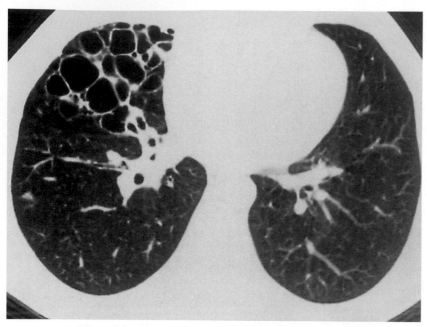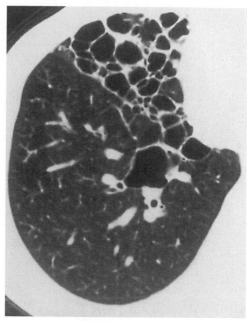

A
B

FIG. 8-7. A,B: Cystic bronchiectasis largely limited to the right middle lobe in a patient who has a history of tuberculosis.

at spaced intervals in a noncontiguous fashion. As discussed in this book, this has clear implications for optimizing scan technique in patients who have suspected airways disease.

Visualization of Peripheral Airways

Another frequently cited manifestation of bronchiectasis is the visibility of airways in the lung periphery (Table 8-2) [4,64]. The smallest airways normally visible using HRCT techniques have a diameter of approximately 2 mm and a wall thickness of 0.2 to 0.3 mm [70]; in normal subjects, airways in the peripheral 2 cm of lung are uncommonly seen because their walls are too thin [71]. Peribronchial fibrosis and bronchial wall thickening in patients who have bronchiectasis, in combination with dilatation of the bronchial lumen, allow the visualization of small airways in the lung periphery, and this finding can be very helpful in diagnosing the presence of an airway abnormality. In a study by Kang et al. [4], bronchi visualized within 1 cm of pleura were seen in 21 of 47 (45%) bronchiectatic lobes.

Kim et al. have further assessed the value of this sign in the diagnosis of bronchiectasis [64], pointing out that although normal bronchi are not visible within 1 cm of the costal pleural surfaces, bronchi may be seen within 1 cm of the mediastinal pleural surfaces in normal subjects; visible bronchi were identified within 1 cm of the mediastinal pleura in 40% of normal subjects [64]. These authors found that visible bronchi within 1 cm of the pleural surface or bronchi touching the mediastinal pleural surfaces were visible in 81% and 53%, respectively, of HRCT interpretations in patients who had clinical or pathologic evidence of cylindrical bronchiectasis (Figs. 8-4A, 8-6, and 8-7).

Bronchial Wall Thickening

Although bronchial wall thickening is a nonspecific finding, it is usually present in patients who have bronchiectasis (Table 8-2) (Figs. 8-3, 8-4, and 8-7 through 8-9). Generally accepted criteria for determining abnormal bronchial wall thickening have yet to be established.

Airways divide by asymmetric dichotomous branching, with approximately 23 generations of branches from the trachea to the alveoli. Anatomically, second- to fourth-generation segmental airways have mean diameters of between 5 and 8 mm, corresponding to a wall thickness of approximately 1.5 mm; sixth- to eighth-generation airways have mean diameters measuring between 1.5 and 3 mm with walls of approximately 0.3 mm; and eleventh- to thirteenth-generation airways have diameters measuring 0.7 to 1 mm, with walls of 0.1 to 0.15 mm [72]. The wall thickness of conducting airways distal to the segmental level is approximately proportional to their diameter. In general, the thickness of the wall of a bronchus or bronchiole smaller than 5 mm in diameter should measure from one-sixth to one-tenth of its diameter [73]; however, precise measurement of the wall thickness of small bronchi or bronchioles is difficult, as wall thickness approximates pixel size [70].

Precise definitions of bronchial wall thickening have been proposed by several investigators, relying on the visual assessment or measurement of the ratio between bronchial wall thickness and the diameter of adjacent pulmonary arteries or nearby normal airways (Fig. 8-9) [57,67,74,75]. Proposed techniques include determining the ratio of airway wall thickness to the outer airway diameter, as well as the percentage wall area defined as (wall area/total airway area) × 100. Using these parameters, Awadh et al. have shown that there is a

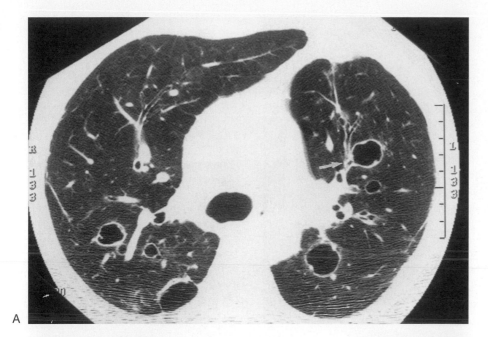

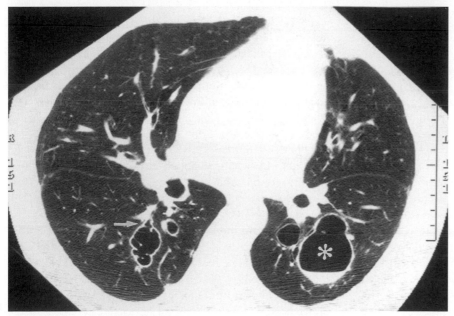

FIG. 8-8. Cystic bronchiectasis. **A,B:** Sections through the carina and mid lungs, respectively, show isolated foci of cystic bronchiectasis. Bronchi are dilated and thick-walled. Note that some of these clearly communicate with proximal airways (*arrows* in **A** and **B**); others have clearly defined air-fluid levels (*asterisk* in **B**).

clearly definable gradient in bronchial wall thickness between normal subjects and asthmatic patients of varying severity [76]. The relationship between wall thickness and bronchial diameter has also been assessed by Kim et al. [58], using the bronchial lumen ratio (BLR). At the subsegmental level, the BLR, defined as the inner diameter of the bronchus divided by its outer diameter, was measured at the subsegmental level on a display console. Considerable variation in the BLR was found, averaging 0.66 ± 0.06 with a range of 0.51 to 0.86 [58]. It has also been suggested that bronchial wall thickening may be diagnosed if the airway wall is at least 0.5 times the width of an adjacent vertically oriented pulmonary artery (Table 8-2).

Identification of thickened bronchial walls for the purposes of interpretation of clinical scans remains largely sub-

jective (Fig. 8-9) [4,36]. Because bronchiectasis and bronchial wall thickening are often multifocal rather than diffuse and uniform, a comparison of one lung region to another can be helpful in making this diagnosis. It must be emphasized that using consistent window settings is very important in the diagnosis of bronchial wall thickening; bronchial walls can vary significantly in apparent thickness with different CT window settings (see Chapter 1).

Although estimates of airway wall thickening are subjective, it has been shown that visual assessment of wall thickening may be reliable when sequential scans are assessed. Using a visual estimation of wall thickness, Diederich et al. [57] found acceptable levels of agreement among three readers as to the presence or absence of bronchial wall thickening

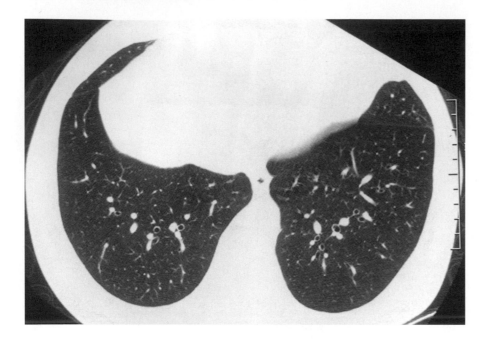

FIG. 8-9. Bronchial wall thickening. HRCT section through the lung bases shows evidence of subtle bronchial wall thickening. Although this is usually diagnosed by visual inspection, it has been suggested that bronchial wall thickening should not be diagnosed until the airway wall is at least one-half the width of an adjacent vertically oriented pulmonary artery. By this criterion, the airway walls in the present example should not be considered abnormal in the absence of careful clinical correlation.

($\kappa = 0.64$). It should be emphasized, however, that interobserver agreement in itself might be a misleading statistic in assessing the validity of HRCT measurements. Bankier et al. [77], in a study of normal and abnormal airways evaluated by three independent observers before and after a training period, showed that although interobserver variability improved significantly on second readings, training had no effect on sensitivity. Sensitivity in detecting abnormal bronchi was 46% before and 44% after training, and specificity measured 71% and 72%, respectively [77]. Although these results are disappointing, it should be emphasized that the airway abnormalities evaluated in this study were extremely subtle, with abnormal segmental and subsegmental wall thickness measuring 1.77 mm and 0.95 mm, respectively, as compared with normal segmental and subsegmental airways measuring 1.14 mm and 0.46 mm. Furthermore, individual airways were assessed individually on targeted reconstructed images only. Nonetheless, a statistically significant difference ($p = .001$) between measured wall thickness of normal and pathologic bronchi was found [77].

Mucoid Impaction

The presence of mucus- or fluid-filled bronchi may be helpful in confirming a diagnosis of bronchiectasis (Table 8-2). The HRCT appearance of fluid- (Fig. 8-8) or mucus-filled airways is dependent both on their size and orientation relative to the scan plane. Larger mucus-filled airways result in abnormal lobular or branching structures when they lie in the same plane as the CT scan (Figs. 8-10 through 8-15). Although these may be confused with abnormally dilated vessels, in most cases, the recognition of dilated, fluid-filled airways is simplified by the identification of other areas of bronchiectasis in which the bronchi are air-filled; these are usually present if carefully sought (Figs. 8-10A

and 8-11). In problematic cases, a distinction between larger fluid-filled bronchi and dilated blood vessels is easily made by rescanning patients after the bolus injection of intravenous contrast medium (Fig. 8-13). Alternatively, with the introduction of newer-generation scanners, it is now possible to obtain high quality multiplanar and maximum-intensity projection images in a variety of imaging planes as a means for further evaluation (Figs. 8-14 and 8-15).

Although commonly associated with bronchiectasis and infection, dilated mucus-filled airways in the central lung can also result from congenital bronchial abnormalities, such as bronchopulmonary sequestration or bronchial atresia (Fig. 8-15) [78–83].

It should also be emphasized that the finding of dilated mucus-filled airways, especially when central or predominantly segmental or lobular in distribution, should alert one to the possibility of central endobronchial obstruction, resulting either from tumor or foreign body aspiration. As previously discussed, the use of intravenous contrast media in this setting may allow differentiation between central tumor and fluid-filled peripheral airways.

As is discussed in greater detail in the section on Bronchiolitis, mucus- or pus-filled small airways in the lung periphery are usually identifiable either as branching structures within the center of secondary lobules, aptly described as having a tree-in-bud (TIB) appearance [27,84] or as ill-defined centrilobular nodules (Table 8-2) [70,85–88] (Figs. 8-4, 8-11, 8-16, and 8-17). These are frequently identified in association with bronchiectasis and usually indicate infection. For example, in patients who have diffuse panbronchiolitis (DPB) [89], bronchiolectasis results in small, ring-shaped, round, or branching opacities in the peripheral lung. These opacities correspond to abnormalities of distal airways, including terminal and respiratory bronchioles [86–88].

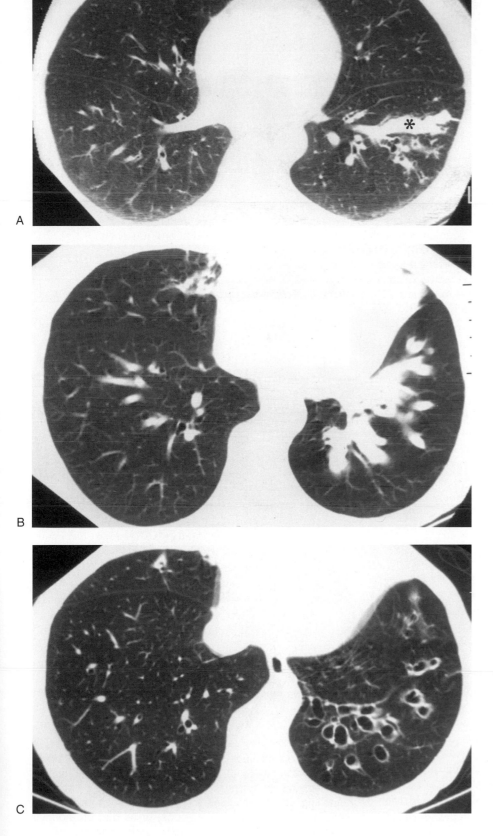

FIG. 8-10. Mucoid impaction. **A:** Section through the lower lobes shows typical appearance of mucoid impaction, appearing as a tubular branching density (*asterisk*) associated with adjacent air-filled dilated airways. **B:** Section through the lower lobes in a different patient than **A** shows typical findings of mucoid impaction with linear branching densities throughout the left lower lobe. A focal area of ill-defined consolidation is also present in the medial tip of the middle lobe. **C:** Section at the same level as in **B**, after a course of antibiotic therapy and postural drainage. After clearing of retained secretions, cystic bronchiectasis is now easily identified.

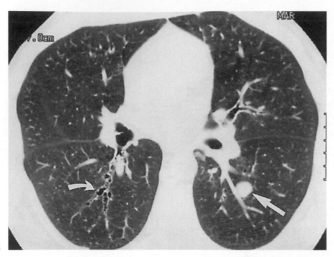 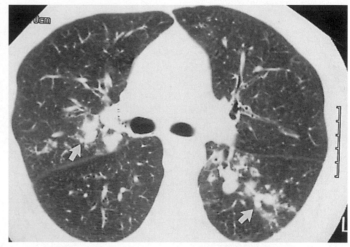

FIG. 8-11. Varicose bronchiectasis in allergic bronchopulmonary aspergillosis. **A:** HRCT at the level of the middle lobe bronchus in a patient who has proven allergic bronchopulmonary aspergillosis. The proximal portion of the superior segmental bronchus of the right lower lobe is dilated and has a distinctly beaded appearance (*curved arrow*). Varicose bronchiectasis can only be diagnosed when involved bronchi course horizontally within the plane of the CT section. The rounded opacity on the left (*straight arrow*) is the result of mucoid impaction within a vertically coursing bronchus. **B:** HRCT in the same patient just below the carina. At this level, the predominant finding is mucoid impaction, recognizable as lobulated linear or branching densities extending toward the lung periphery (*arrows*).

Mosaic Perfusion and Air-Trapping

Over the past several years it has become increasingly apparent that in most cases, patients who have bronchiectasis also show evidence of small airway pathology. Kang et al., for example, in their study of 47 resected lobes with documented bronchiectasis, found pathologic evidence of bronchiolitis in 85% [4]. These included six lobes with obliterative bronchiolitis, 18 with inflammatory or suppurative bronchiolitis, and 16 with both obliterative and inflammatory bronchiolitis. HRCT findings consistent with bronchiolitis were identified in 30 of 47 (75%) lobes, including a pattern of mosaic perfusion (n = 21) (Fig. 8-18); bronchiolectasis (n = 17); and centrilobular nodular or branching opacities, or both (i.e., TIB) (n = 10) (Figs. 8-4 and 8-16) [4].

In particular, the findings of mosaic perfusion on inspiratory scans and focal air-trapping on expiratory scans may prove of special interest in the early diagnosis of bronchiolitis associated with large airways disease (Table 8-2) (Figs. 8-18 and 8-19). In one study of 70 patients [90] who had HRCT evidence of bronchiectasis visible in 52% of lobes evaluated, areas of decreased attenuation (i.e., mosaic perfusion) were visible on inspiratory scans in 20% of lobes, and on expiration (air-trapping) in 34%. Although areas of decreased attenuation on expiratory scans were more prevalent in lobes with severe (59%) or localized (28%) bronchiectasis, in 17% of lobes, air-trapping was identified in the absence of associated bronchiectasis. This has led to speculation that evidence of bronchiolar disease may in fact precede and even lead to the development of bronchiectasis [7,90,91].

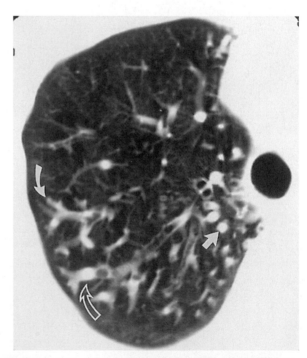

FIG. 8-12. Bronchiectasis with mucoid impaction. Target-reconstructed HRCT through the right upper lobe. mucus-filled airways can be recognized as lobulated linear or branching structures when they course horizontally in the plane of the section (*curved arrows*) or as discrete nodular opacities when they course vertically (*straight arrow*).

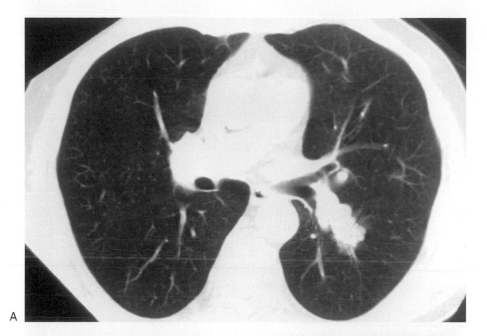

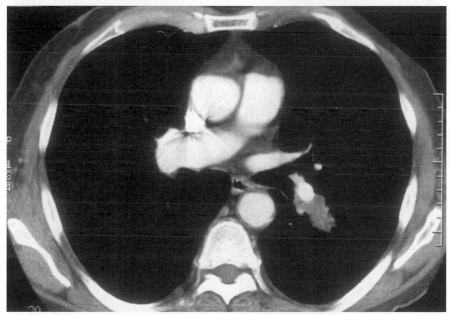

FIG. 8-13. Mucoid impaction—contrast enhancement. **A:** Section through the left upper lobe spur shows central mucoid impaction, with some distortion of the adjacent superior segmental bronchus identified. There is no evidence of peripheral air-trapping on this inspiratory scan. **B:** Section at the same level as in **A** after a bolus of intravenous contrast material shows no evidence of enhancement, confirming the diagnosis of mucoid impaction. Despite the absence of an apparent central tumor, this appearance is consistent with a focal endobronchial lesion. Bronchoscopically confirmed small central carcinoid tumor.

In this same study [90], the presence of decreased attenuation on expiratory scans was also associated with mucoid impaction. This finding was seen in 73% of lobes with large mucous plugs and in 58% of those with centrilobular mucous plugs. These same authors noted a correlation ($r = 0.40$; $p < .001$) between the total extent and severity of bronchiectasis and the extent of decreased attenuation shown on expiratory CT. Not surprisingly, in 55 patients who had pulmonary function tests, the extent of expiratory attenuation abnormalities proved inversely related to measures of airway obstruction, such as forced expiratory volume in one second (FEV_1) and FEV_1/forced vital capacity (FVC) [90].

Associated Bronchial Artery Hypertrophy

Normal bronchial arteries extend along the central airways to a level a few generations proximal to the terminal bronchioles and are the main blood supply for the bronchi. Arising directly from the proximal descending thoracic aorta, these typically measure less than 2 mm and, in addition to supplying the central airways, supply blood to the esophagus and mediastinal lymph nodes. Enlarged bronchial arteries can be identified pathologically in most cases of bronchiectasis and, when severe, usually account for the occurrence of hemoptysis in these patients. With HRCT, it has proved possible to identify both normal and abnormal bronchial arteries in select cases, especially after a bolus of intravenous contrast [92,93].

Song et al. were able to demonstrate good correlation between non–contrast enhanced HRCT images and corresponding CT angiograms for demonstrating hypertrophied bronchial arteries in patients who had bronchiectasis [94]. Specifically, these authors showed that the finding of tubular or nodular areas of soft-tissue attenuation, distinct from blood vessels within the mediastinum and adjacent to the central airways, correctly predicted bronchial artery hypertrophy in 88% and 53% of cases, respectively. Although the diagnosis of bronchiectasis rarely is dependent on demonstrating bronchial artery hypertrophy, identification of focal bronchial wall abnormalities due to enlarged bronchial arter-

ies is important before attempted bronchoscopy, as inadvertent biopsy may lead to significant hemorrhage [94].

Classification of Bronchiectasis

Traditionally, bronchiectasis has been classified into three types, depending on the severity of bronchial dilatation. These three types are *cylindrical*, *varicose*, and *cystic* [95]. Although a distinction between these three types of bronchiectasis is sometimes helpful in diagnosis and correlates with the severity of the anatomic and functional abnormality [67], their differentiation is generally less important clinically than is a determination of the extent and distribution of the airways disease. Evaluating the

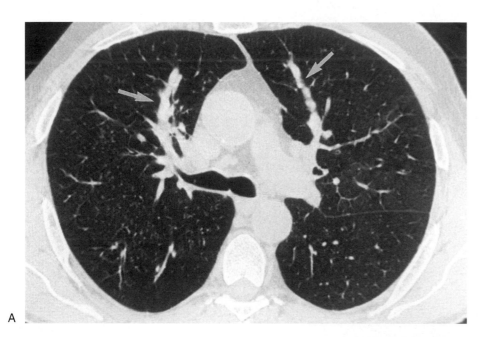

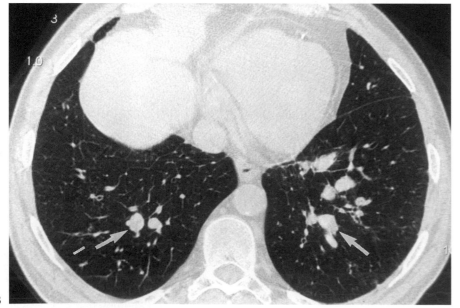

FIG. 8-14. Mucoid impaction—value of retrospective reconstructions. **A,B:** Select axial images through the upper and lower lobes, respectively, acquired in a single breath-hold period on a multidetector-row CT scanner using 1-mm detectors, show evidence of central mucoid impaction in both upper lobes (*arrows* in **A**) and both lower lobes (*arrows* in **B**). *Continued*

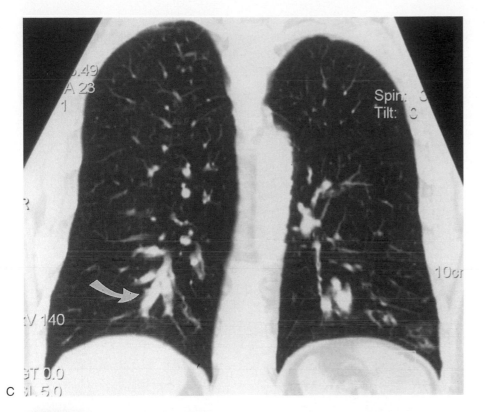

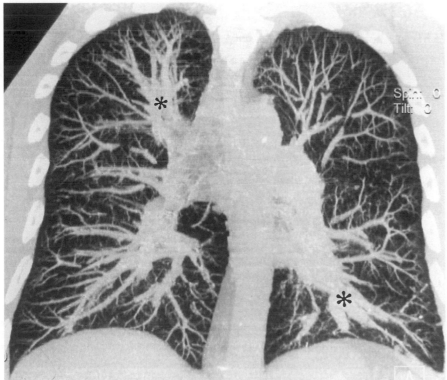

FIG. 8-14. *Continued* **C:** Multiplanar coronal reconstruction through the posterior aspect of the lower lobes shows to better advantage the appearance of branching densities in both lower lobes (*curved arrow*). **D:** Maximum intensity projection image in the coronal plane using five adjacent 1-mm sections also shows the extent of mucoid impaction in the lower lobes and right upper lobe to better advantage (*asterisks*).

extent of bronchiectasis is particularly important, as surgery is only rarely performed in patients who have involvement of multiple lung segments [23,24,96].

In CT scoring systems for bronchiectasis [67], the severity of bronchiectasis, in part, is related to its diameter relative to adjacent pulmonary artery branches, as less than two times the artery diameter, from two to three times the artery diameter, or more than three times the artery diameter. Although these three measurements of bronchial size have no specific relationship to the type of bronchiectasis defined pathologically, they may be reasonable clinical correlates with the terms *cylindrical*, *varicose*, and *cystic*, respectively.

Cylindrical Bronchiectasis

Mild or cylindrical bronchiectasis is diagnosed if the dilated bronchi are of relatively uniform caliber and have roughly parallel walls (Fig. 8-2). The appearance of cylindri-

cal bronchiectasis varies depending on whether the abnormal bronchi have a horizontal or vertical course relative to the scan plane. When horizontal, bronchi are visualized along their length and are recognizable as branching tram tracks that fail to taper as they extend peripherally and are visible more peripherally than is normal. When cylindrically dilated bronchi are oriented in a vertical direction, they are scanned in cross section and appear as thick-walled, circular lucen-

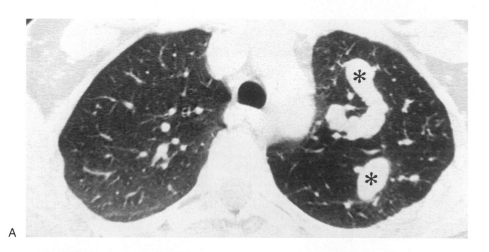

A

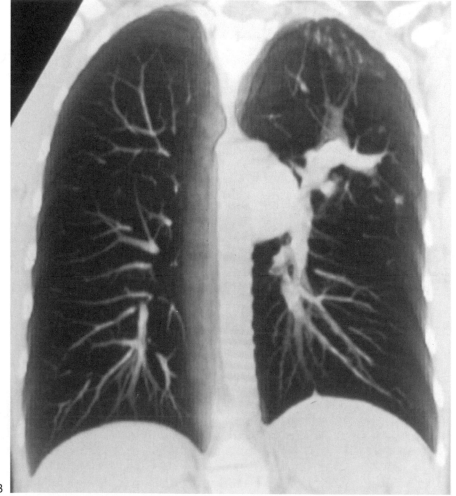

B

FIG. 8-15. Complex congenital disease—bronchial atresia and bronchogenic cyst. **A:** Axial section through the upper lobes, acquired in a single breath-hold period on a multidetector-row CT scanner using 1-mm collimation, shows classic appearance of mucoid-impacted airways in the left upper lobe (*asterisks*), associated with peripheral decreased lung attenuation. **B,C:** Volumetric rendering in the coronal plane and maximum intensity projection image in the sagittal plane, respectively, confirm the presence of extensive mucoid impaction restricted to the left upper lobe associated with peripheral air-trapping, findings characteristic of bronchial atresia. *Continued*

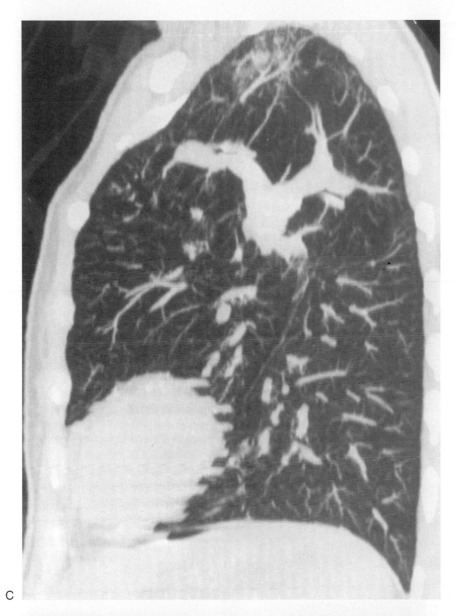

C

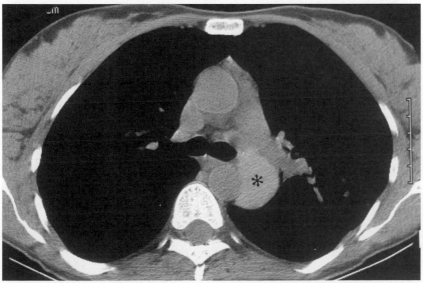

D

FIG. 8-15. *Continued* **D:** Axial section obtained without intravenous contrast media shows a high attenuation bronchogenic cyst insinuated between the descending thoracic aorta and the left main pulmonary artery (*asterisk*). Combinations of congenital airway anomalies should not be considered rare.

cies. In most cases, dilated bronchi seen in cross section can easily be distinguished from emphysematous blebs or other causes of lung cysts by identifying the signet ring sign and the continuity of the dilated bronchus on adjacent scans.

Varicose Bronchiectasis

With increasingly severe abnormalities of the bronchial wall, bronchi may assume a beaded configuration referred to as *varicose bronchiectasis*. This diagnosis can be made consistently

only when the involved bronchi course horizontally in the plane of scan (Figs. 8-3, 8-11, and 8-16). Varicose bronchiectasis is much less frequent than cylindrical bronchiectasis.

Cystic Bronchiectasis

With severe or cystic bronchiectasis, involved airways are cystic or saccular in appearance and may extend to the pleural surface (Figs. 8-4 and 8-6 through 8-8). On HRCT, cystic bronchiectasis may be associated with the presence of (i) air-

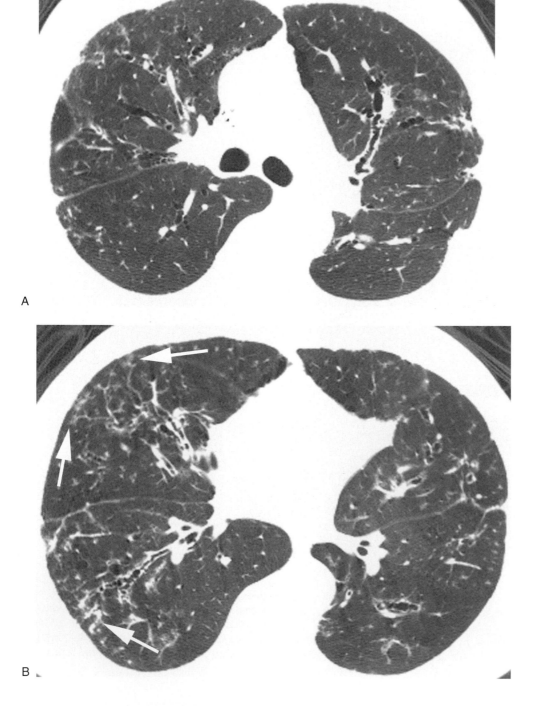

A

B

FIG. 8-16. A–C: Varicose bronchiectasis associated with chronic airway infection by *Haemophilus influenzae*. Irregularly dilated and thick-walled bronchi are typical of varicose bronchiectasis. Ill-defined branching structures (tree-in-bud) and small centrilobular nodules (*arrows*, **B** and **C**) are also visible. *Continued*

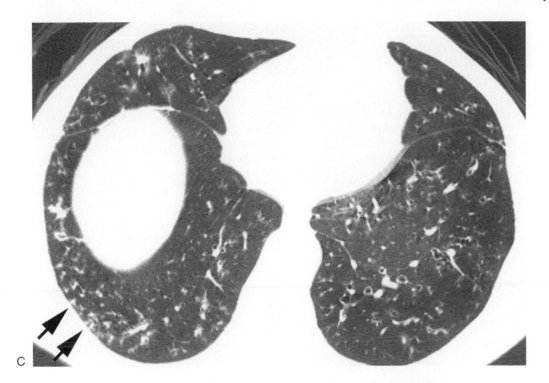

FIG. 8-16. *Continued*

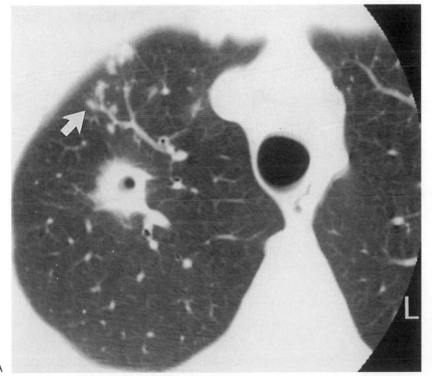

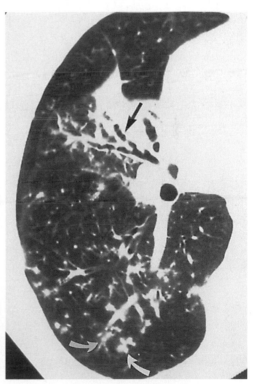

FIG. 8-17. Bronchiectasis associated with endobronchial spread of mycobacteria. **A:** Target-reconstructed HRCT section through the right upper lobe in a patient who has documented active cavitary tuberculosis. Note the presence of a focal cluster of small nodules anterior to the cavity, and adjacent to peripheral pulmonary artery branch (*arrow*). This has been called a *tree-in-bud* appearance and results from mucus or infected material within small peripheral airways. This finding is associated with endobronchial spread of infection. **B:** Target-reconstructed HRCT image through the right lung in a different patient shows marked volume loss and varicose bronchiectasis throughout the middle lobe (*straight arrow*). In addition, note the presence of mucous plugging with a tree-in-bud appearance in the right lower lobe (*curved arrows*). In the appropriate clinical setting, this constellation of findings should suggest the possibility of mycobacterial infection, specifically *Mycobacterium avium* complex, which was subsequently documented.

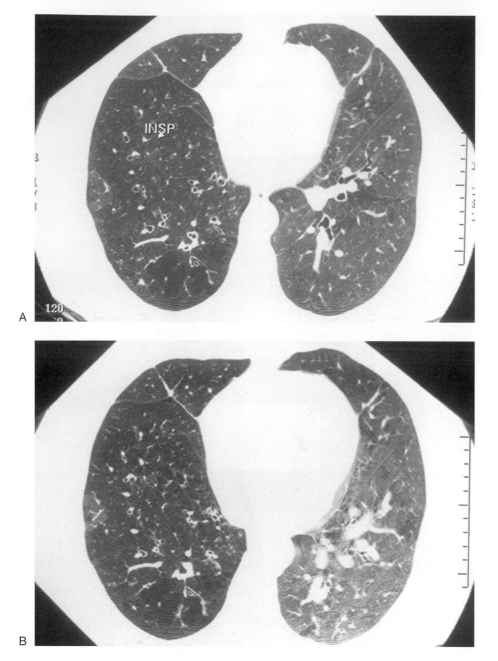

FIG. 8-18. Bronchiolitis obliterans and bronchiectasis. **A,B:** Sections through the lower lobes in inspiration (INSP) and expiration, respectively. Moderately severe bronchiectasis is present in the right lower lobe, resulting in mild bronchial dilatation and wall thickening. Whereas mosaic attenuation is apparent on the inspiratory scan, air-trapping is more definitively identified on the expiration scan. Areas of low density in regions of bronchiectasis have been shown to be due to bronchiolitis obliterans, which may in fact precede the development of bronchiectasis.

fluid levels caused by retained secretions in the dependent portions of the dilated bronchi (Fig. 8-8), (ii) a string of cysts, caused by sectioning irregularly dilated bronchi along their length, or (iii) a cluster of cysts (Figs. 8-7 and 8-20), caused by multiple dilated bronchi lying adjacent to each other. Clusters of cysts are most frequently seen in atelectatic lobes (Fig. 8-20), presumably as a result of chronic infection such as commonly occurs in patients who have pulmonary tuberculosis. In general, the dilated airways in patients who have cystic bronchiectasis are thick-walled; however, cystic bronchiectasis may also appear thin-walled (Fig. 8-6). Recognition of some combination of dilated bronchi, air-fluid levels, and strings or clusters of cysts should be diagnostic of cystic bronchiectasis [97].

Assessment of Bronchiectasis Extent and Severity

It has been shown that CT classification of the type of bronchiectasis may be useful as an index of disease severity. As documented by Lynch et al. [98] in a study of 261 patients who had symptomatic and functionally significant bronchiectasis, excluding patients who had cystic fibrosis (CF), allergic bronchopulmonary aspergillosis (ABPA), or fungal or mycobacterial infections, there was significant correlation between the severity and extent of bronchiectasis with FEV_1 and FVC. Furthermore, those who had cystic bronchiectasis were more likely to have purulent sputum, especially due to *Pseudomonas*, than patients who had cylindrical or varicose bronchiectasis.

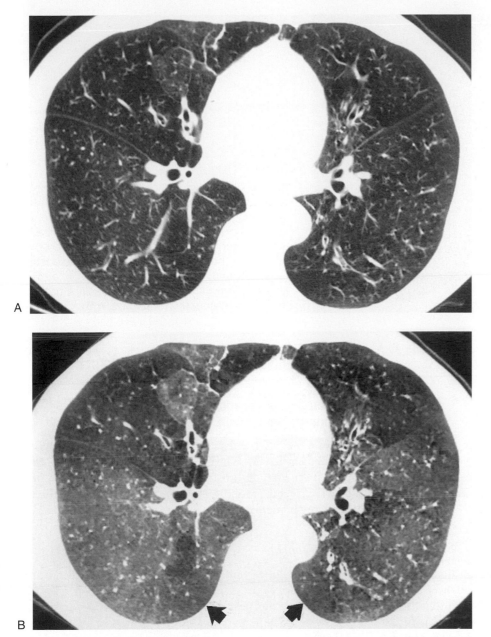

FIG. 8-19. Mosaic perfusion in bronchiectasis and bronchiolitis: assessment with minimum-intensity projection images. **A:** HRCT section through the midlungs shows evidence of mild bronchial dilatation and subtle mosaic perfusion in this patient who has known obliterative bronchiolitis. **B:** Corresponding minimum-intensity projection image using five contiguous 1-mm sections shows to better advantage the extent of mosaic perfusion (*arrows*).

Although visual estimates of disease severity and extent are commonly used, it is apparent that a more accurate approach to disease assessment requires some degree of quantification. Given the importance that has traditionally been placed on the radiographic and clinical scoring of abnormalities in patients who have CF, it is not surprising that CT scoring systems have been most carefully evaluated in this population. Bhalla et al., in the most widely cited method, used nine separate variables, including the extent of mucous plugging, peribronchial thickening, generations of bronchial divisions involved, number of bullae, and the presence of emphysema to calculate a global CT score [74]. Based on this approach, these authors found CT to be a valuable tool for objectively evaluating the extent and severity of bronchiectasis in patients who have CF.

Subsequent modifications of this system have been proposed by a number of authors [55,67,99–103]. Although similar in scope, there are important differences among these approaches. These include differences in the definition of bronchial dilatation and bronchial wall thickening and the extent of bronchiectasis. For example, although Bhalla et al. [74] assessed segments in their scoring system, Smith et al. [55] assessed lobes using a five-point scale based on the visual assessment of the number of abnormal bronchi (as less than 25%, 25 to 49%, 50 to 74%, or greater than 75%). Although this approach has the benefit of relative simplicity, its adequacy has been questioned by Diederich et al. [57], who reported only moderate interobserver agreement among three readers ($\kappa = 0.58$) for assessing disease severity.

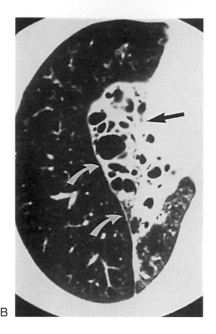
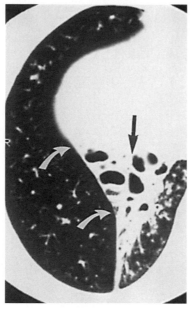

A, B

FIG. 8-20. Cystic bronchiectasis. **A,B:** Target-reconstructed HRCT images through the right lower lung field show the characteristic appearance of a cluster-of-grapes sign. This sign typically results when bronchiectasis occurs in atelectatic lung. Note that in this case both the middle lobe (*arrow*, **A**) and the right lower lobe (*straight arrow*, **B**) are collapsed, causing marked displacement of the oblique fissure (*curved arrows*, **A,B**).

Other differences among scoring systems include the methods of describing the axial extent of disease. Some investigators assess the number of generations of airways involved [74,102,103], whereas others use descriptive schema based on the identification of abnormal airways either in the peripheral half or one-third of the lung [67,99,100] or describe the overall extent of disease as assessed regionally by lobe and zone [101]. More recent scoring systems have also emphasized the inclusion of centrilobular nodules and mosaic perfusion as additional signs of airways disease [99,100,102,103].

These differences notwithstanding, most reports have documented good correlation between HRCT assessment of bronchiectasis extent and severity of disease when compared with more traditional radiographic, clinical, or functional evaluations [55,74,100,102,103]. For example, Smith et al. [55] found correlations between the extent of bronchiectasis and both dyspnea and FEV_1. In patients who had CF, Shah et al. [100] found that HRCT severity scores in symptomatic and asymptomatic patients correlated with FVC ($r = 0.44$; $p = .01$) and FEV_1 ($r = 0.34$; $p = .04$), whereas severity of bronchiectasis correlated with FVC ($r = 0.50$; $p = .004$) and FEV_1 ($r = 0.40$; $p = .02$). In symptomatic patients, improvement in HRCT score correlated with changes in FEV_1/FVC ($r = 0.39$; $p = .049$). In a study by Roberts et al. [91], the extent and severity of bronchiectasis and the severity of bronchial wall thickening correlated strongly with the severity of airflow obstruction. The severity of bronchial dilatation was negatively associated with airflow obstruction.

Nonetheless, given the lack of general clinical acceptance for the use of CT scoring systems to quantitatively assess and monitor patients, especially those who have chronic diseases such as CF, the need for a standardized scoring system is apparent not only for accurate assessment of response to therapy, but also to ensure valid comparisons between studies of differing populations. Such a system derived from existing published reports is proposed in Table 8-3.

Technical Considerations in the High-Resolution Computed Tomography Diagnosis of Airways Disease

Given the range and subtlety of abnormalities that can be identified in patients who have airways disease, it is apparent that an accurate diagnosis requires meticulous attention to both scan technique and scan protocols. These techniques are discussed in more detail in Chapter 1.

Scan Technique

A number of technical factors need to be considered in assessing airway pathology. As discussed in Chapter 1, these include slice thickness, slice spacing, field of view (FOV), and reconstruction algorithm. Using an FOV of 13 cm × 13 cm provides the maximum spatial resolution, with resulting pixels measuring approximately 0.25 mm × 0.25 mm [104]. If 1-mm collimation is used, voxel size is 0.25 mm × 0.25 mm × 1.00 mm, equal to 0.06 mm^3 [105]. Although a small FOV is rarely used in routine clinical imaging, the ability to obtain target-reconstructed images through select areas may enhance visualization of fine parenchymal detail and be of value in select cases with airways disease.

Most important for accurate airway evaluation is the use of appropriate window levels and windows, especially in those cases for which quantitative information is sought (see Fig. 1-13). As first shown by Webb and coworkers using phantoms composed of lucite cylinders, an optimal window level for assessing the airway lumen and walls is –450 Hounsfield units (HU) [106]. A similar conclusion has been reached by McNamara et al., also by using a reference phantom [105,107]. In distinction, others have suggested that window

TABLE 8-3. *HRCT bronchiectasis scoring system[a]*

Category	Score			
	0	1	2	3
Severity				
Bronchiectasis[b,d]	Normal	<2×	2–3×	>3×
Bronchial wall thickening[b,d,f]	Normal	<0.5× or <10 mm	0.5–1× or 10–15 mm	>1× or >15 mm
Mosaic perfusion[h]	Normal	1–5 segments	6–9 segments	>9 segments
Sacculations/abscesses[e]	Normal	1–5 segments	6–9 segments	>9 segments
Extent				
Bronchiectasis[e]	Normal	1–5 segments	6–9 segments	>9 segments
Axial distribution[g]	Normal	Central[c]	Peripheral[c]	Mixed
Mucous plugging/centrilobular nodules[h]	Normal	1–5 segments	6–9 segments	>9 segments
Optional				
Severity of emphysema[e]	Normal	1–5 segments	>5 segments	
Severity of bullae[e]	Normal	Unilateral (<4)	Bilateral (<4)	>4
Severity of consolidation/atelectasis[f]	Normal	1–3 segments	4–6 segments	>7 segments

[a]Total score: without options, from 0 to 21; with options, from 0 to 29.
[b]Compared to the diameter of an adjacent pulmonary artery.
[c]Peripheral defined as the outer 50% of the lung parenchyma in axial section.
[d]From Reiff DB, Wells AU, Carr DH, et al. CT findings in bronchiectasis: limited value in distinguishing between idiopathic and specific types. *AJR Am J Roentgenol* 1995;165:261.
[e]From Bhalla M, Turcios N, Aponte V, et al. Cystic fibrosis: scoring system with thin-section CT. *Radiology* 1991;179:783.
[f]From Shah RM, Sexauer W, Ostrum BJ, et al. High-resolution CT in the acute exacerbation of cystic fibrosis: evaluation of acute findings, reversibility of those findings, and clinical correlation. *AJR Am J Roentgenol* 1997;169:375.
[g]From Cartier Y, Kavanagh PV, Johkoh T, et al. Bronchiectasis: accuracy of high-resolution CT in the differentiation of specific diseases. *AJR Am J Roentgenol* 1999;173:47.
[h]From Helbich TH, Heinz-Peer G, Eichler I, et al. Evolution of CT findings in patients with cystic fibrosis. *AJR Am J Roentgenol* 1999;173:81.

width is as important as or more important than window level in airway measurements. Bankier et al. [108], using inflation-fixed lungs to evaluate the effect of window width and levels on bronchial wall thickness confirmed by planimetry, concluded that an optimal window width should vary between 1,000 and 1,400 HU, whereas window levels could vary as much as between –250 and –700 HU. In our experience, for practical purposes, these windows and levels are adequate for routine visual assessment (see Fig. 1-13).

Scan Protocols

Following the report of Grenier et al., the use of HRCT sections acquired every 10 mm in deep inspiration has become standard for diagnosing bronchiectasis [109]. Using this protocol, Grenier et al. [109] have found a very high accuracy for HRCT in diagnosing bronchiectasis as compared to bronchography. Subsequent reports have further confirmed the value of these techniques for establishing the diagnosis of bronchiectasis [62,110].

Based on the results of these studies and several others, the following technique is recommended for patients who have suspected bronchiectasis (see Chapter 1). In patients in whom there are no specific clinical or radiographic signs to help localize disease, 1- to 1.5-mm high-resolution images should be obtained every 10 mm from the lung apices to bases. Despite the lack of contiguous scanning, this technique allows adequate assessment of the bronchial tree in nearly all cases. Although the routine use of thick sections is not indicated, in select cases, especially those in whom mild cylindrical bronchiectasis is suspected, selected thick sections within a limited range of interest may be of value [38].

This approach can be modified to reflect varying clinical presentations. For example, in patients presenting with hemoptysis, it is usually necessary to rule out occult central endobronchial lesions in addition to detecting bronchiectasis. This is best accomplished by obtaining 1- to 1.5-mm-thick sections every 10 mm through the upper- and lower-lung zones, and contiguous 3- to 5-mm-thick sections from the carina to the level of the inferior pulmonary veins [50]. Using this protocol, in a retrospective study of 59 patients evaluated both by CT and fiberoptic bronchoscopy, CT proved abnormal in all cases in which fiberoptic bronchoscopy depicted focal airway pathology [50]. Alternatively, when available, helical or spiral scanning can be substituted for the routine 5-mm axial images through the central airways. These have

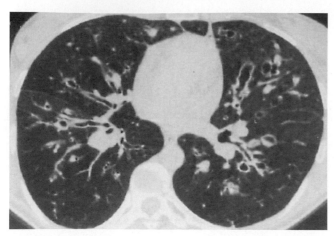

FIG. 8-21. Cystic fibrosis evaluation with low-dose CT. HRCT section through the midlung in a patient who has diffuse bronchiectasis due to cystic fibrosis. Note that central bronchi are involved to a greater degree than peripheral bronchi. Although cylindrical bronchiectasis predominates, small cystic lucencies are also present, reflecting cystic bronchiectasis or abscess cavities. This 2-second scan was performed using 120 kV(p) and 20 mA. In select patients for whom repeated follow-up CT scans may be indicated, high-quality images can be obtained using a low-dose technique. (Courtesy of Minnie Bhalla, M.D., Massachusetts General Hospital, Boston, Massachusetts.)

the advantage of eliminating misregistration artifacts as well as allowing high quality three-dimensional or multiplanar reconstructions to be performed.

Additional scan techniques have also been advocated. As suggested by Remy-Jardin et al. [111], visualization of bronchiectatic segments may be enhanced by use of 20-degree cranial angulation of the CT gantry (see Fig. 1-19). Although unnecessary in most patients, this technique may be of value in equivocal cases, especially for those airways that normally course obliquely, such as the middle lobe and lingular bronchi.

The use of low-dose HRCT techniques for performing routine follow-up scans in patients who have severe chronic disease has also been suggested [74,112]. Bhalla et al. [74], evaluating scans obtained using both 70 and 20 mA, showed that high-quality HRCT images of bronchiectatic airways could be obtained in patients who had CF (Fig. 8-21).

The introduction of spiral CT scanning has led to a reconsideration of optimal scan protocols in patients who have airways disease. In a study by van der Bruggen-Bogaarts et al. [113], spiral CT was found to have a high sensitivity (91%) and specificity (99%) in the diagnosis of bronchiectasis detected using HRCT. In this study, 30 patients and 177 lobes were evaluated with spiral CT (slice thickness, 5 mm; pitch, 1; reconstructed at 2 mm) and HRCT (1.5 mm, 10 mm scan spacing). At HRCT, 14 patients showed signs of bronchiectasis in 32 lobes: Spiral CT con-

firmed the presence in 29 lobes. In one lobe, spiral CT was falsely positive. In a study by Lucidarme et al. [6] of 50 consecutive patients who had suspected bronchiectasis, 1.5-mm HRCT sections obtained at 10-mm intervals were compared to a single 24-second volumetric acquisition using 3-mm collimation. These authors found volumetric data acquisition to be more accurate than routine HRCT for the identification of bronchiectasis. Although helical CT failed to identify bronchiectasis in seven segments in which the disease was diagnosed with HRCT, in four cases a diagnosis of subsegmental cylindrical bronchiectasis was made only with helical CT. In comparison, there were no patients in whom a diagnosis of bronchiectasis was established by HRCT alone.

Spiral CT shows greatest promise in the diagnosis of subtle cylindrical bronchiectasis. Evaluation of the finding of lack of bronchial tapering is difficult using noncontiguous 1-mm sections, effectively reducing the value of this sign to those bronchi that course within the plane of the CT scan. As documented by Giron et al. [110], in a study of 54 patients who had bronchographic evidence of bronchiectasis, obtaining 1-mm sections every 10 mm, three cases were missed and all had mild cylindrical bronchiectasis.

The introduction of multidetector-row spiral CT scanners promises to greatly improve our ability to diagnose airway pathology (see Fig. 1-23; Figs. 8-14, 8-15, and 8-22). The ability to scan the entire thorax in a single breath hold, using 1- to 1.25-mm detector width, and enabling sections of varying thickness to be prospectively and retrospectively reconstructed at any level, is of great value in the diagnosis of airways disease. As indicated in Chapter 1, this technique may fundamentally change the manner in which HRCT is obtained, at least in some patients. The use of reconstruction techniques such as maximum- and minimum-intensity projection images and precise internal and external volumetric renderings of the airways (see Fig. 1-23; Figs. 8-14, 8-15, 8-19, and 8-22) is of potential value. Although many of these techniques are best suited to evaluating small airways disease, potential applications also extend to the larger airways. Of particular interest is the potential to generate CT bronchograms (Fig. 8-22) [8,114].

Given these options, it is apparent that choice of scan technique depends on the type of scanner available, as well as available postprocessing capabilities. It is also likely that specific protocols will continue to evolve with continued clinical experience. Our current recommendation for single-detector scanners calls for an initial series of 1-mm routine axial sections acquired every 10 mm. This may be supplemented with volumetric acquisition of 3-mm sections through the central airways with a pitch of 1.6 to 2, reconstructed every 2 mm [6,115]. Based on our initial experience, a range of potential scan techniques may be applicable to multidetector-row scanners. Using either 1-mm or 1.25-mm detector widths, we reconstruct 3- to 5-mm sections every 2 to 4 mm, as well as contigu-

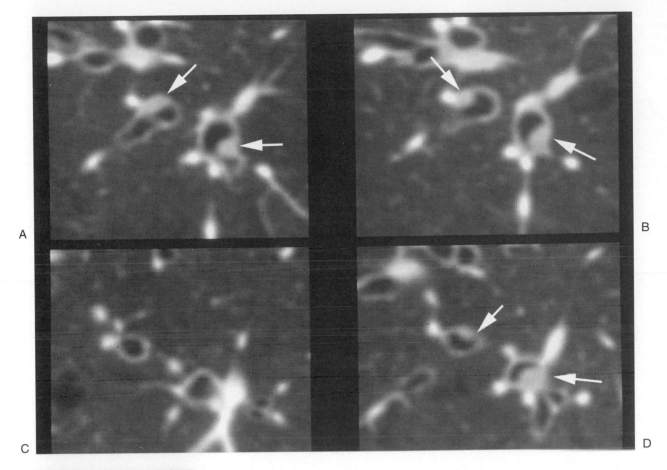

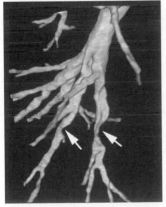

FIG. 8-22. CT bronchography. **A–D:** Sequential axial images through the left lower lobe obtained with a multidetector-row scanner, using 1-mm detectors acquired in a single breath-hold using cardiac gating, show focal filling defects consistent with retained secretions (*arrows*). **E:** External surface rendering of these same airways creating a CT bronchogram: Note the presence of focal airway narrowing corresponding to the same foci identified in **A** through **D** (*arrows*). (Courtesy of Dr. Bernhard Geiger, Siemens Medical Research Inc., Princeton, New Jersey.)

ous 1- to 1.25-mm sections or 1- to 1.25-mm sections every 10 mm.

HRCT may also be used to evaluate the presence of air-trapping in patients who have suspected bronchiectasis (see Figs. 3-148 through 3-153; Fig. 8-18) [11,17,90,91, 116,117]. This may be accomplished by repeatedly acquiring scans at one preselected level during a forced expiration or as two separate acquisitions, first in deep inspiration, followed by scans obtained through the same region in expiration (see Chapters 1 and 2) [9,10,14,90,115, 118,119]. This technique of paired inspiratory and expiratory images may be obtained using HRCT or spiral volumetric techniques. It

should be emphasized that although a variety of strategies for acquiring expiratory scans have been proposed, including 1-mm images obtained at three levels (aortic arch, tracheal carina, and above the diaphragm) are usually sufficient to identify significant air-trapping, even when inspiratory scans are normal [117].

Regardless of the expiratory scan technique used, the resulting images allow the identification of focal areas of air-trapping, as well as changes in the appearance of the airways themselves. In a study of 100 patients who had bronchiectasis having both inspiratory and expiratory scans [91], the extent of decreased attenuation (i.e., air-trapping) on the

TABLE 8-4. *Pitfalls in the HRCT diagnosis of bronchiectasis*

Technical factors[a]
  Respiratory and/or cardiac motion artifacts[a]
  Inappropriate collimation (sections greater than 3 mm)
  Inappropriate window settings (e.g., window width less than 1,000 HU)
Reversible bronchiectasis[a]
  Lung consolidation/pneumonia
  Atelectasis
Pseudobronchiectasis
  (e.g., Langerhans histiocytosis; cavitary metastases; *Pneumocystis carinii* pneumonia)
Traction bronchiectasis[a]
Increased bronchoarterial ratio in normals, asthmatics, or at high altitude[a]

    [a]Most common findings.

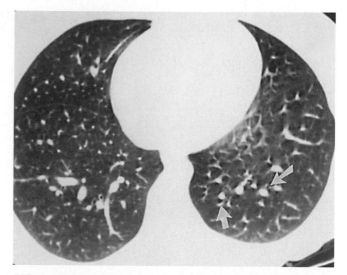

FIG. 8-23. Pseudobronchiectasis. HRCT section through the lung bases in a normal patient. In this case, transmitted cardiac pulsations have caused characteristic stellate artifacts in the left lower lobe that superficially mimic the appearance of bronchiectasis (*arrows*). Note the normal appearance of the lung on the right side by comparison.

expiratory CT scan correlated strongly with the severity of airflow obstruction; the closest relationship ($r = -0.55$; $p = .00005$) was seen between decreased FEV_1.

It is worth noting that in select cases, minimum-intensity projection images may be more sensitive than routine images for detecting subtle regions of air-trapping on expiratory scans (Fig. 8-19) [120–122].

Pitfalls in the Diagnosis of Bronchiectasis

Several potential pitfalls in the diagnosis of bronchiectasis should be avoided (Table 8-4) [1]. Of particular concern are those due to respiratory and cardiac motion artifacts (Fig. 8-23). Transmitted cardiac motion artifacts frequently obscure detail in the left lower lobe and may lead to an erroneous diagnosis of subtle bronchiectasis [123]. Respiratory motion artifacts also cause ghosting that can very closely mimic the appearance of tram tracks. As previously discussed in the section Bronchial Wall Thickening, and in Chapter 1, the appearance of bronchial wall thickening is dependent on the use of appropriate window widths and levels [108]. Furthermore, on expiratory scans, bronchi can appear thicker-walled and narrower than on inspiratory scans.

Bronchiectasis is especially difficult to diagnose in patients who have concurrent parenchymal consolidation or atelectasis, as CT often discloses dilated peripheral airways that will revert to normal after resolution of the lung disease, so-called reversible bronchiectasis (Fig. 8-24) [124]. In such cases, follow-up scans are recommended, pending radiographic resolution. Another potential pitfall related to lung consolidation is the fact that consolidation may obscure vascular anatomy, rendering interpretation of bronchoarterial ratios difficult or impossible [4]. Of course, as emphasized throughout this textbook, visualization of small structures within the lung requires a high-resolution technique. This is especially true when assessing smaller airways (Fig. 8-25).

A number of cystic lung diseases may also be difficult to differentiate from bronchiectasis (Figs. 8-26 and 8-27). Included in this grouping are cavitary nodules in patients who have either widespread bronchoalveolar cell carcinoma or cavitary metastases. Rarely, cystic lesions in patients who have *Pneumocystis carinii* pneumonia (PCP) may superficially simulate bronchiectasis: In these cases, it should be recognized that cystic changes usually occur within areas of ground-glass opacity, simplifying differential diagnosis. In patients who have Langerhans cell histiocytosis, bizarre-shaped cysts are often seen, especially in the upper lobes. As these may appear to branch, their appearance may be suggestive of bronchiectasis, so-called pseudobronchiectasis (Figs. 8-26A and 8-27). In fact, pathologically, some of these cystic abnormalities indeed represent abnormally dilated bronchi, presumably the result of peribronchiolar inflammation.

Bronchiectasis may occur as a component of fibrotic lung diseases or may be seen after radiation therapy. Regardless of the underlying etiology, the result is so-called traction bronchiectasis (Figs. 8-28 and 8-29). This is easily identified, as peripheral bronchi appear irregularly thick-walled or corkscrewed and are invariably found in association with either diffuse reticular changes or honeycombing [125]. Traction bronchiectasis does not represent primary airways disease and is unassociated with symptoms [125].

Utility of High-Resolution Computed Tomography for the Diagnosis of Bronchiectasis

In our experience, most patients studied using HRCT have clinically suspected disease and subtle abnormalities identified on routine radiographs. Symptomatic patients who have

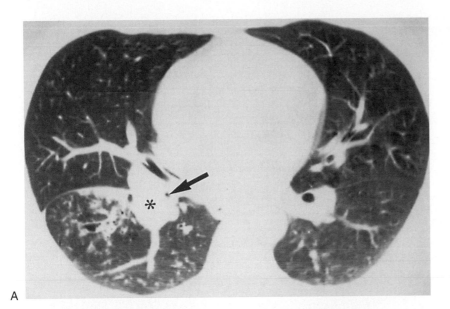

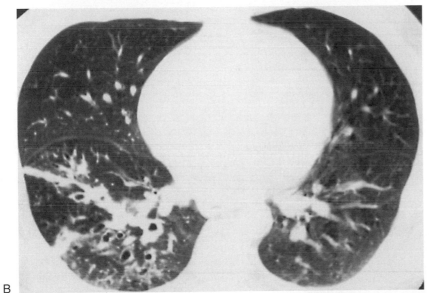

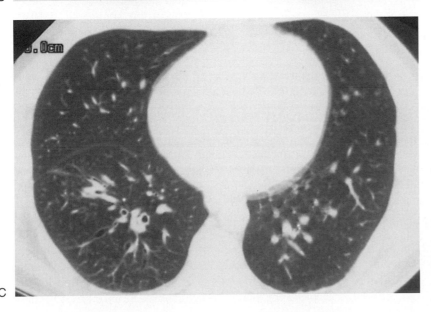

FIG. 8-24. Reversible bronchiectasis. **A,B:** HRCT section shows marked narrowing of the right lower lobe bronchus (*arrow*), with an associated mass in the right hilum (*asterisk*) and apparent bronchiectasis in the right lower lobe, respectively. These findings were interpreted as secondary to a partially obstructing proximal tumor. At bronchoscopy, the right lower lobe bronchus proved to be obstructed by aspirated foreign material (cellulose) without tumor. Nodal enlargement proved to be reactive hyperplasia. **C:** HRCT section at the same level as **B**, obtained 3 months later, shows minimal residual dilatation of the airways. These findings indicate that care should be exercised in diagnosing the presence and severity of bronchiectasis in the presence either of obstruction, atelectasis, or active parenchymal inflammation.

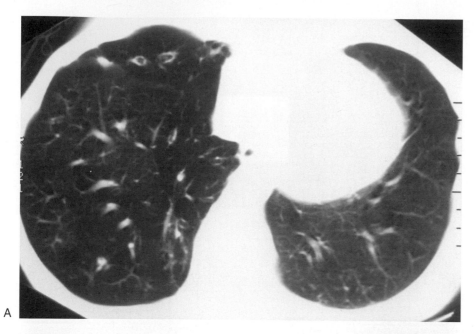

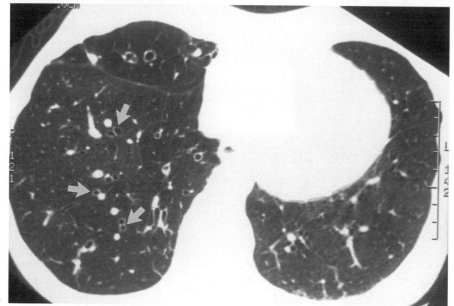

FIG. 8-25. Bronchiectasis: value of HRCT. **A,B:** Corresponding 7- and 1-mm axial images, respectively, obtained through the same level of the lower lobes in a patient who has moderately severe cylindrical bronchiectasis in both the middle and right lower lobes, clearly demonstrate the superiority of HRCT for identifying dilated airways (*arrows*).

entirely normal radiographs are the exception. In a prospective study comparing chest radiographs and HRCT [126], a normal chest radiograph was found to almost always exclude significant bronchiectasis. In this study, 37 patients had a normal radiograph, and 32 of these had a normal HRCT. The other five had mild cylindrical bronchiectasis. In distinction, in the 47 patients who had an abnormal radiograph, 36 had signs of bronchiectasis at HRCT and 11 had a normal HRCT. Thus, in this study, the sensitivity of chest radiography for detecting bronchiectasis diagnosed by HRCT was 88% and the specificity was 74%.

Although its use was initially controversial, HRCT has emerged as the imaging modality of choice for evaluating bronchiectasis; HRCT has all but eliminated the use of bronchography.

Studies assessing the CT diagnosis of bronchiectasis using 10-mm-thick collimation provided low sensitivities, ranging between 60% and 80%, with specificities between 90% and 100% [59–61,127–130]. It quickly became apparent, however, that a significant improvement in diagnostic sensitivity could be achieved by the use of high-resolution 1- and 1.5-mm sections.

Grenier et al. [109], using 1.5-mm-thick sections obtained every 10 mm, retrospectively compared CT and bronchography in 44 lungs in 36 patients and found that CT confirmed the diagnosis of bronchiectasis with a sensitivity of 97% and a specificity of 93%. Young et al. [62] also assessed the reliability of HRCT in the assessment of bronchiectasis as compared to bronchography in 259 segmental bronchi from 70 lobes of 27 lungs. HRCT was positive in 87 of 89 segmental bronchi shown to have bronchiectasis

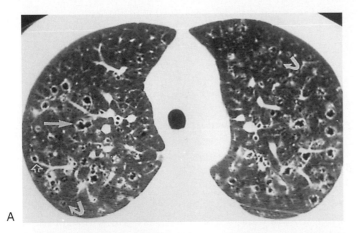

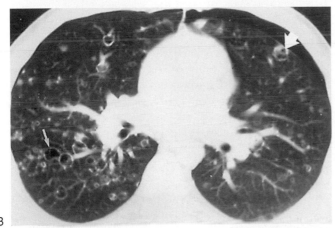

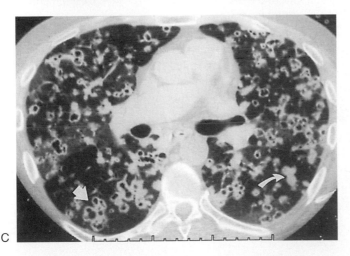

FIG. 8-26. Pitfalls in the diagnosis of bronchiectasis: diffuse cystic lung disease. **A:** Langerhans cell histiocytosis. Section through the middle lungs shows scattered, thick-walled cystic lesions. Although some appear to be branching (*straight arrow*), others are unrelated to any accompanying artery (*curved arrows*), whereas others appear to have feeding vessels (*open arrow*). Note also the presence of few ill-defined subpleural nodules. This constellation of findings is characteristic of Langerhans cell histiocytosis. Although most of these cystic lesions represent cavitating nodules, some likely actually represent abnormally dilated airways. **B:** Cystic *Pneumocystis carinii* pneumonia. Section through the middle lungs shows scattered thin- and thick-walled cysts, some with an apparent branching configuration (*small arrow*). Many of these cysts are unrelated to adjacent arteries, whereas others are clearly subpleural (*large arrow*), accounting in this case for the presence of a small anterior pneumothorax on the left side. **C:** Metastatic adenocarcinoma: 1-mm section in a patient who has adenocarcinoma metastatic to the airways. The bronchi are dilated diffusely and thick-walled (*straight arrow*), without central obstruction. Solid lobular densities (*curved arrow*) represent impacted bronchi.

(sensitivity, 98%). HRCT was negative in 169 of 170 segmental bronchi without bronchiectasis at bronchography (specificity, 99%). Similar results have been reported by Giron et al. [110].

It should be emphasized that despite the excellent sensitivity of HRCT, bronchiectasis may be focal and exceedingly subtle on HRCT scans. Cylindrical bronchiectasis, in particular, can be missed on HRCT, especially if care is not taken to obtain images in deep inspiration [109,110,131]. Giron et al. [110], in a study of 54 patients who had bronchographic

evidence of bronchiectasis, found that they missed three cases, all with mild cylindrical bronchiectasis, using 1-mm-thick slices obtained every 10 mm.

Differentiation of Causes of Bronchiectasis

Although an underlying cause of bronchiectasis is identified in less than 40% to 70% of cases, specific HRCT findings in a number of disease entities have been described. The reliability of CT for distinguishing between these is still debated

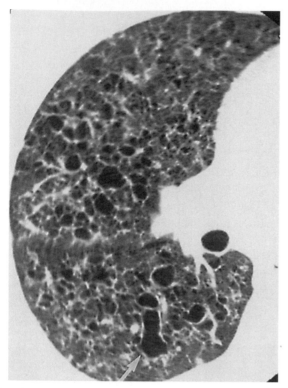

FIG. 8-27. Pseudobronchiectasis in Langerhans cell histiocytosis. Target-reconstructed HRCT image through the right middle lung of a patient who has Langerhans cell histiocytosis shows multiple, variably sized cystic lesions, some with bizarre or branching appearances (*arrow*).

[67,101,132]. Reiff et al. [67] evaluated the HRCT scans of 168 patients who had chronic purulent sputum production suspected of having bronchiectasis. With the exception of a predominant lower lobe distribution in patients who had syndromes of impaired mucociliary clearance, these authors

found no significant difference in lobar distribution between cases of idiopathic bronchiectasis and those with a known etiology. Although central bronchiectasis was more common in patients who had ABPA, the sensitivity of this finding as a diagnostic feature proved to be only 37% [67]. Similarly, although the extent and severity of disease were more pronounced in patients who had both ABPA and CF, these features were of only limited value in individual cases [67].

Lee et al. [132], in a similar study of CT scans in 108 patients who had bronchiectasis from a variety of causes, found that a correct first-choice diagnosis was made by three experienced observers in only 45% of cases; more problematic still, a high confidence level was reached in only 9%, and of these, a correct diagnosis was made in only 35%. Furthermore, interobserver agreement was poor (mean, $\kappa = 0.20$) leading these investigators to conclude that CT was of little value in diagnosing specific etiologies of bronchiectasis. It should be emphasized that CT scans were interpreted in the absence of clinical data [132].

Cartier et al. [101] reported slightly better results in a retrospective study of 82 consecutive patients who had bronchiectasis with documented etiologies. These authors noted that a correct diagnosis was reached by two independent observers in 61% of cases, including a correct diagnosis in 68% of cases of CF, 67% of cases with tuberculosis, and 56% of cases of ABPA [101]. Specifically, in this study, a bilateral upper lobe distribution was most commonly seen in patients who had CF and ABPA, whereas unilateral upper lobe distribution was most common in patients who had tuberculosis, and a lower lobe distribution was most often seen in patients after childhood viral infections.

It should be emphasized that the value of HRCT is considerably enhanced when more focused clinical issues are addressed. Ward et al. [63], for example, assessing the accuracy of HRCT in the diagnosis of ABPA in asthmatic patients, found that a combination of bronchiectasis in more than three

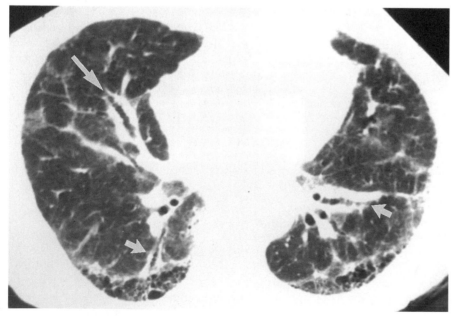

FIG. 8-28. Traction bronchiectasis in interstitial fibrosis. **A:** Section through the lower lobes in a patient who has histologically documented usual interstitial pneumonia (UIP) shows architectural distortion and honeycombing predominantly affecting the peripheral and inferior portions of the lower lobes. Dilated irregular bronchi are apparent bilaterally (*arrows*), associated with peribronchial increased soft tissue, findings characteristic of traction bronchiectasis due to peribronchial cicatrization. *Continued*

A

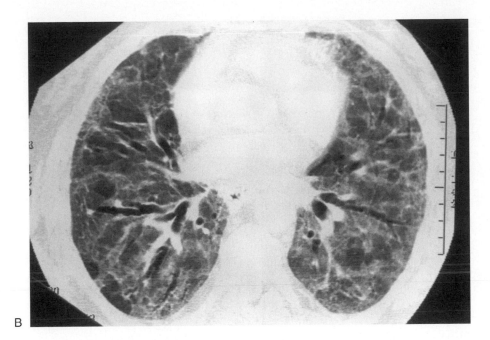

FIG. 8-28. *Continued* B: Section through the lung bases at nearly the same level as in **A**, in a different patient also with histologically proven UIP. Despite the lack of honeycombing, there are marked reticular markings and a suggestion of diffuse ground-glass opacity. Note that the airways are dilated and mildly corkscrewed and fail to taper peripherally. This appearance is consistent with extensive and irreversible parenchymal fibrosis with resultant traction bronchiectasis.

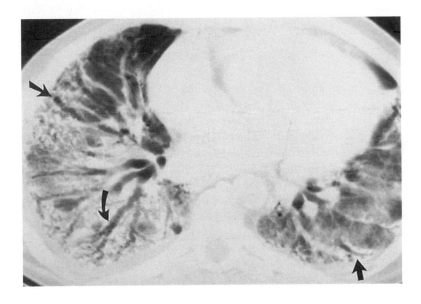

FIG. 8-29. Traction bronchiectasis in interstitial fibrosis. HRCT section through the lower lobes shows evidence of diffuse parenchymal consolidation and ground-glass opacity associated with numerous dilated, tortuous airways both centrally (*curved arrow*) and peripherally (*straight arrows*). An autopsy performed shortly after this study revealed extensive pulmonary fibrosis and traction bronchiectasis without significant inflammation.

lobes, centrilobular nodules, and mucoid impaction could be identified in 95%, 93%, and 67% of cases, respectively, in patients who had ABPA. By comparison, these same findings were present in only 29%, 28%, and 4% of asthmatic controls, leading these investigators to conclude that HRCT is of clinical value in identifying asthmatic patients who have ABPA [63].

DISEASES ASSOCIATED WITH BRONCHIECTASIS

The HRCT appearances of a number of diseases associated with bronchiectasis have been described. In many of these, such as hypogammaglobulinemia [133], HRCT findings are unremarkable as described previously. On the other hand, a few conditions associated with bronchiectasis have been reported to have distinctive HRCT appearances that can aid in their diagno-

sis or are sufficiently common to warrant detailed description. The most important of these are CF, ABPA, and nontuberculous mycobacterial infection. Bronchiectasis in association with lung nodules is characteristic of nontuberculous mycobacterial infection resulting from MAC (Fig. 8-30) and is described in detail in Chapter 5. It should also be recognized that bronchiectasis is a common feature of diseases usually regarded to predominantly involve small airways, such as BO and panbronchiolitis. These are described in detail later in this chapter.

Cystic Fibrosis

CF is the most common cause of pulmonary insufficiency in the first three decades of life [134,135]. It results from an autosomal-recessive genetic defect in the structure of the

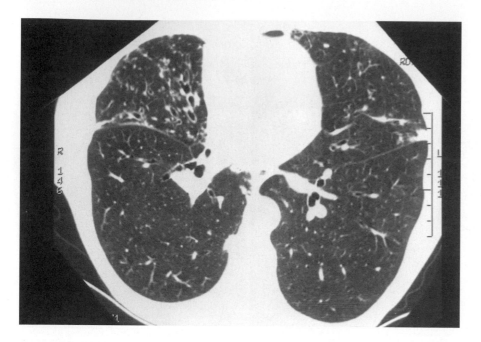

FIG. 8-30. Atypical mycobacterial infection. Section through the middle lungs in a patient who has documented *Mycobacterium avium* infection shows extensive bronchiectasis primarily involving the middle lobe, and, to a lesser degree, the lingula, with near-complete sparing of the lower lobes. Scattered small centrilobular nodules are also apparent. This distribution of disease is characteristic of this infection, especially in elderly women.

cystic fibrosis transmembrane regulator protein, which leads to abnormal chloride transport across epithelial membranes. The mechanisms by which this leads to lung disease are not entirely understood, but an abnormally low water content of airway mucus is at least partially responsible, resulting in decreased mucus clearance, mucous plugging of airways, and an increased incidence of bacterial airway infection. Bronchial wall inflammation progressing to secondary bronchiectasis is universal in patients who have long-standing disease and is commonly visible on chest radiographs [136].

Plain radiographs can be diagnostic in patients who have CF, showing increased lung volumes, accentuated linear opacities in the central or upper lung regions due to bronchial wall thickening or bronchiectasis, central bronchiectasis, and mucoid impaction [136]. However, plain film findings in patients who have early or mild disease may be quite subtle. Hyperinflation, which can represent an early finding, reflects the presence of obstruction of small airways by mucus; thickening of the wall of the right upper lobe bronchus, best seen on the lateral radiograph, can also be an early sign of disease [137]. In adult CF patients and patients who have chronic disease, abnormalities can include cystic regions in the upper lobes, representing cystic bronchiectasis, healed abscess cavities, or bullae; atelectasis, findings of pulmonary hypertension, or cor pulmonale; pneumothorax; and pleural effusion [138]. In the large majority of patients who have an established diagnosis of CF, clinical findings and chest radiographs are sufficient for clinical management. On the other hand, it should be recognized that patients who have CF can have a significant exacerbation of their symptoms with little visible radiographic change [139].

High-Resolution Computed Tomography Findings

HRCT findings in patients who have CF have been well described (Figs. 8-31 through 8-35) [74,99,100,102,103,135,

140–142]. Bronchiectasis is present in all patients who have advanced CF who are studied using HRCT (Table 8-5) [74,99,100,102,103,135,140,141]. Proximal or perihilar bronchi are always involved when bronchiectasis is present, and bronchiectasis is limited to these central bronchi in approximately one-third of the cases, a finding that is referred to as *central bronchiectasis* (Figs. 8-34 and 8-35). Both the central and peripheral bronchi are abnormal in approximately two-thirds of patients [74,140]. All lobes are typically involved, although early in the disease abnormalities are often predominantly upper lobe in distribution, and a right upper lobe predominance may be present in some patients (Fig. 8-32) [74,99,100,102,103,135,140–142].

Cylindrical bronchiectasis is the most frequent pattern seen; it was visible in 94% of lobes in one study of patients who had severe disease [140]. Thirty-four percent of lobes in this study showed cystic bronchiectasis, whereas varicose bronchiectasis was seen in 11%. In another report, cystic lesions representing cystic bronchiectasis or abscess cavities were present in eight of 14 (57%) patients (Fig. 8-21) [74].

Bronchial wall thickening, peribronchial interstitial thickening, or both are also commonly present in patients who have CF (Figs. 8-31 through 8-35) [99,102,103,143]. The thickening is generally more evident than bronchial dilatation in patients who have early disease and may be seen independent of bronchiectasis [74,142]. Thickening of the wall of proximal right upper lobe bronchi was the earliest abnormal feature visible on HRCT in one study of patients who had mild CF [74,142].

Mucous plugging is also common, reported in between one-quarter and one-half of cases [99,102,103], and may be visible in all lobes [74,141]. Collapse or consolidation can be seen in as many as 80% of cases (Figs. 8-31 and 8-33) [74,99,143]. Volume loss was visible in 20% of lobes in patients who had advanced disease [140].

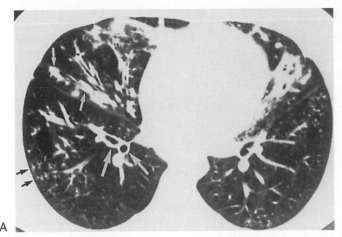
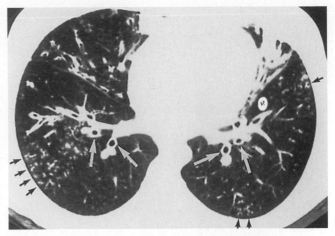

FIG. 8-31. Cystic fibrosis. **A,B:** HRCT at two levels shows extensive bronchial wall thickening (*large white arrows*); bronchiectasis, which is most evident anteriorly in the middle lobe and lingula; and mucous impaction in both large (*small white arrows*) and small (*small black arrows*) airways resulting in a tree-in-bud appearance. Lingular atelectasis is also present. (**A** from Webb WR. High-resolution computed tomography of obstructive lung disease. *Radiol Clin North Am* 1994;32:745–757, with permission.)

Branching or nodular centrilobular opacities (i.e., tree-in-bud) which reflect the presence of bronchiolar dilatation with associated mucous impaction, infection, or peribronchiolar inflammation, can be an early sign of disease (Figs. 8-31 and 8-32) [141]. Focal areas of decreased lung opacity, representing air-trapping or mosaic perfusion, are common (Figs. 8-33 through 8-35). These can be seen to correspond to pulmonary lobules or subsegments and may appear to surround dilated, thick-walled, or mucous-plugged bronchi [141] in as many as two-thirds of patients [102]. Air-trapping can often be seen on expiratory scans (Fig. 8-35) [140].

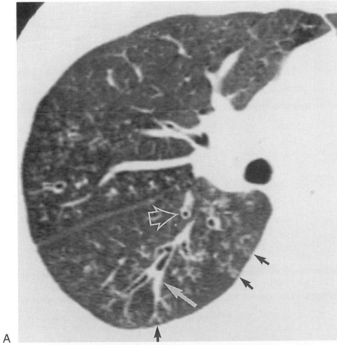
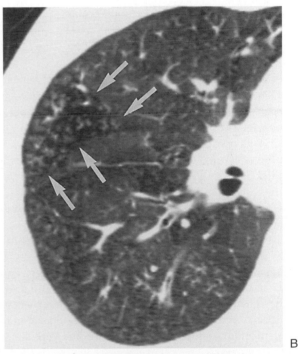

FIG. 8-32. Cystic fibrosis with early abnormalities in a boy with a normal sweat chloride test. **A:** HRCT at the level of the middle and lower lobes shows bronchial wall thickening (*open arrow*), bronchiectasis with mucous impaction (*large arrow*), and small airway impaction with a tree-in-bud appearance (*small arrows*). **B:** At a slightly higher level, a region of the middle lobe (*arrows*) shows extensive bronchiolar impaction with a characteristic tree-in-bud appearance. This region also appears relatively lucent compared to surrounding lung as a result of mosaic perfusion.

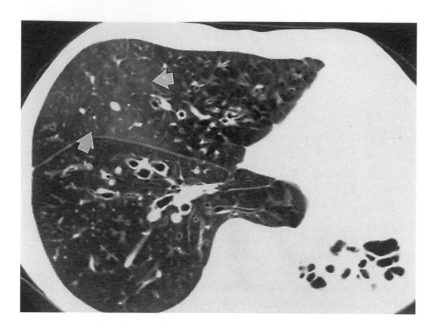

FIG. 8-33. Cystic fibrosis. Atelectasis of the left lung is associated with extensive bronchiectasis. Bronchial wall thickening and bronchiectasis are visible on the right. A region of relatively increased attenuation (*arrows*) anteriorly reflects mosaic perfusion. Note that bronchiectasis is not visible in this region, and vessels appear larger than in lucent lung regions. (From Webb WR. High-resolution computed tomography of obstructive lung disease. *Radiol Clin North Am* 1994;32:745–757, with permission.)

Lung volumes may appear increased on CT, although this diagnosis is rather subjective and may be better assessed on chest radiographs [140]. Cystic or bullous lung lesions can also be visible and typically predominate in the subpleural regions of the upper lobes [74,140]. Hilar or mediastinal lymph node enlargement and pleural abnormalities can also be seen, largely reflecting chronic infection. Pulmonary artery dilatation resulting from pulmonary hypertension can also be seen in patients who have long-standing disease.

Utility of High-Resolution Computed Tomography

HRCT can demonstrate morphologic abnormalities in patients who have early CF who are asymptomatic, have normal pulmonary function, have normal chest radiographs, or a combination of these. In a study of 38 patients who had mild CF with normal pulmonary function [142], chest radiographs were normal in 17 (45%), showed mild bronchial wall thickening in 17, and showed mild bronchiectasis in four (10%). On HRCT in this group, features of bronchiectasis were present in 77% of all patients and in 65% of those with normal chest radiographs; only three patients had a normal HRCT [142]. In another study of HRCT findings in 12 largely asymptomatic pediatric patients who had early CF, chest radiographs were normal in seven, whereas HRCT was normal in only two. HRCT findings not visible on radiographs included bronchial wall thickening, bronchiectasis, centrilobular small airway abnormalities, and lobular or segmental inhomogeneities representing mosaic perfusion or air-trapping [141].

In patients who have more advanced disease, HRCT can also show abnormalities not visible on chest radiographs. In a study of 14 patients who had CF [74], HRCT was found to be superior to chest radiographs in detecting bronchiectasis and mucous plugging. Of a total of 162 segments assessed,

bronchiectasis was detected in 124 segments using HRCT, whereas only 71 segments were considered to show this finding on chest radiographs. Mucous plugs were detected on HRCT in 38 segments, whereas they were seen on radiographs in only four segments. In a study by Hansell et al. [140], bronchiectasis was considered to be present on HRCT in 124 of 126 lobes; on chest radiographs, only 84 of 102 lung zones were considered to show this finding. Chest radiographs also underestimated the extent of bronchiectasis. Bronchiectasis was considered to be both central and peripheral in only 31% of lung zones on chest radiographs, whereas a diffuse distribution was seen in 59% of lobes using HRCT.

Despite numerous reports detailing the range of abnormalities identified in patients who have CF, few if any of these find-

---

TABLE 8-5. *HRCT findings in adult cystic fibrosis*

Bronchiectasis[a,b]

  Central bronchi and upper lobes involved in all cases[a,b]

  Sometimes severe (varicose and cystic) and widespread (5–6 lobes)[b]

Bronchial wall thickening[a,b]

  Central and upper lobe distribution[a,b]

  Right upper lobe first involved[b]

Mucous plugging[a,b]

Branching or linear centrilobular opacities (tree-in-bud)[a,b]

Large lung volumes[a,b]

Areas of atelectasis[a]

Mosaic perfusion[a]

Air-trapping on expiration[a]

[a]Most common findings.
[b]Findings most helpful in differential diagnosis.

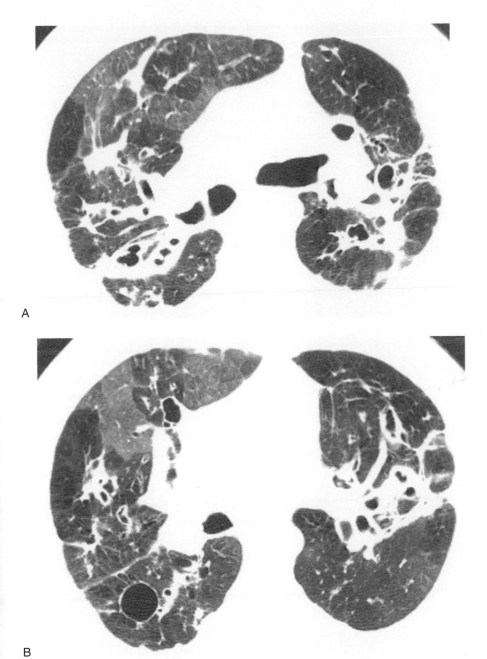

A

B

FIG. 8-34. A,B: Cystic fibrosis in an adult. HRCT scans through the upper lung zones show central bronchiectasis and inhomogeneous opacity due to mosaic perfusion. Note the presence of decreased vessel size and abnormal bronchi in the relatively lucent lung regions. A cyst is visible in the posterior right lung.

ings are specific. Reiff et al., in an assessment of 168 patients who had suspected bronchiectasis from a variety of etiologies, found that patients who had adult CF tended to have more widespread involvement than idiopathic bronchiectasis (p <.01) [67]. In patients who have early disease, abnormalities are often predominantly upper lobe in distribution, with a right upper lobe predominance. Despite these findings, as reported by Lee et al. and Cartier et al., a specific diagnosis of adult CF was made in only 38% and 68% of cases, respectively [101,132].

The routine clinical evaluation of CF makes use of clinical and radiograph-based scoring systems. Several authors have also suggested the use of an HRCT scoring system [74,99,144]; these are described in detail above. It is hypothesized that such a scoring system may facilitate the objective evaluation of existing and newly developed therapeutic regimens [74]. One scoring system [74], based on an assessment of the degree and extent of bronchiectasis, bronchial wall thickening, mucous plugging, atelectasis, emphysema, and other findings, showed a statistically significant correlation to the percent ratios of FEV_1/FVC ($r = 0.69$; $p = .006$) [74]. In another study based on assessment of bronchiectasis and mucous plugging [144], CT scores correlated highly with clinical ($r = 0.88$; p <.0001) and radiographic ($r = 0.93$; p <.0001) scores and several pulmonary function tests. The best correlation was with bronchiectasis.

Several reports have shown that CT offers a reliable alternative to routine radiographic and clinical methods for monitoring disease status and progression, as well as assessing response to treatment [74,103,144,145]. These studies consistently document close correlation between HRCT findings and clinical and pulmonary functional evaluation of these patients.

HRCT may be used to closely monitor potentially reversible morphologic changes as a means for monitoring disease progression and treatment therapy. Shah et al., using a modification of the scoring system proposed by Bhalla et al. [74], reported findings in 19 symptomatic patients who had adult

CF evaluated initially and after 2 weeks of therapy, compared to a control group of eight asymptomatic CF patients [100]. Reversible findings included air-fluid levels in bronchiectatic cavities, centrilobular nodules, mucous plugging, and peribronchial thickening. Significantly, whereas severity of bronchiectasis was found to correlate with FVC ($p = .004$) and FEV_1 ($p = .02$), no correlation was identified between pulmonary function test (PFT) parameters and either mucous

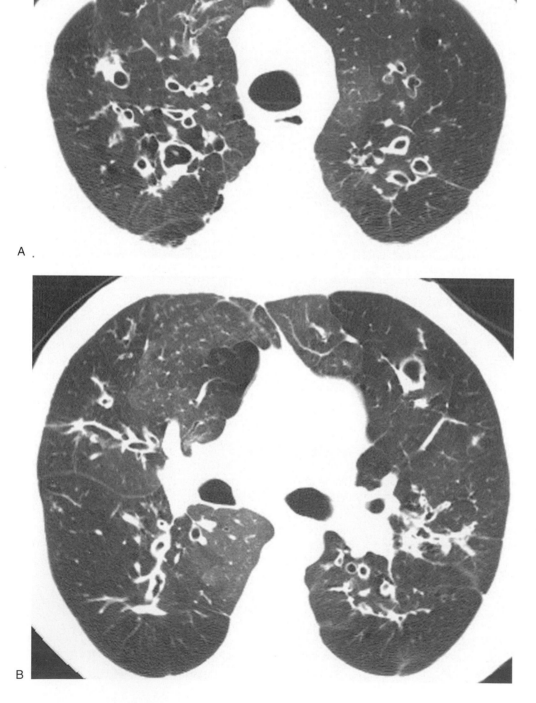

FIG. 8-35. A–D: Cystic fibrosis in an adult patient who has bronchiectasis, mosaic perfusion, and air-trapping on an expiratory scan. HRCT scans through the upper **(A)**, middle **(B)**, and lower **(C)** lung zones show multiple thick-walled and dilated bronchi. Bronchiectasis is most evident in the central lung regions, a finding typical of cystic fibrosis and termed *central bronchiectasis. Continued*

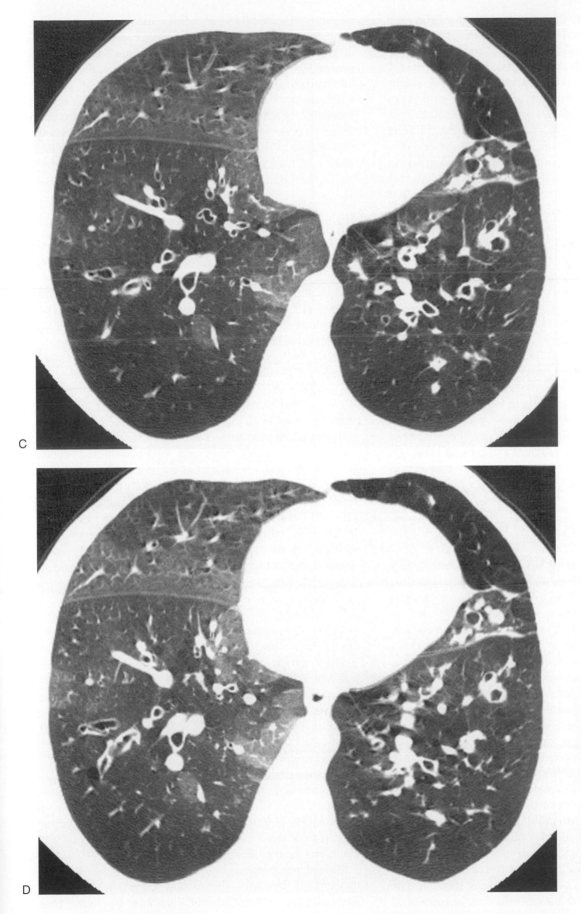

FIG. 8-35. *Continued* On the inspiratory scans **(A–C)**, the lung appears inhomogeneous in opacity, with decreased vessel size and abnormal bronchi visible in the lucent lung regions. This is typical of mosaic perfusion secondary to air-trapping. An expiratory scan **(D)**, obtained at the same level as **C**, shows air-trapping in lucent lung regions.

plugging or centrilobular nodules, suggesting that PFTs were an insensitive means for identifying potentially reversible and hence treatable disease [100].

In a related study, Helbich et al. [103] evaluated serial CT studies obtained at various time intervals of up to 48 months in 107 patients to determine both the evolution of findings and optimal time intervals for sequential CT evaluation. These authors found that 6 to 18 months of follow-up were valuable for identifying potentially reversible morphologic changes, in particular, the presence of mucous plugging. In distinction, bronchiectasis and mosaic perfusion progressed at a significantly slower rate, rendering them less useful as a means for monitoring therapeutic interventions. Of particular interest was the finding that although CT correlated significantly with PFTs and clinical scores, these same parameters by comparison with CT were relatively insensitive means for identifying either improvement or disease progression [103]. Whereas mucous plugging could be identified in 25% of patients reexamined by CT within 18 months, for example, only minor changes could be identified by PFTs.

These findings lend support to the notion that HRCT should be incorporated into follow-up regimens of patients who have CF. In distinction, it has been reported that CT may play only a limited role in the preoperative assessment of patients who have CF before lung transplantation [146]. In a retrospective review of 26 patients who had CF who subsequently underwent bilateral lung transplantation, in no case was an unsuspected malignancy identified [146]. Of particular surgical interest, CT proved of little value in predicting the presence of pleural adhesions, a potential concern before transplantation.

Asthma

Asthma is characterized by airway inflammation, largely reversible airway obstruction, and hyperreactivity of the airways to various stimuli [66,147]. Pathologically, patients who have asthma show bronchial wall thickening, caused by inflammation and edema, and excess mucus production, which can result in mucous plugging [148]. Bronchiectasis may be seen in some patients who have long-standing asthma.

Radiographic findings associated with asthma include increased lung volume, increased lung lucency, mild bronchial wall thickening, and mild prominence of hilar vasculature due to transient pulmonary hypertension [149–152]. Bronchial wall thickening is visible in approximately half of patients [38,152]. Bronchiectasis is not usually recognized, but small mucous plugs can sometimes be seen. Associated complications of asthma, although uncommon, include pneumonia, atelectasis, pneumomediastinum, and pneumothorax [151]. Radiographic abnormalities are generally more common and more severe in children with asthma [150,151].

Plain radiographs are uncommonly used to make a diagnosis of asthma; radiographs are often normal, and visible abnormalities in this disease are usually nonspecific [66,150]. The usefulness of radiography in patients who have an established diagnosis of asthma who experience an acute attack is also limited. A correlation between the severity of radiographic findings and the severity or reversibility of an asthma attack is generally poor [149–151], and radiographs provide significant information that alters treatment in 5% or fewer of patients who have acute asthma [153,154]. Although it is difficult to generalize regarding the role of radiographs in adults and children with acute asthma, chest films are often used to exclude the presence of associated pneumonia or other complications when significant symptoms, appropriate clinical or laboratory findings, or both, are suggestive [149–151,153].

High-Resolution Computed Tomography Findings

HRCT is uncommonly indicated in the routine assessment of patients who have asthma, but it is sometimes used when complications, particularly ABPA, are suspected [36], and in documenting the presence of emphysema in smokers with asthma [155,156]. ABPA is associated with more severe bronchiectasis than that typically seen in patients who have uncomplicated asthma.

HRCT findings in patients who have uncomplicated asthma include mild bronchial dilatation. Mild bronchial dilatation has been reported in from 15% to 77% of patients who have uncomplicated asthma (Fig. 8-5) [36,38,65,152,157]. In a study by Lynch et al. [38], bronchi were defined as dilated if their internal diameters exceeded those of accompanying pulmonary arteries. Using this criteria, 77% of asthmatic patients and 153 (36%) of 429 bronchi assessed in asthmatic patients were considered dilated (Fig. 8-5). In a study by Grenier et al., bronchiectasis was found in 28.5% of the asthmatic subjects, primarily involving subsegmental and distal bronchi. As noted by Lynch and others [38,66], bronchial dilatation in asthmatic patients may partially reflect reduction in pulmonary artery diameter, due to changes in blood volume or local hypoxia, or may be physiologic; Lynch suggests caution in diagnosing mild bronchiectasis in this patient population [66].

Experimental studies in dogs [14] and asthmatic subjects [13,158] have measured bronchial luminal diameter using HRCT before and during a histamine or methacholine-induced episode of bronchospasm. These studies have found a significant reduction in the luminal diameter of small bronchi in association with acute asthma. Also, a significant decrease in lung attenuation due to air-trapping was seen in association with induced bronchospasm in these subjects [13].

Bronchial wall thickening, mucoid impaction, and centrilobular bronchiolar abnormalities such as tree-in-bud, patchy areas of lucency, and regional air-trapping on expiratory scans may also be identified on HRCT in patients who have uncomplicated asthma. Bronchial wall thickening has been reported in from 16% to 92% of patients [38,65,152,157], and there appears to be some tendency for the degree of bronchial wall thickening to correlate with the severity of disease [65,76].

Mucoid impaction has been reported in as many as 21% of cases [152]; this abnormality may clear after treatment. Branching or nodular centrilobular opacities have been

TABLE 8-6. *HRCT findings in allergic broncho-pulmonary aspergillosis*

Central bronchiectasis[a,b]
  Typically severe and widespread[a]
Mucous plugging[a]
High-density mucus[a,b]
Linear or branching centrilobular opacities (tree-in-bud)
Atelectasis
Peripheral consolidation or diffuse ground-glass opacity
Mosaic perfusion[a]
Air-trapping on expiration[a]

  [a]Most common findings.
  [b]Findings most helpful in differential diagnosis.

reported to be present in as many as 10% to 21% of patients, sometimes manifested as tree-in-bud. These likely reflect bronchiolar wall thickening or inflammation, with or without mucoid impaction. However, this finding is absent or tends to be inconspicuous in most patients who have asthma.

Focal or diffuse hyperlucency has been observed on inspiratory scans in from 18% to 31% of cases [38,157,159], undoubtedly due to air-trapping and mosaic perfusion. Expiratory CT can show evidence of patchy air-trapping in asthmatic patients (see Figs. 3-149 and 3-151) [160]. In a study by Park et al. [65], air-trapping involving more than a segment was seen in 50% of asthmatic patients. In some patients, air-trapping may be seen in the absence of morphologic abnormalities visible on inspiratory scans [117,161].

Allergic Bronchopulmonary Aspergillosis

ABPA reflects a hypersensitivity reaction to *Aspergillus* species and is characteristically associated with eosinophilia;

symptoms of asthma, such as wheezing and findings of central or proximal bronchiectasis, usually associated with mucoid impaction; atelectasis; and sometimes consolidation similar to that seen in patients who have eosinophilic pneumonia. It occurs in asthmatics, but ABPA has also been noted to occur in between 2% and 10% of patients who have CF [162,163].

ABPA results from both type I and type III (IgE and IgG) immunologic responses to the endobronchial growth of fungal (*Aspergillus*) species. The immune reactions result in central bronchiectasis, which is usually varicose or cystic in appearance, and the formation of mucous plugs, which contain fungus and inflammatory cells. The acronym ARTEPICS has been proposed as an aid for remembering the primary criteria for ABPA, which include A for asthma, R for radiologic evidence of pulmonary disease, T for positive skin test for *Aspergillus fumigatus*, E for eosinophilia, P for precipitating antibodies to *A. fumigatus*, I for elevated IgE, C for central bronchiectasis, and S for elevated *A. fumigatus* serum-specific IgE and IgG [162]. A diagnosis of ABPA is nearly certain when six of these eight criteria are fulfilled. Secondary criteria include the presence of *A. fumigatus* in sputum, a history of expectoration of mucous plugs, and delayed cutaneous reactivity to *Aspergillus* antigen [162].

It has been suggested that disease progression be divided into five separate phases. These include: (i) an acute phase, which usually leads to (ii) resolution, during which time pulmonary infiltrates clear and serum IgE declines; resolution is followed by (iii) remission, when all diagnostic criteria recur, evolving to (iv) a phase of dependence on corticosteroids and, finally, leading in some cases to (v) diffuse pulmonary fibrosis [162].

High-Resolution Computed Tomography Findings

HRCT findings in patients who have ABPA have been well described (Table 8-6) (Fig. 8-11 and Figs. 8-36 through 8-39) [36,37,63,66,67,101,132,164–169]. A characteristic finding of

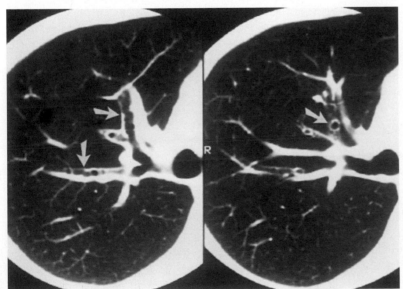

A,B

FIG. 8-36. Allergic bronchopulmonary aspergillosis (ABPA) with early changes. **A,B:** Sequential target-reconstructed HRCT images through the right upper lobe bronchus in a patient who has ABPA. The proximal portions of the anterior and posterior segmental bronchi are mildly dilated and have a distinctly beaded, irregular, and varicose appearance (*arrows*, **A**). Branches of the apical segmental bronchus are also dilated (*arrow*, **B**). Central bronchiectasis is typical of ABPA.

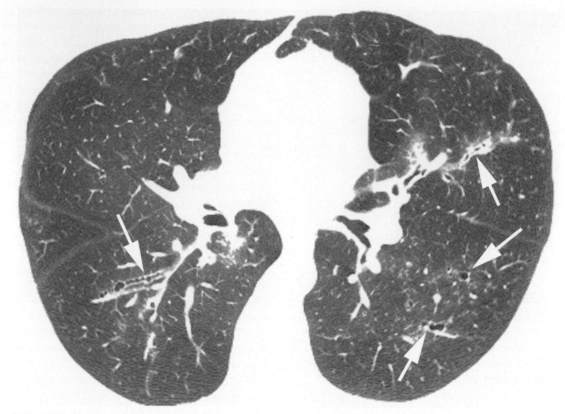

FIG. 8-37. Allergic bronchopulmonary aspergillosis with central bronchiectasis. Irregular, thick-walled, and mildly dilated bronchi (*arrows*) are visible in both lungs.

central bronchiectasis can be identified in nearly all cases. As documented by Panchal et al. in their study of 23 patients who had ABPA, central bronchiectasis could be identified in 85% of lobes and 52% of lung segments using 4- and 8-mm-thick sections [169]. Central bronchiectasis typically occurred in

association with bronchial occlusion due to mucous plugging; air-fluid levels in dilated, cystic airways; and bronchial wall thickening.

In addition to widespread and severe central bronchiectasis, a number of ancillary findings have been reported to

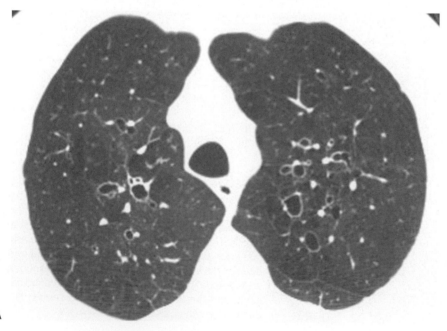

A

FIG. 8-38. A–C: Allergic bronchopulmonary aspergillosis with mild central bronchiectasis. Thick-walled and dilated bronchi are visible diffusely, but with an upper lobe predominance. Mild inhomogeneity of lung attenuation reflects mosaic perfusion. *Continued*

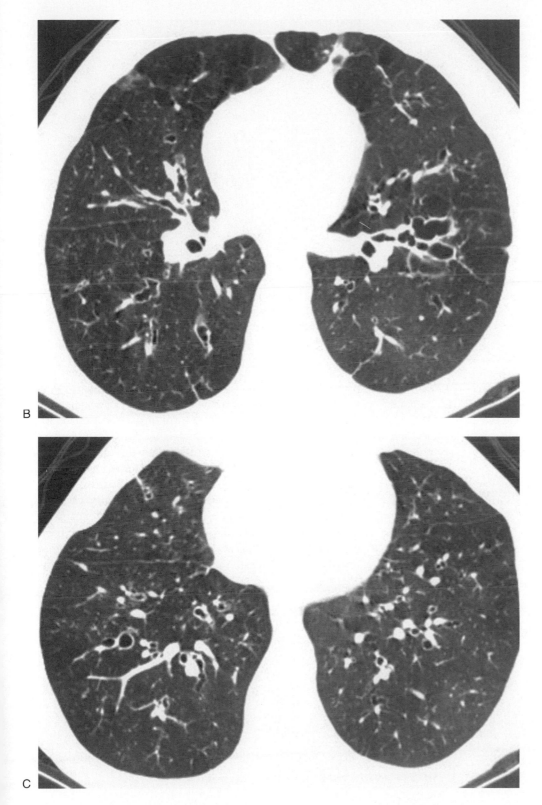

B

C

FIG. 8-38. *Continued*

occur in patients who have ABPA. As noted by Webb et al., disease involving the small airways is often present resulting in either a tree-in-bud appearance due to mucus-filled bronchioles or mosaic perfusion, and air-trapping due to bronchiolar obstruction (Figs. 8-11 and 8-39) [161].

The finding of aspergillomas in ectatic airways in patients who have ABPA has also been reported [170]. Additional parenchymal abnormalities, including consolidation, collapse, cavitation, and bullae, may be identified, especially in the upper lobes in as many as 43% of cases [169]. An identi-

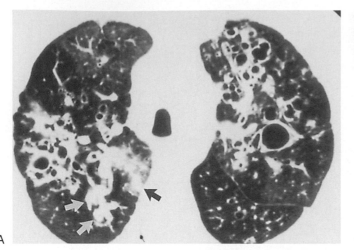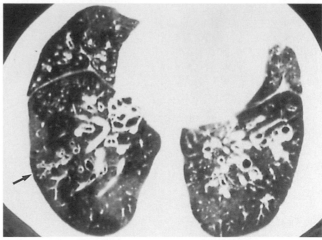

FIG. 8-39. Allergic bronchopulmonary aspergillosis with extensive bronchiectasis. **A:** HRCT scan through the upper lobes shows bilateral cystic bronchiectasis. mucous-plugged bronchi (*white arrows*) are visible and ill-defined foci of parenchymal consolidation are also present (*black arrow*). **B:** HRCT near the lung bases shows extensive bronchiectasis. In some regions, dilated bronchioles (*arrow*) are visible in the lung periphery. Lung attenuation is inhomogeneous as a result of mosaic perfusion.

cal percentage of cases also had evidence of pleural abnormalities, especially focal pleural thickening. Masslike foci of eosinophilic pneumonia may also be seen in ABPA patients who have acute exacerbations [171,172].

Of particular interest is the finding of high-attenuation mucoid impaction (Fig. 8-40) [173,174]. First described in association with chronic fungal sinusitis, high-density mucus presumably represents the presence of calcium ions, metallic ions, or both, within viscous mucus [175]. The prevalence of this finding has been noted to be as high as 28% in one series, and when present should be considered characteristic [174].

ABPA should be distinguished from both angioinvasive and airway-invasive aspergillosis [176]. These latter enti-

ties occur almost exclusively in severely immunosuppressed individuals—for example, after bone marrow or renal transplantation or in patients who have leukemia. By definition, the airway-invasive form of the disease is associated with the presence of organisms deep to the airway basement membrane. In distinction to the angioinvasive form of disease, airway-invasive aspergillosis may occur clinically even when the degree of immunosuppression is mild. Radiologically, airway-invasive aspergillosis most often manifests as patchy areas of parenchymal consolidation. On HRCT scans, the majority of patients have been reported to have a distinct peribronchial or peribronchiolar distribution of disease, ranging from patchy areas of con-

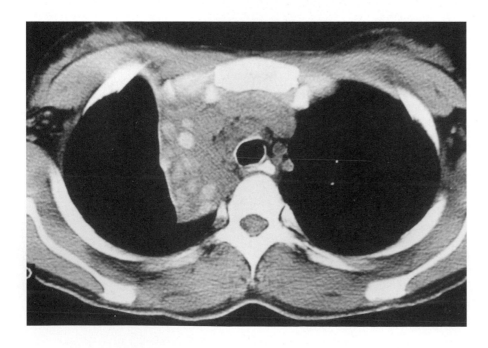

FIG. 8-40. Allergic bronchopulmonary aspergillosis (ABPA): high-density mucoid impaction. Noncontrast-enhanced CT section through the upper lung shows atelectasis of the right upper lobe. Within are numerous high-density foci representing dilated airways. This finding is characteristic of long-standing ABPA and presumably represents the presence of calcium, metallic, or both, types of ions within viscous mucus.

solidation to poorly defined centrilobular nodules [176]. In one study, sequential CT studies showed that airway-invasive aspergillosis resulted in bronchiectasis in cases without prior airway dilatation [176].

Utility of High-Resolution Computed Tomography

Although ABPA is classically associated with central bronchiectasis, this finding in itself is nonspecific and insensitive [67,132]. For example, Reiff et al. [67], in a study of 168 patients who had chronic sputum production [67], patients who had ABPA were significantly more likely than patients who had other diseases to have central bronchiectasis ($p < .005$), and bronchiectasis was more likely to be varicose or cylindrical morphologically ($p < .01$); however, the sensitivity of central bronchiectasis in this same study proved to only be 37% in diagnosing ABPA. Similarly, in a retrospective study of 82 consecutive patients who had bronchiectasis with known etiologies, Cartier et al. found that in only five (56%) of nine cases was a diagnosis of ABPA specifically suggested [101].

CT may be valuable in the early identification of lung damage in patients who have ABPA and thus help in planning treatment [164,165]. HRCT is more sensitive than plain radiographs in detecting abnormalities associated with ABPA [166]. In one study, narrow-section (3-mm) CT and plain chest radiography were compared in ten patients who had ABPA [164]. Bronchiectasis was reported in 31 of 60 lobes on CT scans but was visible in only 15 lobes on plain chest radiographs; CT was also more sensitive in detecting central bronchiectasis. In another study, CT with 8-mm collimation was compared to bronchography in two pediatric patients who had ABPA [165]; CT was able to identify 24 of 27 segments that showed central bronchiectasis.

As previously mentioned, whereas ABPA occurs exclusively in asthmatics, this diagnosis may be difficult to make in a general population of asthmatics on clinical grounds alone; many of the features of asthma and ABPA overlap. In addition to the finding of bronchiectasis, these include serum precipitins to *A. fumigatus* in up to 10% of asthmatics, a positive skin test to *Aspergillus* in up to 25% of asthmatics, and elevated IgE levels and eosinophilia. In a study by Neeld et al. [36], the HRCT findings in patients who had ABPA were compared to those in patients who had uncomplicated asthma. Bronchial dilatation was seen in 41% of lobes in the patients who had ABPA as compared to 15% of lobes in the patients who had asthma.

In the most extensive evaluation to date, Ward et al. retrospectively assessed the accuracy of CT in the diagnosis of ABPA in asthmatic patients [63]. Comparing the CT findings in 44 patients who had documented ABPA with 36 asthmatic controls, these authors noted a clear distinction in the frequency of a number of CT findings in patients who had ABPA, including the following: bronchiectasis in 95% of cases, versus 29% of asthmatics; centrilobular nodules in 93% of cases, versus 28% of asthmatics; and mucoid impac-

tion in 67% of cases, versus 4% of asthmatics. Furthermore, as noted by others, patients who had ABPA consistently had more severe and extensive disease compared with asthmatics, especially when present in three or more lobes [63]. It should be noted that the prevalence of bronchiectasis in this study far exceeds that reported in most other studies. In comparison to patients who have CF who often have diffuse cylindrical bronchiectasis, those with ABPA more typically show bronchiectasis that is cystic in appearance [140].

Tracheobronchomegaly

Also referred to as *Mounier-Kuhn syndrome*, the term *tracheobronchomegaly* is used to describe a heterogeneous group of patients who have marked dilatation of the trachea and mainstem bronchi, frequently in association with tracheal diverticulosis, recurrent lower respiratory tract infections, and bronchiectasis [177–179]. The etiology of this disorder is controversial. Findings in favor of a congenital etiology include histopathologic evidence of deficiency of tracheobronchial muscle fibers and absence of the myenteric plexus, as well as an association with other congenital or connective tissue disorders, including ankylosing spondylitis, Marfan's syndrome, CF, Ehlers-Danlos syndrome, and cutis laxa in children [180,181]. In distinction, findings in favor of an acquired etiology include the fact that tracheobronchomegaly most often is diagnosed in men in their third and fourth decades without an antecedent history of respiratory tract infection, often in association with chronic cigarette smoking [180,181]. An association between tracheomegaly and diffuse pulmonary fibrosis has also been reported, presumably the result of increased traction on the tracheal wall due to increased elastic recoil pressure in both lungs [180,181].

CT findings in patients who have tracheobronchomegaly have been described (Fig. 8-41) [182–184]. Using a tracheal diameter of greater than 3 cm and measured 2 cm above the aortic arch, and diameters of 2.4 and 2.3 cm for the right and left main bronchi, respectively, the diagnosis of tracheobronchomegaly is relatively straightforward [182]. Additional findings include tracheal scalloping, diverticulae, or both, diverticulae being especially common along the posterior tracheal wall. Also common is the finding of a marked tracheal flaccidity, identifiable as a marked decrease in the diameter of the trachea on expiration, even to the point of airway occlusion, indicative of tracheomalacia [10].

The importance of tracheomegaly lies in its association with distal airway inflammation. In a study of 75 consecutive patients referred for CT evaluation of possible bronchiectasis, Roditi and Weir [180] found that overall, 12% of their patients proved to have dilated tracheas, including seven (17%) of 42 patients who had CT evidence of bronchiectasis as well as three (6%) of 32 without. These data suggest that tracheomegaly may play a causative role in the development of bronchiectasis as a result of a predisposition to infection resulting from abnormal mucous clearance in patients who have inefficient cough and stagnant mucus.

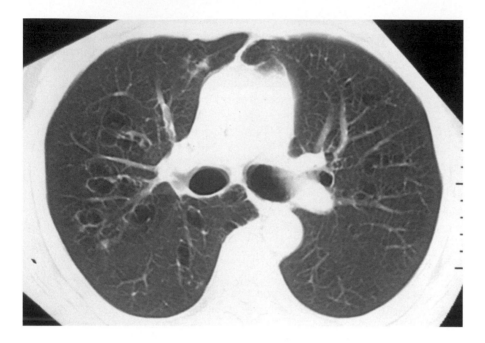

FIG. 8-41. Tracheobronchomegaly with bronchiectasis. Section through the carina shows massive enlargement of both the right and left main bronchi, associated with thin-walled cystic bronchiectasis bilaterally. Bronchiectasis frequently can be identified in patients with tracheobronchomegaly.

Williams-Campbell Syndrome

Williams-Campbell syndrome is a rare type of cystic bronchiectasis that is due to defective cartilage in the fourth- to sixth-order bronchi. HRCT can show areas of central cystic bronchiectasis with distal regions of abnormal lucency, probably related to air-trapping or bronchiolitis. These findings are useful in differentiating Williams-Campbell syndrome from other causes of cystic bronchiectasis (Fig. 8-42) [185]. Ballooning of central bronchi on inspiration and collapse on expiration have also been reported [186].

Alpha-1-Antitrypsin Deficiency

In addition to emphysema, bronchiectasis is also frequently identified in patients who have alpha-1-antitrypsin deficiency. King et al., in a study of 14 patients who had alpha-1-antitrypsin deficiency, found evidence of bronchiectasis in six (43%) [187]. This correlates well with the fact that approximately 50% of patients who have this deficiency manifest symptoms of airways disease, in particular chronic sputum production. Surprisingly, a frequent association between bronchiectasis and other forms of emphysema has not been well documented [187].

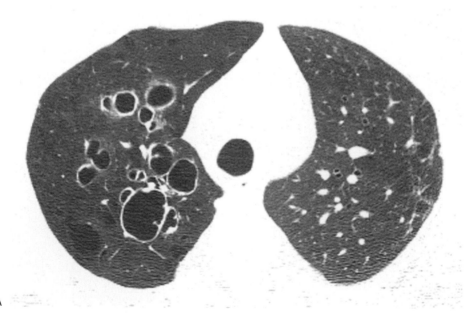

FIG. 8-42. A–C: Williams-Campbell syndrome with bronchiectasis in a patient who had left lung transplantation. Histologic evaluation of the resected lung revealed deficient cartilage in central bronchi. HRCT at three levels shows marked dilatation of bronchi within central lung regions. Peripheral lung appears lucent, particularly when compared to the normal left lung transplant. This lucency reflects air-trapping and mosaic perfusion. *Continued*

A

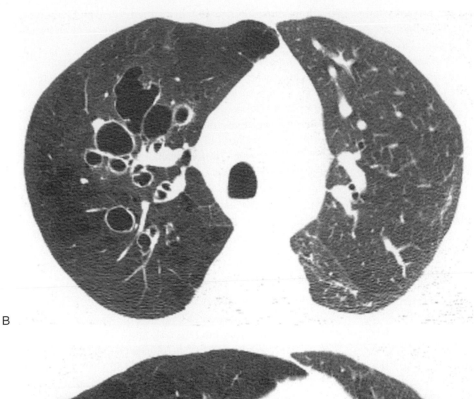

B

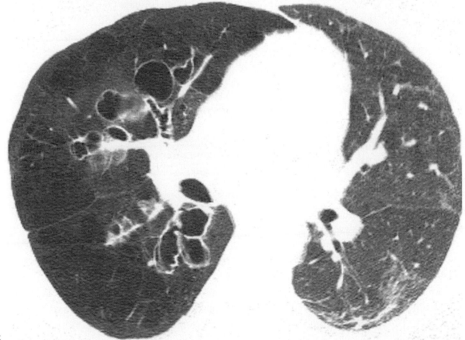

C

FIG. 8-42. *Continued*

Bronchiectasis Associated with Systemic Diseases

Bronchiectasis may be an important finding in a number of major systemic diseases. Of particular interest is the association between bronchiectasis and both rheumatologic diseases and inflammatory bowel disease.

Collagen-Vascular Disease

Rheumatoid arthritis (RA) may be associated with a variety of parenchymal abnormalities, including pulmonary fibrosis, bronchiolitis obliterans organizing pneumonia (BOOP), respiratory tract infections (including tuberculosis), and necrobiotic nodules. Airways disease, including both bronchiectasis and bronchiolectasis, is often overlooked as an association with RA [188]. Although airways disease was previously reported to occur in 5% to 10% of patients who have RA, since the introduction of HRCT, it has been estimated that bronchiectasis occurs in up to 35% of all patients who have this disease [189–192]. McDonagh et al., for example, in an evaluation of 20 patients who had clinical and radiologic evidence of RA, found that bronchiectasis could be identified in six patients, including two previously thought to have diffuse interstitial lung disease, on the basis of chest radiographs [190]. In this same study, bronchiectasis was also identified in four of 20 asymptomatic control patients who had documented RA and normal chest radiographs. In a study of 38 patients who had documented RA reported by Remy-Jardin et al., there was evidence of either bronchiectasis or bronchiolectasis in 23 (30%) including 8% of asymptomatic patients, with additional features suggestive of small airways disease in another six patients [189]. These findings included linear or branching centrilobular opacities, or both, believed by these authors to represent BO [189]. Whereas this included seven patients who had traction bronchiectasis in areas of honeycombing, in the remaining 16 patients bronchiectasis was seen in the absence of CT evidence of lung fibrosis.

More recently, it has been shown that in a select population of RA patients who have normal radiographs, the prevalence of airways disease may be considerably higher than previously thought. In a study of 50 RA patients who did not have radiographic evidence of lung disease, Perez et al. [192] reported findings of both direct and indirect bronchial and/or bronchiolar disease in 35 (70%), including air-trapping on expiratory scans in 32%, cylindrical bronchiectasis in 30%, mosaic attenuation on inspiratory scans in 20%, and centrilobular nodules in 6%. Importantly, HRCT depicted features of small airways disease in 20 of 33 patients who had normal pulmonary function tests.

It has long been observed that airway obstruction is especially common in patients who have RA [193], leading to speculation by some to a possible etiologic relationship between bronchiectasis and RA. It has been suggested, for example, that chronic bacterial infections may trigger an immune reaction in genetically predisposed individuals, leading to autoimmune disease [188]. In this regard, it has been observed that bronchiectasis may precede the development of RA by several decades. However, in distinction, it has also been suggested that steroid therapy or related treatment, especially with immunosuppressive therapy itself, may lead to an increased incidence of respiratory infections. It has also been suggested that the association between RA and bronchiectasis may reflect a shared genetic predisposition, although this remains controversial [191]. More recently, it has been suggested that airway obstruction in RA patients is only secondarily related to bronchiectasis and in fact primarily reflects the presence of BO [189,194].

Regardless of the precise role played by bronchiectasis in the etiology of RA, it has been shown that although there is no evidence to suggest that patients who have coexisting bronchiectasis have more severe RA, these individuals appear to have decreased survival. Swinson et al. [195], in a case-control study of the 5-year survival of 32 patients who had both RA and bronchiectasis matched for age, gender, and disease duration with 32 patients who had RA alone, and an additional 31 patients who had bronchiectasis alone, found that patients who had both RA and bronchiectasis were 7.3 times as likely to die than the general population,

five times more likely to die than patients who had RA alone, and 2.4 times more likely to die than patients who had bronchiectasis alone.

Similar to the unexpectedly high incidence of bronchiectasis in patients who have RA, it has been shown that bronchiectasis may be identified in up to 20% of patients who have systemic lupus erythematosus (SLE) [196]. Banker et al., in a prospective study of 45 patients who had documented SLE and normal radiographs, found abnormal CT findings in 38%, including bronchial wall thickening in 20% and bronchial dilatation in another 18% [197]; bronchiectasis has usually not been considered a manifestation of SLE [188]. A similarly unexpected high prevalence of airway pathology has also been noted in patients who have primary Sjögren's syndrome [198].

Ulcerative Colitis

A wide range of airway abnormalities has been identified in patients who have ulcerative colitis. In addition to BOOP and diffuse interstitial lung disease, these include subglottic stenosis, chronic bronchitis, and chronic suppurative inflammation of both large and small airways [188]. Similar to what is seen in patients who have RA, chronic suppurative airways disease may precede, coexist with, or follow, the development of inflammatory bowel disease. Of particular interest is the fact that, unlike other causes of bronchiectasis, chronic suppurative airways disease associated with ulcerative colitis frequently responds to treatment with inhaled steroids [188].

Human Immunodeficiency Virus– and Acquired Immunodeficiency Syndrome–Related Airways Disease

A number of reports have documented an increase in the prevalence of airway-related infections in HIV-positive/AIDS patients [31,34,199–202]. Paralleling a marked decrease in the incidence of PCP due to routine prophylaxis, lower respiratory tract infections, including bacterial pneumonia and bronchitis, have superseded PCP as the most common infections in the lungs of AIDS patients [203–205]. Wallace et al., for example, in a study of more than 1,000 HIV-positive patients who did not have an AIDS-defining illness, found a significantly higher incidence of acute bronchitis compared to HIV-negative subjects [205]. Most commonly, they result from organisms such as *Haemophilus influenzae*, *Pseudomonas aeruginosa*, *Streptococcus viridans*, or *Streptococcus pneumoniae*, and in fact a wide range of infectious agents has been described affecting the airways, including both mycobacterial and fungal infections [199].

First reported by Holmes et al. [201], and later confirmed by McGuinness et al. [31], an accelerated form of bronchiectasis appears to occur in HIV-positive patients. Although the etiology is unclear, it is likely that bronchiectasis results from recurrent bacterial infections affecting airways, possibly made more susceptible due to the

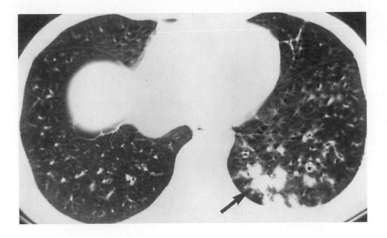

FIG. 8-43. Acquired immunodeficiency syndrome (AIDS)–associated bronchiectasis: 1.5-mm axial image in a 32-year-old AIDS patient who has productive cough and left lower lobe infiltrate. Evidence of focal rounded and tubular densities in the posteriobasilar segment of the left lower lobe (*arrow*) is consistent with mucoid impaction in the absence of parenchymal consolidation. At bronchoscopy, the bronchial mucosa was inflamed, and the lumen was packed with inflammatory material and hyphae, identified as *Aspergillus.*

direct effects of HIV infection on the pulmonary immune system. A correlation has also been shown between airway dilatation identified by CT and the presence of elevated levels of neutrophils on bronchoalveolar lavage (BAL). In a study comparing BAL findings in 50 HIV-positive subjects with 11 HIV-negative individuals, King et al. showed that patients who had bronchial dilatation on CT had significantly higher BAL neutrophil counts ($p = .014$) as well as significantly lower diffusing capacity ($p = .003$) [34]. As noted by these authors, neutrophils are an important mediator of pulmonary damage, possibly due to the action of human neutrophil elastase.

AIDS-related airways disease is manifested by a variety of HRCT abnormalities, a fact that reflects the number of organisms that may be involved. Findings include bronchial wall thickening, bronchiectasis, bronchial or bronchiolar impaction with tree-in-bud, endoluminal masses or nodules, and consolidation [199]. A lower lobe predominance is typical. The common finding of air-trapping in HIV-positive patients has also been stressed [206], suggesting that small airways disease may be a significant contributor to pulmonary function decline and may precede more obvious findings of airways disease. Gelman et al. [206] evaluated the HRCT scans of 59 subjects using inspiratory and expiratory HRCT, 48 of whom were HIV-positive and 11 of whom were HIV-negative. Expiratory CT revealed focal air-trapping in 33 subjects, 30 of whom were HIV-positive and three of whom were HIV-negative ($p = .0338$). The mean values of FEV_1, forced mid-expiratory flow, and diffusion capacity were significantly lower for subjects with focal air-trapping than for those with normal findings on CT ($p = .001$, $p = .021$, and $p = .003$, respectively).

It should also be noted that although less common than bacterial or viral infections, the airways may also be the site of fungal infections, especially due to *Aspergillus* (Fig. 8-43). Typically occurring late in the course of HIV infection, and usually in association with other risk factors, including corticosteroid use and granulocytopenia, approximately 10% of all reported cases of aspergillosis in AIDS patients will affect the airways [199]. Whereas several distinct subtypes of aspergillosis of the airways have been described, including

necrotizing acute tracheobronchitis, obstructing bronchial aspergillosis, and chronic cavitary parenchymal aspergillosis, it is likely that these represent a single spectrum of fungal disease potentially affecting the airways [207–209].

On one end of the spectrum is obstructing bronchial aspergillosis. Representing a stage before frank tissue invasion, obstructing bronchial aspergillosis typically presents acutely with fever, dyspnea, and progressive cough associated with the expectoration of fungal casts and is characterized on CT by the presence of mucoid impaction typically involving the lower lobe airways [209]. It has been suggested that this form of disease is unique to AIDS patients. Rarely, aspergillosis primarily affects the small airways again in the absence of bronchial inflammation. Described in only two patients who had AIDS, this form of infection has been termed *chronic cavitary parenchymal aspergillosis* and results in necrotic debris and fungi filling respiratory bronchioles with extension into adjacent alveolar spaces in the absence of bronchial invasion [210]. In distinction, necrotizing tracheobronchial aspergillosis (also referred to as *diffuse, ulcerative,* and *pseudomembranous tracheobronchitis*) is associated with frank tissue invasion resulting on CT in a range of abnormalities, from subtle focal irregularity and nodularity of airway walls to airway obstruction with or without accompanying parenchymal infiltrates.

BRONCHIOLITIS

Bronchiolitis is a nonspecific term used to describe inflammation of the small airways. Although a number of classifications have been proposed to encompass the wide spectrum of clinicopathologic conditions associated with bronchiolar inflammation, none has gained widespread acceptance [211]. At least partially, this is because there is all too frequently little correspondence between histologic findings and specific diseases. For example, patients who have RA may develop BO, BOOP, follicular bronchiolitis, or panbronchiolitis. Perhaps most confusing is the fact that even within the narrower confines of histologic and etiologic or clinical classifications, there is still little agreement concerning appropriate terminology.

TABLE 8-7. *Bronchiolar disease: pathologic classification*

Cellular bronchiolitis
Common
  Infectious bronchiolitis
  Hypersensitivity pneumonitis
Rare
  Follicular bronchiolitis
  Panbronchiolitis
Respiratory bronchiolitis
Common
  Respiratory bronchiolitis
  Respiratory bronchiolitis–interstitial lung disease
Rare
  Desquamative interstitial pneumonia
Constrictive bronchiolitis
Common
  Secondary (i.e., associated with infection, drugs, collagen-vascular disease, transplantation)
Rare
  Idiopathic
Bronchiolitis obliterans with intraluminal polyps
Common
  Idiopathic
  Secondary (i.e., associated with infection, drugs, collagen-vascular disease, transplantation)

Pathologic Classification of Bronchiolitis

Histologically, bronchiolitis may be classified in different ways, but several entities are consistently recognized by different authors [21,212]. These include *cellular bronchiolitis, respiratory bronchiolitis, constrictive bronchiolitis,* and *bronchiolitis obliterans with intraluminal polyps* (Table 8-7). In some classifications, respiratory bronchiolitis is classified with cellular bronchiolitis, and constrictive bronchiolitis and BO with intraluminal polyps are considered subtypes of BO.

Cellular Bronchiolitis

Included in the category of cellular bronchiolitis is a diverse set of diseases characterized in common by the presence of inflammatory cellular infiltrates involving both the bronchiolar lumen and wall and some degree of fibrosis. Further characterized as acute or chronic, and by the predominant cell type, this classification most commonly includes (i) infectious bronchiolitis (bacterial, viral, mycoplasma, and fungal), (ii) follicular bronchiolitis in collagen-vascular diseases, (iii) panbronchiolitis, (iv) aspiration bronchiolitis, (v) bronchiolitis associated with hypersensitivity pneumonitis, and (vi) asthma. Nonspecific cellular bronchiolitis is also frequently identified in patients who have bronchiectasis and chronic obstructive pulmonary disease.

Respiratory Bronchiolitis

Respiratory bronchiolitis is part of a spectrum of smoking-related diseases of the airways and lungs, characterized by the accumulation of pigmented macrophages within respiratory bronchioles and alveoli. This spectrum includes respiratory bronchiolitis (RB), respiratory bronchiolitis–interstitial lung disease (RB-ILD), and desquamative interstitial pneumonitis (DIP), also known as *alveolar macrophage pneumonia* [213–217]. Although RB is typically identified as an incidental finding in asymptomatic smokers, it has been recognized that some smokers present with both signs and symptoms of diffuse interstitial lung disease, so-called RB-ILD. Histologically, these patients are considered to have an exaggerated form of RB with evidence of inflammation and fibrosis away from respiratory bronchioles and into adjacent alveolar septa. In distinction, patients who have DIP have more diffuse involvement with a greater likelihood of developing parenchymal fibrosis and progressive lung disease. It has been suggested that RB, RB-ILD, and DIP be further classified as one of a larger group of smoking-related diseases, aptly termed *smoking-related interstitial lung diseases*, that also includes centrilobular emphysema and Langerhans cell histiocytosis [216]. Support for this classification stems from a possible association between respiratory bronchiolitis and the development of centrilobular emphysema [216,217].

Constrictive Bronchiolitis (Bronchiolitis Obliterans)

Constrictive bronchiolitis is defined histologically by the presence of concentric fibrosis predominantly between the bronchiolar epithelium and the muscularis mucosa, resulting in marked narrowing or obliteration of bronchioles, or both, in the absence of intraluminal granulation tissue polyps or surrounding parenchymal inflammation. Clinically, constrictive bronchiolitis is associated with marked airflow obstruction that usually is not responsive to steroid therapy [218,219]. Radiographically, little if any abnormality apart from hyperinflation is apparent. This pathologic entity is associated with the clinical syndrome often referred to as BO. It may result from a variety of diseases or conditions, described below in detail.

Bronchiolitis Obliterans with Intraluminal Polyps

BO with intraluminal polyps, also known as *BOOP* or *cryptogenic organizing pneumonia* (COP), is defined by the presence of granulation tissue polyps within respiratory bronchioles and alveolar ducts (Masson bodies) associated with patchy organizing pneumonia [220–222]. Because in the majority of cases the predominant histologic abnormality is the presence of organizing pneumonia, the terms *BOOP* and *COP* are usually used to describe this entity.

Two distinct patterns of intraluminal fibrosis or Masson bodies have been described [223]. Type 1 Masson bodies are

TABLE 8-8. *Bronchiolar disease: etiologic classification*

Common

Infection (bacteria, fungi, mycoplasma, viruses, parasites)

Smoking

Immunologic disease

Organ transplantation

Connective tissue disease

Hypersensitivity pneumonitis

Irradiation

Chronic aspiration

Rare

Inhalational disease (gases, fumes, dusts)

Drugs and chemicals, including *Sauropus androgynus* ingestion

Neuroendocrine cell hyperplasia

Wegener's granulomatosis

Ulcerative colitis

Acute and chronic eosinophilic pneumonia

those that show abundant myxoid matrix, sparse fibrosis, and little or no fibrin and presumably represent immature mesenchymal cells. In distinction, Type 2 Masson bodies contain fibrin and have histochemical properties of myofibroblasts. This distinction may be of importance, as in at least one study patients who had Type 1 disease showed good response to steroid therapy, whereas those who had Type 2 disease generally failed to respond to treatment [223].

Although the majority of cases of BOOP are idiopathic, similar findings may be seen in association with a variety of clinical conditions. As described by Katzenstein [219], BOOP may be classified into three separate categories. In the first, BOOP is the primary cause of respiratory illness. This includes idiopathic BOOP as well as BOOP resulting from RA, toxic inhalants, drug toxicity, and collagen-vascular diseases; prior infection, both viral and bacterial; and acute radiation pneumonitis [219,224]. In the second category are cases in which BOOP is found as a nonspecific reaction along the periphery of unrelated pathologic processes, including neoplasms, infectious granulomas, vasculitis, and even infarcts. Finally, BOOP may also be identified as a minor component of other diseases, including hypersensitivity pneumonitis, nonspecific interstitial pneumonitis, and Langerhans cell histiocytosis, among others [219]. It is for this reason that the finding of features consistent with BOOP on transbronchial biopsy is of only limited value in the absence of detailed clinical and radiologic correlation (Fig. 8-52 and 8-53) [219].

Reflecting not only the presence of intraluminal polyps, but also more extensive inflammatory changes involving alveolar ducts and alveoli, BOOP characteristically results in predominantly restrictive lung disease manifested radiographically as ill-defined areas of parenchymal consolidation [211,218,219,225]. BOOP is described in Chapter 6.

Clinical and Etiologic Classification of Bronchiolitis

It is also possible to classify bronchiolitis by known etiology or clinical association (Table 8-8). Etiologies of bronchiolitis include (i) diverse infections, including viruses, bacteria, mycoplasma, fungi, and parasites; (ii) inhalation of fumes, gases, and dusts, including cigarette smoke and asbestos; (iii) inhalation of organic material with hypersensitivity pneumonitis; (iv) exposure to a wide variety of drugs and chemicals (e.g., amiodarone, paraquat, and *Sauropus androgynus*); (v) a wide range of immunologic diseases, including connective tissue diseases; and (vi) as a complication of bone marrow, heart-lung, or lung transplantation. Bronchiolitis is also commonly identified in a number of miscellaneous conditions that affect the lung including vasculitides, eosinophilic lung syndromes, inflammatory bowel diseases, and chronic aspiration [226]. BO has also been described in patients who have neuroendocrine cell hyperplasia [227].

Computed Tomography Classification of Bronchiolitis

It is not an exaggeration to say that the introduction of HRCT has revolutionized our ability to diagnose small airways disease [3,18,19,27,85,88,89,161,228–237]. Reflecting the lack of reliable plain radiologic or physiologic methods for diagnosing small airways disease, bronchiolitis is uncommonly diagnosed or even suspected clinically. As a consequence, small airways pathology has usually required histologic confirmation. However, HRCT findings are frequently suggestive, if not diagnostic, of small airways disease. In our experience, CT findings are frequently the first indication of the presence of small airways pathology. Equally important, HRCT provides the most reliable assessment of both the extent and severity of disease, and provides a reliable, noninvasive method for assessing response to therapy without the need for repeated histologic evaluation.

Anatomic Considerations

Airways distal to those containing identifiable cartilage in their walls are termed *bronchioles*. Terminal bronchioles are the last purely conductive airways, varying in length from 0.8 to 2.5 mm, and are usually found between the sixth and twenty-third airway generations. Respiratory bronchioles lie distal to terminal bronchioles and are defined as airways in which the ciliated epithelial lining is interrupted by alveoli [148,238]. Along with alveolar ducts and sacs, respiratory bronchioles comprise the gas-exchanging unit of the lung. A number of different cell types can be identified in normal bronchioles. These include special columnar secretory stem cells, known as *Clara cells*, as well as neuroendocrine or Kulchitsky cells. In distinction, mucus-secreting goblet cells and bronchus-associated lymphoid tissue are only rarely identified in nonsmokers.

Along with their accompanying pulmonary artery branches, bronchioles lie within the center of secondary pulmonary lobules. Normally, individual airways can only be identified when their walls are larger than 300 microns, corresponding to bronchi between 1.5 and 2 mm in size. As a consequence, normal bronchioles with luminal diameters of approximately 0.6 mm cannot be identified on HRCT.

Although the term *small airways disease* is usually used synonymously with bronchiolar disease, this term as originally defined was used to describe inflammatory changes in peripheral airways in smokers resulting in moderate to severe airflow obstruction [239]. Subsequently defined by Macklem and colleagues [240] to indicate an idiopathic syndrome of chronic airflow obstruction in patients having no evidence of underlying emphysema or chronic bronchitis, this concept of small airways disease is essentially physiologic and is associated with abnormalities involving airways between 2 and 3 mm in diameter. The distinction between anatomic and physiologic definitions is significant, as small airways contribute only approximately 10% of total airway resistance. As a consequence, numerous small airways can be damaged before conventional measurements of lung function, in particular measurements of airway resistance, become abnormal.

Although normal intralobular bronchioles cannot usually be identified, direct and indirect signs of bronchiolar disease have been described [18,19,161]. Direct signs result from the presence of bronchiolar secretions, peribronchiolar inflammation, or, less commonly, bronchiolar wall thickening. Characteristically, these result in either branching or Y-shaped linear densities (Figs. 8-17 and 8-44), or poorly defined centrilobular nodules (Fig. 8-45). Less commonly, bronchiolar inflammation results in the finding of small centrilobular lucencies due to bronchiolectasis [3,70,85,89].

Indirect signs have also been described, the most important of which are the findings of mosaic perfusion on inspiratory scans and areas of lucency and air-trapping, either focal or global, on scans obtained at end expiration [116,161,241,242].

Using a combination of HRCT findings, it is possible to classify bronchiolitis into one of four basic HRCT patterns based on the predominant abnormality (Table 8-9). These include (i) bronchiolar diseases associated with a tree-in-bud appearance, (ii) bronchiolar diseases associated with poorly-defined centrilobular opacities, (iii) bronchiolar diseases associated with areas of decreased lung attenuation, and (iv) bronchiolar diseases associated with focal or diffuse ground-glass opacity, consolidation, or both. Use of this classification in conjunction with clinical findings frequently allows precise diagnoses even in the absence of histologic correlation.

Bronchiolar Diseases Associated with a Tree-in-Bud Pattern

The hallmark of this group of diseases is the finding of dilated, mucus-filled bronchioles resulting in a pattern of centrilobular nodular, branching, or Y-shaped densities that has been aptly referred to as simulating a TIB appearance or the children's toy jacks (Figs. 8-17, 8-31, 8-32, 8-44, and 8-46 through 8-48) [84–86]. A TIB appearance is most typ-ical of cellular bronchiolitis. In our experience this appearance is almost always the result of acute or chronic infection (Table 8-9). The differential diagnosis of TIB is discussed in greater detail in Chapter 3.

Aquino et al. [84] found that a TIB pattern could be identified on HRCT in 25% of patients who had bronchiectasis (including patients who had CF and ABPA) and 17% of patients who had acute infectious bronchitis or pneumonia. On the other hand, this pattern was not identified in any of 141 HRCT studies in patients who had noninfectious airways diseases, including emphysema, RB, constrictive bronchiolitis, BOOP, and hypersensitivity pneumonitis, among others.

Infectious Bronchiolitis

The finding of a TIB pattern is nearly always due to acute infectious bronchiolitis, regardless of the underlying disease (Figs. 8-17 and 8-47A). As documented by Im et al. [27], in patients who had tuberculosis, the TIB pattern correlates pathologically with the presence of secretions within dilated terminal and respiratory bronchioles (Fig. 8-44). These are characteristically centrilobular in distribution and are most easily identified in the lung periphery. Ill-defined buds associated with the branching airway reflect the presence of peribronchiolar granulomas, a finding especially common in patients who have chronic infection due to MAC (Fig. 8-30) [84] or peribronchiolar inflammation. Poorly defined centrilobular nodules or rosettes of nodules are almost always visible in patients who have TIB; these may be seen if images show distended centrilobular bronchioles in cross section. In our experience, however, these are always ancillary to the main finding of linear or branching densities. Additional findings include areas of ground-glass opacity, consolidation, or both. With healing, a distinctive pattern of branching or V-shaped densities associated with secondary lobular emphysema may be identified, presumably the result of bronchial, bronchiolar, or both types of obstruction.

Infectious bronchiolitis is usually reversible and is most often caused by *Mycoplasma pneumoniae*, *Haemophilus influenzae*, and *Chlamydia* species and viral infections, especially respiratory syncytial virus. Infectious bronchiolitis is common in infants and children and is being increasingly diagnosed in adults, especially those who have atypical mycobacterial infections or other causes of chronic airways disease [28,29], AIDS [34,199], or a combination of both. Although histologic examination typically shows necrosis of respiratory epithelium with a mixed cellular infiltrate usually in association with accompanying pneumonitis, it is, in fact, rarely necessary to obtain biopsies in these patients. In our experience, HRCT findings in conjunction with clinical findings are usually sufficient to allow presumptive therapy with antibiotics, pending the results of sputum culture.

It should be emphasized that an appearance similar to that of TIB has also been reported in association with noninfectious etiologies. Numerous reports, for example, have documented linear or branching centrilobular densities in patients

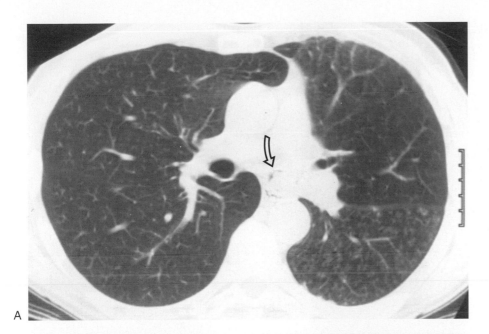

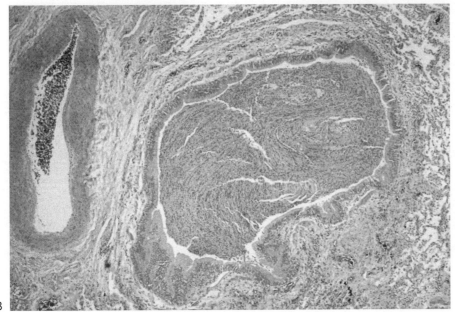

FIG. 8-44. Infectious bronchiolitis: *Chlamydia* pneumonia. **A:** A 5-mm section through the middle lung shows a central endobronchial lesion partially obstructing the distal left main stem bronchus (*open arrow*). Throughout the superior segment of the left lower lobe are ill-defined nodules clustered around peripheral vessels, an appearance aptly described as resembling tree-in-bud. These fail to reach the pleural surface, a finding characteristic of centrilobular, as opposed to perilymphatic, distribution. Centrilobular nodules with a tree-in-bud appearance are diagnostic of infectious bronchiolitis, in this case resulting from a central carcinoid tumor. **B:** Histologic section obtained in **A** after lobectomy shows inspissated infected secretions within bronchioles.

who had RA or Sjögren's syndrome [189,192,198,243]. Although usually attributed to either follicular bronchiolitis [244–246] or BO, many of the patients have coexisting productive cough and other clinical signs indicative of possible infection. In this regard, Hayakawa et al. correlated HRCT findings with histologic findings identified on open lung biopsy in 14 RA patients who had documented bronchiolitis [247]. Whereas linear or branching centrilobular nodules could be identified in five of seven patients who had follicular bronchiolitis and three of seven who had BO, as noted by the authors, 73% of patients had chronic sinusitis, and 93% of patients had chronic cough with sputum. Furthermore, bacterial cultures were positive in 50% and 71% of patients who had follicular bronchiolitis and BO, respectively.

Panbronchiolitis

In Asia, especially in Japan, a form of diffuse panbronchiolitis termed *DPB* is common (Figs. 8-63 and 8-65) [89]. DPB has been defined as a clinicopathologic entity, characterized by symptoms of chronic cough, sputum, and dyspnea; associated with abnormal PFTs, usually indicating mild to moderate airway obstruction and radiographic evidence of ill-defined nodular infiltrates typically basilar in distribution [248]. Histologically, DPB is characterized by chronic inflammation with mononuclear cell proliferation and foamy macrophages predominantly involving the walls of respiratory bronchioles, adjacent alveolar ducts, and alveoli, constituting the so-called unit lesion of panbronchiolitis [248]. Inclusion of this entity in the

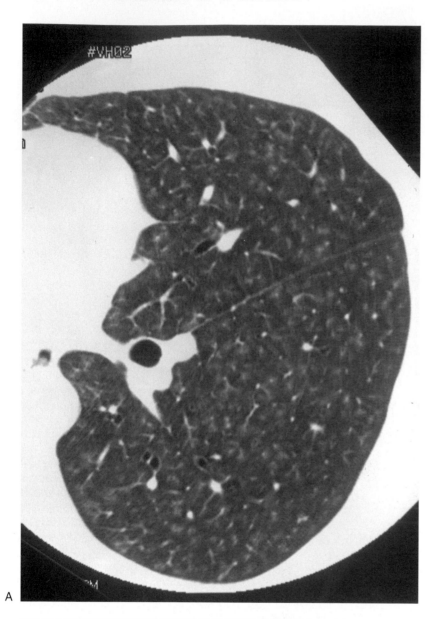

A

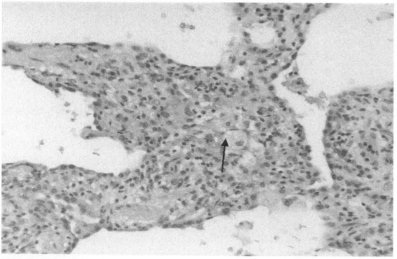

B

FIG. 8-45. Centrilobular nodules—hypersensitivity pneumonitis. **A:** Target-reconstructed HRCT image through the left middle lung shows typical appearance of centrilobular nodules. Although some of these seem to branch, the vast majority is best described as poorly defined ground-glass opacity nodules without evidence of branching. Diffuse distribution is characteristic of subacute hypersensitivity pneumonitis. **B:** Open lung biopsy in a different patient than in **A** also with hypersensitivity pneumonitis shows foam cells in the interstitium (*arrow*). *Continued*

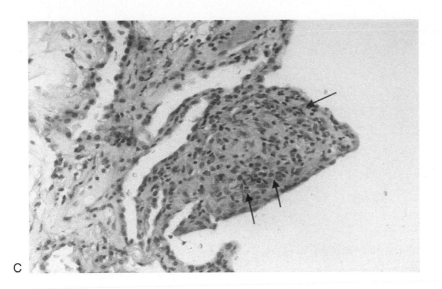

C

FIG. 8-45. *Continued* **C:** Different section from the same patient as **B** shows an ill-defined, noncaseating granuloma (*arrows*). These histologic features are characteristic of hypersensitivity pneumonitis.

category of infectious etiologies of bronchiolitis is justified, as nearly all patients develop superinfection with *Pseudomonas*. On HRCT, a characteristic diffuse TIB pattern is invariably seen, predominantly affecting the lung bases, that has been shown to disappear after treatment with erythromycin (Fig. 8-64) [249]. Despite initial improvement, DPB is usually considered a progressive disease, with 5- and 10-year survival rates reported to be in the range of 60% and 30%, respectively [248]. DPB is described in further detail below.

Bronchiolar Diseases Associated with Poorly Defined Centrilobular Nodules

The hallmark of this group of diseases is the finding of ill-defined centrilobular nodules without associated TIB or branching densities (Table 8-9). As indicated by Gruden et al. [85,86], although the finding of ill-defined centrilobular nodules in patients who have bronchiolar disease usually results from peribronchiolar inflammation or fibrosis, in the absence of airway impaction with secretions, a similar CT appearance may also be the result of perilymphatic or perivascular disease. Not surprisingly, this pattern is associated with a wide range of pathologic entities (see Chapter 3). Diseases associated with primarily peribronchiolar abnormalities include RB and RB-ILD, hypersensitivity pneumonitis, follicular bronchiolitis, pneumoconioses (e.g., asbestosis, silicosis, and coal worker's pneumoconiosis), Langerhans cell histiocytosis, and, rarely, BOOP.

Despite the large number of diseases included in this category, in most cases, differential diagnosis is simplified by detailed clinical correlation, including careful occupational and environmental exposure histories. A few entities are sufficiently characteristic to warrant special attention.

Respiratory Bronchiolitis

RB is a smoking-related disease of the airways and lungs characterized by the accumulation of pigmented macrophages within respiratory bronchioles and alveoli [213–216]. RB is typ-

ically identified as an incidental finding in asymptomatic smokers; if symptoms are associated, this disease is termed *RB-ILD*.

HRCT findings in RB and RB-ILD have been described, and are discussed in detail in Chapter 6 (Fig. 8-49). In most patients who have documented RB, the lungs appear either normal or show evidence of poorly defined, predominantly middle and upper lobe centrilobular ground-glass opacities, with or without accompanying areas of diffuse ground-glass opacity [235]. Findings in the few reported series published to date in patients who had RB-ILD have proven more variable. First reported in five patients by Holt et al., findings ranged from normal lungs to either ill-defined centrilobular and/or diffuse ground-glass opacity, or bibasilar areas of atelectasis and/or scarring [250]. In another study of eight patients evaluated by HRCT reported by Moon et al., five of the eight had evidence of both areas of ground-glass opacity and mild reticulation, whereas one case showed evidence of only diffuse ground-glass opacity. In all, six cases were interpreted as consistent with either RB-ILD or DIP. Interestingly, in two cases there was also evidence of diffuse centrilobular emphysema [216].

Hypersensitivity Pneumonitis

Hypersensitivity pneumonitis is associated with a chronic, nonspecific, predominantly interstitial lymphocytic pneumonitis that early in its course is primarily distributed around respiratory bronchioles with relative sparing of intervening lung [219]. This pattern may persist even later in the course of disease. Additionally, in nearly two-thirds of cases, there is also evidence of nonnecrotizing granulomas, again typically localized to the peribronchiolar interstitium. Foci of BOOP may also be identified in some cases, with characteristic findings of intraluminal fibrous plugs.

Together, these findings result in a pattern of diffuse, poorly defined centrilobular nodular opacities, especially in the subacute phase of disease (Figs. 8-45 and 8-50) [251–257]. These nodules are typically uniform in distribution. On occasion, their proliferation is so widespread as to result in diffuse ground-glass opacity. Close inspection, however, invariably discloses

TABLE 8-9. *Bronchiolar disease: HRCT classification by predominant abnormality*

Bronchiolar diseases with tree-in-bud pattern

Common

  Mycobacterium tuberculosis

  Atypical mycobacterial infections (*Mycobacterium avium* complex)

  Bacterial infections [e.g., cystic fibrosis; HIV(+)/acquired immunodeficiency syndrome (AIDS) patients]

Uncommon

  Viral and fungal infections, (e.g., cytomegalovirus, *Pneumocystis carinii* pneumonia)

  Asiatic panbronchiolitis

  Collagen-vascular diseases (follicular bronchiolitis or infection)

  Asthma

  Allergic bronchopulmonary aspergillosis

Bronchiolar diseases with poorly defined centrilobular nodules

Common

  Subacute hypersensitivity pneumonitis

  Respiratory bronchiolitis with interstitial lung disease

Uncommon

  Lymphocytic interstitial pneumonitis in AIDS patients

  Follicular bronchiolitis

  Mineral dust–induced bronchiolitis

  Collagen-vascular diseases

  Sarcoidosis

Bronchiolar disease associated with decreased lung attenuation

Common

  Constrictive bronchiolitis after lung and/or bone marrow transplantation

  Postinfectious (e.g., Swyer-James syndrome)

  Toxic fume inhalation (e.g., smoke inhalation)

Uncommon

  Idiopathic

  Associated with collagen-vascular diseases

  Consumption of *Sauropus androgynus*

  Constrictive bronchiolitis associated with neuroendocrine hyperplasia

  Sarcoidosis

Bronchiolar disease associated with ground-glass opacity and/or consolidation

Common

  Idiopathic bronchiolitis obliterans organizing pneumonia (BOOP)

  BOOP associated with toxic fume inhalation

  Collagen-vascular diseases

  Prior infection

  Radiation therapy

Uncommon

  BOOP associated with unrelated pathologic processes (e.g., neoplasm, infectious granulomas, and vasculitides)

  BOOP as a component of other diseases (e.g., hypersensitivity pneumonitis, Langerhans cell histiocytosis)

Adapted from Müller NL, Miller RR. Diseases of the bronchioles: CT and histopathologic findings. *Radiology* 1995;196:3.

the presence of innumerable centrilobular ground-glass nodules accounting for this appearance. Findings in hypersensitivity pneumonitis are described in greater detail in Chapter 6.

Another feature described in these patients is the finding of focal air-trapping, frequently restricted to secondary pulmonary lobules. Whereas this may be the result of inhomogeneous distribution of inhaled causative agents resulting in sparing of individual pulmonary lobules, it has alternatively been speculated that air-trapping may represent associated obliterative bronchiolitis [117,257].

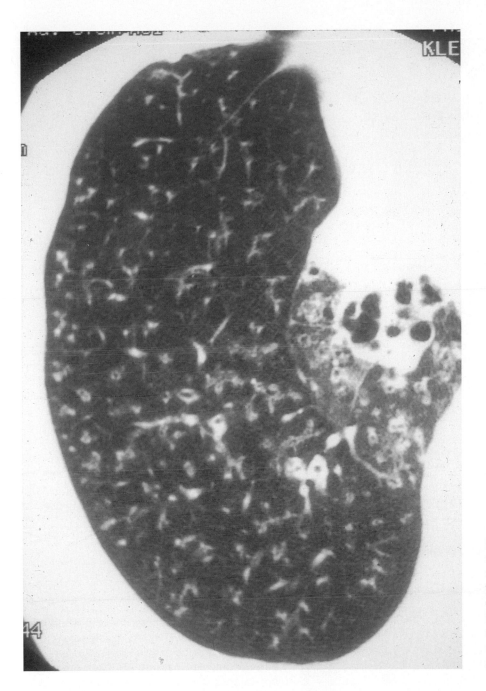

FIG. 8-46. Infectious bronchiolitis. Target-reconstructed HRCT section through the right lower lobe shows innumerable centrilobular linear and branching structures consistent with the clinical diagnosis of infection. Note that these densities do not extend to the pleural surface. Follow-up confirmed complete resolution after antibiotic therapy.

Follicular Bronchiolitis

Follicular bronchiolitis represents nonspecific lymphoid hyperplasia of the bronchus-associated lymphoid tissue. Histologically, follicular bronchiolitis is characterized by the finding of hyperplastic lymphoid follicles with reactive germinal centers, typically characteristically distributed along bronchioles, and, to a lesser extent, bronchi. Extension into the lung interstitium with resulting pulmonary infiltrates is generally not considered a feature of follicular bronchiolitis [258]. Most cases are associated with underlying disorders, most often collagen-vascular diseases, in particular RA [189,245,247] and Sjögren's syndrome, immunodeficiency disorders, and hypersensitivity reactions [259]. In children, the disease typically occurs in the first 6 to 8 weeks of life, results in respiratory distress and fever, and is usually unresponsive to either bronchodilator therapy or steroids [258].

CT findings in adult patients who have follicular bronchiolitis have been described in a few small series [189,244,260]. Cardinal features include bilateral centrilobular, peribronchial, or both types of ground-glass opacity nodules measuring 3 to 12 mm in diameter, corresponding histologically with bronchial and peribronchial lymphoid infiltration (see Fig. 5-14). Areas of ground-glass opacity may also be identified, but never in isolation. In the majority of cases, although characteristic, definitive diagnosis requires histologic confirmation. Interestingly, CT findings in one report of individuals with RA and documented follic-

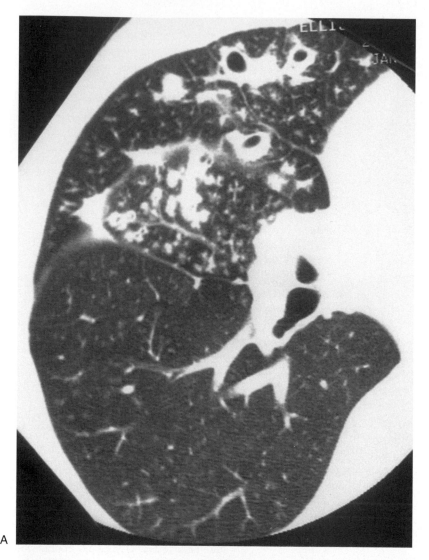

A

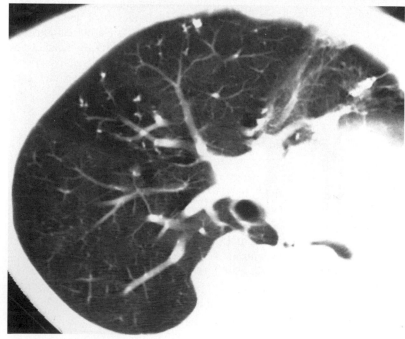

B

FIG. 8-47. Infectious bronchiolitis: endobronchial tuberculosis (TB). **A:** Enlargement of a section through the middle lobe in a patient who has documented cavitary TB. Note the typical appearance of a tree-in-bud pattern, resulting from endobronchial spread of TB. **B:** A 1-mm section through the right middle lung in a patient who has long-standing chronic TB, resulting in complete atelectasis of the left lung. Small, well-defined nodules are identified adjacent to peripheral branching vessels, around which a distinct zone of hyperlucency can be identified. This appearance correlates with healed endobronchial spread of TB with focal emphysema resulting from prior bronchial and bronchiolar obstruction. (Reprinted from Naidich DP, Webb WR, Müller NL, et al. *Computed tomography and magnetic resonance imaging of the thorax*, 3rd ed. Philadelphia: Lippincott-Raven, 1999.)

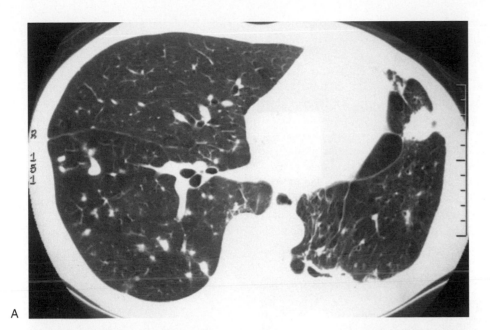

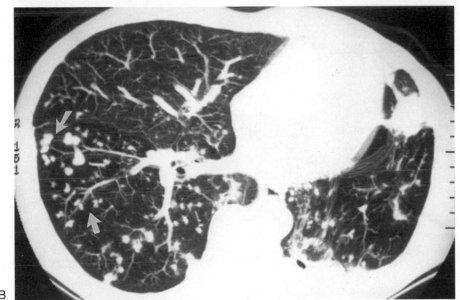

FIG. 8-48. Infectious bronchiolitis: use of maximum-intensity projection images. **A:** A 1-mm axial image through the lower chest shows well-defined nodular densities in the right lower lobe associated with mosaic attenuation. This appearance is nonspecific. Architectural distortion is apparent in the left base. **B:** Corresponding maximum intensity projection image using five contiguous 1-mm sections shows to better advantage that the nodules in the right lower lobe have a tree-in-bud configuration characteristic of infectious bronchiolitis (*arrows*, **B**).

ular bronchiolitis showed that in all cases in which both branching and poorly defined centrilobular nodules were evident, the disease was either stabilized or reversed after treatment with erythromycin, reinforcing the notion that a TIB pattern likely reflects underlying infection [247].

Similar CT findings have been identified in patients who have lymphocytic interstitial pneumonitis (LIP), especially in HIV-positive and AIDS patients (Fig. 8-51) [33]. Characterized by an interstitial infiltrate of mature lymphocytes, LIP is part of the spectrum of hyperplasia of bronchus-associated lymphoid tissue that also includes follicular bronchiolitis. Although characterized by more diffuse interstitial involvement, histologic differentiation between follicular bronchiolitis and LIP may be difficult, raising the possibility that the poorly defined centrilobular nodules identified on CT in most cases of LIP diagnosed by transbronchial biopsy actually represent follicular bronchiolitis.

Bronchiolitis Obliterans Organizing Pneumonia

BOOP is characterized histologically by the presence of granulation tissue polyps within respiratory bronchioles and alveolar ducts associated with patchy organizing pneumonia [220–222]. Ill-defined centrilobular nodules reflecting bronchiolitis and focal organizing pneumonia may be seen. BOOP more often results in patchy consolidation.

Bronchiolar Diseases Associated with Decreased Lung Attenuation

In this category are patients who have BO (i.e., constrictive bronchiolitis or obliterative bronchiolitis). BO is defined histologically by the presence of concentric fibrosis involving the submucosal and peribronchial tissues of terminal and respiratory bronchioles exclusively, with resulting bronchial narrowing or obliteration (Fig. 8-54F). This process is typically nonuniform and, as the surrounding parenchyma is normal, may be difficult to identify even on open lung biopsy. Clinically, whereas these patients may be relatively asymptomatic, in most cases there is progressive airways obstruction, resulting in severe respiratory compromise that is usually unresponsive to steroid therapy.

Conditions associated with constrictive bronchiolitis include heart-lung or lung transplantations, chronic allograft rejection, allogeneic bone marrow transplantation with chronic graft-versus-host disease, and collagen-vascular diseases, especially RA [211]. Also known as the *Swyer-James syndrome*, BO frequently occurs as the sequela of childhood respiratory tract infections, most often viral [261]; similar findings may also be seen in children after infection with mycoplasma. Constrictive bronchiolitis is only rarely idiopathic. Obliterative bronchiolitis has also been linked to consumption of *S. androgynus* [242,262], a small, lowland shrub found in Asia consumed in the form of an uncooked juice as a means of weight reduction, especially in Taiwan. An HRCT pattern of mosaic perfusion has also been reported in association with neuroendocrine hyperplasia in patients who had carcinoid tumorlets [227,263].

BO is characterized by patchy areas of decreased attenuation due to mosaic perfusion and air-trapping on expiratory scans. Ancillary findings include bronchial wall thickening, bronchiectasis, atelectasis, and mucous plugging. The HRCT appearance of BO is described in detail below.

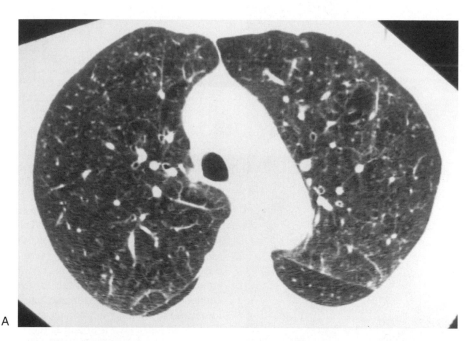

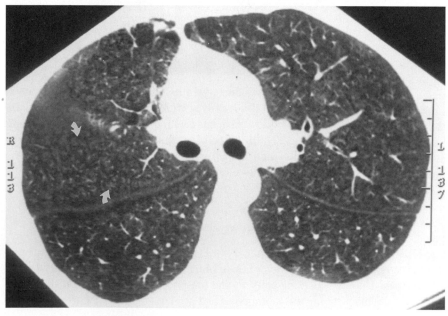

FIG. 8-49. Respiratory bronchiolitis-interstitial lung disease (RB-ILD). **A–C:** Sections through the upper, middle, and lower lungs show diffuse centrilobular ground-glass opacity nodules without evidence of significant bronchial dilatation (*arrows*, **B**). Mild bronchial wall thickening is identified in the lower lobes, accentuated by the use of narrow windows to target centrilobular changes. Note the absence of reticular densities, architectural distortion, or tubular or branching structures. This appearance is consistent with the diagnosis of RB-ILD in a known cigarette smoker with mildly obstructive pulmonary function test results. *Continued*

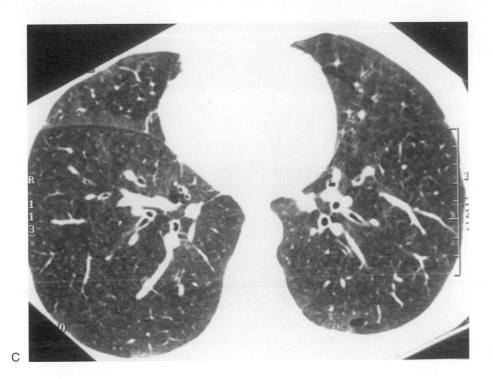

C

FIG. 8-49. *Continued*

Bronchiolar Diseases Associated with Focal Ground-Glass Opacity, Consolidation, or Both

This pattern of presentation is characteristic of BOOP [211,218]. BOOP is characterized histologically by the presence of granulation tissue polyps within respiratory bronchioles and alveolar ducts (Masson bodies) associated with patchy organizing pneumonia [220–222].

Clinically, patients who have idiopathic BOOP usually present with a 1- to 3-month history of nonproductive cough, low-grade fever, and increasing shortness of breath [220–222,264,265]. A variety of radiographic patterns have been described [266]. Most often radiographs show patchy, nonsegmental, unilateral, or bilateral foci of airspace consolidation [221,222,264,265]; however, in a smaller number of cases, focal nodules as well as irregular, predominantly basilar reticular densities have been described. Honeycombing is rare. Whereas the majority of patients who have ill-defined areas of patchy airspace consolidation respond to treatment with corticosteroids, the response in patients who have interstitial infiltrates has been noted to be worse [266].

Several studies have reviewed the CT and HRCT findings in patients who have BOOP; these are described in detail in Chapter 6 (see Figs. 3-76 and 3-77; Fig. 8-52 and 8-53)

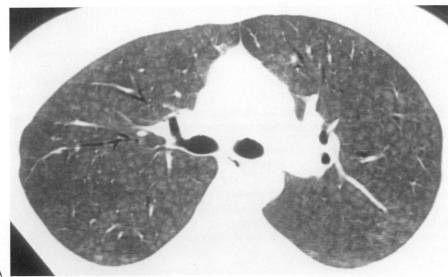

A

FIG. 8-50. A,B: Sections through the carina and lower lobes, respectively, show innumerable ill-defined centrilobular ground-glass opacity nodules, characteristic of subacute hypersensitivity pneumonitis. Note the absence of linear or branching structures, suggestive of infectious bronchiolitis. There is evidence of mild and probably physiologic airway dilatation. Note that there are also foci of relative sparing associated with air-trapping (*arrows*, **B**), likely due to inhomogeneous distribution of inhaled agents. *Continued*

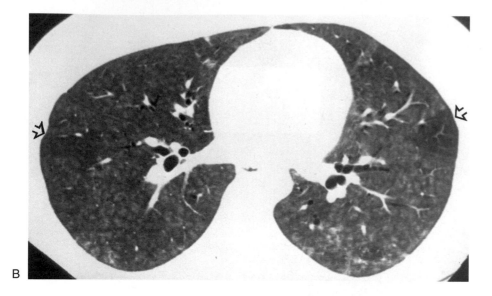

B

FIG. 8-50. *Continued*

[229,267,268]. The most common abnormality consists of patchy bilateral consolidation, seen in approximately 80% of cases, which frequently has a predominantly peribronchial and subpleural distribution (Figs. 8-52 and 8-53). Bronchial wall thickening and dilatation are commonly present in the areas with consolidation. Although small (1- to 10-mm), ill-defined, predominately peribronchial or peribronchiolar nodules are seen in 30% to 50% of cases, the finding of a TIB pattern is distinctly unusual [3,84].

Areas of ground-glass opacity may be seen in up to 60% of immunocompetent patients who have BOOP, but they are seldom the predominant abnormality in these patients. These are seen more commonly in immunocompromised patients who have BOOP and may be the predominant or only abnormality seen in these patients [267]. Small nodules are also seen more commonly in immunocompromised patients; nodules 1 to 10 mm in diameter were observed in 6 of 11 (55%) immunocompromised patients as compared to seven of 32 (22%) immunocompetent patients who had idiopathic BOOP reported by Lee et al. [267].

In a minority of cases, BOOP may present as multiple, large (1- to 5-cm) nodules or masses. In a report by Akira

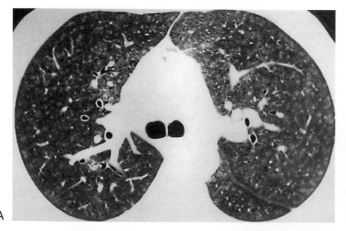

A

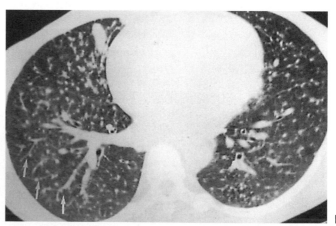

B

FIG. 8-51. Lymphoproliferative disorders in acquired immunodeficiency syndrome (AIDS). **A:** A 44-year-old mildly dyspneic woman with AIDS contracted from a blood transfusion. Her CD$_4$ cell count was 123 cells per mm^3. A 1.5-mm section shows innumerable centrilobular nodules 2 to 4 mm in diameter. These nodules are poorly marginated and of a hazy, ground-glass attenuation. At biopsy, poorly formed granulomas secondary to lymphocytic interstitial pneumonitis were identified. **B:** Denser nodules in the same size range are seen on the 1.5-mm sections in a 36-year-old man who has atypical lymphoproliferative disorder. Nodules are identified throughout the interstitium; the peribronchovascular distribution results in nodular vascular margins (*arrows*).

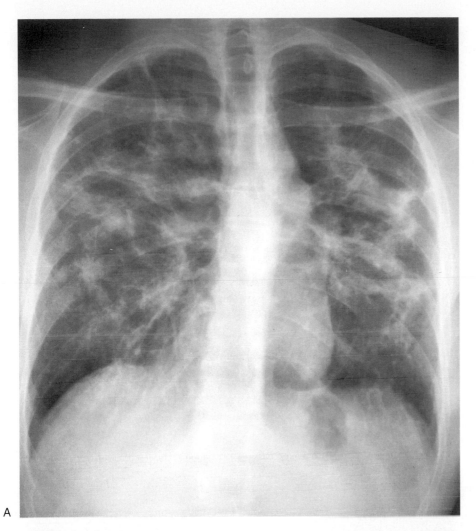

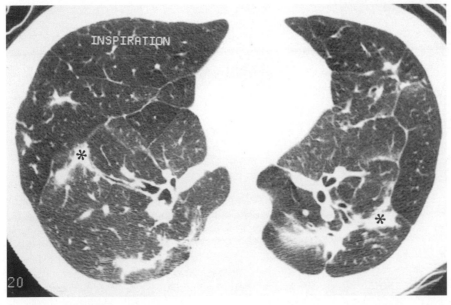

FIG. 8-52. Bronchiolitis obliterans organizing pneumonia (BOOP). **A:** Pulmonary artery radiograph shows bilateral, patchy, and poorly defined areas of parenchymal consolidation. **B,C:** Sections through the lung bases on inspiration and expiration, respectively, show evidence of bilateral, slightly nodular areas of parenchymal consolidation with a distinctly lower lobe and peribronchovascular distribution (*asterisks*, **B,C**). In addition, there is evidence of air-trapping most pronounced in the middle lobe on expiration. This combination of findings is nonspecific: differential diagnosis includes, among others, chronic eosinophilic pneumonia. Open lung biopsy confirmed the diagnosis of idiopathic BOOP. *Continued*

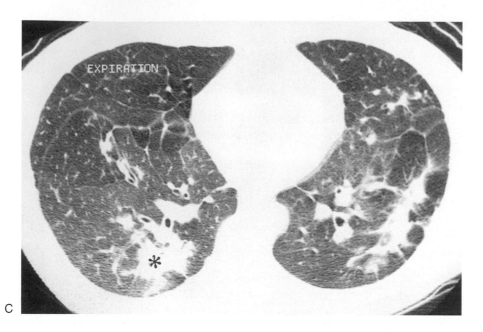

C

FIG. 8-52. *Continued*

et al. [269], 12 of 50 (20%) patients who had BOOP presented with multiple nodules or masses as the predominant finding. Of a total of 60 lesions, 88% proved to have irregular margins, 45% were associated with air bronchograms, and 38% had pleural tags. The finding of an irregular mass-like area of consolidation adjacent to pleural surfaces, in particular, proved suggestive. Similar findings have been reported by Bouchardy et al., who also found nodular or masslike opacities to be a frequent finding, occurring in 5 of 12 (42%) patients [229].

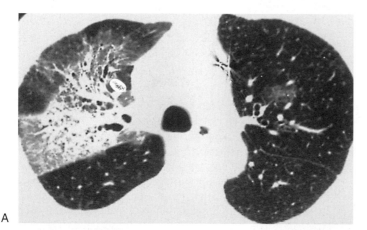

A

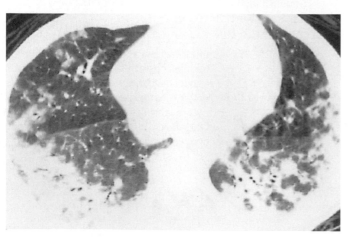

B

FIG. 8-53. **A:** Bronchiolitis obliterans organizing pneumonia (BOOP). Most commonly bibasilar and peribronchial in distribution, BOOP is frequently associated with mild bronchial wall thickening. BOOP may also appear predominantly unilateral, lobar, or even nodular. These findings are nonspecific: Identical findings may be seen, especially in patients with eosinophilic pneumonia. However, in distinction to diseases resulting in interstitial fibrosis, evidence of reticulation, architectural distortion, or traction bronchiectasis is unusual. **B:** BOOP in a 27-year-old man with polymyositis. HRCT demonstrates peribronchial and subpleural areas of consolidation and ill-defined nodular opacities involving mainly the lower lobes.

DISEASES ASSOCIATED WITH BRONCHIOLITIS

Bronchiolitis may be associated with a number of diseases (Table 8-8), including those described above in the section Bronchiectasis. In several diseases, the predominant abnormality is bronchiolitis. These are discussed in detail below.

Bronchiolitis Obliterans (Constrictive Bronchiolitis)

BO (constrictive bronchiolitis) represents a nonspecific reaction that may be caused by a variety of insults. It is characterized by concentric fibrosis involving the submucosal and peribronchial tissues of terminal and respiratory bronchioles, with resulting bronchiolar narrowing or obliteration of the bronchiolar lumen. BO may be classified by etiology [211,219], as (i) postinfectious BO, due to bacterial, mycoplasmal, or viral (especially respiratory syncytial virus, adenovirus, influenza, parainfluenza, and cytomegalovirus) infection, or as a sequela of PCP, HIV viral infection, or both in AIDS patients [218,261,270–274]; (ii) toxic fume BO, resulting from exposure to gases such as nitrogen dioxide (silo-filler's lung), sulfur dioxide, ammonia, chlorine, phosgene, and ozone [218,270,275–278] (Fig. 8-54); (iii) idiopathic [279,280]; (iv) BO associated with connective tissue diseases, particularly RA and polymyositis [218,236,281–284]; (v) BO associated with drug therapy (e.g., penicillamine or gold) [218]; and (vi) BO as a complication of lung or bone marrow transplantation [39,40,44 46,285–289]. Obliterative bronchiolitis has also been linked to consumption of *S. androgynus* [242,262], a small, lowland shrub found in Asia, consumed in the form of an uncooked juice as a means of weight reduction, especially in Taiwan. BO has also been reported in association with neuroendocrine hyperplasia, especially in patients who have carcinoid tumors [227,263]. In may also be present in children surviving bronchopulmonary dysplasia [290].

The radiologic manifestations of the various forms of BO were described by Gosink et al. [270] and have been reviewed by McLoud [291]. The chest radiograph in BO is often normal. In some patients, mild hyperinflation, subtle peripheral attenuation of the vascular markings [292], and evidence of central airway dilatation may be seen [19,39,41,42].

High-Resolution Computed Tomography Findings

The HRCT appearance of BO has been described in a number of studies (Table 8-10) [18,20,39,43,87,141,230,234, 242,293,294], and characteristic abnormalities have been reported in patients who have both idiopathic and secondary BO [18,230,234,294]. HRCT findings are similar regardless of the cause of disease (Fig. 8-54).

The most obvious HRCT finding is often that of focal, sharply defined areas of decreased lung attenuation associated with vessels of decreased caliber (Fig. 8-54A and C). These changes represent a combination of air-trapping and oligemia, typically occurring in the absence of parenchymal consolidation, and termed *mosaic perfusion* [230]. Bronchiectasis, both central and peripheral, may be present as well (Fig. 8-54A) [42]. Rarely, 2- to 4-mm centrilobular branching opacities, representing inspissated secretions within distal airways or ill-defined centrilobular opacities, may be the predominant finding [85,234], but recognizable small airway abnormalities are usually inconspicuous in patients who have BO.

Air-trapping is commonly visible on expiratory HRCT in patients who have BO (Fig. 8-54B, D, and E). In fact, the presence of air-trapping on expiratory scans may be the only abnormal HRCT finding in patients who have BO (Fig. 8-55) [117]. In a study by Arakawa and Webb of 45 patients who had air-trapping found on routine expiratory HRCT scans [117], nine patients had normal inspiratory HRCT findings; five of these nine patients had BO.

Abnormal findings are far more evident on HRCT than on chest radiographs in patients who have BO. For example, in one study of patients who had BO [294], chest radiographs were normal in one-third of patients and showed mild hyperinflation and vascular attenuation in the remaining two-thirds. CT, on the other hand, showed widespread and conspicuous abnormalities in lung attenuation in nearly 90% of the patients.

Postinfectious Bronchiolitis Obliterans and the Swyer-James Syndrome

Chang et al. [261] assessed the long-term clinical, imaging, and pulmonary function sequelae of postinfectious BO in 19 children. Clinical follow-up averaging 6.8 years revealed a high incidence of continuing problems, largely relating to asthma and bronchiectasis. Fixed airway obstruction was the most common pulmonary function abnormality. Chest radiographs showed five patterns: (i) unilateral hyperlucency of increased volume, (ii) complete collapse of the affected lobe, (iii) unilateral hyperlucency of a small or normal-sized lung, (iv) bilateral hyperlucent lungs and a mixed pattern of persistent collapse, and (v) hyperlucency and peribronchial thickening.

Lynch et al. [141] reported the HRCT findings of postinfectious BO in six children. The most striking finding in these patients was the presence of focal areas of decreased lung opacity, which usually had sharp margins. These areas of decreased opacity corresponded to segments or lobules, and the pulmonary vessels within these areas appeared to be reduced in size. Four of these six had bronchiectasis visible on HRCT (Fig. 8-56), and in all four the abnormal bronchi were in areas of lung showing decreased opacity. It is likely that the areas of decreased opacity represent regions of lung that are poorly ventilated and perfused. Areas of increased lung opacity containing vessels that were normal or large in size were also seen in this series; these areas of increased opacity reflect well-perfused areas of lung or mosaic perfusion.

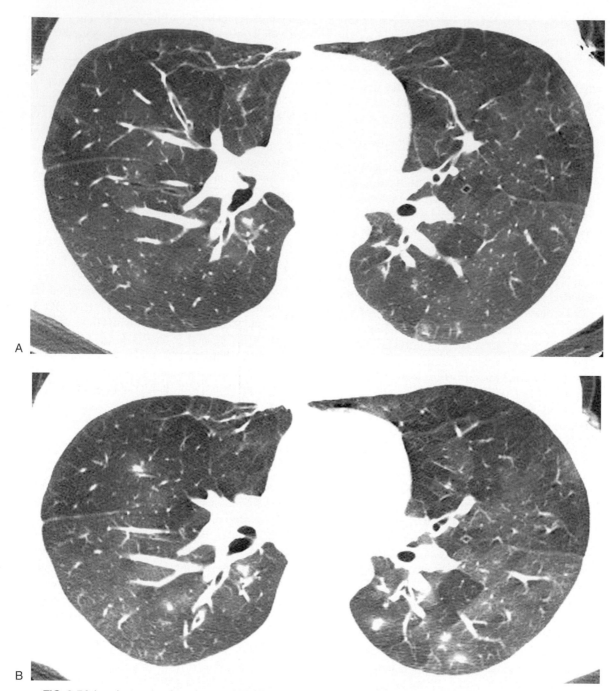

FIG. 8-54. Inspiratory and expiratory HRCT in a young woman with bronchiolitis obliterans resulting from smoke inhalation. **A:** Inspiratory scan shows mild bronchiectasis bilaterally, associated with a distinct pattern of mosaic perfusion, manifested by sharply marginated areas of inhomogeneous lung opacity. **B:** A postexpiratory scan at the same level shows an accentuation of the mosaic appearance as a result of air-trapping. *Continued*

Zhang et al. [295] performed a prospective study to define the HRCT features of 31 pediatric patients who had postinfectious BO. All patients had chest radiographs and lung perfusion scans, and 27 of the 31 patients had HRCT of the lung. The most common abnormal features shown on CT included bronchial wall thickening (100%), bronchiectasis (85%, graded as moderate or severe in 30%), and areas of increased and decreased attenuation (82%), likely due to mosaic perfusion secondary to air-trapping. Perfusion defects on radionuclide imaging were found in all patients. Lobular, segmental, or subsegmental atelectasis was also common, being seen in 70% of cases.

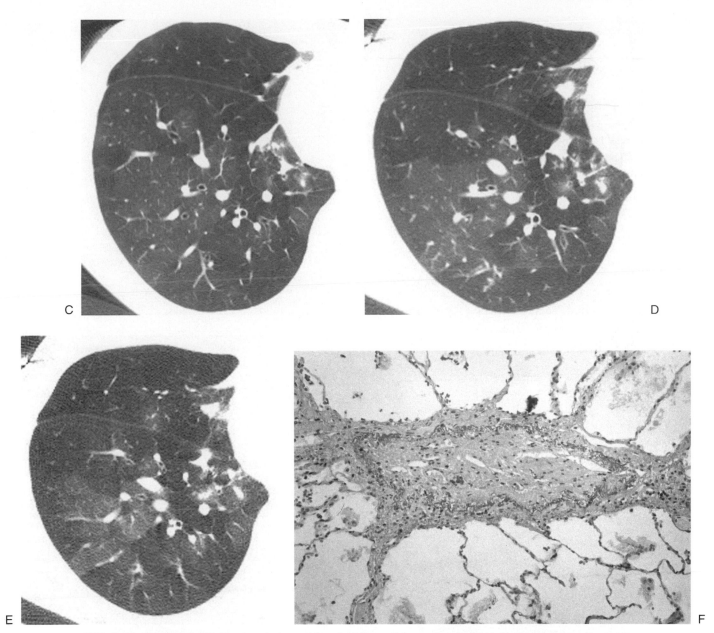

FIG. 8-54. *Continued* **C:** Targeted view of the right lower lobe on inspiration shows findings of mosaic perfusion with reduced vessel size in lucent lung regions. **D:** Postexpiratory scan at this level shows air-trapping. **E:** This appearance is further accentuated on a dynamic expiratory scan. **F:** Histologic section from an open-lung biopsy in a different patient shows typical histologic findings of constrictive bronchiolitis, with concentric fibrosis and narrowing of a bronchiole in the absence of associated parenchymal disease.

In this study [295], HRCT showed a higher sensitivity than chest radiography in detecting pulmonary abnormalities. Although bronchial wall thickening was seen on radiographs in all cases showing this finding on HRCT, areas of decreased opacity were seen in only 59% of HRCT-positive cases, and bronchiectasis was seen in only 35%.

BO is a major component of Swyer-James or MacLeod syndrome [296,297]. In patients who have Swyer-James syndrome,

BO is the result of lower respiratory tract infection, usually viral, occurring in infancy or early childhood. Damage to the terminal and respiratory bronchioles leads to incomplete development of their alveolar buds. The radiographic hallmark of this syndrome is unilateral hyperlucent lung with reduced lung volume on inspiration and air-trapping on expiration (Figs. 8-56 and 8-57). Although previously necessitating confirmation either by bronchography (to demonstrate extensive bronchiecta-

TABLE 8-10. *HRCT findings in bronchiolitis obliterans (constrictive bronchiolitis)*

Mosaic perfusion, usually patchy in distribution[a,b]
Bronchiectasis[a]
Air-trapping on expiration, usually patchy in distribution[a]
Air-trapping on expiration with normal inspiratory scans[a,b]
Areas of consolidation or increased lung opacity
Reticulonodular opacities (rare)
Tree-in-bud (rare)

[a]Most common findings.
[b]Findings most helpful in differential diagnosis.

sis), or arteriography (to demonstrate a small central pulmonary artery and decreased peripheral vascularity), these procedures have been all but obviated by HRCT.

Marti-Bonmati et al. [293] described the CT findings in nine patients who had Swyer-James syndrome. On CT, the affected lung showed decreased opacity in eight patients (Figs. 8-56 and 8-57); in the one remaining patient, the affected lung was very small but of normal attenuation. Lung volume on the affected site was reduced in six patients and normal in three; one patient showed normal lung opacity on chest radiographs but decreased opacity on CT. In all patients, the size of the affected lung did not change on CT scans obtained during inspiration and expiration.

All nine patients had CT findings of bronchiectasis [293]. In each, cylindrical bronchiectasis was present, but two also had cystic bronchiectasis and three had varicose bronchiectasis. The lower lobes were affected in eight patients, the middle lobes or lingula in seven patients, and the upper lobes in three patients. Parenchymal abnormalities were present in eight patients.

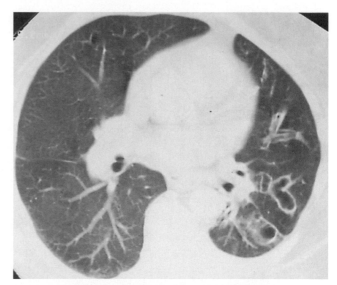

FIG. 8-56. Bronchiolitis obliterans (constrictive bronchiolitis) in the Swyer-James syndrome. On HRCT, the lungs appear asymmetric, with marked volume loss on the left. The left lung appears relatively lucent, with diminished vascular markings and extensive cystic bronchiectasis. These findings are characteristic of the Swyer-James syndrome. CT scans through the left hilum (not shown) confirmed the presence of a hypoplastic left pulmonary artery. Currently asymptomatic, this patient recalled a history of childhood pneumonia.

Idiopathic Bronchiolitis Obliterans

Idiopathic BO usually affects middle-aged women and has a relentless downhill course despite steroid therapy. A more benign course has been described in a limited number of patients who have more stable disease, suggesting a wider range of clinical presentations than previously appreciated [280].

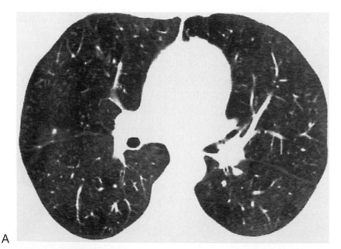
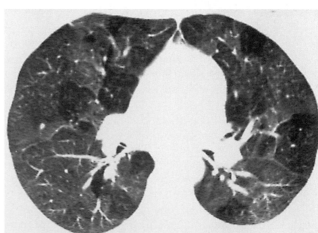

A   B

FIG. 8-55. Bronchiolitis obliterans (constrictive bronchiolitis) with air-trapping on expiratory HRCT. **A:** HRCT at full inspiration shows minimal lung inhomogeneity as a result of bronchiolitis obliterans. No bronchiectasis is visible, and the chest radiograph was normal. **B:** On a postexpiratory HRCT, marked lung inhomogeneity is visible as a result of air-trapping.

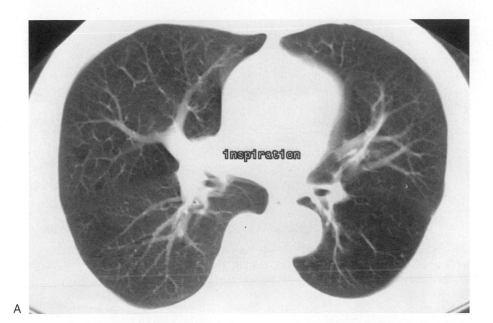

A

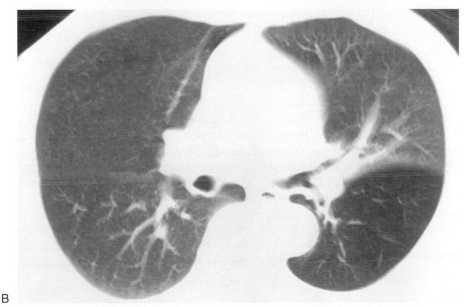

B

FIG. 8-57. Air-trapping in the Swyer-James syndrome. **A:** Section through the midlung fields in deep inspiration in an asymptomatic patient shows homogeneous decreased lung density in the left lower lobe in the absence of endobronchial obstruction or evidence of bronchiectasis. **B:** Section at the same level as **(A)** in expiration confirms that there is air-trapping in the left lower lobe. In this case, the patient recalled having had a severe childhood pneumonia.

Sweatman et al. [294] described the CT findings in 15 patients who had idiopathic BO. The chest radiograph was normal in five patients and showed mild hyperinflation and vascular attenuation in the remaining ten. CT showed widespread abnormalities in 13 of the 15 patients (87%), consisting of patchy irregular areas of high and low attenuation in variable proportions (Fig. 8-58). These changes were accentuated on expiration.

Bronchiolitis Obliterans Associated with Rheumatoid Arthritis

The pulmonary manifestations of RA include bronchiolar diseases such as follicular bronchiolitis and BO [247]. BO is an uncommon manifestation, being seen in one of 29 patients suspected of having lung disease studied by Akira et al. [243]. The HRCT and expiratory CT findings of two patients who had RA

and BO have been reported by Aquino et al. [194]. Both had been treated using penicillamine and gold. Plain film findings were limited to large lung volumes, but HRCT showed similar findings in both patients, with evidence of bronchiectasis and regional lung inhomogeneities (mosaic perfusion) (Fig. 8-59). In both, dynamic expiratory CT showed air-trapping on expiratory scans. Among 77 patients who had RA studied by Remy-Jardin et al. using HRCT, four of 16 with bronchiectasis were considered to have BO based on PFTs [189].

Bronchiolitis Obliterans Associated with Heart-Lung or Lung Transplantation

BO is the major long-term complication of lung transplantation, occurring in 25% to 50% of transplant recipients, and its presence or absence usually determines long-term sur-

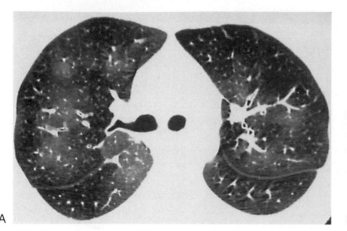
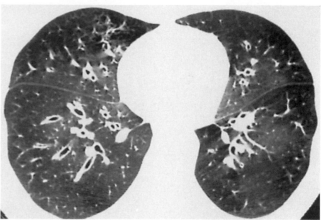

FIG. 8-58. Bronchiolitis obliterans (constrictive bronchiolitis). HRCT sections through the right upper **(A)** and lower **(B)** lobes, in a young woman presenting with progressive dyspnea. Pulmonary function tests disclosed severe obstructive lung disease. Corresponding chest radiograph (not shown) was interpreted as normal. HRCT sections obtained in deep inspiration show geographic areas of low attenuation interspersed with areas of relatively increased opacity. Dilated thick-walled bronchi are easily identified throughout the lower lobes, middle lobe, and lingula. This constellation of clinical and CT findings is characteristic of patients with idiopathic constrictive bronchiolitis (cryptogenic bronchiolitis obliterans). This patient is currently awaiting lung transplantation.

vival [298–301]. It rarely develops in the first 3 months after transplantation, and instead usually occurs at the end of or after the first postoperative year [302]. The prompt diagnosis of BO is important, as appropriate immunosuppressive treatment may be helpful in the maintenance of lung function [303]. Of patients developing BO, between 25% and 40% die as a direct result.

Although most likely due to immunologically mediated injury of the pulmonary endothelial and bronchial epithelial cells, other etiologies have been implicated, including vascu-

lar insufficiency and infection. The primary risk factor for posttransplantation constrictive bronchiolitis appears to be the frequency and severity of acute cellular rejection that nearly always occurs in patients in the early postoperative setting [304]. Histologically, BO reflects chronic rejection and is characterized by submucosal and intraepithelial lymphocytic and histiocytic infiltrates primarily affecting the distal small airways, associated with dense submucosal eosinophilic scar tissue. Intraluminal fibrous plaques also occur, leading to either partial or complete bronchiolar obstruction [289].

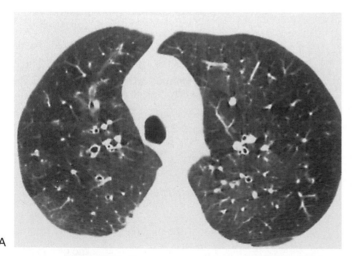
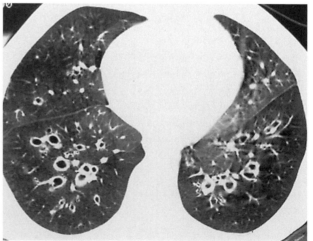

FIG. 8-59. Bronchiolitis obliterans (constrictive bronchiolitis) in a patient who has rheumatoid arthritis treated with penicillamine. HRCT at two levels **(A,B)** shows bronchiectasis and patchy lung opacity as a result of air-trapping. (**B** from Webb WR. High-resolution computed tomography of obstructive lung disease. *Radiol Clin North Am* 1994;32:745–757, with permission.)

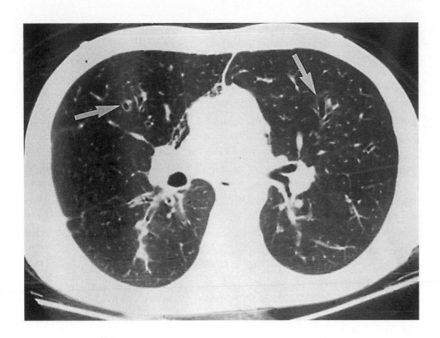

FIG. 8-60. Bronchiolitis obliterans (constrictive bronchiolitis) after heart-lung transplantation. Note that there is moderate dilatation of the central bronchi bilaterally (*arrows*). This may be an early finding in patients with bronchiolitis obliterans. (Case courtesy of Denise Aberle, M.D., University of California, Los Angeles, UCLA Medical Center.)

Clinically, the earliest manifestation of chronic rejection is nonproductive cough, which may progress to a cough productive of purulent but sterile sputum. Later, the course is dominated by increasingly severe dyspnea. Pulmonary function tests show progressive obstruction. In accordance with definitions proposed by the International Society of Heart Lung Transplantation, the term *bronchiolitis obliterans* is reserved for patients having a biopsy diagnosis [305]. However, because a histologic diagnosis of BO may be difficult to make, particularly by transbronchial biopsy, the term *bronchiolitis obliterans syndrome* (BOS) has been proposed to describe a clinical constellation of findings consistent with this diagnosis [304]. BOS is used to refer to patients who have a progressive deterioration of graft function secondary to airways disease, but not explained by other factors such as infection, acute rejection, or anastomotic complications [305]. Using criteria established by the International Society of Heart Lung Transplantation, the diagnosis of BOS is established by a decrease in FEV_1 by 20% or more from previous baseline PFT studies obtained at least one month previously [305]. A decrease in $FEF_{25-75\%}$ to less than 70% of predicted has also been suggested as a more sensitive criterion in patients who have undergone a bilateral lung transplantation [232,289,298,299,306]. However, in patients who have undergone a single lung transplant for emphysema, $FEF_{25-75\%}$ is usually abnormal regardless of graft function, and this criterion is difficult to apply.

Radiographic findings in transplant patients who have BO are often nonspecific. In most, chronic rejection is associated with a normal-appearing radiograph, or an appearance suggestive of CF with mild to extensive bronchiectasis. Skeens et al. [39] described the radiologic findings in 11 patients who had BO after heart-lung transplantation. In all patients, the chest radiographs showed parenchymal abnormalities consisting of reticulonodular, nodular, or airspace opacities. Radio-

graphic evidence of central bronchiectasis was present in 9 of the 11 patients. Chest CT scans performed in two patients confirmed the radiographic findings of bronchiectasis.

HRCT findings in patients who have BO after lung transplantation include both central and peripheral bronchiectasis (Fig. 8-60); focal lucencies, presumably the result of air-trapping and mosaic perfusion; and localized parenchymal consolidation [39–44,307,308]. Bronchiectasis is commonly reported in these series but should be considered a relatively late finding of BO in patients who had undergone transplantation; the sensitivity of this finding in the detection of early disease is limited. In a study by Worthy et al. [309], 80% of patients who had proven BO after lung transplantation showed bronchial dilatation, whereas 27% were believed to have bronchial wall thickening; in a control group of normal patients, bronchial wall dilatation was felt to be present in 22%. Lentz et al. [42] found a close correlation between the percentage of bronchi in the lower lobes that appeared dilated on HRCT and PFT findings of airway obstruction. They concluded that dilatation of lower lobe bronchi is a good indicator of BO in this population, and that the percentage of dilated bronchi generally increases with increasing pulmonary dysfunction [42].

The relatively low sensitivity of the HRCT finding of bronchiectasis, however, has been emphasized by others [310]. In a study by Leung et al. [311] in patients who had an established diagnosis of BO, bronchiectasis was visible on HRCT in 4 of 11 (36%) patients who had BO and two of ten (20%) patients who did not have BO. In this study, the sensitivity, specificity, and accuracy of bronchiectasis in making the diagnosis of BO were 36%, 80%, and 57%, respectively. Others have suggested that this finding may predict the development of BO. In a study by Loubeyre et al. [308], bronchiectasis visible on HRCT was found to be a predictor of the development of clinical BO with a sensitivity of 14%, a specificity of 77%, a positive predictive value of 25%, and a negative predictive value of 63%. Bronchiectasis appeared concomitantly with symptoms of BO in 8 of 12 (67%) patients.

Hruban et al. [43] reported the HRCT findings seen in seven lung specimens obtained from patients who received a heart-lung transplant. The lungs were fixed using a method that allows direct one-to-one pathologic-radiologic correlation. They examined two lungs from patients who had clinical, pathologic, and HRCT evidence of chronic rejection; both lungs showed severe BO associated with bronchiectasis and peribronchial fibrosis.

Mosaic perfusion due to BO and abnormal lung ventilation is commonly seen in patients who have obliterative bronchiolitis, but the accuracy of this finding in predicting the presence of BO is limited, particularly in patients who have early disease [310]. In a study by Worthy et al. [309], mosaic perfusion was visible in 40% of patients who had proven BO after lung transplantation and in 22% of controls. In the study by Leung et al. of patients who had known disease [311], the presence of mosaic perfusion was present in 7 of 11 (64%) patients who had BO, and one of ten (10%) patients who did not have BO (p <.05). In this study, the sensitivity, specificity, and accuracy of mosaic perfusion for diagnosing BO were 64%, 90%, and 70%, respectively.

The presence of air-trapping on expiratory HRCT may be of the most value in making the diagnosis of BO [309,311], but the accuracy of this finding may be limited in patients who have early disease [310]. In the study by Worthy et al. [309], air-trapping, diagnosed on expiratory scans if a total area of more than one segment appeared abnormal, was seen in four of five (80%) patients who had biopsy-proven BO and expiratory scans, and in none of three patients who had a negative biopsy. In a study by Leung et al. [311], air-trapping was found in ten of 11 patients who had biopsy-diagnosed BO, compared to two of ten patients who did not have biopsy-diagnosed BO or PFT abnormalities. Thus, air-trapping was found to have a sensitivity of 91%, a specificity of 80%, and accuracy of 86% for diagnosing BO. However, the patients who had BO in this study had established disease; the mean time from lung transplantation to CT in their study was 4.8 years, and the mean duration of a known diagnosis of BO was 1.3 years.

In a study by Lee et al. [310], HRCT including expiratory scans was reviewed in consecutive normal lung transplant patients and patients first diagnosed as having BO or BOS (i.e., early disease). The frequency of significant air-trapping in patients who had BO or BOS was significantly higher than in patients who had a normal biopsy and PFTs. However, the sensitivity of significant air-trapping on expiratory CT was only 74%; its specificity was 67%, and its accuracy was 71%.

The role of repeated HRCT scans in monitoring the development of BOS after lung transplantation has also been assessed by Ikonen et al. [312]. In a study of 13 lung transplant recipients who underwent a total of 126 HRCT scans during a mean follow-up period of 23 months, 8 of the 13 patients developed BOS. The authors demonstrated that the HRCT findings occurred concurrently with the development of BOS. Making use of a combination of abnormalities for diagnosis, the overall sensitivity of HRCT for the diagnosis of BO was 93% and the specificity was 92% [312].

The HRCT appearance of posttransplantation BOS has been reviewed by Lau et al. [313] in six infants and young children with BOS (age range, 2 months to 5.5 years) and in 15 control patients who did not have obstructive airways disease (age range, 2 months to 7 years). HRCT scans were obtained during quiet sleep at a median of 24 months (range, 6 to 36 months) after transplantation. The HRCT findings in the six patients who had clinically proven BOS were mosaic perfusion in five (83%), bronchial dilation in three (50%), and bronchial wall thickening in one (17%). Of the 15 control patients who had normal PFT results, six (40%) were believed to have findings of mosaic perfusion, whereas none had bronchial dilatation or bronchial wall thickening. Mucous plugging was not seen in either group. Only the association of bronchial dilatation with BOS was significant (p = .02).

Bronchiolitis Obliterans Associated with Bone Marrow Transplantation

BO is one of several pulmonary complications of bone marrow transplantation, occurring in approximately 10% of patients [46,314–316]. Other complications include infection (bacterial, viral, and fungal—in particular, invasive aspergillosis); pulmonary edema; drug and radiation toxicity; and metastatic tumor. A syndrome of diffuse pulmonary hemorrhage has also been described, occurring within the first two weeks after bone marrow transplantation [317]. Determining the cause of pulmonary disease in these patients is frequently problematic, as biopsies are usually contraindicated due to severe thrombocytopenia.

BO is usually identified in patients after allogeneic transplants, presumably the result of chronic graft-versus-host disease (GVHD) (Figs. 8-61 and 8-62) [45,46,218,285,318]. Histologically, BO (constrictive bronchiolitis) is the predominant abnormality, characterized both by neutrophilic and lymphocytic peribronchiolar inflammation. Importantly, histologic evidence of BOOP/COP (or proliferative bronchiolitis) with extension into alveolar ducts and alveoli is distinctly unusual as a cause of airway obstruction in this population [46]. Typically, these patients also have evidence of GVHD involving the skin, liver, and gastrointestinal tract. Patients also frequently have evidence of chronic sinusitis. In fact, bronchiolitis has also been identified in patients after autologous bone marrow transplants, leaving the true etiology of bronchiolitis unexplained [46].

Clinically, patients may present with cough, wheezing, or dyspnea between 1 and 10 months after transplantation [46]. Alternatively, evidence of airways obstruction may be present physiologically in otherwise asymptomatic patients. In either setting, the key to diagnosing bronchiolitis in these patients are serial PFTs. The hallmark of this disease is a decrease in the FEV_1/FVC ratio of less than 70% predicted, often in association with an increased residual volume. In

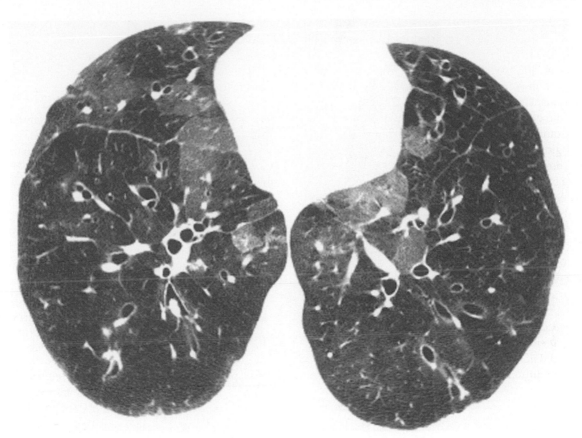

FIG. 8-61. Bronchiolitis obliterans in a bone marrow transplant patient. Extensive bronchiectasis is associated with patchy areas of mosaic perfusion.

most institutions, in distinction to patients who have lung or heart-lung transplantations, pulmonary function testing is considered diagnostic even in the absence of histologic verification. BAL is indicated only in those patients who can tolerate this procedure, in whom concomitant infection is suspected. Despite aggressive therapy with steroids, bronchodilators, or azathioprine, nearly 50% of patients die from progressive respiratory insufficiency.

In the absence of infection, radiographs typically are normal or show only mild hyperinflation, similar to changes identified in other conditions associated with constrictive bronchiolitis. HRCT shows typical findings of BO, with evidence of bronchiectasis, mosaic perfusion, and air-trapping. In an early stage, ill-defined peribronchiolar, centrilobular opacities have been identified [85]. In a study by Ooi et al. [319], HRCT was performed in nine patients who had moderately severe irreversible airflow obstruction and a clinical diagnosis of BOS (persistent lung function deterioration, with FEV_1 of less than 80% of baseline values) after bone marrow transplantation. Two patients had normal HRCT scans. In the remaining seven patients, 7 of 11 HRCT scans were abnormal, with nonspecific findings of bronchial dilatation (one patient), consolidation (two patients), areas of decreased opacity (four patients), and vascular attenuation (four patients).

It should be emphasized that constrictive bronchiolitis represents only one of a wide range of potential pulmonary abnormalities that can occur after bone marrow transplantation [316]. Not surprisingly, the range of CT findings that can be identified primarily reflects the patient's clinical status. Graham et al. [45], in a broad-based study of 18 patients who had 21 episodes of intrathoracic complications after allogeneic bone marrow transplantation, showed that CT disclosed diagnostically relevant findings not apparent on chest radiographs in more than 50% of cases. These included a ground-glass pattern in five patients who had early pneumonia; a peripheral distribution of abnormalities, including bronchiectasis, in four patients who had BO, eosinophilic lung disease, or both; and cavitating lesions or hemorrhagic infarcts in one case each of PCP and invasive aspergillosis, respectively [45]. In comparison, a much narrower range of findings has been described when only febrile patients are evaluated. In this setting, CT has been advocated as a noninvasive means for diagnosing invasive fungal infections. Mori et al. [320], in a retrospective study of 33 febrile bone marrow transplant recipients, documented 21 episodes of fungal infection. In 20 of 21 of these cases, CT showed nodules most of which proved either cavitary, poorly defined, or had associated characteristic halo signs. In distinction, in nine patients who had bacteremia, CT failed to disclose any abnormalities, suggesting that the source of infection was outside the lungs.

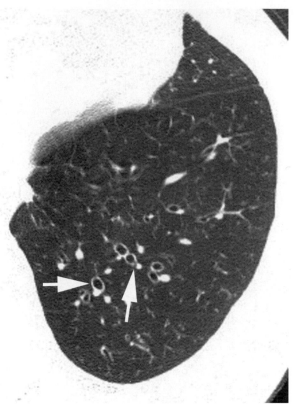
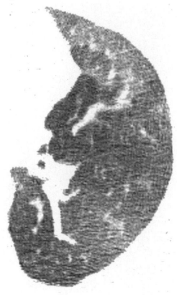

A,B

FIG. 8-62. Bronchiolitis obliterans in a bone marrow transplant patient. **A:** Targeted image of the left lower lobe shows mild bronchiectasis with the signet ring sign (*arrows*). **B:** Dynamic low-dose expiratory scan shows patchy air-trapping.

Diffuse Panbronchiolitis

DPB is a unique syndrome described almost exclusively in Asia, especially in Japan and Korea [88,89,218,321–323]. This entity typically affects middle-aged men. Patients present with the subacute development of airways obstruction, and in nearly three-fourths of patients, there is associated sinusitis. The disease is progressive, marked by frequent episodes of superimposed infection, typically with *Pseudomonas aeruginosa*. In nearly 20% of cases, death occurs within 5 years of the onset of the disease, with another 30% dying within ten years. Current therapy requires long-term low-dose administration of erythromycin.

Histologically, characteristic findings of this disease include centrilobular peribronchiolar infiltrates of acute and chronic inflammatory cells, principally at the level of the respiratory bronchioles, associated with bronchiolar dilatation and intraluminal inflammatory exudates (Fig. 8-63). A striking accumulation of interstitial foam cells and lymphoid hyperplasia is also commonly seen. This combination of findings has been referred to as the *unit lesion* of panbronchiolitis and is considered unique to this syndrome [218]. Although the disease characteristically involves respiratory bronchioles, terminal bronchioles may be involved. In a minority of cases, there is also evidence of peripheral bronchiectasis. Chest radiographs in patients who have DPB are nonspecific and usually show small nodular shadows throughout both lungs and, often, increased lung volumes.

High-Resolution Computed Tomography Findings

HRCT findings in patients who have DPB have been extensively described (Table 8-11) [88,89,248,249,321,322]. As initially shown by Akira et al. [89], the most important findings, in order of severity, are poorly defined centrilobular

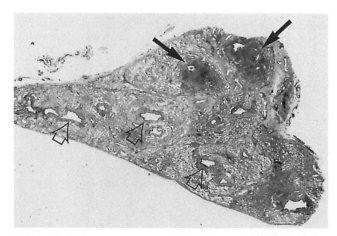

FIG. 8-63. Diffuse panbronchiolitis. Open lung biopsy specimen shows centrilobular peribronchiolar infiltrates of acute and chronic inflammatory cells (*solid arrows*), principally at the level of the respiratory bronchioles, associated with bronchiolar dilatation (*open arrows*). (From Gruden JF, Webb WR, Warnock M. Centrilobular opacities in the lung on high-resolution CT: diagnostic considerations and pathologic correlation. *AJR Am J Roentgenol* 1994;162:569–574, with permission.)

TABLE 8-11. *HRCT findings in diffuse panbronchiolitis*

Centrilobular branching opacities, tree-in-bud[a,b]
Bronchiolectasis[a,b]
Bronchiectasis[a]
Diffuse distribution/basilar predominance[a]
Large lung volumes
Mosaic perfusion
Air-trapping on expiration[a]

[a]Most common findings.
[b]Findings most helpful in differential diagnosis.

nodules, centrilobular branching opacities or TIB, and branching thick-walled centrilobular lucencies (see Fig. 3-75; Fig. 8-64). As confirmed by Nishimura et al. [88], these findings correspond to, respectively, peribronchiolar inflammation and fibrosis, dilated bronchioles with inflammatory wall thickening and intraluminal secretions, and dilated, air-filled bronchioles (Fig. 8-65) [88]. The finding of small, peripheral peribronchiolar nodules is particularly characteristic, resulting in a TIB appearance.

In addition to these findings, patients who have DPB usually show evidence of air-trapping with large lung volumes and decreased attenuation of peripheral lung parenchyma [88]. As documented by Murata et al. [322], in a study comparing positron emission tomography and CT in seven patients who had DPB, CT attenuation values were considerably lower in the periphery of the lung as compared with the central portions, a finding indicative of extensive peripheral air-trapping. Such stratified distribution of ventilatory impairment may be considered characteristic of diffuse bronchiolar narrowing.

Utility of High-Resolution Computed Tomography

Although the course of this disease is typically monitored clinically, HRCT may play a role in select cases. As documented by Akira et al. [321], in a study of 19 patients randomly assigned either to therapy with low-dose erythromycin or to follow-up without treatment, centrilobular nodular and branched opacities decreased in number and size in treated patients, suggesting a positive response to therapy. In distinction, among untreated patients, similar densities observed initially were found to have progressed with resultant dilatation of the proximal airways. Similar results have been shown by Ichikawa et al. [249]. These findings suggest a potential role for HRCT for monitoring as well as for predicting the outcome of therapy.

It should be noted that the finding of nodular or branching centrilobular opacities may be seen in a number of different diseases in which bronchiolar abnormalities are present [70,85]. Linear or branching centrilobular opacities result from bronchiolar dilatation with intraluminal accumulation of mucus, fluid, or pus. As noted previously, this has been termed the *TIB* appearance and can be identified in patients who have CF [141]; endobronchial spread of tuberculosis [27] or nontuberculous mycobacteria; lobular pneumonia or bronchopneumonia, including those with PCP or cytomegalovirus pneumonia; bronchiectasis of any cause; and other airways diseases that result in the accumulation of mucus or pus in small bronchi. The differential diagnosis of centrilobular opacities is described in detail in Chapter 3.

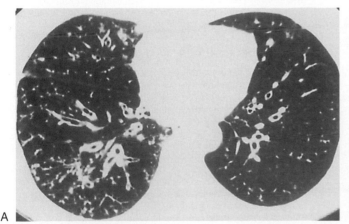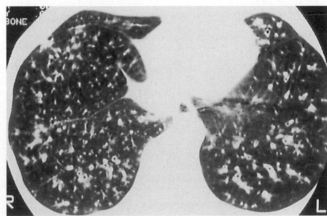

FIG. 8-64. Diffuse panbronchiolitis. HRCT at two levels shows findings of poorly defined centrilobular nodules in the lung periphery, centrilobular branching opacities or tree-in-bud, and bronchiectasis. (Courtesy of Shin-Ho Kook, M.D., Koryo General Hospital, Seoul, Korea.)

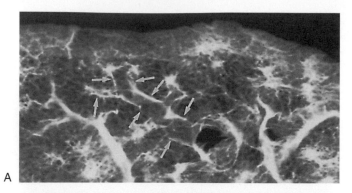

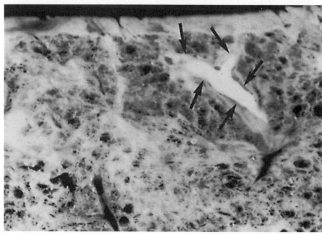

FIG. 8-65. Diffuse panbronchiolitis. **A:** Radiograph of a 1-mm slice of lung obtained from a patient who has panbronchiolitis. A dilated air-filled bronchiole (*arrows*) is visible in the lung periphery, extending to within 5 mm of the pleural surface. **B:** Photomicrograph shows a dilated bronchiole (*arrows*) in the subpleural lung filled with secretions. (From Nishimura K, Kitaichi M, Isum T, et al. Diffuse panbronchiolitis: correlation of high-resolution CT and pathologic findings. *Radiology* 1992;184:779–785, with permission.)

REFERENCES

1. McGuinness G, Naidich DP, Leitman BS, et al. Bronchiectasis: CT evaluation. *AJR Am J Roentgenol* 1993;160:253–259.
2. Grenier P, Cordeau MP, Beigelman C. High-resolution computed tomography of the airways. *J Thorac Imag* 1993;8:213–229.
3. Hartman TE, Primack SL, Lee KS, et al. CT of bronchial and bronchiolar diseases. *Radiographics* 1994;14:991–1003.
4. Kang EY, Miller RR, Müller NL. Bronchiectasis: comparison of preoperative thin-section CT and pathologic findings in resected specimens. *Radiology* 1995;195:649–654.
5. Worthy SA, Flower CD. Computed tomography of the airways. *Eur Radiol* 1996;6:717–729.
6. Lucidarme O, Grenier P, Coche E, et al. Bronchiectasis: comparative assessment with thin-section CT and helical CT. *Radiology* 1996;200:673–679.
7. Hansell D. Bronchiectasis. *Rad Clin North Am* 1998;36:107–128.
8. Remy-Jardin M, Remy J, Artaud D, et al. Tracheobronchial tree: assessment with volume rendering—technical aspects. *Radiology* 1998;208:393–398.
9. Webb WR, Stern EJ, Kanth N, et al. Dynamic pulmonary CT: findings in normal adult men. *Radiology* 1993;186:117–124.
10. Stern EJ, Webb WR. Dynamic imaging of lung morphology with ultrafast high-resolution computed tomography. *J Thorac Imag* 1993;8:273–282.
11. Stern EJ, Webb WR, Gamsu G. Dynamic quantitative computed tomography: a predictor of pulmonary function in obstructive lung diseases. *Invest Radiol* 1994;29:564–569.
12. Goldin JG, Aberle DR. Functional imaging of the airways. *J Thorac Imag* 1997;12:29–37.
13. Goldin JG, McNitt-Gray MF, Sorenson SM, et al. Airway hyperreactivity: assessment with helical thin-section CT. *Radiology* 1998;208:321–329.
14. Herold CJ, Brown RH, Mitzner W, et al. Assessment of pulmonary airway reactivity with high-resolution CT. *Radiology* 1991;181:369–374.
15. Brown RH, Zerhouni E. New techniques and developments in physiologic imaging of airways. *Radiol Clin North Am* 1998;36:211–230.
16. Brown RH, Zerhouni EA, Mitzner W. Variability in the size of individual airways over the course of one year. *Am J Respir Crit Care Med* 1995;151:1159–1164.
17. Lucidarme O, Coche E, Cluzel P, et al. Expiratory CT scans for chronic airways disease: correlation with pulmonary function test results. *AJR Am J Roentgenol* 1998;170:301–307.
18. Lynch DA. Imaging of small airways disease. *Clin Chest Med* 1993;14:623–634.
19. Müller NL, Miller RR. Diseases of the bronchioles: CT and histopathologic findings. *Radiology* 1995;196:3–12.
20. Hwang JH, Kim TS, Lee KS, et al. Bronchiolitis in adults: pathology and imaging. *J Comput Assist Tomogr* 1997;21:913–919.
21. Worthy SA, Müller NL. Small airways diseases. *Rad Clin North Am* 1998;36:163–173.
22. Essadki O, Grenier P. Bronchiolitis: computed tomographic findings. *J Radiol* 1999;80:17–24.
23. Barker AF, Bardana EJ. Bronchiectasis: update on an orphan disease. *Am Rev Resp Dis* 1988;137:969–978.
24. Stanford W, Galvin JR. The diagnosis of bronchiectasis. *Clin Chest Med* 1988;9:691–699.
25. Davis AL, Salzman SH. Bronchiectasis. In: Cherniack NS, ed. *Chronic obstructive pulmonary disease*. Philadelphia: W. B. Saunders, 1991:316–338.
26. Nicotra MB, Rivera M, Dale AM, et al. Clinical, pathophysiologic, and microbiologic characterization of bronchiectasis in an aging cohort [see comments]. *Chest* 1995;108:955–961.
27. Im JG, Itoh H, Shim YS, et al. Pulmonary tuberculosis: CT findings—early active disease and sequential change with antituberculous therapy. *Radiology* 1993;186:653–660.
28. Hartman TE, Swensen SJ, Williams DE. Mycobacterium avium-intracellulare complex: evaluation with CT. *Radiology* 1993;187:23–26.
29. Swensen SJ, Hartman TE, Williams DE. Computed tomography in diagnosis of Mycobacterium avium-intracellulare complex in patients with bronchiectasis. *Chest* 1994;105:49–52.
30. Moore EH. Atypical mycobacterial infection in the lung: CT appearance. *Radiology* 1993;187:777–782.
31. McGuinness G, Naidich DP, Garay SM, et al. AIDS associated bronchiectasis: CT features. *J Comput Assist Tomogr* 1993;17:260–266.
32. Amorosa JK, Miller RW, Laraya-Cuasay L, et al. Bronchiectasis in children with lymphocytic interstitial pneumonia and acquired immune deficiency syndrome: plain film and CT observations. *Pediatr Radiol* 1992;22:603–606.
33. McGuinness G, Scholes JV, Jagirdar JS, et al. Unusual lymphoproliferative disorders in nine adults with HIV or AIDS: CT and pathologic findings. *Radiology* 1995;197:59–65.
34. King MA, Neal DE, St. John R, et al. Bronchial dilatation in patients with HIV infection: CT assessment and correlation with pulmonary function tests and findings at bronchoalveolar lavage. *AJR Am J Roentgenol* 1997;168:1535–1540.
35. McGuinness G, Naidich DP. Bronchiectasis: CT/clinical correlations. *Semin Ultrasound CT MR* 1995;16:395–419.
36. Neeld DA, Goodman LR, Gurney JW, et al. Computerized tomography in the evaluation of allergic bronchopulmonary aspergillosis. *Am Rev Respir Dis* 1990;142:1200–1206.
37. Kullnig P, Pongratz M, Kopp W, et al. Computerized tomography in the diagnosis of allergic bronchopulmonary aspergillosis. *Radiologe* 1989;29:228–231.
38. Lynch DA, Newell JD, Tschomper BA, et al. Uncomplicated asthma in adults: comparison of CT appearance of the lungs in asthmatic and healthy subjects. *Radiology* 1993;188:829–833.

39. Skeens JL, Fuhrman CR, Yousem SA. Bronchiolitis obliterans in heart-lung transplantation patients: radiologic findings in 11 patients. *AJR Am J Roentgenol* 1989;153:253–256.

40. O'Donovan P. Imaging of complications of lung transplantation. *Radiographics* 1993;13:787–796.

41. Morrish WF, Herman SJ, Weisbrod GL, et al. Bronchiolitis obliterans after lung transplantation: findings at chest radiography and high-resolution CT. *Radiology* 1991;179:487–490.

42. Lentz D, Bergin CJ, Berry GJ, et al. Diagnosis of bronchiolitis obliterans in heart-lung transplantation patients: importance of bronchial dilatation on CT. *AJR Am J Roentgenol* 1992;159:463–467.

43. Hruban RH, Ren H, Kuhlman JE, et al. Inflation-fixed lungs: pathologic-radiologic (CT) correlation of lung transplantation. *J Comput Assist Tomogr* 1990;14:329–335.

44. Herman S, Rappaport D, Weisbrod G, et al. Single-lung transplantation: imaging features. *Radiology* 1989;170:89–93.

45. Graham NJ, Müller NL, Miller RR, et al. Intrathoracic complications following allogeneic bone marrow transplantation: CT findings. *Radiology* 1991;181:153–156.

46. Crawford SW, Clark JG. Bronchiolitis associated with bone marrow transplantation. *Clin Chest Med* 1993;14:741–749.

47. Haponik F, Britt EJ, Smith PL, et al. Computed chest tomography in the evaluation of hemoptysis. *Chest* 1987;91:80–85.

48. Currie DC, Cooke JC, Morgan AD, et al. Interpretation of bronchograms and chest radiographs in patients with chronic sputum production. *Thorax* 1987;42:278–284.

49. Millar A, Boothroyd A, Edwards D, et al. The role of computed tomography (CT) in the investigation of unexplained hemoptysis. *Resp Med* 1992;86:39–44.

50. Naidich DP, Funt S, Ettenger NA, et al. Hemoptysis: CT-bronchoscopic correlations in 58 cases. *Radiology* 1990;177:357–362.

51. Gudjberg CE. Roentgenologic diagnosis of bronchiectasis: an analysis of 112 cases. *Acta Radiol (Stockh)* 1955;43:209–226.

52. Woodring JH. Improved plain film criteria for the diagnosis of bronchiectasis. *J Ky Med Assoc* 1994;92:8–13.

53. Naidich DP, McCauley DI, Khouri NF, et al. Computed tomography of bronchiectasis. *J Comput Assist Tomogr* 1982;6:437–444.

54. McNitt-Gray MF, Goldin JG, Johnson TD, et al. Development and testing of image-processing methods for the quantitative assessment of airway hyperresponsiveness from high-resolution CT images. *J Comput Assist Tomogr* 1997;21:939–947.

55. Smith IE, Jurriaans E, Diederich S, et al. Chronic sputum production: correlations between clinical features and findings on high resolution computed tomographic scanning of the chest. *Thorax* 1996;51:914–918.

56. Kim JS, Müller NL, Park CS, et al. Bronchoarterial ratio on thin section CT: comparison between high altitude and sea level. *J Comput Assist Tomogr* 1997;21:306–311.

57. Diederich S, Jurriaans E, Flower CD. Interobserver variation in the diagnosis of bronchiectasis on high-resolution computed tomography. *Eur Radiol* 1996;6:801–806.

58. Kim SJ, Im JG, Kim IO, et al. Normal bronchial and pulmonary arterial diameters measured by thin section CT. *J Comput Assist Tomogr* 1995;19:365–369.

59. Joharjy IA, Bashi SA, Abdullah AK. Value of medium-thickness CT in the diagnosis of bronchiectasis. *AJR Am J Roentgenol* 1987;149:1133–1137.

60. Cooke JC, Currie DC, Morgan AD, et al. Role of computed tomography in diagnosis of bronchiectasis. *Thorax* 1987;42:272–277.

61. Silverman PM, Godwin JD. CT/bronchographic correlations in bronchiectasis. *J Comput Assist Tomogr* 1987;11:52–56.

62. Young K, Aspestrand F, Kolbenstvedt A. High resolution CT and bronchography in the assessment of bronchiectasis. *Acta Radiol* 1991;32:439–441.

63. Ward S, Heyneman L, Lee MJ, et al. Accuracy of CT in the diagnosis of allergic bronchopulmonary aspergillosis in asthmatic patients. *AJR Am J Roentgenol* 1999;173:937–942.

64. Kim JS, Müller NL, Park CS, et al. Cylindric bronchiectasis: diagnostic findings on thin-section CT. *AJR Am J Roentgenol* 1997;168:751–754.

65. Park CS, Müller NL, Worthy SA, et al. Airway obstruction in asthmatic and healthy individuals: inspiratory and expiratory thin-section CT findings. *Radiology* 1997;203:361–367.

66. Lynch DA. Imaging of asthma and allergic bronchopulmonary mycosis. *Rad Clin N Amer* 1998;36:129–142.

67. Reiff DB, Wells AU, Carr DH, et al. CT findings in bronchiectasis: limited value in distinguishing between idiopathic and specific types. *AJR Am J Roentgenol* 1995;165:261–267.

68. Desai SR, Wells AU, Cheah FK, et al. The reproducibility of bronchial circumference measurements using CT. *Br J Radiol* 1994;67:257–262.

69. Seneterre E, Paganin F, Bruel JM, et al. Measurement of the internal size of bronchi using high resolution computed tomography (HRCT). *Eur Respir J* 1994;7:596–600.

70. Murata K, Itoh H, Todo G, et al. Centrilobular lesions of the lung: demonstration by high-resolution CT and pathologic correlation. *Radiology* 1986;161:641–645.

71. Webb WR, Stein MG, Finkbeiner WE, et al. Normal and diseased isolated lungs: high-resolution CT. *Radiology* 1988;166:81–87.

72. Weibel ER. High resolution computed tomography of the pulmonary parenchyma: anatomical background. Presented at: Fleischner Society Symposium on Chest Disease, Scottsdale, Arizona; 1990.

73. Weibel ER, Taylor CR. Design and structure of the human lung. In: Fishman AP, ed. *Pulmonary diseases and disorders*. New York: McGraw-Hill, 1988:11–60.

74. Bhalla M, Turcios N, Aponte V, et al. Cystic fibrosis: scoring system with thin-section CT. *Radiology* 1991;179:783–788.

75. Remy-Jardin M, Remy J, Boulenguez C, et al. Morphologic effects of cigarette smoking on airways and pulmonary parenchyma in healthy adult volunteers: CT evaluation and correlation with pulmonary function tests. *Radiology* 1993;186:107–115.

76. Awadh N, Müller NL, Park CS, et al. Airway wall thickness in patients with near fatal asthma and control groups: assessment with high resolution computed tomographic scanning. *Thorax* 1998;53:248–253.

77. Bankier AA, Fleischmann D, De Maertelaer V, et al. Subjective differentiation of normal and pathologic bronchi on thin-section CT: impact of observer training. *Eur Respir J* 1999;13:781–786.

78. Naidich DP, Rumancik WM, Ettenger NA, et al. Congenital anomalies of the lungs in adults: MR diagnosis. *AJR Am J Roentgenol* 1988;151:13–19.

79. Pugatch RD, Gale ME. Obscure pulmonary masses: bronchial impaction revealed by CT. *AJR Am J Roentgenol* 1983;141:909–914.

80. Rappaport DC, Herman SJ, Weisbrod GL. Congenital bronchopulmonary diseases in adults: CT findings. *AJR Am J Roentgenol* 1994;162:1295–1299.

81. Ikezoe J, Murayama S, Godwin JD, et al. Bronchopulmonary sequestration: CT assessment. *Radiology* 1990;176:375–379.

82. Finck S, Milne ENC. A case report of segmental bronchial atresia: radiologic evaluation including computed tomography and magnetic resonance. *J Thorac Imag* 1988;3:53–58.

83. Ward S, Morcos SK. Congenital bronchial atresia—presentation of three cases and a pictorial review. *Clin Radiol* 1999;54:144–148.

84. Aquino SL, Gamsu G, Webb WR, et al. Tree-in-bud pattern: frequency and significance on thin section CT. *J Comput Assist Tomogr* 1996;20:594–599.

85. Gruden JF, Webb WR, Warnock M. Centrilobular opacities in the lung on high-resolution CT: diagnostic considerations and pathologic correlation. *AJR Am J Roentgenol* 1994;162:569–574.

86. Gruden JF, Webb WR. Identification and evaluation of centrilobular opacities on high-resolution CT. *Semin Ultrasound CT MR* 1995;16:435–449.

87. Murata K, Khan A, Herman PG. Pulmonary parenchymal disease: evaluation with high-resolution CT. *Radiology* 1989;170:629–635.

88. Nishimura K, Kitaichi M, Izumi T, et al. Diffuse panbronchiolitis: correlation of high-resolution CT and pathologic findings. *Radiology* 1992;184:779–785.

89. Akira M, Kitatani F, Lee Y-S, et al. Diffuse panbronchiolitis: evaluation with high-resolution CT. *Radiology* 1988;168:433–438.

90. Hansell DM, Wells AU, Rubens MB, et al. Bronchiectasis: functional significance of areas of decreased attenuation at expiratory CT. *Radiology* 1994;193:369–374.

91. Roberts HR, Wells AU, Milne DG, et al. Airflow obstruction in bronchiectasis: correlation between computed tomography features and pulmonary function tests. *Thorax* 2000;55:198–204.

92. Furuse M, Saito K, Kunieda E, et al. Bronchial arteries: CT demonstration with arteriographic correlation. *Radiology* 1987;162:393–398.

93. Murayama S, Hashiguchi N, Murakami J, et al. Helical CT imaging of bronchial arteries with curved reformation technique in comparison with selective bronchial arteriography: preliminary report. *J Comput Assist Tomogr* 1996;20:749–755.

94. Song JW, Im JG, Shim YS, et al. Hypertrophied bronchial artery at thin-section CT in patients with bronchiectasis: correlation with CT angiographic findings. *Radiology* 1998;208:187–191.

95. Reid LM. Reduction in bronchial subdivision in bronchiectasis. *Thorax* 1950;5:233–236.

96. Annest LS, Kratz JM, Crawford FA. Current results of treatment of bronchiectasis. *J Thorac Cardiovasc Surg* 1982;83:546–550.

97. Naidich DP. High-resolution computed tomography of cystic lung disease. *Semin Roentgenol* 1991;26:151–174.

98. Lynch DA, Newell J, Hale V, et al. Correlation of CT findings with clinical evaluations in 261 patients with symptomatic bronchiectasis. *AJR Am J Roentgenol* 1999;173:53–58.

99. Maffessanti M, Candusso M, Brizzi F, et al. Cystic fibrosis in children: HRCT findings and distribution of disease. *J Thorac Imag* 1996;11:27–38.

100. Shah RM, Sexauer W, Ostrum BJ, et al. High-resolution CT in the acute exacerbation of cystic fibrosis: evaluation of acute findings, reversibility of those findings, and clinical correlation. *AJR Am J Roentgenol* 1997;169:375–380.

101. Cartier Y, Kavanagh PV, Johkoh T, et al. Bronchiectasis: accuracy of high-resolution CT in the differentiation of specific diseases. *AJR Am J Roentgenol* 1999;173:47–52.

102. Helbich TH, Heinz-Peer G, Eichler I, et al. Cystic fibrosis: CT assessment of lung involvement in children and adults. *Radiology* 1999;213:537–544.

103. Helbich TH, Heinz-Peer G, Fleischmann D, et al. Evolution of CT findings in patients with cystic fibrosis. *AJR Am J Roentgenol* 1999;173:81–88.

104. Mayo JR, Webb WR, Gould R, et al. High-resolution CT of the lungs: an optimal approach. *Radiology* 1987;163:507–510.

105. King GG, Müller NL, Pare PD. Evaluation of airways in obstructive pulmonary disease using high-resolution computed tomography. *Am J Respir Crit Care Med* 1999;159:992–1004.

106. Webb WR, Gamsu G, Wall SD, et al. CT of a bronchial phantom: factors affecting appearance and size measurements. *Invest Radiol* 1984;19:394–398.

107. McNamara AE, Muller NL, Okazawa M, et al. Airway narrowing in excised canine lungs measured by high-resolution computed tomography. *J Appl Physiol* 1992;73:307–316.

108. Bankier AA, Fleischmann D, Mallek R, et al. Bronchial wall thickness: Appropriate window settings for thin-section CT and radiologic-anatomic correlation. *Radiology* 1996;199:831–836.

109. Grenier P, Maurice F, Musset D, et al. Bronchiectasis: assessment by thin-section CT. *Radiology* 1986;161:95–99.

110. Giron J, Skaff F, Maubon A, et al. The value of thin-section CT scans in the diagnosis and staging of bronchiectasis: comparison with bronchography in a series of fifty-four patients. *Ann Radiol* 1988;31:25–33.

111. Remy-Jardin M, Remy J. Comparison of vertical and oblique CT in evaluation of the bronchial tree. *J Comput Assist Tomogr* 1988;12:956–962.

112. Zwirewich CV, Mayo JR, Müller NL. Low-dose high-resolution CT of lung parenchyma. *Radiology* 1991;180:413–417.

113. van der Bruggen-Bogaarts BA, van der Bruggen HM, van Waes PF, et al. Assessment of bronchiectasis: comparison of HRCT and spiral volumetric CT. *J Comput Assist Tomogr* 1996;20:15–19.

114. Remy-Jardin M, Remy J, Artaud D, et al. Volume rendering of the tracheobronchial tree: clinical evaluation of bronchographic images. *Radiology* 1998;208:761–770.

115. Naidich DP, Gruden JF, McGuinness G, et al. Volumetric (helical/spiral) CT (VCT) of the airways. *J Thorac Imag* 1997;12:11–28.

116. Arakawa H, Webb WR. Expiratory high-resolution CT scan. *Radiol Clin North Am* 1998;36:189–209.

117. Arakawa H, Webb WR. Air-trapping on expiratory high-resolution CT scans in the absence of inspiratory scan abnormalities: correlation with pulmonary function tests and differential diagnosis. *AJR Am J Roentgenol* 1998;170:1349–1353.

118. Stern EJ, Graham CM, Webb WR, et al. Normal trachea during forced expiration: dynamic CT measurements. *Radiology* 1993;187:27–31.

119. Gotway MB, Lee ES, Reddy GP, et al. Low-dose, dynamic expiratory high-resolution CT using a spiral scanner. *J Thorac Imag (in press)*.

120. Remy-Jardin M, Remy J, Gosselin B, et al;. Sliding thin slab, minimum intensity projection technique in the diagnosis of emphysema: histopathologic-CT correlation. *Radiology* 1996;200:665–671.

121. Fotheringham T, Chabat F, Hansell DM, et al. A comparison of methods for enhancing the detection of areas of decreased attenuation on CT caused by airways disease. *J Comput Assist Tomogr* 1999;23:385–389.

122. Wittram C, Rappaport DC. Case report: expiratory helical CT scan minimum intensity projection imaging in cystic fibrosis. *Clin Radiol* 1998;53:615–616.

123. Tarver RD, Conces DJ, Godwin JD. Motion artifacts on CT simulate bronchiectasis. *AJR Am J Roentgenol* 1988;151:1117–1119.

124. Mansour Y, Beck R, Danino J, et al. Resolution of severe bronchiectasis after removal of long-standing retained foreign body. *Pediatr Pulmonol* 1998;25:130–132.

125. Westcott JL, Cole SR. Traction bronchiectasis in end-stage pulmonary fibrosis. *Radiology* 1986;161:665–669.

126. van der Bruggen-Bogaarts BA, van der Bruggen HM, van Waes PF, et al. Screening for bronchiectasis: a comparative study between chest radiography and high-resolution CT. *Chest* 1996;109:608–611.

127. Phillips MS, Williams MP, Flower CDR. How useful is computed tomography in the diagnosis and assessment of bronchiectasis? *Clin Rad* 1986;37:321–325.

128. Müller NL, Bergin CJ, Ostrow DN, et al. Role of computed tomography in the recognition of bronchiectasis. *AJR Am J Roentgenol* 1984;143:971–976.

129. Mootoosamy IM, Reznek RH, Osman J. Assessment of bronchiectasis by computed tomography. *Thorax* 1985;40:920–924.

130. Munro NC, Cooke JC, Currie DC, et al. Comparison of thin section computed tomography with bronchography for identifying bronchiectatic segments in patients with chronic sputum production. *Thorax* 1990;45:135–139.

131. Grenier P, Lenoir S, Brauner M. Computed tomographic assessment of bronchiectasis. *Semin Ultrasound CT MR* 1990;11:430–441.

132. Lee PH, Carr DH, Rubens MB, et al. Accuracy of CT in predicting the cause of bronchiectasis. *Clin Radiol* 1995;50:839–841.

133. Curtin JJ, Webster AD, Farrant J, et al. Bronchiectasis in hypogammaglobulinaemia—a computed tomography assessment. *Clin Radiol* 1991;44:82–84.

134. Wood BP. Cystic fibrosis: 1997. *Radiology* 1997;204:1–10.

135. Stern RC. The diagnosis of cystic fibrosis. *N Engl J Med* 1997;336:487–491.

136. Friedman PJ. Chest radiographic findings in the adult with cystic fibrosis. *Semin Roentgenol* 1987;22:114–124.

137. Reinig JW, Sanchez FW, Thomason DM, et al. The distinctly visible right upper lobe bronchus on the lateral chest: a clue to adolescent cystic fibrosis. *Pediatr Radiol* 1985;15:222–224.

138. Schwartz EE, Holsclaw DS. Pulmonary involvement in adults with cystic fibrosis. *AJR Am J Roentgenol* 1974;122:708–718.

139. Greene KE, Takasugi JE, Godwin JD, et al. Radiographic changes in acute exacerbations of cystic fibrosis in adults: a pilot study. *AJR Am J Roentgenol* 1994;163:557–562.

140. Hansell DM, Strickland B. High-resolution computed tomography in pulmonary cystic fibrosis. *Br J Radiol* 1989;62:1–5.

141. Lynch DA, Brasch RC, Hardy KA, et al. Pediatric pulmonary disease: assessment with high-resolution ultrafast CT. *Radiology* 1990;176:243–248.

142. Santis G, Hodson ME, Strickland B. High resolution computed tomography in adult cystic fibrosis patients with mild lung disease. *Clin Radiol* 1991;44:20–22.

143. Taccone A, Romano L, Marzoli A, et al. Computerized tomography in pulmonary cystic fibrosis. *Radiol Med (Torino)* 1991;82:79–83.

144. Nathanson I, Conboy K, Murphy S, et al. Ultrafast computerized tomography of the chest in cystic fibrosis: a new scoring system. *Pediatr Pulmonol* 1991;11:81–86.

145. Shah RM, Friedman AC, Ostrum BJ, et al. Pulmonary complications of cystic fibrosis in adults. *Crit Rev Diagn Imaging* 1995;36:441–477.

146. Marom EM, McAdams HP, Palmer SM, et al. Cystic fibrosis: usefulness of thoracic CT in the examination of patients before lung transplantation. *Radiology* 1999;213:283–288.

147. American Thoracic Society. Standards for the diagnosis and care of patients with chronic obstructive pulmonary disease (COPD) and asthma. *Am Rev Respir Dis* 1987;136:225–243.

148. Jeffery PK. Comparative morphology of the airways in asthma and chronic obstructive pulmonary disease. *Am J Respir Crit Care Med* 1994;150:S6–S13.

149. Hodson ME, Simon G, Batten JC. Radiology of uncomplicated asthma. *Thorax* 1974;29:296–303.

150. Zieverink SA, Harper AP, Holden RW, et al. Emergency room radiology in asthma: an efficacy study. *Radiology* 1982;145:27–29.

151. Blair DN, Coppage L, Shaw C. Medical imaging in asthma. *J Thorac Imag* 1986;1:23–35.

152. Paganin F, Trussard V, Seneterre E, et al. Chest radiography and high resolution computed tomography of the lungs in asthma. *Am Rev Respir Dis* 1992;146:1084–1087.

153. Sherman S, Skoney JA, Ravikrishnan KP. Routine chest radiographs in exacerbations of chronic obstructive pulmonary disease: diagnostic value. *Arch Intern Med* 1989;149:2493–2496.

154. Gershel JC, Goldman HS, Stein REK, et al. The usefulness of chest radiographs in first asthma attacks. *N Engl J Med* 1983;309:336–339.

155. Kinsella M, Müller NL, Staples C, et al. Hyperinflation in asthma and emphysema: assessment by pulmonary function testing and computed tomography. *Chest* 1988;94:286–289.

156. Kondoh Y, Taniguchi H, Yokoyama S, et al. Emphysematous change in chronic asthma in relation to cigarette smoking: assessment by computed tomography. *Chest* 1990;97:845–849.

157. Grenier P, Mourey-Gerosa I, Benali K, et al. Abnormalities of the airways and lung parenchyma in asthmatics: CT observations in 50 patients and inter- and intraobserver variability. *Eur Radiol* 1996;6:199–206.

158. Kee ST, Fahy JV, Chen DR, et al. High-resolution computed tomography of airway changes after induced bronchoconstriction and bronchodilation in asthmatic volunteers. *Acad Radiol* 1996;3:389–394.

159. Park JW, Hong YK, Kim CW, et al. High-resolution computed tomography in patients with bronchial asthma: correlation with clinical features, pulmonary functions and bronchial hyperresponsiveness. *J Investig Allergol Clin Immunol* 1997;7:186–192.

160. Newman KB, Lynch DA, Newman LS, et al. Quantitative computed tomography detects air-trapping due to asthma. *Chest* 1994;106:105–109.

161. Webb WR. High-resolution computed tomography of obstructive lung disease. *Rad Clin N Am* 1994;32:745–757.

162. Zhaoming W, Lockey RF. A review of allergic bronchopulmonary aspergillosis. *J Investig Allergol Clin Immunol* 1996;6:144–151.

163. Geller DE, Kaplowitz H, Light MJ, et al. Allergic bronchopulmonary aspergillosis in cystic fibrosis: reported prevalence, regional distribution, and patient characteristics. Scientific Advisory Group, Investigators, and Coordinators of the Epidemiologic Study of Cystic Fibrosis. *Chest* 1999;116:639–646.

164. Currie DC, Goldman JM, Cole PJ, et al;. Comparison of narrow section computed tomography and plain chest radiography in chronic allergic bronchopulmonary aspergillosis. *Clin Radiol* 1987;38:593–596.

165. Shah A, Pant CS, Bhagat R, et al. CT in childhood allergic bronchopulmonary aspergillosis. *Pediatr Radiol* 1992;22:227–228.

166. Sandhu M, Mukhopadhyay S, Sharma SK. Allergic bronchopulmonary aspergillosis: a comparative evaluation of computed tomography with plain chest radiography. *Australas Radiol* 1994;38:288–293.

167. Angus RM, Davies ML, Cowan MD, et al. Computed tomographic scanning of the lung in patients with allergic bronchopulmonary aspergillosis and in asthmatic patients with a positive skin test to Aspergillus fumigatus. *Thorax* 1994;49:586–589.

168. Panchal N, Pant C, Bhagat R, et al. Central bronchiectasis in allergic bronchopulmonary aspergillosis: comparative evaluation of computed tomography with bronchography. *Eur Respir J* 1994;7:1290–1293.

169. Panchal N, Bhagat R, Pant C, et al. Allergic bronchopulmonary aspergillosis: the spectrum of computed tomography appearances. *Respir Med* 1997;91:213–219.

170. Roberts CM, Citron KM, Strickland B. Intrathoracic aspergilloma: role of CT in diagnosis and treatment. *Radiology* 1987;165:123–128.

171. Logan PM, Muller NL. CT manifestations of pulmonary aspergillosis. *Crit Rev Diagn Imaging* 1996;37:1–37.

172. Logan PM, Muller NL. High-resolution computed tomography and pathologic findings in pulmonary aspergillosis: a pictorial essay. *Can Assoc Radiol J* 1996;47:444–452.

173. Goyal R, White CS, Templeton PA, et al. High attenuation mucous plugs in allergic bronchopulmonary aspergillosis: CT appearance. *J Comput Assist Tomogr* 1992;16:649–650.

174. Logan PM, Müller NL. High-attenuation mucous plugging in allergic bronchopulmonary aspergillosis. *Can Assoc Radiol J* 1996;47:374–377.

175. Zinreich SJ, Kennedy DW, Malat J, et al. Fungal sinusitis: diagnosis with CT and MR imaging. *Radiology* 1988;169:439–444.

176. Logan PM, Primack SL, Miller RR, et al. Invasive aspergillosis of the airways: radiographic, CT, and pathologic findings. *Radiology* 1994;193:383–388.

177. Choplin RH, Wehunt WD, Theros EG. Diffuse lesions of the trachea. *Semin Roentgenol* 1983;18:38–50.

178. Schwartz M, Rossoff L. Tracheobronchomegaly. *Chest* 1994;106:1589–1590.

179. Dunne MG, Reiner B. CT features of tracheobronchomegaly. *J Comput Assist Tomogr* 1988;12:388–391.

180. Roditi GH, Weir J. The association of tracheomegaly and bronchiectasis. *Clin Radiol* 1994;49:608–611.

181. Woodring JH, Barrett PA, Rehm SR, et al. Acquired tracheomegaly in adults as a complication of diffuse pulmonary fibrosis. *AJR Am J Roentgenol* 1989;152:743–747.

182. Shin MS, Jackson RM, Ho KJ. Tracheobronchomegaly (Mounier-Kuhn syndrome): CT diagnosis. *AJR Am J Roentgenol* 1988;150:777–779.

183. Kwong JS, Müller NL, Miller RR. Diseases of the trachea and mainstem bronchi: correlation of CT with pathologic findings. *Radiographics* 1992;12:647–657.

184. Webb EM, Elicker BM, Webb WR. Using CT to diagnose nonneoplastic tracheal abnormalities: appearance of the tracheal wall. *AJR Am J Roentgenol* 2000;174:1315–1321.

185. Kaneko K, Kudo S, Tashiro M, et al. Computed tomography findings in Williams-Campbell syndrome. *J Thorac Imag* 1991;6:11–13.

186. Watanabe Y, Nishiyama Y, Kanayama H, et al. Congenital bronchiectasis due to cartilage deficiency: CT demonstration. *J Comput Assist Tomogr* 1987;11:701–703.

187. King MA, Stone JA, Diaz PT, et al. Alpha 1-antitrypsin deficiency: evaluation of bronchiectasis with CT. *Radiology* 1996;199:137–141.

188. Cohen M, Sahn SA. Bronchiectasis in systemic diseases. *Chest* 1999;116:1063–1074.

189. Remy-Jardin M, Remy J, Cortet B, et al. Lung changes in rheumatoid arthritis: CT findings. *Radiology* 1994;193:375–382.

190. McDonagh J, Greaves M, Wright AR, et al. High resolution computed tomography of the lungs in patients with rheumatoid arthritis and interstitial lung disease. *Br J Rheumatol* 1994;33:118–122.

191. Hassan WU, Keaney NP, Holland CD, et al. High resolution computed tomography of the lung in lifelong non-smoking patients with rheumatoid arthritis. *Ann Rheum Dis* 1995;54:308–310.

192. Perez T, Remy-Jardin M, Cortet B. Airways involvement in rheumatoid arthritis: clinical, functional, and HRCT findings. *Am J Respir Crit Care Med* 1998;157:1658–1665.

193. Geddes DM, Webley M, Emerson PA. Airways obstruction in rheumatoid arthritis. *Ann Rheum Dis* 1979;38:222–225.

194. Aquino SL, Webb WR, Golden J. Bronchiolitis obliterans associated with rheumatoid arthritis: findings on HRCT and dynamic expiratory CT. *J Comput Assist Tomogr* 1994;18:555–558.

195. Swinson DR, Symmons D, Suresh U, et al. Decreased survival in patients with coexistent rheumatoid arthritis and bronchiectasis. *Br J Rheumatol* 1997;36:689–691.

196. Fenlon HM, Doran M, Sant SM, et al. High-resolution chest CT in systemic lupus erythematosus. *AJR Am J Roentgenol* 1996;166:301–307.

197. Bankier AA, Kiener HP, Wiesmayr MN, et al. Discrete lung involvement in systemic lupus erythematosus: CT assessment. *Radiology* 1995;196:835–840.

198. Franquet T, Giménez A, Monill JM, et al. Primary Sjögren's syndrome and associated lung disease: CT findings in 50 patients. *AJR Am J Roentgenol* 1997;169:655–658.

199. McGuinness G, Gruden JF, Bhalla M, et al. AIDS-related airways disease. *AJR Am J Roentgenol* 1997;168:67–77.

200. Verghese A, al-Samman M, Nabhan D, et al. Bacterial bronchitis and bronchiectasis in human immunodeficiency virus infection. *Arch Intern Med* 1994;154:2086–2091.

201. Holmes AH, Trotman-Dickenson B, Edwards A, et al. Bronchiectasis in HIV disease. *Q J Med* 1992;85:875–882.

202. Moskovic E, Miller R, Pearson M. High resolution computed tomography of Pneumocystis carinii pneumonia in AIDS. *Clin Radiol* 1990;42:239–243.
203. Hirschtick RE, Glassroth J, Jordan MC, et al. Bacterial pneumonia in persons infected with the human immunodeficiency virus: Pulmonary Complications of HIV Infection Study Group [see comments]. *N Engl J Med* 1995;333:845–851.
204. Markowitz GS, Concepcion L, Factor SM, et al. Autopsy patterns of disease among subgroups of an inner-city Bronx AIDS population. *J Acquir Immune Defic Syndr Hum Retrovirol* 1996;13:48–54.
205. Wallace JM, Hansen NI, Lavange L, et al. Respiratory disease trends in the Pulmonary Complications of HIV Infection Study cohort: Pulmonary Complications of HIV Infection Study Group. *Am J Respir Crit Care Med* 1997;155:72–80.
206. Gelman M, King MA, Neal DE, et al. Focal air-trapping in patients with HIV infection: CT evaluation and correlation with pulmonary function test results. *AJR Am J Roentgenol* 1999;172:1033–1038.
207. Klapholz A, Salomon N, Perlman DC, et al. Aspergillosis in the acquired immunodeficiency syndrome. *Chest* 1991;100:1614–1618.
208. Denning DW. Aspergillus tracheobronchitis [letter; comment]. *Clin Infect Dis* 1994;19:1176–1177.
209. Staples CA, Kang EY, Wright JL, et al. Invasive pulmonary aspergillosis in AIDS: radiographic, CT, and pathologic findings. *Radiology* 1995;196:409–414.
210. Wright JL, Lawson L, Chan N, et al. An unusual form of pulmonary aspergillosis in two patients with the acquired immunodeficiency syndrome. *Am J Clin Pathol* 1993;100:57–59.
211. King TE. Overview of bronchiolitis. *Clin Chest Med* 1993;14:607–610.
212. Colby TV. Bronchiolitis. Pathologic considerations. *Am J Clin Pathol* 1998;109:101–109.
213. Myers J. Respiratory bronchiolitis with interstitial lung disease. *Sem Resp Med* 1992;13:134–139.
214. Yousem SA, Colby TV, Gaensler EA. Respiratory bronchiolitis-associated interstitial lung disease and its relationship to desquamative interstitial pneumonia. *Mayo Clin Proc* 1989;64:1373–1380.
215. Heyneman LE, Ward S, Lynch DA, et al. Respiratory bronchiolitis, respiratory bronchiolitis-associated interstitial pneumonia: different entities or part of the spectrum of the same disease process? *AJR Am J Roentgenol* 1999;173:1617–1622.
216. Moon J, du Bois RM, Colby TV, et al. Clinical significance of respiratory bronchiolitis on open lung biopsy and its relationship to smoking-related interstitial lung disease. *Thorax* 1999;54:1009–1014.
217. Niewoehner DE, Kleinerman J, Rice DB. Pathologic changes in the peripheral airways of young cigarette smokers. *N Engl J Med* 1974;291:755–758.
218. Myers JL, Colby TV. Pathologic manifestations of bronchiolitis, constrictive bronchiolitis, cryptogenic organizing pneumonia and diffuse panbronchiolitis. *Clin Chest Med* 1993;14:611–623.
219. Katzenstein AL. *Katzenstein and Askin's surgical pathology of non-neoplastic lung disease*, 3rd ed. Philadelphia: WB Saunders, 1997.
220. Davidson AG, Heard BE, McAllister WC, et al. Cryptogenic organizing pneumonitis. *Q J Med* 1983;52:382–393.
221. Epler GR, Colby TV, McLoud TC, et al. Bronchiolitis obliterans organizing pneumonia. *N Engl J Med* 1985;312:152–158.
222. Epler GR. Bronchiolitis obliterans organizing pneumonia: definition and clinical features. *Chest* 1992;102(S):2–6.
223. Yoshinouchi T, Ohtsuki Y, Kubo K, et al. Clinicopathologic study on two types of cryptogenic organizing pneumonitis. *Respir Med* 1995;89:271–278.
224. King TE Jr. BOOP: an important cause of migratory pulmonary infiltrates? [editorial; comment]. *Eur Respir J* 1995;8:193–195.
225. Colby TV, Myers JL. The clinical and histologic spectrum of bronchiolitis obliterans including bronchiolitis obliterans organizing pneumonia (BOOP). *Semin Respir Dis* 1992;13:119–133.
226. Matsuse T, Oka T, Kida K, et al. Importance of diffuse aspiration bronchiolitis caused by chronic occult aspiration in the elderly. *Chest* 1996;110:1289–1293.
227. Miller RR, Muller NL. Neuroendocrine cell hyperplasia and obliterative bronchiolitis in patients with peripheral carcinoid tumors. *Am J Surg Pathol* 1995;19:653–658.
228. Bartter T, Irwin RS, Nash G, et al. Idiopathic bronchiolitis obliterans organizing pneumonia with peripheral infiltrates on chest roentgenogram. *Arch Intern Med* 1989;149:273–279.
229. Bouchardy LM, Kuhlman JE, Ball WC, et al. CT findings in bronchiolitis obliterans organizing pneumonia (BOOP) with radiographic, clinical, and histologic correlation. *J Comput Assist Tomogr* 1993;17:352–357.
230. Garg K, Newell JD, King TE, et al. Proliferative and constrictive bronchiolitis: classification and radiologic features. *AJR Am J Roentgenol* 1994;162:803–808.
231. Hansell DM. What are bronchiolitis obliterans organizing pneumonia (BOOP) and cryptogenic organizing pneumonia (COP)? *Clin Radiol* 1992;45:369–370.
232. Keller CA, Cagle PT, Brown RW, et al. Bronchiolitis obliterans in recipients of single, double, and heart-lung transplantation. *Chest* 1995;107:973–980.
233. Nishimura K, Itoh H. High-resolution computed tomographic features of bronchiolitis obliterans organizing pneumonia. *Chest* 1992;102:26S–31S.
234. Padley SPG, Adler BD, Hansell DM, et al. Bronchiolitis obliterans: high-resolution CT findings and correlation with pulmonary function tests. *Clin Radiol* 1993;47:236–240.
235. Remy-Jardin M, Remy J, Gosselin B, et al. Lung parenchymal changes secondary to cigarette smoking: pathologic-CT correlations. *Radiology* 1993;186:643–651.
236. Wells AU, duBois RM. Bronchiolitis in association with connective tissue diseases. *Clin Chest Med* 1993;14:655–666.
237. Webb WR. Radiology of obstructive pulmonary disease. *AJR Am J Roentgenol* 1997;169:637–647.
238. Jeffery PK. The development of large and small airways. *Am J Respir Crit Care Med* 1998;157:S174–S180.
239. Hogg JC, Macklem PT, Thurlbeck WM. Site and nature of airway obstruction in chronic obstructive lung disease. *N Engl J Med* 1968;278:1355–1360.
240. Macklem PT, Mead J. Resistance of central and peripheral airways measured by a retrograde catheter. *J Appl Physiol* 1967;22:395–401.
241. Desai SR, Hansell DM. Small airways disease: expiratory computed tomography comes of age. *Clin Radiol* 1997;52:332–337.
242. Yang CF, Wu MT, Chiang AA, et al. Correlation of high-resolution CT and pulmonary function in bronchiolitis obliterans: a study based on 24 patients associated with consumption of *Sauropus Androgynus*. *AJR Am J Roentgenol* 1997;168:1045–1050.
243. Akira M, Sakatani M, Hara H. Thin-section CT findings in rheumatoid arthritis-associated lung disease: CT patterns and their courses. *J Comput Assist Tomogr* 1999;23:941–948.
244. Howling SJ, Hansell DM, Wells AU, et al. Follicular bronchiolitis: thin-section CT and histologic findings. *Radiology* 1999;212:637–642.
245. Kinoshita M, Higashi T, Tanaka C, et al. Follicular bronchiolitis associated with rheumatoid arthritis. *Intern Med* 1992;31:674–677.
246. Oh YW, Effmann EL, Redding GJ, et al. Follicular hyperplasia of bronchus-associated lymphoid tissue causing severe air-trapping. *AJR Am J Roentgenol* 1999;172:745–747.
247. Hayakawa H, Sato A, Imokawa S, et al. Bronchiolar disease in rheumatoid arthritis. *Am J Respir Crit Care Med* 1996;154:1531–1536.
248. Iwata M, Colby TV, Kitaichi M. Diffuse panbronchiolitis: diagnosis and distinction from various pulmonary diseases with centrilobular interstitial foam cell accumulations. *Hum Pathol* 1994;25:357–363.
249. Ichikawa Y, Hotta M, Sumita S, et al. Reversible airway lesions in diffuse panbronchiolitis: detection by high-resolution computed tomography. *Chest* 1995;107:120–125.
250. Holt RM, Schmidt RA, Godwin JD, et al. High resolution CT in respiratory bronchiolitis-associated interstitial lung disease. *J Comput Assist Tomogr* 1993;17:46–50.
251. Silver SF, Müller NL, Miller RR, et al. Hypersensitivity pneumonitis: evaluation with CT. *Radiology* 1989;173:441–445.
252. Adler BD, Padley SP, Müller NL, et al. Chronic hypersensitivity pneumonitis: high-resolution CT and radiographic features in 16 patients. *Radiology* 1992;185:91–95.
253. Akira M, Kita N, Higashihara T, et al. Summer-type hypersensitivity pneumonitis: comparison of high-resolution CT and plain radiographic findings. *AJR Am J Roentgenol* 1992;158:1223–1228.
254. Buschman DL, Gamsu G, Waldron JA, et al. Chronic hypersensitivity pneumonitis: use of CT in diagnosis. *AJR Am J Roentgenol* 1992;159:957–960.
255. Lynch DA, Rose CS, Way D, et al. Hypersensitivity pneumonitis: sensitivity of high-resolution CT in a population-based study. *AJR Am J Roentgenol* 1992;159:469–472.

256. Remy-Jardin M, Remy J, Wallaert B, et al. Subacute and chronic bird breeder hypersensitivity pneumonitis: sequential evaluation with CT and correlation with lung function tests and bronchoalveolar lavage. *Radiology* 1993;198:111–118.

257. Hansell DM, Wells AU, Padley SP, et al. Hypersensitivity pneumonitis: correlation of individual CT patterns with functional abnormalities. *Radiology* 1996;199:123–128.

258. Bramson RT, Cleveland R, Blickman JG, et al. Radiographic appearance of follicular bronchitis in children. *AJR Am J Roentgenol* 1996;166:1447–1450.

259. Yousem SA, Colby TV, Carrington CB. Follicular bronchitis/bronchiolitis. *Hum Pathol* 1985;16:700–706.

260. Remy-Jardin M, Remy J, Wallaert B, et al. Pulmonary involvement in progressive systemic sclerosis: sequential evaluation with CT, pulmonary function tests, and bronchoalveolar lavage. *Radiology* 1993;188:499–506.

261. Chang AB, Masel JP, Masters B. Post-infectious bronchiolitis obliterans: clinical, radiological and pulmonary function sequelae. *Pediatric Radiology* 1998;28:23–29.

262. Chang H, Wang JS, Tseng HH, et al. Histopathologic study of *Sauropus androgynus*-associated constrictive bronchiolitis obliterans: a new cause of constrictive bronchiolitis obliterans [see comments]. *Am J Surg Pathol* 1997;21:35–42.

263. Brown MJ, English J, Müller NL. Bronchiolitis obliterans due to neuroendocrine hyperplasia: high-resolution CT—pathologic correlation. *AJR Am J Roentgenol* 1997;168:1561–1562.

264. Epler GR, Colby TV, McLoud TC, et al. Idiopathic bronchiolitis obliterans with organizing pneumonia. *N Engl J Med* 1985;312:152–159.

265. Müller NL, Guerry-Force ML, Staples CA, et al. Differential diagnosis of bronchiolitis obliterans with organizing pneumonia and usual interstitial pneumonia: clinical, functional, and radiologic findings. *Radiology* 1987;162:151–156.

266. Cordier JF, Loire R, Brune J. Idiopathic bronchiolitis obliterans organizing pneumonia. *Chest* 1989;96:999–1005.

267. Lee KS, Kullnig P, Hartman TE, et al. Cryptogenic organizing pneumonia: CT findings in 43 patients. *AJR Am J Roentgenol* 1994;162:543–546.

268. Müller NL, Staples CA, Miller RR. Bronchiolitis obliterans organizing pneumonia: CT features in 14 patients. *AJR Am J Roentgenol* 1990;154:983–987.

269. Akira M, Yamamoto S, Sakatani M. Bronchiolitis obliterans organizing pneumonia manifesting as multiple large nodules or masses. *AJR Am J Roentgenol* 1998;170:291–295.

270. Gosink BB, Friedman PJ, Liebow AA. Bronchiolitis obliterans: roentgenographic-pathologic correlation. *AJR Am J Roentgenol* 1973;117:816–832.

271. Laraya-Cuasay LR, DeForest A, Huff D, et al. Chronic pulmonary complications of early influenza virus infection in children. *Am Rev Respir Dis* 1977;116:617–625.

272. Nikki P, Meretoja O, Valtonen V, et al. Severe bronchiolitis probably caused by varicella-zoster virus. *Crit Care Med* 1982;10:344–346.

273. Ezri T, Kunichezky S, Eliraz A, et al. Bronchiolitis obliterans—current concepts. *Q J Med* 1994;87:1–10.

274. Penn CC, Liu C. Bronchiolitis following infection in adults and children. *Clin Chest Med* 1993;14:645–654.

275. Epler GR, Colby TV. The spectrum of bronchiolitis obliterans. *Chest* 1983;83:161–162.

276. Lowry T, Schuman LM. "Silo-filler's disease" — a syndrome caused by nitrogen dioxide. *JAMA* 1956;162:153–158.

277. Cornelius EA, Betlach EH. Silo-filler's disease. *Radiology* 1960;74:232–235.

278. Charan NB, Myers CG, Lakshminarayan S, et al. Pulmonary injuries associated with acute sulfur dioxide inhalation. *Am Rev Respir Dis* 1979;119:555–560.

279. St. John RC, Dorinsky PM. Cryptogenic bronchiolitis. *Clin Chest Med* 1993;14:667–675.

280. Kraft M, Mortenson R, Colby TV, et al. Cryptogenic constrictive bronchiolitis. *Am Rev Resp Dis* 1993;148:1093–1101.

281. Geddes DM, Corrin B, Brewerton DA, et al. Progressive airway obliteration in adults and its association with rheumatoid disease. *Q J Med* 1977;46:427–444.

282. Epler GR, Snider GL, Gaensler EA, et al. Bronchiolitis and bronchitis in connective tissue disease. *JAMA* 1979;242:528–532.

283. Herzog CA, Miller RR, Hoidal JR. Bronchiolitis and rheumatoid arthritis. *Am Rev Respir Dis* 1979;119:555–560.

284. Schwarz MI, Matthay RA, Sahn SA, et al. Interstitial lung disease in polymyositis and dermatomyositis: an analysis of six cases and review of the literature. *Medicine* 1976;55:89–104.

285. Ostrow D, Buskard N, Hills RS, et al. Bronchiolitis obliterans complicating bone marrow transplantation. *Chest* 1985;87:828–830.

286. Roca J, Granena A, Rodriguez-Roisin J, et al. Fatal airways disease in an adult with chronic graft-versus-host disease. *Thorax* 1982;37:77–78.

287. Stein-Streilen J, Lipscomb MF, Hart DA, et al. Graft-versus-host reaction in the lung. *Transplantation* 1981;32:38–44.

288. Burke CM, Theodore J, Dawkins KD, et al. Post transplant obliterative bronchiolitis and other late lung sequelae in human heart-lung transplantation. *Chest* 1984;86:824–829.

289. Paradis I, Yousem S, Griffith B. Airway obstruction and bronchiolitis obliterans after lung transplantation. *Clin Chest Med* 1993;14:751–763.

290. Aquino SL, Schechter MS, Chiles C, et al. High-resolution inspiratory and expiratory CT in older children and adults with bronchopulmonary dysplasia. *AJR Am J Roentgenol* 1999;173:963–967.

291. McLoud TC, Epler GR, Colby TV, et al. Bronchiolitis obliterans. *Radiology* 1986;159:1–8.

292. Breatnach E, Kerr I. The radiology of cryptogenic obliterative bronchiolitis. *Clin Radiol* 1982;33:657–661.

293. Marti-Bonmati L, Ruiz PF, Catala F, et al. CT findings in Swyer-James syndrome. *Radiology* 1989;172:477–480.

294. Sweatman MC, Millar AB, Strickland B, et al. Computed tomography in adult obliterative bronchiolitis. *Clin Radiol* 1990;41:116–119.

295. Zhang L, Irion K, da Silva Porto N, et al. High-resolution computed tomography in pediatric patients with postinfectious bronchiolitis obliterans. *J Thorac Imaging* 1999;14:85–89.

296. MacLeod EM. Abnormal transradiancy of one lung. *Thorax* 1954;9:147–153.

297. Swyer PR, James GCW. A case of unilateral pulmonary emphysema. *Thorax* 1953;8:133–136.

298. Reichenspurner H, Girgis RE, Robbins RC, et al. Obliterative bronchiolitis after lung and heart-lung transplantation. *Ann Thorac Surg* 1995;60:1845–1853.

299. Reichenspurner H, Girgis RE, Robbins RC, et al. Stanford experience with obliterative bronchiolitis after lung and heart-lung transplantation. *Ann Thorac Surg* 1996;62:1467–1472; discussion 1472–1473.

300. Nathan SD, Ross DJ, Belman MJ, et al. Bronchiolitis obliterans in single-lung transplant recipients [see comments]. *Chest* 1995;107:967–972.

301. Kramer MR, Stoehr C, Whang JL, et al. The diagnosis of obliterative bronchiolitis after heart-lung and lung transplantation: low yield of transbronchial lung biopsy. *J Heart Lung Transplant* 1993;12:675–681.

302. Yousem SA, Berry GJ, Cagle PT, et al. Revision of the 1990 working formulation for the classification of pulmonary allograft rejection: Lung Rejection Study Group. *J Heart Lung Transplant* 1996;15:1–15.

303. Chamberlain D, Maurer J, Chaparro C, et al. Evaluation of transbronchial lung biopsy specimens in the diagnosis of bronchiolitis obliterans after lung transplantation. *J Heart Lung Transplant* 1994;13:963–971.

304. Dauber JH. Posttransplant bronchiolitis obliterans syndrome. Where have we been and where are we going? [editorial; comment]. *Chest* 1996;109:857–859.

305. Cooper JD, Billingham M, Egan T, et al. A working formulation for the standardization of nomenclature and for clinical staging of chronic dysfunction in lung allografts. International Society for Heart and Lung Transplantation. *J Heart Lung Transplant* 1993;12:713–716.

306. Patterson GM, Wilson S, Whang JL, et al. Physiologic definitions of obliterative bronchiolitis in heart-lung and double lung transplantation: a comparison of the forced expiratory flow between 25% and 75% of the forced vital capacity and forced expiratory volume in one second. *J Heart Lung Transplant* 1996;15:175–181.

307. Shepard JA. Imaging of lung transplantation. *Clin Chest Med* 1999;20:827–844.

308. Loubeyre P, Revel D, Delignette A, et al. Bronchiectasis detected with thin-section CT as a predictor of chronic lung allograft rejection. *Radiology* 1995;194:213–216.

309. Worthy SA, Park CS, Kim JS, et al. Bronchiolitis obliterans after lung transplantation: high resolution CT findings in 15 patients. *AJR Am J Roentgenol* 1997;169:673–677.

310. Lee ES, Gotway MB, Reddy GP, et al. Expiratory high-resolution CT: accuracy for the diagnosis of early bronchiolitis obliterans following lung transplantation. *Radiology* (in press).

311. Leung AN, Fisher K, Valentine V, et al. Bronchiolitis obliterans after lung transplantation: detection using expiratory HRCT. *Chest* 1998;113:365–370.
312. Ikonen T, Kivisaari L, Harjula AL, et al. Value of high-resolution computed tomography in routine evaluation of lung transplantation recipients during development of bronchiolitis obliterans syndrome. *J Heart Lung Transplant* 1996;15:587–595.
313. Lau DM, Siegel MJ, Hildebolt CF, et al. Bronchiolitis obliterans syndrome: thin-section CT diagnosis of obstructive changes in infants and young children after lung transplantation. *Radiology* 1998;208:783–788.
314. Soubani AO, Miller KB, Hassoun PM. Pulmonary complications of bone marrow transplantation. *Chest* 1996;109:1066–1077.
315. Palmas A, Tefferi A, Myers JL, et al. Late-onset noninfectious pulmonary complications after allogeneic bone marrow transplantation. *Br J Haematol* 1998;100:680–687.
316. Worthy SA, Flint JD, Müller NL. Pulmonary complications after bone marrow transplantation: high-resolution CT and pathologic findings. *Radiographics* 1997;17:1359–1371.
317. Witte R, Gurney J, Robbins R, et al. Diffuse pulmonary alveolar hemorrhage after bone narrow transplantation: radiographic findings in 39 patients. *AJR Am J Roentgenol* 1991;157:461–464.
318. Wright JL, Cagle P, Churg A, et al. Diseases of the small airways. *Am Rev Respir Dis* 1992;146:240–262.
319. Ooi GC, Peh WC, Ip M. High-resolution computed tomography of bronchiolitis obliterans syndrome after bone marrow transplantation. *Respiration* 1998;65:187–191.
320. Mori M, Galvin JR, Barloon TJ, et al. Fungal pulmonary infections after bone marrow transplantation: evaluation with radiography and CT. *Radiology* 1991;178:721–726.
321. Akira M, Higashihara T, Sakatani M, et al. Diffuse panbronchiolitis: follow-up CT examination. *Radiology* 1993;189:559–562.
322. Murata K, Itoh H, Senda M, et al. Stratified impairment of pulmonary ventilation in "diffuse panbronchiolitis": PET and CT studies. *J Comput Assist Tomogr* 1989;13:48–53.
323. Sugiyama Y. Diffuse panbronchiolitis. *Clin Chest Med* 1993;14:765–772.

CHAPTER 9

Pulmonary Hypertension and Pulmonary Vascular Disease

Pulmonary hypertension (PH) and pulmonary vascular disease (PVD) are often associated with nonspecific symptoms of respiratory dysfunction and nonspecific pulmonary function test findings. PH may result from cardiac or pulmonary abnormalities, or vascular diseases primarily affecting the small arteries or veins. In most cases, PVD and PH are assessed using techniques and imaging modalities other than high-resolution computed tomography (HRCT). However, in some patients, HRCT may be performed to determine whether lung disease is present as a cause of the patient's disability or to evaluate specific small vessel diseases. If vascular disease is suspected, assessment of the lung using multidetector-row spiral HRCT with contrast infusion is an ideal technique (see Figs. 1-26 and 1-27). Furthermore, in patients who have known PH, HRCT may be performed when the etiology of the vascular disease is unclear. Only those vascular diseases commonly assessed using HRCT are described in this chapter.

HIGH-RESOLUTION COMPUTED TOMOGRAPHY FINDINGS OF PULMONARY VASCULAR DISEASE

PH and PVD may be associated with a number of findings on HRCT [1]. These include alterations in the size of large or small pulmonary arteries; mosaic perfusion, commonly seen in patients who have pulmonary vascular obstruction of various causes (see Chapter 3); pulmonary edema and hemorrhage (see Chapter 6); and cardiac abnormalities.

Pulmonary Artery Abnormalities

Of primary importance in making the diagnosis of PVD is the recognition of increased or decreased pulmonary artery (PA) diameter. The diameters of main, right and left, and intrapulmonary artery branches can be determined on HRCT obtained without contrast infusion in most cases, because these arteries are usually outlined by mediastinal fat or air-containing lung.

Increased Artery Diameter

Dilatation of the main PA usually indicates the presence of PH and can be an important finding in recognizing the presence of PVD on HRCT (Fig. 9-1). Even when HRCT scans are obtained at 2-cm intervals, at least one image traverses the main PA, allowing its measurement on soft-tissue window scans.

The main PA measures up to 30 mm in diameter in normal subjects. This measurement is best made at a right angle to the long axis of the PA, lateral to the ascending aorta, and near the level of its bifurcation. In a CT study of normal subjects by Guthaner et al. [2], the main PA diameter was found to average 28 ± 3 mm. Kuriyama et al. [3] measured PA diameters in both normal subjects and patients who have PH. In normals, the main PA averaged 24.2 ± 2.2 mm in diameter at a level near its bifurcation [3]. Based on this data, the authors concluded that 28.6 mm (mean plus 2 standard deviations) should be considered the upper limit of normal for main PA diameter; this value was found to accurately distinguish patients who have PH from normals. Also, Kuriyama et al. [3] found that the main PA diameter correlated well with PA pressure.

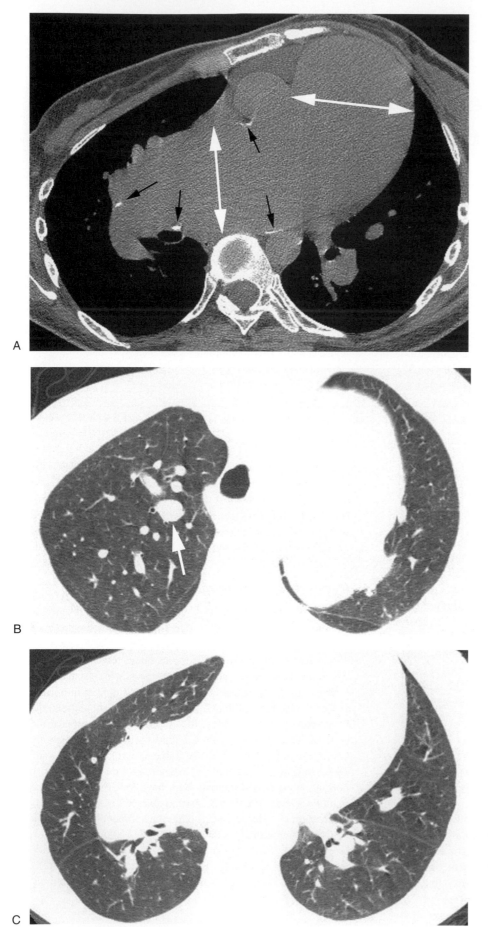

FIG. 9-1. A–C: Pulmonary hypertension in a patient with Eisenmenger's syndrome associated with congenital heart disease. HRCT was performed to exclude lung disease. **A:** Marked dilatation of the main pulmonary artery and right pulmonary artery is visible (*white arrows*). The main pulmonary artery is significantly larger than the aorta. Calcification of the artery wall (*black arrows*) reflects atherosclerosis. **B:** Enlargement of central pulmonary artery branches is also visible (*arrow*). **C:** Despite marked enlargement of central arteries, peripheral pulmonary vessels appear normal or reduced in diameter.

In a study of patients who had chronic lung disease or PVD [4] who were awaiting lung or heart-lung transplantation, considerably more overlap in PA diameter was seen between patients who had normal or elevated PA pressures. Main PA diameter measured 28 ± 7 mm in patients having normal PA pressure (less than or equal to 18 mm Hg) and 33 ± 11 mm in those who have PH (pressure greater than 18 mm Hg).

The diameter of the main PA may also be compared to that of the aorta; this is quickly and easily done on HRCT. In normals, the PA is usually smaller than the adjacent aorta. In a study by Ng et al. [5], the ratio of the diameter of the main PA to the aortic diameter (A) was measured using HRCT in 50 patients who had a variety of pulmonary and cardiovascular diseases, and also had PA pressures measured at right heart catheterization. Measurement of vessel diameters was made at the level at which the right PA traverses the mediastinum. Both the diameter of the PA and the PA/A ratio were significantly related to PA pressure ($r = 0.74$; $p < .0005$) [5]. For patients younger than 50 years, PA pressure correlated more closely to PA/A ($r = 0.77$; $p < .00005$) than to PA diameter ($r = 0.59$; $p < .005$); for patients older than 50 years, the opposite was true. More important, a PA diameter to aortic diameter ratio of more than 1 strongly suggests PH (Fig. 9-1A) [5]. In this study [5], the specificity and positive predictive value of this finding were 92% and 96%, respectively. The sensitivity and negative predictive value were lower, measuring 70% and 52%, respectively. Thus, a PA/A of less than 1 does not necessarily mean PA pressure is normal.

Dilatation of main pulmonary arteries may also be seen in the presence of PH. The right and left pulmonary arteries should be of approximately equal size, although the left PA appears slightly larger in most subjects. In the study by Kuriyama et al. [3], the proximal right PA measured 18.7 ± 2.8 mm in diameter in normals, and the left PA averaged 21.0 ± 3.5 mm. In the study

by Haimovici et al. of transplantation patients [4], the left PA averaged 21 ± 5 mm in those who have normal PA pressure.

Within the lung, the diameter of a small PA and its neighboring bronchus should be approximately equal, although vessels may appear slightly larger than their accompanying bronchus, particularly in dependent lung regions. In patients who have PH or increased blood volume or blood flow [6], significant dilatation of these small vessels relative to adjacent bronchi may be seen (Fig. 9-1B) [7].

Decreased Artery Diameter

Decreased diameter of intrapulmonary arteries is common in patients who have PH or regional decrease in pulmonary blood flow (Fig. 9-2). This abnormality is usually recognized in association with inhomogeneous lung attenuation (i.e., mosaic perfusion) (Figs. 9-2C and D) [8–10]. An abrupt decrease in size of a PA along its course, visible on lung window scans, is suggestive of chronic pulmonary thromboembolism (CPTE) as the cause of PH or PVD. Asymmetry in the size of pulmonary arteries in the right and left lungs visible on lung window scans may also be seen in patients who have CPTE.

Pulmonary Artery Obstruction

Obstruction of large or small PA branches by thrombus or another substance is important in the diagnosis of several abnormalities, most commonly acute or CPTE [11–13], but also including PA sarcoma [14] and tumor embolization [15]. CT techniques for making the diagnosis of PA obstruction involve the use of spiral or electron beam scanners and the injection of a contrast agent. Usually, spiral scanning with 3-mm collimation and a pitch of 1.7 to 2 is used for making this diagnosis. This technique results in an

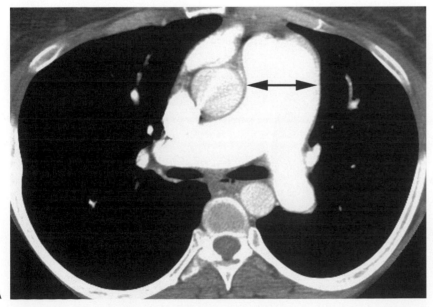

FIG. 9-2. A–D: Chronic pulmonary embolism. **A:** On a contrast-enhanced mulitdetector-row spiral HRCT, marked enlargement of the main pulmonary artery (*arrow*) and right pulmonary artery is present. *Continued*

A

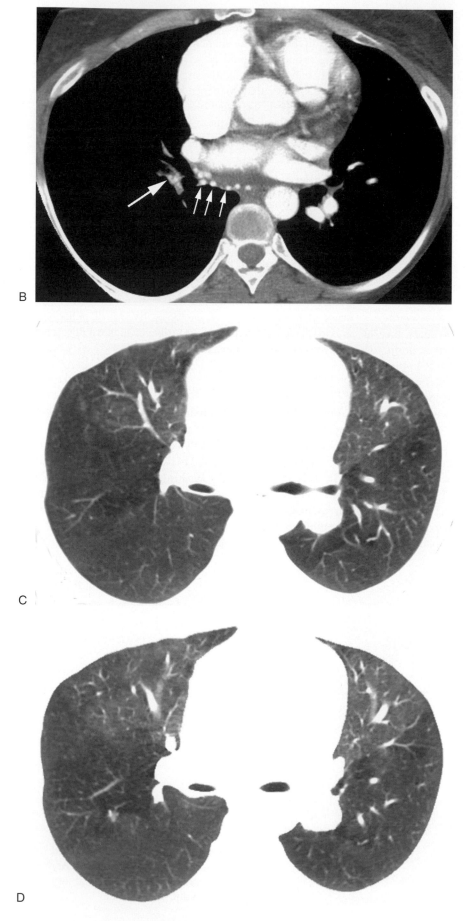

FIG. 9-2. *Continued* **B:** The right interlobular pulmonary artery (*large arrow*) is reduced in diameter compared to the left side and bronchial artery dilatation is present (*small arrows*). **C,D:** Lung window scans show reduced vessel size in the posterior lungs, particularly on the right, associated with reduced lung attenuation (i.e., mosaic perfusion). The patient was treated using embolectomy.

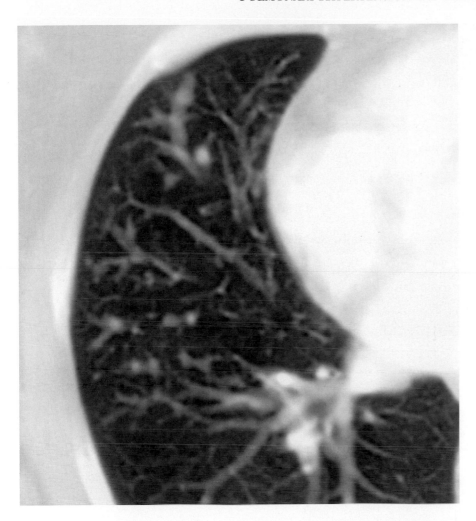

FIG. 9-3. Intravascular tumor emboli. Magnified view of CT scan at the level of the lingula demonstrates beaded appearance of the peripheral pulmonary arteries. The findings were due to intravascular tumor emboli from breast carcinoma. (Courtesy of Drs. Lynn Broderick and Robert Tarver, Indiana University Medical Center, Indianapolis, IN.)

effective slice thickness of approximately 3.9 mm, adequate for the diagnosis of pulmonary embolism (PE), but not sufficient for the HRCT diagnosis of lung disease. However, with a multidetector-row spiral CT scanner, contrast-enhanced evaluation of pulmonary arteries may be obtained using a detector width of 1.25 mm and a nominal slice thickness of 1.6 mm. Thus, with a multidetector-row spiral CT scanner, evaluation of the pulmonary arteries for acute or chronic emboli can be combined with spiral HRCT evaluation of distal PA branches, abnormalities of lung attenuation (i.e., mosaic perfusion), and pulmonary parenchymal abnormalities. Such a protocol would be valuable in patients who have nonspecific symptoms of dyspnea in whom PVD, PE, and lung disease are all considered diagnostic possibilities.

In some patients who have PA occlusion by clot or tumor, a focal increase in diameter of pulmonary arteries may be visible on CT (Fig. 9-3). This finding likely reflects impaction of the artery lumen by the embolic material. In patients who have tumor embolism [15], findings visible on CT included multifocal dilatation and beading of peripheral pulmonary arteries, primarily in a subsegmental distribution, and presumably related to the presence of intravascular nodules of tumor.

Mosaic Perfusion and Mosaic Lung Attenuation

Mosaic perfusion refers to decreased lung attenuation resulting from decreased blood flow [8–10]. It may result from vascular disease (e.g., CPTE) or airways disease (see Chapter 3). Mosaic perfusion is commonly associated with decreased size of pulmonary vessels within relatively lucent lung regions (Figs. 9-2 and 9-4). If this combination of decreased vessel size and decreased lung attenuation is visible, a diagnosis of mosaic perfusion is easily made. However, patients who have PVD may show inhomogeneous lung opacity without a clear-cut decrease in vessel size. This occurrence may be referred to as *mosaic lung attenuation* and is less specific [8,10].

In patients who have PH, mosaic lung attenuation is seen significantly more often in patients who have PH due to vascular disease than in patients who have PH due to cardiac or lung disease, and CPTE is the most common disease responsible for this finding. The frequency with which mosaic lung attenuation is seen on CT in patients who have various causes of PH has been studied by Sherrick et al. [8]. In this study, 23 patients had PH due to vascular disease, 17 patients had PH due to cardiac disease, and 21 patients had PH due to lung disease. Of the 23 patients with PH due to vascular disease, 17 (74%) had

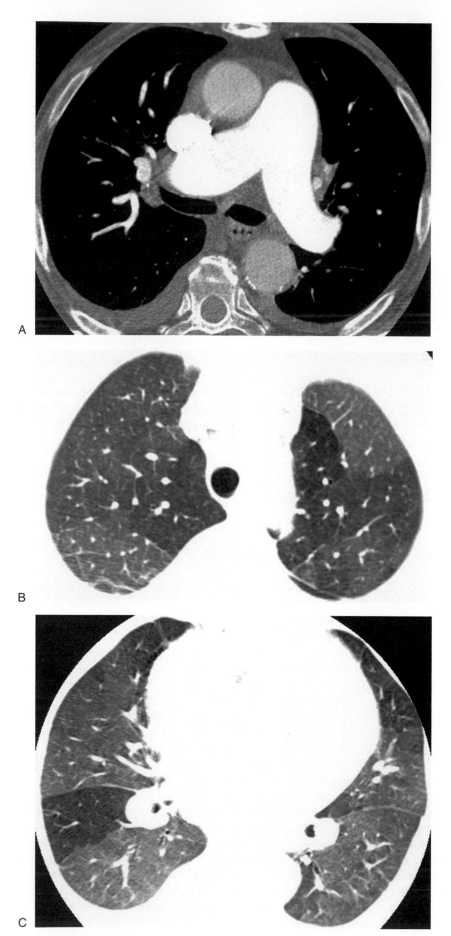

FIG. 9-4. A–C: Pulmonary hypertension and mosaic perfusion in a patient with chronic pulmonary embolism. **A:** On a contrast-enhanced multidetector-row spiral HRCT obtained using 1.25-mm detector width, the main pulmonary arteries appear dilated. **B,C:** At lung window settings, areas of decreased opacity reflect mosaic perfusion. Vessels within the lucent regions are reduced in size.

mosaic lung attenuation. Twelve of the 17 patients with mosaic lung attenuation due to vascular disease had CPTE, two had idiopathic or primary PH, two had pulmonary venoocclusive disease, and one had fibrosing mediastinitis associated with vascular obstruction. Among the 17 patients with PH due to cardiac disease, only two patients (12%) had a mosaic pattern of lung attenuation [8]. Of the 21 patients with PH due to lung disease, one patient (5%) had mosaic lung attenuation.

Pulmonary Edema and Hemorrhage

Hydrostatic pulmonary edema may be associated with PVD [16,17]. It is manifested by ground-glass opacity, interlobular septal thickening, or a combination of these. Pulmonary hemorrhage may be associated with small vessel disease and may also result in diffuse pulmonary abnormalities [18]. Pulmonary edema and pulmonary hemorrhage are discussed in Chapter 6.

Centrilobular Opacities

Processes resulting in a vascular and perivascular inflammation, including vasculitis [19] and reaction to injected substances, such as talc [20–22], can produce ill-defined centrilobular opacities visible on HRCT. Ill-defined centrilobular opacities may also be seen in patients who have PH associated with proliferation of small vessels [23,24], lobular mosaic perfusion, pulmonary hemorrhage, or cholesterol granulomas [25].

Cardiac Abnormalities

Enlargement of the right ventricle and right atrium is common in patients who have PH, being seen in all patients who had PH studied by Bergin et al. [26]. Findings of right atrial or right ventricular enlargement may be largely subjective. Flattening of the ventricular septum is a finding of value in making the diagnosis of right ventricular enlargement, but contrast infusion is needed for diagnosis. Enlargement of the right atrium may be associated with dilatation of the inferior vena cava and right atrial thrombus, which may calcify [12,26]. Pericardial thickening or effusion may also be present.

DISEASES ASSOCIATED WITH PULMONARY HYPERTENSION

PH may have a variety of causes, and its treatment may vary considerably depending on its etiology. The treatment of PH in different diseases may require pharmacologic intervention, embolectomy, or lung transplantation.

The assessment of patients who have PH usually involves techniques other than HRCT. However, HRCT may be performed (i) to assess patients who have PH related to lung disease (i.e., emphysema or pulmonary fibrosis), (ii) in patients having PH of unknown cause, (iii) in patients thought to have vasculitis or small vessels disease, or (iv) in patients being evaluated for lung transplantation. Also, patients who have

PH occurring because of CPTE often have CT for diagnosis, and a knowledge of CT findings in these patients is helpful.

PH associated with a specific disease is usually referred to as *secondary pulmonary hypertension*. It is most commonly associated with lung disease (e.g., emphysema, chronic obstructive pulmonary disease, idiopathic pulmonary fibrosis) and cardiac disease (e.g., chronic left-to-right shunts, left heart failure, mitral valve lesions), but other diseases (e.g., drug use, embolism of foreign material, obesity, sleep apnea, pericardial disease) may also result in PH [8]. The term *primary pulmonary hypertension* is used to refer to PH of obscure cause, and as defined by the World Health Organization, this group usually includes several entities: CPTE, plexogenic arteriopathy, and pulmonary venoocclusive disease. In clinical practice, however, primary PH is more commonly used to describe idiopathic causes of plexogenic arteriopathy.

Pulmonary Hypertension Associated with Lung Disease

In patients who have PH resulting from lung disease, a pulmonary abnormality should be easily visible on HRCT (Fig. 9-5). Common lung diseases resulting in PH include emphysema, pulmonary fibrosis related to idiopathic pulmonary fibrosis or other fibrotic lung diseases, and chronic obstructive pulmonary disease. The absence of a recognizable lung abnormality on HRCT in a patient who has known PH or dyspnea should suggest other causes, most specifically PVD.

Chronic Thromboembolic Pulmonary Hypertension

The diagnosis of CPTE as a cause of PH [27] is often difficult, as symptoms and pulmonary function test results are usually nonspecific [28]. Also, CPTE is a relatively rare cause of PH [26]. Although contrast-enhanced spiral CT is most appropriate in the assessment of patients who have suspected CPTE, allowing the diagnosis of thromboembolic vascular obstruction, HRCT may be obtained as the initial examination in such patients because of unexplained dyspnea or other nonspecific symptoms [29]. Furthermore, with multidetector-row spiral CT scanners, CT for the diagnosis of CPTE may be obtained with thin collimation (e.g., 1.25 mm), and a knowledge of HRCT findings in such patients may be helpful in diagnosis (Figs. 9-2 and 9-4).

HRCT findings in patients who have CPTE reflect variable obstruction of large and small arteries, and include (i) symmetric or asymmetric dilatation of the central pulmonary arteries, with a diameter often exceeding that of the ascending aorta, (ii) reduced diameter of segmental arteries, which thus appear smaller than their accompanying bronchi, (iii) abruptly truncated segmental arteries, (iv) variation in the size of arteries, and (v) mosaic perfusion (Figs. 9-2 and 9-4) (Table 9-1). Calcification of the walls of central arteries or thrombus may be seen (Fig. 9-6).

Inhomogeneous lung attenuation representing mosaic perfusion is common in patients who have CPTE, and decreased vessel size in less opaque regions is commonly visible (Figs. 9-2 and 9-4). In the absence of airways abnormalities and air-trapping, this combination of findings is strongly suggestive of CPTE. In a study of pulmonary parenchymal abnormalities in 75 patients who had CPTE, 58 patients (77.3%) showed mosaic perfusion with normal or dilated arteries in areas of relative increased attenuation [30]. In a study of patients who had PH due to CPTE, PH of other causes, and a variety of other pulmonary diseases, HRCT was thought to show mosaic perfusion in all patients who had CPTE [26]. Considerably more variation in the size of segmental vessels in different lung regions was also visible in the patients who had CPTE as compared to patients who had other lung diseases, and this was the most accurate finding in making the correct diagnosis [26]. Overall, HRCT had a sensitivity of 94% to 100% and a specificity of 96% to 98% in diagnosing CPTE based on these findings [26].

Peripheral wedge-shaped, pleural-based opacities suggest the presence of infarcts in patients who have PE [30]

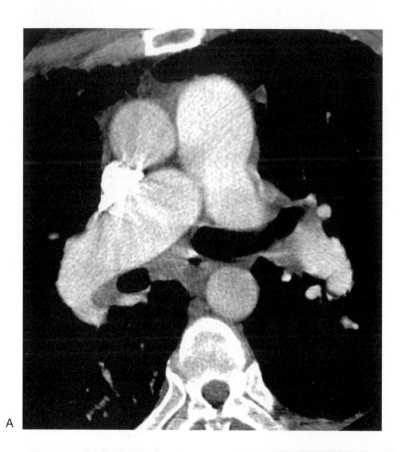

A

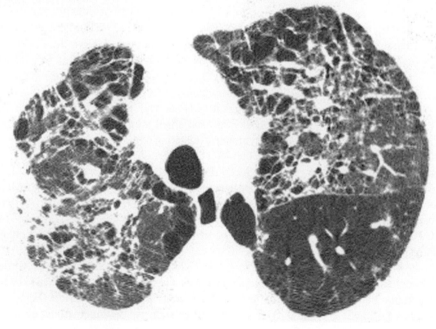

B

FIG. 9-5. A–C: Pulmonary hypertension associated with end-stage sarcoidosis. **A:** On a contrast-enhanced spiral CT, enlargement of the main pulmonary artery to a diameter greater than that of the aorta is visible, as is dilatation of the right pulmonary artery. **B:** Extensive lung disease with pulmonary fibrosis is visible at a lung window setting. *Continued*

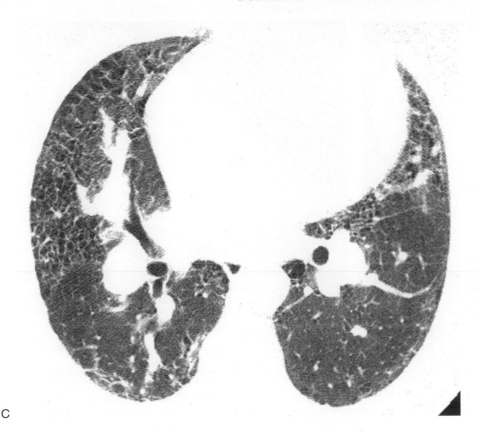

C

FIG. 9-5. *Continued* **C:** At a lower level, dilatation of the hilar pulmonary arteries is associated with findings of lung disease.

but are nonspecific and uncommon in patients who have chronic disease [26]. On the other hand, scars from prior pulmonary infarction are commonly seen on CT in patients who have CPTE, appearing as parenchymal bands or irregular linear opacities [12,26]. These were identified in the majority of patients who had CPTE in one study, but they were also seen in 22% to 26% of patients who had PH of other cause [26].

Radionuclide imaging also has a high sensitivity and specificity in making the diagnosis of CPTE [26]. In one study, it identified 94% of patients with this diagnosis. However, specificity in this study was only 75%, which was lower than that of HRCT.

Plexogenic Arteriopathy

The term *plexogenic arteriopathy* refers to a proliferation of small muscular arteries commonly seen in patients who have primary PH; it may also be referred to as *pulmonary hypertensive arteriopathy* [31]. Although usually idiopathic, a similar histologic abnormality may occur as a result a variety of causes of PH, including drug use (Fig. 9-7), acquired immunodeficiency syndrome (see Fig. 1-26), liver disease, and collagen-vascular disease.

Idiopathic plexogenic arteriopathy is most common in patients in their thirties, and women are affected more often than men. Symptoms include the insidious onset of dyspnea on exertion. Progressive symptoms, cor pulmonale, and death within a few years are typical [32].

In one study, HRCT in five patients who have plexogenic arteriopathy showed enlargement of central pulmonary arteries, normal lung parenchyma (n = 3), or a mosaic pattern of lung attenuation (n = 2) without evidence of centrilobular nodules or septal thickening (Figs. 9-8 and 9-9) (Table 9-2) [23].

Ill-defined centrilobular opacities may occasionally be seen in patients who have plexogenic arteriopathy. This finding may represent patchy mosaic perfusion or vascular proliferation, or may be the result of hemorrhage (Fig. 9-9). Also, cholesterol granulomas may result in small ill-defined centrilobular nodules in patients who have PH. In one study, histopathologic evidence of cholesterol granulomas was found in five (25%) of 20 patients with severe PH [25]. In three of these five patients, the granulomas were visible on HRCT as small centrilobular nodules.

TABLE 9-1. *HRCT findings in chronic pulmonary thromboembolism*

Symmetric or asymmetric dilatation of the central pulmonary arteries
Abruptly truncated segmental arteries
Variation in the size of arteries[a,b]
Mosaic perfusion[a,b]
Intravascular filling defects on contrast-enhanced CT[a,b]
Peripheral wedge-shaped opacities

[a]Most common findings.
[b]Finding(s) most helpful in differential diagnosis.

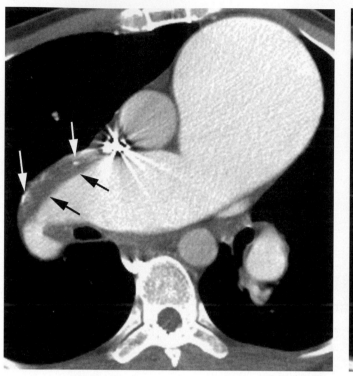
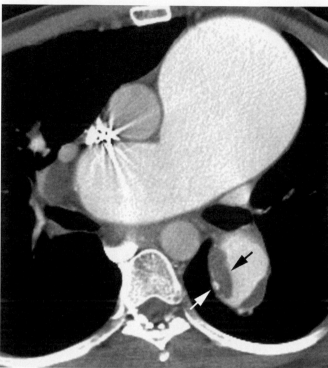

A

B

FIG. 9-6. A,B: Chronic pulmonary embolism. On a contrast-enhanced spiral HRCT, marked enlargement of the main pulmonary artery is present, with its diameter exceeding that of the aorta. Thrombus (*black arrows*) layers against walls of the pulmonary artery. Calcification of the vessel wall or thrombus (*white arrows*) is also visible.

Pulmonary Hypertension Associated with Collagen-Vascular Disease

PAH occurring in the absence of lung disease may be seen in patients who have systemic disorders such as scleroderma, mixed connective tissue disease, rheumatoid disease, and systemic lupus erythematosus. Generally, the histologic and HRCT findings are those of plexogenic arteriopathy.

Capillary Hemangiomatosis

Capillary hemangiomatosis is a rare cause of PH, most often occurring in young adults and associated with dyspnea and hemoptysis [33]. Slow progression is typical. Pathologically, this disease represents a patchy interstitial proliferation of thin-walled capillary-sized blood vessels. The vessels appear to invade the walls of veins and arteries and are asso-

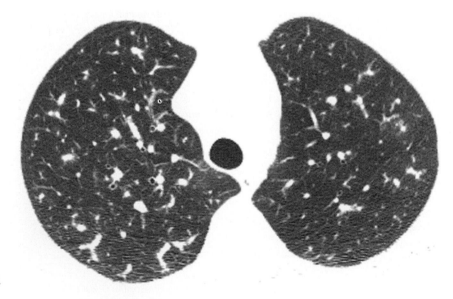

A

FIG. 9-7. A–C: Pulmonary hypertension associated with use of anorectic drugs. Enlargement of the main pulmonary artery is associated with marked variation in the size of small pulmonary arteries. In general, arteries in the right lung appear larger than the left. *Continued*

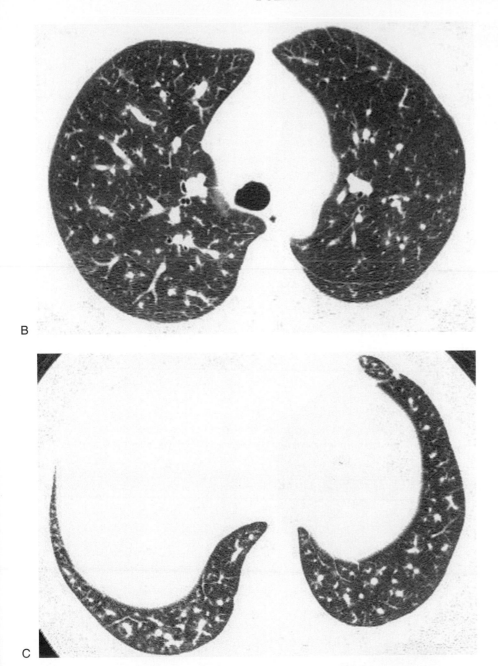

FIG. 9-7. *Continued*

ciated with intimal fibrosis, vascular stenosis, interstitial edema, and hemorrhage [34]. The nature of this disease is uncertain, and it may represent a low-grade malignancy of pulmonary endothelial cells or a metastatic angiosarcoma [24,33]. Chest radiographs may be normal, except for findings of PH, or may show small nodular opacities.

HRCT findings have been reported in a few patients who have this disease. Generally, patchy, lobular, or centrilobular areas of ground-glass opacity are most common (Table 9-3). HRCT in two patients who had capillary hemangiomatosis showed mediastinal and hilar lymph node enlargement and enlargement of pulmonary arteries, occurring as a result of PH, and pleural effusions [23]. In both patients [23], and in one other reported patient [24], HRCT showed smooth thick-

ening of interlobular septa, small ill-defined centrilobular nodules, and focal regions of lobular or centrilobular ground-glass opacity (Fig. 9-10). Pathologic correlation in these cases showed proliferations of small capillary-sized vessels resulting in thickening of interlobular septa and vascular congestion with intraalveolar hemosiderin-laden macrophages.

Pulmonary Venoocclusive Disease

Pulmonary venoocclusive disease is a rare disorder in which gradual obliteration of the pulmonary veins by intimal fibrosis leads to PH [35,36]. The disease has multiple causes, including viral infections, inhaled toxins, deposition of immune complexes in the lung, genetic predisposition,

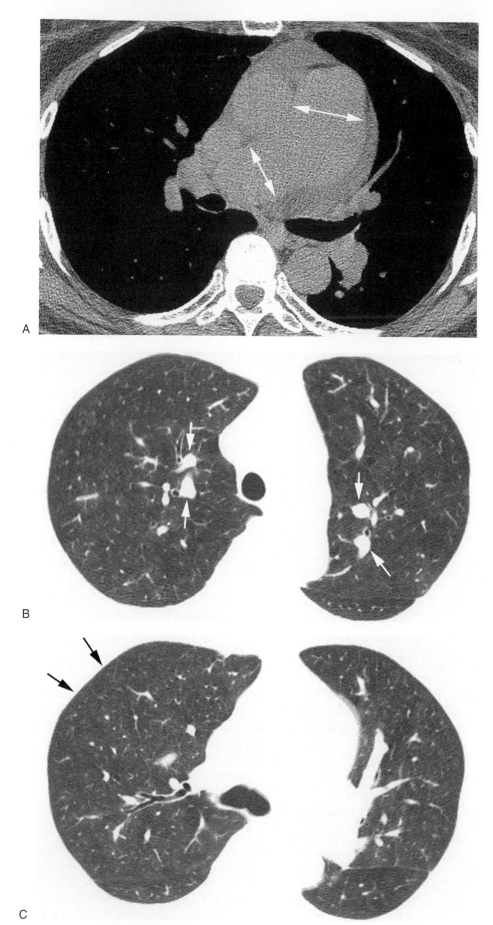

A

B

C

FIG. 9-8. A–C: Idiopathic pulmonary hypertension with plexogenic arteriopathy. **A:** Enlargement of the main pulmonary artery and right pulmonary arteries is visible at tissue windows (*arrows*). A small pericardial effusion is present. **B:** At a lung window, central pulmonary artery branches (*arrows*) are increased in diameter, and appear much larger than their adjacent bronchi. **C:** Pulmonary arteries appear relatively small in the lung periphery (*arrows*). Lung parenchyma shows a slightly inhomogeneous attenuation, likely due to mosaic perfusion.

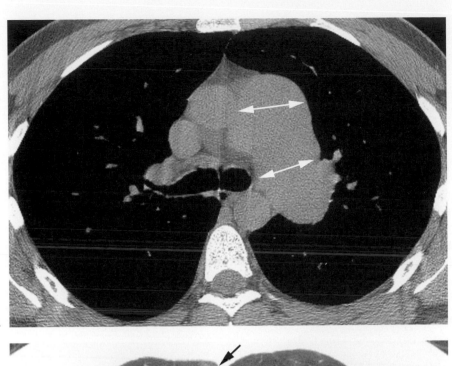

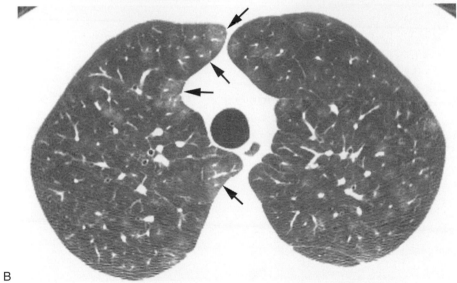

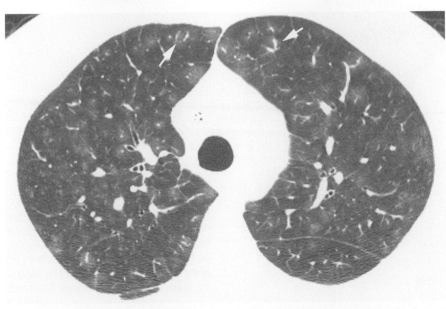

FIG. 9-9. A–C: Idiopathic pulmonary hypertension with plexogenic arteriopathy. **A:** Enlargement of the main and left pulmonary artery is visible at tissue windows (*arrows*). **B,C:** Lung window scans through the upper lobes show inhomogeneous lung attenuation with a lobular or centrilobular distribution. Relatively large vessel size in areas of increased attenuation (*arrows*) suggests mosaic perfusion as the cause of inhomogenous opacity. A similar appearance was visible in the lower lobes. Histologic examination of the lungs after removal for lung transplantation showed plexogenic arteriopathy.

TABLE 9-2. *HRCT findings in plexogenic arteriopathy*

Symmetric dilatation of the central pulmonary arteries[a]
Mosaic perfusion
Ill-defined centrilobular opacities

[a]Most common findings.

TABLE 9-3. *HRCT findings in capillary hemangiomatosis*

Dilatation of the central pulmonary arteries[a]
Patchy or centrilobular ground-glass opacities[a]
Interlobular septal thickening
Lymph node enlargement
Pleural effusion

[a]Most common findings.

acquired immunodeficiency syndrome, and use of contraceptive or cytotoxic chemotherapeutic agents. In addition, radiation injury has been proposed as a possible cause. The disease is generally fatal within a few years.

CT findings have been described in a small number of patients [23,35,37]. The most common findings include smooth interlobular septal thickening, diffuse multifocal regions of

ground-glass opacity, pleural effusions, enlarged central pulmonary arteries, and pulmonary veins of normal caliber; these findings are highly suggestive of pulmonary venoocclusive disease (Table 9-4) [37]. In the largest study [37], seven of eight patients had interlobular septal thickening. All eight patients

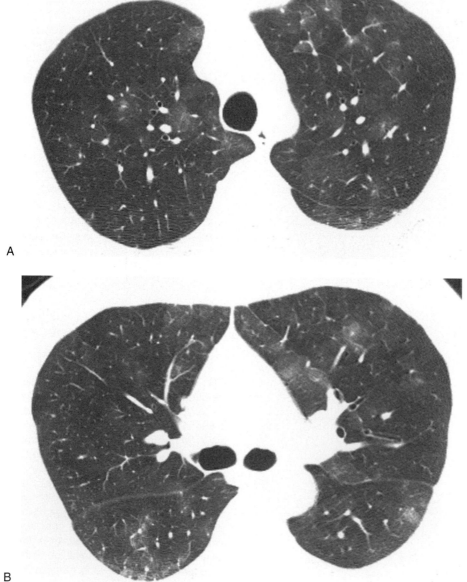

A

B

FIG. 9-10. A–C: Capillary hemangiomatosis. HRCT at three levels shows patchy areas of ground-glass opacity, a common finding in this disease. This appearance is nonspecific. The diagnosis was made at lung biopsy. *Continued*

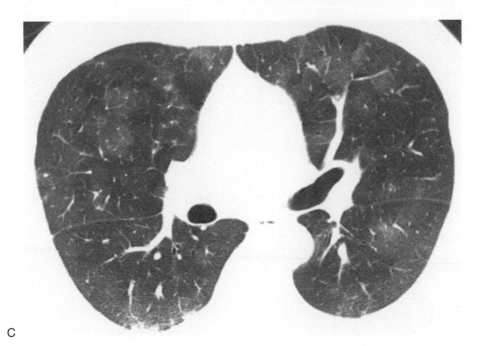

C

FIG. 9-10. *Continued*

had regions of ground-glass opacity (Fig. 9-11). Central pulmonary arteries were considered to be enlarged in seven of eight cases. Four of the eight patients had a mosaic pattern of lung attenuation. Five patients had bilateral pleural effusions [37].

Histologic correlation with CT findings [37] showed that thickened interlobular septa corresponded to the presence of septal fibrosis and venous sclerosis. Ground-glass opacity may be related to alveolar wall thickening or pulmonary edema.

Nonthromboembolic Pulmonary Embolism

In addition to pulmonary thromboembolism, embolism of a variety of materials may result in similar symptoms and radiographic findings. These include embolism of injected substances, embolism of parasites, such as occurs in *Schistosomiasis*, and pulmonary tumor embolism. None of these is common, although injection of foreign substances may be seen in drug abusers.

Talcosis

Talcosis secondary to intravenous injection of talc is seen almost exclusively in drug users who inject crushed oral medications, including talc (magnesium silicate) [38,39]. The injected talc particles result in small vascular granulomas composed of multinucleated giant cells surrounded by a small amount of fibrous tissue [40,41]. Talcosis is described in Chapter 5.

HRCT findings in patients who have talcosis include (i) nodules as small as 1 mm in diameter, which may be diffuse or centrilobular, (ii) diffuse ground-glass opacities, (iii) confluent perihilar masses resembling progressive massive fibrosis, and (iv) panlobular emphysema with a basal predominance (see Fig. 5-58) [20,22,40,42]. The confluent masses may appear

high in attenuation because of contained talc. Emphysema is usually associated with patients injecting crushed methylphenidate [methylphenidate hydrochloride (Ritalin)] tablets [40,42].

Pulmonary Artery Tumor Embolism

The diagnosis of pulmonary arterial tumor emboli is difficult to establish clinically [43]. Symptoms include progressive dyspnea due to PH and cor pulmonale or a more acute presentation that mimics pulmonary thromboembolism. Most often, patients have a known history of neoplasm, but tumor emboli may occasionally be the first manifestation of disease. Four cases of intravascular pulmonary metastases were reported by Shepard et al. [15]. All four patients had invasive tumors (atrial myxoma, renal cell carcinoma, osteosarcoma, chondrosarcoma). Three cases had histopathologic documentation of PA tumor emboli. At CT, all the patients demonstrated multifocal dilatation and beading of peripheral pulmonary arteries, pri-

TABLE 9-4. *HRCT findings in pulmonary venoocclusive disease*

Dilatation of the central pulmonary arteries[a]
Normal pulmonary veins[a]
Interlobular septal thickening[a]
Patchy ground-glass opacities[a]
Combination of first four findings[a,b]
Mosaic perfusion
Pleural effusion

[a]Most common findings.
[b]Findings most helpful in differential diagnosis.

marily in a subsegmental distribution and involving multiple lobes (Fig. 9-3). In two cases, small, peripheral wedge-shaped opacities distal to some abnormal pulmonary arteries suggested pulmonary infarction. A CT appearance of multiple subpleural opacities, some wedge-shaped, has also been reported by Kim et al. [44] in a woman who had carcinoma of the cervix and histologic confirmation of intravascular emboli and distal areas of lung infarction.

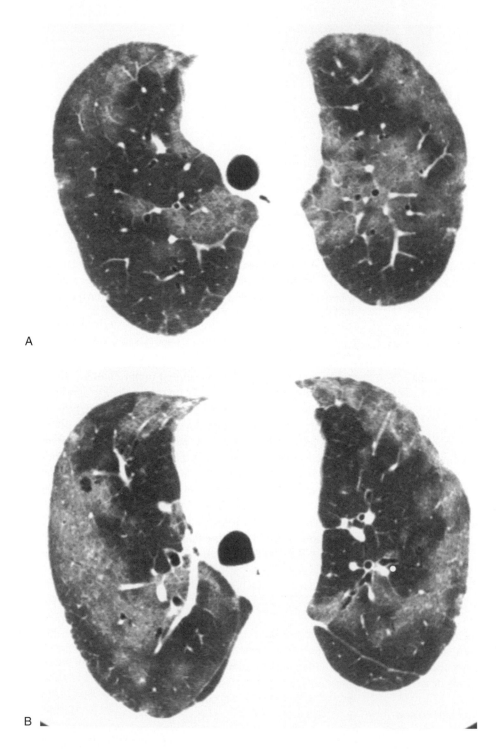

A

B

FIG. 9-11. A–C: Pulmonary venoocclusive disease. HRCT at three levels shows patchy areas of ground-glass opacity, with a predominantly peripheral distribution. Some intralobular interstitial thickening is visible in the areas of ground-glass opacity, but interlobular septal thickening is not clearly visible. *Continued*

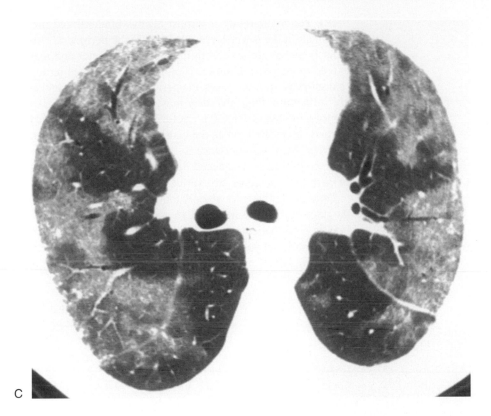

C

FIG. 9-11. *Continued*

OTHER PULMONARY VASCULAR DISEASES

Pulmonary Vasculitis

A number of collagen-vascular diseases or embolic processes may result in pulmonary vasculitis [20,22,45]. Although patients who have pulmonary vasculitis may show normal HRCT findings, HRCT in some patients shows ill-defined centrilobular perivascular opacities, correlating with the presence of perivascular inflammation or hemorrhage. Connolly et al. [19] reported hazy or fluffy centrilobular, perivascular opacities in eight children with vasculitis, including five with Wegener's granulomatosis, one with systemic lupus erythematosus, one with scleroderma-polymyositis overlap syndrome, and one with Churg-Strauss syndrome. In these eight children, centrilobular opacities were associated with the onset of active disease or an exacerbation of preexisting disease. In four of five patients, this abnormality disappeared on treatment.

In the case of Churg-Strauss vasculitis, HRCT demonstrated enlarged, irregular, and stellate-shaped arteries, and small patchy opacities were present in the pulmonary parenchyma. On open lung biopsy, arteries appeared enlarged due to eosinophilic infiltration in the vessel walls and the adjacent lymphatics were dilated [46].

Hepatopulmonary Syndrome

Hepatopulmonary syndrome (HPS) is defined by the triad of hepatic dysfunction, intrapulmonary vascular dilatation, and abnormal arterial oxygenation (hypoxemia) [47–49]. Clinically, HPS typically manifests with progressive dyspnea and hypoxemia in a patient who has cirrhosis. It may also be associated with platypnea and orthodeoxia, defined respectively as dyspnea and hypoxemia occurring when upright and relieved when recumbent [47,48]. PA pressure is normal or reduced.

Although the pathogenesis of vascular dilatation is unknown, some investigators have suggested that nitric oxide associated with portal hypertension might influence the autoregulation of peripheral pulmonary vasculature, resulting in vasodilatation [49]. Although it would seem logical that the hypoxemia of HPS is due to a right-to-left shunt through dilated pulmonary vessels, this is not usually the case. Hypoxemia in patients who have HPS has multiple complex causes and is thought to occur primarily because of a limitation in oxygen diffusion occurring because of vascular dilatation (diffusion-perfusion impairment) [47]. In patients who have diffusion-perfusion impairment, the use of 100% oxygen results in a decrease in the size of the apparent shunt with significant improvement in oxygenation. In patients who have arteriovenous fistulas, this does not occur.

Based primarily on arteriographic findings, Krowka et al. [48,49] have classified the lesions of HPS into two types. The type 1 (minimal) pattern is most common (85%); it is associated with a spidery appearance of peripheral vessels and, usually, a good response to treatment with 100% oxygen. Type 2 lesions (15%) represent small, discrete pulmonary arteriovenous fistulas; type 2 lesions are associated with a poor response to 100% oxygen.

The radiologic manifestations of HPS have been recently reviewed [7,50]. Radiographic findings in patients who have

TABLE 9-5. *HRCT findings in hepatopulmonary syndrome*

Dilatation of peripheral pulmonary vessels[a,b]
Lower lobe predominance[a,b]

[a]Most common findings.
[b]Findings most helpful in differential diagnosis.

HPS may include bibasilar nodular or reticular opacities on chest radiographs and peripheral arteriolar dilatation on pulmonary angiography [50]. Mild enlargement of central pulmonary arteries may also be seen [50].

CT and HRCT findings in HPS include vascular dilatation in the peripheral lungs associated with an abnormally large number of visible terminal artery branches (Table 9-5) (Fig.

9-12). The abnormality is almost always bilateral and predominant in the lower lobes. On HRCT, the peripheral vascular branches are several millimeters in diameter and may extend to the pleural surface [50], a finding not seen in normal subjects. In some cases, the peripheral vascular branches are sufficiently large that they may be seen to opacity after contrast infusion. HRCT is useful in excluding pulmonary fibrosis or emphysema as the cause of the plain film abnormalities. Also of importance in the CT diagnosis of HPS is the recognition of associated hepatic disease, with findings of cirrhosis, splenomegaly, varices, and ascites [50].

The extent of the vascular dilatation tends to correlate with the degree of hypoxemia [50]. In one study [7], HRCT findings in eight patients with HPS were compared to those of eight healthy subjects and in four patients with normoxic cirrhosis. On HRCT, the ratio of segmental arterial diameter to

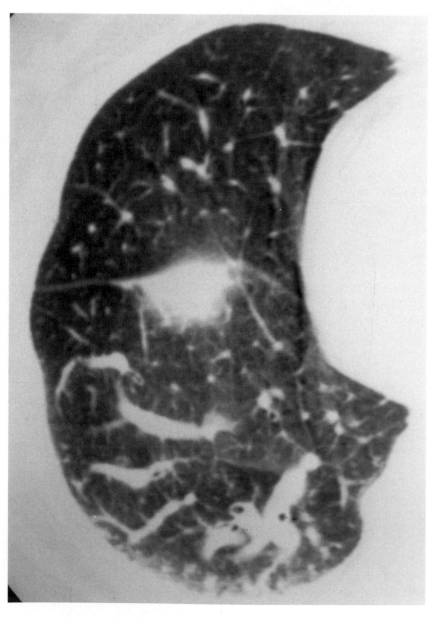

A

FIG. 9-12. Hepatopulmonary syndrome in a 68-year-old woman. **A:** HRCT shows dilatation of the right basal pulmonary arteries; the ratio of segmental artery to accompanying bronchus is increased. *Continued*

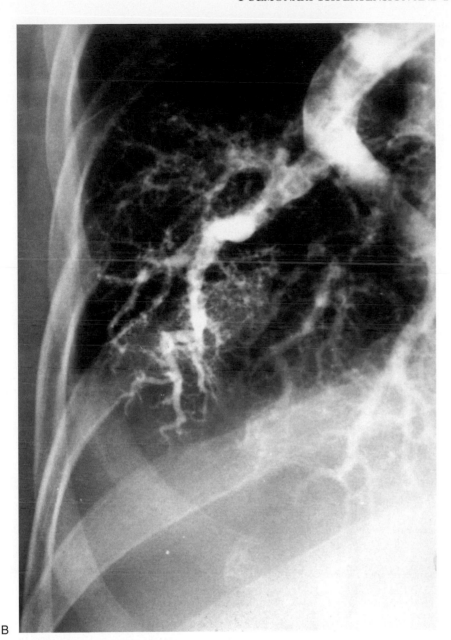

B

FIG. 9-12. *Continued* B: Pulmonary angiography shows dilated and tortuous peripheral pulmonary arteries. [Reproduced from Lee KN, Lee HJ, et al. Hypoxemia and liver cirrhosis (hepatopulmonary syndrome) in eight patients: comparison of the central and peripheral pulmonary vasculature. *Radiology* 1999; 211:549, with permission.]

adjacent bronchial diameter in the right lower lobe was significantly increased in HPS patients compared to control subjects and patients who had normoxic cirrhosis ($p = .002$). The diameter of peripheral pulmonary arteries in the right lower lobe was 7.3 mm ± 1.6, compared to 4 mm ± 0.4 in patients who had normoxic cirrhosis. The ratio of arterial diameter to adjacent bronchial diameter was 2.0 ± 0.2 in patients who had HPS, compared to 1.2 ± 0.2 in patients who had normoxic cirrhosis ($p <.05$) [7].

Sickle Cell Anemia

Pulmonary abnormalities associated with sickle cell anemia include pneumonia, acute chest syndrome (ACS), cor pulmonale, and pulmonary fibrosis. ACS is characterized by fever, cough, chest pain, hypoxia, prostration, and pulmonary opacities on chest radiographs. It is likely related to sickling of red blood cells with pulmonary microvascular occlusion and infarction, although pneumonia has also been implicated in the pathogenesis of this syndrome. Infarction and pneumonia are not easily differentiated using chest radiography or ventilation-perfusion scintigraphy.

HRCT findings in patients who have ACS [51] include patchy airspace consolidation likely related to edema or infarction, ground-glass opacity, and vascular attenuation. In one study of patients who have ACS, Bhalla et al. [51] assessed the ability of HRCT to diagnose small vessel abnormalities, thus helping to distinguish vascular obstruction from pneumonia as a cause of symptoms. In nine of ten patients with moderate to severe ACS, HRCT was thought to show findings of microvascular occlusion (i.e., paucity or absence of small vessels) and areas of ground-glass attenuation, probably due to hemorrhagic edema. In all patients, the degree of hypoxia was out of proportion to the extent of consolidation evident at chest radiography.

The end result of repeated episodes of pneumonia or ACS in patients who have sickle cell anemia is termed *sickle cell lung disease* [52]. Its prevalence in patients who have sickle cell anemia is 4%. Postmortem examinations have shown pulmonary fibrosis and obliteration of pulmonary arterioles [53]. HRCT findings in 29 patients with a history of one or more episodes of ACS were also reported by Aquino et al. and are most consistent with fibrosis and infarction [54]. Twelve of the 29 patients (41%) had significant multifocal interstitial lung disease, including interlobular septal thickening, parenchymal bands, traction bronchiectasis, and architectural distortion. Mosaic perfusion with decreased vessel size, likely as a result of vascular obstruction, was seen in two patients, both with PH. A correlation was found between the extent of abnormalities and the number of episodes of ACS ($p = .02$) [54].

REFERENCES

1. Primack SL, Müller NL, Mayo JR, et al. Pulmonary parenchymal abnormalities of vascular origin: high-resolution CT findings. *Radiographics* 1994;14:739–746.
2. Guthaner DF, Wexler L, Harell G. CT demonstration of cardiac structures. *AJR Am J Roentgenol* 1979;133:75–81.
3. Kuriyama K, Gamsu G, Stern RG, et al. CT-determined pulmonary artery diameters in predicting pulmonary hypertension. *Invest Radiol* 1984;19:16.
4. Ackman Haimovici JB, Trotman-Dickenson B, Halpern EF, et al. Relationship between pulmonary artery diameter at computed tomography and pulmonary artery pressures at right-sided heart catheterization. *Acad Radiol* 1997;4:327–334.
5. Ng CS, Wells AU, Padley SP. A CT sign of chronic pulmonary arterial hypertension: the ratio of main pulmonary artery to aortic diameter. *J Thorac Imag* 1999;14:270–278.
6. Herold CJ, Wetzel RC, Robotham JL, et al. Acute effects of increased intravascular volume and hypoxia on the pulmonary circulation: assessment with high-resolution CT. *Radiology* 1992;183:655–662.
7. Lee KN, Lee HJ, Shin WW, et al. Hypoxemia and liver cirrhosis (hepatopulmonary syndrome) in eight patients: comparison of the central and peripheral pulmonary vasculature. *Radiology* 1999;211:549–553.
8. Sherrick AD, Swensen SJ, Hartman TE. Mosaic pattern of lung attenuation on CT scans: frequency among patients with pulmonary artery hypertension of different causes. *AJR Am J Roentgenol* 1997;169:79–82.
9. Arakawa H, Webb WR, McCowin M, et al. Inhomogeneous lung attenuation at thin-section CT: diagnostic value of expiratory scans. *Radiology* 1998;206:89–94.
10. Austin JH, Müller NL, Friedman PJ, et al. Glossary of terms for CT of the lungs: recommendations of the Nomenclature Committee of the Fleischner Society. *Radiology* 1996;200:327–331.
11. Greaves SM, Hart EM, Brown K, et al. Pulmonary thromboembolism: spectrum of findings on CT. *AJR Am J Roentgenol* 1995;165:1359–1363.
12. King MA, Bergin CJ, Yeung DWC, et al. Chronic pulmonary thromboembolism: detection of regional hypoperfusion with CT. *Radiology* 1994;191:359–363.
13. Roberts HC, Kauczor HU, Schweden F, et al. Spiral CT of pulmonary hypertension and chronic thromboembolism. *J Thorac Imag* 1997;12:118–127.
14. Cook DJ, Tanser PH, Dobranowski J, et al. Primary pulmonary artery sarcoma mimicking pulmonary thromboembolism. *Can J Cardiol* 1988;4:393–396.
15. Shepard JA, Moore EH, Templeton PA, et al. Pulmonary intravascular tumor emboli: dilated and beaded peripheral pulmonary arteries at CT [see comments]. *Radiology* 1993;187:797–801.
16. Ketai LH, Godwin JD. A new view of pulmonary edema and acute respiratory distress syndrome. *J Thorac Imag* 1998;13:147–171.
17. Storto ML, Kee ST, Golden JA, et al. Hydrostatic pulmonary edema: high-resolution CT findings. *AJR Am J Roentgenol* 1995;165:817–820.
18. Primack SL, Miller RR, Müller NL. Diffuse pulmonary hemorrhage: clinical, pathologic, and imaging features. *AJR Am J Roentgenol* 1995;164:295–300.
19. Connolly B, Manson D, Eberhard A, et al. CT appearance of pulmonary vasculitis in children. *AJR Am J Roentgenol* 1996;167:901–904.
20. Gruden JF, Webb WR, Warnock M. Centrilobular opacities in the lung on high-resolution CT: diagnostic considerations and pathologic correlation. *AJR Am J Roentgenol* 1994;162:569–574.
21. Akira M, Higashihara T, Yokoyama K, et al. Radiographic type p pneumoconiosis: high-resolution CT. *Radiology* 1989;171:117–123.
22. Padley SPG, Adler BD, Staples CA, et al. Pulmonary talcosis: CT findings in three cases. *Radiology* 1993;186:125–127.
23. Dufour B, Maitre S, Humbert M, et al. High-resolution CT of the chest in four patients with pulmonary capillary hemangiomatosis or pulmonary venoocclusive disease. *AJR Am J Roentgenol* 1998;171:1321–1324.
24. Eltorky MA, Headley AS, Winer-Muram H, et al. Pulmonary capillary hemangiomatosis: a clinicopathologic review. *Ann Thorac Surg* 1994;57:772–776.
25. Nolan RL, McAdams HP, Sporn TA, et al. Pulmonary cholesterol granulomas in patients with pulmonary artery hypertension: chest radiographic and CT findings. *AJR Am J Roentgenol* 1999;172:1317–1319.
26. Bergin CJ, Rios G, King MA, et al. Accuracy of high-resolution CT in identifying chronic pulmonary thromboembolic disease. *AJR Am J Roentgenol* 1996;166:1371–1377.
27. Fedullo PF, Auger WR, Channick RN, et al. Chronic thromboembolic pulmonary hypertension. *Clin Chest Med* 1995;16:353–374.
28. Chapman PJ, Bateman ED, Benatar SR. Primary pulmonary hypertension and thromboembolic pulmonary hypertension—similarities and differences [see comments]. *Respir Med* 1990;84:485–488.
29. King MA, Ysrael M, Bergin CJ. Chronic thromboembolic pulmonary hypertension: CT findings. *AJR Am J Roentgenol* 1998;170:955–960.
30. Schwickert HC, Schweden F, Schild HH, et al. Pulmonary arteries and lung parenchyma in chronic pulmonary embolism: preoperative and postoperative CT findings. *Radiology* 1994;191:351–357.
31. Wagenvoort CA. Plexogenic arteriopathy. *Thorax* 1994;49:S39–S45.
32. Hughes JD, Rubin LJ. Primary pulmonary hypertension: n analysis of 28 cases and a review of the literature. *Medicine (Baltimore)* 1986;65:56–72.
33. Masur Y, Remberger K, Hoefer M. Pulmonary capillary hemangiomatosis as a rare cause of pulmonary hypertension [published erratum appears in *Pathol Res Pract* 1996 Jun;192(6):646]. *Pathol Res Pract* 1996;192:290–295; discussion 296–299.
34. Faber CN, Yousem SA, Dauber JH, et al. Pulmonary capillary hemangiomatosis: a report of three cases and a review of the literature. *Am Rev Respir Dis* 1989;140:808–813.
35. Cassart M, Genevois PA, Kramer M, et al. Pulmonary venoocclusive disease: CT findings before and after single-lung transplantation. *AJR Am J Roentgenol* 1993;160:759–760.
36. Wagenvoort CA, Wagenvoort N, Takahashi T. Pulmonary venoocclusive disease: involvement of pulmonary arteries and review of the literature. *Hum Pathol* 1985;16:1033–1041.
37. Swensen SJ, Tashjian JH, Myers JL, et al. Pulmonary venoocclusive disease: CT findings in eight patients. *AJR Am J Roentgenol* 1996;167:937–940.
38. Pare JA, Fraser RG, Hogg JC, et al. Pulmonary "mainline" granulomatosis: talcosis of intravenous methadone abuse. *Medicine (Baltimore)* 1979;58:229–239.
39. Pare JP, Cote G, Fraser RS. Long-term follow-up of drug abusers with intravenous talcosis. *Am Rev Respir Dis* 1989;139:233–241.
40. Ward S, Heynman LE, Reittner P, et al. Talcosis secondary to IV abuse of oral medications: CT findings. *AJR Am J Roentgenol* 2000;174(3):789–793.
41. Schmidt RA, Glenny RW, Godwin JD, et al. Panlobular emphysema in young intravenous Ritalin abusers. *Am Rev Respir Dis* 1991;143:649–656.
42. Stern EJ, Frank MS, Schmutz JF, et al. Panlobular pulmonary emphysema caused by i.v. injection of methylphenidate (Ritalin): findings on chest radiographs and CT scans. *AJR Am J Roentgenol* 1994;162:555–560.

43. von Herbay A, Illes A, Waldherr R, et al. Pulmonary tumor thrombotic microangiopathy with pulmonary hypertension. *Cancer* 1990;66:587–592.

44. Kim AE, Haramati LB, Janus D, et al. Pulmonary tumor embolism presenting as infarcts on computed tomography. *J Thorac Imag* 1999;14:135–137.

45. Prakash UB. Respiratory complications in mixed connective tissue disease. *Clin Chest Med* 1998;19:733–746, ix.

46. Buschman DL, Waldron JA, Jr., King TE, Jr. Churg-Strauss pulmonary vasculitis: high-resolution computed tomography scanning and pathologic findings. *Am Rev Respir Dis* 1990;142:458–461.

47. Lange PA, Stoller JK. The hepatopulmonary syndrome. *Ann Intern Med* 1995;122:521–529.

48. Krowka MJ, Cortese DA. Hepatopulmonary syndrome: current concepts in diagnostic and therapeutic considerations. *Chest* 1994;105:1528–1537.

49. Castro M, Krowka MJ. Hepatopulmonary syndrome: a pulmonary vascular complication of liver disease. *Clin Chest Med* 1996;17:35–48.

50. McAdams HP, Erasmus J, Crockett R, et al. The hepatopulmonary syndrome: radiologic findings in 10 patients. *AJR Am J Roentgenol* 1996;166:1379–1385.

51. Bhalla M, Abboud MR, McLoud TC, et al. Acute chest syndrome in sickle cell disease: CT evidence of microvascular occlusion. *Radiology* 1993;187:45–49.

52. Powars D, Weidman JA, Odom-Maryon T, et al. Sickle cell chronic lung disease: prior morbidity and the risk of pulmonary failure. *Medicine (Baltimore)* 1988;67:66–76.

53. Powars DR. Sickle cell anemia and major organ failure. *Hemoglobin* 1990;14:573–598.

54. Aquino SL, Gamsu G, Fahy JV, et al. Chronic pulmonary disorders in sickle cell disease: findings at thin-section CT. *Radiology* 1994;193:807–811.

Clinical Utility of High-Resolution Computed Tomography

The clinical assessment of a patient who has suspected diffuse lung disease can be a difficult and perplexing problem. Similar symptoms and, in some cases, similar chest radiographic findings can result from a variety of acute or chronic lung diseases affecting the lung interstitium, airways, or airspaces. Diffuse infiltrative lung disease (DILD) represents a strikingly heterogeneous group of diseases. Although sarcoidosis and various causes of pulmonary fibrosis account for between one-third and one-half of all cases of DILD seen in clinical practice [1,2], more than one hundred different causes of DILD have been described [1,3,4]. Similarly, acute diffuse lung diseases in immunocompetent patients, or in association with acquired immunodeficiency syndrome (AIDS) or other causes of immunosuppression, can have a number of infectious or noninfectious causes, and their differentiation on clinical and radiographic findings can be difficult.

Furthermore, diffuse lung diseases are far more common than generally perceived. As estimated in a 1972 Respiratory Diseases Task Force report from the National Institutes of Health, patients who have DILD represent as many as 15% of all patients referred to pulmonologists for evaluation [5]. Using a population-based registry of 2,936 patients who had interstitial lung diseases, Coultas et al. [3] reported the yearly incidence of interstitial disease as 31.5 and 26.1 per 100,000 people, in men and women, respectively. Also, in a review of autopsy results, these authors found that undiagnosed or preclinical interstitial lung disease was present in 1.8% of all cases [3]. Although acute lung disease in the AIDS population is declining due to increased use of antiviral agents, diffuse lung disease in this population, as well as other immunocompromised groups, especially those undergoing organ transplantation, remains an important clinical problem.

Tests used in diagnosing diffuse lung disease are numerous, with the final diagnosis, or differential diagnosis, often based on a combination of laboratory tests, physiologic studies, radiographic examinations, and invasive procedures, including fiberoptic bronchoscopy with transbronchial biopsy (TBB), bronchoalveolar lavage (BAL), or both, or open-lung biopsy [6]. It is in this context that high-resolution CT (HRCT) has assumed an increasingly important role in assessing patients who have undiagnosed diffuse lung disease. HRCT should not generally be used by itself in an attempt to diagnose lung disease; it should be part of a comprehensive clinical evaluation, and should be interpreted in light of clinical findings.

In previous chapters, we reviewed the utility of HRCT in regard to the diagnosis of a number of specific diseases. The purpose of this chapter is to summarize our current understanding of the clinical utility of HRCT in diagnosing diffuse lung disease and the clinical indications for performing HRCT in patients suspected of having a diffuse abnormality. Special emphasis will be placed on answering the following questions:

1. How sensitive and specific is HRCT for diagnosing diffuse lung disease, both in relation to chest radiographs and conventional CT?
2. What is the diagnostic accuracy of HRCT in diagnosing diffuse lung diseases, both chronic and acute?
3. Can HRCT findings be sufficiently diagnostic of specific disease entities that lung biopsy may be avoided?
4. Is there a role for HRCT in assessing disease activity and prognosis?
5. Of what value is HRCT in planning lung biopsy?

SENSITIVITY AND SPECIFICITY OF HIGH-RESOLUTION COMPUTED TOMOGRAPHY IN THE DIAGNOSIS OF DIFFUSE LUNG DISEASE

Chest radiographs are important in the assessment of patients suspected of having diffuse lung disease; they are

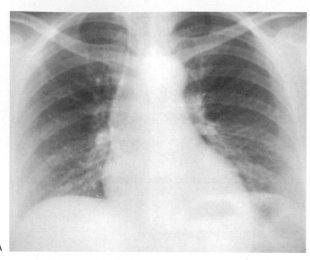
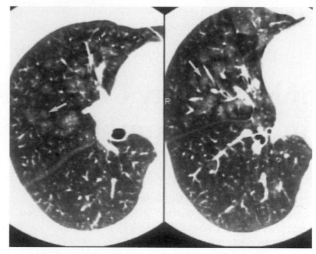

A

B,C

FIG. 10-1. Abnormal HRCT in a patient who had a normal chest radiograph. **A:** Posteroanterior radiograph in a patient who presented with recurrent episodes of hemoptysis. No abnormality is visible. **B,C:** Target-reconstructed HRCT images through the right lung obtained the same day as the chest radiograph in **A** show evidence of focal areas of ground-glass opacity, especially in the anterior segment of the right upper lobe and the middle lobes (*arrows*, **B,C**). At bronchoscopy, no discrete endobronchial lesion was identified, although there was extensive blood within the airways on the right side. The HRCT appearance is compatible with the aspiration of blood, identification of which is obviously more apparent with CT than the corresponding radiograph.

inexpensive, readily available, and can display a wide range of abnormalities. In some patients, chest radiographs can provide information sufficient for diagnosis and management. Furthermore, in those patients who have acute or progressive symptoms for whom prior films are available, radiographs often provide an accurate assessment of the course of disease. It is difficult to imagine a physician evaluating a patient who has diffuse lung disease without using chest radiographs in an attempt to detect lung disease, assess its type and extent, and to monitor the effects of treatment.

It is well-documented that chest radiographs are limited in both their sensitivity and specificity in patients who have diffuse lung disease (Figs. 10-1 and 10-2) [7–9]. For example, in a study by Epler et al. [7] of 458 patients who had histologically confirmed DILD, 44 patients, or nearly 10%, had normal chest radiographs. Similarly, Gaensler and Carrington [8] reported that nearly 16% of patients who had pathologic proof of interstitial lung disease had normal chest radiographs. Padley et al. [9] reviewed the plain radiographs of 86 patients who had biopsy-proven DILD and 14 normal subjects; in keeping with previous reports, 10% of the patients who had DILD were thought to have normal chest radiographs. Chest radiographs are even less sensitive in diagnosing airway abnormalities such as bronchiectasis, with 30% to 50% of patients who have proven bronchiectasis having normal chest films, and in patients who have emphysema, radiographs are normal in 20% or more of cases [10–13].

An equally important limitation of chest radiographs is their susceptibility to over-interpretation; it is easy to overcall the presence of diffuse pulmonary disease on chest radiographs in normal subjects [14]. It has been shown that between 10% and

20% of patients who have DILD suspected on chest radiographs subsequently prove to have normal lung biopsies [7,8]. In the study by Padley et al. [9], 18% of normal subjects were interpreted as having abnormal chest radiographs.

The sensitivity of CT and HRCT for detecting lung disease has been compared to that of plain radiography in a number of studies. Without exception, these have shown that CT, and particularly HRCT, is more sensitive than chest radiography for detecting diffuse lung diseases, although the relative sensitivity of plain films and HRCT varies with the type of abnormality present and whether it is acute or chronic [10,15–26]. Averaging the results of several studies, the sensitivity of HRCT for detecting chronic infiltrative pulmonary disease is approximately 94%, as compared to 80% for chest radiographs [14].

HRCT has been shown to be more sensitive than chest radiographs in every study of diffuse lung disease in which the two have been compared (Figs. 10-1 and 10-2) (Table 10-1). Furthermore, it should be noted that the increased sensitivity of HRCT is not achieved at the expense of decreased specificity or diagnostic accuracy [9,27,28]. A specificity of 96% for HRCT, as compared to 82% for chest radiographs, was reported by Padley et al. [9] in patients who had DILD. Similar high sensitivity (97% to 98%) and specificity (93% to 99%) values have been shown for HRCT in the diagnosis of bronchiectasis [29,30]. HRCT can further be of value in diagnosing the presence or absence of lung disease in patients who have subtle or questionable plain radiographic findings associated with acute or chronic disease (Fig. 10-3).

Although HRCT is clearly more sensitive than chest radiographs, its sensitivity in detecting lung disease is not 100%, and a negative HRCT cannot generally be used to rule out

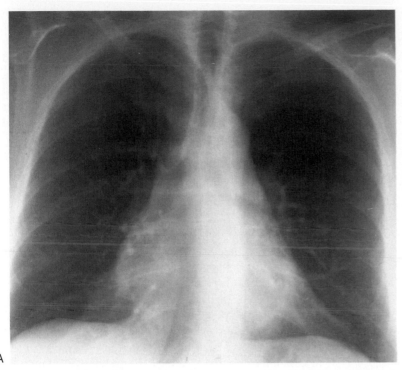
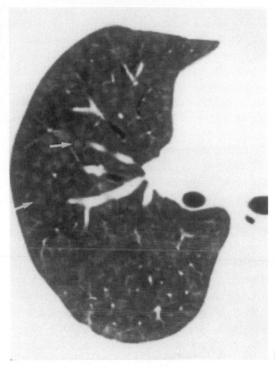

A

B

FIG. 10-2. Abnormal HRCT in a patient who had a normal chest radiograph. **A:** Chest radiograph in a patient who has progressive dyspnea appears normal, even in retrospect. **B:** HRCT through the right middle lung obtained at the same time as the radiograph in **A** is distinctly abnormal, showing numerous, ill-defined centrilobular nodules of ground-glass opacity (*arrows*). This appearance is suggestive of hypersensitivity pneumonitis; the patient had a history of exposure to birds.

lung disease, particularly in patients who have DILD. In the largest series reported to date, Padley et al. [9] evaluated HRCT studies in 100 patients, including 86 patients who had DILD and 14 normal controls. In this study, although HRCT had very high sensitivity and specificity values, 4% of subjects with biopsy-proven lung disease were interpreted as having a normal HRCT. Similar results in patients who had

early or subtle DILD have been reported by others [15,39]. In a study of eleven patients who had histologically proven hypersensitivity pneumonitis (HP), Lynch et al. [15] found that ten patients had normal chest radiographs, and six patients (55%) had a normal HRCT. Among 24 patients and six lungs with pathologic evidence of asbestosis studied by Gamsu et al. [39], five had normal HRCT scans.

TABLE 10-1. *Diseases in which HRCT has been shown to be more sensitive than plain radiographs*

Idiopathic pulmonary fibrosis [31–33]	Tuberculosis (cavitation, endobronchial spread, miliary) [46–48]
Rheumatoid lung disease [34]	Nontuberculous mycobacterial infections [49]
Scleroderma [35]	Infections in immunosuppressed patients [50]
Drug-induced lung disease [36]	Septic embolism [51]
Radiation-induced lung disease [37,38]	Hypersensitivity pneumonitis [15,52]
Asbestosis [21,22,39]	Desquamative interstitial pneumonitis [49]
Lymphangitic spread of carcinoma [19]	Respiratory bronchiolitis [53]
Hematogenous metastases [40]	*Pneumocystis carinii* pneumonia [24,25,54,55]
Bronchioloalveolar carcinoma (diffuse) [41]	Langerhans cell histiocytosis [56–58]
Sarcoidosis [17,42]	Lymphangioleiomyomatosis [18,59,60]
Berylliosis [43]	Emphysema [61,62]
Silicosis [44]	Bronchial abnormalities and bronchiectasis [29,30]
Coal worker's pneumoconiosis [45]	Cystic fibrosis [63,64]
Community-acquired pneumonia [23]	Bronchiolitis obliterans and the Swyer-James syndrome [65,66]

HRCT may also be advantageous in patients who have acute lung diseases. For example, in patients with clinical symptoms and signs suspicious for community-acquired pneumonia, HRCT identified 44% more cases than did chest radiographs [23]. Furthermore, it has been estimated that up to 10% of immunosuppressed patients who have acute diffuse lung disease have normal radiographs [67]. Thus, in immunosuppressed patients having a high clinical suspicion of disease, HRCT may be used to detect a pulmonary abnormality despite the presence of normal chest films. For example, HRCT has been shown to have a high sensitivity and specificity in the diagnosis of pulmonary complications in AIDS patients [26,68,69]. In one study, the sensitivity and specificity of CT measured 100% and 98%, respectively, in this setting [69]. In another study of patients who had AIDS [26], of 106 patients who had intrathoracic complications, 90% were correctly identified by two observers on chest radiographs, whereas 96% were identified using CT. Of 33 patients who did not have intrathoracic disease, 73% were correctly identified using chest radiographs, and 86% were correctly called normal on CT. Similarly, Hartman et al. [68], in an assessment of HRCT findings in 102 AIDS patients who had proven intrathoracic complications, and 20 human immunodeficiency virus (HIV)–positive patients who did not have active intrathoracic disease, found that one observer detected all 102 cases of active disease, whereas a second observer detected all but one. More specifically, in AIDS patients who have suspected *Pneumocystis carinii* pneumonia and normal or equivocal chest radiographs [24], the sensitivity of HRCT has been shown to be 100% in making this diagnosis, whereas the speci-

ficity was 89%. Similar accuracy in excluding disease has been reported by Mori et al. [50] in a study of 55 pairs of chest radiographs and CT studies obtained in 33 bone marrow transplant patients who had fever. On the one hand, these authors found that CT proved a reliable method for detecting fungal infection, with nodules being seen in 20 of 21 cases. On the other hand, a negative CT study suggested that the underlying cause of fever most likely was due to a bacteremia or nonfilamentous fungal infection of nonpulmonary origin [50].

The sensitivity of HRCT has also proven superior to that of conventional CT obtained with thicker collimation (Figs. 10-4 and 10-5) [21,70,71]. Remy-Jardin et al. [71] assessed 150 patients using both conventional CT (10-mm collimation) and HRCT (1.2-mm collimation), with sections obtained at identical levels; they found that HRCT was clearly superior to conventional CT in identifying a number of abnormalities, including septal and nonseptal lines, nodular and linear interfaces, small cystic airspaces, bronchiectasis, and pleural thickening. Furthermore, these authors found that reliable identification of ground-glass opacity required the use of HRCT. Conventional CT proved superior to HRCT only in the detection of small nodules, and even here, nearly 15% of small nodules could only be seen using HRCT. Similarly, in a study of patients who had asbestosis, Aberle et al. [21] were able to identify subtle parenchymal reticulation on HRCT in 96% of cases, as compared to only 83% of cases with conventional CT. As another example, studies comparing the accuracy of HRCT to bronchography in diagnosing bronchiectasis [29,30]

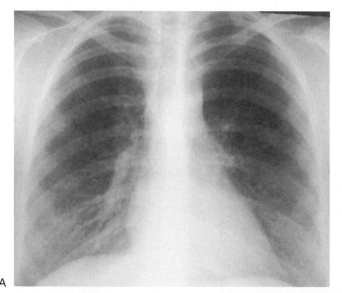

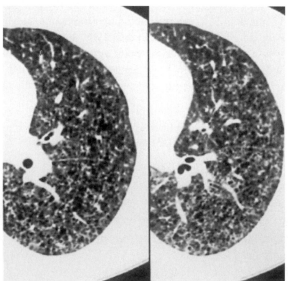

A   B,C

FIG. 10-3. Abnormal HRCT in a patient who has questionable radiographic abnormalities. **A:** Routine posteroanterior radiograph in an asymptomatic patient shows a subtle diffuse increase in lung markings difficult to characterize. It would be difficult to say that this radiograph is definitely abnormal. **B,C:** Target-reconstructed HRCT images through the left lung show the presence of thin-walled cysts, evenly spaced throughout the lungs associated with a few small, poorly defined nodules. These findings are characteristic of Langerhans cell histiocytosis. Although the differential diagnosis includes lymphangiomyomatosis, the presence of nodules and the fact that the patient is asymptomatic make this diagnosis much less likely. The diagnosis was subsequently confirmed by transbronchial biopsy.

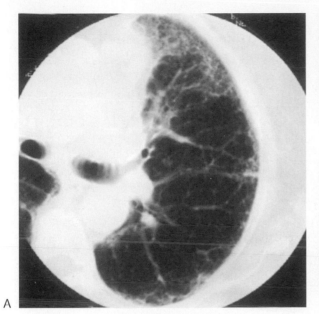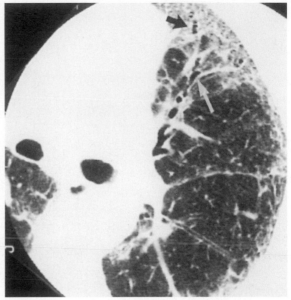

A
B

FIG. 10-4. HRCT versus routine CT in the evaluation of diffuse lung disease. **A,B:** Target reconstructions of a routine 10-mm-thick section **(A)** and a 1.5-mm-thick HRCT section **(B)** obtained at the same level through the left midlung in a patient who has biopsy-proven idiopathic pulmonary fibrosis. The presence of reticular opacities is far easier to assess with HRCT. In particular, note the presence of bronchiectasis involving the anterior segmental bronchus (*arrows* in **B**), visible only on the HRCT section.

have found sensitivity values of 97% to 98%, and a specificity of 93% to 99%; previous studies of conventional CT with 10-mm collimation reported sensitivities ranging from 60% to 80% [72,73].

Because of its excellent sensitivity, we consider that HRCT is indicated to detect lung disease in patients who have normal or questionable radiographic abnormalities, and symptoms or pulmonary function findings suggestive of acute or chronic

diffuse lung disease (Table 10-2). This includes patients who have unexplained dyspnea in whom chronic DILD is suspected; symptomatic patients who have known exposures to inorganic dusts such as silica and asbestos, organic antigens, or drugs; immunosuppressed patients who have unexplained dyspnea or fever; patients who have unexplained hemoptysis; and patients who have dyspnea or other symptoms and suspected airways or obstructive lung disease [14,74].

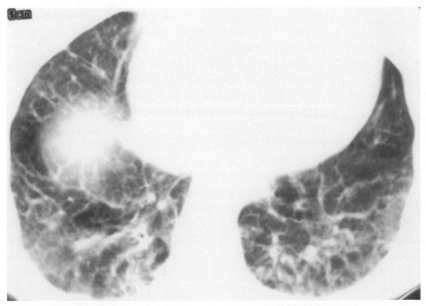

A

FIG. 10-5. Conventional CT (10-mm collimation) versus HRCT. Sections at identical levels through the lung bases in a patient who has proven lymphangitic carcinomatosis, obtained with 10-mm **(A)** and 1.5-mm **(B)** collimation. Note that identification of fine architectural details, including secondary lobular anatomy and peribronchial infiltration, can only be appreciated with high-resolution imaging. *Continued*

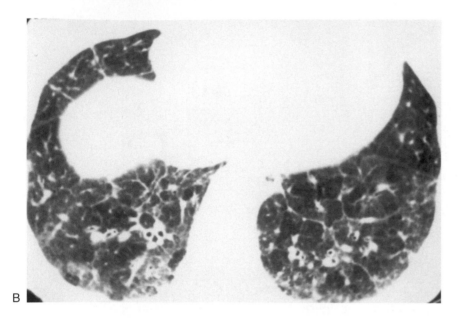

B

FIG. 10-5. *Continued*

TABLE 10-2. *Indications for the use of HRCT in patients who have suspected diffuse lung disease*

Chronic disease

To detect lung disease in patients who have normal or questionable radiographic abnormalities, who have symptoms or pulmonary function findings suggestive of diffuse lung disease

To make a specific diagnosis, or limit the differential diagnosis, in patients who have abnormal chest radiographs, in whom the clinical and radiographic findings are nonspecific, and further evaluation is considered appropriate

To assess disease activity

As a guide for the need or optimal site and type of lung biopsy

Acute disease

To detect lung disease in patients who have symptoms of acute lung disease and normal or nondiagnostic chest radiographs, particularly in immunosuppressed patients

To exclude specific diseases (e.g., *Pneumocystis carinii* pneumonia), based on HRCT findings

To suggest specific diagnoses or a list of possible diagnoses to determine subsequent evaluation (e.g., using bronchoscopy)

To evaluate otherwise unexplained hemoptysis

As a guide for the need or optimal site for lung biopsy

DIAGNOSTIC ACCURACY OF HIGH-RESOLUTION COMPUTED TOMOGRAPHY

Even in the presence of definite abnormalities, chest radiographs have limited diagnostic accuracy in patients who have diffuse lung disease. Because of superimposition of structures and relatively low contrast resolution, it is often difficult to accurately characterize chest radiographic abnormalities (Figs. 10-6 and 10-7). Although a pattern recognition approach to the diagnosis of lung disease can be helpful in interpreting chest radiographs, it has well-documented limitations, and correlation with histologic findings is often poor [75–77].

In an attempt to improve diagnostic accuracy, McLoud and coworkers [78] used a semi-quantitative approach to the plain film diagnosis of diffuse lung disease based on a modification of the International Labor Office and Union Internationale Contre le Cancer classification of plain film abnormalities [78]. In an evaluation of 365 patients who had open-lung biopsy–confirmed DILD, these investigators found that their first two diagnostic choices corresponded to the histologic diagnosis in only 50% of patients, improving to 78% when the first three choices were included. Furthermore, there was only 70% interobserver agreement as to the predominant type of parenchymal abnormality or its extent. These results clearly show how difficult the precise interpretation of chest films can be, even for the experienced observer. Even as seemingly simple a diagnosis as identification of focal consolidation in patients who have clinical evidence of pneumonia is associated with considerable interobserver variation, which furthermore may be independent of level of interpreter expertise [79].

Similar limitations in the diagnostic accuracy of chest radiography have been observed [9,27,28]. In a study by Mathieson et al. [27], the accuracy of chest radiographs in 118 consecutive patients who had chronic diffuse lung disease were assessed; radiographs were assessed independently by three observers who listed their three most likely diagnoses in order of probability, as well as their degree of confidence in these diagnoses. A confident diagnosis was reached radiographically in only 23% of cases; a correct first-choice diagnosis was made in only 57%, and in 73% the correct diagnosis was among the first three choices. In a similarly designed study by Grenier et al. [28], the diagnostic accuracy of chest radiographs determined in 140 consecutive patients

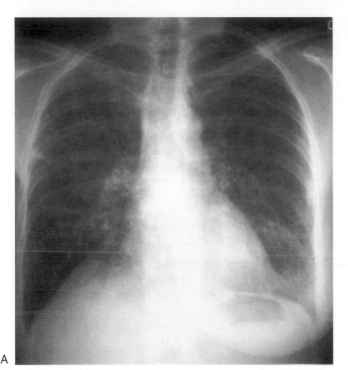
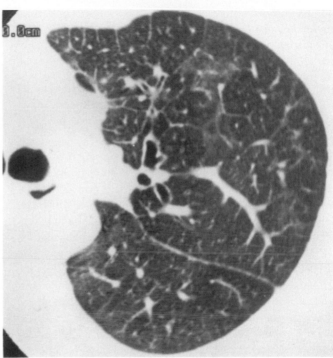

FIG. 10-6. HRCT-radiographic correlation in a patient who has lymphangitic carcinomatosis. **A:** Posteroanterior chest radiograph in a middle-aged woman, following a right mastectomy. Increased reticular markings are visible but nonspecific; although these findings could be due to lymphangitic carcinomatosis, their differential diagnosis also includes radiation or drug-related pneumonitis, or both, viral pneumonia, and even pulmonary edema. **B:** Targeted HRCT through the left upper lobe shows characteristic findings of lymphangitic carcinomatosis, including slightly nodular interlobular septal thickening.

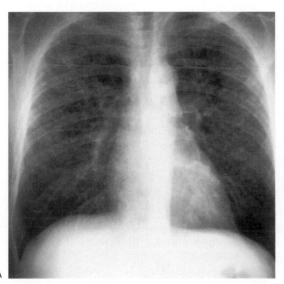
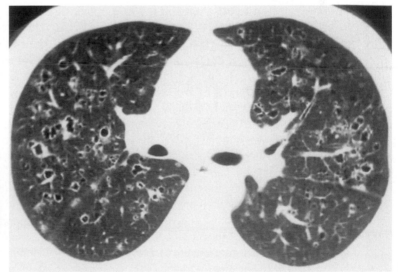

FIG. 10-7. HRCT-radiographic correlation in a patient who has Langerhans cell histiocytosis. **A:** Routine posteroanterior radiograph in an asymptomatic young male smoker shows diffuse increased markings throughout both lungs, with relative sparing of the lung bases. **B:** HRCT through the middle lungs shows unusually shaped cysts and a few small peripheral nodules, in the absence of reticulation. These findings are characteristic of patients who have Langerhans cell histiocytosis, subsequently verified by transbronchial biopsy. In this case, HRCT clearly enhances diagnostic accuracy, as compared with the corresponding chest radiograph.

who had proven diffuse chronic lung disease was 64% for a first-choice diagnosis, and 78% if the top three choices were considered. These data substantiate that the accurate radiographic interpretation of DILD represents something of an art, relatively difficult to perform as well as to teach [76].

Given the precision with which HRCT can delineate lung morphology, it is not surprising that there is a close correlation between cross sectional imaging findings and gross pathology. As noted by Colby and Swensen [80], many interstitial diseases preferentially affect certain anatomic compartments that may be appreciated at low-power microscopic evaluation. These include diseases that are primarily broncho- or bronchiolocentric, angiocentric, perilymphatic, peripheral acinar, septal, and diffuse interstitial, among others, which are distributions of disease also recognizable on HRCT. For example, of particular value for the interpretation of HRCT is recognition of diseases that primarily affect the secondary pulmonary lobule, especially those characterized by centrilobular disease [81–84]. Close equivalence between lung morphology and HRCT has been documented for a number of diseases, including pulmonary fibrosis of varying causes (including the idiopathic interstitial pneumonias, asbestosis, and collagen-vascular diseases, among others), sarcoidosis, Langerhans cell histiocytosis (LCH), HP, lymphangitic carcinomatosis, lymphangiolieomyomatosis (LAM), as well as the various patterns of bronchiectasis, and emphysema [80,85–87].

Numerous reports have shown that HRCT is significantly more accurate than are plain radiographs in diagnosing both acute and chronic diffuse lung disease, usually allows a more confident diagnosis, and is subject to considerably less interobserver variation in its interpretation (Figs. 10-6 through 10-9) [9,14,27,28,67–69,71,88–92]. These studies consistently show that the accuracy of HRCT in the diagnosis of diffuse lung disease is superior to that of chest radiography, with a diagnostic advantage averaging 10% to 20% regardless of the criteria used (Table 10-3). Nonetheless, although their overall conclusions are not in doubt, many of these studies suffer from important design flaws, some unavoidable, which limit their precision [93]. Given the importance of these studies for assessing the impact of HRCT on clinical practice, these are reviewed in depth.

In an early retrospective study reported by Mathieson et al. [27], the accuracy of chest radiographs, and both conventional and HRCT images in making specific diagnoses were compared in 118 cases imaged over a 4-year period. A confident diagnosis was reached more than twice as often with CT and HRCT than with chest radiographs (49% and 23%, respectively). More important, a correct diagnosis was made in 93% of the first-choice CT interpretations, as compared to 77% of the first-choice plain film interpretations ($p < .001$). It should be noted, however, that the number of diseases assessed was limited. Also, the degree of high "confidence" assessed by these authors was never defined. Furthermore, images were interpreted without the benefit of clinical history, additionally limiting diagnostic accuracy. Equally as

important, as with most subsequent reports, a patient referral bias likely existed because many of the patients in this study had forms of interstitial lung disease that tended to have specific HRCT appearances [93].

Similar findings have been reported by Padley et al. [9]. In this retrospective study of 86 patients who had DILD, comprising 15 different lung diseases and 14 normal subjects, a confident diagnosis was reached more often with CT using 3-mm collimation (49%) than with chest radiography (41%), the diagnoses were more often correct with HRCT (82%) than with chest radiographs (69%), and HRCT interpretations were associated with less interobserver disagreement. However, as with Mathieson et al. [27], images were interpreted without supporting clinical data, and a confident diagnosis was not clearly defined. In this study, the overall accuracy of HRCT proved less than that reported by Mathiesen et al. In part, this may reflect differences in the mix of cases; for example, only three cases of lymphangitic carcinoma were included in this study (an easy diagnosis to make), compared with seven cases of bronchiolitis obliterans organizing pneumonia (BOOP), for which HRCT is less diagnostic [94]. Furthermore, although the accuracy of HRCT for diagnosing usual interstitial pneumonia (UIP) and LCH proved greater than 90%, the accuracy rates for sarcoidosis and HP were considerably lower, possibly reflecting differences in the stages in which these diseases were evaluated [9].

In the first such study to use state-of-the-art HRCT, with 1-mm images obtained every 10 mm, Grenier et al. also confirmed the superior diagnostic accuracy of HRCT compared with plain radiographs [28]. In this retrospective study of 140 patients who had 18 different causes of DILD, interpreted by three independent observers without clinical history, a correct first-choice diagnosis overall was made in 64% of cases with radiographs versus 76% with HRCT, regardless of the confidence level. When a confident first-choice diagnosis was made, defined as a greater than 75% chance of being correct, HRCT proved accurate overall in 53% of cases, compared to 27% for chest radiographs ($p < .001$). In this study, a correct high-probability diagnosis was made in 59% to 88% of cases of LCH, 64% to 72% with sarcoidosis, 30% to 67% with UIP, and 27% to 55% with silicosis, indicating the presence of considerable interobserver variability, although significantly less than for the interpretation of corresponding radiographs [28].

In an attempt to further assess the role of HRCT, these authors also evaluated chest radiographic and HRCT findings by ranked stepwise discriminant analysis of five separate groups [28]. These groups included patients who had sarcoidosis, pulmonary fibrosis, LCH, silicosis, and miscellaneous diseases. Analyzed in this fashion, the four findings that were most discriminant in distinguishing these groups were HRCT findings, and included intralobular reticular lines, thin-walled cysts, a peripheral distribution of abnormalities, and traction bronchiectasis. Similarly, eight of the most discriminant 12 findings were on HRCT.

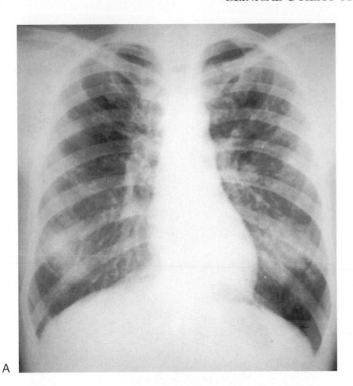

A

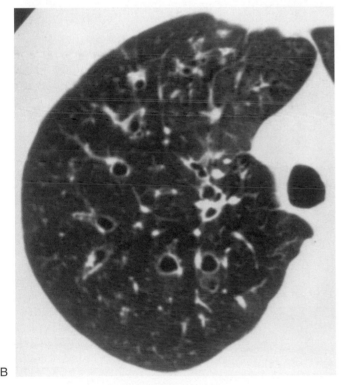

B

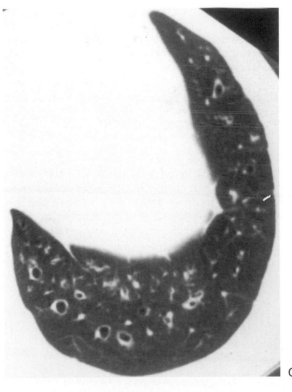

C

FIG. 10-8. HRCT-radiographic correlation in a patient who has diffuse bronchiectasis. **A:** Posteroanterior chest radiograph shows nonspecific increased lung markings in both upper lobes, with a suggestion of focal, poorly defined lucencies in the upper lobes. **B,C:** Targeted HRCT through the right upper lobe **(B)** and left lower lobe **(C)** shows characteristic findings of cystic bronchiectasis, in the absence of lung fibrosis.

Nishimura et al. reported their findings comparing HRCT with plain radiographs in 134 cases of both acute and chronic diffuse lung disease, representing 21 different entities read without history by 20 different physicians [88]. These authors also confirmed the higher diagnostic accuracy of HRCT as compared to chest radiographs, although slightly less convincingly than previous authors. Overall, a correct first-choice diagnosis was made radiographically in 38% of cases versus 46% of cases using HRCT ($p < .01$), whereas the correct diagnosis was listed among the first three choices in 49% of cases radiographically and in 59% of cases with HRCT. It is worth noting that diffuse infectious diseases [endobronchial spread of both tuberculosis (TB) and nontuberculous mycobacteria, and *Mycoplasma* pneumonia] were included in this study, likely accounting for the slightly lower accuracy of HRCT in this study as compared to others.

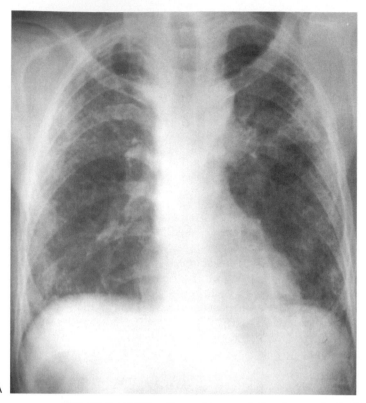
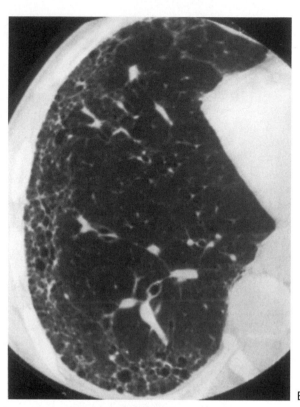

A

B

FIG. 10-9. HRCT-radiographic correlation in a patient who has idiopathic pulmonary fibrosis. **A:** Posteroanterior radiograph shows diffuse increased reticular markings throughout both lung fields. Although this appearance is suggestive of parenchymal fibrosis, the pattern is nonspecific. **B:** Retrospectively targeted HRCT through the right lower lobe shows characteristic findings of honeycombing, with irregularly thick-walled cystic spaces, mild traction bronchiolectasis, and a strikingly peripheral distribution. Ground-glass opacity and nodules are absent. In this case, HRCT findings strongly mitigate against the need either for transbronchial or open-lung biopsy.

TABLE 10-3. *Comparative accuracy of chest radiographs and HRCT in patients with diffuse lung disease*

Study	Confident first-choice diagnosis		Correct first-choice diagnosis when confident		Correct first-choice diagnosis		Correct diagnosis in first three choices	
	Chest x-ray (%)	HRCT (%)	Chest x-ray (%)	HRCT (%)	Chest x-ray (%)	HRCT (%)	Chest x-ray (%)	HRCT (%)
Mathieson et al.[a]	23	49	77	93	57	72	73	89
Padley et al.[b]	41	49	69	82	47	56	72	81
Grenier et al.[c]	—	—	27	53	64	76	78	83
Nishimura et al.[d]	—	—	60	63	38	46	49	59
Average	32	49	58	73	52	63	67	78

[a]Mathieson JR, Mayo JR, Staples CA, et al. Chronic diffuse infiltrative lung disease: comparison of diagnostic accuracy of CT and chest radiography. *Radiology* 1989;171:111–116.
[b]Padley SPG, Hansell DM, Flower CDR, et al. Comparative accuracy of high resolution computed tomography and chest radiography in the diagnosis of chronic diffuse infiltrative lung disease. *Clin Radiol* 1991;44:222–226.
[c]Grenier P, Valeyre D, Cluzel P, et al. Chronic diffuse interstitial lung disease: diagnostic value of chest radiography and high-resolution CT. *Radiology* 1991;179:123–132.
[d]Nishimura K, Izumi T, Kitaichi M, et al. The diagnostic accuracy of high-resolution computed tomography in diffuse infiltrative lung diseases. *Chest* 1993;104:1149–1155.

In an attempt to focus on problematic cases for whom surgical biopsy was deemed necessary, Swensen et al. retrospectively reviewed CT scans from 85 patients [58 (68%) of whom had HRCT images available] who had documented DILD [95]. Diagnoses were reached by consensus, with the three most likely reported in order of probability. Similar to most prior studies, images were interpreted without clinical history or knowledge of the specific diseases included in the study; confidence levels were reported only as definite, probable, or possible. In 79 cases (93%), the correct diagnosis proved to be one of the three suggested diagnoses. In 54 cases (64%), the correct diagnosis proved to be the first suggested. Although a high level of confidence was reached in only 20 cases (24%), the diagnosis in such cases proved accurate in 18 of those patients (90%). It should be emphasized that these results were intentionally biased by patient selection. Only those who had unexplained disease requiring biopsy were selected. Importantly, only a single case each of sarcoidosis and lymphangitic carcinomatosis were included, reflecting the practice in this institution of making these diagnoses either clinically or by TBB. In distinction, a total of 13 cases of proved lung infections were included, diagnoses that may have been suggested by CT with the appropriate clinical history. Similarly, this study also included three cases of diffuse alveolar damage that the authors themselves noted likely would have been diagnosed with appropriate clinical correlation.

Low-dose HRCT techniques have also been shown to be more accurate than chest radiographs in diagnosing diffuse lung disease (Fig. 10-10). In a study by Lee et al. [90], the diagnostic accuracies of chest radiographs, low-dose HRCT (80 mA; 120 kilovolt peak [kV(p)], 40 mA, 2 seconds), and conventional-dose HRCT [340 mAs; 120 kV(p), 170 mA, 2 seconds] were compared in ten normal controls and 50 patients who had chronic infiltrative lung disease. For each HRCT technique, only three images were used, obtained at the levels of the aortic arch, tracheal carina, and 1 cm above the right hemidiaphragm. A correct first-choice diagnosis was made significantly more often with either HRCT technique than with radiography; the correct diagnosis was made in 65% of cases using radiographs, 74% of cases with low-dose HRCT ($p < .02$), and 80% of conventional HRCT ($p < .005$). A high confidence level in making a diagnosis was reached in 42% of radiographic examinations, 61% of the low-dose ($p < .01$), and 63% of the conventional-dose HRCT examinations ($p < .005$), which were correct in 92%, 90%, and 96% of the studies, respectively. Although conventional-dose HRCT was more accurate than low-dose HRCT, this difference was not significant, and both techniques were felt to provide quite similar anatomic information (see Figs. 1-7 and 1-8; Fig. 10-7) [90].

The diagnostic accuracy of HRCT has also been assessed relative to that of conventional CT. In one study [70], the authors randomly compared three HRCT sections with conventional CT scans obtained at the same three levels and a complete conventional CT study of the lungs in 75 patients who had proven diffuse lung disease. In each case, observers provided their most likely diagnoses, as well as their degrees

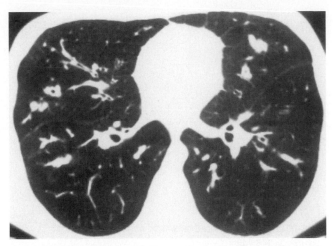

FIG. 10-10. Low-dose HRCT. A 1.5-mm section through the middle lungs in a patient who has cystic fibrosis and evidence of diffuse bronchiectasis and mucoid impaction. Although this study was performed using 40 mA, morphologic detail in the lung is comparable to most routine HRCT images. (Courtesy of Minnie Bhalla, M.D., New York University Medical Center, New York, New York.)

of confidence. Although no significant difference in diagnostic accuracy was identified, the highest confidence level in diagnosis (49%) was reached using the three available HRCT sections. By comparison, the highest confidence level was only recorded in 31% of cases for interpretation based on the corresponding three 10-mm sections, and 43% of cases for interpretations based on a complete set of contiguous conventional CT sections through the thorax. Based on these data, the authors concluded that in patients who have diffuse lung disease, the correct diagnosis may be suggested by only a limited number of HRCT scans, eliminating the need for a complete conventional CT examination [70].

In an attempt to address the problem of a lack of clinical and radiologic correlation in HRCT interpretation, Grenier et al. used Bayesian analysis to determine the relative value of clinical data, chest radiographs, and HRCT in patients who had chronic DILD [96]. For this study, two samples from the same population of patients who had 27 different diffuse lung diseases were consecutively assessed: an initial, retrospectively evaluated set of training cases (n = 208), and a subsequent prospectively evaluated set of test cases (n = 100) for validation. This approach enabled the assignment of diagnostic probabilities based on clinical, radiologic, and CT variables. The results showed that for the test group, an accurate diagnosis could be made in 27% of cases based on clinical data only, increasing to 53% of cases ($p < .0001$) with the addition of chest radiographs, and to 61% of cases ($p = .07$) with the further addition of HRCT scans. Assessed for individual diseases, HRCT made the greatest contribution to the diagnosis of sarcoidosis, LCH, HP, lymphangitic carcinomatosis, and to a lesser degree, silicosis (Table 10-4). Although only minor improvement was seen in the diagnosis of pulmo-

TABLE 10-4. *Diseases in which HRCT is advantageous*

Disease	Mathieson et al.[a]	Grenier et al.[b]	Grenier et al.[c]	Nishimura et al.[d]	Padley et al.[e]
Sarcoidosis	X	X	X	X	
Usual interstitial pneumonia	X			X	
Langerhans cell histiocytosis	X	X	X		X
Hypersensitivity pneumonitis			X	X	
Lymphangitic carcinomatosis	X		X		X
Silicosis	X		X	X	
Alveolar proteinosis				X	X
Lymphangioleiomyomatosis				X	X
Bronchiolitis obliterans organizing pneumonia/cryptogenic organizing pneumonia				X	X

[a]Mathieson JR, Mayo JR, Staples CA, et al. Chronic diffuse infiltrative lung disease: comparison of diagnostic accuracy of CT and chest radiography. *Radiology* 1989;171:111–116.

[b]Grenier P, Valeyre D, Cluzel P, et al. Chronic diffuse interstitial lung disease: diagnostic value of chest radiography and high-resolution CT. *Radiology* 1991;179:123–132.

[c]Grenier P, Chevret S, Beigelman C, et al. Chronic diffuse infiltrative lung disease: determination of the diagnostic value of clinical data, chest radiography, and CT with Bayesian analysis. *Radiology* 1994;9:383–390.

[d]Nishimura K, Izumi T, Kitaichi M, et al. The diagnostic accuracy of high-resolution computed tomography in diffuse infiltrative lung diseases. *Chest* 1993;104:1149–1155.

[e]Padley SPG, Hansell DM, Flower CDR, et al. Comparative accuracy of high resolution computed tomography and chest radiography in the diagnosis of chronic diffuse infiltrative lung disease. *Clin Radiol* 1991;44:222–226.

nary fibrosis, as the authors themselves noted, this probably reflected a population with advanced disease, as virtually all of these patients presented with diffuse radiographic abnormalities. Not surprisingly, the value of HRCT diminished with uncommon diseases; 23 of 34 (68%) misdiagnosed patients in this study had diseases classified as miscellaneous.

It should be noted that for the first time, these authors also report the occurrence of incorrect high confidence diagnoses in both the retrospective and prospective portions of their study [96]. In the retrospective portion, incorrect high confidence diagnoses occurred in 4% of patients. Many of these incorrect diagnoses could be considered spurious: rheumatoid lung misclassified as idiopathic pulmonary fibrosis (IPF), for example, or hematogenous metastases mistaken for lymphangitic carcinomatosis [93]. More problematic, however, is the fact that in the prospective part of this study, two patients who had lymphangitic carcinomatosis were misdiagnosed as having sarcoidosis or HP, and four patients who had silicosis were diagnosed as having sarcoidosis. These misdiagnoses likely reflect, at least in part, unavoidable assumptions regarding the prevalence of various diseases: sarcoidosis being more common than silicosis, for example. Furthermore, in this study, important designators such as "centrilobular" were excluded, no doubt accounting for the fact that in no case was a diagnosis of HP made [93].

It is apparent that despite the overall similarity of the results of these cited studies, important limitations apply, accounting for differences in the reported accuracies of HRCT in diagnosing specific infiltrative diseases (Tables 10-3 and 10-4). In addition to differences in scan techniques, these limitations include retrospective design, failure to account for a wide range of interpretive skill, lack of clinical correlation, marked variation in case mix (referral bias), lack of correlation with disease stage, and inconsistent definition of degrees of confidence. Furthermore, it is also important to consider baseline probabilities for diagnostic decision making, as this could vary considerably. Clearly, optimal use of HRCT requires integration of clinical and radiologic data as part of a broader team approach involving pulmonologists, surgeons, pathologists, and radiologists.

Recent experience with HRCT in diagnosing obstructive disease, airways disease, and emphysema also supports the utility of HRCT in making these diagnoses. Large airways diseases, small airways diseases of various types, and emphysema are all accurately diagnosed [10,74,92,97–112].

HRCT is very accurate in the diagnosis of large airways disease and bronchiectasis (Fig. 10-8) [29,30,111,113]. Furthermore, although HRCT is of some value in distinguishing among the common causes of bronchiectasis, at least to the extent that further appropriate evaluation may be suggested, results of studies assessing its accuracy have been mixed [114–116]. Lee et al. [115], in a study of CT scans in 108 patients who had bronchiectasis from a variety of causes [including idiopathic bronchiectasis, allergic bronchopulmonary aspergillosis (ABPA), impaired mucociliary clearance, hypogammaglobulinemia, and adult cystic fibrosis (CF)] found that HRCT was of limited accuracy in the diagnosis of the specific etiology of the airway abnormality. They found that a correct first-choice diagnosis was made by three experienced observers in only 45% of cases, and a high confidence

TABLE 10-5. *Accuracy of HRCT in patients with acquired immunodeficiency syndrome–related lung disease*

	Correct diagnosis listed in top 3 (%)	Correct first choice diagnosis (%)	Confident diagnosis made (%)	Confident diagnosis correct (%)
Pneumocystis carinii pneumonia	84	83	73	94
Kaposi's sarcoma	92	83	75	90
Tuberculosis/*Mycobacterium avium* complex	77	44	15	88
Pyogenic infection	50	29	7	100
Fungal infection	86	41	18	100
Lymphoma	70	20	0	—
Lung carcinoma	75	75	0	—
Nocardia	50	0	0	—
Toxoplasmosis	0	0	0	—

Modified from Hartman TE, Primack SL, Müller NL, et al. Diagnosis of thoracic complications in AIDS: accuracy of CT. *AJR Am J Roentgenol* 1994;162:547–553.

level was reached in only 9% of cases. Of these, a correct diagnosis was reached in only 35% of cases, and poor interobserver agreement (mean κ = 0.20) was also found. It should be emphasized, however, that in this study, CT scans were interpreted in the absence of clinical data [115]. Cartier et al. [116] reported better results in a retrospective study of 82 consecutive patients who had various causes of bronchiectasis. These authors noted that a correct diagnosis was reached by two independent observers in 61% of cases, including a correct diagnosis in 68% of cases of CF, 67% of cases with TB, 56% of cases of ABPA, and 43% of cases of previous childhood infection, with moderate agreement between the observers for correct diagnoses (κ = 0.53) [116]. It should be emphasized that the value of HRCT in patients who have large airways disease is significantly better if clinical information is also assessed, and the presence or absence of specific findings is sought. Ward et al. [117], for example, assessing the accuracy of HRCT in the diagnosis of ABPA in asthmatic patients, found that a combination of bronchiectasis in more than three lobes, centrilobular nodules, and mucoid impaction could be identified in 95%, 93%, and 67% of cases, respectively, in patients who had ABPA, but were present in only 29%, 28%, and 4% of asthmatic controls [117]. Similarly, Swensen et al. [118] tested the hypothesis that bronchiectasis and multiple small lung nodules seen on chest CT are indicative of *Mycobacterium-avium* complex infection or colonization by reviewing the CT scans of 100 patients with a CT diagnosis of bronchiectasis. The authors found a sensitivity of 80%, a specificity of 87%, and an accuracy of 86% in predicting positive cultures for *M. avium* complex based on these HRCT findings. Similar findings were documented by Tanaka et al. [119].

HRCT is also accurate in diagnosing emphysema, a fact that has been recognized since the introduction of this technique. For example, in a retrospective review of HRCT findings in patients who had pathologically proven cystic lung diseases, including LCH, LAM, and emphysema [92], HRCT allowed two radiologists to be confident of the diag-

nosis of pulmonary emphysema in 95% of cases. When confident, the observers were correct in 100% of the cases. However, it should be pointed out that the number of patients and diseases evaluated in this study were limited.

HRCT findings may also be of value in the diagnosis of acute lung disease in AIDS patients [24,25,68,120–124]. In patients who had AIDS and acute lung disease studied by Hartman et al. [68] using HRCT, the correct first-choice diagnosis, regardless of the degree of confidence, was made in 66% of the cases. A confident diagnosis was made in 48% of all cases, and the observers were correct in 92% of those cases. The interpretations of CT scans were most often accurate in the confident diagnosis of *Pneumocystis carinii* pneumonia (94%) and Kaposi's sarcoma (90%) (Table 10-5). Similarly, in a study by Kang et al. [121] of 89 patients who had a single proved thoracic complication, two observers were confident in their first-choice diagnosis in 61 of 178 (34%) interpretations using chest radiographs, and in 83 of 178 (47%) interpretations using CT. The diagnosis was correct in 67% (41 of 61) of confident radiographic interpretations, as compared with 87% (72 of 83) of interpretations at CT (*p* <.01). These studies also suffer from some of the limitations described above.

In other clinical situations, HRCT findings in patients who have suspected pneumonia can be sufficiently accurate to determine presumptive treatment or subsequent diagnostic evaluation. For example, in patients who have suspected *Pneumocystis carinii* pneumonia and normal or equivocal radiographic findings, HRCT can be quite helpful in selecting patients who have a high likelihood of this disease; in a study by Gruden et al., HRCT had a sensitivity of 100% and a specificity of 89% in diagnosing *Pneumocystis carinii* pneumonia [24]. In this study, 18 of 51 patients were managed according to the HRCT interpretation and followed clinically without the need for bronchoscopy.

CT has been found to be superior to chest radiography in the differential diagnosis of acute pulmonary complications in immunocompromised patients who do not have AIDS [69]. In a study comparing the abilities of CT and radiography for detecting and diagnosing acute pulmonary complications in this group, the CT scans and radiographs of 45 immunocompromised non-AIDS patients who had proven pulmonary disease and 20 normal controls were independently assessed by two observers, without knowledge of clinical or pathologic data. The observers listed the three most likely diagnoses and their degree of confidence in the first-choice diagnosis on a three-point scale. The sensitivity and specificity in detecting pulmonary complications were 100% and 98% for CT, respectively, compared to 98% and 93%, respectively, for chest radiography. In the immunocompromised patients, the first-choice diagnosis was correct in 44% of CT scans and 30% of radiograph readings ($p < .01$). The correct diagnosis was among the top three diagnoses for 70% of CT scans and 53% of radiograph readings ($p < .01$). Confidence level one (definite) was reached in 33% of CT scans and 10% of chest radiographs ($p < .001$). Diseases with a dominant nodular pattern had a higher occurrence of correct first-choice diagnosis (62% vs. 34%; $p < .02$) and level one confidence ratings (53% vs. 13%; $p < .001$) than diseases with ground-glass opacity, consolidation, or irregular linear opacities.

CT may also play an important role in assessing acute parenchymal disease in immunocompetent patients. In a study of HRCT findings in 90 patients who had acute parenchymal diseases assessed without the benefit of clinical history, Tomiyama et al. showed that two independent observers were 90% accurate in classifying diseases as infectious or noninfectious, although the types of infections studied were limited. Furthermore, the observers made a correct first-choice diagnosis in an average of 55 of 90 (61%) cases [125]. This included 50% of cases with bacterial pneumonia, 62% of cases with *Mycoplasma* pneumonia, 90% of cases with acute interstitial pneumonitis (AIP), 72% of cases with HP, 30% of cases with acute eosinophilic pneumonia, and 28% of cases with pulmonary hemorrhage. One can only speculate how much greater the accuracy of CT would have been if clinical histories had been provided. On the other hand, a more inclusive list of infections would likely reduce accuracy below that reported in this study.

DIAGNOSTIC APPEARANCES ON HIGH-RESOLUTION COMPUTED TOMOGRAPHY

HRCT is often indicated in patients who have an abnormal chest radiograph, when radiographic and clinical findings are nonspecific, and when further evaluation is considered appropriate (Table 10-2). In this setting, HRCT findings can often be used to limit the differential diagnosis to a few possibilities, and this can be of considerable value in determining the subsequent diagnostic evaluation. More important, HRCT appearances can be diagnostic in select cases, or else so strongly suggestive that lung biopsy can be avoided. In our judgment, there are some diseases in which information derived from HRCT can be sufficiently characteristic to allow a specific or presumptive

TABLE 10-6. Diseases for which HRCT can be diagnostic in the appropriate clinical setting
Pulmonary fibrosis
Idiopathic (usual interstitial pneumonia/idiopathic pulmonary fibrosis)
Associated with collagen-vascular diseases; asbestosis
Sarcoidosis
Lymphangitic/hematogenous metastases
Subacute hypersensitivity pneumonitis
Silicosis or coal worker's pneumoconiosis
Langerhans cell histiocytosis
Lymphangioleiomyomatosis/tuberculous sclerosis
Emphysema
Bronchiectasis
Infectious bronchiolitis
Pneumocystis carinii pneumonia[a]
Kaposi's sarcoma[a]
[a]In human immunodeficiency virus–positive/acquired immunodeficiency syndrome patients.

diagnosis to be made in the absence of histologic verification in the appropriate clinical setting (Table 10-6). Several examples are reviewed below.

HRCT findings of diffuse centrilobular ground-glass opacities, for example, suggest the diagnosis of subacute HP; this diagnosis can usually be confirmed by the clinical history and appropriate serologic tests, precluding lung biopsy (Figs. 10-2 and 10-11) [126,127]. Indeed, in our experience, HRCT findings not infrequently lead to the first suspicion of the diagnosis of HP.

Similarly, in the appropriate clinical setting, the diagnosis of sarcoidosis also can be confidently made based on a combination of clinical, radiographic, and CT findings [93,95]. Although a number of other diseases, most notably lymphangitic carcinomatosis, may result in a perilymphatic distribution of disease typical of sarcoidosis, differentiation is usually easily made even in the absence of clinical correlation. For example, in a study comparing CT scans in 40 patients who had lymphangitic carcinomatosis with 41 patients who had sarcoidosis, Honda et al. showed that findings of thickened interlobular septa and extensive involvement of the subpleural interstitium were significantly more common in patients who had lymphangitic carcinomatosis ($p < .0001$), whereas bilateral distribution of disease was significantly more common in patients who had sarcoidosis ($p < .001$) [128]. Nonetheless, as proposed in a Joint Statement of the American Thoracic Society (ATS), recommendations for the initial evaluation of patients suspected of having sarcoidosis include a history and physical examination, chest radiographs, pulmonary function tests (PFTs), peripheral blood counts, serum chemistries, urine analysis, ophthalmologic examination, an electrocardiogram, and tuberculin skin testing, but omit HRCT [129]. In our opinion, the finding of

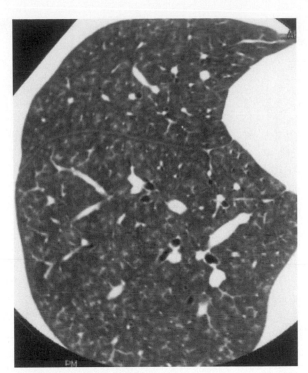

FIG. 10-11. Hypersensitivity pneumonitis with suggestive HRCT findings. Retrospectively targeted HRCT through the right middle and lower lobes shows a pattern of poorly defined centrilobular nodules evenly distributed throughout the lungs, in the absence of reticular changes or ground-glass opacity. Although this pattern can be seen in a number of diseases, it is most characteristic of subacute hypersensitivity pneumonitis. In this case, the patient was scanned prior to bronchoscopy for evaluation of otherwise nonspecific infiltrates on chest radiographs (not shown). Based on the HRCT findings, a specific diagnosis of hypersensitivity pneumonitis was suggested, leading to the appropriate diagnosis without a necessity for histologic confirmation.

clusters of ill-defined peribronchovascular and subpleural nodules, especially when bilateral, predominantly upper lobe, and associated with central airways abnormalities, in the appropriate clinical setting, should allow a definitive diagnosis of sarcoidosis to be made without the necessity for histologic confirmation (Fig. 10-12) [16,17,130–132]. Also, as shown by Gruden et al. [104] and others [130], the anatomic distribution of multinodular lung disease may be accurately determined using HRCT for a variety of diseases other than sarcoidosis, a finding of great value in differential diagnosis.

Likewise, when the HRCT features are highly suggestive of pneumoconiosis and there is a well-documented history of prior occupational exposure, lung biopsy is seldom required. This is especially true of patients who have silica and asbestos exposure [39].

HRCT can also prove diagnostic in patients who have LAM (see Fig. 7-13), LCH (Fig. 10-7; see Fig. 7-3), lymphangitic carcinomatosis (Fig. 10-6), emphysema (see Fig. 7-19), and bronchiectasis (Fig. 10-8) provided the HRCT

shows characteristic abnormalities in the appropriate clinical setting [10,27,28,85,86,92,96,133].

The finding of tree-in-bud on HRCT is diagnostic of small airways disease [81,82,134] and is most typical of cellular bronchiolitis, almost always resulting from either acute or chronic infection. Aquino et al. [134] found that a tree-in-bud pattern could be identified in 25% of patients who had bronchiectasis and also had HRCT performed (including patients with CF and ABPA), and 17% of patients who had acute infectious bronchitis or pneumonia. On the other hand, this pattern was not identified in any of 141 HRCT studies in patients who had noninfectious airway diseases, including emphysema, respiratory bronchiolitis, constrictive bronchiolitis, BOOP, and HP, among others. Thus, the presence of tree-in-bud is not only highly suggestive of an infectious cause of disease, it suggests the most appropriate method of diagnosis (i.e., sputum analysis or bronchoscopy) (see Figs. 8-17 and 8-47A).

More controversial is the use of HRCT to diagnose IPF. HRCT findings have been shown as highly accurate in making a diagnosis of pulmonary fibrosis (Fig. 10-9) [33,89,135]. As a consequence, HRCT is now considered an integral part in the diagnostic work-up of patients who have suspected IPF. As proposed in a Joint Statement of the ATS and the European Respiratory Society, in the absence of open-lung biopsy confirmation, HRCT should be considered one of the four major criteria necessary for the diagnosis of IPF, along with exclusion of other known causes of diffuse pulmonary disease, established both by history and either TBB or BAL, and abnormal PFTs (Table 10-7) [6]. In addition, for diagnosis, three of four minor criteria also must be met, including age older than 50 years, a clinical history of insidious onset of dyspnea, disease duration greater than 3 months, and bibasilar rales on auscultation.

Interestingly, despite numerous studies documenting that the accuracy of a confident diagnosis of IPF is approximately 90% based on HRCT findings of basilar, peripheral honeycombing or reticulation, traction bronchiectasis, and histologic evidence of fibrosis [27,28,33,88,136], HRCT is not considered, in itself, sufficient to establish a diagnosis of IPF [6]. Patients who have sarcoidosis [137], idiopathic BOOP [33], nonspecific interstitial pneumonitis (NSIP) [94], or HP may occasionally mimic IPF.

In the most extensive study published assessing the role of HRCT in diagnosing IPF, Hunninghake et al. prospectively evaluated 91 patients who had suspected IPF [138]. Of the 54 patients subsequently proved to have IPF at open-lung biopsy, a confident HRCT diagnosis of IPF was correctly made in 26 of 27 (96%) cases, despite a lack of clinical correlation. Using multivariate analysis to assess clinical, physiological, and radiologic findings most strongly associated with the diagnosis of IPF, the most important findings were lower lobe honeycombing on CT (odds ratio of 8.1) and chest radiographic findings consistent with honeycombing (odds ratio of 7.2). Based on these data, it would seem that in select cases, a confident diagnosis of IPF by experienced

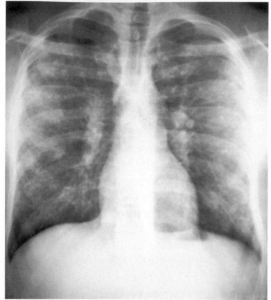

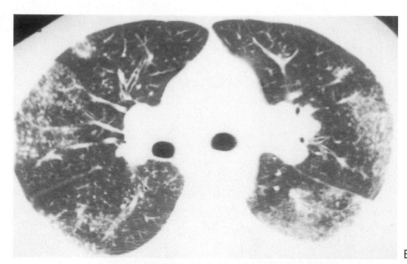

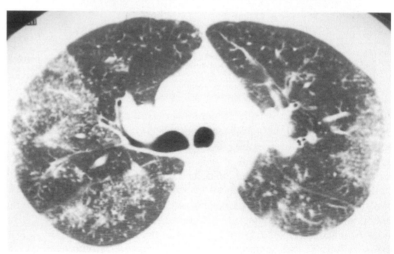

FIG. 10-12. Sarcoidosis with diagnostic HRCT findings. **A:** Posteroanterior radiograph in an asymptomatic 20-year-old man shows symmetric bilateral hilar and mediastinal lymphadenopathy associated with bilateral, ill-defined reticulonodular opacities. **B,C:** HRCT through the mid- and upper lung fields, respectively, confirms the presence of diffuse, poorly defined parenchymal nodules, clustered in a predominantly peribronchovascular distribution. In this case, the combination of clinical, radiographic, and HRCT findings were sufficiently characteristic to warrant empiric therapy without the need for biopsy confirmation.

observers should obviate biopsy, despite the recommendations of an ATS Consensus Statement (Fig. 10-9) [6], and in clinical practice, this is largely the case. It is unusual for a patient who has HRCT findings of basal honeycombing to have a lung biopsy. The use of TBB and BAL, in particular, seems unwarranted given that the accuracy of these procedures for diagnosing diffuse lung disease is extremely limited [139].

On the other hand, a study by Johkoh et al. [94] of pathologically proven cases of idiopathic interstitial pneumonias showed considerable overlap in the HRCT appearances of these entities. In this study, HRCT scans were independently evaluated by two observers. The correct diagnosis was made on average in 25 cases (71%) of UIP, 19 cases (79%) of BOOP, 14.5 cases (63%) of desquamative interstitial pneumonia (DIP), 13 cases (65%) of AIP, and 2.5 cases (9%) of NSIP. As with numerous previous

TABLE 10-7. *Diagnostic criteria for the diagnosis of idiopathic pulmonary fibrosis[a]*

Major criteria	Minor criteria
Exclusion of other diseases by history	Age >50 yr
Abnormal pulmonary function tests	Insidious onset of dyspnea
Abnormal HRCT >6 mo	Disease >3 mo duration
Transbronchial biopsy/bronchoalveolar lavage to exclude other disease	Bibasilar rales

[a]Diagnosis requires all four major and three of four minor criteria.
Adapted from Idiopathic pulmonary fibrosis: diagnosis and treatment. International consensus statement. *Am J Respir Crit Care Med* 2000;161:646–664.

reports, HRCT scans were interpreted without corresponding clinical data, lessening their overall accuracy, and because all cases had lung biopsy, some selection bias for atypical appearances seems likely. Patients who had obvious honeycombing typical of UIP and IPF were likely excluded.

As documented by Primack et al., HRCT is of value in differentiating among the various causes of end-stage lung disease. In this study of 61 consecutive patients, observers made a correct first-choice diagnosis in an average of 87% of cases, including 100% of cases with silicosis and LCH, 90% of patients who had asbestosis, and 88% of patients who had UIP [89]. More recently, it has been shown that distinctive patterns of fibrosis may also be recognized in patients who have sarcoidosis [140]. These include a pattern of predominantly central bronchial distortion, peripheral honeycombing, and diffuse linear reticulation and architectural distortion that are easily distinguished (see Figs. 5-46 through 5-48) [140]. Conventional wisdom to the contrary [141], these data taken together strongly suggest that open-lung biopsy may be unnecessary to distinguish some causes of diffuse pulmonary fibrosis.

ASSESSMENT OF DISEASE ACTIVITY AND PROGNOSIS WITH HIGH-RESOLUTION COMPUTED TOMOGRAPHY

In addition to being more sensitive, specific, and accurate than chest radiographs, HRCT may also play a critical role in the evaluation of disease activity in patients who have diffuse lung disease. Available data suggest that, in certain cases, HRCT may be used to determine the presence or absence, and extent, of abnormalities likely to be reversible (acute or active) lung disease, as compared to irreversible (fibrotic) lung disease. Furthermore, because HRCT may accurately identify subtle active lung disease, it can be used to follow patients who are being treated, to monitor the success or failure of the treatment that is being used [42,142–148].

Although a number of HRCT findings have been described as indicative of active or reversible lung disease in patients who have different disease entities with different pathologic findings (Table 10-8), most attention has focused on the potential significance of ground-glass opacity in patients who have

TABLE 10-8. *HRCT findings and histologic abnormalities associated with active diffuse lung disease*

Diagnosis	HRCT findings	Histologic findings
Usual interstitial pneumonia	Ground-glass opacity (uncommon)	Alveolar septal inflammation; intraalveolar histiocytes; fibrosis
Nonspecific interstitial pneumonia	Ground-glass opacity (common)	Varying proportions of interstitial inflammation and fibrosis
Desquamative interstitial pneumonia	Ground-glass opacity	Alveolar macrophages predominant; interstitial inflammation
Lymphocytic interstitial pneumonia	Ground-glass opacity	Mature lymphocytic and plasma cell infiltrates
Respiratory bronchiolitis	Ground-glass opacity, centrilobular nodules	Pigment containing alveolar macrophages
Bronchiolitis obliterans organizing pneumonia/cryptogenic organizing pneumonia	Consolidation, ground-glass opacity, nodules	Alveolar septal inflammation; alveolar cellular desquamation
Sarcoidosis, berylliosis	Nodules, less often ground-glass opacity	Numerous small granulomas
Hypersensitivity pneumonitis	Ground-glass opacity	Alveolitis, poorly defined granulomas, cellular bronchiolitis
Alveolar proteinosis	Ground-glass opacity, septal thickening	Intraalveolar and septal lipo-protein
Acute interstitial pneumonia	Ground-glass opacity, consolidation	Interstitial inflammatory exudate; edema; diffuse alveolar damage
Pneumocystis carinii pneumonia	Ground-glass opacity	Alveolar inflammatory exudate, alveolar septal thickening
Eosinophilic pneumonia	Consolidation, ground-glass opacity	Eosinophilic interstitial infiltrate; alveolar eosinophils and histiocytes
Tuberculosis	Small nodules, centrilobular opacities, tree-in-bud, consolidation	Miliary spread, endobronchial spread of infection, pneumonia
Nontuberculous mycobacterial infection	Bronchiectasis, centrilobular opacities, tree-in-bud	Chronic infection, endobronchial spread of infection
Cytomegalovirus infection	Ground-glass opacity, consolidation, reticulation	Diffuse alveolar damage, interlobular and intralobular thickening
Langerhans cell histiocytosis	Nodules	Granulomas containing Langerhans histiocytes and eosinophils

chronic DILD [149]. This finding has been reported in a wide range of DILDs (see Chapter 6), including IPF and other causes of UIP, NSIP, DIP, lymphocytic interstitial pneumonitis, sarcoidosis, HP (Figs. 10-2 and 10-11), alveolar proteinosis, BOOP, respiratory bronchiolitis, and chronic eosinophilic pneumonia [149]. Ground-glass opacity also has been described in patients who have neoplasms, in particular bronchioloalveolar carcinoma, as well as a wide variety of acute lung processes, such as AIP, bacterial, fungal, *Mycoplasma* (Fig. 10-15), viral, and *P. carinii* infections, pulmonary hemorrhage syndromes, and congestive heart failure and other causes of pulmonary edema (see Chapter 6). Ground-glass opacity has even been described in such unusual diseases as extramedullary hematopoiesis, and in patients who have metastatic pulmonary calcification [150,151].

Although ground-glass opacity is a nonspecific finding and reflects various histologic abnormalities in patients with chronic DILDs (see Chapter 6), ground-glass opacity often represents, or is associated with, active parenchymal inflammation (Table 10-8). As reported by Remy-Jardin et al. [152] in a study of 26 patients who had DILD, in whom histologic correlation was obtained, biopsies demonstrated that ground-glass opacity corresponded to inflammation in 24 cases (65%), whereas in eight additional cases (22%), inflammation was present but fibrosis predominated; in only five cases (13%) was fibrosis the sole histologic finding. Similarly, Leung et al., in a study of 22 patients with a variety of chronic infiltrative lung diseases and evidence of ground-glass opacity either as a predominant or exclusive HRCT finding, showed that 18 patients (82%) had potentially active disease identified on lung biopsy [153]. As discussed in detail in Chapters 3 and 6, ground-glass opacity is a nonspecific finding in patients who have DILD and does not always represent alveolitis or lung inflammation, but has a variety of correlates. Ground-glass opacity may also be seen in the presence of interstitial fibrosis without disease activity [149,153]. To strongly suggest that ground-glass opacity indicates active disease, this finding should generally be unassociated with HRCT findings of fibrosis [149,153].

In general, HRCT is indicated in the assessment of disease activity in patients who have chronic diffuse lung disease, and in the detection of active disease in some patients who have suspected acute lung disease and normal or nonspecific chest radiographs (Table 10-2). In patients who have chronic lung disease, the assessment of disease activity is most clearly indicated in patients who have suspected chronic idiopathic interstitial pneumonia (e.g., UIP, NSIP, DIP, BOOP), HP, or sarcoidosis, at least partially because of their common occurrence in the general population [1], but HRCT's utility in demonstrating HRCT findings of active disease in other chronic diseases cannot be disputed.

Disease Activity and Prognosis in Idiopathic Pulmonary Fibrosis

The significance of ground-glass opacity as a potential marker of disease activity and as an indicator of prognosis has been most thoroughly evaluated in patients who have IPF; this disease is relatively common, and its clinical course is notoriously difficult to predict [142,154–157]. Traditional methods of assessing disease activity, including TBB, BAL, or both, chest radiographs, gallium scintigraphy, and PFTs have all proved to be unreliable indicators of both disease activity and prognosis in patients who have IPF [6]. As a consequence, open-lung biopsy has remained the gold standard both for the diagnosis of IPF as well as assessment of disease activity [6,158].

Initial studies have shown good correlation between HRCT findings in patients who have IPF and the development of pulmonary fibrosis [159], the patient's prognosis [142,145,147,155,156,160], and the likelihood of response to therapy [142,145,147,157]. Although initial studies suggested good correlation between the presence of ground-glass attenuation and pathologic evidence of alveolitis [154], other studies have shown that ground-glass opacity usually represents patchy fibrotic thickening of alveolar septa and intraalveolar granulation tissue, especially in patients who have evidence of traction bronchiectasis and extensive reticulation or honeycombing, or both [32,149,152]. Furthermore, although ground-glass attenuation is often reversible in other diffuse interstitial lung diseases such as DIP, for example, this has been shown to occur less frequently in patients who have IPF [159].

Nonetheless, the presence of ground-glass attenuation has proved of value as a predictor both of response to therapy as well as overall prognosis. This may not be so surprising, given evidence suggesting that the main focus of disease activity in these patients are so-called fibrogenic foci and not active inflammation per se [161].

In an early study, Wells et al. [160] found that the presence of ground-glass opacity and its extent, relative to findings of fibrosis, was related to prognosis and likelihood of response to treatment. In this study, CT abnormalities were interpreted as predominantly ground-glass opacity (group 1), mixed ground-glass and reticular opacities (group 2), or opacities that were predominantly reticular in nature (group 3). Four-year survival was highest in patients who had predominantly ground-glass opacity, and higher in patients who had mixed opacities than in those who had reticular abnormalities, independent of the duration of symptoms or severity of pulmonary function abnormalities ($p <.001$). Similarly, response to therapy in previously untreated patients was significantly greater in patients who had predominantly ground-glass opacity, and greater in group 2 than in group 3 [160]. In retrospect, it is apparent that the HRCT findings in group 1 patients described by Wells et al. bear a striking resemblance to HRCT findings in patients who had NSIP [94,162–165] or DIP [166,167], raising the possibility that the improved survival in at least some of the patients in this group is related to variations in the underlying pathology (Fig. 10-13) [160,166].

In the most careful study to date attempting to identify factors predicting response to therapy and survival in patients who had IPF, Gay et al. assessed 38 patients who had open-lung biopsy–proven IPF. In each case, a pretreatment clini-

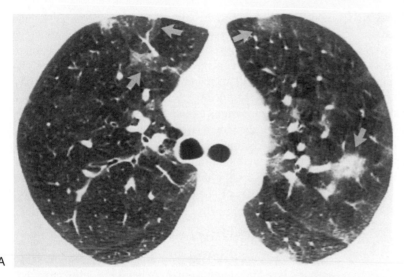

A

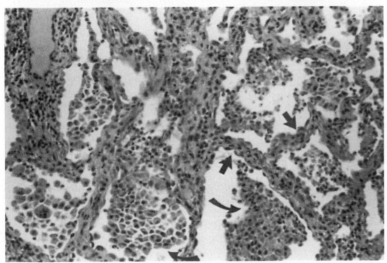

B

FIG. 10-13. Ground-glass opacity—HRCT pathologic correlation. **A:** HRCT at the level of the carina in a 40-year-old man who has desquamative interstitial pneumonia shows patchy areas of ground-glass opacity (*arrows*) highly suggestive of active disease. **B:** Corresponding histologic section from an open-lung biopsy demonstrates intraalveolar macrophages (*curved arrows*) and alveolar septal inflammation (*straight arrows*). The combination of septal inflammation and intraalveolar macrophages accounts for the ground-glass opacity seen on HRCT. The histologic findings indicate an active process.

cal, radiographic, and physiologic score (CRP) was generated. CT scans also were obtained before the initiation of steroid therapy and assessed by four independent observers for the presence and extent of ground-glass opacity (so-called CT-alveolitis) and linear opacities (CT-fibrosis), using a five-point scale ranging from 0 to 4. After 3 months of steroid therapy, patients were reassessed and assigned to one of three groups: responders (those with a greater than 10-point drop in their CRP (n = 10); those who remained stable (n = 14); and nonresponders [those with an increase of greater than 10 on their CRP; (n = 13)]. Consistent with prior reports, responders had higher CT-alveolitis scores and lower CT-fibrosis scores than either nonresponders or patients who remained stable. However, it was also found that ground-glass opacity had only a weak correlation with pathologic evidence of alveolitis. More importantly, of all parameters evaluated, only CT-fibrosis scores ($p = .009$) and fibrosis scores obtained from open-lung biopsies ($p = .004$) were able to predict mortality. Stated otherwise, CT-fibrosis scores greater than or equal to 2 had a sensitivity of 80% and a specificity of 85% in predicting survival [147].

Zisman et al. has extended the observations of Gay et al. [147] by prospectively assessing IPF patients receiving treatment with cyclophosphamide in whom prior steroid therapy had proved unsuccessful [148]. A total of 19 patients were evaluated using both CRP and HRCT scores, including one responder, seven patients who remained stable, and 11 who deteriorated. Of a total of 11 parameters evaluated, including age, CRP score, year of onset, and a variety of PFTs, only HRCT-fibrosis score ($p = .07$) and percentage of lymphocytes on BAL ($p = .04$) proved significant predictors of response to cyclophosphamide therapy. Similarly, HRCT-fibrosis score was one of the few parameters to be a significant predictor of survival ($p = .03$), along with BAL lymphocytosis, level of dyspnea, and CRP score. Although only limited conclusions could be drawn from the sole responder, interestingly, this patient had the lowest HRCT-alveolitis score and the shortest duration of symptoms. Based on these data, these authors concluded not only that cyclophosphamide therapy was of limited value for the treatment of IPF, but that in patients who had high HRCT-fibrosis scores, the prognosis was sufficiently poor to warrant withholding therapy [148].

These cumulative data suggest that HRCT should play a decisive role both in the diagnosis and assessment of disease activity and prognosis in patients who have suspected idiopathic interstitial pneumonia before biopsy and treatment. HRCT findings of a predominantly fibrotic pattern as represented by a basal distribution of traction bronchiectasis and bronchiolectasis, honeycombing, or both, is highly predictive of IPF and a poor prognosis and response to treatment. In this setting, open-lung biopsy is not often obtained, although bronchoscopy may be performed to exclude other diseases (Fig. 10-9) [6]. On the other hand, the absence of such findings of fibrosis and a predominance of ground-glass opacity makes entities such as NSIP more likely, prognosis and response to treatment are likely to be better, and open-lung biopsy is often obtained.

Disease Activity in Sarcoidosis

HRCT has been used to assess disease activity as well as the likelihood of response to therapy in patients who have sarcoidosis [42,143,168–170]. In most series of patients who have sarcoidosis, the main HRCT determinant of disease activity has been the presence and, to a lesser degree, the extent and distribution of small nodules. The finding of ground-glass opacity has proved to be of lesser diagnostic or prognostic significance [170]; although ground-glass opacity has been identified in a small subset of patients who have sarcoidosis, in most cases this finding probably results from conglomerates of small nodules below the resolution of HRCT [168]. Generally speaking, nodules and areas of parenchymal consolidation or ground-glass opacity decrease or disappear after treatment; in distinction, little if any change can usually be identified after treatment in patients who show parenchymal reticulation and cystic airspaces or architectural distortion, or both, on HRCT (Fig. 10-14) [42,143].

Unfortunately, despite this distinction between reversible and irreversible HRCT findings in patients who have sarcoidosis, the utility of HRCT in patient management has yet to be clearly defined. Unlike patients who have IPF, in most patients who have sarcoidosis, a combination of clinical, radiographic, scintigraphic, or bronchoscopic findings are usually adequate for successful diagnosis and management [171]. Furthermore, as documented by Remy-Jardin et al. [170], no significant correlation could be found between the presence of nodules on HRCT and disease activity as measured by serum angiotensin converting enzyme activity, lymphocytosis, or both at BAL [170]. However, it must be pointed out that these measures of disease activity do not necessarily reflect the activity of sarcoid granulomas in the lung [168]. In another study [170], only the profusion of septal lines correlated with serum angiotensin converting enzyme activity, lymphocytosis, or both at BAL, and the authors concluded that HRCT findings were of no value in predicting the evolution of lung changes over time.

Leung et al. correlated HRCT findings in 29 patients who had documented sarcoidosis with other standard methods of assessing disease activity including scintigraphy, BAL, and serum angiotensin-converting enzyme (SACE) levels. The extent of nodules and consolidation correlated with the intensity of lung gallium uptake ($r = 0.46$; $p < .02$), BAL lymphocytosis ($r = 0.50$; $p < .01$), and SACE levels ($r = 0.38$, $p < .05$). However, no significant correlation could be identified between these measures of disease activity and either the finding of ground-glass attenuation or linear opacities [146].

Given the seemingly contradictory results of these studies, it is apparent that a definitive conclusion regarding the role of HRCT in assessing disease activity in patients who have sarcoidosis remains to be determined.

Disease Activity in Hypersensitivity Pneumonitis

The significance of HRCT findings in assessing disease activity has also been shown in patients who have HP [52]. The stage of disease may be related to the HRCT appearance. Those patients in whom the primary HRCT abnormalities included diffuse small ill-defined nodules, ground-glass opacity, and focal air-trapping in the absence of diffuse reticulation, honeycombing, or both uniformly improved after cessation of exposure, whereas those who had a predominantly fibrotic pattern showed little if any change.

Acute Lung Diseases

In addition to assessing disease activity in patients who have chronic DILDs, HRCT has also proved to be of value in assessing disease activity in patients who have acute lung diseases, especially those associated with infection (Fig. 10-15). Clinically, this has been most useful in the evaluation of immunocompromised patients, and particularly those patients who have AIDS. As shown by Hartman et al. in a review of CT scans from 102 AIDS patients who had intrathoracic abnormalities, and 20 HIV-positive patients who did not have intrathoracic disease, acute disease was correctly diagnosed in more than 99% of cases [68].

In patients who have acute lung disease, ground-glass opacity has been shown to accurately reflect the presence of airspace consolidation, especially in patients who have pneumonia due to such organisms as *P. carinii*, although other findings can also be indicative of active infectious disease [54,67,68,122,172,173]. As documented by Gruden et al., especially in patients who have equivocal chest radiographs, HRCT may play an important role by excluding the presence of ground-glass opacity, thus effectively eliminating the possibility of *P. carinii* pneumonia. Furthermore, identifying bronchiolar inflammation resulting in characteristic centrilobular branching densities can indicate the need for routine antibiotics [24].

HRCT may play a pivotal role in assessing disease activity in patients who have mycobacterial infections, with or without a history of immune compromise. Im et al. evaluated sequential HRCT scans before and after antitu-

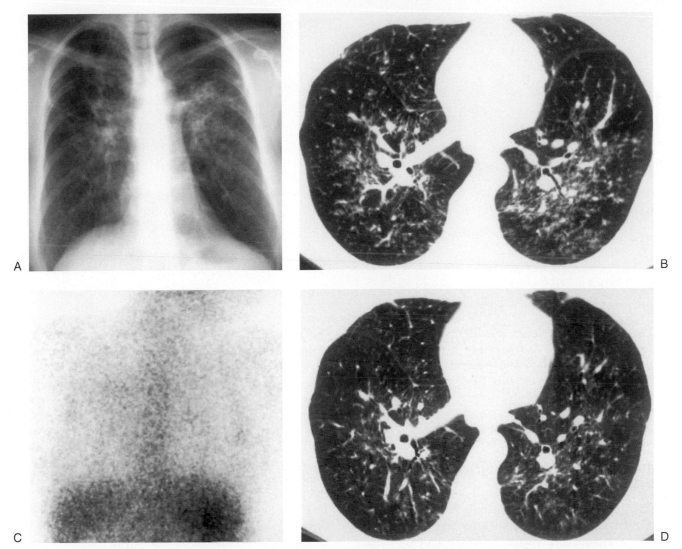

FIG. 10-14. Disease activity in sarcoidosis. **A:** Posteroanterior chest radiograph shows findings of stage 3 sarcoidosis. **B:** HRCT through the lower lobes obtained at the same time as the chest radiograph shows poorly defined peribronchovascular nodules typical of sarcoidosis, and the presence of granulomas. **C:** Anteroposterior scintigraphic image obtained 48 hours after administration of ^{67}Ga citrate shows scant evidence of abnormal activity. **D:** HRCT obtained at the same level as **B** following 6 weeks of steroid therapy. Note that there is a marked reduction in the number of nodules identifiable in both lungs. This change is consistent with regression of parenchymal granulomas.

berculous chemotherapy in a total of 26 patients who had documented active TB [46]. On HRCT examination, the most common finding was the presence of centrilobular nodules, linear branching structures (tree-in-bud), or both, corresponding pathologically to the presence of small airways filled with infected material; in virtually all cases, sequential studies showed these opacities to be reversible within 5 months after the start of treatment. Furthermore, in 11 of 12 patients who had recent reactivation, HRCT accurately differentiated old fibrotic lesions from new active ones [46]. Based on this data, the authors concluded that HRCT was a reliable method for determining disease activity in patients who had mycobacterial infection.

CT may also be of value by differentiating disease progression from those cases in which there is evidence of transient radiographic progression after initiation of therapy [174]. In the latter case, foci of ground-glass opacity, consolidation, or both typically are seen either at the site of the original parenchymal involvement or in a subpleural distribution, in the same and distant lobes. In distinction, in most patients who have disease progression, CT reveals the presence of centrilobular branching densities, likely the result of endobronchial spread of disease.

Despite HRCT findings, definitive diagnosis and treatment of mycobacterial infection in most cases still requires that organisms be cultured. Although HRCT is not routinely recommended for evaluating patients who have suspected TB, it

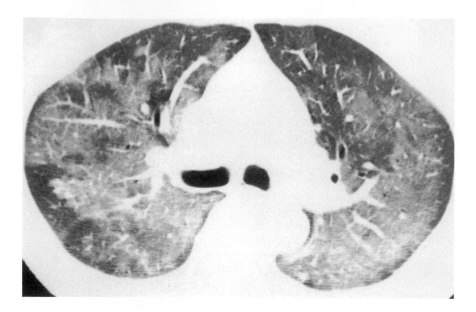

FIG. 10-15. Ground-glass opacity in acute lung disease. HRCT at the level of the carina in a febrile patient who has mycoplasmal pneumonia. HRCT shows a pattern of diffuse ground-glass opacity. In this case, these changes are primarily the result of diffuse airspace disease.

may provide the initial clue to the diagnosis, especially in patients who have AIDS. As reported by Bissuel et al. [175] in a retrospective study of 57 HIV-infected patients presenting with fever of unknown origin, CT examination proved to be the one test that contributed most to the diagnosis of mycobacterial infection by disclosing otherwise unsuspected adenopathy in seven of 18 (38%) scans performed.

DETERMINATION OF LUNG BIOPSY SITE AND TYPE

Among the many indications for using HRCT, perhaps the most important is as a potential guide for lung biopsy (Table 10-2). Many diffuse lung diseases are quite patchy in distribution, with areas of abnormal lung frequently interspersed among relatively normal areas of lung parenchyma. Furthermore, both active and fibrotic disease can be present in the same lung [141,156,160]. To establish a specific diagnosis and assess the clinical significance of the abnormalities present, it is critically important to selectively sample those portions of the lung that are abnormal and most likely to be active. This can be accomplished by using HRCT. Also, as a direct consequence of its ability to visualize, characterize, and determine the distribution of parenchymal disease, HRCT also provides a unique insight into the likely efficacy of TBB or open-lung biopsy (via thoracotomy or video-assisted thoracoscopy) in patients who have either acute or chronic diffuse lung disease.

Lung Biopsy in Chronic Infiltrative Lung Disease

To date, there is little consensus as to the best method for establishing a diagnosis in patients who have suspected DILD [176]. Available methods include fiberoptic bronchoscopy with TBB or BAL, or both, or open-lung biopsy.

Although TBB is frequently used in an attempt to diagnose diffuse lung disease, the limitations of TBB for establishing

the etiology of diffuse pulmonary disease have been well documented. In a classic study, Wall et al. showed that TBB was diagnostic in only 20 of 53 (38%) patients presenting with radiographic evidence of diffuse lung disease [139]. In the remaining 33 cases, TBBs were reported either as normal or nonspecific, whereas open-lung biopsies resulted in specific diagnoses in 92%. Similar results have been reported by Wilson et al. [177] in a study of 127 patients with a variety of parenchymal abnormalities. They found that TBB allowed a specific diagnosis in only 52% of patients who had diffuse infiltrative processes. Also, diagnoses suggested by TBB may bear little relationship to diagnoses subsequently made on open biopsy [139], and a nonspecific TBB diagnosis, such as interstitial pneumonia or interstitial fibrosis should be considered as potentially misleading [141].

In patients who have chronic diffuse lung disease, TBB is most accurate in patients who have sarcoidosis or lymphangitic carcinomatosis [139]; these entities preferentially involve peribronchial tissues and therefore are most accessible to TBB (Fig. 10-16) [131,139]. Although the accuracy of TBB has improved over the past decade, especially in establishing such diagnoses as LCH, pulmonary alveolar proteinosis, eosinophilic lung disease, Goodpasture's syndrome, and Wegener's granulomatosis, these entities represent a distinct minority of cases [3,178]. More importantly, there has been little improvement in the ability of TBB or BAL to assess patients who have pulmonary fibrosis [141].

Open-lung biopsy is often diagnostic, with accuracies greater than 90% generally reported [8,139,179]. This procedure is also subject to sampling error, as biopsies taken from a small region of lung may not reflect the state of the diseased lung as a whole. This point has been emphasized in a study of 91 patients referred for evaluation for possible IPF; nearly 15% remained without a specific diagnosis even after open-lung biopsy [138]. As a further example, it is somewhat controversial at present as to whether NSIP diagnosed patho-

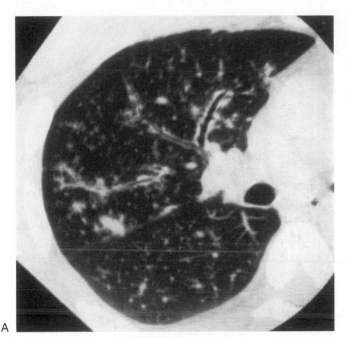
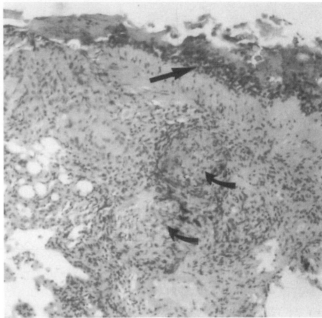

A B

FIG. 10-16. HRCT-bronchoscopic correlation in sarcoidosis. **A:** Retrospectively targeted HRCT through the right upper lobe shows peribronchial nodules associated with narrowing and irregular thickening of bronchial walls. This appearance is characteristic of sarcoidosis. **B:** Photomicrograph of a specimen obtained following transbronchial biopsy clearly shows the intimate relationship between the bronchial mucosa (*straight arrow*) and noncaseating granulomata (*curved arrows*). Not surprisingly, transbronchial biopsies are most accurate in diseases such as sarcoid or lymphangitic carcinomatosis that preferentially involve the bronchial wall. These entities also produce characteristic changes easily identified with HRCT.

logically represents a specific disease entity or is nonspecific simply because insufficient lung was sampled to make a specific diagnosis of other disease such as UIP, HP, or BOOP.

Sampling error at open-lung biopsy is also important when attempts are made to assess disease activity in patients who have diffuse fibrotic lung diseases such as IPF or collagen-vascular disease [141]. It has been emphasized that the role of the surgeon at the time of open-lung biopsy is to obtain representative tissue, while avoiding areas of extensive honeycombing [8]. However, this may be difficult, especially in patients who have IPF, owing to the predominantly subpleural distribution of the fibrosis. Furthermore, as shown by Newman et al. [180], the routine practice of obtaining lingular biopsies may lead to nonspecific findings in patients who have patchy disease, and the lingula may not be a valid biopsy site when compared to biopsy material obtained simultaneously from two other lung segments.

Given the limitations of both transbronchial and open biopsy techniques, it is not surprising that HRCT has emerged as an important tool for assessing patients who have suspected DILD before lung biopsy. HRCT is of considerable value in determining the most appropriate sites for biopsy [69]. As already noted, diffuse pulmonary disease is frequently nonuniform or patchy in distribution, and HRCT can be used to target the lung regions most likely to be active and, therefore, most likely to be diagnostic. Also, using HRCT, areas of end-stage honeycombing can be avoided. Secondly, HRCT can play a

decisive role in selecting among TBB, BAL, or open-lung biopsy as the most efficacious method for obtaining a histologic diagnosis. Of particular value is the identification of peribronchial abnormalities that characteristically occur in patients who have sarcoidosis [16,17,28,140,169,181], and lymphangitic carcinomatosis [27,182,183]. As shown by Lenique et al., the demonstration of abnormal airways in patients who have sarcoidosis clearly correlates with the likelihood of obtaining a histologic diagnosis (Fig. 10-16) [131]. In this study, HRCT findings were compared both with the macroscopic or visual appearance of the airways during fiberoptic bronchoscopy as well as the results of both endo- and transbronchial biopsies; bronchial abnormalities were present in 39 of 60 (65%) patients [131]. There was particularly good correlation between HRCT findings and biopsy results of 39 patients who had evidence of bronchial wall thickening on HRCT, and biopsies showed typical granulomatous changes in 31 patients (80%) (Fig. 10-16). Still more convincingly, 13 of 14 (93%) patients who had HRCT evidence of bronchial luminal abnormalities had positive biopsies. As reliance was placed almost exclusively on the use of endobronchial instead of TBBs to establish the diagnosis in this study, it is likely that a histologic diagnosis would have been still more common if TBBs had been used routinely.

Not surprisingly, HRCT has proved far more efficacious than chest radiographs in predicting the likely efficacy of TBB for diagnosing DILD. Mathieson et al. [27] compared the accuracy of plain radiographs and CT in determining whether TBB or open-lung biopsy would be most appropriate in patients who had chronic infiltrative lung disease. Using CT, three observers correctly predicted that a TBB would be necessary for diagnosis in 87% of patients in which this was appropriate. They correctly predicted the need for open-lung biopsy in 99% of cases. By comparison, plain radiographs proved significantly less valuable (p <.001).

Recently, video-assisted thoracoscopic lung biopsy has gained acceptance as an alternate to thoracotomy for performing an open-lung biopsy. As most studies confirm equivalent diagnostic accuracy, video-assisted thoracoscopic lung biopsy may be the preferred method, given lower cost and morbidity compared with thoracotomy [179,184]. Because the operator's field of view is rather limited when performing this procedure, HRCT has proven extremely helpful in directing the surgeon to the most appropriate biopsy site. Additionally, using CT guidance, needle localization of the biopsy site may be performed before the procedure. Although this technique has been described primarily as a localization technique for resection of lung nodules, it has proved equally applicable to the biopsy of diffuse lung disease.

Lung Biopsy in Acute Lung Disease

In addition to evaluating specific diffuse chronic infiltrative lung diseases before biopsy, HRCT also plays a complementary role to fiberoptic bronchoscopy in the assessment of patients who have acute diffuse lung disease. Although BAL and TBB are generally more accurate in diagnosing acute lung disease than chronic lung disease, there is still considerable controversy concerning appropriate guidelines for the use of these techniques [185,186].

It cannot be overemphasized that meaningful evaluation of the role of both HRCT and fiberoptic bronchoscopy must take into account the clinical and, in particular, the immune status of patients being evaluated [69]. HRCT has been shown to play an especially important potential role in the prebronchoscopic assessment of immunocompromised patients. As documented by Janzen et al., in a retrospective study evaluating 33 consecutive immunocompromised non-AIDS patients (including 20 bone marrow transplant patients) presenting with acute pulmonary disease with both HRCT and bronchoscopy [69], bronchoscopy provided a specific diagnosis in 17 of 33 (52%) patients. Significantly, bronchoscopy proved diagnostic more often in patients who had HRCT disease involving the central one-third of the lungs versus the peripheral one-third of the lungs (70% vs. 23%; p = .02). Results also proved more diagnostic in

patients who had infectious versus noninfectious disease (71% vs. 17%; p <.005). Based on these findings, the authors concluded that HRCT should precede bronchoscopy in immunocompromised patients to determine optimal sites for biopsy as well as predict likely results of bronchoscopy.

Similar studies have also concluded a role for HRCT in evaluating bone marrow transplant patients [50,187]. Mori et al., in a study of 33 febrile bone marrow recipients, found that CT showed nodules in 20 of 21 episodes of documented fungal infection, but none in nine bacteremic episodes [50]. From this data, the authors concluded that CT studies showing the presence of nodules in this population could be taken as presumptive evidence of fungal infection warranting empiric therapy without the need for bronchoscopy. As noted by Leung et al., this is especially important in the first 30 days after bone marrow transplant as fungal infections, especially due to *Aspergillus* species, account for as many as 82% of episodes of infection in this time period [188]. In a similar prospective study of 36 symptomatic episodes in 33 bone marrow transplant patients, Barloon et al. reported that in comparison with plain radiographs, HRCT resulted in a change of management in a total of 11 of 22 (50%) patients, including establishing the need for bronchoscopy, open-lung biopsy, or both in six patients [187].

HRCT may also play a role in the prebronchoscopic assessment of symptomatic patients who have AIDS. As reported by Hartman et al., in an assessment of 102 patients who had AIDS and 20 HIV-positive patients who did not have active intrathoracic disease, HRCT proved especially accurate in the confident diagnosis of *P. carinii* pneumonia (94%) and Kaposi's sarcoma (90%) (Fig. 10-17) [68]. Furthermore, in this same population, HRCT proved 93% accurate in excluding active thoracic disease.

Of even greater potential clinical utility is the potential role of HRCT in evaluating patients presenting with hemoptysis [189–191]. The role of bronchoscopy in the evaluation of patients presenting with hemoptysis has proved controversial [192,193]. In fact, the etiology of hemoptysis most often proves elusive; nearly 50% of cases remain undiagnosed despite radiographic and bronchoscopic evaluation [192,194]. In most reported series to date, HRCT has proved of greatest value in identifying bronchiectasis as a cause of hemoptysis [190,191,194]. As shown by McGuinness et al. [194] in a prospective study of 57 consecutive patients presenting with hemoptysis evaluated both with CT and fiberoptic bronchoscopy, CT identified all cancers; furthermore, the overall diagnostic yield of bronchoscopy was documented to be less than CT (47% compared with 61%, respectively). CT proved especially valuable in diagnosing bronchiectasis, present in 25% of cases.

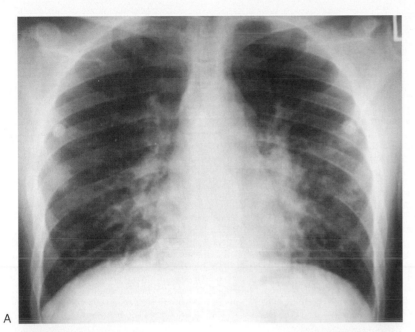

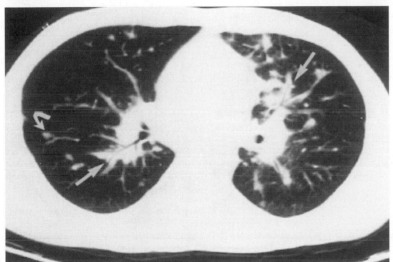

FIG. 10-17. HRCT diagnosis of Kaposi's sarcoma (KS). **A:** Posteroanterior radiograph shows bilateral perihilar nodular infiltrates in a patient who has acquired immunodeficiency syndrome. There is also a suggestion of mediastinal adenopathy in the region of the aorticopulmonary window. These findings are nonspecific. **B:** HRCT section through the hila shows bilateral peribronchial infiltrates emanating from the hila (*straight arrows*) associated with a few peripheral, perivascular nodules (*curved arrow*). This appearance is suggestive of intraparenchymal KS, especially in patients with previously documented cutaneous involvement.

REFERENCES

1. Roelandt M, Demedts M, Callebaut W, et al. Epidemiology of interstitial lung disease (ILD) in flanders: registration by pneumologists in 1992-1994. Working group on ILD, VRGT. Vereniging voor Respiratoire Gezondheidszorg en Tuberculosebestrijding. *Acta Clin Belg* 1995;50:260–268.
2. Schweisfurth H. [Report by the Scientific Working Group for Therapy of Lung Diseases: German Fibrosis Register with initial results]. *Pneumologie* 1996;50:899–901.
3. Coultas DB, Zumwalt RE, Black WC, et al. The epidemiology of interstitial lung diseases. *Am J Respir Crit Care Med* 1994;150:967–972.
4. DeRemee RA. Diffuse interstitial pulmonary disease from the perspective of the clinician. *Chest* 1987;92:1068–1073.
5. U.S. Department of Health, Education and Welfare. Respiratory Diseases Task Force: report of problems, research, approaches, and needs., Washington, D.C., U.S. Government Printing Office, 1976.
6. Idiopathic pulmonary fibrosis: diagnosis and treatment. International consensus statement. *Am J Respir Crit Care Med* 2000;161:646–664.
7. Epler GR, McLoud TC, Gaensler EA, et al. Normal chest roentgenograms in chronic diffuse infiltrative lung disease. *N Engl J Med* 1978;298:801–809.
8. Gaensler EA, Carrington CB. Open biopsy for chronic diffuse infiltrative lung disease: clinical, roentgenographic, and physiologic correlations in 502 patients. *Ann Thorac Surg* 1980;30:411–426.
9. Padley SPG, Hansell DM, Flower CDR, et al. Comparative accuracy of high resolution computed tomography and chest radiography in the diagnosis of chronic diffuse infiltrative lung disease. *Clin Radiol* 1991;44:222–226.
10. Müller NL. Clinical value of high-resolution CT in chronic diffuse lung disease. *AJR Am J Roentgenol* 1991;157:1163–1170.
11. Thurlbeck WM, Simon G. Radiographic appearance of the chest in emphysema. *AJR Am J Roentgenol* 1978;130:429–440.
12. Pratt PC. Role of conventional chest radiography in diagnosis and exclusion of emphysema. *Am J Med* 1987;82:998–1006.
13. Burki NK. Roentgenologic diagnosis of emphysema: accurate or not? *Chest* 1989;95:1178–1179.
14. Padley SPG, Adler B, Müller NL. High-resolution computed tomography of the chest: current indications. *J Thorac Imag* 1993;8:189–199.
15. Lynch DA, Rose CS, Way D, et al. Hypersensitivity pneumonitis: sensitivity of high-resolution CT in a population-based study. *AJR Am J Roentgenol* 1992;159:469–472.
16. Brauner MW, Grenier P, Mompoint D, et al. Pulmonary sarcoidosis: evaluation with high-resolution CT. *Radiology* 1989;172:467–471.

17. Müller NL, Kullnig P, Miller RR. The CT findings of pulmonary sarcoidosis: analysis of 25 patients. *AJR Am J Roentgenol* 1989;152:1179–1182.
18. Müller NL, Chiles C, Kullnig P. Pulmonary lymphangiomyomatosis: correlation of CT with radiographic and functional findings. *Radiology* 1990;175:335–339.
19. Stein MG, Mayo J, Müller N, et al. Pulmonary lymphangitic spread of carcinoma: appearance on CT scans. *Radiology* 1987;162:371–375.
20. Strickland B, Strickland NH. The value of high definition, narrow section computed tomography in fibrosing alveolitis. *Clin Radiol* 1988;39:589–594.
21. Aberle DR, Gamsu G, Ray CS, et al. Asbestos-related pleural and parenchymal fibrosis: detection with high-resolution CT. *Radiology* 1988;166:729–734.
22. Staples CA, Gamsu G, Ray CS, et al. High resolution computed tomography and lung function in asbestos-exposed workers with normal chest radiographs. *Am Rev Respir Dis* 1989;139:1502–1508.
23. Syrjälä H, Broas M, Suramo I, et al. High-resolution computed tomography for the diagnosis of community-acquired pneumonia. *Clin Infect Dis* 1998;27:358–363.
24. Gruden JF, Huang L, Turner J, et al. High-resolution CT in the evaluation of clinically suspected *Pneumocystis carinii* pneumonia in AIDS patients with normal, equivocal, or nonspecific radiographic findings. *AJR Am J Roentgenol* 1997;169:967–975.
25. Richards PJ, Riddell L, Reznek RH, et al. High-resolution computed tomography in HIV patients with suspected *Pneumocystis carinii* pneumonia and a normal chest radiograph. *Clin Radiol* 1996;51:689–693.
26. Kang EY, Staples CA, McGuinness G, et al. Detection and differential diagnosis of pulmonary infections and tumors in patients with AIDS: value of chest radiography versus CT. *AJR Am J Roentgenol* 1996;166:15–19.
27. Mathieson JR, Mayo JR, Staples CA, et al. Chronic diffuse infiltrative lung disease: comparison of diagnostic accuracy of CT and chest radiography. *Radiology* 1989;171:111–116.
28. Grenier P, Valeyre D, Cluzel P, et al. Chronic diffuse interstitial lung disease: diagnostic value of chest radiography and high-resolution CT. *Radiology* 1991;179:123–132.
29. Grenier P, Maurice F, Musset D, et al. Bronchiectasis: assessment by thin-section CT. *Radiology* 1986;161:95–99.
30. Young K, Aspestrand F, Kolbenstvedt A. High resolution CT and bronchography in the assessment of bronchiectasis. *Acta Radiol* 1991;32:439–441.
31. Staples CA, Müller NL, Vedal S, et al. Usual interstitial pneumonia: correlation of CT with clinical, functional, and radiologic findings. *Radiology* 1987;162:377–381.
32. Nishimura K, Kitaichi M, Izumi T, et al. Usual interstitial pneumonia: histologic correlation with high-resolution CT. *Radiology* 1992;182:337–342.
33. Tung KT, Wells AU, Rubens MB, et al. Accuracy of the typical computed tomographic appearances of fibrosing alveolitis. *Thorax* 1993;48:334–338.
34. Fujii M, Adachi S, Shimizu T, et al. Interstitial lung disease in rheumatoid arthritis: assessment with high-resolution computed tomography. *J Thorac Imag* 1993;8:54–62.
35. Schurawitzki H, Stiglbauer R, Graninger W, et al. Interstitial lung disease in progressive systemic sclerosis: high-resolution CT versus radiography. *Radiology* 1990;176:755–759.
36. Padley SPG, Adler B, Hansell DM, et al. High-resolution computed tomography of drug-induced lung disease. *Clin Radiol* 1992;46:232–236.
37. Bell J, McGivern D, Bullimore J, et al. Diagnostic imaging of post-irradiation changes in the chest. *Clin Radiol* 1988;39:109–119.
38. Ikezoe J, Takashima S, Morimoto S, et al. CT appearance of acute radiation-induced injury in the lung. *AJR Am J Roentgenol* 1988;150:765–770.
39. Gamsu G, Salmon CJ, Warnock ML, et al. CT quantification of interstitial fibrosis in patients with asbestosis: a comparison of two methods. *AJR Am J Roentgenol* 1995;164:63–68.
40. Peuchot M, Libshitz HI. Pulmonary metastatic disease: radiologic-surgical correlation. *Radiology* 1987;164:719–722.
41. Metzger RA, Multhern CB, Arger PH, et al. CT differentiation of solitary from diffuse bronchioloalveolar carcinoma. *J Comput Assist Tomogr* 1981;5:830–833.
42. Brauner MW, Lenoir S, Grenier P, et al. Pulmonary sarcoidosis: CT assessment of lesion reversibility. *Radiology* 1992;182:349–354.
43. Newman LS, Buschman DL, Newell JD, et al. Beryllium disease: assessment with CT. *Radiology* 1994;190:835–840.
44. Bégin R, Ostiguy G, Fillion R, et al. Computed tomography scan in the early detection of silicosis. *Am Rev Respir Dis* 1991;3:1.
45. Remy-Jardin M, Degreef JM, Beuscart R, et al. Coal worker's pneumoconiosis: CT assessment in exposed workers and correlation with radiographic findings. *Radiology* 1990;177:363–371.
46. Im JG, Itoh H, Shim YS, et al. Pulmonary tuberculosis: CT findings—early active disease and sequential change with antituberculous therapy. *Radiology* 1993;186:653–660.
47. McGuinness G, Naidich DP, Jagirdar J, et al. High resolution CT findings in miliary lung disease. *J Comput Assist Tomogr* 1992;16:384–390.
48. Kuhlman JE, Deutsch JH, Fishman EK, et al. CT features of thoracic mycobacterial disease. *Radiographics* 1990;10:413–431.
49. Hartman TE, Swensen SJ, Williams DE. Mycobacterium avium-intracellulare complex: evaluation with CT. *Radiology* 1993;187:23–26.
50. Mori M, Galvin JR, Barloon TJ, et al. Fungal pulmonary infections after bone marrow transplantation: evaluation with radiography and CT. *Radiology* 1991;178:721–726.
51. Huang RM, Naidich DP, Lubat E, et al. Septic pulmonary emboli: CT-radiographic correlation. *AJR Am J Roentgenol* 1989;153:41–45.
52. Remy-Jardin M, Remy J, Wallaert B, et al. Subacute and chronic bird breeder hypersensitivity pneumonitis: sequential evaluation with CT and correlation with lung function tests and bronchoalveolar lavage. *Radiology* 1993;198:111–118.
53. Holt RM, Schmidt RA, Godwin JD, Raghu G. High resolution CT in respiratory bronchiolitis-associated interstitial lung disease. *J Comput Assist Tomogr* 1993;17:46–50.
54. Bergin CJ, Wirth RL, Berry GJ, Castellino RA. *Pneumocystis carinii* pneumonia: CT and HRCT observations. *J Comput Assist Tomogr* 1990;14:756–759.
55. Moskovic E, Miller R, Pearson M. High resolution computed tomography of *Pneumocystis carinii* pneumonia in AIDS. *Clin Radiol* 1990;42:239–243.
56. Moore AD, Godwin JD, Müller NL, et al. Pulmonary histiocytosis X: comparison of radiographic and CT findings. *Radiology* 1989;172:249–254.
57. Brauner MW, Grenier P, Mouelhi MM, et al. Pulmonary histiocytosis X: evaluation with high resolution CT. *Radiology* 1989;172:255–258.
58. Brauner MW, Grenier P, Tijani K, et al. Pulmonary Langerhans cell histiocytosis: evolution of lesions on CT scans. *Radiology* 1997;204:497–502.
59. Sherrier RH, Chiles C, Roggli V. Pulmonary lymphangioleiomyomatosis: CT findings. *AJR Am J Roentgenol* 1989;153:937–940.
60. Lenoir S, Grenier P, Brauner MW, et al. Pulmonary lymphangiomyomatosis and tuberous sclerosis: comparison of radiographic and thin-section CT findings. *Radiology* 1990;175:329–334.
61. Thurlbeck WM, Müller NL. Emphysema: definition, imaging, and quantification. *AJR Am J Roentgenol* 1994;163:1017–1025.
62. Klein JS, Gamsu G, Webb WR, et al. High-resolution CT diagnosis of emphysema in symptomatic patients with normal chest radiographs and isolated low diffusing capacity. *Radiology* 1992;182:817–821.
63. Santis G, Hodson ME, Strickland B. High resolution computed tomography in adult cystic fibrosis patients with mild lung disease. *Clin Radiol* 1991;44:20–22.
64. Lynch DA, Brasch RC, Hardy KA, et al. Pediatric pulmonary disease: assessment with high-resolution ultrafast CT. *Radiology* 1990;176:243–248.
65. Sweatman MC, Millar AB, Strickland B, et al. Computed tomography in adult obliterative bronchiolitis. *Clin Radiol* 1990;41:116–119.
66. Marti-Bonmati L, Ruiz PF, Catala F, et al. CT findings in Swyer-James syndrome. *Radiology* 1989;172:477–480.
67. Primack SL, Müller NL. High-resolution computed tomography in acute diffuse lung disease in the immunocompromised patient. *Radiol Clin North Am* 1994;32:731–744.
68. Hartman TE, Primack SL, Müller NL, et al. Diagnosis of thoracic complications in AIDS: accuracy of CT. *AJR Am J Roentgenol* 1994;162:547–553.
69. Janzen DL, Padley SP, Adler BD, et al. Acute pulmonary complications in immunocompromised non-AIDS patients: comparison of diagnostic accuracy of CT and chest radiography. *Clin Radiol* 1993;47:159–165.

70. Leung AN, Staples CA, Müller NL. Chronic diffuse infiltrative lung disease: comparison of diagnostic accuracy of high-resolution and conventional CT. AJR Am J Roentgenol 1991;157:693–696.
71. Remy-Jardin M, Remy J, Deffontaines C, et al. Assessment of diffuse infiltrative lung disease: comparison of conventional CT and high-resolution CT. Radiology 1991;181:157–162.
72. Silverman PM, Godwin JD. CT/bronchographic correlations in bronchiectasis. J Comput Assist Tomogr 1987;11:52–56.
73. Müller NL, Bergin CJ, Ostrow DN, et al. Role of computed tomography in the recognition of bronchiectasis. AJR Am J Roentgenol 1984;143:971–976.
74. Webb WR. High-resolution computed tomography of obstructive lung disease. Radiol Clin North Am 1994;32:745–757.
75. Heitzman ER. Pattern recognition in pulmonary radiology. In: The lung: radiologic-pathologic correlations, 2nd ed. St. Louis: CV Mosby, 1984:70–105.
76. Felson B. A new look at pattern recognition of diffuse pulmonary disease. AJR Am J Roentgenol 1979;133:183–189.
77. Genereux GP. Pattern recognition in diffuse lung disease: a review of theory and practice. Med Radiogr Photog 1985;61:2–31.
78. McLoud TC, Carrington CB, Gaensler EA. Diffuse infiltrative lung disease: a new scheme for description. Radiology 1983;149:353–363.
79. Young M, Marrie TJ. Interobserver variability in the interpretation of chest roentgenograms of patients with possible pneumonia. Arch Intern Med 1994;154:2729–2732.
80. Colby TV, Swensen SJ. Anatomic distribution and histopathologic patterns in diffuse lung disease: correlation with HRCT. J Thorac Imag 1996;11:1–26.
81. Gruden JF, Webb WR, Warnock M. Centrilobular opacities in the lung on high-resolution CT: diagnostic considerations and pathologic correlation. AJR Am J Roentgenol 1994;162:569–574.
82. Gruden JF, Webb WR. Identification and evaluation of centrilobular opacities on high-resolution CT. Semin Ultra CT MR 1995;16:435–449.
83. Murata K, Khan A, Herman PG. Pulmonary parenchymal disease: evaluation with high-resolution CT. Radiology 1989;170:629–635.
84. Murata K, Itoh H, Todo G, et al. Centrilobular lesions of the lung: demonstration by high-resolution CT and pathologic correlation. Radiology 1986;161:641–645.
85. Müller NL, Miller RR. Computed tomography of chronic diffuse infiltrative lung disease: part 1. Am Rev Respir Dis 1990;142:1206–1215.
86. Müller NL, Miller RR. Computed tomography of chronic diffuse infiltrative lung disease: part 2. Am Rev Respir Dis 1990;142:1440–1448.
87. Grenier P, Brauner M, Valeyre D. Computed tomography in the assessment of diffuse lung disease. Sarcoidosis Vasc Diffuse Lung Dis 1999;16:47–56.
88. Nishimura K, Izumi T, Kitaichi M, et al. The diagnostic accuracy of high-resolution computed tomography in diffuse infiltrative lung diseases. Chest 1993;104:1149–1155.
89. Primack SL, Hartman TE, Hansell DM, et al. End-stage lung disease: CT findings in 61 patients. Radiology 1993;189:681–686.
90. Lee KS, Primack SL, Staples CA, et al. Chronic infiltrative lung disease: comparison of diagnostic accuracies of radiography and low- and conventional-dose thin-section CT. Radiology 1994;191:669–673.
91. Aberle DL. HRCT in acute diffuse lung disease. J Thorac Imag 1993;8:200–212.
92. Bonelli FS, Hartman TE, Swensen SJ, et al. Accuracy of high-resolution CT in diagnosing lung diseases. AJR Am J Roentgenol 1998;170:1507–1512.
93. Gruden JF, Naidich DP. High-resolution CT: can it obviate biopsy? Clin Pulm Med 1998;5:23–35.
94. Johkoh T, Müller NL, Cartier Y, et al. Idiopathic interstitial pneumonias: diagnostic accuracy of thin-section CT in 129 patients. Radiology 1999;211:555–560.
95. Swensen SJ, Aughenbaugh GL, Myers JL. Diffuse lung disease: diagnostic accuracy of CT in patients undergoing surgical biopsy of the lung. Radiology 1997;205:229–234.
96. Grenier P, Chevret S, Beigelman C, et al. Chronic diffuse infiltrative lung disease: determination of the diagnostic value of clinical data, chest radiography, and CT with Bayesian analysis. Radiology 1994;191:383–390.
97. Grenier P, Cordeau MP, Beigelman C. High-resolution computed tomography of the airways. J Thorac Imag 1993;8:213–229.
98. Jeffery PK. Comparative morphology of the airways in asthma and chronic obstructive pulmonary disease. Am J Respir Crit Care Med 1994;150:S6–S13.
99. Lamers RJ, Thelissen GR, Kessels AG, et al. Chronic obstructive pulmonary diseases. Evaluation with spirometrically controlled CT lung densitometry. Radiology 1994;193:109–113.
100. Gould GA, Redpath AT, Ryan M, et al. Lung CT density correlates with measurements of airflow limitation and the diffusing capacity. Eur Respir J 1991;4:141–146.
101. Webb WR. Radiology of obstructive pulmonary disease. AJR Am J Roentgenol 1997;169:637–647.
102. Müller NL, Thurlbeck WM. Thin-section CT, emphysema, air trapping, and airway obstruction [editorial]. Radiology 1996;199:621–622.
103. Müller NL, Miller RR. Diseases of the bronchioles: CT and histopathologic findings. Radiology 1995;196:3–12.
104. Gruden JF, Webb WR, Naidich DP, et al. Multinodular disease: anatomic localization at thin-section CT—multireader evaluation of a simple algorithm. Radiology 1999;210:711–720.
105. Arakawa H, Webb WR, McCowin M, et al. Inhomogeneous lung attenuation at thin-section CT: diagnostic value of expiratory scans. Radiology 1998;206:89–94.
106. Arakawa H, Webb WR. Air trapping on expiratory high-resolution CT scans in the absence of inspiratory scan abnormalities: correlation with pulmonary function tests and differential diagnosis. AJR Am J Roentgenol 1998;170:1349–1353.
107. Worthy SA, Müller NL. Small airway diseases. Radiol Clin North Am 1998;36:163–173.
108. Worthy SA, Müller NL, Hartman TE, et al. Mosaic attenuation pattern on thin-section CT scans of the lung: differentiation among infiltrative lung, airway, and vascular diseases as a cause. Radiology 1997;205:465–470.
109. Worthy SA, Flower CD. Computed tomography of the airways. Eur Radiol 1996;6:717–729.
110. Lucidarme O, Coche E, Cluzel P, et al. Expiratory CT scans for chronic airway disease: correlation with pulmonary function test results. AJR Am J Roentgenol 1998;170:301–307.
111. Hansell D. Bronchiectasis. Radiol Clin North Am 1998;36:107–128.
112. McGuinness G, Naidich DP, Leitman BS, et al. Bronchiectasis: CT evaluation. AJR Am J Roentgenol 1993;160:253–259.
113. Grenier P, Lenoir S, Brauner M. Computed tomographic assessment of bronchiectasis. Semin Ultra CT MR 1990;11:430–441.
114. Reiff DB, Wells AU, Carr DH, et al. CT findings in bronchiectasis: limited value in distinguishing between idiopathic and specific types. AJR Am J Roentgenol 1995;165:261–267.
115. Lee PH, Carr DH, Rubens MB, et al. Accuracy of CT in predicting the cause of bronchiectasis. Clin Radiol 1995;50:839–841.
116. Cartier Y, Kavanagh PV, Johkoh T, et al. Bronchiectasis: accuracy of high-resolution CT in the differentiation of specific diseases. AJR Am J Roentgenol 1999;173:47–52.
117. Ward S, Heyneman L, Lee MJ, et al. Accuracy of CT in the diagnosis of allergic bronchopulmonary aspergillosis in asthmatic patients. AJR Am J Roentgenol 1999;173:937–942.
118. Swensen SJ, Hartman TE, Williams DE. Computed tomography in diagnosis of Mycobacterium avium-intracellulare complex in patients with bronchiectasis. Chest 1994;105:49–52.
119. Tanaka E, Amitani R, Niimi A, et al. Yield of computed tomography and bronchoscopy for the diagnosis of Mycobacterium avium complex pulmonary disease. Am J Respir Crit Care Med 1997;155:2041–2046.
120. Edinburgh KJ, Jasmer RM, Huang L, et al. Multiple pulmonary nodules in AIDS: usefulness of CT in distinguishing among potential causes. Radiology 2000;214:427–432.
121. Kang EY, Staples CA, McGuinness G, et al. Detection and differential diagnosis of pulmonary infections and tumors in patients with AIDS: value of chest radiography versus CT. AJR Am J Roentgenol 1996;166:15–19.
122. Naidich DP, Garay SM, Goodman PC, et al. Pulmonary manifestations of AIDS. In: Radiology of acquired immune deficiency syndrome. New York: Raven, 1988:47–77.
123. McGuinness G, Gruden JF, Bhalla M, et al. AIDS-related airway disease. AJR Am J Roentgenol 1997;168:67–77.
124. Naidich DP, McGuinness G. Pulmonary manifestations of AIDS: CT and radiographic correlations. Radiol Clin North Am 1991;29:999–1017.

125. Tomiyama N, Muller NL, Johkoh T, et al. Acute parenchymal lung disease in immunocompetent patients: diagnostic accuracy of high-resolution CT. *AJR Am J Roentgenol* 2000;174:1745–1750.

126. Buschman DL, Gamsu G, Waldron JA, et al. Chronic hypersensitivity pneumonitis: use of CT in diagnosis. *AJR Am J Roentgenol* 1992;159:957–960.

127. Rose C, King TE. Controversies in hypersensitivity pneumonitis [Editorial]. *Am Rev Respir Dis* 1992;145:1–2.

128. Honda O, Johkoh T, Ichikado K, et al. Comparison of high resolution CT findings of sarcoidosis, lymphoma, and lymphangitic carcinoma: is there any difference of involved interstitium? *J Comput Assist Tomogr* 1999;23:374–379.

129. Hunninghake GW, Costabel U, Ando M, et al. ATS/ERS/WASOG statement on sarcoidosis. American Thoracic Society/European Respiratory Society/World Association of Sarcoidosis and Other Granulomatous Disorders. *Sarcoidosis Vasc Diffuse Lung Dis* 1999;16:149–173.

130. Lee KS, Kim TS, Han J, et al. Diffuse micronodular lung disease: HRCT and pathologic findings. *J Comput Assist Tomogr* 1999;23:99–106.

131. Lenique F, Brauner MW, Grenier P, et al. CT assessment of bronchi in sarcoidosis: endoscopic and pathologic correlations. *Radiology* 1995;194:419–423.

132. Lynch DA, Webb WR, Gamsu G, et al. Computed tomography in pulmonary sarcoidosis. *J Comput Assist Tomogr* 1989;13:405–410.

133. Bergin CJ, Coblentz CL, Chiles C, et al. Chronic lung diseases: specific diagnosis using CT. *AJR Am J Roentgenol* 1989;152:1183–1188.

134. Aquino SL, Gamsu G, Webb WR, et al. Tree-in-bud pattern: frequency and significance on thin section CT. *J Comput Assist Tomogr* 1996;20:594–599.

135. Al-Jarad N, Strickland B, Pearson MC, et al. High-resolution computed tomographic assessment of asbestosis and cryptogenic fibrosing alveolitis: a comparative study. *Thorax* 1992;47:645–650.

136. Lynch DA, Newell JD, Logan PM, et al. Can CT distinguish hypersensitivity pneumonitis from idiopathic pulmonary fibrosis? *AJR Am J Roentgenol* 1995;165:807–811.

137. Padley SP, Padhani AR, Nicholson A, et al. Pulmonary sarcoidosis mimicking cryptogenic fibrosing alveolitis on CT. *Clin Radiol* 1996;51:807–810.

138. Hunninghake G, Zimmerman M, Lynch D, et al. Lung CT and the diagnosis of IPF (abstract). American Lung Association/American Thoracic Society Annual Conference 1999: San Diego, CA: April 23–28, 1999.

139. Wall CP, Gaensler EA, Carrington CB, et al. Comparison of transbronchial and open biopsies in chronic infiltrative lung diseases. *Am Rev Respir Dis* 1981;123:280–285.

140. Abehsera M, Valeyre D, Grenier P, et al. Sarcoidosis with pulmonary fibrosis: CT patterns and correlation with pulmonary function. *AJR Am J Roentgenol* 2000;174:1751–1757.

141. Raghu G. Idiopathic pulmonary fibrosis. a rational clinical approach. *Chest* 1987;92:148–154.

142. Terriff BA, Kwan SY, Chan-Yeung MM, et al. Fibrosing alveolitis: chest radiography and CT as predictors of clinical and functional impairment at follow-up in 26 patients. *Radiology* 1992;184:445–449.

143. Murdoch J, Müller NL. Pulmonary sarcoidosis: changes on follow-up CT examinations. *AJR Am J Roentgenol* 1992;159:473–477.

144. Akira M, Higashihara T, Sakatani M, et al. Diffuse panbronchiolitis: follow-up CT examination. *Radiology* 1993;189:559–562.

145. Lee JS, Im JG, Ahn JM, et al. Fibrosing alveolitis: prognostic implication of ground-glass attenuation at high-resolution CT. *Radiology* 1992;184:415–454.

146. Leung AN, Brauner MW, Caillat-Vigneron N, et al. Sarcoidosis activity: correlation of HRCT findings with those of ^{67}Ga scanning, bronchoalveolar lavage, and serum angiotensin-converting enzyme assay. *J Comput Assist Tomogr* 1998;22:229–234.

147. Gay SE, Kazerooni EA, Toews GB, et al. Idiopathic pulmonary fibrosis: predicting response to therapy and survival. *Am J Respir Crit Care Med* 1998;157:1063–1072.

148. Zisman DA, Lynch III JP, Toews GB, et al. Cyclophosphamide in the treatment of idiopathic pulmonary fibrosis: a prospective study in patients who failed to respond to corticosteroids. *Chest* 2000;117:1619–1626.

149. Remy-Jardin M, Remy J, Giraud F, et al. Computed tomography assessment of ground-glass opacity: semiology and significance. *J Thorac Imag* 1993;8:249–264.

150. Wyatt SH, Fishman EK. Diffuse pulmonary extramedullary hematopoiesis in a patient with myelofibrosis: CT findings. *J Comput Assist Tomogr* 1994;18:815–817.

151. Greenberg S, Suster B. Metastatic pulmonary calcifications: appearance on high resolution CT. *J Comput Assist Tomogr* 1994;18:497–499.

152. Remy-Jardin M, Giraud F, Remy J, et al. Importance of ground-glass attenuation in chronic diffuse infiltrative lung disease: pathologic-CT correlation. *Radiology* 1993;189:693–698.

153. Leung AN, Miller RR, Müller NL. Parenchymal opacification in chronic infiltrative lung diseases: CT-pathologic correlation. *Radiology* 1993;188:209–214.

154. Müller NL, Staples CA, Miller RR, et al. Disease activity in idiopathic pulmonary fibrosis: CT and pathologic correlation. *Radiology* 1987;165:731–734.

155. Wells AU, Rubens MB, du Bois RM, et al. Serial CT in fibrosing alveolitis: prognostic significance of the initial pattern. *AJR Am J Roentgenol* 1993;161:1159–1165.

156. Wells AU, Hansell DM, Corrin B, et al. High resolution computed tomography as a predictor of lung histology in systemic sclerosis. *Thorax* 1992;47:508–512.

157. Akira M, Sakatani M, Ueda E. Idiopathic pulmonary fibrosis: progression of honeycombing at thin-section CT. *Radiology* 1993;189:687–691.

158. Raghu G. Interstitial lung disease: a diagnostic approach. Are CT scan and lung biopsy indicated in every patient? *Am J Respir Crit Care Med* 1995;151:909–914.

159. Hartman TE, Primack SL, Kang EY, et al. Disease progression in usual interstitial pneumonia compared with desquamative interstitial pneumonia. Assessment with serial CT. *Chest* 1996;110:378–382.

160. Wells AU, Hansell DM, Rubens MB, et al. The predictive value of appearances of thin-section computed tomography in fibrosing alveolitis. *Am Rev Respir Dis* 1993;148:1076–1082.

161. Katzenstein AL, Myers JL. Idiopathic pulmonary fibrosis: clinical relevance of pathologic classification. *Am J Respir Crit Care Med* 1998;157:1301–1315.

162. Nishiyama O, Kondoh Y, Taniguchi H, et al. Serial high resolution CT findings in nonspecific interstitial pneumonia/fibrosis. *J Comput Assist Tomogr* 2000;24:41–46.

163. Cottin V, Donsbeck AV, Revel D, et al. Nonspecific interstitial pneumonia. Individualization of a clinicopathologic entity in a series of 12 patients. *Am J Respir Crit Care Med* 1998;158:1286–1293.

164. Kim TS, Lee KS, Chung MP, et al. Nonspecific interstitial pneumonia with fibrosis: high-resolution CT and pathologic findings. *AJR Am J Roentgenol* 1998;171:1645–1650.

165. Kim EY, Lee KS, Chung MP, et al. Nonspecific interstitial pneumonia with fibrosis: serial high-resolution CT findings with functional correlation. *AJR Am J Roentgenol* 1999;173:949–953.

166. Hartman TE, Primack SL, Swensen SJ, et al. Desquamative interstitial pneumonia: thin-section CT findings in 22 patients. *Radiology* 1993;187:787–790.

167. Heyneman LE, Ward S, Lynch DA, et al. Respiratory bronchiolitis, respiratory bronchiolitis-associated interstitial lung disease, and desquamative interstitial pneumonia: different entities or part of the spectrum of the same disease process? *AJR Am J Roentgenol* 1999;173:1617–1622.

168. Müller NL, Miller RR. Ground-glass attenuation, nodules, alveolitis, and sarcoid granulomas [editorial]. *Radiology* 1993;189:31–32.

169. Bergin CJ, Bell DY, Coblentz CL, et al. Sarcoidosis: correlation of pulmonary parenchymal pattern at CT with results of pulmonary function tests. *Radiology* 1989;171:619–624.

170. Remy-Jardin M, Giraud F, Remy J, et al. Pulmonary sarcoidosis: role of CT in the evaluation of disease activity and functional impairment and in prognosis assessment. *Radiology* 1994;191:675–680.

171. Austin JHM. Pulmonary sarcoidosis: what are we learning from CT? *Radiology* 1989;171:603–604.

172. Kuhlman JE, Kavuru M, Fishman EK, et al. *Pneumocystis carinii* pneumonia: spectrum of parenchymal CT findings. *Radiology* 1990;175:711–714.

173. McGuinness G, Scholes JV, Garay SM, et al. Cytomegalovirus pneumonitis: spectrum of parenchymal CT findings with pathologic correlation in 21 AIDS patients. *Radiology* 1994;192:451–459.

174. Akira M, Sakatani M, Ishikawa H. Transient radiographic progression during initial treatment of pulmonary tuberculosis: CT findings. *J Comput Assist Tomogr* 2000;24:426–431.

175. Bissuel F, Leport C, Perronne C, et al. Fever of unknown origin in HIV-infected patients: a critical analysis of a retrospective series of 57 cases. *J Intern Med* 1994;236:529–535.

176. Smith CM, Moser KM. Management of interstitial lung disease. state of the art. *Chest* 1989;95:676–678.

177. Wilson RK, Fechner RE, Greenberg SD, et al. Clinical implications of a "nonspecific" transbronchial biopsy. *Am J Med* 1978;65:252–256.

178. Shure D. Transbronchial biopsy and needle aspiration. *Chest* 1989;95:1130–1138.

179. Bensard DD, McIntyre Jr RC, Waring BJ, et al. Comparison of video thoracoscopic lung biopsy to open lung biopsy in the diagnosis of interstitial lung disease. *Chest* 1993;103:765–770.

180. Newman SL, Michel RP, Wang NS. Lingular biopsy: is it representative? *Am Rev Respir Dis* 1985;132:1084–1086.

181. Nishimura K, Itoh H, Kitaichi M, et al. Pulmonary sarcoidosis: correlation of CT and histopathologic findings. *Radiology* 1993;189:105–109.

182. Munk PL, Müller NL, Miller RR, et al. Pulmonary lymphangitic carcinomatosis: CT and pathologic findings. *Radiology* 1988;166:705–709.

183. Johkoh T, Ikezoe J, Tomiyama N, et al. CT findings in lymphangitic carcinomatosis of the lung: correlation with histologic findings and pulmonary function tests. *AJR Am J Roentgenol* 1992;158:1217–1222.

184. Ferson PF, Landreneau RJ, Dowling RD, et al. Comparison of open versus thoracoscopic lung biopsy for diffuse infiltrative pulmonary disease. *J Thorac Cardiovasc Surg* 1993;106:194–199.

185. Schluger NW, Rom WN. Current approaches to the diagnosis of active pulmonary tuberculosis. *Am J Respir Crit Care Med* 1994;149:264–267.

186. Tu JV, Biem J, Detsky AS. Bronchoscopy versus empirical therapy in HIV-infected patients with presumptive *Pneumocystis carinii* pneumonia. *Am Rev Resp Dis* 1993;148:370–377.

187. Barloon TJ, Galvin JR, Mori M, et al. High-resolution ultrafast chest CT in the clinical management of febrile bone marrow transplant patients with normal or nonspecific chest roentgenograms. *Chest* 1991;99:928–933.

188. Leung AN, Gosselin MV, Napper CH, et al. Pulmonary infections after bone marrow transplantation: clinical and radiographic findings. *Radiology* 1999;210:699–710.

189. Naidich DP, Funt S, Ettenger NA, et al. Hemoptysis: CT-bronchoscopic correlations in 58 cases. *Radiology* 1990;177:357–362.

190. Millar A, Boothroyd A, Edwards D, et al. The role of computed tomography (CT) in the investigation of unexplained hemoptysis. *Resp Med* 1992;86:39–44.

191. Set PAK, Flower CDR, Smith IE, et al. Hemoptysis: comparative study of the role of CT and fiberoptic bronchoscopy. *Radiology* 1993;189:677–680.

192. Poe RH, Levy PC, Israel RH, et al. Use of fiberoptic bronchoscopy in the diagnosis of bronchogenic carcinoma. A study in patients with idiopathic pleural effusions. *Chest* 1994;105:1663–1667.

193. Rohwedder JJ. Enticements for fruitless bronchoscopy [Editorial]. *Chest* 1989;96:708–710.

194. McGuinness G, Beacher JR, Harkin TJ, et al. Hemoptysis. High-resolution CT/bronchoscopic correlation. *Chest* 1994;105:982–983.

CHAPTER 11

Illustrated Glossary of High-Resolution Computed Tomography Terms

As a quick reference and as an aid to understanding the nomenclature used in this book, we have listed the definitions of a number of useful high-resolution computed tomography (HRCT) terms and their significance and have provided illustrations of their typical appearances. Throughout this book, we have attempted to define HRCT terms relative to their specific anatomic correlates. Purely descriptive terms have been avoided, except in situations in which the findings themselves are nonspecific and cannot be related to particular anatomic abnormalities, when the nonspecific descriptive term is particularly helpful in understanding and recognizing the abnormal finding, or when the term is already widely accepted. The terms defined and the definitions used reflect our personal preferences [1] and incorporate the recommendations of the Nomenclature Committee of the Fleischner Society [2,3].

ACINAR SHADOW (ACINAR NODULE)

See *airspace nodule*.

ACINUS

A unit of lung structure distal to a terminal bronchiole and supplied by first-order respiratory bronchioles. An acinus is the largest lung unit in which all airways participate in gas exchange. Acini average 7 to 8 mm in diameter in adults and range from 6 to 10 mm in diameter (Fig. 11-29) [4–7]. Acini are not visible on HRCT in normal subjects, although acinar arteries can sometimes be seen. Secondary pulmonary lobules are comprised of a varying number of acini, ranging from three to 24 [8].

Equivalent

Pulmonary acinus.

AIRSPACE CONSOLIDATION

See *consolidation*.

AIRSPACE NODULE

A small, nodular opacity, usually ranging from a few millimeters to 1 centimeter in diameter, that can be seen in patients who have airspace diseases. It represents a focal area of peribronchiolar inflammation or airspace consolidation [9–12]. Airspace nodules are typically ill-defined and often appear centrilobular in location (Fig. 11-1). However, HRCT findings are unreliable in distinguishing small nodules that are primarily airspace in origin from those that are primarily interstitial; thus, a description of the size, appearance, and distribution of nodules is usually more appropriate when interpreting HRCT. See *centrilobular*; *nodule*. This term is preferred to *acinar shadow* and *acinar nodule*.

AIR-TRAPPING

Abnormal retention of gas (i.e., air) within a lung or part of a lung, especially during or after expiration, as a result of airway obstruction or abnormalities in lung compliance. It is diagnosable if lung parenchyma remains lucent on postexpiratory CT scans, shows a less than normal increase in attenuation after expiration, or shows little change in cross-sectional area (Fig. 11-2) [3,13–20]. Air-trapping is difficult to diagnose on inspiratory scans; lung inhomogeneity on inspiratory scans in patients who have airways disease should usually be referred to as *mosaic perfusion*.

Equivalent

Gas trapping.

ARCHITECTURAL DISTORTION

A manifestation of lung disease in which abnormal displacement of pulmonary structures, including bronchi, vessels, fissures, and interlobular septa, results in a distorted appearance of lung anatomy [1,3]. This finding is commonly seen in the presence of fibrosis or volume loss.

BAND

See *parenchymal band*.

BEADED SEPTUM SIGN

Nodular septal thickening that suggests the appearance of a row of beads. This finding is most common in patients who have lymphangitic spread of neoplasm [21] and sarcoidosis.

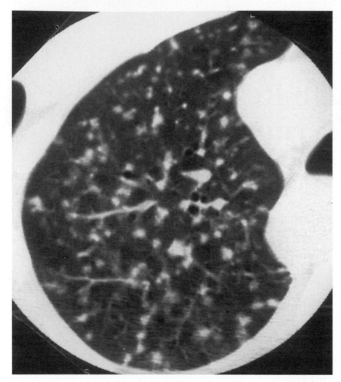

FIG. 11-1. Airspace nodule. In this patient who has endobronchial spread of tuberculosis, small, ill-defined, centrilobular nodules reflect the presence of peribronchiolar inflammation and consolidation. As is typical of centrilobular nodules, some are associated with small arteries, and many are centered 5 to 10 mm from the pleural surfaces.

BLEB

A gas-containing space within the visceral pleura [2]. Radiologically, this term is sometimes used to describe a focal thin-walled lucency, contiguous with the pleura, usually at the lung apex. However, a distinction between *bleb* and *bulla* is of little practical significance and is seldom justified. On HRCT, a bleb and bulla cannot be distinguished, and the term *bulla* is usually preferred [2].

BRONCHIECTASIS

Localized or diffuse, irreversible bronchial dilatation, usually resulting from chronic infection, airway obstruction by tumor, stricture, impacted material, inherited bronchial abnormalities, or fibrosis (see *traction bronchiectasis*). Although the definition of this term indicates that abnormalities must be irreversible, this is difficult to establish in the absence of serial examinations and is not required for diagnosis. Bronchiectasis can be classified into three types (cylindric, varicose, and cystic) depending on the appearances of the abnormal bronchi (Figs. 11-3, 11-4, 11-10B, 11-30, and 11-34). Although bronchial dilatation is the primary feature of bronchiectasis, bronchial

wall thickening, fluid retention within the bronchi, and small airway abnormalities are also commonly visible on HRCT.

BRONCHIOLAR IMPACTION

See *bronchiolectasis* and *tree-in-bud sign*.

BRONCHIOLE

Small airways that lack cartilage in their walls. The largest bronchioles measure approximately 3 mm in diameter and have walls approximately 0.3 mm in thickness.

BRONCHIOLECTASIS

Dilatation of bronchioles. Bronchiolectasis can occur as a result of airways disease (Fig. 11-4), or in the presence of lung fibrosis (see *traction bronchiolectasis*). Dilated bronchioles can be air- or fluid-filled. Dilated fluid-filled bronchioles are often described using the terms *bronchiolar impaction* or *tree-in-bud* [22–26], or may be visible as centrilobular nodular opacities.

BRONCHOVASCULAR BUNDLE

See *peribronchovascular interstitium*.

BULLA

A sharply demarcated area of emphysema, measuring 1 cm or more in diameter and possessing a wall less than 1 mm in thickness (Figs. 11-5, 11-12, and 11-24) [2]. To make the diagnosis of a bulla on HRCT, other areas of emphysema should also be visible. Subpleural bullae are commonly the result of paraseptal emphysema [27–29].

BULLOUS EMPHYSEMA

Emphysema in which bullae are the predominant feature (Fig. 11-5) [30].

CENTRILOBULAR

An adjective describing a structure (e.g., centrilobular bronchiole), HRCT finding (e.g., centrilobular nodule), or disease process that involves the center of the lobule. It is also used to describe abnormal findings seen in relation to centrilobular structures such as bronchioles or small arteries, but that cannot be precisely localized to the centers of lobules (Figs. 11-1, 11-6, and 11-22). On HRCT, a centrilobular abnormality can appear as an opacity or lucency centered within the lobule or as a group of opacities or lucencies surrounding centrilobular arteries [9,22,23]. It can reflect inflammation, airspace consolidation, airways disease, interstitial fibrosis, or emphysema.

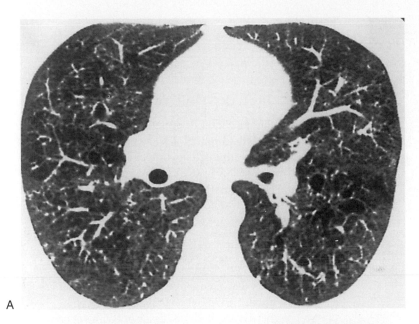

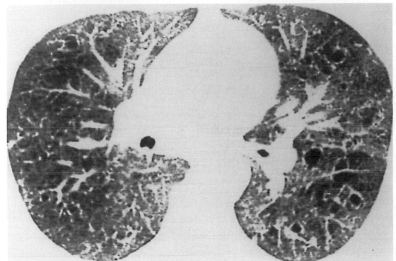

A

B

FIG. 11-2. Air-trapping on expiratory HRCT. **A:** Inspiratory scan in a patient who has histiocytosis obtained as part of a dynamic expiratory HRCT. Some cystic lesions are visible, but lung parenchyma is relatively homogeneous in attenuation. **B:** On an expiratory scan, some lung regions remain lucent as a result of air-trapping, whereas more normal lung regions increase in attenuation. (From Stern EJ, Webb WR, et al. Cystic lung disease associated with eosinophilic granuloma and tuberous sclerosis: air-trapping at dynamic ultrafast high-resolution CT. *Radiology* 1992;182:325, with permission.)

Equivalent

Lobular core.

CENTRILOBULAR EMPHYSEMA

Emphysema that predominantly affects the respiratory bronchioles in the center of acini, and therefore predominantly involves the central portion of secondary lobules [27–29]. Common in the upper lobes and in smokers. Usually visible on HRCT as multifocal areas of lucency that lack visible walls, although thin walls can sometimes be seen (Figs. 11-5, 11-7, and 11-12). Occasionally, the lucencies can be seen to surround the centrilobular artery.

Equivalents

Proximal acinar emphysema, centriacinar emphysema.

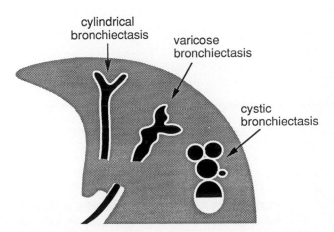

FIG. 11-3. Bronchiectasis. Classification of bronchiectasis based on morphology and HRCT appearance.

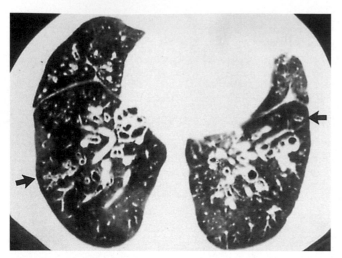

FIG. 11-4. Bronchiolectasis. In a patient who has allergic bronchopulmonary aspergillosis, there is extensive bronchiectasis bilaterally, manifested by bronchial dilatation and bronchial wall thickening. Dilated air-filled bronchioles in the peripheral lung (*arrows*) reflect bronchiolectasis. Also note lung inhomogeneity due to mosaic perfusion.

CENTRILOBULAR INTERSTITIAL THICKENING

Thickening of the centrilobular peribronchovascular interstitium that surrounds centrilobular bronchioles and vessels. It is recognizable by an increase in prominence of centrilobular structures.

CENTRILOBULAR INTERSTITIUM

The peripheral, centrilobular extension of the peribronchovascular interstitium. Part of the axial fiber network described by Weibel [5].

Equivalents

Centrilobular peribronchovascular interstitium; axial interstitium [2].

CENTRILOBULAR STRUCTURES

Structures in the center of pulmonary lobules, most notably the centrilobular bronchioles and arteries. Centrilobular arteries and their immediate branches measure approximately 1 mm and 0.5 to 0.7 mm in diameter, respectively [3,31], and are normally visible on HRCT. Centrilobular bronchioles have a wall measuring approximately 0.15 mm in thickness and are not normally visible on HRCT.

CONGLOMERATE MASS

A large opacity that often surrounds and encompasses bronchi and vessels, usually in the central or perihilar lung (Fig. 11-8). It often represents a mass of fibrous tissue or confluent nodules. It is most common in silicosis (Fig. 11-20), coal worker's pneumoconiosis, and sarcoidosis (Figs. 11-8 and 11-33).

Equivalent in Pneumoconiosis Patients

Complicated pneumoconiosis, progressive massive fibrosis.

CONSOLIDATION

An increase in lung opacity, discernible on plain radiographs or HRCT, that results in obscuration of underlying vessels (Figs. 11-8 and 11-9). This finding usually indicates the replacement of alveolar air or filling of airspaces by fluid, cells, or tissue [11] but can also be seen with extensive interstitial disease. On HRCT, it should be differentiated from

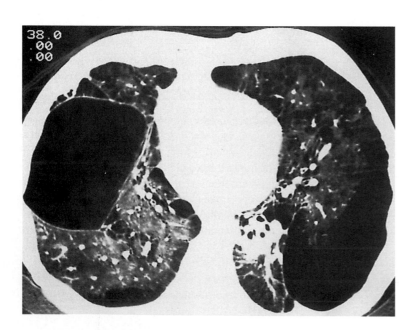

FIG. 11-5. Bullae. Large thin-walled subpleural bullae are visible bilaterally, in association with centrilobular emphysema. Because of the predominance of bullae in this patient, the term *bullous emphysema* could be used to describe this appearance.

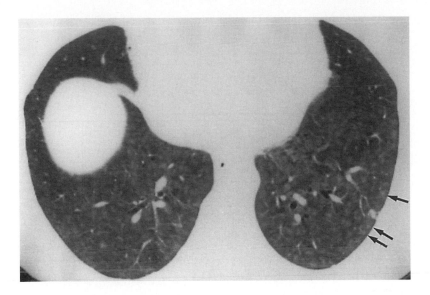

FIG. 11-6. Centrilobular nodules. Centrilobular nodules (*arrows*) of ground-glass opacity in a patient who has hypersensitivity pneumonitis. The nodules can be localized to the centrilobular region because of their relationship to centrilobular arteries. The nodules appear to be centered 5 to 10 mm from the pleural surface.

ground-glass opacity, in which underlying vessels are not obscured by increased lung opacity.

Equivalents

Airspace consolidation, airspace opacification, airspace attenuation.

CRAZY-PAVING

The superimposition of ground-glass opacity and a reticular pattern, often having the appearance of interlobular septal thickening [32–34]. This pattern was first recognized in patients who had pulmonary alveolar proteinosis (PAP) [35] (see Figs. 3-11 and 3-96), and is quite typical of PAP, but may also be seen in patients who have a variety of other diseases. In patients who have crazy-paving, ground-glass opacity may reflect the presence of airspace or interstitial abnormalities [33,34]; the reticular opacities may represent interlobular septal thickening, thickening of the intralobular interstitium, irregular areas of fibrosis, or a preponderance of an airspace filling process at the periphery of lobules or acini [33].

CYST

A nonspecific term describing the presence of a thin-walled (usually less than 3 mm thick), well-defined and circumscribed, air- or fluid-containing lesion, 1 cm or more in

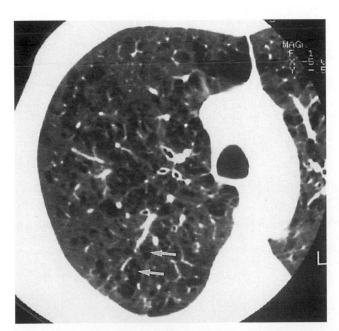

FIG. 11-7. Centrilobular emphysema. Multiple areas of low attenuation without distinct walls are visible bilaterally. Some of the areas of emphysema (*arrows*) surround visible centrilobular arteries.

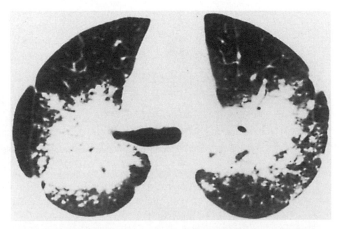

FIG. 11-8. Conglomerate mass. Bilateral upper lobe masses obscuring the perihilar vessels in a patient who has active sarcoidosis. Air bronchograms are visible within the masses. These conglomerate masses reflect a multitude of confluent granulomas. This appearance could also be referred to as *consolidation*.

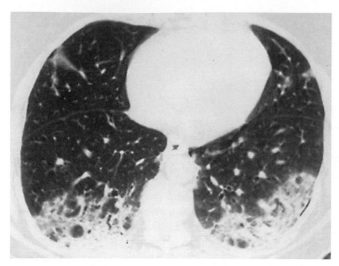

FIG. 11-9. Consolidation. A patient who has bronchiolitis obliterans organizing pneumonia shows bilateral consolidation. Pulmonary vessels are invisible in the densest areas, and air bronchograms are visible.

diameter, that has an epithelial or fibrous wall (Fig. 11-10) [1,2]. On HRCT, the term *cyst* is usually used to refer to an air-containing lesion or air-filled cyst. Air-filled cysts are commonly seen in patients who have Langerhans histiocytosis, lymphangiomyomatosis, sarcoidosis, and lymphocytic interstitial pneumonia [36–40], but can be seen in other diseases as well. Honeycombing also results in the presence of cysts (i.e., honeycomb cyst). The term *cyst* can be used to described the dilated bronchi seen in patients who have cys-

tic bronchiectasis (Fig. 11-10B), although the latter term is preferred. This term is not used to refer to focal lucencies associated with emphysema; *bulla* is preferred.

CYSTIC AIRSPACE

An enlarged airspace surrounded by a wall of varying thickness, which may be thin, as in emphysema or lymphangiomyomatosis, or thick, as in honeycombing. See also *bulla, cyst, honeycomb cyst,* and *pneumatocele.*

DEPENDENT INCREASED ATTENUATION

See *dependent opacity.*

DEPENDENT OPACITY

An ill-defined subpleural opacity, ranging from a few millimeters to a centimeter or more in thickness, that is only visible in dependent lung regions and disappears when the lung region is nondependent (Fig. 11-11) [2,41]. Dependent opacity represents normal dependent atelectasis. It is visible in the posterior lung when the subject is supine and disappears in the prone position. This normal finding may also appear as a *subpleural line* (Fig. 11-32), although this term is best used to refer to a thin, sharply defined opacity that persists in the nondependent lung.

Equivalent

Dependent density.

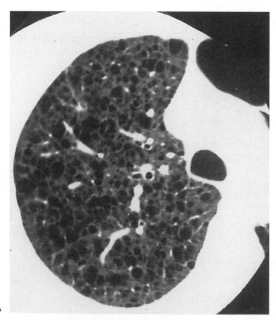

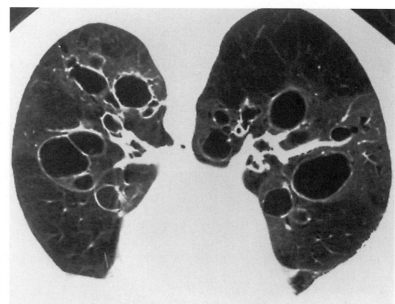

A

B

FIG. 11-10. Cysts. **A:** Multiple lung cysts in a patient who has lymphangiomyomatosis. The low attenuation air-filled cysts are marginated by thin walls. **B:** Lung cysts in this patient reflect cystic bronchiectasis. Although the cysts are thin-walled, thick-walled bronchi are visible centrally. Bronchiolitis obliterans was also present in this patient, manifested by decreased lung attenuation and hypervascularity.

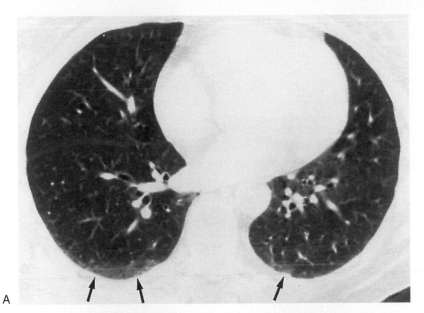

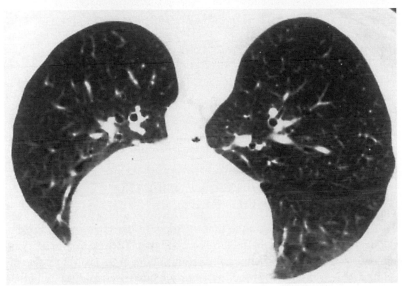

FIG. 11-11. Dependent opacity. **A:** Ill-defined opacities (*arrows*) are visible in the posterior lungs, more evident on the right than the left. **B:** At the same level with the patient positioned prone, the posterior lungs appear normal.

DISTAL ACINAR EMPHYSEMA

See *paraseptal emphysema.*

DYNAMIC EXPIRATORY HRCT

HRCT scans performed during expiration to diagnose air-trapping or airway collapse (Fig. 11-2) [13,14,18,42].

EMPHYSEMA

Permanent, abnormal enlargement of airspaces distal to the terminal bronchiole, accompanied by the destruction of their walls [27,43]. Previous definitions of emphysema have included the caveat "without obvious fibrosis" [28], but recent observations have established that some associated fibrosis is not uncommon [27,43]. Visible on HRCT as areas of low attenuation, usually without visible walls, and classified morphologically relative to the pulmonary lobule as centrilobular, panlobular, or paraseptal (Fig. 11-12) [31,44]. See also *bulla* (Fig. 11-5), *bullous emphysema, centrilobular emphysema* (Fig. 11-7), *irregular airspace enlargement* (Fig. 11-20), *panlobular emphysema* (Fig. 11-23), and *paraseptal emphysema* (Fig. 11-24).

END-STAGE LUNG

The final stage in progression of a lung disease, usually characterized by fibrosis, alveolar dissolution, bronchiolectasis, and disruption of normal lung architecture. Generally speaking, end-stage lung is considered to be present in patients who have morphologic evidence of honeycombing, extensive cystic changes, or conglomerate fibrosis [45–47]. See *honeycombing.*

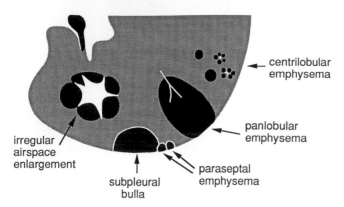

FIG. 11-12. Emphysema. Morphologic classification.

EXPIRATORY HRCT

HRCT scans performed during or after expiration to diagnose air-trapping in patients who have obstructive lung disease (Fig. 11-2) [13,15,18,20]. Scans can be obtained after expiration, can be gated to spirometry [48–50], or can be obtained dynamically during forced expiration [13,18,42] (see *dynamic expiratory HRCT*).

GROUND-GLASS ATTENUATION

See *ground-glass opacity*.

GROUND-GLASS OPACITY

A hazy increase in lung opacity on HRCT that is not associated with obscuration of underlying vessels and can therefore be differentiated from airspace consolidation (Fig. 11-13). This finding is nonspecific and can reflect the presence of minimal interstitial thickening, partial airspace filling, a combination of both interstitial and airspace abnormality, partial collapse of alveoli (i.e., dependent opacity), or increased capillary blood volume [3,12,51–53]. In many different diseases, and to varying degrees, this finding suggests an active or acute disease [51–53]. Ground-glass opacity visible on CT scans obtained with thick collimation (greater than 5 mm) is much less specific because of volume averaging, and it has been recommended that this term be applied only to HRCT [52]. Ground-glass opacity can be diffuse, patchy, or nodular (Fig. 11-6). When possible, it should be distinguished from *mosaic perfusion*, which can have a similar appearance.

HALO SIGN

A halo of ground-glass opacity surrounding a nodule or mass. It is nonspecific. It may be seen in patients who have invasive aspergillosis (representing hemorrhage), other infections, neoplasms (adenocarcinoma, bronchioloalveolar carcinoma, Kaposi sarcoma, metastases), Wegener granulomatosis, or other processes [54–57].

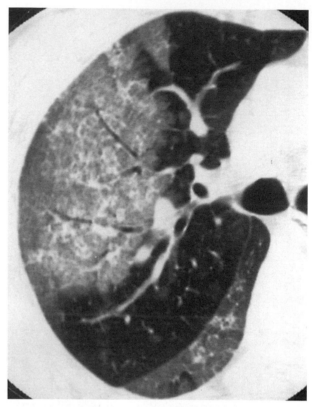

FIG. 11-13. Ground-glass opacity. In a patient who has pulmonary hemorrhage, focal areas of increased attenuation represent ground-glass opacity. Note that vessels are visible within the area of increased opacity. Air bronchograms are visible.

HIGH-RESOLUTION COMPUTED TOMOGRAPHY (HRCT)

A CT technique that attempts to optimize spatial resolution in visualizing lung parenchyma. The use of thin sections (e.g., 1- to 2-mm collimation) and a high–spatial frequency (sharp) reconstruction algorithm are essential [58], but other modifications of CT technique also can enhance spatial resolution. This term is preferable to *thin-section CT*, which takes into account only the use of narrow collimation.

HONEYCOMB CYSTS

Cystic airspaces, usually ranging from 3 to 10 mm in diameter, but up to several cm in size, associated with *honeycombing*.

HONEYCOMBING

A process characterized by the presence of cystic airspaces, ranging from several millimeters to several centimeters in diameter and characterized by thick, clearly definable fibrous walls lined by bronchiolar epithelium. Honeycombing results from, and is associated with, pulmonary fibrosis with lung destruction, dissolution of alveoli, and the loss of acinar architecture. The cystic airspaces of honeycombing commonly are clustered and share walls, are predominantly

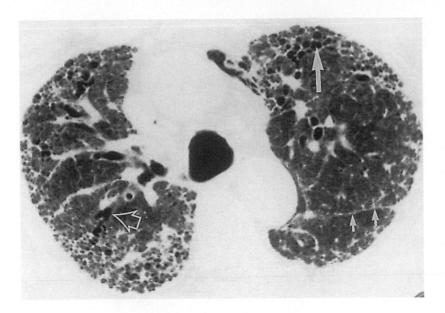

FIG. 11-14. Honeycombing. In a 73-year-old man who has end-stage idiopathic pulmonary fibrosis, honeycombing is visible predominantly in the subpleural lung regions (*large arrow*). The cystic airspaces show clearly definable walls, and adjacent cysts tend to share walls. Also note irregular interfaces at the pleural surfaces, traction bronchiectasis (*open arrow*), interlobular interstitial thickening, and subpleural interstitial thickening (*small arrows*) adjoining the left major fissure.

subpleural, and occur in several layers at the pleural surface (Figs. 11-14 and 11-15).

Equivalents

Honeycomb lung [46,59,60], *honeycomb cysts.*

INTERFACE SIGN

The presence of irregular interfaces at the edges of pulmonary parenchymal structures, such as vessels or bronchi, or at the pleural surfaces of lung (Figs. 11-14 and 11-15)

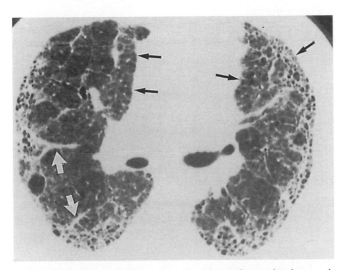

FIG. 11-15. The interface sign. In this patient who has pulmonary fibrosis and honeycombing, irregular interfaces at the edges of pulmonary vessels (*white arrows*) and bronchi, and at the pleural surfaces (*black arrows*) are indicative of the interface sign. As in this patient, it is not necessary to rely on this sign for diagnosis, as other abnormalities (e.g., honeycombing) are also evident.

[61,62]. A nonspecific finding usually indicative of interstitial thickening. Other, more specific, HRCT abnormalities are always or almost always visible, and a diagnosis of disease should rarely be based on this finding.

INTERLOBULAR SEPTAL THICKENING

Abnormal thickening of interlobular septa usually resulting from fibrosis, edema, or infiltration by cells or other material (Figs. 11-17, 11-25, and 11-33). Thickening can be smooth, nodular, or irregular in different diseases. See also *beaded-septum sign.*

Equivalents

Septal thickening; *septal lines.*

INTERLOBULAR SEPTUM

A connective tissue septum that marginates part of a secondary pulmonary lobule and contains pulmonary veins and lymphatics. It represents an inward extension of the peripheral interstitium, described by Weibel [5], which extends over the surface of the lung beneath the visceral pleura. Septa measure approximately 100 μ (0.1 mm) in thickness and are occasionally visible in normal subjects (Fig. 11-16).

INTERSTITIAL NODULE

A small nodule, usually ranging from a few millimeters to 1 cm in diameter, that is predominantly interstitial in location. Interstitial nodules are often well defined and can be seen when quite small (Fig. 11-18). This term should generally be avoided in interpreting HRCT, as HRCT findings are unreliable in making this diagnosis. See *nodule.*

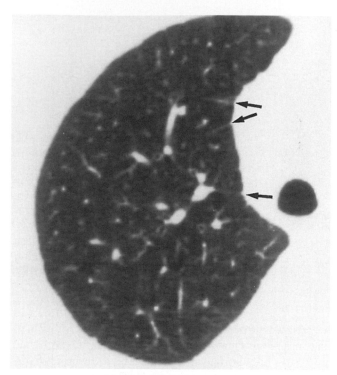

FIG. 11-16. Interlobular septa. A few septa are visible in this normal subject. These are most evident along the mediastinal pleural surface (*arrows*).

INTERSTITIUM

The fibrous supporting structure of the lung.

INTRALOBULAR INTERSTITIAL THICKENING

Thickening of the intralobular interstitium, resulting in a fine reticular, or meshlike appearance to the lung parenchyma (Fig. 11-19) [31]. It is an early sign of fibrosis in a number of lung diseases or may be associated with lung infiltration, as in pulmonary edema or hemorrhage.

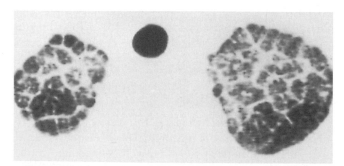

FIG. 11-17. Interlobular septal thickening. Marked thickening of septa is present in the upper lobes of this patient who has lymphangitic spread of carcinoma.

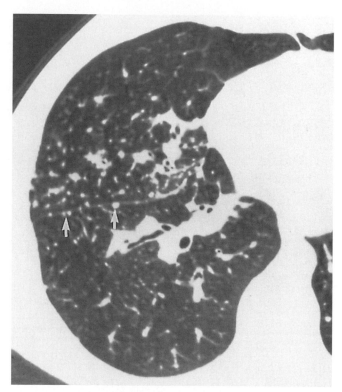

FIG. 11-18. Interstitial nodules. Small, sharply defined nodules (*arrows*) in a patient who has sarcoidosis are primarily interstitial in origin. In this patient, nodules show a perilymphatic distribution, being predominantly subpleural (*arrows*), septal, and peribronchovascular.

INTRALOBULAR INTERSTITIUM

The interstitial network, excluding the interlobular septa, that supports structures of the pulmonary lobule. It is not normally visible but can be seen on HRCT when abnormally thickened. This term refers primarily to the fine network of very thin connective tissue fibers within the alveolar walls (the septal fibers described by Weibel [4,5] or the parenchymal interstitium [2]).

INTRALOBULAR LINES

See *intralobular interstitial thickening* [3,31].

IRREGULAR AIRSPACE ENLARGEMENT

Emphysema or lung destruction that occurs adjacent to areas of pulmonary fibrosis (Figs. 11-12 and 11-20) [28,29].

Equivalent

Paracicatricial or irregular emphysema.

IRREGULAR LINEAR OPACITY

Any abnormal linear opacity of irregular thickness (1 to 3 mm) that does not represent a specific abnormality such as

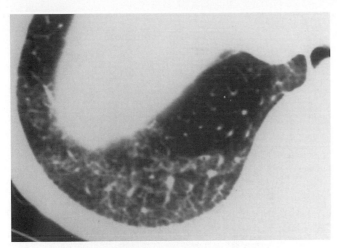

FIG. 11-19. Intralobular interstitial thickening. In this patient who has pulmonary fibrosis, a fine reticular pattern visible posteriorly reflects intralobular interstitial thickening. Note the presence of irregular interfaces at the posterior pleural surface.

interlobular septal thickening or peribronchovascular interstitial thickening [3]. It may be intralobular or extend through several adjacent pulmonary lobules.

LINEAR OPACITY

Any elongated, thin line of soft-tissue attenuation [3].

LOBULAR CORE

The central portion of a secondary lobule [63] containing the pulmonary artery and bronchiolar branches that supply

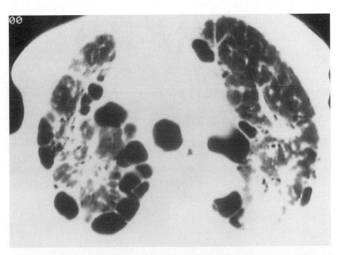

FIG. 11-20. Irregular airspace enlargement. In this patient who has silicosis and progressive massive fibrosis, areas of emphysema adjacent to the fibrotic masses reflect irregular airspace enlargement or irregular emphysema.

the lobule, as well as supporting peribronchovascular or axial connective tissue [5]. The term *centrilobular* is preferred.

LOBULAR CORE STRUCTURES

See *centrilobular structures.*

LOBULE

See *secondary pulmonary lobule.*

LOW-DOSE HRCT

An HRCT technique in which radiation dose is reduced by using reduced milliamperes (mA). This technique results in some decrease in resolution and diagnostic accuracy and is most suitable for screening or follow-up of patients. Appropriate technical factors for low-dose HRCT are 120 kV(p) and 40 to 80 mA [64–66].

LUNG CYST

See *cyst.*

MICRONODULE

A discrete, small, focal, rounded opacity of at least soft-tissue attenuation with a diameter of no more than 7 mm [3,67–70]. Some authors have used this term to refer to nodules smaller than 3 mm in diameter [71]. Others simply use the term *small nodule*. In this book, nodules are classified on the basis of their size as small (less than 1 cm) or large (greater than 1 cm).

MIDLUNG WINDOW

A relatively avascular region in the right middle lung, corresponding to the location of the minor fissure and adjacent lung [72].

MOSAIC OLIGEMIA

See *mosaic perfusion.*

MOSAIC PERFUSION

Regional differences in lung perfusion resulting in visible attenuation differences on inspiratory HRCT. This finding can reflect vascular obstruction or abnormal ventilation. It is most common in patients who have airways disease [1]. Vessels in the lucent regions of lung characteristically appear smaller than in denser lung regions (Figs. 11-4 and 11-21). *Mosaic perfusion* is preferred to *mosaic oligemia* [73] in most cases [1], as it is a more inclusive term, recognizing that areas of increased perfusion may also be present. Expiratory HRCT is of value in diagnosing mosaic perfusion resulting from airways disease.

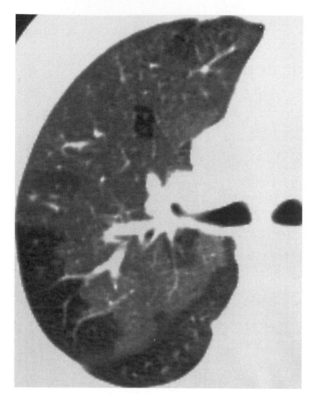

FIG. 11-21. Mosaic perfusion. In a child who has bronchiolitis obliterans, focal regions of lucency reflect airway obstruction and decreased perfusion. Vessels in the lucent regions appear smaller, a characteristic finding.

NODULE

A focal, rounded opacity of varying size, which can be well or ill defined. In this book, nodules have been classified on the basis of their size as small (smaller than 1 cm) or large (larger than 1 cm). *Micronodule* may be used to describe nodules 7 mm or less in diameter [3,67–70]. Nodules are also classified as well or ill defined and by location (e.g., random, perilymphatic, centrilobular) (Figs. 11-1, 11-6, 11-18, and 11-22). The terms *airspace nodule* and *interstitial nodule* should generally be avoided; airspace and interstitial nodules can be difficult to distinguish on HRCT. See also *micronodule, interstitial nodule,* and *air space nodule.*

OPACIFICATION

A term indicating an increase in lung attenuation, as in parenchymal opacification [51,74]. It may or may not result in obscuration of pulmonary vessels. When possible, use of the more specific terms *consolidation* (vessels obscured) and *ground-glass opacity* (vessels not obscured) is preferred [3]. This term is not usually used to refer to increased lung attenuation that reflects mosaic perfusion.

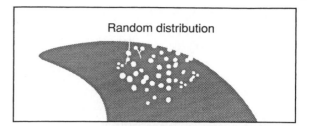

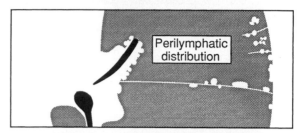

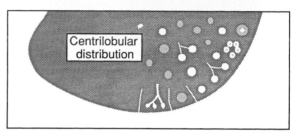

FIG. 11-22. Nodules. Nodules with a random distribution can be seen in relation to small vessels, interlobular septa, and the pleural surfaces, but appear to be diffuse and uniformly distributed. Perilymphatic nodules predominate in the perihilar peribronchovascular regions, the centrilobular regions, and in relation to interlobular septa and the pleural surfaces. Centrilobular nodules are widely distributed, mimicking the appearance of random nodules, but spare the pleural surfaces and interlobular septa.

OPACITY

A term indicating a focal increase in lung attenuation. It can indicate the presence of airspace consolidation or ground-glass opacity.

PANACINAR EMPHYSEMA

See *panlobular emphysema.*

PANLOBULAR EMPHYSEMA

Emphysema that more or less uniformly involves all the components of the acinus, and therefore involves the entire lobule [28]. It predominates in the lower lobes and is classically associated with alpha-1-protease inhibitor (alpha-1-antitrypsin) deficiency. HRCT usually shows uniformly reduced parenchymal attenuation and a paucity of vascular markings and is usually unassociated with focal lucencies or bullae (Figs. 11-12 and 11-23). Severe

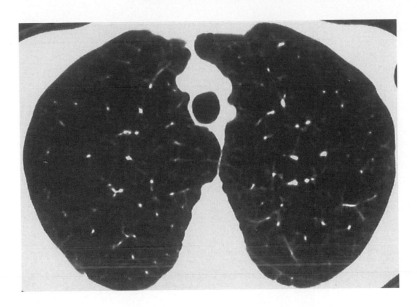

FIG. 11-23. Panlobular emphysema. Emphysema that more or less uniformly involves the pulmonary lobule is termed *panlobular*. As in this patient, HRCT usually shows large regions of lucency and a paucity of vascular markings.

centrilobular emphysema may be indistinguishable from panlobular emphysema.

PARASEPTAL EMPHYSEMA

Emphysema that predominantly involves the alveolar ducts and sacs [28]. It is typically subpleural in location, and associated with intact interlobular septa, and it is commonly associated with subpleural bullae (Figs. 11-12 and 11-24). It

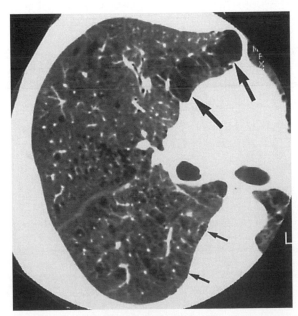

FIG. 11-24. Paraseptal emphysema. In this patient who has centrilobular emphysema, subpleural lucencies (*small arrows*) represent paraseptal emphysema. These areas of emphysema may be marginated by interlobular septa. When larger than 1 cm, areas of paraseptal emphysema are called *bullae* (*large arrows*).

can be seen as an isolated abnormality and may be associated with spontaneous pneumothorax. It is commonly associated with centrilobular emphysema (Fig. 11-24).

Equivalent

Distal acinar emphysema.

PARENCHYMAL BAND

The term *parenchymal band* has been used to describe linear opacities several millimeters thick and from 2 to 5 cm in length, which can be seen in patients who have pulmonary fibrosis or other causes of interstitial thickening [3,41,75]. They are often peripheral and generally contact the pleural surface. Parenchymal bands can represent contiguous thickened interlobular septa, peribronchovascular fibrosis, coarse scars, or atelectasis associated with lung or pleural fibrosis (Figs. 11-25 and 11-33) [76,77]. They are most common in patients who have asbestos exposure and sarcoidosis.

PARENCHYMAL OPACIFICATION

See *opacification*.

PERIBRONCHOVASCULAR INTERSTITIAL THICKENING

Thickening of the peribronchovascular interstitium that surrounds the perihilar bronchi and vessels [12,78–80]. This is recognizable by an apparent thickening of the bronchial wall and an apparent increase in size or nodular appearance of the pulmonary arteries (Fig. 11-26) [79]. This term is generally used to describe interstitial thickening in relation to relatively large airways. In a centrilobular location, peribronchovascular interstitial thickening may be referred to

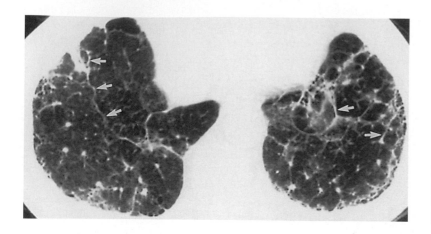

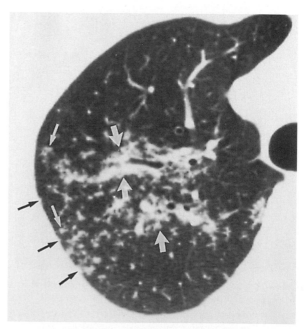

FIG. 11-25. Parenchymal bands. In a 66-year-old patient who has asbestosis, interlobular septal thickening is associated with numerous parenchymal bands (*small arrows*).

as *centrilobular interstitial thickening* on HRCT, and it is recognized by increased prominence of the centrilobular arteries or bronchioles. It can be irregular, smooth (Fig. 11-26), or nodular (Fig. 11-27) and represent fibrosis or interstitial infiltration, as in lymphangitic spread of carcinoma or sarcoidosis.

Equivalents

Peribronchial cuffing, thickening of the bronchovascular bundle.

PERIBRONCHOVASCULAR INTERSTITIUM

The strong connective tissue sheath that encloses the bronchi and hilar vessels and extends from the level of the pulmonary hila into the peripheral lung. Part of the axial fiber network described by Weibel [5].

Equivalents

Axial interstitium; bronchovascular interstitium [2], *bronchovascular bundle.*

PERILYMPHATIC

A term that refers to a distribution of abnormalities (e.g., nodules) corresponding to the location of lymphatics in the lung [67,81,82]. Nodules that predominate in relation to the perihilar peribronchovascular interstitium, the centrilobular interstitium, and interlobular septa and in a subpleural location are typical of a perilymphatic distribution (Figs. 11-22 and 11-27), and are most commonly seen in patients who have sarcoidosis, silicosis and coal worker's pneumoconiosis, and lymphangitic spread of tumor [67,81,82].

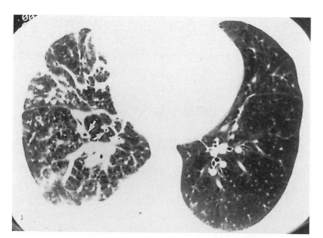

FIG. 11-26. Peribronchovascular interstitial thickening. In a patient with unilateral lymphangitic carcinomatosis, smooth peribronchovascular interstitial thickening is visible in the right middle and lower lobes. The bronchial walls (*arrows*) appear thicker than on the left, and vessels in the right lower zone appear larger than left-sided vessels. Subpleural interstitial thickening is present on the right, making the right major fissure appear thickened.

FIG. 11-27. Perilymphatic nodules. In this patient who has sarcoidosis, nodules predominate in the peribronchovascular regions (*large white arrows*), subpleural regions (*black arrows*), and in the centrilobular regions (*small white arrows*).

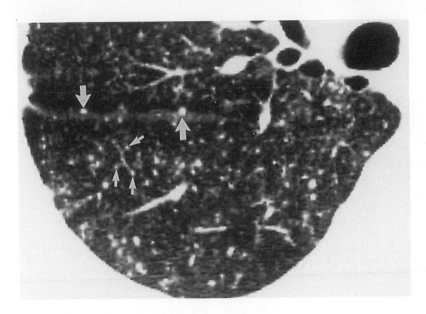

FIG. 11-28. Random nodules. A patient who has miliary mycobacterial disease shows numerous, widely distributed, small nodules. Some are visible in relation to small vessels (*small arrows*) and the pleural surfaces (*large arrows*).

PERIPHERAL

Refers to pulmonary structures within 1 to 2 cm of the pleural surface. See *subpleural.*

PNEUMATOCELE

A thin-walled, gas-filled cystic space within the lung, usually occurring in association with acute pneumonia and almost invariably transient [2]. Pneumatoceles have an appearance similar to lung cyst or bulla on HRCT and cannot be distinguished on the basis of HRCT findings. However, the association of such an abnormality with acute pneumonia would suggest the presence of a pneumatocele.

PSEUDOPLAQUES

A grouping of small subpleural nodules, several millimeters thick, that form a bandlike subpleural opacity simulating the appearance of an asbestos-related parietal pleural plaque [67]. Most common in sarcoidosis (Fig. 11-27) and silicosis.

PULMONARY LOBULE

See *secondary pulmonary lobule.*

RANDOM DISTRIBUTION

A term that refers to a random distribution of nodules relative to secondary lobular and lung structures [67,81,82]. A random distribution is often seen in metastatic neoplasm, miliary tuberculosis, and miliary fungal infections, although nodules in histiocytosis and silicosis can also show this distribution. Nodules appear to be diffuse but can be seen in relation to interlobular septa, the pleural surfaces, and small vessels (Figs. 11-22 and 11-28).

RESPIRATORY BRONCHIOLE

The largest bronchiole with alveoli arising from its walls. Thus, the largest bronchiole that participates in gas exchange. An acinus is supplied by one or more respiratory bronchioles.

RETICULAR PATTERN

See *reticulation.*

RETICULATION

Innumerable, interlacing line shadow suggesting a mesh or net. A descriptive term usually associated with interstitial lung disease. Reticulation may be more specifically characterized as representing *interlobular septal thickening*, *intralobular septal thickening*, *honeycombing*, or resulting from *parenchymal bands* or *irregular linear opacities.*

SECONDARY PULMONARY LOBULE

This term is defined differently by Miller and Reid (Fig. 11-29).
1. According to Miller [4,83], the smallest unit of lung structure marginated by connective tissue septa. Secondary pulmonary lobules are variably delineated by interlobular septa containing veins and lymphatics and are supplied by arterial and bronchiolar branches in the lobular core. Using this definition, a secondary pulmonary lobule is usually made up of a dozen or fewer acini, appears irregularly polyhedral in shape, and measures approximately 1 to 2.5 cm on each side [4–8,83]. Miller's definition is most appropriate to interpretation of HRCT, because interlobular septa, arteries, and septal veins can be seen using this technique.

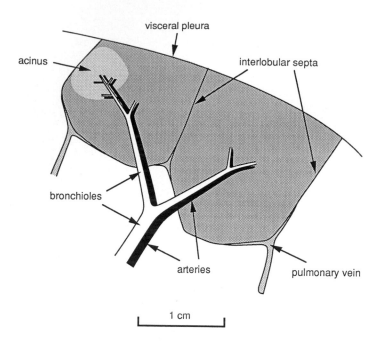

visceral pleura

acinus

interlobular septa

bronchioles

arteries

pulmonary vein

1 cm

FIG. 11-29. Secondary pulmonary lobule. According to Miller's definition.

2. According to Reid, the unit of lung supplied by any bronchiole that gives off three to five terminal bronchioles [63,84,85]; these lobules are approximately 1 cm in diameter and contain three to five acini. This definition does not necessarily describe lung units equivalent to secondary lobules as defined by Miller or marginated by interlobular septa [8,84]. Reid's definition is most appropriate to interpretation of bronchograms.

Equivalents

Lobule, secondary lobule, pulmonary lobule.

SEPTAL LINE

See *interlobular septal thickening.*

SEPTAL THICKENING

See *interlobular septal thickening.*

SEPTUM

See *interlobular septum.*

SIGNET RING SIGN

A ring shadow (representing a dilated, thick-walled bronchus) associated with a small, soft-tissue opacity (the adjacent pulmonary artery) that together have the appearance of a signet ring (Fig. 11-30). Diagnostic of bronchiectasis [86,87]. Distinguish from *peribronchovascular interstitial thickening* or peribronchial cuffing, in which the bronchus is not dilated.

SMALL AIRWAYS

Airways 3 mm or less in diameter, the vast majority of which represent bronchioles [88,89]. *Small airway* is a more general term than *bronchiole.*

SMALL AIRWAYS DISEASE

A term referring to diseases involving small airways. This term was originally used to describe a functional abnormal-

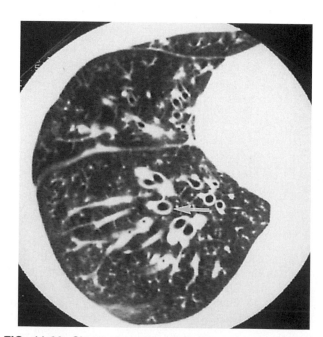

FIG. 11-30. Signet ring sign. A patient who has cylindric bronchiectasis shows several examples of the signet ring sign (*arrow*) in the right lower lobe.

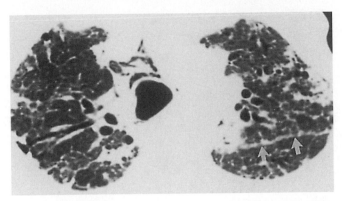

FIG. 11-31. Subpleural interstitial thickening. Apparent thickening of the left major fissure (*arrows*) in this patient who has pulmonary fibrosis represents subpleural interstitial thickening. An incidental pneumomediastinum is also present.

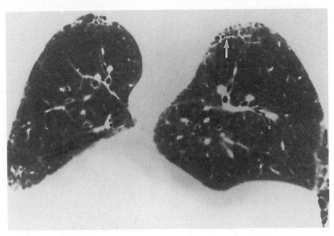

FIG. 11-32. Subpleural line. An irregular subpleural line (*arrow*) is visible on the right on a prone scan in a patient who has rheumatoid arthritis, pulmonary fibrosis, and early honeycombing.

ity but may be used on HRCT to describe a variety of diseases involving airways 3 mm or smaller in diameter [88,89]. Large airway abnormalities often coexist.

SUBPLEURAL

Refers to structures that are adjacent to the visceral pleural surfaces.

SUBPLEURAL INTERSTITIAL THICKENING

Abnormal thickening of the subpleural interstitium. Most easily seen on HRCT adjacent to the fissures, giving the appearance of thickening of the fissures (Fig. 11-31). Commonly associated with interlobular septal thickening. *Subpleural interstitial thickening* is preferred to *fissural thickening*.

SUBPLEURAL INTERSTITIUM

The interstitial fiber network that lies beneath the visceral pleura and envelops the lung in a fibrous sac. It extends over the surface of the lung and in relation to the interlobar fissures. Along with the interlobular septa, the subpleural interstitium represents a portion of the peripheral fiber system described by Weibel [5].

SUBPLEURAL LINE

A thin, curvilinear opacity a few millimeters or less in thickness, usually less than 1 cm from the pleural surface and paralleling the pleura (Fig. 11-32) [90]. This is a nonspecific term and may be used to describe dependent opacity (a normal finding), dependent and transient atelectasis, or fibrosis. A subpleural line that persists when nondependent often reflects fibrosis or honeycombing, and other findings of fibrosis will usually be visible.

TARGETED RECONSTRUCTION

Reconstruction of the CT image, using a smaller field of view than used to scan the patient, to reduce the image pixel size and increase spatial resolution [58,91].

TERMINAL BRONCHIOLE

The last purely conducting airway that does not participate in gas exchange. Approximately 0.7 mm in diameter, it gives rise to respiratory bronchioles.

TRACTION BRONCHIECTASIS

Bronchial dilatation and irregularity occurring in patients who have pulmonary fibrosis because of traction by fibrous tissue on the bronchial wall (Fig. 11-33) [31,92]. Visible on HRCT as bronchiectasis that is commonly irregular in contour. The term *traction bronchiolectasis* applies to intralobular bronchioles, and is usually diagnosed if dilated airways are visible in the lung periphery.

TRACTION BRONCHIOLECTASIS

See *traction bronchiectasis, bronchiolectasis*.

TREE-IN-BUD SIGN

Bronchiolar dilatation and filling by mucus, pus, or fluid, resembling a branching or budding tree and usually somewhat nodular in appearance [22–26]. Usually visible in the lung periphery, this finding is indicative of airways disease, and is particularly common in endobronchial spread of infection (e.g., tuberculosis), cystic fibrosis, diffuse panbronchiolitis, and chronic airways infection (Fig. 11-34) [22–26].

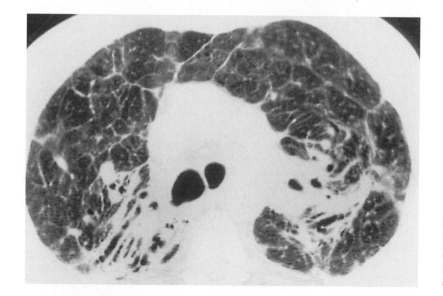

FIG. 11-33. Traction bronchiectasis. In a patient who has end-stage sarcoidosis, dilated bronchi are associated with perihilar conglomerate masses of fibrosis. Also note septal thickening and parenchymal bands anteriorly.

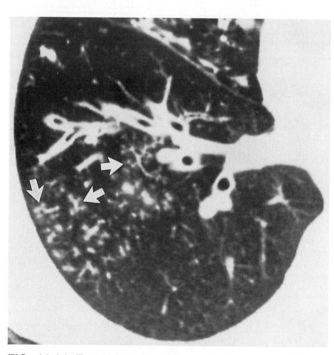

FIG. 11-34. Tree-in-bud. A patient who has cystic fibrosis shows numerous examples of tree-in-bud. Several of these are indicated by arrows. This appearance reflects the presence of dilated, branching, mucus-filled bronchioles. Also noted is central bronchial wall thickening.

REFERENCES

1. Webb WR, Müller NL, Naidich DP. Standardized terms for high-resolution computed tomography of the lung: a proposed glossary. *J Thorac Imag* 1993;8:167–185.
2. Tuddenham WJ. Glossary of terms for thoracic radiology: recommendations of the Nomenclature Committee of the Fleischner Society. *AJR Am J Roentgenol* 1984;143:509–517.
3. Austin JH, Müller NL, Friedman PJ, et al. Glossary of terms for CT of the lungs: recommendations of the Nomenclature Committee of the Fleischner Society. *Radiology* 1996;200:327–331.
4. Weibel ER, Taylor CR. Design and structure of the human lung. In: Fishman AP, ed. *Pulmonary diseases and disorders*. New York: McGraw-Hill, 1988:11–60.
5. Weibel ER. Looking into the lung: what can it tell us? *AJR Am J Roentgenol* 1979;133:1021–1031.
6. Raskin SP. The pulmonary acinus: historical notes. *Radiology* 1982;144:31–34.
7. Osborne DR, Effmann EL, Hedlund LW. Postnatal growth and size of the pulmonary acinus and secondary lobule in man. *AJR Am J Roentgenol* 1983;140:449–454.
8. Itoh H, Murata K, Konishi J, et al. Diffuse lung disease: pathologic basis for the high-resolution computed tomography findings. *J Thorac Imag* 1993;8:176–188.
9. Murata K, Itoh H, Todo G, et al. Centrilobular lesions of the lung: demonstration by high-resolution CT and pathologic correlation. *Radiology* 1986;161:641–645.
10. Murata K, Herman PG, Khan A, et al. Intralobular distribution of oleic acid–induced pulmonary edema in the pig: evaluation by high-resolution CT. *Invest Radiol* 1989;24:647–653.
11. Naidich DP, Zerhouni EA, Hutchins GM, et al. Computed tomography of the pulmonary parenchyma: part 1. Distal airspace disease. *J Thorac Imag* 1985;1:39–53.
12. Webb WR. High-resolution CT of the lung parenchyma. *Radiol Clin North Am* 1989;27:1085–1097.
13. Stern EJ, Webb WR. Dynamic imaging of lung morphology with ultrafast high-resolution computed tomography. *J Thorac Imag* 1993;8:273–282.
14. Stern EJ, Webb WR, Gamsu G. Dynamic quantitative computed tomography: a predictor of pulmonary function in obstructive lung diseases. *Invest Radiol* 1994;29:564–569.
15. Webb WR. Radiology of obstructive pulmonary disease. *AJR Am J Roentgenol* 1997;169:637–647.
16. Webb WR, Stern EJ, Kanth N, et al. Dynamic pulmonary CT: findings in normal adult men. *Radiology* 1993;186:117–124.
17. Webb WR. High-resolution computed tomography of obstructive lung disease. *Rad Clin N Am* 1994;32:745–757.
18. Arakawa H, Webb WR. Expiratory high-resolution CT scan. *Radiol Clin North Am* 1998;36:189–209.
19. Chen D, Webb WR, Storto ML, et al. Assessment of air-trapping using postexpiratory high-resolution computed tomography. *J Thorac Imag* 1998;13:135–143.
20. Lucidarme O, Coche E, Cluzel P, et al. Expiratory CT scans for chronic airway disease: correlation with pulmonary function test results. *AJR Am J Roentgenol* 1998;170:301–307.
21. Ren H, Hruban RH, Kuhlman JE, et al. Computed tomography of inflation-fixed lungs: the beaded septum sign of pulmonary metastases. *J Comput Assist Tomogr* 1989;13:411–416.
22. Gruden JF, Webb WR. Identification and evaluation of centrilobular opacities on high-resolution CT. *Semin Ultra CT MR* 1995;16:435–449.

23. Gruden JF, Webb WR, Warnock M. Centrilobular opacities in the lung on high-resolution CT: diagnostic considerations and pathologic correlation. *AJR Am J Roentgenol* 1994;162:569–574.

24. Akira M, Kitatani F, Lee Y-S, et al. Diffuse panbronchiolitis: evaluation with high-resolution CT. *Radiology* 1988;168:433–438.

25. Im JG, Itoh H, Shim YS, et al. Pulmonary tuberculosis: CT findings—early active disease and sequential change with antituberculous therapy. *Radiology* 1993;186:653–660.

26. Aquino SL, Gamsu G, Webb WR, et al. Tree-in-bud pattern: frequency and significance on thin section CT. *J Comput Assist Tomogr* 1996;20:594–599.

27. Snider GL. Pathogenesis and terminology of emphysema. *Am J Respir Crit Care Med* 1994;149:1382–1383.

28. Snider GL, Kleinerman J, Thurlbeck WM, et al. The definition of emphysema: report of a National Heart, Lung, and Blood Institute, Division of Lung Diseases workshop. *Am Rev Respir Dis* 1985;132:182–185.

29. Thurlbeck WM. *Chronic airflow obstruction in lung disease.* Philadelphia, WB Saunders, 1976:12–30.

30. Stern EJ, Webb WR, Weinacker A, et al. Idiopathic giant bullous emphysema (vanishing lung syndrome): imaging findings in nine patients. *AJR Am J Roentgenol* 1994;162:279–282.

31. Webb WR, Stein MG, Finkbeiner WE, et al. Normal and diseased isolated lungs: high-resolution CT. *Radiology* 1988;166:81–87.

32. Franquet T, Giménez A, Bordes R, et al. The crazy-paving pattern in exogenous lipoid pneumonia: CT-pathologic correlation. *AJR Am J Roentgenol* 1998;170:315–317.

33. Johkoh T, Itoh H, Müller NL, et al. Crazy-paving appearance at thin-section CT: spectrum of disease and pathologic findings. *Radiology* 1999;211:155–160.

34. Murayama S, Murakami J, Yabuuchi H, et al. "Crazy-paving appearance" on high resolution CT in various diseases. *J Comput Assist Tomogr* 1999;23:749–752.

35. Murch CR, Carr DH. Computed tomography appearances of pulmonary alveolar proteinosis. *Clin Radiol* 1989;40:240–243.

36. Brauner MW, Grenier P, Mouelhi MM, et al. Pulmonary histiocytosis X: evaluation with high resolution CT. *Radiology* 1989;172:255–258.

37. Moore AD, Godwin JD, Müller NL, et al. Pulmonary histiocytosis X: comparison of radiographic and CT findings. *Radiology* 1989;172:249–254.

38. Aberle DR, Hansell DM, Brown K, et al. Lymphangiomyomatosis: CT, chest radiographic, and functional correlations. *Radiology* 1990;176:381–387.

39. Lenoir S, Grenier P, Brauner MW, et al. Pulmonary lymphangiomyomatosis and tuberous sclerosis: comparison of radiographic and thin-section CT findings. *Radiology* 1990;175:329–334.

40. Müller NL, Chiles C, Kullnig P. Pulmonary lymphangiomyomatosis: correlation of CT with radiographic and functional findings. *Radiology* 1990;175:335–339.

41. Aberle DR, Gamsu G, Ray CS, et al. Asbestos-related pleural and parenchymal fibrosis: detection with high-resolution CT. *Radiology* 1988;166:729–734.

42. Gotway MB, Lee ES, Reddy GP, et al. Low-dose, dynamic expiratory thin-section CT of the lungs using a spiral scanner. *J Thorac Imag* 2000;15:168–172.

43. Cardoso WV, Thurlbeck WM. Pathogenesis and terminology of emphysema. *Am J Respir Crit Care Med* 1994;149:1383.

44. Naidich DP. High-resolution computed tomography of cystic lung disease. *Semin Roentgenol* 1991;26:151–174.

45. Hogg JC. Benjamin Felson lecture. Chronic interstitial lung disease of unknown cause: a new classification based on pathogenesis. *AJR Am J Roentgenol* 1991;156:225–233.

46. Genereux GP. The end-stage lung: pathogenesis, pathology, and radiology. *Radiology* 1975;116:279–289.

47. Snider GL. Interstitial pulmonary fibrosis. *Chest* 1986;89[Suppl]:115–121.

48. Kalender WA, Fichte H, Bautz W, et al. Semiautomatic evaluation procedures for quantitative CT of the lung. *J Comput Assist Tomogr* 1991;15:248–255.

49. Kalender WA, Rienmuller R, Seissler W, et al. Measurement of pulmonary parenchymal attenuation: use of spirometric gating with quantitative CT. *Radiology* 1990;175:265–268.

50. Robinson TE, Leung AN, Moss RB, et al. Standardized high-resolution CT of the lung using a spirometer-triggered electron beam CT scanner. *AJR Am J Roentgenol* 1999;172:1636–1638.

51. Leung AN, Miller RR, Müller NL. Parenchymal opacification in chronic infiltrative lung diseases: CT-pathologic correlation. *Radiology* 1993;188:209–214.

52. Remy-Jardin M, Remy J, Giraud F, et al. Computed tomography assessment of ground-glass opacity: semiology and significance. *J Thorac Imag* 1993;8:249–264.

53. Remy-Jardin M, Giraud F, Remy J, et al. Importance of ground-glass attenuation in chronic diffuse infiltrative lung disease: pathologic-CT correlation. *Radiology* 1993;189:693–698.

54. Gaeta M, Volta S, Stroscio S, et al. CT "halo sign" in pulmonary tuberculoma. *J Comput Assist Tomogr* 1992;16:827–828.

55. Hruban RH, Meziane MA, Zerhouni EA, et al. Radiologic-pathologic correlation of the CT halo sign in invasive pulmonary aspergillosis. *J Comput Assist Tomogr* 1987;11:534–536.

56. Primack SL, Hartman TE, Lee KS, et al. Pulmonary nodules and the CT halo sign. *Radiology* 1994;190:513–515.

57. Kuriyama K, Seto M, Kasugai T, et al. Ground-glass opacity on thin-section CT: value in differentiating subtypes of adenocarcinoma of the lung. *AJR Am J Roentgenol* 1999;173:465–469.

58. Mayo JR, Webb WR, Gould R, et al. High-resolution CT of the lungs: an optimal approach. *Radiology* 1987;163:507–510.

59. Genereux GP. The Fleischner lecture: computed tomography of diffuse pulmonary disease. *J Thorac Imag* 1989;4:50–87.

60. Primack SL, Hartman TE, Hansell DM, et al. End-stage lung disease: CT findings in 61 patients. *Radiology* 1993;189:681–686.

61. Zerhouni EA, Naidich DP, Stitik FP, et al. Computed tomography of the pulmonary parenchyma: part 2. Interstitial disease. *J Thorac Imag* 1985;1:54–64.

62. Zerhouni E. Computed tomography of the pulmonary parenchyma: an overview. *Chest* 1989;95:901–907.

63. Heitzman ER, Markarian B, Berger I, et al. The secondary pulmonary lobule: a practical concept for interpretation of radiographs. I. Roentgen anatomy of the normal secondary pulmonary lobule. *Radiology* 1969;93:508–513.

64. Zwirewich CV, Mayo JR, Müller NL. Low-dose high-resolution CT of lung parenchyma. *Radiology* 1991;180:413–417.

65. Lee KS, Primack SL, Staples CA, et al. Chronic infiltrative lung disease: comparison of diagnostic accuracies of radiography and low- and conventional-dose thin-section CT. *Radiology* 1994;191:669–673.

66. Majurin ML, Valavaara R, Varpula M, et al. Low-dose and conventional-dose high resolution CT of pulmonary changes in breast cancer patients treated by tangential field radiotherapy. *Eur J Radiol* 1995;20:114–119.

67. Remy-Jardin M, Beuscart R, Sault MC, et al. Subpleural micronodules in diffuse infiltrative lung diseases: evaluation with thin-section CT scans. *Radiology* 1990;177:133–139.

68. Remy-Jardin M, Degreef JM, Beuscart R, et al. Coal worker's pneumoconiosis: CT assessment in exposed workers and correlation with radiographic findings. *Radiology* 1990;177:363–371.

69. Remy-Jardin M, Remy J, Deffontaines C, et al. Assessment of diffuse infiltrative lung disease: comparison of conventional CT and high-resolution CT. *Radiology* 1991;181:157–162.

70. Remy-Jardin M, Remy J, Wallaert B, et al. Subacute and chronic bird breeder hypersensitivity pneumonitis: sequential evaluation with CT and correlation with lung function tests and bronchoalveolar lavage. *Radiology* 1993;198:111–118.

71. Grenier P, Valeyre D, Cluzel P, et al. Chronic diffuse interstitial lung disease: diagnostic value of chest radiography and high-resolution CT. *Radiology* 1991;179:123–132.

72. Goodman LR, Golkow RS, Steiner RM, et al. The right mid-lung window. *Radiology* 1982;143:135–138.

73. Martin KW, Sagel SS, Siegel BA. Mosaic oligemia simulating pulmonary infiltrates on CT. *AJR Am J Roentgenol* 1986;147:670–673.

74. Müller NL, Staples CA, Miller RR, et al. Disease activity in idiopathic pulmonary fibrosis: CT and pathologic correlation. *Radiology* 1987;165:731–734.

75. Aberle DR, Gamsu G, Ray CS. High-resolution CT of benign asbestos-related diseases: clinical and radiographic correlation. *AJR Am J Roentgenol* 1988;151:883–891.

76. Akira M, Yamamoto S, Yokoyama K, et al. Asbestosis: high-resolution CT-pathologic correlation. *Radiology* 1990;176:389–394.
77. Lynch DA, Gamsu G, Ray CS, et al. Asbestos-related focal lung masses: manifestations on conventional and high-resolution CT scans. *Radiology* 1988;169:603–607.
78. Stein MG, Mayo J, Müller N, et al. Pulmonary lymphangitic spread of carcinoma: appearance on CT scans. *Radiology* 1987;162:371–375.
79. Munk PL, Müller NL, Miller RR, et al. Pulmonary lymphangitic carcinomatosis: CT and pathologic findings. *Radiology* 1988;166:705–709.
80. Bergin CJ, Müller NL. CT in the diagnosis of interstitial lung disease. *AJR Am J Roentgenol* 1985;145:505–510.
81. Colby TV, Swensen SJ. Anatomic distribution and histopathologic patterns in diffuse lung disease: correlation with HRCT. *J Thorac Imag* 1996;11:1–26.
82. Gruden JF, Webb WR, Naidich DP, et al. Multinodular disease: anatomic localization at thin-section CT—multireader evaluation of a simple algorithm. *Radiology* 1999;210:711–720.
83. Miller WS. *The lung.* Springfield, IL: Charles C Thomas Publisher, 1947:203.
84. Reid L. The secondary pulmonary lobule in the adult human lung, with special reference to its appearance in bronchograms. *Thorax* 1958;13:110–115.
85. Reid L, Simon G. The peripheral pattern in the normal bronchogram and its relation to peripheral pulmonary anatomy. *Thorax* 1958;13:103–109.
86. Naidich DP, McCauley DI, Khouri NF, et al. Computed tomography of bronchiectasis. *J Comput Assist Tomogr* 1982;6:437–444.
87. Grenier P, Maurice F, Musset D, et al. Bronchiectasis: assessment by thin-section CT. *Radiology* 1986;161:95–99.
88. Müller NL, Miller RR. Diseases of the bronchioles: CT and histopathologic findings. *Radiology* 1995;196:3–12.
89. Worthy SA, Müller NL. Small airway diseases. *Radiol Clin North Am* 1998;36:163–173.
90. Yoshimura H, Hatakeyama M, Otsuji H, et al. Pulmonary asbestosis: CT study of subpleural curvilinear shadow. Work in progress. *Radiology* 1986;158:653–658.
91. Murata K, Khan A, Herman PG. Pulmonary parenchymal disease: evaluation with high-resolution CT. *Radiology* 1989;170:629–635.
92. Westcott JL, Cole SR. Traction bronchiectasis in end-stage pulmonary fibrosis. *Radiology* 1986;161:665–669.

Subject Index

Note: Numbers followed by *f* indicate figures; numbers followed by *t* indicate tables.